CLINICAL GYNECOLOGIC ONCOLOGY

EIGHTH EDITION

PHILIP J. DI SAIA, MD

The Dorothy J. Marsh Chair in Reproductive Biology
Director, Division of Gynecologic Oncology
Professor, Department of Obstetrics and Gynecology
University of California–Irvine College of Medicine
Orange, California

WILLIAM T. CREASMAN, MD

J. Marion Sims Professor
Department of Obstetrics and Gynecology
Medical University of South Carolina
Charleston, South Carolina

ASSOCIATE EDITORS

ROBERT S. MANNEL, MD
Professor and James A. Merrill Chair
Department of Obstetrics and Gynecology
University of Oklahoma Health Sciences Center
Oklahoma City, Oklahoma

D. SCOTT MCMEEKIN, MD
Presbyterian Foundation Presidential Professor
University of Oklahoma Health Sciences Center
Oklahoma City, Oklahoma

DAVID G. MUTCH, MD
Judith and Ira Gall Professor of Gynecologic Oncology
Obstetrics and Gynecology Division Chief
Washington University School of Medicine
St. Louis, Missouri

ELSEVIER
SAUNDERS

ELSEVIER
SAUNDERS

1600 John F. Kennedy Blvd.
Ste 1800
Philadelphia, PA 19103-2899

Notices

Knowledge and best practice in this field are constantly changing. As new research and experience broaden our understanding, changes in research methods, professional practices, or medical treatment may become necessary.

Practitioners and researchers must always rely on their own experience and knowledge in evaluating and using any information, methods, compounds, or experiments described herein. In using such information or methods, they should be mindful of their own safety and the safety of others, including parties for whom they have a professional responsibility.

With respect to any drug or pharmaceutical products identified, readers are advised to check the most current information provided (i) on procedures featured or (ii) by the manufacturer of each product to be administered, to verify the recommended dose or formula, the method and duration of administration, and contraindications. It is the responsibility of practitioners, relying on their own experience and knowledge of their patients, to make diagnoses, to determine dosages and the best treatment for each individual patient, and to take all appropriate safety precautions.

To the fullest extent of the law, neither the Publisher nor the authors, contributors, or editors assume any liability for any injury and/or damage to persons or property as a matter of products liability, negligence or otherwise, or from any use or operation of any methods, products, instructions, or ideas contained in the material herein.

Previous editions copyrighted 2007, 2002, 1997, 1993, 1989, 1984, 1981

Library of Congress Cataloging-in-Publication Data
Clinical gynecologic oncology / [edited by] Philip J. Di Saia, William T. Creasman ; associate editors, Robert S. Mannel, D. Scott McMeekin, David G. Mutch. – 8th ed.
    p. ; cm.
  Rev. ed. of: Clinical gynecologic oncology / Philip J. Di Saia, William T. Creasman. 7th ed. 2007.
  Includes bibliographical references and index.
  ISBN 978-0-323-07419-3 (hardcover : alk. paper)
  I. Di Saia, Philip J., 1937-   II. Creasman, William T., 1934- III. Di Saia, Philip J., 1937- Clinical gynecologic oncology.
  [DNLM: 1. Genital Neoplasms, Female. WP 145]
616.99'465—dc23
                                            2011047871

Senior Content Strategist: Stefanie Jewell-Thomas
Senior Content Development Specialist: Deidre Simpson
Publishing Services Manager: Anne Altepeter
Senior Project Manager: Cheryl A. Abbott
Design: Ellen Zanolle
Marketing Manager: Carla Holloway

Printed in China
Last digit is the print number: 9 8 7 6 5 4 3 2 1

Working together to grow
libraries in developing countries

www.elsevier.com | www.bookaid.org | www.sabre.org

ELSEVIER   BOOK AID International   Sabre Foundation

Cognizant of our major sources of support and comfort,
we wish to dedicate this work to our loving wives,
Patti Di Saia, Erble Creasman, Becky Mannel, Cathy McMeekin, and
Lynn Mutch; to our children, John Di Saia,
Steven Di Saia, Dominic Di Saia, Vincent Di Saia, Valrie Creasman-Duke,
Scott Creasman, David Mannel, Lisa Mannel, Brian Mannel,
Charlotte McMeekin, Jackson McMeekin, Remy McMeekin,
David Mutch, and Adrienne Mutch; and to our students,
residents, and fellows, who we learn from each day.

A note of deepest gratitude to all the women, past and present,
who have trusted us with their care.
These women nurtured the tree of knowledge contained in this book.
The roots of this tree have been founded on the courage of these women
and intertwined with their lives.

Contributors

MICHAEL A. BIDUS, MD
Portsmouth Naval Medical Center, Residency Program Director; Vice Chair, Department of Obstetrics and Gynecology, Portsmouth, Virginia
Fallopian Tube Cancer; Germ Cell, Stromal, and Other Ovarian Tumors

WENDY R. BREWSTER, MD, PhD
Associate Professor, Division of Gynecologic Oncology, University of North Carolina School of Medicine, Chapel Hill, North Carolina
Epidemiology and Commonly Used Statistical Terms and Analysis of Clinical Studies

DANA M. CHASE, MD
Associate Professor, Creighton University School of Medicine, St. Joseph's Hospital and Medical Center, Phoenix, Arizona
Palliative Care and Quality of Life

CHRISTINA S. CHU, MD
Assistant Professor, Gynecologic Oncology, Division of Gynecologic Oncology, Hospital of the University of Pennsylvania, Philadelphia, Pennsylvania
Basic Principles of Chemotherapy

DANIEL L. CLARKE-PEARSON, MD
Robert A. Ross Professor of Obstetrics and Gynecology, University of North Carolina, Chapel Hill, North Carolina
Complications of Disease and Therapy

DAVID E. COHN, MD
Associate Professor, Obstetrics/Gynecology, Division of Gynecologic Oncology, The Ohio State University, Columbus, Ohio
Role of Minimally Invasive Surgery in Gynecologic Malignancies

ROBERT L. COLEMAN, MD
Professor, University of Texas, MD Anderson Cancer Center, Department of Gynecologic Oncology, Houston, Texas
Invasive Cancer of the Vagina; Targeted Therapy and Molecular Genetics

LARRY J. COPELAND, MD
Professor and Chair, William Greenville Pace III and Joann Norris Collins-Pace Chair, Department of Obstetrics and Gynecology, James Cancer Hospital, The Ohio State University, Columbus, Ohio
Epithelial Ovarian Cancer

WILLIAM T. CREASMAN, MD
J. Marion Sims Professor, Department of Obstetrics and Gynecology, Medical University of South Carolina, Charleston, South Carolina
Adenocarcinoma of the Uterine Corpus; Preinvasive Disease of the Cervix

PHILIP J. DI SAIA, MD
The Dorothy J. Marsh Chair in Reproductive Biology; Director, Division of Gynecologic Oncology; Professor, Department of Obstetrics and Gynecology, University of California–Irvine College of Medicine, Orange, California
The Adnexal Mass; Genes and Cancer: Genetic Counseling and Clinical Management

ERIC L. EISENHAUER, MD
Assistant Professor, Department of Obstetrics and Gynecology, James Cancer Hospital, The Ohio State University, Columbus, Ohio
Epithelial Ovarian Cancer

JOHN C. ELKAS, MD
Associate Clinical Professor, Department of Obstetrics and Gynecology, Virginia Commonwealth University, Inova Campus, Falls Church, Virginia
Germ Cell, Stromal, and Other Ovarian Tumors

JEFFREY M. FOWLER, MD
Professor, Department of Obstetrics and Gynecology; Director, Division of Gynecologic Oncology, James Cancer Hospital, The Ohio State University, Columbus, Ohio
Role of Minimally Invasive Surgery in Gynecologic Malignancies

MARY L. GEMIGNANI, MD
Associate Attending Surgeon, Department of Surgery/Breast Service/Gynecologic Oncology, Memorial Sloan-Kettering Cancer Center, New York, New York
Breast Diseases

EMILY M. KO, MD
Fellow, Division of Gynecologic Oncology, Department of Obstetrics and Gynecology, University of North Carolina School of Medicine, Chapel Hill, North Carolina
Gestational Trophoblastic Disease

LISA M. LANDRUM, MD
Assistant Professor of Obstetrics and Gynecology, University of Oklahoma Health Sciences Center, Oklahoma City, Oklahoma

ROBERT S. MANNEL, MD
Professor and James A. Merrill Chair, Department of Obstetrics and Gynecology, University of Oklahoma Health Sciences Center, Oklahoma City, Oklahoma
The Adnexal Mass; Role of Minimally Invasive Surgery in Gynecologic Malignancies

CARA A. MATHEWS, MD
Fellow, Gynecologic Oncology, Department of Obstetrics and Gynecology, University of Oklahoma Health Sciences Center, Oklahoma City, Oklahoma
Preinvasive Disease of the Vagina and Vulva and Related Disorders

G. LARRY MAXWELL, MD
Professor, Department of Obstetrics and Gynecology, Uniformed Services, University of the Health Sciences; Chief, Division of Gynecologic Oncology, Walter Reed Army Medical Center, Washington, District of Columbia
Fallopian Tube Cancer

D. SCOTT McMEEKIN, MD
Presbyterian Foundation Presidential Professor, University of Oklahoma Health Sciences Center, Oklahoma City, Oklahoma
The Adnexal Mass; Sarcoma of the Uterus

DAVID SCOTT MILLER, MD
Director and Dallas Foundation Chair in Gynecologic Oncology, University of Texas Southwestern, Dallas, Texas
Adenocarcinoma of the Uterine Corpus

BRADLEY J. MONK, MD
Professor, Creighton University School of Medicine, St. Joseph's Hospital and Medical Center, Phoenix, Arizona
Invasive Cervical Cancer; Palliative Care and Quality of Life

DAVID G. MUTCH, MD
Judith and Ira Gall Professor of Gynecologic Oncology; Obstetrics and Gynecology Division Chief, Washington University School of Medicine, St. Louis, Missouri
Genes and Cancer: Genetic Counseling and Clinical Management

G. SCOTT ROSE, MD
Director, Division of Gynecologic Oncology, Walter Reed Army Medical Center, Washington, District of Columbia
Germ Cell, Stromal, and Other Ovarian Tumors; Fallopian Tube Cancer

STEPHEN C. RUBIN, MD
Franklin Payne Professor and Chief, Division of Gynecologic Oncology, Hospital of the University of Pennsylvania, Philadelphia, Pennsylvania
Basic Principles of Chemotherapy

RITU SALANI, MD
Assistant Professor, Department of Obstetrics and Gynecology, James Cancer Hospital, The Ohio State University, Columbus, Ohio
Epithelial Ovarian Cancer

JEANNE M. SCHILDER, MD
Associate Professor, Division of Gynecologic Oncology, Indiana University Medical Center, Indianapolis, Indiana
Invasive Cancer of the Vulva

BRAIN M. SLOMOVITZ, MD
Professor, Department of Obstetrics and Gynecology, Morristown Memorial Hospital Women's Cancer Center, Morristown, New Jersey
Invasive Cancer of the Vulva

ANIL K. SOOD, MD
Professor and Director, Ovarian Cancer Research, Gynecologic Oncology and Reproductive Medicine, The University of Texas, MD Anderson Cancer Center, Houston, Texas
Targeted Therapy and Molecular Genetics

JOHN T. SOPER, MD
Professor of Obstetrics and Gynecology, Division of Gynecologic Oncology, University of North Carolina School of Medicine, Chapel Hill, North Carolina
Gestational Trophoblastic Disease

FREDERICK B. STEHMAN, MD
The Clarence E. Ehrlich Professor and Chair, Department of Obstetrics and Gynecology, University Hospital, Indianapolis, Indiana
Invasive Cancer of the Vagina

KRISHNANSU S. TEWARI, MD
Associate Professor, University of California–Irvine College of Medicine, Division of Gynecologic Oncology, Orange, California
Cancer in Pregnancy; Invasive Cervical Cancer

JOAN L. WALKER, MD
Professor of Gynecologic Oncology, Department of Obstetrics and Gynecology, University of Oklahoma Health Sciences Center, Oklahoma City, Oklahoma
Endometrial Hyperplasia, Estrogen Therapy, and the Prevention of Endometrial Cancer; Preinvasive Disease of the Vagina and Vulva and Related Disorders

LARI B. WENZEL, PhD
Associate Professor, University of California–Irvine, Center for Health Policy Research, Irvine, California
Palliative Care and Quality of Life

SHANNON N. WESTIN, MD, MPH
Assistant Professor, Gynecologic Oncology and Reproductive Medicine, University of Texas, MD Anderson Cancer Center, Houston, Texas
Targeted Therapy and Molecular Genetics

SIU-FUN WONG, MD
Clinical Professor of Medicine, Division of Hematology/Oncology, University of California–Irvine; Professor, Oncology, Department of Pharmacotherapy and Outcome Science, School of Pharmacy, Loma Linda University, Loma Linda, California
Palliative Care and Quality of Life

CATHERYN M. YASHAR, MD
Univeristy of California, San Diego, Moores Cancer Center, Radiation Oncology, La Jolla, California.
Basic Principles in Ggynecologic Radiotherapy

ROSEMARY E. ZUNA, MD
Associate Professor of Pathology, Pathology Department, University of Oklahoma Health Sciences Center, Oklahoma City, Oklahoma
Endometrial Hyperplasia, Estrogen Therapy, and the Prevention of Endometrial Cancer

Preface

The first seven editions of *Clinical Gynecologic Oncology* were stimulated by a recognized need for a readable text on gynecologic cancer and related subjects addressed primarily to the community physician, resident, and other students involved with these patients. The practical aspects of the clinical presentation and management of these problems were heavily emphasized in the first seven editions, and we have continued that style in this text. As in every other textbook, the authors interjected their own biases on many topics, especially in those areas where more than one approach to management has been utilized. On the other hand, most major topics are treated in depth and supplemented with ample references to current literature so that the text can provide a comprehensive resource for study by the resident, fellow, or student of gynecologic oncology and serve as a source for review material.

We continued the practice of placing an outline on the first page of each chapter as a guide to the content for that section. The reader will notice that we included topics not discussed in the former editions and expanded areas previously introduced. Some of these areas include new guidelines for managing the dying patient; current management and reporting guidelines for cervical and vulvar cancer; current management and reporting guidelines for breast cancer; expanded discussion on the basic principles of genetic alterations in cancer; techniques for laparoscopic surgery in treatment of gynecologic cancers; and new information on breast, cervical, and colon cancer screenings and detection. The seventh edition contained, for the first time, color photographs of key gross and microscopic specimens for the reader's review. In addition, Drs. Di Saia and Creasman have included several other authors for most of the chapters, as well as three new associate editors. Much more information is included to make the text as practical as possible for the practicing gynecologist. In addition, key points are highlighted for easy review.

Fortunately, many of the gynecologic malignancies have a high "cure" rate. This relatively impressive success rate with gynecologic cancers can be attributed in great part to the development of diagnostic techniques that can identify precancerous conditions, the ability to apply highly effective therapeutic modalities that are more restrictive elsewhere in the body, a better understanding of the disease spread patterns, and the development of more sophisticated and effective treatment in cancers that previously had very poor prognoses. As a result, today a patient with a gynecologic cancer may look toward more successful treatment and longer survival than at any other time. This optimism should be realistically transferred to the patient and her family. Patient denial must be tolerated until the patient decides that a frank conversation is desired. When the prognosis is discussed, some element of hope should always be introduced within the limits of reality and possibility.

The physician must be prepared to treat the malignancy in light of today's knowledge and to deal with the patient and her family in a compassionate and honest manner. The patient with gynecologic cancer needs to feel that her physician is confident and goal oriented. Although, unfortunately, gynecologic cancers will cause the demise of some individuals, it is hoped that the information collected in this book will help to increase the survical rate of these patiemts by bringing current practical knowledge to the attention of the primary care and specialized physician.

Our ideas are only intellectual instruments which we use to break into phenomena; we must change them when they have served their purpose, as we change a blunt lancet that we have used long enough.

Claude Bernard (1813-1878)

Some patients, though conscious that their condition is perilous, recover their health simply through their contentment with the goodness of their physician.

Hippocrates (440-370 BC)

Philip J. Di Saia, MD
William T. Creasman, MD
Robert S. Mannel, MD
D. Scott McMeekin, MD
David G. Mutch, MD

Acknowledgments

We wish to acknowledge the advice given and contributions made by several colleagues, including, Michael A. Bidus, Wendy R. Brewster, Dana Chase, Christina S. Chu, Daniel L. Clarke-Pearson, Robert L. Coleman, Larry J. Copeland, Eric Eisenhauer, Jeffrey Fowler, Mary L. Gemignani, Emily M. Ko, Robert S. Mannel, Cara Mathews, D. Scott McMeekin, David Miller, Bradley J. Monk, David G. Mutch, G. Scott Rose, Stephen C. Rubin, Ritu Salani , Jeanne Schilder, Brian M. Slomovitz, John T. Soper, Frederick B. Stehman, Krishnansu S. Tewari, Joan Walker, Lari B. Wenzel, Siu-Fun Wong, Catheryn Yashar, and Rosemary E. Zuna. We give special thanks to Lucy DiGiuseppe and, especially, Lisa Kozik for their diligent administrative support in preparing the manuscript and also to David F. Baker, Carol Beckerman, Richard Crippen, Susan Stokskopf, and David Wyer for their excellent and creative contributions to many of the illustrations created for this book.

We are grateful to the sincere and diligent efforts of Stefanie Jewell-Thomas, Dee Simpson, Ellen Zanolle, and Cheryl Abbott from Elsevier in bringing this book to fruition. Through their deliberate illumination and clearing of our path, this material has traversed the far distance from mere concept to a compelling reference book.

Contents

Preinvasive Disease of the Cervix

William T. Creasman

CERVICAL INTRAEPITHELIAL NEOPLASIA

Screening Guidelines

The unique accessibility of the cervix to cell and tissue study and to direct physical examination has permitted intensive investigation of the nature of malignant lesions of the cervix. Although our knowledge is incomplete, investigations have shown that most of these tumors have a gradual, rather than explosive, onset. Their preinvasive precursors may exist in a reversible phase of surface or in situ disease for some years, although this may not be in some patients.

According to data from the Third National Cancer Survey, published by Cramer and Cutler, the mean age of patients with carcinoma in situ (CIS) was 15.6 years younger than that of patients with invasive squamous cell carcinoma, exceeding the 10-year difference found by others. This difference is, at best, a rough approximation of the duration of intraepithelial carcinoma in its assumed progression to clinical invasive cancer. Data such as these serve to emphasize the essential nature of cytologic screening programs, even when performed on less than an annual basis.

Although these early phases may be asymptomatic, they can be detected by currently available methods.

This concept of development of cervical malignancy has convinced many that control of this disease is well within grasp in the foreseeable future. It is possible to eradicate most deaths resulting from cervical cancer by use of the diagnostic and therapeutic techniques now available.

There is convincing evidence that cytologic screening programs are effective in reducing mortality from carcinoma of the cervix. The extent of the reduction in mortality achieved is related directly to the proportion of the population that has been screened. In fact, all studies worldwide show that screening for cancer not only decreases mortality but also probably does so by decreasing the incidence. The incidence of cervical cancer has not decreased without a screening program being implemented.

Numerous papers and lengthy discussions have focused on the optimal screening interval. Unfortunately, numerous recommendations during the last decade and a half have resulted in a confused public and dissatisfied professionals. In 1988 the American College of Obstetricians and Gynecologists (ACOG) and the American Cancer Society (ACS) agreed on the recommendation that has subsequently been accepted by other organizations. That recommendation was changed in 2002 and again in 2009 (Table 1-1).

Screening has decreased the incidence and death rate from cervical cancer, but it also has identified many

TABLE 1-1   American College of Obstetricians and Gynecologists Recommendations for Screening of the Cervix, 2009

- Women from age 21 to 29 should be screened every 2 years using either the standard Pap or liquid-based cytology.
- Women 30 years or older who have had three consecutive negative cervical cytology test results may be screened once every 3 years with either standard Pap or liquid-based cytology.
- Ca-testing using combination of cytology plus HPV DNA testing is appropriate for women older than 30 years. Any woman 30 years or older at low risk who has negative cytology and HPV DNA testing can be rescreened at 3-year intervals.
- Cervical cancer screening can be discontinued between the ages of 65 and 70 years in women who have had three or more negative consecutive test results and no abnormal test results in the past 10 years.
- Cervical cancer screening is not recommended in women before 21 years of age.
- Women with certain risk factors may need more frequent screening, including those with HIV; those who are immunosuppressed; those exposed to DES in utero; and those who have been treated for CIN II, CIN III, or cervical cancer.

women with preinvasive neoplasia (which is the role of screening, not to diagnose cancer). It is estimated that 50% of cervical cancer diagnosed is in women who have never had a Pap smear and as many as one third have had a Pap smear, but it may have been years ago. As many as 4 million women per year will have an abnormal Pap smear result in the United States. This represents 5% to 7% of cervical smears, with 90% or more having atypical squamous cells of undetermined significance (ASCUS) or low-grade squamous intraepithelial lesions (LGSIL). In addition, women who have been screened but subsequently developed cervical cancer usually have an earlier stage of disease. In the United States death rates from cervical cancer have dropped from number 1 among all cancers in women to number 12. The American Cancer Society estimates that 11,270 cervical and 4070 cancer deaths occurred in the United States in 2009. Approximately 55,000 new cases of CIS invasive carcinoma in situ also were diagnosed. Although it has not been proved in a prospective randomized study, all investigators credit screening as a major contributor to this reduction in death rate. In contrast to the industrialized world, cancer of the cervix remains the primary cancer killer in women in Third World countries. Approximately 500,000 cervical cancers will be diagnosed this year worldwide, representing 12% of all cancers diagnosed in women, and almost half will die of their cancer. Because this is a poor woman's disease, not much political pressure has been brought to bear to improve the situation for this group.

The rationale for the change and recommendation concerning commencement of screening guidelines are several. It is well recognized that infection with human papillomavirus (HPV) is required for the development of cervical neoplasia. It is also appreciated that most women with HPV will not develop cervical neoplasia. Sexually transmitted, high-risk types of HPV (Table 1-2) cause disease to develop in the transformation zone. The transformation zone is that area on the cervix that undergoes squamous metaplasia, which develops mainly during the adolescent years. Fortunately for most women, particularly those who are young, their immune system is effective and clears the infection. In most, they are cleared within 1 to 2 years without producing neoplastic changes. The risk of neoplasia increases in those women in whom the infection persists.

There does appear to be a high prevalence of the infection in teenagers, peaking in the 30s with subsequent decrease. In a study by Wright and colleagues of 10,090 Pap tests in 12- to 18-year-old females, only about 5% were reported as LSIL and <1% were high-grade squamous intraepithelial lesions (HSIL). Most lesions present in teenagers spontaneously regress. In another study, Moscicki and colleagues followed 187 women, 18 to 22 years of age, with LSIL and found 61% regressed spontaneously at 1 year and 91% at 3 years. Only 3% progressed to cervical intraepithelial neoplasia grade III (CIN III).

In addition, even though there is a high prevalence of HPV in teenagers, invasive cancer is rare in women younger than 21. Only 0.1% of cervical cancer is diagnosed in women 21 years old or younger. The SEER database estimates the incidence rates of females 15 to 19 years old to be 1 to 2 cases per 1 million women. Therefore, the recommendation to start screening at 21 years is based on the low incidence of cancer in young women regardless of when they become sexually active. The potential adverse effects of aggressive management of these young women with abnormal screening results may be appreciable. A recent review and meta-analysis note a considerable increase in premature births in women who previously were treated with excisional procedures for dysplasia.

It is important to follow the guidelines if screening is to be stopped at 70 years. Studies have shown that the older patient is at increased risk for cervical cancer. Mandelblatt and colleagues reported that 25% of all cervical cancers and 41% of all deaths from cancer occurred in women older than 65 years of age. The prevalence of abnormal Pap smears is high in this group (16 in 1000). The chance of developing an invasive cancer is not necessarily related to prior screening habits in this age group. Another study noted that increasing age is associated with more advanced disease, yet when stage of disease was controlled, there was no effect of age on disease-free survival. Women aged 65 and older have a cervical cancer incidence of 16.8 per 100,000 compared to 7.4 in younger women. The mortality rate for those

65 and older is 9.3 compared to 2.2 for younger women. African-American women older than age 65 have a higher incidence rate and mortality rate for cervical cancer than white women of the same age. It is estimated that about 10% of women receive no regular cytology screening and as many as 82% of women in the United States were screened in the past 3 years. In women 65 and older, 25% have no regular screening and 15% are screened at 3-year intervals. This increases as the women age to 50% and 20%, respectively. It is estimated that half of women who do develop cervical cancer had never been screened for cervical cancer and an additional 10% have not been screened in the previous 5 years. Although screened less frequently, they have the same number of recent physician visits as do younger women. The need to educate older women and their health care providers about the importance of Pap smear screening is evident. A National Omnibus survey was conducted to ascertain women's knowledge, attitudes, and behavior with regard to Pap screening. Of women 18 years or older, 82% believed the Pap smear is very important. Among women who believed that the Pap smear was important, 82% stated it was to identify cancer. Among those aged 18 to 24, only 61% understood that the Pap smear was to detect cancer. Of this same age group, 35% believed the Pap smear was important to detect vaginal infections and sexually transmitted diseases. More than one fourth of those who believed that Pap smears were important did not have a Pap test during the previous year. The older and lower-income women were less likely than others to say that Pap smears are very important, yet they had regular physical examinations. Only 51% of women stated that Pap smears identified cervical and endometrial cancers. Seven percent believed breast cancer was found on the Pap smear. Risk factors for cervical cancer were poorly understood. Approximately two thirds of women identified a family history as a cervical cancer risk factor. One in five women could not name any risk factors for cervical cancer. Women believed that physicians did not sufficiently explain the reasons for Pap smears and the results from these tests. The need for better communication between physicians and women should be obvious.

Screening patterns to some degree appear to be changing, although some habits apparently do not. The number of women who had health insurance, a higher level of education, and current employment was related to Pap smear usage. Of interest is that recently, black women have substantially increased the use of the Pap smear, with rates now exceeding those of white women. This is age-related: Screening is similar for blacks and whites up to age 29, but from 30 to 49 years, blacks are significantly more compliant. Among those older than 70 years of age, compliance among white women is greater. Although screening rates appear to be higher in black women, the mortality rate is lower for white women. Age is also important in that younger women are more compliant than older women. The highest-risk group in the United States appears to be Hispanics, particularly if they speak only Spanish. Approximately 1.6 million Hispanics are not screened in the United States. This is the fastest-growing segment of our population, which may explain why they are not screened. The following reasons were given for noncompliance: It was unnecessary, no problems, procrastination, physicians' nonrecommendation, having a hysterectomy, and costs. One study noted that 72% of all women had a Pap smear within the last year. Yet almost 80% of women who did not have a Pap smear reported contact with medical facilities during the past 2 years, whereas more than 90% reported making contact during the last 5 years. Organized screening programs over the last 40 to 50 years have decreased the incidence of cervical cancer by 75%. Although cervical cancer is a potentially preventable disease, some 4000 women in the United States will die from cervical cancer. This is mainly a result of the fact that a significant (1 million or more) number of women have not been screened for cervical neoplasia. About 60% of women with cervical cancer have not been screened in the past 5 years or longer. These women tend to have low incomes, have little education, be unmarried, and lack insurance; however, a study of women in long-term, prepaid health plans reviewed similar characteristics: older age, residence in a high poverty area, and low education levels. More than half of these women with cervical cancer have not had a Pap smear in the last 3 years even though 81% had seen a doctor and 63% had three or more visits during this time interval. Obvious education about screening to older women and health care providers would be of benefit. The new screening guidelines appear appropriate; unfortunately, a large segment of our population has not satisfied these guidelines.

Another important consideration is that there is a relatively high false-negative Pap smear rate in the United States. Several studies in the United States and abroad have shown that an alarming number of patients were found to have invasive carcinoma of the cervix within a relatively short time after a reportedly normal Pap smear. A study from Seattle indicates that 27% of patients with stage I carcinoma of the cervix had a normal Pap smear within 1 year of the time of diagnosis. Bearman noted that after 3 years from last screen, women who develop cervical cancer have the same incidence of advanced disease as do women who have never been screened. The false-negative rate of Pap smears is really unknown. Cervicography and colposcopic studies have suggested that the majority of women identified with CIN by these two techniques had normal Pap smears at the time of diagnosis. False-negative Pap smear results may occur from sampling errors in that cells are not obtained with the Pap smear and the lack of recognition of abnormal cells in the laboratory. As many as 30% of new cases of cervical cancer each year are the result of false-negative test results. Cytology remains an art to a certain extent in that there is an inconsistency in the interpretation by cytologists. Only negative LSILs had greater than 50% consistency when cytologic specimens were reviewed by quality-control pathologists. On review, most were downgraded to a lesser diagnosis. Of those reported as atypical cells of undetermined significance, 39% were thought to be negative. Even in those originally diagnosed as HSIL, more than half were reinterpreted as LSIL, ASC-US, or negative.

Although Pap smear screening has decreased the incidence of cervical cancer, it is apparent that sensitivity could be improved. The role of HPV testing compared to Pap smear screening has been reported. These have led to combining Pap smears with HPV testing as a routine for women older than 30 years old.

In a study performed in Canada, HPV testing was compared to conventional Pap smears. More than 10,000 women were randomly assigned to testing. Both tests were performed on all women in a randomly assigned sequence at the same session. The sensitivity of the Pap smear on HPV testing for CIN II+ was 94.6% and 96.8%, respectively. The sensitivity of both tests used together was 100%, and the specificity was 92.5%.

In a Finnish study of more than 58,000 women, they assessed the performance of HPV DNA screening with cytology triage compared with conventional cytology on CIN III, adenocarcinoma in situ (AIS), and cervical cancer. The relative rate of CIN III in the HPV arm versus the conventional Pap was 1.44 (CI 1.01-2.05) in those invited to screening and 1.77 (1.16-2.74) among those who attended.

Epidemiology

Numerous epidemiologic studies reported in the literature have established a positive association between cancer of the cervix and multiple, interdependent social factors. A greater incidence of cervical cancer is observed among blacks and Mexican-Americans, and this is undoubtedly related to their lower socioeconomic status. Increased occurrence of cancer of the cervix in multiparous women is probably related to other factors, such as age at first marriage and age at first pregnancy. These facts, combined with the high incidence of the disease in prostitutes, lead to a firm conclusion that first coitus at an early age and multiple sexual partners increase the probability of developing CIN. Even socioeconomic status is interrelated because an association has long been noted between relative poverty and early marriage and youthful childbearing. The final common factors appear to be onset of regular sexual activity as a teenager

and continued exposure to multiple sexual partners. Indeed, cervical cancer is rare in celibate groups such as nuns, and many have labeled cancer of the cervix a "venereal disease."

Much has been made about the sexual activity of a woman because it may affect her risk for developing CIN. Increasing data suggest that a woman may also be placed at increased risk by her sexual partner, even though she does not satisfy the requirements of early intercourse and multiple partners. The sexual history of her partner may be as important as hers. In a study by Zunzunegui and colleagues, patients with cervical cancer were compared with selected controls. Both populations came from a low socioeconomic group of recent Hispanic migrants to California. All were married. Sexual histories were obtained from both sexes. Among the women the age of first coitus was earlier among the cases than among the controls (19.5 years vs 21.7 years). The average number of lifetime sexual partners did not differ between cases and controls. Of note, case husbands had more sexual partners than did control husbands; they had first intercourse at an earlier age and also a much greater history of venereal diseases. Visits to prostitutes were equal between the two groups, but the case husbands tended to have frequented prostitutes more often than did the husbands in the control group. Husbands in the case group smoked more than the husbands in the control group. If the number of sexual partners of the husband was greater than 20, the risk of cervical cancer increased in the wife five times more than that of a woman whose husband had fewer than 20 sexual partners. This may be related to the "infectious" agent obtained by the husband and, in turn, to the duration of exposure by the woman. (Note the following section on HPV and the male factor.)

The interaction of the carcinogen with the cervix depends on the specific woman at risk. The epidemiologic data strongly suggest that the adolescent is at risk. The probable reason is that active metaplasia is occurring on the cervix. Because there is active proliferation of cellular transformation from columnar to squamoid epithelium, the potential for interaction between the carcinogen and the cervix is increased. Once this process of metaplasia is complete, the cervix may no longer be at high risk, although CIN certainly can occur in patients who are virginal until after this process has been completed. Smoking is now considered a high-risk factor for carcinoma of the cervix, and this observation correlates with distribution of other smoking-related cancers. An increased, excess risk of preinvasive and invasive disease appears to exist among smokers, particularly among current, long-term users, high-risk intensity smokers, and users of nonfiltered cigarettes. Smoking appears to be an independent risk factor, even after controlling for sexual factors. In a case-control study, the risk of HSIL increased with increasing years and pack-years of exposure. The association is for squamous cell cancers only, and no relationship with adenocarcinomas has been noted. Studies have found mutagens in cervical mucus, some of which are many times higher than those found in the blood.

One study evaluated whether smoking caused DNA modification (addicts) in cervical epithelium. Smokers had a higher level of DNA addicts than did nonsmokers. Women with abnormal Pap smear results had a significantly higher number of DNA addicts than those with normal Pap smear results. Women with a higher proportion of addicts may have an increased susceptibility to cervical cancer. This suggests direct biochemical evidence of smoking as a cause of cervical cancer.

It has been suggested that vitamin deficiency may have a role in certain malignancies, including cervical cancer. Butterworth evaluated 294 patients with dysplasia and 170 controls defined by cytology and colposcopy. Multiple known risk factors for cervical neoplasia were evaluated along with 12 nutritional indices on nonfasting blood specimens. Plasma nutrient levels were generally not associated with risks; however, red blood cell folate levels at or below 660 nmol/L interacted with HPV-16 infections. Chemoprevention with vitamin A may prevent some cancers. Vitamin A derivatives, particularly retinoids in vitro and in vivo, modulate the growth of normal epithelial cells, usually by inhibiting proliferation and allowing differentiation and maturation of cells to occur. Meyskens, in a randomized prospective study, treated a group of patients with CIN II and III with all-*trans* retinoic acid or a similar placebo delivered directly to the cervix. Retinoic acid patients with CIN II had a complete histologic regression of 43% versus 27% for the placebo group ($P = 0.041$). No treatment difference was noted for the patient with CIN III. The results of this study and others suggest a chemoprevention role in the prevention of cervical neoplasia.

Human Papillomavirus

Epidemiologic studies have identified the association of cervical neoplasia with sexual activity. The initial study suggests this relationship is more than 150 years old. The sexually transmitted agent that could be related to the initiation or promotion of cervical neoplasia has been sought for many years. Essentially every substance found in the genital tract has been implicated over the years. These have included sperm, smegma, spirochetes, *Trichomonas*, fungus, herpes simplex virus type II (HSV-2), and HPV. During the 1970s, HSV-2 was studied extensively in an attempt to develop a possible etiologic link. These endeavors mainly used case-control studies, which showed a significant higher prevalence of HSV-2

in cancer cases compared with controls. These studies encountered problems with cross-reactivity between HSV-1 and HSV-2 and standardization of assays. It could not be determined if the infection with the virus preceded the cancer. When controlled for high-risk factors, many studies found no difference among patients and controls in the prevalence of HSV-2 antibody. Most investigators today do not consider HSV-2 to be a serious candidate as an etiologic agent for cervical neoplasia, although some have postulated that it may in some way be a cofactor.

Since the mid-1970s there has been an explosion of information concerning HPV. It was actually in the mid-1970s when zur Hausen suggested that HPV was a likely candidate as a sexually transmitted agent that may result in genital tract neoplasias. This work resulted in a Nobel Prize in medicine. Later in that decade Meisel published a series of articles that described a new virus-induced condylomatous lesion of the cervix. Although koilocytosis had previously been described, these workers noted the presence of intranuclear HPV in koilocytotic cells associated with CIN. In contrast to the long-identified typical cauliflower condyloma, it was noted that HPV also produced a flat, white lesion, best recognized colposcopically, that was thought to be a precursor of cervical neoplasia. The development of immunoperoxidase techniques that can identify the HPV confirmed these original observations. Subsequently, HPV has been isolated from genital lesions; with the use of hybridization techniques, HPV DNA can be typed.

About 20 million Americans and 630 million people worldwide are infected with HPV. In the United States, about 6.2 million will acquire a new infection every year. Rates are highest in sexually active women 25 years old or younger. In young HPV-negative women, the accumulative incidence for first HPV infection has been estimated at 32% at 24 months and 43% at 36 months. Of the approximately 35 HPV subtypes that infect the genital track, HPV-16 and HPV-18 are said to be present in about 70% of all squamous cervical cancers and 80% of all adenocarcinomas.

The oncogenic link, particularly of HPV-16 and -18, is well established. In a large 20,000 women study, 10% of women with HPV-16 and 5% of those with HPV-18 at enrollment developed CIN III within 36 months. Those negative for HPV at enrollment developed 1% accumulative incidence of CIN III or cervical cancer. At 10 years, 10% with HPV-16 and 14% with HPV-18 develop CIN III or cancer. In another study among Seattle college students, those infected with HPV-16 or -18 at study onset had CIN II or III and 27% over the 36-month study. Median time to detection of CIN II or III from discovery of HPV infection was 14 months.

The lifetime risk of acquiring a genital HPV infection is about 80%. Most infections, particularly in young women, are cleared by her immune system. It is believed that subsequent clearance of an HPV subtype protects one against reinfection of the same type. Clinical regression usually takes place within 6 to 12 months. There is a question of whether there is a latency period in which the virus is undetected. Women have been observed to be HPV negative before an organ transplant and then become positive after transplantation and immunosuppression. In most women, it is thought that those who become infected with a specific HPV type will later show no evidence of that type and can be assured that later reinfection is uncommon with the same HPV subtype. The time from new infection to occurrence of a clinical lesion can vary from 4 weeks for genital warts and up to 2 years for CIN. Most lesions will clear usually within 2 years. HPV-6 and -11 (low-risk type) are mainly responsible for genital warts, and the vast majority of cases are laryngeal papillomas (also called recurrent respiratory papillomatosis or RRP). It is estimated that 1.4 million men and women in the United States have genital warts requiring up to 900,000 office visits a year. RRP is rare but potentially fatal and is the result of HPV-6 and -11 infections. It is mainly seen in the first 5 years of life but may occur in adults. It is felt that transmission is from mother to child during childbirth. It is difficult to treat and, in many instances, treatment is only palliative in nature.

HPV is one of the easiest viruses to transmit. It is estimated that the probability of transmission per active intercourse is about 40% (based on computer modeling). The use of condoms to reduce the risk of HPV transmission is controversial. Most studies suggest condoms have not reduced the risk, although a recent study that followed a group of young women over an average of 34 months reported that women whose partners used condoms 100% of the time had 70% reduction in the rate of HPV acquisition compared to women whose partner used condoms less than 5% of the time.

HPV type distribution notes 70% of cervical cancer results from types 16 and 18 and another 20% results from types 45, 31, 32, 58, 52, and 35. For HSIL, most cases are caused by HPV types 16, 31, 58, 18, 33, 52, 35, 51, 56, 45, 39, 66, and 6 (in the order of increasing prevalence). In LSIL, 80% in 13 studies done in North America were positive for HPV, although it was lower in other countries. About a quarter of HPV-positive cases are type 16. For ASCUS, HPV positivity depends on age. In the ASCUS-LSIL Triage Study (ALTS), 61% of cases tested positive for HPV. The baseline prevalence of HPV-16 was 24% and HPV-18 was 8%. HPV-16 and -18 positivity was 35% for ages 18 to 24 and 19% in women ages 35 and older.

To date, about 120 different types of HPV have been isolated and characterized (Table 1-2). The identity of a new subtype has usually been based on the description

TABLE 1-2   Gynecologic Lesions Associated with Human Papilloma Virus

	Common HPV Types	Less Common HPV Types
Condyloma acuminata	6, 11	2, 16, 30, 40, 41, 42, 44, 45, 54, 55, 61
CIN, VIN, VAIN	16, 18, 31	6, 11, 30, 34, 35, 39, 40, 42-45, 51, 52, 56-59, 61, 62, 64, 66, 67, 69
Cervical cancer	16, 18, 31, 45	6, 10, 11, 26, 33, 35, 39, 51, 52, 55, 56, 58

From Evans H, Walker PG: Infection and cervical intraepithelial neoplasia. Cont Clin Gynecol Obstet 2:217, 2002.
CIN, Cervical intraepithelial neoplasia; VIN, vulvar intraepithelial neoplasia; VAIN, vaginal intraepithelial neoplasia.

of the DNA genome compared with the known HPV prototypes. A new type must share less than 50% DNA homology to any known HPV. Classification depends on the composition of DNA. About 30 HPV types primarily infect the squamous epithelium of the lower anogenital tracts of both males and females. So-called low-risk types (6, 11, 42, 43, 44) are mainly associated with benign lesions such as condyloma, which rarely progress to a malignancy. The high-risk types (16, 18, 31, 33, 35, 39, 45, 51, 52, 56, 58) are detected in intraepithelial and invasive cancers. More than 85% of all cervical cancers are said to contain high-risk HPV sequences. In benign precursor lesions, the HPV DNA is episomal (has extra chromosomal replication). In cancers, the DNA is integrated into the human genome. All HPVs contain at least seven early genes (E1-E7) and two late genes (L1 and L2) (Figure 1-1).

The integration usually occurs in the E1 and E2 region, resulting in disrupting gene integrity and expression. These open reading frames encode DNA-binding proteins that regulate viral transcription and replication. With HPV-16 and -18, the E2 protein represses the promoter from which the E6 and E7 genes are transcribed. Because of integration, the E6 and E7 genes are expressed in HPV-positive cervical cancer. It appears that E6 and E7 are the only viral factors necessary for immortalization of human genital epithelial cells. These two oncoproteins form complexes with host regulatory proteins such as p53 and retroblastoma susceptibility gene (pRB). High-risk HPV E6, on binding with p53, caused rapid degradation of the protein, thus preventing p53 normal function from responding to DNA damage induced by radiation or chemical mutagens. Without this binding, increased levels of p53 growth arrest of cells may occur, which allows repair of damaged DNA to take place or apoptosis (programmed cell death) to occur. E7 protein may bind to several cellular proteins, including pRB. This interaction may inactivate pRB and push the cell

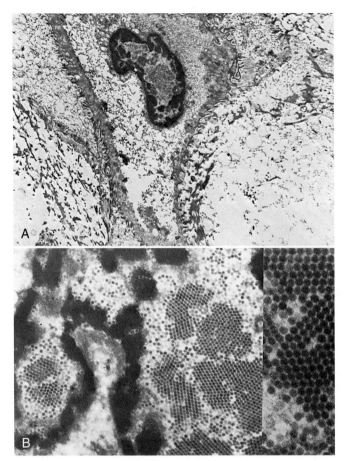

FIGURE 1-1 **A,** Koilocytotic cells with intranuclear virions (×6900). **B,** Human papillomavirus particles. Note the intranuclear crystalline array ("honeycomb") arrangement of virions (×20,500). See the *insert* (×80,000). *(Courtesy Alex Ferenczy, MD, Montreal, Canada.)*

cycle into the S phase and induce DNA synthesis. Other regulatory genes such as c-*myc* may also be involved. Other factors are obviously important because only a small percentage of women infected with high-risk HPV develop cancer. For instance, HPV-immortalized human keratinocyte cell lines will be manifest in nude mice only after transfection with additional oncogenes such as *ras*. In humans, the immunologic response may contribute to this complicated scenario.

HPVs carry their genetic information within a cellular double-stranded DNA molecule. Infections caused by these viruses are usually not systemic but result in local infections manifested as warty papillary condylomatous lesions. HPV-infected cells contain both the fully formed viral particles and their DNA. Replication of the virus occurs only in the cell nuclei, in which DNA synthesis is low. Mature HPV particles are never found in replicating basal or parabasal cells; they are found in the koilocytotic cells in the superficial layer. HPV, like HSV-2, may also have a latent intranuclear form in which only fragments of the viral DNA are expressed.

Initially, it was suggested that in all cancers the HPV DNA was integrated, whereas in CIN lesions the HPV DNA was episomal. This suggested the role of a more virulent type of HPV (i.e., 16 and 18). More recently, an increased number of cancers with episomal HPV DNA have been reported. Integration has been noted in CIN lesions; therefore it appears that integration is not a constant finding in cancers. Although integration of HPV-16 has been demonstrated, the importance of this finding in the development of cancer has not been determined.

HPV-18 may be more virulent than HPV-16 and may be a prognostic factor. Kurman and associates noted a deficit of HPV-18 in CIN compared with cancer, whereas there was no significant difference in the distribution of HPV-16 in CIN compared with cancer. These authors postulated that this deficit of HPV-18 in CIN could represent a rapid transit time through the preinvasive phase. Obviously, this is conjecture at this time. Walker and colleagues noted that patients with cervical cancer and HPV-18 had a worse prognosis than did similar-staged patients with HPV-16. One other study noted that the prognosis was worse in patients with cervical cancer if no HPV subtype was identified than if any HPV type was present. Today it is generally accepted that type 18 is more frequently associated with adenocarcinoma of the cervix and type 16 with squamous cancer.

A difference in sexual behavior and reproductive risk factors between the two histotypes also is apparent. There is a positive association of high gravidity and squamous cancer and an inverse association with adenocarcinoma. Age of first intercourse and number of sexual partners is of greater risk for squamous carcinoma than for adenocarcinoma. Over the past several years, many studies worldwide attempted to characterize HPV DNA with regard to specific types and correlate these findings with the cervical neoplastic process. Although the laboratory evidence of the role of HPV DNA in the carcinogenesis was being established, the epidemiologic studies were lacking. Many studies, which used testing that was considered appropriate just a few years ago, are today considered inadequate because of the test's insensitivity in light of current technology. For many years the Southern blot analysis for HPV DNA was considered to be the gold standard. Because it is very laboratory and personnel intense, and difficult to replicate between different laboratories, other techniques were developed. The filter in situ hybridization and dot blot test were developed; the latter was used in the commercially available Vira-Pap and Vira-type kits. Both techniques were insensitive. The HPV Profile kit was developed to increase the number of HPV types tested (from 7 to 14), but it is labor intense and uses radiolabeling. This was introduced in 1993 but was replaced by *hybrid capture,* which is said to have greater sensitivity, requires less time, and uses a chemiluminescence substrate instead of radiolabeling. The hybrid capture second generation (HC2) is FDA approved for HPV testing of the cervix. Both high- and low-risk HPV types can be identified but require separate RNA probes. Testing for low-risk types is not recommended. The high-risk probe can identify types 16, 18, 31, 33, 35, 39, 45, 51, 52, 56, 58, 59, and 68. A semiquantitative measure of the viral load can be obtained based on the intensity of light emitted by the sample. In many instances, more than one subtype may be present.

With our current knowledge, HPV typing is offered as part of our routine screening and triage. This implies that we know the answer to several other questions (e.g., the incidence or prevalence in the "normal" population; what affects the positive rate; which technique is considered to be the gold standard; whether HPV DNA detection can predict future cervical neoplasia). Some investigators have stated that HPV DNA is ubiquitous and endemic. The most common method of transmittal appears to be sexual; however, nonsexual transfer is not rare. Jenison found that 28% to 65% of children younger than 10 years old had antibodies HPV-6, -16, or -18 fusion proteins, and 20% had polymerase chain reaction (PCR) detection of HPV-6 or 16 in oral mucosa. The prevalence of HPV DNA detection appears to increase during pregnancy, and transmission from the mother to the child during delivery is accepted as a possible transfer mechanism. Although the prevalence of HPV DNA does appear to be related to sexual activity, detection of the DNA has been found in coed virgins. It appears that HPV DNA is detected most often in women without evidence of CIN in the 15- to 25-year age range. Studies of sexually active adolescents noted that detection of HPV DNA varied from 15% to 38%. The HPV detection rate was usually higher in women with more sexual partners; however, one study noted that the rate decreased significantly as the number of sexual partners increased (>10 partners). The rate of detection did not correlate with the years of sexual activity. These usually decreased with age when other factors were controlled. Mao and associates evaluated 516 sexually active university students (18-24 years old). They collected genital specimens for HPV testing every 4 months for up to 4 years. During the study, more than 4000 study visits were completed, and at about 20% of the visits HPV positivity other than 6 and 11 was noted. Only 5% were positive for 6 and 11. Except for those with 6 and 11, all other HPV subtypes identified, the women were asymptomatic.

Ho and colleagues followed 608 college women at 6-month intervals for 3 years. The accumulative 30-month incidence of HPV infection was 43%. The increased risk was associated with younger age, increased number of vaginal sex partners, high frequency of vaginal sex, and partners with an increase of sexual partners. The median duration of new infections was 8 months. The persistence of HPV for 6 months or longer was related to older age, type of HPV, and multiple subtypes of HPV. The risk of an abnormal Pap smear result increased with persistent HPV infection, particularly high-risk types.

Woodman and associates recruited 2001 women, 15 to 19 years old, who had recently become sexually active. The researchers took cervical smears every 6 months. In 1075 women who were cytologically normal and HPV negative at recruitment, the accumulative risk for any HPV infection was 44%. The accumulative 3-year risk of a different HPV type than present initially was 26%. Of the women, 246 had abnormal smear results and 28 progressed to high-grade CIN. This risk was highest in women who were positive for HPV-16, but 40% tested negative for HPV and another 33% tested positive for first time only at the visit as the abnormal smear result. Five women who progressed to high-grade CIN consistently tested negative for HPV.

Moscicki and colleagues followed a small group of HPV DNA–positive women for longer than 2 years with several visits in which HPV DNA using both PCR and dot blot technique were tested. Twelve of 27 tested positive for HPV-16 or -18. More than half of the women had negative results spontaneously (defined as two or more negative test results) for the original HPV type detected during the first visit. The data suggested that the number of virions decreased over a relatively short period and that the infection was presumed terminated. When a new HPV type was identified, most reported acquiring a new sexual partner since the last visit. This probably reflects a new infection and not reactivation. Rosenfeld and colleagues found that more than 50% of young urban patients tested positive for HPV either at an initial visit or at follow-up 6 to 36 months later using the Southern blot test. Therefore, the prevalence and incidence of HPV DNA appear to vary greatly, depending on age, sexual activity, the number of times tested, and the laboratory technique used. More than 1 million people are estimated to seek medical attention each year in the United States because of virus-induced lesions. The incidence therefore appears to be high for finding HPV DNA in the female genital tract. Even with the high-risk HPV types, infections commonly cause only mild transient cytologic changes and rarely lead to significant CIN or invasive cancer. Therefore the use of routine screening using HPV DNA probes does not appear to be clinically indicated in the young patient.

HPV testing has been evaluated as an adjunct to primary cervical screening. Cuzick and associates obtained HPV testing for types 16, 18, 31, and 33 using a semiquantitative type-specific PCR test. In 1980 their study was done on evaluable women who had never been treated for CIN and who had not had an abnormal Pap smear result during the previous 3 years. Cytologic abnormality or high concentrations of HPV were obtained in 11.6% (231 patients) and 4% (81 patients) had CIN II or III, respectively. The positive predictive value (PPV) of HSIL cytology in identifying CIN II or III was 66%. HPV testing detected 61 cases of CIN II or III (sensitivity 75% and PPV of 42%). Of the 81 cases of CIN II or III, cytology was negative in 33 and 20 had no evidence of any of the HPV types tested. Although sensitivity and PPV were noted, specificity and the negative predictive value (NPV) were not.

Recently cell proliferation pathways have been evaluated in regard to HPV. This has led to evaluation of genes and growth factors. Data have suggested that the progression of CIN to cancer can lead to an upregulation of epidermal growth factor receptor (EGF-R). This upregulation is common to all squamous cell cancers; however, in cervical cancer EGF-R upregulation leads to a specific upregulation of insulin-like growth factor-II (IGF-II). IGF-I levels, but not IGF-II levels, are elevated in other gynecologic, breast, and prostate cancers. It has been suggested that IGF-II levels could be used as a monitor for CIN and cervical cancers post therapy. Increased serum IGF-II levels in cervical cancer are accompanied by a significantly reduced level of serum IGF-binding protein-3 (IGF-BP3). IGF-BP3 appears to be a cell regulatory and pro-apoptotic agent, and an increase in its level offers an excellent prognosis for cervical cancer regression through its down-regulating effects on EGF-R, IGF-II, and vascular-endothelial growth factor (VEGF). VEGF-B is known to be elevated during metastatic spread of many cancers. A reduction in IGF-BP3 levels has been observed upon treatment with VEGF in HPV-positive and negative cell lines. VEGF-C has been found to be significantly elevated in women with persistent cervical cancer or HSIL and appears to be effective in early diagnosis of metastatic cervical cancer. VEGF-C appears to be unique to cervical cancer in that it interacts with IGF-II and IGF-BP3 through EGF-R. It is interesting that VEGF-C is upregulated by nicotine in cervical cancer cell lines. This translational research may not only lead to a better understanding of cervical cancer and its precursors, but also may increase our ability to predict which CIN may progress, monitor cervical cancer post treatment, and identify persistence or recurrence at an earlier time than currently available.

It has been suggested that the sexual partners of women with CIN and HPV infection should be treated to control the infectious process among women. Campion and colleagues evaluated 140 women who presented for treatment of biopsy-proven CIN. As a control group, 280 females matched for age and disease severity (two control patients for each study patient) were identified. HPV typing was performed on each control and case. The atypical TZ was destroyed with the laser in each. Repeat HPV typing was done at 6 months. In the study group, the current sexual partners were evaluated and all HPV lesions were treated. The male partners of the control group were not treated. The primary cure rate of CIN was the same in the two groups (92% study vs 94% control group). The role of controlling disease in the male sexual partner does not appear to be helpful.

It is now generally accepted that the virus itself cannot be eliminated with any known therapy. Not only is HPV commonly found in as many as 80% of normal (non-CIN) patients, but after treatment for CIN, HPV was found in 100% of 20 females with CIN who were successfully treated with laser. Riva and associates treated 25 women with koilocytotic atypia, CIN, vaginal intraepithelial neoplasia (VAIN), or vulval intraepithelial neoplasia (VIN). All patients had laser therapy of the cervix, vagina, and vulva in continuity. Morbidity was significant. Histologic persistence of subclinical HPV infection was documented in 88% of patients after treatment. Neither treatment of male sexual consorts nor sexual abstinence significantly improved treatment outcome.

Vaccines

Two HPV vaccines currently are FDA approved and available in the United States. One is a quadrivalent vaccine with HPV types 6, 11, 16, and 18, and the other is a bivalent vaccine with types 16 and 18. Both vaccines consist of a viruslike particle that is an empty viron shell that contains no HPV DNA. These are identical to the capsid surrounding the naturally occurring viral DNA yet contains no genetic material. Because there is no genetic material in these viruslike particles, this removes any possibility that the vaccine could induce HPV manifestations, including cancer. The bivalent vaccine is produced in a baculovirus, and the quadrivalent is produced in yeast. The adjuvants are also different. The bivalent contains an ASO4 adjuvant, whereas the quadrivalent vaccine contains an alum adjuvant. There is also a slight difference in treatment regimens, although both recommend three vaccinations over a 6-month time frame. The FDA recommendation for the vaccine is in females from 9 to 26 years for both vaccines. Recently the quadrivalent vaccine was also approved for males.

Several large phase II and III studies have been completed and have shown efficacy for the HPV vaccine. The FUTURE I and II studies evaluated the quadrivalent vaccine in more than 16,000 women who were followed for 3 years. The end point was CIN II–positive and AIS. The efficacy of the vaccine in preventing these high-grade neoplasias associated with vaccine-targeted HPV types in the two trials was 98% and 100% among the per protocol population. In the "intent to treat" population, which included all women in the study regardless of HPV status at time of enrollment, at 3 years the vaccine reduced high-grade neoplasia associated with the vaccine-targeted HPV types by only 29% and 50% in the two trials. In the "intent to treat" population there were a number of women already infected with the vaccine-targeted HPV at the time of enrollment. Some of these developed CIN II and III associated with the vaccine-targeted HPV strains during the first 18 months of the trial, although with longer follow-up the cumulative number of cases plateaued in the vaccinated women, whereas it continued to rise in the placebo arm. Thus, with longer follow-up, the vaccine efficacy did improve. Therefore, the recommendation is that all sexually active adolescents and young women be vaccinated through 26 years of age. A recent publication updated the cases of more than 17,000 women ages 15 to 26 enrolled in the FUTURE I and II study. This was investigated in the population of sexually naïve women, in that they were negative to 14 HPV types and were in a mixed population of HPV-exposed and HPV-unexposed women (the "intent to treat" group). With an average follow-up of 3.6 years (maximum 4.9 years), in the population negative to the 14 HPV subtypes there was 100% effectiveness from the vaccination in reducing the risk of HPV-16 and -18–related high-grade cervical, vulva, and vaginal lesions and of HPV-6 and -11–related genital warts. In the "intent to treat" group, vaccinations also reduced the risks of high-grade lesions 19%, vulvar and vaginal lesions 50.7%, genital warts 62%, Pap smear abnormalities 11% reduction, and cervical definitive therapy 23%, irrespective of the causal HPV type. All of these reductions were statistically significant. The 14 HPV types were 12 high risk and 2 low risk in patients who had normal cytology at baseline.

A phase III trial evaluating the bivalent vaccine in more than 15,000 women has recently been updated. The end point in this study was CIN II+ or greater, and the efficacy in women 15 to 25 years of age naïve for HPV-16 and 18, was more than 93%. The efficacy in HPV-16 and -18–associated ASCUS was 88%. The data were similar in young women 15 to 17 years of age from the same study.

There does appear to be HPV cross protection. In the bivalent study, efficacy against CIN II+ of 37.4% was seen for any oncogenic type except HPV-16 or -18. If coinfections with HPV-16 or -18 were included, the efficacy was 54%. Cross protection against HPV-31 and -33 and 45 were noted for prevention of infection with HPV-3-45 and 28% for HPV-31, -33, -45, -52, and -58 if naïve for these types at time of vaccination.

Adverse effects have been reported after HPV vaccination. Of these, more than 90% have been considered to be nonserious, including such things as dizziness, syncope, nausea, pain at injection site, headache, fever, and rash. A small number of serious events including Guillain-Barré syndrome, venous thromboembolism, and death have been reported; however, the U.S. Centers for Disease Control and Prevention (CDC) and the FDA have concluded that these were not causally linked to the vaccination. The duration of immunogenesis and clinical efficacy is unknown. As further experience is obtained with long-term follow-up of the programs reported, this information should be available. The efficacy of the vaccination in men is not well defined; however, the immunologic response to the quadrivalent vaccine is equal in males and females.

The vaccine is contraindicated in pregnant women. If the vaccination has been started before the knowledge of the pregnancy, subsequent doses are recommended to be withheld until after completion of the pregnancy. A woman can be immunized immediately following delivery and during lactation because there is no vaccine-related risk to the baby. Patients with immunosuppression can receive the vaccine; however, the immune response may be weaker than in individuals who are immunocompromised.

HIV and Cervical Neoplasia

Human immune deficiency virus (HIV) is an ever-increasing disease affecting all our citizens. Initially thought to be limited to homosexual males and intravenous (IV) drug users, more and more women are being diagnosed with HIV and acquired immunodeficiency virus (AIDS). At the end of 2006, an estimated 1,106,400 persons in the United States were living with HIV, including more than 468,000 with AIDS and 21% of them undiagnosed. In 2006 the CDC estimated about 56,000 persons were newly infected with HIV, of which 27% were women and more than 60% were African-American women. Historically, more than 56% of HIV infection in women was transmitted by high-risk heterosexual contact and 42% from drug injection use. In 2007, 74% of women who contracted HIV infection acquired the infection via high-risk heterosexual contact. On January 1, 1993, the CDC expanded the case definition of AIDS to include HIV-positive women with invasive cervical cancer. This inclusion remains controversial because it apparently was based on preliminary data. These data suggested that in HIV-positive patients, there was a high incidence of CIN, Pap smear results were unreliable, and other diagnostic procedures (i.e., colposcopy) should be part of routine evaluation of these patients. Some have voiced their opinions that this designation should be eliminated. Their rationale is the low incidence of cervical cancer in HIV-positive women and the fact that the incidence has not decreased with the use of highly active antiretroviral therapy (HAART). This is in contrast to Kaposi's sarcoma and non-Hodgkin's lymphoma, in which the relationship with AIDS is well established.

In comparison to HIV-negative women, HIV-positive individuals are at a higher risk for cervical cytologic abnormalities. It appears that HPV infection is more common in women with HIV. Initially it was felt that cervical cancer was increased in women with HIV; however, the Women's Interagency HIV Study (WIHS), the largest study of women with HIV in the United States, found no significant increase in the risk for invasive cervical cancer. Studies from other countries have also noted the same findings.

As a part of the WIHS, Massad and colleagues reported an ongoing multicenter cohort study of the natural history of HIV and related health conditions in women seropositive for HIV compared to at-risk uninfected women. This report included 2623 women who were followed over a median of 8.4 years with 23,843 Pap tests from 1931 HIV-positive women and 533 HIV-negative women. The incidences of abnormal Pap smear results were significantly increased in HIV-positive women compared to HIV-negative women (RR 2.4, CI 2.0-2.8). The incidence of HSIL or cancer was also increased (RR 3.4, CI 1.2-9.5). Although the risk of abnormal cervical cytology in HIV-positive women was significantly increased in this group of regularly screened women, over time the incidence of abnormal Pap smear results decreased. Even so, the abnormal Pap smear rate remains higher than 25% in this study. Among women followed for at least 10 years, 77% had had at least one abnormal Pap test result, and at every visit more than 25% of HIV-positive women had abnormal Pap results.

Other studies noted similar results. Ellerbrock and associates found that 91% of abnormal Pap results in HIV-positive women were low grade and no cancers were found. Delmore and colleagues found only 3% with high-grade lesions. Cubie and colleagues, and also Schuman and colleagues, also found that the vast majority of abnormal Pap results in HIV-positive women were low grade. It appears that, although there is an increased risk of LSIL and HSIL, the absolute incidence remains low (about 4/1000 for HSIL), suggesting that the majority of Pap test abnormalities reflect opportunistic infection with HPV.

Treatment of CIN- and HIV-positive women appears to have a high failure rate regardless of modality use. It appears that persistence and recurrence are particularly high in those patients treated with destructive therapy; however, recurrence after loop electrosurgical excision procedure (LEEP) mirrors results of ablation therapy. Those individuals treated with excisional therapy are more likely to have margin involvement than women who are HIV negative. Even with conization of the cervix or hysterectomy, there is a much higher chance of having a recurrent disease in HIV-positive women compared with those who are HIV negative. Massad and colleagues reported two prospective cohort studies from the WIHS and Heart and Estrogen/Progestin Replacement Study (HERS) studies. These individuals were followed for 6 months after every treatment for CIN with HPV testing and cytology along with colposcopy as indicated. If abnormality was identified within 6 months of treatment, it was defined as treatment failure; those recurring after 6 months were defined as recurrence. Disease persisted at 6 months in 45% of the women. Most failures were low grade, even those initially treated for high-grade disease. Of women with oncogenic HPV before treatment, 67% had the same type at diagnosis of treatment persistence. HIV positivity combined with low CD4 lymphocyte count and the detection of HPV DNA at treatment were the only factors associated with a higher degree of probability of treatment failure in multivariant analysis. Of 101 women who had negative cytology 6 months after treatment, 56 subsequently experienced recurrence of disease, with 49 being low-grade and 7 being high-grade disease. The authors noted that many women with failures and recurrence after treatment do not have the same lesion returning but instead have a new HPV infection associated with low-grade changes. Time to recurrence after initial negative follow-up was associated with HPV status, CD stratum detection of oncogenic HPV, and CIN grade. Because of a high failure rate irrespective of treatment received, it is apparent that close follow-up of these patients is required.

Natural History

The natural history of CIN has been evaluated by reviewing the literature on the subject and by conducting meta-analysis. This information may be used as a guideline in clinical management. In a review of the literature of almost 14,000 patients followed for less than 1 year up to 20 years, Östör noted that in CIN I, 60% will regress and only 10% will progress to CIS. In patients with CIN III, one third will regress to normal. The initial diagnosis was by cytology, biopsy, or a combination of the two. In more than 15,000 patients, 1.7% progressed to invasive cancer, with CIN I doing so in 1% compared with 12% of patients with CIN III. In a meta-analysis of almost 28,000 patients, Melnikow and colleagues found that ASCUS progressed to HSIL at 24 months in 7.3% and LSIL in 21%. Progression to cancer was 0.25% with ASCUS, 0.15% with LSIL (LGSIL), and 1.44% with HSIL. Regression to normal occurred in 68% in ASCUS, 47% in LSIL, and 35% in HSIL.

The average age of patients with CIS reproducibly is 10 to 15 years younger than the average age of patients with invasive cancer of the cervix. However, there are many exceptions; in the past two decades, CIS and invasive disease have been reported in an increasing number of patients in their late teens and early 20s. Whether all invasive carcinomas begin as in situ lesions is unknown, but Peterson reported that in one third of 127 untreated patients, invasive carcinoma developed subsequent to CIS at the end of 9 years. Masterson and colleagues found that 28% of 25 untreated patients demonstrated invasive carcinoma at the end of 5 years.

CIS is usually asymptomatic, and on routine examination the lesion is frequently not observed. Recognition of the lesion is assisted considerably by the use of cytologic testing and colposcopy. The mucous membrane sometimes bleeds easily on contact, and erosion or a superficial defect of the ectocervix is relatively common in patients with CIS, but these findings are not pathognomonic. The diagnosis must always be confirmed by histologic sections of a biopsy specimen.

What happens to a patient with early CIN in regard to its natural history is important because it relates to management. A review of the literature of the past 40 years suggests that more advanced lesions (CIN III) are more likely to persist or progress than CIN I. CIN III can regress spontaneously, but more important, it is suggested that progression to cancer occurs more than 15% of the time, whereas CIN I progresses to cancer only 1% of the time. The regression and persistence of CIN I and II appear to be similar. If the eventual outcome of a given patient with an abnormal Pap smear result could be predicted, the problem of management would be greatly simplified. Certainly, not all patients with abnormal cervical cells develop cancer of the cervix or even progression of CIN.

Unfortunately, most of the studies performed on the natural history of this disease were carried out in the absence of the current diagnostic techniques—namely, colposcopy. Most studies used cytologic tests or biopsy as the diagnostic tools, resulting in varying progression/regression rates. Kessler reviewed many of the studies on the biologic behavior of cervical dysplasia. The occurrence of the progression of CIN lesions to either a more severe form or invasive cancer ranges from 1.4% to 60%. Of interest is that the two most variant studies used cytologic tests alone to follow patients. The problems of definitive diagnosis using this technique have been studied in detail, and considerable variation even in the best of hands has been noted. When biopsies are performed, particularly if the lesion is small, the natural history of the disease may be disrupted, further complicating the evaluation of this entity. Even studies on the biologic behavior of cervical CIS are varied, with progression to invasive cancer being reported in up to 50% of cases. The differences in these findings may very well be a result of the length of follow-up once the diagnosis of CIS was established. Some patients with CIN develop invasive cancer, whereas others, even though followed for many years, do not progress either to a more severe form of CIN or to invasive cancer.

Rapid-onset cancer in patients with normal cytology is a phenomenon that is often discussed; however, when evaluated, the cytology appears to be infrequently documented. In a study from Canada, the authors found that more than 95% of so-called rapid-onset cancers (appearing within 3 years of a "normal" Pap) were a result of inadequate and false-negative smear results and failure to evaluate an abnormal test result. In an Italian study of 115 cervical cancer patients, 70% had never had a Pap smear; 7% were diagnosed at their first test; and 10% had false-negative cytology. The other patients had either poor compliance or inadequate evaluation.

It has become apparent from recent studies that CIN is being diagnosed at a much younger age. In our material, the median age for CIS of the cervix has decreased from approximately 40 to 28 years of age. This may reflect only that screening of high-risk patients is done at an earlier time, resulting in a diagnosis at a younger age. Because most of these women desire children and in many cases have not started to have families, preservation of the integrity of the cervix and the uterus is important. In an analysis of approximately 800 patients with CIN at the Duke University Medical Center, 30% were 20 years of age or younger when the diagnosis was established. Nulliparity was seen in about one fourth of the population, and 60% had one child or none. More than 95% of the patients had had intercourse by the age of 20, and half had become sexually active by 16 years of age. More than half of these patients had three or more sexual partners. About half of these patients had the diagnosis of CIN established within 5 years of the beginning of their sexual activity. Screening these patients at an early age, when they seek contraception or other medical attention, was previously routine; however, with recent data on the natural history of CIN, new guidelines have been adopted.

It is not at all unusual to see patients in their early 20s with carcinoma in situ of the cervix. Therefore, the lesion may be identified early in the spectrum of disease, and a patient may continue with CIN for a prolonged period, even after reaching the level of a CIN III lesion. Table 1-3 presents the transition time of CIN in our patients. Those patients whose disease progresses to carcinoma in situ do so within a very short time. After that level of abnormality is reached, stabilization may occur in many of the patients. To date, no method is available to predict which patient will remain within the CIN category, which will progress to a more severe form of CIN or to invasive cancer, or within what time frame this transition will occur.

TABLE 1-3 Transition Time of Cervical Intraepithelial Neoplasia

Stages	Mean Years
Normal to mild-to-moderate dysplasia	1.62
Normal to moderate-to-severe dysplasia	2.2
Normal to carcinoma in situ	4.51

The American Society for Colposcopy and Cervical Pathology (ASCCP) in 2001 developed consensus guidelines for management of women with CIN. As a part of that deliberation, the literature was reviewed in regard to the natural history of cervical neoplasia. The natural history of CIN I was reviewed for 4504 patients and noted spontaneous regression in 57% of patients, whereas 11% progressed to CIN II, CIN III, or cancer. The rate of progression to cancer was 0.3%. A meta-analysis of natural history of CIN I noted similar conclusions.

Cytology

As has already been noted, genital cytology has had a major impact on the incidence of and death rate from cervical cancer. Despite general agreement about this finding, one of the problems with cervical cytology is the false-positive and false-negative rate. A major concern of clinicians has been the ever-changing terminology, which has resulted in a lack of meaning with regard to clinical relevance. The Pap classification has been changed so many times that the numbers have no constant meaning. Many cytologists changed to a descriptive term (dysplasia or, more recently, CIN) to indicate their diagnostic impression of the smear. In most cases, this terminology was clinically useful; however, there was an increasing tendency to use terms such as inflammatory atypia, squamous atypia but not dysplasia, which did not necessarily convey any clinical implications. In an attempt to clarify the varied terminology, the Bethesda System was developed in 1988. This new system was subsequently used in an increasing number of cytology laboratories, mainly because of federal mandates. It became apparent within a short time that the Bethesda System had confusing nomenclature and classification with conflicting impressions to the clinician. As a result, a 2001 Bethesda System and new terminology was developed and reported in 2002. This is currently the cytology reporting system used in the United States today. This update has been generally accepted as an improvement and eliminated those categories that led to different interpretations. The 2001 Bethesda System has only two categories: satisfactory for evaluation and unsatisfactory for evaluation (specify reason). The initial general categorization listed "within normal limits" and "benign cellular changes," which were combined in 2001 as "negative for intraepithelial lesion or malignancy." These and other changes have improved the communication to the clinician.

One of the major changes was made in the epithelial cell abnormality designation (Table 1-4). The previous category of ASCUS represented by far the largest number of abnormal Pap smear results reported each year in the United States (about 3 million). The vast majority of these ASCUS smears on evaluation found no cervical epithelial

TABLE 1-4 Bethesda 2001 Classification

Interpretation/Results
Negative for intraepithelial lesion or malignancy
Organisms may be identified
Other non-neoplastic findings may be noted
Inflammation
Radiation changes
Atrophy
Glandular cells status post hysterectomy
Atrophy
Epithelial cell abnormalities
Squamous cells
Atypical squamous cells (ASC)
Of undetermined significance (ASCUS)
Cannot exclude HSIL (ASC-H)
Low-grade squamous intraepithelial lesions (LSIL)
HPV, CIN I
High-grade squamous intraepithelial lesions (HSIL)
CIN II, CIN III
Squamous cell carcinoma
Glandular cell
Atypical glandular cells (AGC)—specify origin
Atypical glandular cells favor neoplastic—specify origin
Endocervical adenocarcinoma in situ (AIS)
Adenocarcinoma

abnormalities, although a small number did harbor CIN II or III. Cytologists were encouraged to qualify ASCUS as to whether this was a reactive process or favored SIL, but these smears were mainly classified as ASCUS not otherwise specified (NOS), which was not helpful to the clinicians. The 2001 classification redefines this category and renamed it as ASC (atypical squamous cells) with the subclassification of ASCUS (of undetermined significance) and ASC-H (cannot exclude HSIL). The latter represents about 5% to 10% of all ASC, which can eliminate the vast majority of women with ASC undergoing unwarranted more extensive and expensive evaluation. The low-grade SIL (HPV, CIN I) and high-grade SIL (CIN II and CIN III) classifications remain the same.

Under glandular cells, the previous AGUS was interpreted by many clinicians as a similar process of ASCUS and managed accordingly (repeat Pap smear). The AGUS smear carried a much greater risk of having a significant number of cervical and endometrial lesions including cancer. The 2001 Bethesda System has designated new categories under glandular cells: atypical glandular cells (AGC) in which the cytologist should specify origin; endocervical, endometrium, or not otherwise specified; atypical glandular cells, favor neoplastic; and endocervical AIS and adenocarcinoma.

Although the Pap smear has reduced dramatically the incidence of deaths from cervical cancer, false-negative smear results are known to occur with various imprecise numbers being highlighted by the large financial amounts awarded in lawsuits. It is well recognized

TABLE 1-5   Causes of Abnormal Papanicolaou Smears

Invasive cancer
Cervical intraepithelial neoplasia
Atrophic changes
Flat condyloma
Inflammation, especially trichomoniasis and chronic cervicitis
Regeneration after injury (metaplasia)
Vaginal cancer
Vulvar cancer
Upper genital tract cancer (endometrium, fallopian tube, ovary)
Previous radiation therapy

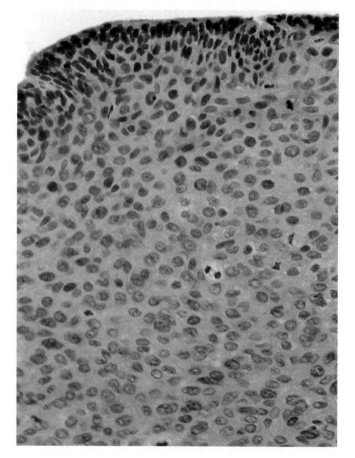

FIGURE 1-2   A cervical intraepithelial neoplasia lesion with multiple mitotic figures.

that the rate of accuracy of the Pap smear is not 100%, as in any test, although the law apparently so adjudicated it as being absolutely accurate (Table 1-5) As a result, newer technology has been developed in an attempt to decrease the present false-negative rate. As has been previously noted, the incidence of mortality would be greatly reduced if all women were screened at regular intervals and appropriate evaluations were performed.

Fluid-based, thin-layer preparations have been developed in an attempt to present to the cytologist a uniform, well-distributed layer of cells that are less likely to be distorted or obscured by blood, mucus, or inflammatory debris. The collection device, instead of being directly applied to the slide, is rinsed in a vial containing a buffered alcohol solution. The cell suspension is put through a filter system where blood and debris are removed, and a sample of cells is placed on a slide in a 20-mm–diameter specimen. This preparation is much cleaner than that normally seen. This ThinPrep (TP) technique has been approved by the FDA.

It is appreciated that most cytology done today in the United States uses the liquid technique, which has replaced the conventional Pap smear. Initial data suggested that accuracy with liquid base was improved compared to conventional method; however, recent meta-analysis found the two methods are comparable. Several countries have dictated that conventional Pap smears are preferred because the liquid base is more expensive and therefore not cost effective.

Pathology

Cervical intraepithelial neoplasia (or CIN) is the term now used to encompass all epithelial abnormalities of the cervix. The epithelial cells are malignant but confined to the epithelium. The older terminology using dysplasia and CIS connotes a two-tier disease process that, at least in the past, has influenced therapy—that is, if only dysplasia was present, no or limited treatment was needed. If CIS was diagnosed, in many cases

a hysterectomy was recommended. This concept is inappropriate, particularly when the cervical epithelium may be no thicker than 0.25 mm. Although CIN has been arbitrarily divided into three subdivisions, it does suggest that CIN is a single neoplastic continuum. The histologic criteria for a CIN diagnosis depend on the findings of nuclear aneuploidy, abnormal mitotic figures, and a loss of normal maturation of the epithelium (Figure 1-2). CIN is divided into grade I, II, or III, depending on the extent of cellular stratification aberration within the epithelium. In CIN I, the cells in the upper two thirds of the epithelium, although showing some nuclear abnormalities, have undergone cytoplasmic differentiation. The cells in the lower one third lack evidence of cytoplasmic differentiation or normal maturation (loss of polarity of the cells). Mitotic figures are few and, if present, are normal. In CIN II the abnormal changes of CIN I involve the lower two thirds of the epithelium. The CIN III lesions have full-thickness changes with undifferentiated nonstratified cells. Nuclear pleomorphism is common, and mitotic figures are abnormal. On the basis of nuclear DNA studies, some investigators have suggested that most lesions diagnosed as CIN I are, in fact, flat condyloma that contain human papilloma viruses 6/11 (groups). It should be remembered that HPV-16 and -18 are more frequently found in CIN I than other subtypes, including HPV-6 and -11. The impression is that these lesions, by and large, are not significant relative to this neoplastic process and have a very low risk for progressing to cancer compared with lesions containing HPV-16 and -18. As the epithelium becomes more involved with this intraepithelial neoplasia, there is a greater probability for HPV-16 and -18 identified with potential for invasion. HPV-16 and -18 can be present in CIN I and HPV-6 and -11 is present in higher-grade CIN.

Evaluation of an Abnormal Cervical Cytology

As noted previously, cervical cytology is a screening test. Much has been written about the reliability and the reproducibility of cervical cytology even though this has been credited with the significant decrease in cervical cancer and cervical cancer mortality that has occurred in the Western world over the last several decades. In the ALTS study, 4948 monolayer cytologic slides were obtained from patients entering into the study. This was from 3488 women who had participated in comparing alternative strategies for the initial management of women with ASCUS. Four clinical centers participated in this study. Cytology was interpreted in the individual institutions and then sent for central review. These specimens were independently reviewed by the pathology quality control (QC) group. This review was done in a blinded fashion. Of the 1473 original interpretations of ASCUS, the QC reviewers concurred in only 43%, rendering less severe readings for most of the rest. Interobserver variation also occurred in the more significant cytologic interpretations, as in those who had HSILs, concurrence was present in only 47.1%, with 22% and 22.6% of the remainder interpreted at LSIL or ASCUS by the QC reviewers. Of further interest is the fact that histologic interpretative reducibility on the biopsies was really no better than cytologic reproducibilities.

Even with the problems of reproducibility in regard to cytology, the ALTS gave some important information as far as management of abnormalities obtained on Pap smears. As a result of these studies, a consensus conference was held in Bethesda, MD in the fall of 2001 sponsored by the American Society for Colposcopy and Cervical Pathology (ASCCP). It was thought that because about 7% of all Pap smears obtained in the United States were diagnosed with some degree of cytologic abnormality with the vast majority noting only minor changes, generalized guidelines for management should be developed to make the most responsible use of

time and resources. These guidelines may aid the clinician in the management of patients with an abnormal cytology.

Atypical Squamous Cells

As previously noted, the 2001 Bethesda system subdivided ASC into two categories: ASCUS and ASC-H. The patients who have ASCUS have a 5% to 17% chance of having CIN II or III confirmed by biopsy, whereas with ASC-H, CIN II or III is identified in 24–94% of women. The risk of invasive cancer with ASC is low (approximately 0.1-0.2%).

Several approaches have been used in the management of a woman who has ASC. Repeat cytology has been widely used with a sensitivity of a single test for detecting CIN II and III between 0.67 and 0.85. Colposcopy has also been used. Its advantage is that immediately the woman can be informed of the presence or absence of a significant disease. Sensitivity for distinguishing normal from abnormal tissue on the cervix by colposcopy was 0.96 and with a weighted mean specificity of 0.48. Several large studies have now been performed using the DNA testing as a triage mechanism for the management of women with ASC. The sensitivity of HPV DNA testing for detection of biopsy-proven CIN II and III has been said to be 0.83 to 1.0. The negative predictive value for high-risk types of HPV is generally reported to be 0.98 or greater. Between 31% and 60% of all women with ASC will have high-risk types of HPV, with the amount decreasing with increasing age. Recent data suggest that young women (≤20 years old in one study and ≤29 years old in another) will have a high-risk HPV type in up to 80% of individuals. This makes HPV DNA testing as part of the triage less applicable. So-called "reflex" HPV DNA testing also has been used in the triage mechanism. This uses liquid-based cytology using the leftover liquid subsequent to the return of ASC cytology. With the aforementioned as a background, the following represents the 2006 consensus guidelines for cervical cytologic abnormalities.

ASCUS

Acceptable methods for managing women with ASCUS may be repeat cervical cytology testing, colposcopy, or DNA testing for high-risk types of HPV. When liquid-based cytology is used, then reflex testing is felt to be the preferred management. Women with ASCUS who test negative for high-risk HPV DNA can then be followed with repeat cytologic testing in 12 months. Suggested options for those individuals who are positive for high-risk types of HPV but do not have biopsy-confirmed CIN include repeat cytologic testing at 6 and 12 months with referral back to colposcopy if the results of ASCUS or greater is obtained or if HPV DNA

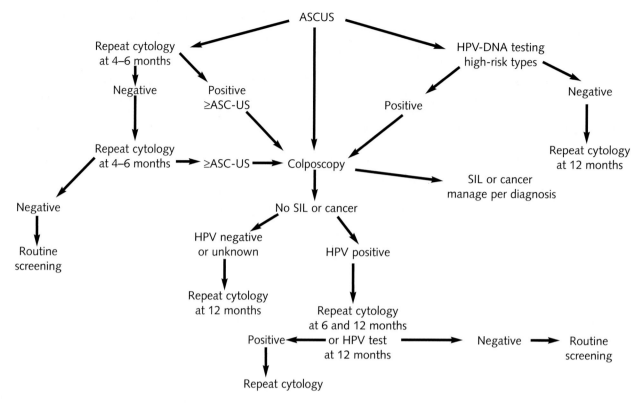

FIGURE 1-3   Management of Women with ASCUS Cytology. ASC-US, Atypical squamous cells of unknown significance; SIL, Squamous intraepithelial lesion.

testing at 12 months returns high-risk positive types (Figure 1-3).

Repeat cervical cytology testing is done at 4–6-month intervals until two consecutive "negative for intraepithelial lesions or malignancy" are obtained. Women with ASCUS or greater on repeat tests should be referred for colposcopy. If two repeat negative smear results are obtained, then the woman can be returned to routine cytologic screening. When immediate colposcopy is used, individuals not found to have CIN should be followed with repeat cytologic testing at 12 months. It was strongly recommended that diagnostic excisional procedures such as LEEP should not be routinely used to treat women with ASC in the absence of biopsy-confirmed CIN.

Certain special circumstances in women with ASCUS should be taken into consideration.

Adolescent women: Although the new guidelines for screening do not recommend routine screening before the age of 21, there will be some adolescent women who will have had an abnormal Pap smear result, usually ASCUS. Prospective studies of adolescents with LSIL have shown that spontaneous regression to normal occurs at a higher rate, up to 91% at 36 months. As a result, these individuals should be treated conservatively. If ASCUS is present, an annual Pap smear is recommended. At the 12-month follow-up, adolescents with only HSIL or greater on repeat cytology should be referred to colposcopy. HPV DNA testing and colposcopy are not recommended for adolescents with ASCUS. LEEP is contraindicated as a diagnostic procedure in these young and nulliparous women.

Postmenopausal women: In women with ASCUS or who have cytologic evidence of atrophy, local intravaginal estrogen can be used for several days and then about a week after completion of therapy repeat cytology can be carried out. If the result is negative, the test should be repeated in 4 to 6 months. If the abnormality remains, the patient should be referred for colposcopy.

Immunosuppressed women: Referral to colposcopy is recommended in all who have ASCUS. This includes women infected with HIV, irrespective of the CD4 cell count, HIV viral load, or antiretroviral therapy.

Pregnant patient: ASC-US should be managed as for the nonpregnant patient.

ASC-H

Because women with ASC-H have an appreciable higher chance of having CIN II and III compared with women with ASCUS, all individuals should be referred for colposcopic evaluation. When no lesion is identified, it is suggested that a review of the cytology, colposcopy, and

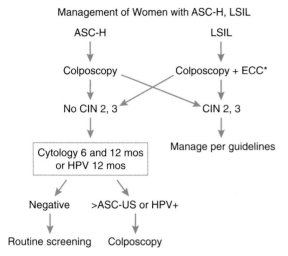

Management of Women with ASC-H, LSIL

*Preferred if no lesions identified or unsatisfactory colposcopy

FIGURE 1-4 Evaluation and management schema for a patient with ASC-H (atypical squamous cells–cannot exclude HSIL) and LSIL (low-grade squamous intraepithelial lesion).

histological results be performed. If on review a revised interpretation is submitted, then management should be to follow guidelines for the revised interpretation. If cytological interpretation of ASC-H is upheld, then follow-up in 6 to 12 months with cytology or HPV DNA testing at 12 months is acceptable. Women who are found to have ASC-H or greater on repeat cervical cytology testing or who test positive for high-risk HPV DNA should be referred for colposcopy (Figure 1-4).

Low-Grade Squamous Intraepithelial Lesions

In most laboratories, the median rate of LSIL is 1.6%; however, this may be as high as 7% to 8% in laboratories serving high-risk populations. Approximately 15% to 30% of women with LSIL will have CIN II or III identified on subsequent cervical biopsies. In the ALTS study, 83% of women referred for evaluation of an LSIL cytology tested positive for high-risk HPV. With this high incidence, using HPV DNA as part of the triage in the management of LSIL is not recommended because essentially all of these individuals would be referred for colposcopy based on the positive HPV test result. Colposcopy is the recommended management option for these women. Management then depends on whether a lesion is identified, whether the colposcopy is satisfactory, or whether the patient is pregnant. The routine use of diagnostic excisional procedures or ablative procedures is unacceptable for the initial management of these patients with LSIL in the absence of biopsy-confirmed CIN. In an individual with a satisfactory colposcopy, endocervical sampling is acceptable for the nonpregnant patient but is preferred for the nonpregnant patient in whom no lesions are identified. If the aforementioned

CIN is not confirmed, acceptable management includes follow-up with repeat cytology at 6 and 12 months and referral for colposcopy if a result of ASCUS or greater is obtained. Follow-up with HPV DNA testing at 12 months with referral colposcopy if testing is positive for high-risk HPV is also an option.

In those nonpregnant patients with unsatisfactory colposcopy results, endocervical sampling is preferred. If a biopsy fails to confirm CIN and colposcopy is unsatisfactory, accepted management can include repeat cytology at 6 to 12 months with referral for colposcopy if results of ASC-US or greater is obtained or with HPV DNA testing at 12-month intervals if testing is positive.

If CIN is identified, then management can be performed as per the guidelines, as noted later in this chapter.

High-Grade Squamous Intraepithelial Lesions

A cytology diagnosis of HSIL accounts for only about 0.5% of cytological interpretations in 1996. Women with HSIL have a 70% to 75% chance of having biopsy confirmed CIN II and III and a 1% to 2% chance of having invasive cervical cancer. Traditionally in women with HSIL, colposcopy with endocervical assessment has been considered the best management. When a high-grade cervical or vaginal lesion is not identified after colposcopy, it is recommended that, when possible, review of cytology, colposcopy, and histological results be performed. If cytologic interpretation of HSIL is upheld, a diagnostic excisional procedure is preferred by many in the nonpregnant patient. Ablation is unacceptable. In an individual with HSIL in whom colposcopy suggests a high-grade lesion, initial evaluation using a diagnostic excisional procedure is also an acceptable option. Triage using either a program of repeat cytology or HPV testing is unacceptable.

In the pregnant patient, colposcopy is preferred but carried out after the middle portion of the second trimester. Biopsy of lesions thought to be high grade or cancerous is preferred; however, endocervical curettage should not be carried out in the pregnant woman. Unless invasive cancer is identified, treatment can be postponed until postpartum. An excisional diagnostic procedure is recommended only if invasion is suspected. Reevaluation with cytology and colposcopy is recommended no sooner than 6 weeks postpartum.

In the young woman of reproductive age, when biopsy-confirmed CIN II and III is not identified, observation with colposcopy and cytology at 4- to 6-month intervals for a year is accepted provided that the colposcopic findings are satisfactory and the endocervical sampling is negative. If HSIL cytology persists, then further evaluation with colposcopy and excisional biopsy is indicated.

Atypical Glandular Cells and Adenocarcinoma In Situ

As previously noted, atypical glandular cells have been redefined in the 2001 Bethesda System. If a report of AGC is obtained, then biopsy-confirmed high-grade lesions or invasive cancer have been found in 9% to 41% with AGC NOS compared with 27% to 96% with women with AGC "favored neoplasia." The cytologic finding of AIS is associated with a very high risk of women having either AIS (48% to 69%) or invasive cervical adenocarcinoma (38%). In all women with either AGC or AIS, further evaluation is needed. Repeat cervical cytology is usually not recommended. CIN is the most common form of neoplasia identified in women with AGC; therefore, inclusion of colposcopy in the initial portion of the workup of women is recommended. Endocervical sampling should also be performed at the same time. There is a higher risk of CIN II or III in AIS in premenopausal women compared with postmenopausal women. About half the women with biopsy-confirmed AIS also have a coexistent squamous abnormality.

As noted, colposcopy with endocervical sampling is recommended for all women with all subcategories of AGC (Figure 1-5). If atypical endometrial cells are also present, endometrial sampling should be performed. Endometrial sampling should be performed in connection with the colposcopy in all women with AGC or AIS who are 35 years of age or older. Management of a program of repeat cervical cytology is unacceptable. The role of HPV DNA testing in the management of patients with AGC or AIS is inconclusive at the present time. If invasive disease is not identified during the initial workup, it is recommended that women with AGC "favored neoplasia" or AIS undergo a diagnostic excisional procedure. A cold knife conization is preferred over a LEEP procedure. If no neoplasia is identified during the initial workup of the woman with AGC NOS, she can be followed with repeat cervical cytology at

4- to 6-month intervals until four consecutive negative results are obtained, after which she may return to routine screening. If an abnormality is noted on repeat Pap smear, acceptable options include repeat colposcopic examinations or referral to a clinician experienced in the management of complex cytologic situations.

CERVICAL GLANDULAR CELL ABNORMALITIES

Cervical glandular cell abnormalities are being identified cytologically and histologically in increasing numbers. In 1979 Chrisopherson, based on a large population-based series, estimated a 1:239 ratio of cervical AIS to squamous cell CIS. Since then, the incidence of adenocarcinoma of the cervix has been increasing in relationship to squamous cancers. Most likely the preinvasive glandular abnormalities are also increasing. AIS is frequently associated with CIN. Most data would suggest that 50% or more cases of AIS are seen with CIN. Although the entire endocervical canal may be involved, more than 95% of AIS occurs at the squamocolumnar junction. Several studies suggest that abnormal glandular elements are associated with HPV-18. This includes AIS and adenocarcinoma. Whether epidemiologic factors associated with squamous CIN are the same for AIS is suggested but unknown. When cytology indicative of glandular abnormalities is present, the canal must be evaluated. Cytology should include the canal with a brush or similar device. Even though AGUS may be present, a considerable number of patients will have more significant disease on histologic evaluation. Although colposcopic findings may not be classic and subtle changes can be missed, most suggest that this is a worthwhile procedure. Colposcopic findings may include areas of whitened villi lying within immature metaplasia. The villi are thicker and more blunt than normal. Long, unbranched horizontal vessels may be present. Invasive disease (either involving adenocarcinoma or squamous cells) may be suspected and confirmed with biopsies. The findings on endocervical curettage (ECC) may help in the diagnosis, and this procedure is encouraged. Most investigators think that conization is the diagnostic technique of choice, unless invasion is proved earlier in the workup. More and more data suggest that conization of the cervix may be adequate therapy for adenoCIS or less particularly if surgical margins are free. Muntz found that one twelfth of women with uninvolved margins and seven tenths of women with positive margins had residual disease in the hysterectomy specimen. They followed 18 women for a median interval of 3 years (1.5-5 years) who had uninvolved cone margins, and none recurred. Other data from the literature note the same findings.

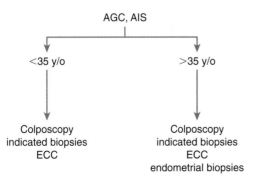

FIGURE 1-5   Management of Papanicolaou smears of atypical glandular cells of undetermined significance (AGUS). (ECC, endocervical curettage.)

Hitchcock and colleagues followed 21 patients with cervical glandular atypia, including AIS, after conization with cytology and pelvic examinations. After 13 years, none developed abnormal cytology or invasive carcinoma, even though 13 conizations contained abnormalities that appeared to be incompletely resected. Others, however, have been more pessimistic. Poynor evaluated 28 patients with a diagnosis of AIS made by conization. Only nine (43%) had a glandular lesion diagnosed on ECC before conization. Four of 10 patients with negative cone margins were found to have residual AIS, either in the hysterectomy or on repeat cone specimens. Four of 8 patients with positive cone margins had residual disease in the second surgical specimen (3 with AIS and one with invasive adenocarcinoma). Seven of 15 patients managed conservatively with close follow-up or repeat cone have had a recurrence; 2 patients had invasive adenocarcinoma. An increasing amount of data suggest that patients who desire future fertility may in fact be managed with cold knife conization only if surgical margins are not involved. The persistence rate is approximately 8% in these circumstances compared with a rate as high as 60% if margins are involved. In situations in which fertility is desired and positive margins are present, reconization may be considered. In patients suspected of having ACIS, the cold knife conization appears to be a better procedure than large loop excision of transformation zone because the latter tends to have a larger number with positive margins and a higher recurrence rate. In patients who are not interested in future fertility, a simple hysterectomy is suggested as definitive therapy for AIS by many. Current practice mandates further evaluation of an abnormal Pap smear result (dysplasia or CIN), initially with colposcopy biopsies and ECC. Further evaluation (conization) may be indicated, depending on these preliminary results.

Colposcopy

With the advent of colposcopy, a conservative schema and treatment plan for the patient with an abnormal Pap test result have been generally accepted. This schema is safe only if the steps are rigorously followed. This is particularly critical when the ECC findings are positive, even though the lesion is completely seen. In this situation, only an expert colposcopist should proceed with local treatment; otherwise, a diagnostic conization must be performed. The possibility of a coexisting unsuspected endocervical adenocarcinoma must also be considered. Omission of any of the diagnostic procedures in the evaluation may lead to the tragedy that results when invasive cancer is missed. A report by Sevin and associates of eight such cases, out of which three patients died, emphasizes the hazards of a less than optimal workup of patients before cryotherapy.

Colposcopy was introduced by Hinselman in 1925 (in Hamburg, Germany) as a result of his efforts to devise a practical method of more minute and comprehensive examination of the cervix. Hinselman and others during his era believed that cervical cancer began as miniature nodules on the surface epithelium and that these lesions could be detected with increased magnification and illumination. The meticulous examination of thousands of cases enabled him to clearly define the multiple physiologic and benign changes in the cervix and to correlate atypical changes with preinvasive and early invasive cancer. Unfortunately, Hinselman was primarily a clinician with very little pathology background, and this factor, in conjunction with the encumbrance of the tumor nodule theory, led to the development of confusing concepts and terminology associated with the use of the colposcope.

In the early 1930s initial efforts were made to introduce colposcopy in the United States as a method of early cervical cancer detection. Because of the cumbersome terminology present at that time, the method was generally ignored; and with the introduction of reliable cytologic testing in the 1940s, North American physicians lost interest in colposcopy. The interest was renewed in the 1950s and early 1960s, but acceptance was slow because of the competitive nature of cytologic examinations, which were more economical and easier to perform and had, for the novice, a lower false-negative rate. Over the last three decades the technique has gained long-awaited popularity and has been recognized as an adjunctive technique to cytologic testing in the investigation of genital tract epithelium. The popularity of colposcopy has been enhanced by the discovery of a scientific basis for most morphologic changes and the acceptance of a logical and simplified terminology for these changes.

The colposcope consists, in general, of a stereoscopic, binocular microscope with low magnification. It is provided with a center illuminating device and mounted on an adjustable stand with a transformer in the base. Several levels of magnification are available, the most useful being between 8× and 18×. A green filter is placed between the light source and the tissue to accentuate the vascular patterns and color tone differences between normal and abnormal patterns. Examination of the epithelium of the female genital tract by colposcopy usually takes no more than a few minutes.

Colposcopy is based on study of the transformation zone (Figure 1-6). The transformation zone is that area of the cervix and vagina that was initially covered by columnar epithelium and, through a process referred to as metaplasia, has undergone replacement by squamous epithelium. The wide range and variation in the colposcopic features of this tissue make up the science of colposcopy. The inheritance of variable vascular

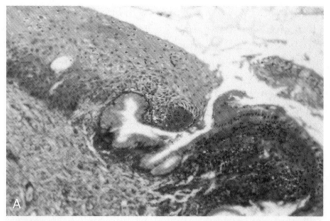

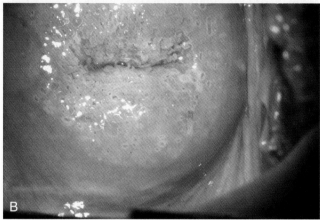

FIGURE 1-6   **A,** Squamocolumnar junction (transformation zone). **B,** Large transformation zone.

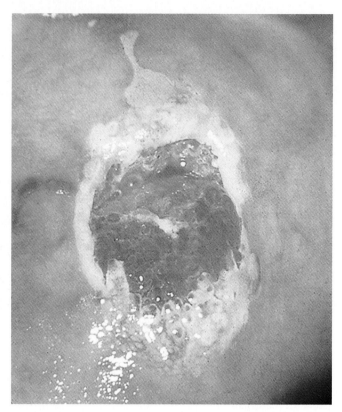

FIGURE 1-7   White epithelium at the cervical os (a colposcopic view).

TABLE 1-6   Abnormal Colposcopic Findings

Atypical transformation zone
Keratosis
Aceto–white epithelium
Punctation
Mosaicism
Atypical vessels
Suspect frank invasive carcinoma
Unsatisfactory colposcopic findings

patterns, as along with the fate of residual columnar glands and clefts, determines the great variety of patterns in this zone. It had been generally taught that the cervix was normally covered by squamous epithelium and that the presence of endocervical columnar epithelium on the ectocervix portio was an abnormal finding. Studies by Coppleson and associates have established that columnar tissue can initially exist on the ectocervix in at least 70% of young women and extend into the vaginal fornix in an additional 5%. This process of transition from columnar to squamous epithelium probably occurs throughout a woman's lifetime. However, it has been demonstrated that this normal physiologic transformation zone is most active during three periods of a woman's life: fetal development, adolescence, and her first pregnancy. The process is enhanced by an acid pH environment and is influenced greatly by estrogen and progesterone levels.

The classification of colposcopic findings has been improved and simplified (Table 1-6), facilitating the recognition of abnormal patterns: white epithelium (Figure 1-7), punctation (Fig. 1-7), mosaic structure (Figure 1-9), and atypical vessels (Figure 1-10). The term *leukoplakia* is generally reserved for the heavy, thick, white lesion that can frequently be seen with the naked eye. White epithelium, mosaic structure, and punctation herald atypical epithelium (CIN) and provide the target for directed biopsies. The pattern of atypical vessels is associated most often with invasive cancer, and biopsies should be performed liberally in areas with these findings. Although the abnormal colposcopic patterns reflect cytologic and histologic alterations, they are not specific enough for final diagnosis, and a biopsy is necessary. The greatest value of the colposcope is in directing the biopsy to the area that is most likely to yield the most significant histologic pattern.

When colposcopy is performed, a standard procedure is followed. First, the cervix is sampled for cytologic

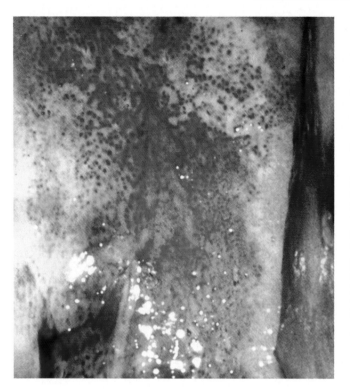

FIGURE 1-8 A punctation pattern is seen clearly above a mosaic structure (a colposcopic view).

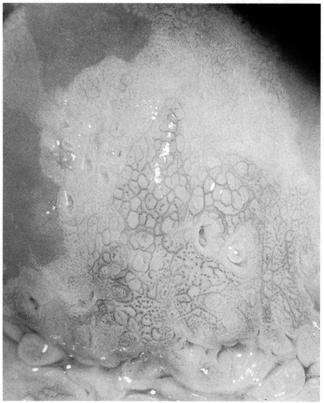

FIGURE 1-9 A large anterior lip lesion with white epithelium punctation and mosaic patterns.

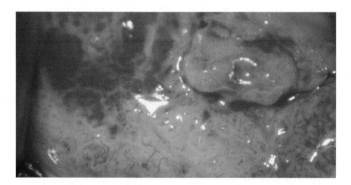

FIGURE 1-10 Many atypical ("corkscrew," "hairpin") vessels indicative of early invasive cancer. (*Courtesy Kenneth Hatch, MD, Tucson, Arizona.*)

screening, and then it is cleansed with a 3% acetic acid solution to remove the excess mucus and cellular debris. The acetic acid also accentuates the difference between normal and abnormal colposcopic patterns. The colposcope is focused on the cervix and the transformation zone, including the squamocolumnar junction, and the area is inspected in a clockwise fashion. In most cases, the entire lesion can be outlined, and the most atypical area can be selected for biopsy. If the lesion extends up the canal beyond the vision of the colposcopist, the patient will require a diagnostic conization to define the

disease. ECC is performed when the lesion extends up the canal, and if invasive cancer is found at any time, plans for a cone biopsy are abandoned. This plan of investigation is based on the assumption that there are no areas of CIN higher up in the canal if indeed the upper limits of the lesion can be seen colposcopically. In other words, CIN begins in the transformation zone and extends contiguously to other areas of the cervix such that if the upper limits can be seen, one can be assured that additional disease is not present higher in the canal. The colposcope can only suggest an abnormality; final diagnosis must rest on a tissue examination by a pathologist. Selected spot biopsies in the areas showing atypical colposcopic patterns, under direct colposcopic guidance and in combination with cytologic testing, give the highest possible accuracy in the diagnosis and evaluation of the cervix. Probably the greatest value of colposcopy is that in most cases a skilled colposcopist can establish and differentiate invasive cancer from CIN by direct biopsy and thus avoid the necessity of surgical conization of the cervix. This is especially valuable in the young nulliparous woman desirous of childbearing for whom cone biopsy of the cervix may result in problems of impaired fertility. The avoidance of conization is also valuable in reducing the risk to the patient from anesthesia and the additional surgical procedure with its prolonged hospitalization.

In all nonpregnant patients undergoing colposcopic examination, an ECC is recommended by many, even if the entire lesion is seen. This gives objective proof of the absence of disease in the endocervical canal. It is believed that if the ECC had been done in several of the patients who had been reported in the literature as having invasive cancer diagnosed after outpatient therapy, the cancer would have been identified at an earlier time, and inappropriate therapy would not have been given.

ECC is performed from the internal os to the external os. The external os is the structure that is created by the opening of the bivalve speculum. A speculum as large as can be tolerated should be used to evaluate the patient with an abnormal Pap smear result. During curettage, it is best to curet the entire circumference of the canal without removing the curet. This is done twice. Short, firm motions in a circumferential pattern are the most satisfactory. Patients experience some discomfort early in the procedure, but rarely does the physician have to stop because of discomfort. It is desirable to obtain endocervical stroma in the specimen if possible. On completion of the curettage, all blood, mucus, and cellular debris must be collected and placed on a 2- × 2-inch absorbent paper towel or something similar. The material is then folded into a mound and, along with the absorbent paper towel, placed into fixative. If any neoplastic tissue is found by the pathologist in the curettings, the results are considered positive. Directed punch biopsies of the cervix are done after the curettage. Using the colposcopic findings as a guide, the physician obtains punch biopsy specimens with a Kevorkian-Younge cervical biopsy instrument (or a similar tool that contains a basket in which the biopsy specimen may be collected). Biopsy specimens should be placed on a small piece of paper towel with proper orientation to minimize tangential sectioning of the specimen.

The goal of any evaluation of a patient with abnormal cervical cytologic findings is to rule out invasive cancer. Diagnostic studies may be done using outpatient facilities or may require hospitalization. No single diagnostic technique can effectively rule out invasive cancer in all patients, but with multiple diagnostic procedures the risk of missing invasive cancer is essentially eliminated. Even conization of the cervix by itself can miss an invasive cancer. Therefore cytologic screening, colposcopy, colposcopically directed biopsies, ECC, and pelvic examination must *all* rule out invasive cancer. Under certain circumstances, conization is indicated, even after the full outpatient evaluation has been performed. Most important, if invasive cancer has not been ruled out by the outpatient evaluation, conization must be performed. Patients who have a positive ECC also require conization. If cytologic testing, biopsies, or colposcopic examination indicates microinvasive carcinoma of the cervix, conization must be performed to fully evaluate the extent of the invasion, which in turn determines appropriate therapy. The postmenopausal patient with abnormal cytologic findings frequently requires conization of the cervix because her lesion is usually located within the endocervical canal and cannot be adequately evaluated with outpatient techniques. The use of local estrogen for several days before colposcopy and biopsy in the postmenopausal patient will augment these diagnostic procedures tremendously.

In patients in whom conization must be done, colposcopy can aid in tailoring the conization to the individual's specific need. If the lesion extends widely onto the portio, the lateral extensions might be missed with a "standard" cone but would be included if colposcopically directed. Occasionally, the disease will extend into the vaginal fornix, and colposcopy can identify this patient so that appropriate margins may be obtained. If, however, the concern is the endocervical canal, and the portio is clean, a narrow conization can be done to remove the endocervical canal only. The use of Lugol solution as a substitute for colposcopy to determine the extent of the disease on the cervix is inappropriate and can be misleading. Both false-positive and false-negative staining with Lugol's solution can occur in identifying CIN. The application of Lugol's solution may be helpful to evaluate the cervix and vagina before conization. The colposcopic lesion and the nonstaining area of Lugol's solution should match. Failure of matching indicates that appropriate adjustments must be made at the time of conization.

This evaluation schema permits triage of patients based on the colposcopic findings (plus the results of the colposcopically directed biopsies) and ECC findings. If the results of curettage of the canal are negative and only preinvasive neoplasia is found on directed biopsy, the patient has been adequately evaluated and treatment can begin. The method of therapy chosen depends on the patient's age, desire for fertility, and reliability for follow-up and the histologic appearance and extent of her lesion. Cryosurgery using the double-freeze technique or destruction of the lesion with a laser beam can be performed in some patients who wish to retain their childbearing capacity but who have disease that is more extensive than can adequately be treated with a simple excisional biopsy in the office. Hysterectomy, either simple vaginal or abdominal, without preceding conization may be recommended for patients who desire sterilization. No effort is made in the performance of the hysterectomy to excise additional vaginal cuff unless there is evidence of abnormal epithelium extending to the vagina; this occurs in less than 3% of patients. A final possibility for treatment is to perform a shallow conization or ring biopsy of the cervix (Figures 1-11 and 1-12).

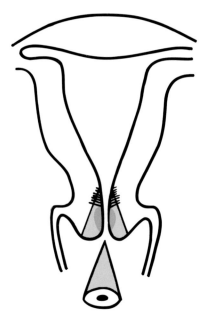

FIGURE 1-11 Cone biopsy for endocervical disease. Limits of the lesion were not seen colposcopically.

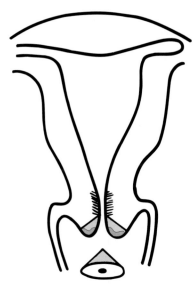

FIGURE 1-12 Cone biopsy for cervical intraepithelial neoplasia of the exocervix. Limits of the lesion were identified colposcopically

As noted in the schema that we have presented for evaluation of the abnormal Pap smear, we prefer that an ECC is performed on all nonpregnant patients. It is appreciated that there are data to suggest an ECC is not required if an adequate colposcopy is present. There also are data that suggest endocervical brush cytology is equivalent to an ECC. Diagnostic conization must be done when ECC shows malignant cells or when colposcopic examination is unsatisfactory (the entire lesion is not seen). Because curettage is performed from the internal os to the external os, the lesion that extends only slightly into the canal is often picked up by the curet, resulting in a number of false-positive ECC results.

Colposcopic evaluation of the cervix in the patient with an abnormal cervical smear has dramatically altered the management of the patient afflicted during pregnancy. The schema previously outlined is closely followed in pregnancy, when the transformation zone is everted, making visualization of the entire lesion almost a certainty. Cone biopsy is rarely indicated during pregnancy. If punch biopsy suggests microinvasion, further evaluation is needed. In many cases, a "wedge" resection of the suspicious area confirms the diagnosis of microinvasion, and conization is unnecessary. If not, then cone biopsy to allow proper management may be considered. Pregnant patients with a firm diagnosis of preinvasive or microinvasive disease of the cervix should be allowed to deliver vaginally, and further therapy can be tailored to their needs after delivery. The cervix is very vascular during pregnancy; thus avoiding a cone biopsy is in the best interest of both the mother and the fetus. *Small* biopsies of the *most* colposcopically abnormal areas are recommended in an effort to minimize bleeding in the diagnostic evaluation. When a patient is in the second or third trimester and the result of the colposcopic examination is negative for any suspicion of invasion, many colposcopists will defer all biopsies to the postpartum period. Lurain and Gallup reported on 131 pregnant patients with abnormal Pap smear results managed in this manner with excellent results, and no invasive cancers were missed.

Roberts and colleagues noted that only two patients had CIN III on cervical biopsies during pregnancy and had microinvasion (stage IA1) on cold knife conization postpartum. Whether this is progression or sampling error is unknown. Post and associates noted CIN II and III in 279 antepartum biopsies. Regression of 68% and 78%, respectively, among patients with CIN II and III was noted postpartum. No progression to cancer was noted. Regression rates did not depend on vaginal deliveries compared with cesarean deliveries. Complete reevaluation postpartum appears to be indicated so that overtreatment does not occur.

Treatment Options

Women with CIN I can be followed without definitive treatment. This is particularly true if the preceding Pap smear result shows ASCUS, ASC-H, or LSIL. These women can be followed with either HPV-DNA testing every 12 months or repeat cytology at 6- to 12-month intervals. If abnormal results remain, further follow-up

TABLE 1-7 Treatment Options for Cervical Intraepithelial Neoplasia

Observations
Local excision
Electrocautery
Cryosurgery
Laser
Cold coagulation
Loop electrosurgical excision procedure (LEEP)
Conization
Hysterectomy

TABLE 1-8 Conservative Treatment for Cervical Intraepithelial Neoplasia

Method (Based on Single Treatment)	Failures (%)
Electrocoagulation[1]	47/1734 (2.7)
Cryosurgery[2]	540/6143 (8.7)
Laser[3]	119/2130 (5.6)
Cold coagulator (CIN III)[4]	110/1628 (6.8)
LEEP[5]	95/2185 (4.3)

[1]Chanen W, Rome RM: Electrocoagulation diathermy for cervical dysplasia and carcinoma in situ: a 15-year survey. Obstet Gynecol 61:673, 1983.
[2]Richart RM et al: An analysis of "long-term" follow-up results in patients with cervical intraepithelial neoplasia treated by cryosurgery. Am J Obstet Gynecol 137:823, 1980; Benedet JL, Nickerson KG, Anderson GH: Cryotherapy in the treatment of cervical intraepithelial neoplasia. Obstet Gynecol 58:72, 1981.
[3]Parashevadis E, Jandial L, Mann EMF et al: Patterns of treatment failure following laser for cervical intraepithelial neoplasia: implications for follow up protocol. Obstet Gynecol 78:80, 1991.
[4]Gordon HK, Duncan ID: Effective destruction of cervical intraepithelial neoplasia (CIN)3 at 100°C using the Semm cold coagulator: 14 years' experience. Br J Obstet Gynaecol 98:14, 1991.
[5]Bigrigg MA, Haffenden DK, Sheehan AL et al: Efficacy and safety of large-loop excision of the TZ. Lancet 343:32, 1994.
CIN, Cervical intraepithelial neoplasia; LEEP, loop electrosurgical excision procedure.

with repeat colposcopy and treatment if abnormality persists or further observation is acceptable. In women with CIN II or III therapy is indicated. For those with CIN I observation is an appropriate option. Many treatment options are available to the patient today (Table 1-7). Essentially all of these options should be considered definitive. The decision about the choice of therapy for CIN depends on many factors, including the patient's desire and the experience of the physician involved. Probably the most compelling reasons for choosing an outpatient modality over inpatient surgery are the patient's age and desire for subsequent fertility. The recommendation that CIS in a teenager or woman in her early 20s must be treated with a hysterectomy is outdated. No therapy is 100% effective; the risk to benefit ratio to the patient should be explained so that she is fully informed, and a reasonable decision can be made concerning her therapy and well-being.

Observation in selected, highly individualized patients may be an option, particularly if the lesion is small and histologically CIN I. Also, some patients have a small lesion that may be completely removed with the biopsy forceps. Elimination of the disease with this technique has occurred in some patients, although some investigators believe that the entire transformation zone should be destroyed. Obviously, the use of observation and local excision can be made only by the experienced physician and must be highly individualized, depending on the patient's needs, desires, and ability to be followed appropriately.

Outpatient Management

ELECTROCAUTERY

Several modalities of treatment for the patient with CIN can be performed on an outpatient basis. If in fact these modalities are as effective as a surgical procedure accomplished in the operating room, the cost-effectiveness is important. Electrocautery has been used for many years to eradicate cervical epithelium. It was fashionable historically to destroy the "abnormal" tissue found on the cervix after delivery. Actually, this was columnar

epithelium, or the transformation zone of the cervix. Some uncontrolled studies suggest that electrocautery decreased the appearance of CIN lesions in patients thus treated. Electrocautery has been shown to be effective in the treatment of CIN. The popularity of this treatment is more apparent in Europe and Australia than in the United States. In a small, controlled study Wilbanks and associates showed that electrocautery was effective in destroying early CIN compared with tetracycline vaginal suppositories used in a control group of patients. Ortiz and colleagues treated all forms of CIN with electrocautery. In CIN I and II lesions, no failures were noted. In CIN III disease, the failure rate was approximately 13%. The failure rate in patients with CIS did not differ regardless of whether the glands were involved. All the patients were treated on an outpatient basis. Chanen and Rome have used this technique extensively in Australia. Table 1-8 illustrates the excellent results that they reported. They treated more than 1700 patients, and the failure rate was only 3%. Cervical stenosis has not been a problem. Dilatation and curettage (D&C) is done at the same time that the electrocautery is performed. The patient is admitted to the hospital, and while she is under anesthesia, electrocautery is performed in the operating room to burn the tissue deep enough to destroy disease that might be present in glands. Chanen and Rome believe this is necessary to obtain excellent results. Electrocautery, of course, is painful if the tissue is burned deeply. If a patient needs to be anesthetized to obtain these results, this negates any benefits that a lesser procedure than conization would obtain. The cost of hospitalization, even on an ambulatory service, would be much higher than that of outpatient treatment.

CRYOSURGERY

Considerable experience with cryosurgery has been obtained in the treatment of CIN. The side effects of electrocautery, mainly pain during treatment, are not present with cryosurgery, and thus it is an ideal outpatient modality in terms of patient comfort.

Ample experience with cryosurgery has now been reported in the literature. In 1980 Charles and Savage reviewed the literature and reported the experience of 16 authors with approximately 3000 patients. The success rate was noted to be between 27% and 96%. Many factors accounted for the wide variation and results, including the experience of the operator; the number of patients treated; criteria established to determine a cure; and freezing techniques, equipment, and the refrigerant used. Subsequently, several studies have been reported in the literature (see Table 1-8). Total failure for the entire group irrespective of the histologic grade was 8%. Results of cryosurgery are essentially the same as those reported for electrocautery, the advantage being that cryosurgery is essentially pain-free and is effectively performed on an outpatient basis.

Ample experience has been obtained in the long-term follow-up of patients who have been treated with cryosurgery. Richart and associates noted that the recurrence rate was less than 1% in almost 3000 patients with CIN who were treated with cryosurgery and followed for 5 years or more. Almost one half of the recurrences were noted within the first year after cryosurgery, and to a certain extent they probably represent persistence and not a true recurrence. No cases of invasive cancer have developed in these patients. The initial failure rate can be reduced even further by a "recycling" of the patient and appropriate re-treatment with cryosurgery or some other outpatient modality. Townsend states that all of the failures in the CIN I category were re-treated successfully with cryosurgery, and the failure rate for the re-treated patients who failed the first treatment lowered the overall failure rate to 3% for CIN II and 7% for CIN III. Although the techniques of cryosurgery are simple, several important technical points must be kept in mind to have an optimal freeze. Carbon dioxide or nitrous oxide can be used as a refrigerant for cryosurgery. The larger "D" tank is preferred over the narrow "E" tank, particularly if cryosurgery is performed on several patients over a short time interval. The pressure in the smaller tank can drop because of the cooling in the gas, even though there may be adequate volume within the tank. Pressure is important for obtaining a satisfactory freeze. If the pressure drops below 40 kg/cm^2 during the freezing process, the treatment should be stopped, tanks should be changed, and the treatment should be started again. A thin layer of water-soluble lubricant over the tip of the probe will allow a more uniform and rapid freeze of the cervix. This allows a better heat-transfer

TABLE 1-9 Cryosurgery Technique

1. N_2O or CO_2
2. K-Y jelly on probe
3. Double-freeze
   a. 4-5 mm iceball
   b. Thaw
   c. 4-5 mm iceball

mechanism to take place between the probe and the cervix. This is particularly important in the case of a woman who may have an irregular cervix, which is common in the parous patient. The probe should cover the entire lesion, and a 4- to 5-mm iceball around the probe is required for an adequate freeze. This should be obtained within 1.5 to 2 minutes with most cryosurgery units today. If the 4- to 5-mm iceball is not obtained within this time, equipment is probably functioning incorrectly and the problem must be identified. We prefer the double-freeze technique. The cervix is allowed to thaw for 4 to 5 minutes and is then refrozen using the same technique (Table 1-9). There is usually a watery discharge for 10 to 14 days. The patient is instructed to refrain from intercourse and to use an external pad if necessary during the time of the watery discharge. She is then seen in 4 months for re-evaluation with a Pap smear. If the result of the Pap smear is positive, the abnormality may be a result of the healing process, and the Pap smear is then repeated in 4 to 6 weeks. If cytologic findings remain abnormal 6 months after cryosurgery, cryosurgery must be considered a failure; the patient should then be re-evaluated and re-treated.

Attention has been drawn to the fact that several patients have been reported to have invasive carcinoma of the cervix after cryosurgery. A report from Miami details eight patients who were treated by cryosurgery for various indications and were found subsequently to have invasive cancer. Only five of the patients had abnormal cervical cytologic findings; three had colposcopic examinations; two had colposcopically directed biopsies; and only one had an ECC.

Townsend and Richart reported on 66 similar patients of members of the Society of Gynecologic Oncologists. Again, an inappropriate precryosurgery evaluation was noted in most of these patients. Invasive cancer has also been reported in patients who are treated with other outpatient modalities, again emphasizing the importance of a proper evaluation before outpatient therapy.

LASER SURGERY

The term *laser* is an acronym for "light amplification by stimulated emission of radiation." The carbon dioxide laser beam is invisible and is usually guided by a second laser that emits visible light. The energy of the laser is absorbed by water with a high degree of efficiency, and the tissue is destroyed principally by vaporization. The laser is mounted on a colposcope, and the laser beam is directed under colposcopic control. Most instruments have a considerable power range and operate by pulse or continuous mode. The spot size may be fixed but usually can be varied. The amount of power delivered to the tissue depends on the spot size and the wattage. Because there is a high-efficiency laser beam absorption by the tissue, and the opportunity to precisely direct the beam, the laser is unique. It also has the ability to control the depth of destruction. Because the tissue is destroyed by vaporization, the base of destruction is clean, with little necrotic tissue and rapid healing. As experience is gained with this modality, changes in technique take place. Because the laser can precisely direct the beam, at first it was thought that only the abnormal area needed to be destroyed with the laser. This prevented the destruction of normal cervical tissue. With this technique, the failure rate was excessive, and, as a result, it was suggested that the entire transformation zone be destroyed. Masterson and colleagues noted that their change in technique from destroying the lesion to ablating the entire transformation zone did not appreciably increase their success rate. The depth of destruction appears to be important in that the failure rate was considerable when only minimal destruction (1-2 mm) was achieved. As the depth of destruction increased, the number of failures decreased. Most lasers now advocate the destruction to a depth of 5 to 7 mm. Burke, Lovell, and Antoniolo concluded that successful treatment was not related to the severity of the histologic grade but to the size of the lesion. A continuous beam gave a better result than an intermittent beam. The depth of destruction was important and must include the lamina propria. Involvement of the endocervical crypt did not preclude success (Table 1-10). Certain precautions must be taken while using the carbon dioxide laser, including avoiding the use of flammable agents, protecting the eyes with appropriate glasses, and using nonreflective surfaces. As the beam is transferred, the tissue vaporizes, filling the vagina with smoke and steam, which are evacuated by a suction tube attached to the speculum. Complications with the laser include pain, which is greater than with cryosurgery but usually

tolerable. Bleeding can be a problem, although spotting is more frequent than significant bleeding. Bleeding increases as the depth of tissue destruction increases, and larger vessels may be reached with the laser beam. Because 5 to 7 mm of tissue is destroyed, increased bleeding will probably occur more frequently.

Two disadvantages to the laser that have not been experienced with cryosurgery follow:

1. The process is more painful for the patient who has the procedure done in the physician's office than for the patient who has cryosurgery.
2. The destruction of all but the smallest of lesions requires much more time for both the patient and the physician.

Although the data suggest that the laser is effective in destroying CIN, it appears to be no better than other available outpatient methods, and one must question the cost-effectiveness of this modality compared with cryosurgery.

In 1983 Townsend and Richart reported a study by alternating cases randomly, as much as possible, on the basis of CIN histologic grade and lesion size to compare the efficacy of cryotherapy and carbon dioxide laser therapy. In their study, 100 patients were treated with laser therapy and 100 patients were treated with cryotherapy. There were seven failures in the cryotherapy group and 11 failures in the group treated with carbon dioxide laser therapy. These authors found no significant differences in the cure rates between the two modalities. They thought that "if the therapeutic results are equivalent, it is logical to choose the modality that provides an equivalent grade of care for the least possible cost, and, at least in an office setting, this would seem to favor cryotherapy over laser therapy."

Mitchell and associates performed a prospective randomized trial of cryosurgery, laser vaporization, and LEEP excision in 390 patients with biopsy-proven CIN. The degree of CIN, lesion size, number of quadrants involved, age, smoking history, and HPV status were similar in all treatment groups. No statistical difference in complications, persistence, or recurrence among the three modalities was seen. They noted that the risk of persistence was higher in those with large lesions. The rate of recurrence was higher among women 30 years of age or older, those with HPV-16 or -18, and those who were previously treated for CIN.

In an evaluation by Parashevadis and associates of 2130 patients treated by laser therapy, these authors noted that failures were higher in women older than 40 years of age and in those with CIN III. CIN III lesions accounted for 75% of the failures, whereas only 7% were originally CIN I. Three cases of invasive cancer were diagnosed within 2 years of laser therapy. There

TABLE 1-10 CO_2 Laser Vaporization—Cervix

Instruments	CO_2 laser, colposcope, micromanipulator
Power output	20-25 W
Power density	800-1400 W/cm^2
Spot size	1.5-2 mm diameter
Operating mode	Continuous
Depth of destruction	6-7 mm measured
Width of destruction	4-5 mm beyond the visible lesion
Bleeding control	Defocus, power density: 800 W/cm^2
Anesthesia	May need a paracervical block
Analgesia	Antiprostaglandins

were 119 (5.6%) treatment failures. Of the failures, 18% had a second lesion detected colposcopically in the presence of negative cytology after laser therapy. Today it appears that the use of laser to treat CIN has decreased considerably over the years and is probably rarely used today.

COLD COAGULATOR

Duncan has reported experience with a Semm cold coagulator in the treatment of CIN III. Over a 14-year period, 1628 women were treated, and the primary success rate was 95% at 1 year and 92% at 5 years, which was similar for all age groups. There were 226 pregnancies following therapy, and the rates for miscarriage, preterm, or operative delivery were not increased.

The cold coagulator essentially coagulates at a lower temperature (100°C). Therapy is performed by overlapping applications of the thermal probe so that the transformation zone and the lower endocervix are destroyed. In most cases, two to five applications were required, taking less than 2 minutes (20 seconds per application).

The exact depth of destruction is difficult to accurately ascertain. Several investigators found destruction up to 4 mm. These data suggest that this depth of destruction is adequate in patients with CIN III lesions. If this is the case, one wonders why 6 to 7 mm of destruction is required for adequate therapy when laser therapy is used. Even in the hands of an experienced colposcopist, subsequent carcinomas were noted in this series, as with every other treatment used in outpatient management. Microinvasion was found in two patients, and invasive cancer was found in four patients. This technique is inexpensive, quick, and essentially pain-free and has very few side effects. Efficacy is excellent (see Table 1-8). One wonders why this technique has not been evaluated and used in the United States.

LOOP ELECTROSURGICAL EXCISION PROCEDURE

A new approach to an old instrument has become popular. If cryosurgery was the "in" treatment of the 1970s and laser surgery was the "in" treatment of the 1980s, LEEP became the instrument of the 1990s and continues today (Table 1-11). LEEP use has grown tremendously within a short time. After colposcopy and if the entire transformation zone is identified, it is excised with a low-voltage diathermy loop under local anesthesia. Usually less than 10 mL of local anesthesia, with epinephrine or vasopressin added to help decrease blood loss, is injected into the cervix at 12, 3, 6, and 9 o'clock. After 3 to 5 minutes, excision can be performed with a loop size that will excise the complete lesion.

An electrosurgical generator is used with wattage set at 25 to 50, depending on loop size (the larger the loop, the higher will be the wattage) and blended cut or coagulated. A disposable grounding plate is used, as in the

TABLE 1-11 LEEP Technique

1. Do a colposcopy of the cervix and outline the lesion.
2. Ensure the patient is grounded with a pad return electrode.
3. Inject anesthetic solution just beneath and lateral to the lesion (at the excision site).
4. Turn on the machine and set cut/blend to 25-50 W (the larger the loop, the higher wattage is needed).
5. Set coagulation to 60 W for ball electrode use.
6. After adequate time for anesthesia to take effect, excise the lesion using the LEEP.
7. Coagulate the base of the cone, even if there is no apparent bleeding.
8. Place ferric subsulfate paste on the base.

LEEP, Loop electrosurgical excision procedure.

operating room. The cutting loop consists of an insulated shaft with a wire loop attached. The sterilized steel wire is 0.2 mm in diameter and comes in various sizes. LEEP can be performed under colposcopy or after Lugol's application (and if it matches colposcopy findings) as a guide for excision. If Lugol's solution is used, saline should be applied to the cervix before LEEP because Lugol's solution tends to dehydrate the tissue. Care should be taken to avoid the vaginal walls with the loop. A smoke evacuator, as used with laser, is recommended. In some cases, the 1.5-cm loop is too small to remove the entire lesion, and an additional "pass" or two is required to remove the remaining abnormal epithelium. Depth of the excised tissue varies, but 5 to 8 mm is the usual depth. This allows tissue for adequate evaluation. The base of the excised tissue is then coagulated with a ball electrode, and Monsel's paste is applied.

This technique has several advantages. The procedure can be done on an outpatient basis. Tissue is available for study. Diagnosis and therapy are done at one time and during the same visit. In essentially all large studies reported to date, several early invasive lesions were identified that had not been recognized on colposcopy examination. This technique tends to negate this inherent problem of destructive techniques.

Side effects are mainly secondary hemorrhage (initially reported at 10% but with experience found to be in the 1% to 2% range). Long-term effects such as those on pregnancy are not known, but one report noted 48 pregnancies in 1000 after LEEP. Some studies report increased preterm labor after LEEPs, whereas others note an increase in premature births.

Results of one large study of 1000 patients noted that 897 women were managed with only one visit. The other 103 required more than one visit, including 9 women who had microinvasion or invasion. Cervical cytology at 4 months after treatment was performed in 969 women, and 41 (4.1%) were found to be abnormal. Of the 9 women with invasion, only 4 were suspected on cervical smear and colposcopy (see Table 1-8).

LEEP appears to be the current treatment of choice. It has been estimated that many thousands of LEEPs have been performed in the United States. Several comments are probably in order. See, diagnose, and treat at one time is a philosophy that has been popularized by some, particularly our European colleagues. In some cases, LEEP has been used before colposcopy or other diagnostic procedures. As noted earlier in its guidelines for management of abnormal cervical cytology, the researchers at the National Cancer Institute–sponsored workshop stated, "Routine electroexcision of the transformation zone of nonstaining areas as a method of evaluating a positive Pap smear diagnosed as LSIL or ASCUS is not recommended." The indiscriminate use of LEEP should not be condoned. In essentially all studies that have addressed the subject, as many as half of LEEP specimens show no epithelial abnormalities (most studies show 15% to 25% with negative histology). It appears that many patients with ASCUS or LSIL on cytology are having LEEPs done that do not appear warranted. The "see and treat" fashion for patients with these degrees of abnormalities on Pap smears should not be encouraged.

Initially, it was said that LEEP caused stenosis, occurring in approximately 1% of cases. More recent data suggest that stenosis may be present four times more often than preliminary data suggested. This is still a low figure (comparable to cryosurgery and laser). Anecdotal experience has suggested that the increasing number of LEEPs being done will lead to an increase in infertility or preterm labor. Many patients with CIN are young and desire to be fertile. In the United Kingdom, where LEEP is the most frequently used therapy for CIN, 1000 patients who underwent large loop excisions of the transformation zone were evaluated for subsequent pregnancy. There were 149 women who had a singleton pregnancy progressing past 20 weeks of gestation and were matched to controls with regard to age, parity, height, father's social class, and smoking. Of women progressing to at least 37 weeks, their newborns' mean birth weights were equal. Following LEEP, 9.4% of deliveries were preterm (<37 weeks) compared with 5% in the control group (not statistically significant). In a small study comparing fertility after LEEP with patients treated with a conization (79 in each group), 11 of 12 women desiring pregnancy did so in the LEEP group compared with all 17 who desired pregnancy in the cone group.

In a retrospective study (Kennedy), 2315 women were treated with LEEP. Only 15 of the 924 new patients attending the university infertility clinic were treated with LEEP. Of the 15 patients, only 10 had good-quality cervical mucus at midcycle, and 3 other patients had spontaneous conception.

Many physicians are reluctant to use LEEP in the young, nulliparous patient because the cervix is small and a considerable amount of the cervix can be removed very quickly with this procedure. In our practice, we have seen several young patients in whom the cervix is flush with the vagina. In this subset, fertility and preterm labor have not been evaluated to any extent.

Preliminary data on large series suggested a low persistence/recurrence rate, but follow-up time was short—only 4 months in many patients. Bigrigg has subsequently reported a longer follow-up period in 250 women out of the original 1000 treated with LEEP. During follow-up, these patients required 68 second treatments because of persistent or recurrent symptoms during their follow-up period.

Several studies have evaluated factors that predict persistence or recurrence after LEEP therapy. Baldauf and colleagues noted that on multivariant analysis, the endocervical location of the initial lesion and incomplete excision predicted treatment failure. Robinson and associates found that positive margins did not identify patients at high risk for a recurrence compared with negative margins. Nor did they find positive ECC that was worse than negative ECCs in predicting a recurrence. These authors saw a high recurrence rate after LEEP (40%). Barnes and colleagues found that only positive ECC after LEEP predicted HSIL on follow-up Pap smears (16 of 219 or 7%). Margin status was not a factor. Experience after cold knife conization has shown that in many patients with positive margins, follow-up found no persistent disease. Whether this is also applicable to patients treated with LEEP will require further evaluation. It is hoped that routine follow-up with cytology will identify those who fail, and additional immediate therapy for positive margins can be tempered.

Thermal artifact, although reported in series to be of minimal concern, in general practice is reported to be unreadable in approximately 10% of specimens, and 20% to 40% have significant coagulation artifact. This is probably related to equipment power setting and technical problems such as "stalling."

Bleeding is reported to occur in approximately 5% of cases, mainly after treatment. Strict adherence to protocol reduces this problem. LEEP done when significant vaginal infection is present will increase the chance of bleeding. In almost all large series, unanticipated microinvasive cancers have been diagnosed when the histologic specimen was evaluated. This has led some authors to suggest that LEEP could be used in place of cold knife conization to evaluate patients in whom cancer has not been ruled out. Murdoch and colleagues noted that 44 of 1143 LEEP specimens contained invasive cancer (18 with stage IA, 17 with stage IB, and 9 with stage IB adenocarcinoma). Thirty-three (75%) of the patients had unsatisfactory results or were suspicious for cancer colposcopy. LEEP was compared with conization in 63 patients with a high suspicion of microinvasion. All patients had a subsequent hysterectomy. The rate of transection of disease with LEEP was significantly higher than with conization (17% vs 0%). The high frequency of tissue fragmentation with multiple passes that were required to remove the entire lesion led to incomplete evaluation using the LEEP. Lesions high in the canal did not lend themselves to management using LEEP.

Two patients with invasion on their LEEP histology were treated with radical hysterectomies and lymphadenectomies because the LEEP histology was inadequate to guide less radical therapy. One of the patients had no evidence of cancer in the hysterectomy specimen. These authors think that LEEP should not be used in place of conization for this purpose.

Conization of the cervix

After the extent of involvement of epithelium on the ectocervix has been clearly demarcated by colposcopy, the limits of the base of the cone biopsy on the cervix can be determined. An incision that is certain to include all the abnormal areas is made into the mucous membrane of the ectocervix. Many believe that blood loss can be reduced by injecting a dilute solution of phenylephrine (Neo-Synephrine) or pitressin into the line of incision before beginning the procedure. This incision does not need to be circular but should accommodate excision of all atypical epithelium. The depth of the incision as it tapers toward the endocervical canal should be determined by the length of the cervical canal and the suspected depth of involvement (see Figure 1-11). Often the entire limits of the lesion have been visualized and a very shallow conization is sufficient (see Figure 1-12). Cervical conization does not need to be a fixed technical procedure for all patients, but it should always consist of adequate excision of all involved areas. Bleeding from the cone bed can usually be controlled by electrocauterization and by placing Monsel's paste on the base. The use of Sturmdorf sutures is probably unnecessary in most cases. Significant cervical stenosis, cervical incompetence, and infertility with a cervical factor are rare complications (Table 1-12) and are functions of the amount of endocervix removed. Several physicians advocate the use of the laser as a cervical tool instead of the knife in conization of the cervix (Table 1-13).

Several studies have now shown that blood loss, infection, and stenosis in laser conization are essentially equal to those occurring in cold knife conization. Some have suggested less dysmenorrhea occurs after laser conization. Complication rates, at least in one study, were equal when laser vaporization was compared with laser conization. Complications after an open cone procedure appear to be similar to those managed with a closed cone procedure (Sturmdorf or other suturing). Although it has been stated that the laser does not distort the cervical margins in regard to pathologic evaluation,

TABLE 1-12 Major Complications of Conization

Immediate	Delayed
Hemorrhage	Bleeding (10-14 days after operation)
Uterine perforation	Cervical stenosis
Anesthetic risk	Infertility
In pregnancy	Incompetent cervix
Rupture of membranes	Increased preterm delivery (low birth weight)
Premature labor	

TABLE 1-13 Laser Conization

Instruments	CO_2 laser, colposcope, micromanipulator
Power output	25-30 W
Power density	1400 W/cm^2
Spot size	0.5 mm
Operating mode	Continuous
Lateral margins	5 mm beyond the lesion
Endocervical margin	Surgically cut
Hemostasis	Lateral sutures, Pitressin infiltration
Anesthesia	General, local

one article suggests this is not the case. The authors reviewed 77 laser conizations, of which 28 (36%) showed extensive epithelial denudization, 10 (13%) contained coagulation artifact that made recognition of CIN extremely difficult or impossible, and 11 (14%) showed laser artifacts that made assessment of margins extremely difficult or impossible.

As has already been indicated, in the United States conization of the cervix is used primarily as a diagnostic tool and secondarily as therapy for patients who are young and desire further fertility. However, in other countries, conization is used as definitive therapy. Extensive experience has been obtained with this operative modality, particularly in the treatment of severe CIN.

In Europe (especially Scandinavia), conization has been used widely to treat patients with CIN, and some interesting data have been published. Bjerre and associates reported on 2099 cases of women with abnormal vaginal smears in whom conization of the cervix had been performed. The frequency of complications was considered low, and cervical CIS was diagnosed in 1500 cases. Conization appeared to be curative in 87% of these 1500 cases. Failure was related to whether the margins of resection were free of pathologic epithelium. If Pap smears were repeatedly negative for the first year after conization, subsequent abnormal smears were found in only 0.4% of the cases. Kolstad and Klem reported on a series of 1121 patients with CIS situ who had been followed for 5 to 25 years. Therapeutic conization had been performed on 795 of these patients, of whom 19 (2.3%) had recurrent CIS and 7 (0.9%) developed invasive

TABLE 1-14   Conization and Hysterectomy as Treatment
for Carcinoma in Situ

	Persistence of CIS	Recurrence of Cancer
Conization (n = 3103)	6.3%	0.6%
Hysterectomy (n = 3729)	0.9%	0.3%

From Boyes, Creasman, Kolstad, Bjerre.

cancer. The corresponding figures for 238 patients treated by hysterectomy were, respectively, 3 (1.2%) and 5 (2.1%). The invasive lesions noted appeared several years later, and the type of initial procedure had no significant influence. Kolstad and Klem emphasized that women who have had CIS of the cervix will always be at some risk and, therefore, should be carefully followed for a much longer time than the conventional period of 5 years (Table 1-14).

If conization has ruled out invasive cancer, those with free surgical margins have almost a 100% disease-free follow-up. The question that is frequently asked is what should management be post conization if surgical margins, particularly the endocervical margins, have disease present? Considerable data in the literature suggest that most will have normal cytology post conization and that no further treatment is necessary. Anderson and colleagues noted 58 patients with positive surgical margins, and only three (5%) had persistent disease. Lopes and colleagues noted in 75 similar patients that 9 (12%) had residual disease. Grundsell found 3 of 21 patients with positive margins with residual disease. Our practice is to follow-up all post conization patients with cytology only irrespective of surgical margin status and intervene only if cytology is abnormal.

Hysterectomy

Traditionally in the United States, a vaginal hysterectomy has been the treatment of choice for patients with CIS. This was particularly true before the establishment of reliable outpatient diagnostic techniques. Hysterectomy is an appropriate method of treatment for the patient with CIN who has completed her childbearing, is interested in permanent sterilization, and has other pathology in which hysterectomy is indicated. CIN as a sole indictor for hysterectomy does not appear to be appropriate with the multiple alternative therapies available today. This decision must be made jointly by the patient, her family, and the physician. For many years the removal of the upper part of the vagina has been advocated in the treatment of CIS, yet there is no basis for this recommendation. In a study by Creasman and Rutledge, the recurrence rate for CIS of the cervix did not depend on the amount of vagina removed with the uterus. Unless vaginal extension of disease can be identified colposcopically (this occurrence is <5%), there is no reason for routine removal of the upper vagina. There appears to be no reason for so-called modified radical hysterectomy in the management of patients with CIN. However, even though hysterectomy is considered to be definitive therapy, patients must be followed in essentially the same manner as patients chosen for outpatient management. Although the chance of subsequent recurrence of invasive disease is small, recurrence can occur, and these patients must be followed indefinitely.

For full reference list, log onto www.expertconsult.com
⟨http://www.expertconsult.com⟩.

2

Preinvasive Disease of the Vagina and Vulva and Related Disorders

Joan L. Walker, MD, and Cara A. Mathews, MD

EMBRYOLOGY

At approximately 12 to 14 weeks, the simple columnar epithelium that lines the vaginal portion of the utero-vaginal canal begins to undergo transformation into stratified müllerian epithelium. This transformation proceeds cranially until it reaches the columnar epithelium of the future endocervical canal. The vagina, which is lined initially by simple columnar epithelium of müllerian origin, now acquires stratified müllerian epithelium. The vaginal plate advances in a caudocranial direction, obliterating the existing vaginal lumen. By caudal cavitation of the vaginal plate, a new lumen is formed, and the stratified müllerian epithelium is replaced by a stratified squamous epithelium, probably from a urogenital sinus origin. Local proliferation of the vaginal plate in the region of the cervicovaginal junction produces the circumferential enlargement of the vagina known as the vaginal fornices, which surround the vaginal part of the cervix.

The administration of diethylstilbestrol (DES) through the 18th week of gestation can apparently result in the disruption of the transformation of columnar epithelium of müllerian origin to the stratified squamous successor (Figure 2-1). This retention of müllerian epithelium gives rise to adenosis. Adenosis may exist in many forms: glandular cells in place of the normal squamous lining of the vagina, glandular cells hidden beneath an intact squamous lining, or mixed squamous metaplasia when new squamous cells attempt to replace glandular cells.

Vaginal adenosis has been observed in patients without a history of DES exposure, but rarely to a clinically significant degree. Adenosis is more common in patients whose mothers began DES treatment early in pregnancy and is not observed if DES administration began after 18 weeks of gestation. At least 20% of women exposed to DES show an anatomic deformity of the upper vagina and cervix; transverse vaginal and cervical ridges, cervical collars, vaginal hoods, and cockscomb cervices have all been described. The transverse ridges and anatomic deformities found in one fifth of women

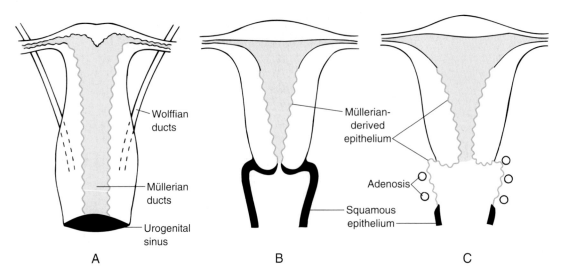

FIGURE 2-1   **A–C,** Schematic representations of the embryologic development of the vagina in unexposed **(A)** and diethylstilbestrol-exposed **(B and C)** women. *(From Stillman RJ: In utero exposure to diethylstilbestrol: adverse effects on the reproductive tract and reproductive performance in male and female offspring. Am J Obstet Gynecol 142(7):905, 1982.)*

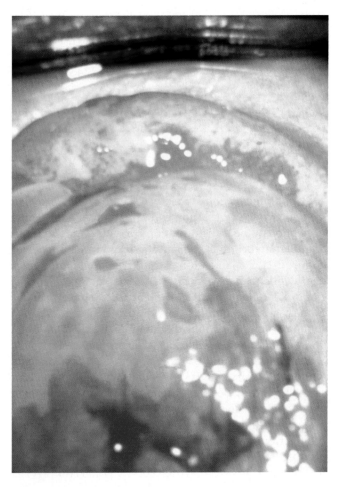

FIGURE 2-2   Hood surrounding the small diethylstilbestrol-exposed cervix, which is completely covered by columnar epithelium (pseudopolyp).

exposed to DES make it difficult to ascertain the boundaries of the vagina and cervix. The cervical eversion causes the cervix grossly to have a red appearance. This coloration is caused by the numerous normal-appearing blood vessels in the submucosa. With a colposcope and application of 3% acetic acid solution, numerous papillae ("grapes") of columnar epithelium are observed, similar to those seen in the native columnar epithelium of the endocervix. The hood (Figure 2-2) is a fold of mucous membrane surrounding the portio of the cervix; it often disappears if the portio is pulled down with a tenaculum or is displaced by the speculum. The cockscomb is an atypical peaked appearance of the anterior lip of the cervix, and vaginal ridges are protruding circumferential bands in the upper vagina that may hide the cervix. A pseudopolyp formation (see Figure 2-2) has been described that occurs when the portio of the cervix is small and protrudes through a wide cervical hood.

The occurrence of vaginal adenosis among young women without in utero DES exposure implies that an event in embryonic development is responsible. The development of the müllerian system depends on and follows formation of the wolffian, or mesonephric, system. The emergence of the müllerian system as the dominant structure appears unaffected by intrauterine exposure to DES when studied in animal systems. However, it is apparent that steroidal and nonsteroidal estrogens, when administered during the proper stage of vaginal embryogenesis in mice, can permanently prevent the transformation of müllerian epithelium into the adult type of vaginal epithelium, thus creating a situation like adenosis. The colposcopic and histologic

TABLE 2-1   Examination of the Female Offspring Exposed to Diethylstilbestrol

1. Inspect the introitus and hymen to assess the patency of the vagina.
2. Palpate the vaginal membrane with the index finger (especially noting non–Lugol-staining areas), noting areas of induration or exophytic lesions, which should be considered for biopsy.
3. Perform a speculum examination with the largest speculum that can be comfortably inserted (virginal-type speculums are often necessary). Adenosis usually appears red and granular (strawberry surface).
4. Obtain cytologic specimens from the cervical os and the walls of the upper third of the vagina.
5. Perform a colposcopic examination or Lugol staining on the initial visit.
6. Do a biopsy of indurated or exophytic areas and colposcopically abnormal areas with a dysplastic Papanicolaou smear.
7. Perform a bimanual rectovaginal examination.

features of vaginal adenosis strongly support the concept of persistent, untransformed müllerian columnar epithelia in the vagina as being the explanation of adenosis.

EXAMINATION AND TREATMENT OF THE FEMALE EXPOSED TO DIETHYLSTILBESTROL

Essentially no diethylstilbestrol has been prescribed to pregnant women since 1971, when the FDA issued an alert regarding the risk of vaginal clear cell adenocarcinoma for females exposed in utero. The youngest women with in utero exposure were born in 1972, and many previously important clinical topics have become less relevant in everyday practice. The associated congenital anomalies and teenage cancers, for example, are no longer being diagnosed. An understanding of the disease process remains essential, however, to care for this cohort of women as they age. Additionally, the evolution and understanding of DES is of great historical importance with many implications and lessons for today's practice.

Approximately 60% of women with in utero DES exposure have vaginal adenosis, cervical-like epithelium in the vagina, which appears red and granular. This is a benign condition that does not require treatment unless symptomatic, and it will generally resolve on its own over time. The premenopausal risk of clear cell adenocarcinoma is approximately 40 times higher among women with in utero DES exposure compared to those without the exposure. In unexposed women, clear cell adenocarcinoma occurs almost exclusively in menopause; in women with in utero exposure, most cases are diagnosed during the late teens and twenties. The oldest reported patient with DES-associated clear cell adenocarcinoma was diagnosed at 51 years. Overall, the incidence of clear cell adenocarcinoma is low in women with in utero exposure (approximately 1.5 cases/1000 women), but the risk is significantly higher than among unexposed women. The etiology of clear cell adenocarcinoma is unclear, and evolution of adenosis to cancer has never been directly observed, only suspected.

Because of an increased risk of clear cell adenocarcinoma of the cervix and vagina and an increased risk of cervical intraepithelial neoplasia (CIN), annual examinations with Pap testing are recommended for the entire lifetime of women with in utero DES exposure. No increased association has been observed between DES and squamous cell cervical cancer.

All DES-exposed females should have an annual gynecologic examination with cytology screening (Table 2-1). Cytology should include separate sampling of the cervix and upper vagina. If suspicious lesions are present, colposcopy and directed biopsies should be performed regardless of the cytology results. If delineations of the vagina, cervix, and endocervix are difficult, Lugol's solution may be helpful in detecting abnormal areas. Colposcopic examination of these patients is hindered by the abnormal patterns seen with squamous metaplasia (Figure 2-3, A,B), which can be confused with neoplastic lesions. Histologic confirmation is essential before any treatment is undertaken. Marked mosaic (Figure 2-4) and punctation patterns that normally herald intraepithelial neoplasia are commonly seen in the vagina of a female exposed to DES as a result of widespread metaplasia. The purpose of regular examination is to permit detection of adenocarcinoma and squamous neoplasia during the earliest stages of development. Although many therapies have been attempted, no recommended treatment plan for vaginal adenosis exists. In most cases, the area of adenosis is physiologically transformed into squamous epithelium during varying periods of observation, and no therapy is necessary.

NON-NEOPLASTIC EPITHELIAL DISORDERS OF THE VULVA

Non-neoplastic epithelial disorders of the vulvar skin and mucosa are often seen in clinical practice. Diagnosis is difficult without a histology result, and multiple changes in terminology over the last 25 years add confusion to the clinical setting. The most recent classification guidelines were published in 2007 by the International Society for the Study of Vulvovaginal Disease (ISSVD)

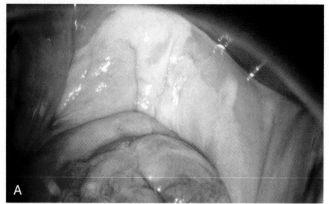

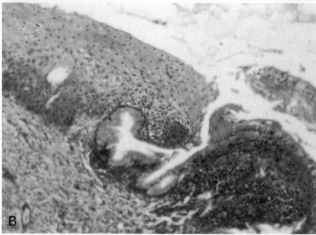

FIGURE 2-3   **A,** Area of white epithelium of squamous metaplasia. **B,** Histologic section of the area in **A** showing metaplasia to the left partially covering the adenosis (columnar epithelium) to the right.

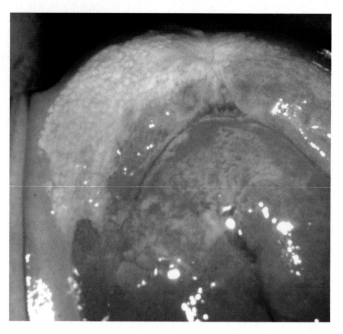

FIGURE 2-4   Heavy mosaic pattern (histologically proven metaplasia) in a hood surrounding the cervix of an offspring exposed to diethylstilbestrol.

TABLE 2-2   2006 World Congress ISSVD Classification of Vulvar Dermatoses

Pathologic Subset	Clinical Correlate
Spongiotic pattern	Atopic dermatitis
	Allergic contact dermatitis
	Irritant contact dermatitis
Acanthotic pattern	Psoriasis
	Lichen simplex chronicus
	Primary (idiopathic)
	Secondary (superimposed on other vulvar disease)
Lichenoid pattern	Lichen sclerosus
	Lichen planus
Dermal homogenization/ sclerosis pattern	Lichen sclerosus
Vesiculobullous pattern	Pemphigoid, cicatrical type
	Linear IgA disease
Acantholytic pattern	Hailey-Hailey disease
	Darier disease
	Papular genitocrural acantholysis
Granulomatous pattern	Crohn's disease
	Melkersson-Rosenthal syndrome
Vasculopathic pattern	Aphthous ulcers
	Behçet disease
	Plasma cell vulvitis

(Table 2-2). The lichenoid pattern subset includes two chronic diseases, lichen sclerosus and lichen planus, which is relevant to this review because of the association of those two diseases with vulvar cancer. Lichen simplex chronicus is not included in the lichenoid subset; it is classified in the acanthotic pattern subset. This is appropriate from an oncology viewpoint because lichen simplex chronicus is not associated with invasive cancer. With similar presenting symptoms and a hyperkeratotic appearance, however, lichen simplex chronicus can be difficult to discriminate from lichen sclerosus and lichen planus on examination (Table 2-3).

Lichen Simplex Chronicus

Lichen simplex chronicus presents in females of all ages, but it is more common in the reproductive and post-menopausal years. Lichen simplex chronicus is a chronic eczematous condition, and most women with this condition also have a history of atopic dermatitis. Pruritus is the most common symptom, and over time scratching leads to epithelial thickening and hyperkeratosis. The status of the skin usually relates to the amount of scratching. Exacerbating agents may include heat, moisture, sanitary or incontinence pads, and topical agents. Lichen simplex chronicus may be seen in conjunction with other processes such as candida infections or lichen sclerosus;

these primary diseases must be treated in order to treat the pruritus leading to scratching and hyperkeratosis.

The locations most often involved on the vulva include the labia majora, interlabial folds, outer aspects of the labia minor, and the clitoris. Changes can also extend to the lateral surfaces of the labia majora or beyond. Areas of lichen simplex chronicus are often localized, elevated, and well delineated, but they may be extensive and poorly defined. The appearance of lesions may vary greatly even in the same patient. The vulva often appears dusky-red when the degree of

hyperkeratosis is slight and may appear thickened and leathery when hyperkeratosis persists. At other times, well-defined white patches may be seen, or a combination of red and white areas may be observed in different locations. Thickening, fissures, and excoriations require careful evaluation because carcinoma may be exhibited by these same features. For this reason, biopsy is essential in ascertaining the correct diagnosis.

Biopsy reveals a variable increase in the thickness of the horny layer (hyperkeratosis) and irregular thickening of the malpighian layer (acanthosis). This latter process produces a thickened epithelium and lengthening and distortion of the rete pegs. Parakeratosis may also be present. The granular layer of the epithelium is usually prominent. An inflammatory reaction is often present within the dermis with varying numbers of lymphocytes and plasma cells.

Lichen Sclerosus

Lichen sclerosus represents a specific disease found in genital and nongenital sites. The vulva is the most common lesion site in women. The age distribution of the disease is bimodal with peaks during the premenarchal and postmenopausal years, but the highest incidence is among postmenopausal women. Although the overall incidence and prevalence are unknown, Leibovitz and colleagues reported the prevalence among elderly women in a nursing home setting as 1 in 30. The mean age in this population was 82 years, 88% were wheelchair bound, and 86% were incontinent (Figures 2-5 and 2-6).

TABLE 2-3 Other Dermatoses

Disorder	Lesion	Genital	Other Locations
Seborrheic dermatitis	Erythema with mild scale oval plaques	Mild scaling, also "inverse type"	Central face, neck, scalp, chest, back
Psoriasis	Annular scaly plaques that bleed easily	Red plaques with gray-white scale	Scalp, elbows, knees, sacrum
Tinea	Annular plaques with central clearing	Common	Skinfolds or single "ringworm" lesion
Lichen simplex chronicus	Lichenified plaques, some dermatitic	Scrotum or labia majora	Nape of the neck, ankle, forearm, antecubital and popliteal fossae
Lichen planus	Flat-topped lilac papules and plaques	White network, erosive aginitis	Volar wrists, shins, buccal mucosa

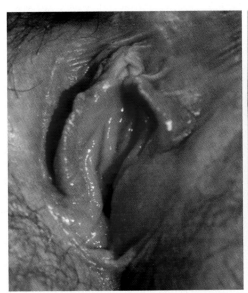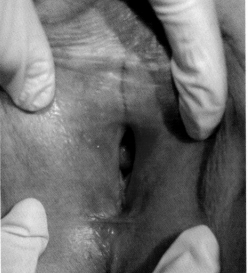

FIGURE 2-5   Progression from early *(left)* to late *(right)* lichen sclerosus, with characteristic loss of labial architecture. *(Courtesy Dr. Lori Boardman, MD, ScM, University of Central Florida College of Medicine.)*

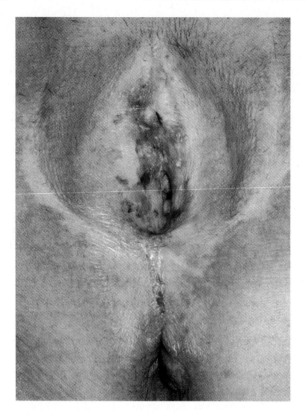

FIGURE 2-6   Lichen sclerosus with stenosis of the introitus, fissuring in the posterior fourchette, and perianal involvement producing the "keyhole appearance." *(Courtesy of Dr. Lori Boardman, MD, ScM, University of Central Florida College of Medicine.)*

Over time, pruritus occurs with essentially all lesions, leading to scratching, which can develop into ecchymosis and ulceration. Symptoms evolve to include burning, tearing, and dyspareunia. Studies have suggested that the epithelium in lichen sclerosus is metabolically active and nonatrophic. A chronic inflammatory, lymphocyte-mediated dermatosis is present. The etiology of the disease is poorly understood, but autoimmune mechanisms appear to be involved.

The microscopic features of lichen sclerosus include hyperkeratosis, epithelial thickening with flattening of the rete pegs, cytoplasmic vacuolization of the basal layer of cells, and follicular plugging. Beneath the epidermis is a zone of homogenized, pink-staining, collagenous-appearing tissue that is relatively acellular. Edema is occasionally seen in this area. Elastic fibers are absent. Immediately below this zone lies a band of inflammatory cells that is consistent with lymphocytes and some plasma cells. Lichen sclerosus is often associated with foci of both hyperplastic epithelium and thin epithelium. Lichen simplex chronicus has been found in 27% to 35% of women with lichen sclerosus after microscopic study of vulvar specimens, likely secondary to pruritus and scratching.

In a well-developed classic lesion, the skin of the vulva is crinkled ("cigarette paper") or appears parchment-like. The process often extends around the anal region in a figure of eight or keyhole configuration, and 30% of women have perianal lesions. At other times, the changes are localized, especially in the periclitoral area or the perineum. Clitoral involvement is usually associated with edema of the foreskin, which may obscure the glans clitoris. Phimosis of the clitoris is often seen late in the course of the disease. As the disease progresses, the labia minora may also completely disappear as a result of atrophy. Synechiae often develop between the edges of the skin in these locations, causing pain and limited physical activity. Fissures also develop in the natural folds of the skin and especially in the posterior fourchette. The introitus may become so strictured or stenosed that intercourse is impossible. Vaginal mucosa is generally spared in this disease, which is helpful in discriminating between lichen sclerosus and lichen planus. In a study by Dalziel, 44 women with lichen sclerosus were evaluated for sexual dysfunction. Apareunia was experienced by 19 women at some point. Dyspareunia and decreased frequency were noted by 80%. Orgasm was altered, and relationships were affected in half. Local steroids improved sexual function in two thirds of these patients.

Lichen sclerosus is a risk factor for invasive vulvar cancer, likely as a result of chronic inflammation and sclerosis. In untreated populations, approximately 5% of patients with lichen sclerosus also have intraepithelial neoplasia. Wallace followed 290 women with lichen sclerosus for an average of 12.5 years and found that 4% (n = 12) developed vulvar cancer. Carlson reported that 4.5% of patients with lichen sclerosus developed vulvar cancer over a mean of 10 years. In treated populations, however, the risk may be lower. Cooper and associates treated 233 women in a vulvar teaching clinic over a 10-year period; 89% of the cohort received superpotent steroid treatment. Invasive vulvar cancer developed in 3% (n = 7), and vaginal intraepithelial neoplasia (VIN) developed in 2% (n = 4). Jones and colleagues reported one case of cancer from a vulvar clinic treating 213 females older than age 8 years. Renaud-Vilmer reported results from an urban dermatology clinic caring for 83 females with no prior treatment of vulvar lichen sclerosus. Invasive cancer was present at the time of presentation in 7% (n = 6) and developed in 2% (n = 2); in those who developed cancer one did not return for follow-up and one did not use the prescribed treatment. In a cohort followed prospectively with repeat vulvar examinations at the University of Florence by Carli and associates, two cases of invasive cancer and one case of VIN developed among 211 women with treated lichen sclerosus. All three cases occurred after more than 3 years of follow-up in the cohort.

The absolute incidence of vulvar cancer is low in women with lichen sclerosus, but 50% to 70% of squamous cell vulvar cancers occur in a background of lichen sclerosus. Currently, there is no diagnostic tool to differentiate between lichen sclerosus that will remain benign versus lichen sclerosus that will evolve into squamous cell carcinoma. Two biomarkers, p53 and monoclonal antibody MIB1, have shown promise in retrospective tissues studies, but further testing is necessary. The standard of care for cancer screening in this population remains serial examination with directed biopsies for new, evolving, or suspicious lesions.

Lichen Planus

Lichen planus is a distinct dermatologic disease that may affect the oral mucosa, esophageal mucosa, skin, scalp, nails, and eyes in addition to the vulva. Approximately 1% of the population likely develops lichen planus; 25% to 50% of women with lichen planus are believed to have vulvar symptoms. Both vulvovaginal-gingival syndrome and penile-gingival syndrome have been described. The disease appears to be a cell-mediated immune disorder causing chronic inflammation. Similar to lichen sclerosus, symptoms are most common in postmenopausal women in their 50s and 60s, usually include pruritus, and can evolve as the disease progresses to include burning, pain, and dyspareunia. Labial agglutination and loss of architecture of the labia and clitoris may occur. The vaginal mucosa is frequently involved, as opposed to lichen sclerosus, which rarely involves the vagina (Figure 2-7).

The relationship between lichen planus and vulvar cancer is not as well-established as the association between lichen sclerosus and cancer. Small studies have suggested an increased risk of vulvar cancer, and subjects with oral lichen planus may also have an increased risk of oral cancer. In the early 1990s, case reports by Franck and Young, Lewis and Harrington, and Dwyer and colleagues reported incidences of vulvar squamous cell carcinoma in subjects with lichen planus and within erosive lichen planus lesions. In a review of 113 patients with erosive vulvar lichen planus followed by Kennedy and colleagues over an 8-year period, one woman developed vulvar cancer. Of interest, two women in this cohort with oral lichen planus were subsequently diagnosed with oral or esophageal cancer, and two additional women were diagnosed with cervical adenocarcinoma in situ and rectal adenocarcinoma. Similar findings were reported by Cooper and associates. Of 114 women with erosive vulvar lichen planus, seven developed VIN, one developed oral squamous cell carcinoma, and two developed anogenital squamous cell carcinomas of the labium minora and perianal area.

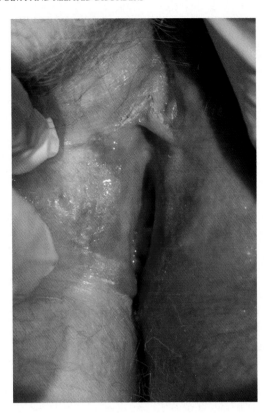

FIGURE 2-7 Erosive lichen planus. *(Courtesy of Dr. Lori Boardman, MD, ScM, University of Central Florida College of Medicine.)*

Diagnosis and Treatment

Biopsies are critical to appropriate management; the exception for biopsy is the pediatric population, which will not be discussed here. Before any treatment is given on a long-term basis, biopsies should be performed from representative areas to ensure the correct diagnosis. Biopsies are focused on sites of fissuring, ulceration, induration, and thick plaques. Patient education regarding hygienic measures for keeping the vulva clean and dry is important; any soaps, perfumes, deodorizers, or other contact irritants should be avoided. A thorough history should be taken to evaluate possible causes of vulvar pruritus. After lesions with malignant potential have been ruled out, local measures for control of symptoms, primarily pruritus, can be instituted (Table 2-4). Additionally, infectious vaginitis should be ruled out with a saline wet preparation, potassium hydroxide (KOH) wet preparation, and yeast culture to evaluate for atypical yeast that may be missed on plain microscopy.

Lichen Simplex Chronicus

Therapy for lichen simplex chronicus is treatment of the underlying cause of irritation and pruritus. All offending environmental agents should be avoided, including wipes, lubricants, sanitary and incontinence pads,

TABLE 2-4   Vulvar Nonneoplastic Epithelial Disorders

Disorder	Treatment
Lichen sclerosus	Topical high-potency steroid ointment
Lichen planus	Topical high-potency steroid ointment
Lichen simplex chronicus	Topical corticosteroid after evaluation and removal of offending environmental agents and treatment of concurrent vaginitis, lichen sclerosus, or lichen planus

detergents, perfumes, and soaps. A thorough history is often necessary to identify possible sources of irritation. Any underlying vaginitis, lichen planus, or lichen simplex requires treatment. For isolated lichen simplex chronicus, a topical steroid ointment such as triamcinolone 0.1% or hydrocortisone 2.5% can be applied daily (after bathing to help seal in moisture) until symptoms are improved, generally in 3 to 4 weeks. If symptoms are particularly severe or a course of low-dose steroids is insufficient, a trial of higher-dose steroid ointment is acceptable. Pruritus is often most severe at night, and short-term use of a pharmacologic sleep aid may be necessary. Lichen simplex chronicus should resolve with removal of the offending agent and treatment; if symptoms persist or recur, the diagnosis and repeat biopsies should be reconsidered.

Lichen Sclerosus

Lichen sclerosus is a chronic condition with no curative treatment; the goal is symptom control. The standard treatment for lichen sclerosus is a topical corticosteroid. Typical regimens begins with a superpotent steroid ointment (i.e., clobetasol proprinate ointment 0.05%) used nightly until resolution of symptoms (usually 8-12 weeks). Because of the chronicity of lichen sclerosus, maintenance therapy is necessary after initial treatment; application one to three times per week is usually sufficient. Many women will stop treatment when their symptoms improve and then present again months later with recurrent symptoms. Therapy can be reinitiated at treatment levels for 6 to 12 weeks, and emphasis is given to maintenance therapy. Theoretically, long-term use of topical steroids may result in striae and thinning of the dermis, but this is infrequently observed in lichen sclerosus. Topical testosterone is no longer the treatment of choice for lichen sclerosus.

A prospective randomized study by Bracco evaluated 79 patients with lichen sclerosus using four different treatment regimens: a 3-month course of testosterone (2%), progesterone (2%), clobetasol propionate (0.05%), and a cream base preparation. Patients experienced greater relief of symptoms with clobetasol (75%) than with testosterone (20%) or other preparations (10%).

Clobetasol therapy was the only treatment in which the gross and histologic evaluation of patients improved after treatment. Recurrences after stopping the steroid occurred, but symptoms were relieved when therapy was resumed. Clobetasol was also more effective than testosterone in the randomized trial performed by Bornstein and colleagues, with a significant improvement in long-term relief experience by clobetasol users. Lorenz and colleagues reported 77% had complete remission of symptoms with clobetasol therapy, but again noted that maintenance therapy was needed after baseline treatment. In the cohort followed by Cooper discussed previously, 65% were symptom free, 31% had a partial response, and 5% has a poor response after steroid use. Improvement was also seen on physical examination; 23% had total resolution, 69% had partial resolution (improvement in purpura, hyperkeratosis, fissures, and erosions, but no change in color and texture), 6% had minor resolution, and 2% had no improvement. Renaud-Vilmer and colleagues noted a different response rate by age group in women treated with 0.05% clobetasol propionate ointment. Complete remission, defined as complete resolution of symptoms, normalization of physical examination, and histologic regression of lichen sclerosus, was observed in 72% of women younger than age 50, 23% of women between 50 and 70, and 0% in women older than 70. Relapse was 84% at 4 years but was not associated with subject age.

Occasionally, vulvar pruritus is so persistent that it cannot be relieved by topical measures. Topical treatment may also fail if significant hyperkeratosis is present. In such cases, intradermal and lesional injection of steroids has been reported to be effective. If lesions persist and symptoms do not improve after a course of superpotent topical steroids, biopsies should be repeated to confirm the initial diagnosis. It is again critical to rule out cancer and VIN to ensure appropriate treatment. Other regimens have been reported for lichen sclerosus recalcitrant to corticosteroids. Specifically, tacrolimus and photodynamic therapy may have some efficacy, but further trials are necessary.

Lichen Planus

Lichen planus is similarly treated with complete evaluation, patient education, and topical steroids. Additionally, the physical examination should exclude the presence of lichen planus on the skin, scalp, nail beds, and oral mucosa. If systemic disease is present, consultation with a dermatologist may be useful. Treatment of vulvar lesions should begin with an ultrapotent steroid ointment (i.e., clobetasol propionate ointment 0.05%) applied nightly for 6 to 8 weeks. If symptoms improve, the frequency of application can be reduced to two to three times weekly for 4 to 8 additional weeks. Cooper and associates reported that in a cohort of 114 women followed and treated for lichen planus, 71% of those treated with ultrapotent topical corticosteroids experienced relief of symptoms with treatment. On examination, 50% experienced healing of erosions but no patients had resolution of scarring. Once lichen planus symptoms are in a prolonged remission, the lowest effective dose is used for maintenance therapy, which may involve less frequent administration and a lower potency steroid. Similar to lichen sclerosus, symptoms will return if maintenance therapy is not used.

Lichen planus does appear more resistant to therapy than lichen sclerosus. In a small series of women with vulvar lichen planus that was nonresponsive to other treatments, Byrd and colleagues at the Mayo Clinic reported that 15 of 16 subjects experienced symptomatic relief after a course of topical tacrolimus. The mean response time was 4 weeks, and 6 subjects experienced mild irritation, burning, or tingling that resolved with persistent use. Tacrolimus therapy was less successful in the subjects followed by Cooper, who were nonresponsive to topical steroid treatment. Of 7 patients treated, 2 had complete symptomatic relief, 3 had some relief, and 2 had no improvement in symptoms.

INTRAEPITHELIAL NEOPLASIA OF THE VAGINA

Clinical Profile

The incidence of vaginal intraepithelial neoplasia (VAIN) is not well described. The first report apparently was by Graham and Meigs in 1952. They reported on three patients with carcinoma of the vagina, two intraepithelial and one invasive, that were discovered 6, 7, and 10 years, respectively, after total hysterectomy for CIS of the cervix. The most recent analysis of the incidence of VAIN in the United States, published in 1977, reported 0.2 to 0.3 cases per 100,000 women. Data published by Joura and colleagues from a large vaccine trial give a more recent estimate; the incidence of high-grade VAIN in the placebo group, women from 24 countries between 16 and 26 years of age who were followed for a mean of 36 months, was 21 cases in 9087 subjects. There may be multiple reasons for the higher incidence observed in the vaccine trial: a true rise in incidence since 1977 similar to the increase seen for VIN, a higher rate of diagnosis because the women were being followed with serial examinations, or a different population from a more heterogeneous international setting. VAIN has many of the same risk factors associated with cervical intraepithelial neoplasia, including smoking, earlier age at first intercourse, increased number of sexual partners, and human papillomavirus (HPV) infection.

CIS of the vagina is much less common than that of the cervix or vulva. For the year 2009, the American Cancer Society estimated that 2160 cases of invasive cancer of the vagina would be diagnosed in the United States. Because of the low prevalence of the disease, routine screening for VAIN and vaginal cancer is not recommended. After hysterectomy for benign disease, the incidence of VAIN is extraordinarily low, and guidelines from the American College of Obstetricians and Gynecology (ACOG) and the American Society for Colposcopy and Cervical Pathology (ASCCP) do not support Pap testing in this population. These guidelines were written in part based on evidence from Pearce and colleagues Noller, and Stokes-Lampard and colleagues showing that a huge number of women would undergo unnecessary cytology screening and colposcopy in order to diagnose a rare outcome. The exceptions to this guideline include women who have a history of in utero DES exposure, are immunosuppressed, or have a history of cervical or vulvar dysplasia. Many women have accepted historical guidelines recommending annual Pap testing and may require counseling and patient education to accept these new guidelines. Rare, unfortunate cases of VAIN or invasive cancer will occasionally be diagnosed in women who have undergone hysterectomy for benign disease, but these exceptional cases cannot drive screening guidelines.

Patients with VAIN tend to have either an antecedent or coexistent neoplasia in the lower genital tract. This is the usual situation in at least half to two thirds of all patients with VAIN. In patients who have been treated for disease in the cervix or vulva, VAIN can appear many years later, necessitating long-term follow-up. First TeLinde, then Gusberg and Marshall, and later Parker and associates indicated that 2%, 1.9%, and 0.9% of patients, respectively, had vaginal recurrences after hysterectomy for a similar lesion in the cervix. More recently, Schockaert and associates were able to follow 94 women who had hysterectomies and concurrently carried a diagnosis of CIN II, CIN III, or FIGO stage Ia1 cervical cancer. In a median interval of 35 months, 7.4% ($n = 7$) developed VAIN II+, including two vaginal cancers. Ferguson and Maclure reported positive cytologic findings in 151 (20.3%) of 633 previously treated patients. This large group included invasive and in situ cancers of the cervix, which were treated by irradiation or hysterectomy. The long-term recurrence rate for CIS of the vagina is uncertain, but it is sufficient to merit continued careful follow-up.

VAIN and invasive cancer are both associated with HPV. HPV positivity reported in the literature ranges from 82% to 94% for VAIN and 60% to 65% for vaginal cancer, and HPV-16 and -18 account for the majority of HPV positivity. In early reports, vaccination appears to be effective at preventing HPV-16– and

HPV-18–associated vaginal lesions in women who receive the vaccination before HPV exposure. HPV mapping has shown identical DNA integration loci between primary lesions of cervical dysplasia and later dysplastic lesions of the vagina and vulva, indicating that later disease may result from monoclonal lesions from the primary cervical dysplasia. Vaginal dysplasia appears to mimic cervical dysplasia with a high prevalence of HPV infection, as opposed to vulvar dysplasia, which displays inconsistent associations.

Isolated lesions can usually be recognized colposcopically (Figure 2-8). The most frequent finding is acetowhite epithelium; mosaicism and punctuation can also be present, and some authors have described a "pink blush" appearance or a slightly granular texture. The diagnosis is confirmed by biopsy. The extent of the lesion can be evaluated with the colposcope or with Lugol's solution. Almost all lesions are asymptomatic, although a patient will occasionally have discharge or postcoital staining. An abnormal Pap smear result usually initiates the diagnostic survey. In almost all series, the upper third of the vagina is most frequently involved (as is the case with the invasive variety), and the posterior wall of the vagina appears more susceptible.

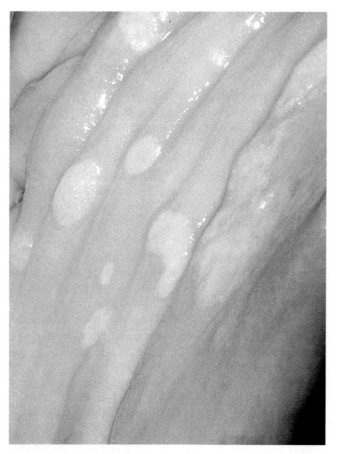

FIGURE 2-8   Carcinoma in situ of the vagina (colposcopic view).

Diagnosis

Patients with an abnormal Pap test who do not have a cervix or patients with an abnormal Pap test result and no cervical abnormality visualized should undergo a careful examination of the vaginal epithelium. Colposcopic examination of the vagina can be difficult to perform. The largest possible speculum should be used and repositioned frequently to allow inspection of all surfaces. Colposcopic findings are similar to those described for the cervix. Each of the four walls should be examined from the apex to the introitus as separate and sequential steps. Small biopsy specimens are taken with a Tischler or Kevorkian–Younge alligator-jaw forceps. Sometimes a sterilized skin-hook for traction at the biopsy site may be helpful. Most patients can tolerate these biopsies without local anesthesia, but the anticipated pain from the biopsies versus pain from a local anesthetic injection should be considered. Lugol's solution is often helpful in delineating lesions of the vagina. Normal vaginal epithelium is stained brown, whereas dysplastic lesions with abnormal glycogen levels remain pale. In the postmenopausal patient, local use of estrogen creams for several weeks helps to highlight the abnormal areas for identification by colposcopy.

The majority of VAIN is multifocal; even if a lesion is identified, one must search the entire vagina for coexisting, multiple lesions. Lesions are more common in the upper third of the vagina, but disease-free skip areas may be encountered with additional VAIN in the lower vagina. In hard-to-locate lesions, selective cytologic methods, such as obtaining Pap smears from different locations in the vagina, can often pinpoint the area of abnormality so that attention can be paid specifically to the area of highest suspicion.

Management

Local excision of the involved area has been the mainstay of therapy. In many cases, a single isolated lesion can be removed easily in the office with biopsy forceps. If larger areas are involved, an upper colpectomy may be necessary if the lesion is to be removed by surgery. A dilute pitressin solution or lidocaine with epinephrine can be injected submucosally at the beginning of the procedure and will greatly facilitate the vaginectomy.

As in CIN, outpatient modalities of therapy have been investigated for VAIN. Many patients have been treated historically with 5-fluorouracil (5-FU), but toxicity has decreased enthusiasm for this option. However, studies by Petrilli and associates and Caglar and colleagues indicate that this modality can be effective. One of the problems with 5-FU is the selection of the best mode of application, dosage, and length of treatment. Several techniques have been suggested with equivalent results. One quarter applicator of 5% 5-FU cream is inserted high in the vagina each night after the patient is in bed. The patient can be instructed to coat the vulva and introitus with white petroleum because the cream leaks out during sleep. A small tampon or cotton ball at the introitus is also helpful to prevent leakage. Because of irritation to the vagina and perineum, the cream should be removed by douching with warm water the next morning. This is done every night for 5 to 8 days, followed by a 10- to 14-day rest period, and then the application cycle is repeated. This usually allows an adequate treatment time without having the patient experience the tremendous local reaction that can occur with prolonged use. Treatment can be repeated if it is not successful after the first cycle. Weekly insertions of 5-FU cream, approximately 1.5 g (one third of an applicator), deep into the vagina once per week at bedtime for 10 consecutive weeks has also been shown to be efficacious. Placement of cotton balls at the introitus and application of a petroleum barrier on the perineum and vaginal introitus help prevent 5-FU contamination of the perineum with resultant skin irritation. Douching the next morning, which is advocated by some, is unnecessary with the weekly instillation. Patient compliance is likely higher and toxicity less with the second approach.

Dungar and Wilkinson noted an interesting finding in the vagina after 5-FU therapy, and it has been confirmed by others. After treatment, a red area suggestive of a lack of squamous epithelium may be present. They found that this represented columnar epithelium consistent with a metaplastic process in which squamous epithelium is replaced with columnar epithelium. They called this finding "acquired vaginal adenosis." These changes are usually found in the upper third of the vagina but may extend into the middle third. The columnar epithelium was of a low cuboidal or mucus-secreting endocervical type. In some cases, squamous epithelium was noted overlying the glandular elements. Marked superficial chronic inflammation was also present. This has also been noted in the vagina after laser therapy.

Cryosurgery has largely fallen out of favor in the treatment of VAIN, and laser therapy is preferred as an ablative technique. In order to give guidance about the depth of vaginal destruction required by the laser, Benedet and associates evaluated 56 patients who ranged from 22 to 84 years of age. Measurement of the epithelium was performed on involved and uninvolved tissue. The involved epithelium had a mean thickness of 0.46 mm (range of 0.1-1.4 mm). Uninvolved tissue was thinner and had a mean thickness of 0.28 mm. No statistical difference was seen in thickness of the involved epithelium in the premenopausal and postmenopausal patient; however, the uninvolved epithelium was thinner in the postmenopausal patient compared with the premenopausal patient (0.25 vs 0.37 mm). Based on this study, the authors believed that destruction of 1 to 1.5 mm would only destroy the epithelium without damaging underlying structures

Over a 6-year period, Townsend and associates treated 36 patients from two large referral hospitals with a CO_2 laser. In 92% of the patients, the lesions were completely removed by the laser without significant side effects. Almost one fourth of the patients, however, required more than one treatment session. Krebs treated 22 patients with topical 5-FU and 37 patients with laser therapy. The success rate was similar for the two treatments. Pain and bleeding have been the main complications but appear to be minimal. Healing is excellent, and impaired sexual function has not been a problem. The optimal technique of laser therapy for vaginal lesions has yet to be determined; whereas some investigators suggest removing only the identified lesions, others advocate treating the entire vagina to avoid missing other lesions. A thorough diagnostic investigation of the vagina to rule out invasive cancer can be difficult, but it is obviously mandatory. Evidence from vaginectomy series shows that invasive cancer may be present concurrently with VAIN. In the 105 patients with VAIN II or VAIN III treated with vaginectomy by Indermaur and colleagues, 12% (n = 13) had invasive cancer on final pathology and 22% (n = 23) had negative findings. Multifocal lesions, particularly posthysterectomy, with deep vaginal angles may be difficult to treat with the laser. Small skin hooks and dental mirrors can be used as adjuncts to successful laser therapy.

More recently, experience with 5% imiquimod cream in the management of VAIN has been reported. In a study by Buck and Guth, 56 women with VAIN (mostly low grade) were treated with 0.25 g placed in the vagina once weekly for 3 weeks. Of 42 women available for follow-up, 36 (86%) were clear of VAIN on colposcopic evaluation 1 week or later after the last treatment. Five patients' disease required two treatment cycles and one needed three treatment cycles before clearing of their lesion. Vulvar or vestibular excoriation was reported in only two individuals. No vaginal ulcerations were noted.

Ultrasonic surgical aspiration has been successfully used by Robinson, von Gruenigen and colleagues, and Matsuo and colleagues, but it is not a technique widely practiced. Some have advocated surface irradiation using an intravaginal applicator, but adverse effects may be severe and include vaginal stenosis, urinary symptoms, and vaginal ulceration. Additionally, vaginal stenosis can make follow-up extremely difficult. Total vaginectomy, with vaginal reconstruction using a split-thickness skin graft, should be reserved for the patient who has failed more conservative therapy because there appears to be no recurrence benefit from the more invasive procedure.

Treated VAIN often recurs, regardless of the treatment method, and there is no clear standard of treatment. In a retrospective series of 121 women treated for VAIN between 1989 and 2000 by Dodge and colleagues, 33% of subjects experienced recurrence of VAIN and 2% progressed to invasive cancer; multifocal lesions were more likely to recur. When stratified by treatment type, VAIN recurred in 0% ($n = 0/13$) of those treated with partial vaginectomy, 38% ($n = 16/42$) of those treated with laser, and 59% ($n = 13/22$) of those treated with 5-FU. However, Indermaur and colleagues noted a higher rate of recurrence in their cohort of patients treated with vaginectomy. Of 52 patients available for follow-up who received vaginectomy as treatment for VAIN II or VAIN III, 6 patients recurred at a mean of 24 months, and 1 was diagnosed with invasive cancer. Sillman and associates reported on 94 patients with VAIN who were treated by various methods. The remission rate was high, but 5% of the cases progressed to invasive disease despite close follow-up.

Incomplete excision of sufficient vaginal cuff with hysterectomy for CIS of the cervix with involvement of the fornices may explain an early recurrence. The finding of CIS in the vaginal cuff area in less than 1 year after hysterectomy makes this explanation likely. Therefore it is important to perform a preoperative evaluation of the upper vagina by Schiller tests or colposcopy at the time of hysterectomy for CIS of the cervix. This allows the surgeon to determine accurately how much of the upper vagina has to be removed. It is also apparent that both CIS and dysplasia may develop in the vagina as primary lesions without an association with a similar process on the cervix or vulva. Still other preinvasive lesions of the vagina may appear after irradiation therapy for invasive carcinoma of the cervix. Data from the MD Anderson Hospital suggest that these postradiation lesions are premalignant and can progress to invasive cancer if they are not treated. Without therapy, approximately 25% of the patients in this series progressed to the invasive state over varying periods of follow-up. Local therapy must be executed with care because of the previous irradiation.

INTRAEPITHELIAL NEOPLASIA OF THE VULVA

Clinical Profile

In 2004 the ISSVD clarified the vulvar intraepithelial neoplasia (VIN) classification system (Table 2-5). Because there was no evidence that VIN I was a precancerous lesion, it was eliminated. The term "VIN" now refers

TABLE 2-5   2003 ISSVD Classification of Vulvar Intraepithelial Neoplasia (VIN)*

A. VIN, usual type
 1. Warty type
 2. Basaloid type
 3. Mixed (warty/basaloid) type
B. VIN, differentiated type

The previous classifications of VIN II and VIN III were consolidated as VIN, and the previous classification of VIN I was eliminated.

TABLE 2-6   VIN Histologic Subtypes and Associations

	Usual (Warty-Basaloid, Differentiated)	Differentiated (Simplex)
Age	Premenopausal women (30-40)	Postmenopausal women (65)
Overall %VIN	Approximately 95%	Approximately 5%
HPV-associated	Yes	No
HPV type	16	N/A
Risk Factors	Smoking, immunosuppression	None identified
Distribution	Multifocal	Unifocal, unicentric
Background histology	Lichen sclerosus	
Progression to	Warty, basaloid squamous cell cancer Invasive cancer	Keratinizing squamous cell cancer (Rare)

only to lesions previously classified as VIN II or III. In the current system, there is no discrimination between VIN II and III, and the two previously distinct classifications are consolidated as "VIN."

Two distinct subtypes of VIN exist: usual type and differentiated type. The two subtypes are different in epidemiology, morphology, and their association with vulvar cancer (Table 2-6). Differentiated type may also be called simplex VIN, whereas usual type may be called warty, basaloid, or undifferentiated VIN. In comparison to usual type, differentiated type tends to occur in older women, be unifocal and unicentric, be found at the edge of vulvar squamous cell carcinoma and in the setting of lichen sclerosus or planus, and be less associated with HPV. Usual type VIN, with warty and basaloid subtypes, is found in younger women, has a strong association with cigarette smoking, is often multifocal, is less frequently found in conjunction with squamous cell cancer, and is usually HPV-associated. There is an association between VIN and vulvar cancer, but the relationship is less clear than the known progression from CIN to invasive cervical squamous carcinoma.

According to a SEER data analysis by Judson and colleagues, the incidence of vulvar CIS increased 411% between 1973 and 2000, whereas the rates of invasive vulvar cancer rose 20%. Several hypotheses regarding the changing incidence of VIN exist: increased physician awareness and evaluation of vulvar disease, increased prevalence of smoking among women, and increased HPV prevalence. Women with a history of preinvasive cervical disease or cervical cancer are at increased risk of preinvasive vulvar dysplasia. HPV is a risk factor for vulvar disease, but the progression from HPV infection to precancer to invasive cancer is poorly understood. In contrast to cervical cancer, which has a peak age in dysplasia incidence followed by a peak age in invasive cancer (after a lag period), there is no similar time course established in vulvar cancer. In fact, the peak incidence of VIN occurs during the mid 40s, followed by a declining incidence, whereas the incidence of invasive vulvar cancer continues to increase and never stabilizes, reaching approximately 13/100,000 women by the age of 80.

Case reports definitively document the development of invasive squamous cell cancers in VIN usual type lesions in patients followed prospectively. In a review of more than 3300 patients with VIN III, van Seters identified occult invasive cancer in 3.2% of subjects at the time of excision, and an additional 3.3% developed cancer during follow-up. Chafe noted that 19% of women who were thoroughly evaluated and thought to have VIN actually had invasive cancer on the vulvectomy specimen. Kagie and associates reported on 66 women with invasive vulvar squamous cell carcinoma; 39 (62%) had synchronous VIN. In other cases, it appears that invasive lesions may arise de novo rather than from precursor VIN lesions.

In a population of 405 women followed for VIN II and III in New Zealand between 1962 and 2003, 2% of cases recurred as invasive cancer at a median time of 2.4 years, and 1.8% of cases recurred as invasive cancer in new fields at a median time of 13.5 years. Additionally, 11.6% of biopsy-proven VIN regressed before treatment (mean age 24.6 years). If observation is considered in young women with small lesions and usual type histology, frequent examinations with directed biopsies are necessary. Barbero and colleagues noted 3 of 55 patients treated with VIN whose condition progressed to carcinoma in 14 months to 15 years. These 3 patients ranged in age from 58 to 74 years. In the New Zealand cohort there were 10 cancers diagnosed in untreated patients; Jones and McLean have previously reported on 5 of the cases diagnosed between 1970 and 1974, and an additional 5 cases were diagnosed between 1983 and 1992. The median interval between VIN and invasive cancer was 3.9 years (range 1.1-7.3 years).

HPV is strongly associated with VIN usual type, but it is less commonly associated with VIN differentiated type. There is a wide variation in the reported presence of HPV in VIN because of the changing terminology and classification of VIN and the improved sensitivity of recent HPV testing. Usual type comprises the majority of VIN, so a high prevalence of HPV positivity would be expected in studies that do not differentiate between the two histologies. In more recently published literature, HPV is present in 61% to 100% of VIN. HPV-16 appears to be the most common type, accounting for as high as 91% of infection in some series. The prevalence of HPV infection in VIN and vulvar cancer decreases with age, probably reflecting a change in the underlying histology. The efficacy of HPV vaccines in preventing vulvar dysplasia and cancer will be determined not only by the vaccine properties, but also by the prevalence of HPV-related vulvar disease in the population.

In initial publications from the vaccine studies, there does appear to be efficacy against VIN. Joura and colleagues report on the vaccine efficacy in reducing specifically HPV-16– or HPV-18–related VIN with a mean duration of follow-up of 36 months. Among subjects who remained HPV negative while receiving the vaccination series, the vaccine was 100% efficacious; 0 cases were diagnosed in 7811 vaccinated women and 8 cases were diagnosed in 7785 women who received placebo. Among subjects who were HPV negative at the time of the first injection but did not necessarily remain HPV negative for the duration of the vaccination series, the vaccine was 95% efficacious; 1 case was diagnosed in 8757 vaccinated women and 20 cases were diagnosed in 8774 women who received placebo. An analysis was also performed on the incidence of VIN, regardless of HPV association, among all subjects, HPV-naïve and HPV-exposed at the time of vaccination, and the rate of VIN II/III was reduced by half in the vaccinated group, but there did not appear to be any benefit for those who were HPV-exposed at the time of vaccination.

The disease is asymptomatic in more than 50% of cases. In the remainder of cases, the predominant symptom is pruritus. The presence of a distinct mass, bleeding, or discharge strongly suggests invasive cancer. The most productive diagnostic technique is careful inspection of the vulva in bright light during a routine pelvic examination followed by biopsies of suspicious lesions. A handheld lens or colposcope can be very helpful, especially after application of 5% acetic acid to the skin and introitus.

Diagnosis

The value of careful inspection of the vulva during routine gynecologic examinations cannot be overstated; this remains the most productive diagnostic technique. The milder forms of VIN first appear clinically as pale areas that vary in density. More severe forms are seen as papules or macules, coalescent or discrete, or single or multiple. Lesions on the cutaneous surface of the vulva usually appear as lichenified or hyperkeratotic plaques—that is, white epithelium (Figures 2-9 and 2-10). By contrast, lesions of mucous membranes are usually macular

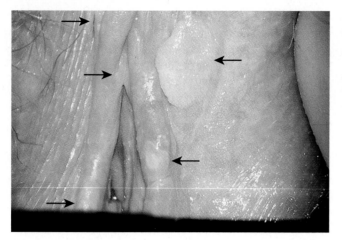

FIGURE 2-9   Multiple white lesions of the vulva caused by vulvar intraepithelial neoplasia.

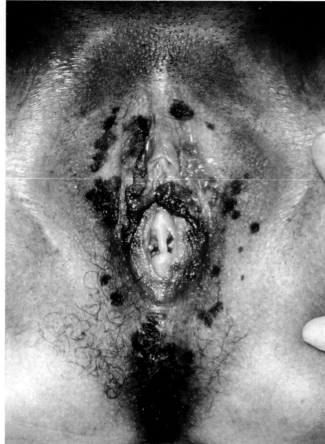

FIGURE 2-11   Pseudopigmented lesions of vulvar carcinoma in situ.

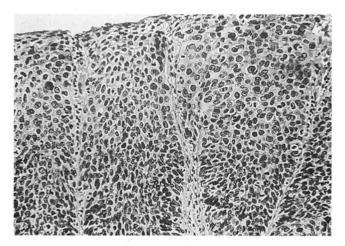

FIGURE 2-10   Histologic section of carcinoma in situ of the vulva.

and pink or red. Vulvar lesions are hyperpigmented in 10% to 15% of patients (Figure 2-11). These lesions range from mahogany to dark brown, and they stand out sharply when observed solely with the naked eye.

The entire vulva, perineum, and perianal area must be evaluated for multifocal lesions. It is not uncommon to find intraepithelial lesions on hemorrhoid tags. The use of acetic acid is helpful in identifying subtle lesions. In contrast to the mucous membrane of the cervix, the keratinized epithelium of the vulva requires application of acetic acid for 5 minutes or longer before many lesions become apparent. Placement of numerous soaked cotton balls or sponges on the vulva for the desired length of time is an effective method. After a lesion has been diagnosed, colposcopic examination of the entire vulva and perianal area should follow to rule out multicentric lesions. A handheld magnifying glass can also be used, which allows greater viewing area at one time compared with

the colposcope. In general, multifocal lesions are more common in premenopausal patients, whereas postmenopausal patients have a higher rate of unifocal disease.

Some investigators prefer to use toluidine blue to identify vulvar lesions. A 1% aqueous solution of the dye is applied to the external genital area. After drying for 2 to 3 minutes, the region is then washed with 1% to 2% acetic acid solution. Suspicious foci of increased nuclear activity become deeply stained (royal blue), whereas normal skin accepts little or none of the dye. Regrettably, hyperkeratotic lesions, even though neoplastic, are only lightly stained, whereas benign excoriations are often brilliant, an observation that accounts for the high false-positive and false-negative rates.

The diagnosis of VIN can be subtle. To avoid delay, the physician must exercise a high degree of suspicion. Vulvar biopsy should be used liberally. It is best accomplished under local anesthesia with a Keyes dermatologic punch (4-6-mm size). This instrument allows removal of an adequate tissue sample and orientation for future sectioning. The biopsy site can be made hemostatic with silver nitrate, Monsel's, or a piece of absorbable gelatin powder (e.g., Gelfoam) cut with the Keyes punch; this is positioned in the skin defect and kept in place with a small dressing for at least 24 hours. Adequate biopsy specimens can also be obtained with a sharp alligator-jaw instrument if one has proper traction on the skin. The problem with ordinary knife biopsies is that only superficial epithelium can be reached. If this technique is used, one must be careful to sample deeper layers.

Pigmented Lesions

Pigmented lesions of the vulva are usually intraepithelial, with the exception of melanoma, which is discussed in Chapter 8. Pigmented lesions account for approximately 10% of all vulvar disease. The most common pigmented lesion is a lentigo, which is a concentration of melanocytes in the basal layer of cells. It can have the clinical appearance of a freckle, although it is more commonly confused with a nevus. The borders are fuzzy, but it is not a raised lesion. A lentigo is benign, and the diagnosis is usually made by inspection with magnification. If there is any doubt, a biopsy should always be performed.

VIN may appear as a pigmented lesion. Friedrich found that CIS of the vulva was more frequent in pigmented lesions than in nevi. Characteristic raised, hyperkeratotic pigmented lesions are suggestive of CIS and should be biopsied.

Bowenoid papulosis is a variant of a pigmented lesion noted by dermatologists for some time. These are small pigmented papules that develop and spread rapidly. According to dermatologists, these papules often regress spontaneously. Histologically, at least on the vulva, these are squamous cell carcinomas in situ. These lesions have been reported to have an aneuploid DNA pattern. Many authorities have not found bowenoid papulosis of the vulva to spontaneously regress. Regardless of the clinical characteristics, if VIN is present histologically, the physician should treat the patient accordingly.

The management of nevi can be conservative. A nevus can often be detected only microscopically. Unfortunately, a simple nevus and an early melanoma cannot be differentiated on clinical evaluation. Excisional biopsy of these raised, smooth, pigmented areas can be done easily in the physician's office. If the nevus changes in color, size, and shape, it should be removed for diagnostic purposes. After a nevus is removed, no further therapy is needed regardless of whether it is a compound, intradermal, or junctional type.

Management

Surgical excision has been the mainstay of therapy for VIN, although laser is a frequently used technique and immune modulators have gained recent prominence. An important advantage of surgical excision is that complete histologic assessment is performed; lesions with early invasion can thus be found. Most localized lesions are managed effectively by wide local excision with end-to-end approximation of the defect. The vulvar skin and mucous membrane are usually very elastic, and cosmetic results are satisfactory after uncomplicated healing. A Cochrane review is currently under way evaluating the benefits and drawbacks for different types of surgical interventions, and the most appropriate treatment for VIN may be clearer in the future.

Excision

Wide local excision is the most commonly performed treatment of VIN. The goal of VIN surgery is to obtain a 5-mm disease-free margin. Margin status and histology results are available on final pathology results, which is a benefit of the excisional procedure. Modesitt and associates reported that recurrences were three times higher (46% vs 17%) when margins were positive for residual VIN II and III. In the New Zealand study discussed earlier, 50% of those with positive margins versus 15% of those with negative margins required further treatment. Hillemanns and colleagues showed an overall recurrence rate of 43% in subjects retrospectively analyzed who had been heterogeneously treated with laser, photodynamic therapy, excision, or vulvectomy. No patients recurred in the vulvectomy group (n = 8). In the natural history review by van Seters and colleagues, 1921 patients were surgically treated. Recurrence was noted in 19% after vulvectomy, 18% after partial vulvectomy, and 22% after local excision. Recurrences were significantly lower after free surgical margins (17%) than after positive surgical margins (47%). Progression to invasive disease occurred in 58 patients, 52% of the time after vulvectomy, and 48% of the time after local excision. In this retrospective review, the surgical approach was likely selected based on individual patient characteristics so that patients considered at higher risk for invasive cancer may have more frequently received vulvectomy. However, there is no definitive evidence or randomized controlled trial to show that vulvectomy is associated with better outcomes and the morbidity associated with the procedure is much greater. Wide local excision is the accepted excisional procedure for VIN.

In the series by Modesitt and colleagues, described earlier, 17 of 73 subjects were diagnosed with invasive cancer at the time of treatment for VIN III. Similarly, 16 of 78 patients undergoing surgical excision for VIN III had invasive cancer in the report by Husseinzadeh and Recinto. To avoid returning to the operating room for deeper re-excision and lymph node dissection, biopsies must be liberally performed preoperatively. Multiple biopsies may be required. Adequate postoperative

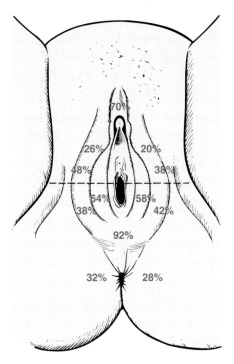

FIGURE 2-12 Plot of lesion locations in 36 patients treated for multifocal carcinoma in situ of the vulva.

follow-up with repeat biopsy for any suspicious lesions is also essential.

Occasionally, a skinning vulvectomy is indicated. With multicentric lesions (Figure 2-12) the involved skin can be excised and substituted with a split-thickness skin graft taken from the buttocks or inner aspect of the thigh. This skinning vulvectomy and skin graft procedure was introduced by Rutledge and Sinclair in 1968 (Fig. 2-13). Its purpose was to replace the skin at risk in the vulvar site with ectopic epidermis from a donor site. Creasman later reported a modification of the procedure with preservation of the clitoris. Any lesions on the glans are scraped off with a scalpel blade, and the epithelium of the glans regenerates without loss of sensation. In more than 100 patients treated, the authors reported no complaints of dyspareunia or diminished sexual responsiveness. The benefits of the skinning vulvectomy and skin graft procedure are preservation of the subcutaneous tissue of the vulva and a better cosmetic and functional result (Figure 2-14). In the elderly patient, simple vulvectomy may be preferred because the skinning vulvectomy and skin graft operation requires prolonged bedrest (6-7 days) to allow the split-thickness graft to adhere to the graft bed. Thus the potential for morbidity is increased. The patient's wishes concerning cosmetic results and sexual function, however, must be taken into account regardless of the person's age.

TABLE 2-7 CO$_2$ Laser Vaporization: Vulva

Instrument	CO$_2$ laser, colposcopic, micromanipulator
Power density	600-1000 W/cm^2
Depth of destruction	Nonhairy areas <1 mm
Hairy areas	>3 mm
Lateral margins	"Brush"
Anesthesia	General, local
Analgesia	Significant postlaser pain: narcotics

Laser

Ablative therapy is an alternative to excision. The disadvantage of ablative therapy is that a necrotic ulcer on the vulva may result and wound healing may be slow. Complete healing may take up to 3 months. The treated area is often very painful for much of that time. Many consider laser therapy the treatment of choice in the management of VIN, particularly for those who have multifocal disease. Townsend and colleagues treated 33 patients with laser therapy and reported success in 31 (94%), but 14 patients required two or more treatments, and two patients required five laser treatments. The results published by Baggish and Dorsey were similar; 32 of 35 patients were believed to have been cured from their disease, 26 of 35 patients required three or more treatments, and 2 women had six treatments. In the review article of the 253 patients treated with laser, 23% recurred.

Only a small portion of the vulva can be treated on an outpatient basis. Patients require general anesthesia if large areas of the vulva are treated at one time. Pain, which is severe in some patients, is the main complication with laser therapy. Bleeding and infection have also been reported. The cosmetic results appear to be excellent. It appears that laser therapy can be an acceptable treatment modality, but patients must be carefully evaluated before treatment to rule out invasive carcinoma (Table 2-7). Greater expertise with the laser is required for this therapy than is needed for cervical vaporization. The depth of destruction must be controlled. Too deep a wound can result in long-term ulcers, which may take some time to heal and cause considerable discomfort. Benedet and colleagues evaluated 165 women with VIN. Of the 122 patients with VIN III, the mean thickness of the epithelium was 0.52 mm (range of 0.1-1.9 mm). In patients with hair follicles involved with VIN, the mean depth of involvement was 1.9 mm (range of 1-3.4 mm). Only 19 patients had appendiceal involvement. Age did not seem to affect the thickness of involved epithelium. Multifocal lesions were present in 64% of all patients. The most common sites were the labia minora, posterior fourchette, and perineum. Based on this study, the authors believe that 1-mm destruction of

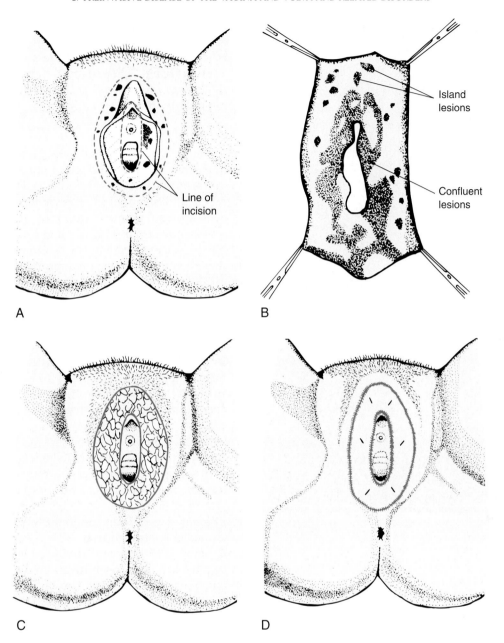

FIGURE 2-13   Skinning vulvectomy and skin graft. **A,** Excise all areas of involvement en bloc. **B,** Lesions may be isolated or confluent. **C,** Preserve all subcutaneous tissue as the graft bed. **D,** Suture the skin graft to the graft bed.

non–hair-bearing epithelium is adequate treatment. If skin appendages are involved, 2.5-3 mm is required (Figure 2-15). When performing excision, do not take the burn level to the subcutaneous fat. Also, wipe the carbon from the surgical site during the procedure and be certain that the shiny white lower dermis is preserved. Reid has defined surgical planes in the vulva as a guide to laser therapy. The first plane is the surface epithelium only, which includes the basement membrane. Opalescent cell debris is noted through the heat char. Healing is rapid, with good cosmetic results. The second plane

involves the dermal papillae, with necrosis extending to the deep papillary area. The appearance is a homogeneous yellow color that resembles a chamois cloth. Again, healing is rapid with good cosmesis. The third plane affects the upper and mid-reticular area where the pilosebaceous ducts are located. Some hypertrophy may appear in this area during the healing process. The fourth plane affects the deep reticular area, and "sand grains" can be visualized. Healing is slow and usually occurs by granulation from the sides. Skin grafting may be required. Destruction to the third plane is adequate

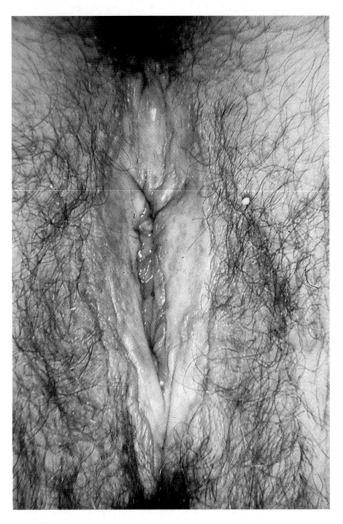

FIGURE 2-14 Excellent cosmetic results are present after superficial vulvectomy and skin graft for vulvar intraepithelial neoplasia (VIN).

for hair-bearing tissue; plane one to two is the depth needed for non–hair-bearing skin.

After laser therapy, the vulva is covered with silvadene. Sitz baths, topical lidocaine, and rinsing of the vulva with water after urination and defecation are important. A hair dryer is then used to dry the area. Repeat application of steroids is used after each washing and drying. A local anesthetic can be applied for mild to moderate pain control. Oral pain medication, including narcotics, may be necessary. The most severe pain is usually evident 3 to 4 days after the laser therapy. Laser therapy is particularly effective around the areas where excision can lead to external sphincter weakening.

Cavitational Ultrasonic Surgical Aspirator

Cavitational ultrasonic surgical aspirator (CUSA) is a less frequently used ablative option. In a randomized prospective trial, von Grueningen and associates compared outcomes from laser ablation versus CUSA. Recurrence was similar in both arms (25% overall), but subjects treated with CUSA had less postoperative pain and less scarring. Other adverse events, including infection, dysuria, adhesions, and discharge, were similar between both groups.

Imiquimod

Imiquimod 5% cream is an immune response modifier with indirect antiviral and antitumor properties. It activates macrophages and dendritic cells to release interferon (IFN)-alpha and other cytokines that provoke an antigen-specific immune response. Imiquimod cream was first shown to be effective and safe in the treatment of HPV-associated genital warts and was subsequently evaluated and has shown great promise in the treatment of VIN. In a phase II trial completed by Le and colleagues, 33 patients with VIN were treated for 16 weeks with 5% imiquimod application; 6 additional subjects were unable to complete the study. At 20 weeks, 21 of 33 subjects had complete response (complete disappearance of the visible lesion and histologic regression), 9 of 33 had a partial response (50% decrease from baseline measurement), and 3 had stable lesions. In a randomized, double-blinded controlled trial, Mathieson and associates treated 21 subjects with 5% imiquimod and 10 with placebo. There was a complete response in 17 of 21 subjects in the treatment group (complete histologic regression) and in 0 of 10 subjects in the placebo group. Because of side effects, the dose was reduced in 14 of 21 women in the treatment group. Van Seters and colleagues report similar results but also include 12-month follow-up from their randomized controlled trial. In 26 subjects treated with imiquimod, histologic and virologic regression was seen in 15 and 14 subjects, respectively. In the 26 subjects who received placebo, histologic and virologic regression was seen in 1 and 2 subjects, respectively. Progression to invasive disease occurred in 1 subject in the treatment arm (who initially had a weak, partial response with imiquimod) and 2 subjects in the placebo arm. Treatment was reduced to once-weekly application in 5 women receiving imiquimod because of severe inflammation. Investigator-reported side effects, including erythema, erosion, vesiculation, and edema, were significantly worse in the treatment group than in the placebo group. At 20 weeks and 12 months, however, self-reported pruritus and pain were significantly better in the treatment group than in the placebo group. Cidofovir, an antiviral agent with activity against HPV, has also been reported as treatment for VIN in a very small sample.

One of the obvious benefits of imiquimod is avoidance of disfiguring surgery. Randomized trials show promise in its use as a primary therapy for VIN and it has been relatively well tolerated, but dose reductions have been necessary in all trials for a considerable

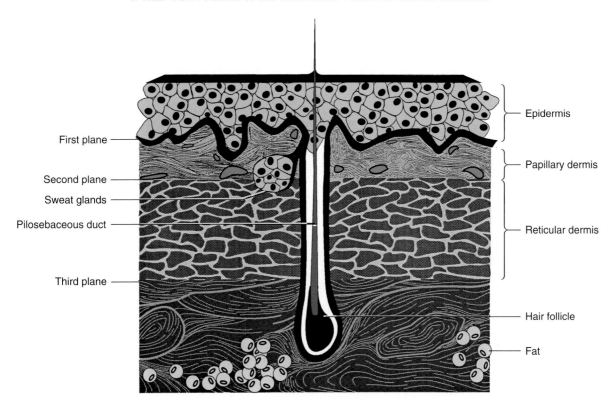

First plane

Second plane

Sweat glands

Pilosebaceous duct

Third plane

Epidermis

Papillary dermis

Reticular dermis

Hair follicle

Fat

FIGURE 2-15   "Planes" for therapy for vulvar intraepithelial neoplasia using a laser.

number of subjects. The trials previously mentioned varied in application frequency from once per week to three times per week when tolerated. Because some of the main benefits are quality-of-life related, it will be important to evaluate the side effects and complications of imiquimod versus excisional procedures. Even in women who did not receive a complete response, a partial response was observed in many. Reduction in lesion size may be another potential application of the therapy, particularly if disease is present in a multifocal, clitoral, or sphincter distribution. Another important question for future trials is whether immune modulators have any effect on non–HPV-associated VIN; it is possible that the treatment of differentiated VIN in older women should not be delayed with a course of imiquimod. Because ISSVD classification has now changed, future trials should specifically evaluate efficacy in usual type VIN versus differentiated type VIN.

In summary, it is important to remember that these lesions often develop in young women who remain asymptomatic. Women should be taught vulvar self-examination to identify early lesions. Physical examination performed by a physician will likely become inadvertently less frequent as Pap screening guidelines continue to evolve, and self-examination may become more important in the future. Postmenopausal women should be instructed in the importance of annual vulvar examinations, even if Pap screening is not required. This could lead to successful therapy that could also be less radical. Early diagnosis depends on careful vulvar examination under a bright light at regular intervals. Biopsy must be done on any suspicious lesions, and if the histologic report confirms intraepithelial neoplasia, an examination for multicentric foci should follow. The therapy of choice depends on the extent of disease, the location of the lesions, and the personal desires of the patient.

For full reference list, log onto www.expertconsult.com
⟨http://www.expertconsult.com⟩

3

Invasive Cervical Cancer

Krishnansu S. Tewari, MD, and Bradley J. Monk, MD

GENERAL OBSERVATIONS

Anatomy

The cervix (Latin for "neck") is a narrow, cylindrical segment of the uterus; it enters the vagina through the anterior vaginal wall and lies, in most cases, at a right angle to it. In the average patient, the cervix measures 2 to 4 cm in length and is contiguous with the inferior aspect of the uterine corpus. The point of juncture of the uterus and the cervix is known as the isthmus; this area is marked by slight constriction of the lumen. Anteriorly, the cervix is separated from the bladder by fatty tissue and is connected laterally to the broad ligament and parametrium (through which it obtains its blood supply). The lower intravaginal portion of the cervix, a free segment that projects into the vault of the vagina, is covered with mucous membrane. The cervix opens into the vaginal cavity through the external os. The cervical canal extends from the anatomic external os to the internal os, where it joins the uterine cavity. The histologic internal os is where there is a transition from endocervical to endometrial glands. The intravaginal portion of the cervix (portio vaginalis, exocervix) is covered with stratified squamous epithelium that is essentially identical to the epithelium of the vagina. The endocervical mucosa is arranged in branching folds (plicae palmatae) and is lined by cylindrical epithelium. The stroma of the cervix consists of connective tissue with stratified muscle fibers and elastic tissue. The elastic tissue is found primarily around the walls of the larger blood vessels.

The stratified squamous epithelium of the portio vaginalis is composed of several layers that are conventionally described as basal, parabasal, intermediate, and superficial. The basal layer consists of a single row of cells and rests on a thin basement membrane. This is the layer in which active mitosis occurs. The parabasal and intermediate layers together constitute the prickle-cell layer, which is analogous to the same layer in the epidermis. The superficial layer varies in thickness, depending on the degree of estrogen stimulation. It consists primarily of flattened cells that show an increasing degree of cytoplasmic acidophilia toward the surface. The thickness and the glycogen content of the epithelium increase following estrogen stimulation and account for the therapeutic effect of estrogens in atrophic vaginitis. The staining of glycogen in the normal epithelium of the portio vaginalis is the basis of the Schiller test.

Epidemiologic Studies

Clinical Profile

In the United States the mortality from cervical cancer in 1945 was 15 of 100,000 females. This had declined to approximately 4.6 of 100,000 by 1986 and 3.4 of 100,000 by 1991. It is unclear whether the mortality from cervical cancer is falling as a result of cervical cytologic screening and intervention at the in situ stage or whether cervical screening has caused an increase in the proportion of early-stage cancer at diagnosis and registration. After therapy for invasive disease, adequate follow-up is the key to early detection of a recurrence (Table 3-1). The yield of examinations such as intravenous pyelography (IVP), computed tomography (CT) scan, and chest radiograph in patients with initial early disease (stages I–IIa) is so low that many have discontinued their routine use. However, frequent Pap tests from the vaginal apex/cervix are recommended.

TABLE 3-1　Optimal Interval Evaluation of Cervical Cancer Following Radiotherapy/Surgery (Asymptomatic Patient*)

Year	Frequency	Examination
1	3 months	Pelvic examination, Pap smear
	6 months	Chest film, CBC, BUN, creatinine
	1 year	IVP or CT scan with contrast
2	4 months	Pelvic examination, Pap smear
	1 year	Chest films, CBC, BUN, creatinine, IVP or CT scan with contrast
3-5	6 months	Pelvic examination, Pap smear

*Symptomatic patients should have appropriate examination where indicated.
BUN, Blood urea nitrogen; CBC, complete blood count; CT, computed tomography; IVP, intravenous pyelogram; Pap, Papanicolaou.

West studied the age of registration and the age of death of women with cervical cancer in South Wales. He found that the observed age at death was very close to 59 years regardless of stage and age at diagnosis. Although the 5-year survival rate of women with localized (early-stage) cervical cancer was much higher than that of women with nonlocalized (late-stage) cancer, the women with localized cancer tended to be younger than those with advanced cancer. Calculations of expected age at death of the whole population suggest that more than half the advantage in survival rate shown by women with early-stage cancers is a result of the diagnosis of the former in younger women.

Christopherson and colleagues reported that the percentage of patients diagnosed as having stage I disease increased by 78% in the population studied from 1953 to 1965. The increase was most remarkable in younger women. The authors concluded that the major problem in cervical cancer control was the screening of older women. Older women had higher incidence rates; the percentage with stage I disease also decreased with each decade, reaching a low of 15% for those 70 years of age and older. These older women with cervical cancer are rarely screened and contribute heavily to the death rate. The initial advanced stage contributes to the patient population with advanced recurrent cervical cancer. These patients, therefore, deserve very close posttreatment observation in an effort to detect a recurrence in its earliest possible form.

In 2011 there were 12,710 new cases of invasive cervical cancer and 4290 deaths from this disease in the United States. It is particularly distressing that more than one third of women diagnosed will die from a disease that is largely preventable by vaccination and screening. There is no other human malignancy for which we have identified the causative agent, have successfully implemented excellent screening programs, and now have efficacious and tolerable prophylactic vaccination available. Oncogenic subtypes of the human

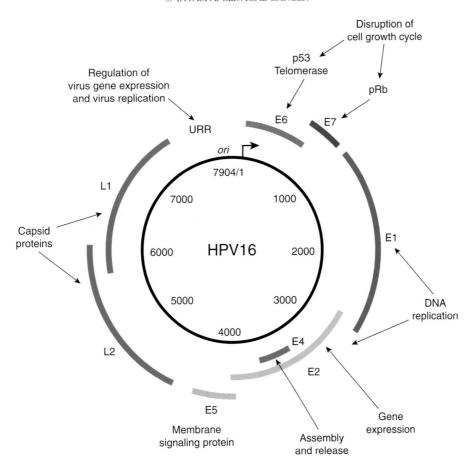

FIGURE 3-1   Human papillomavirus genome. *(From microbiologybytes.com)*

papillomavirus (HPV) have been identified as the etiologic cause of cervical neoplasia (Figure 3-1). The power, consistency, and specificity of the association between subclinical HPV infection and cervical neoplasia raise the strong possibility that this relationship is causal. The biologic plausibility of this is supported by evidence that this sexually transmitted oncogenic virus often produces persistent asymptomatic infection of metaplastic epithelium in the cervical transformation zone.

Epidemiologic surveillance studies performed in the United States during the past two decades have documented decreased incidence rates for invasive cervical cancer. Ethnic and racial disparities, however, still exist. In a Surveillance, Epidemiology and End Results (SEER) analysis of 13 U.S. cancer registries containing cases from 1992 to 2003, Hispanic whites had the highest incidence rate of cervical cancer overall (24 per 100,000), squamous cell carcinoma (18 per 100,000), and adenocarcinoma (5 per 10,000). Non-Hispanic whites had the lowest rates of cervical cancer overall (11 per 100,000) and squamous cell carcinoma (7 per 100,000), whereas African-Americans had the lowest rate of

adenocarcinoma (2 per 100,000). In a recent study using data obtained from the Cancer in North America (CINA) deluxe 1995-2004 database created by the North American Association of Central Cancer Registries (NAACCR), African-American and Hispanic U.S. populations continue to have the highest rates of invasive cervical cancer compared to non-Hispanic whites. Variations in screening utilization and socioeconomic status are thought to account for the majority of the racial/ethnic disparities.

HUMAN PAPILLOMAVIRUS

Prophylactic Vaccination

Targeting groups with the greatest burdens of cervical cancer is of public health importance because we have now officially entered the era of HPV vaccination. There are now two U.S. Food and Drug Administration (FDA)-approved vaccines indicated to prevent cervical cancer (Table 3-2 and Figure 3-2).

TABLE 3-2   HPV Vaccines Available in the United States

	Gardasil	Cervarix
HPV types	6, 11, 16, 18	16, 18
Doses (mcg)	20/40/40/20	20/20
Technology used to produce L1 VLPs	Yeast	Insect cell substrate
Adjuvant	A2HS Amorphous hydoxyphosphate sulfate (Merck and Co., Inc.)	AS04 Aluminum hydroxide + 3 = deacetylated monophosphoryl lipid A (MPL, Corixa/GSK)
Adjuvant dose (mcg)	225	500/50
Dose schedule	0.5 mL IM 0, 2, 6 mos	0.5 mL IM 0, 1-2, 6 mos
Indications	Cervical cancer, CIN, AIS, vulvar cancer, VIN, vaginal cancer, VAIN, anogenital warts Caused by infection caused by HPV 6, -11, -16, and/or -18	Cervical cancer, CIN, AIS Caused by infection by HPV-16 and/or -18
Population approved	Males and females ages 9-26 yr	Females ages 9-25 yr

Quadravalent Vaccine

In 2007 the Females United to Unilaterally Reduce Endo/Ectocervical Disease (FUTURE) II Study Group reported the results from a randomized, double-blind trial of 12,167 women ages 15 to 26 years who received three doses of either quadrivalent HPV-6/-11/-16/-18 viruslike particle (VLP) vaccine (GARDASIL, Merck) or placebo administered intramuscularly at day 1, month 2, and month 6. The primary analysis was performed for a per-protocol susceptible population that included 1565 randomized subjects who had no virologic evidence of infection with HPV-16 or -18 through month 7. The mean follow-up was 3 years and vaccine efficacy for prevention of the primary composite end point (cervical intraepithelial neoplasia [CIN] II, CIN III, adenocarcinoma in situ [AIS], or invasive disease related to HPV-16 or -18) was 98% (95% CI, 86-100) in the per-protocol susceptible population, and 44% (95% CI, 26-58) in an intention-to-treat population of all women who had undergone randomization.

The FUTURE I investigators reported results from their phase III, randomized, double-blind, placebo-controlled trial using the quadrivalent vaccine in 5455 women between the ages of 16 and 24 years. In this trial, the coprimary composite end points were the incidence of genital warts; vulvar intraepithelial neoplasia (VIN)

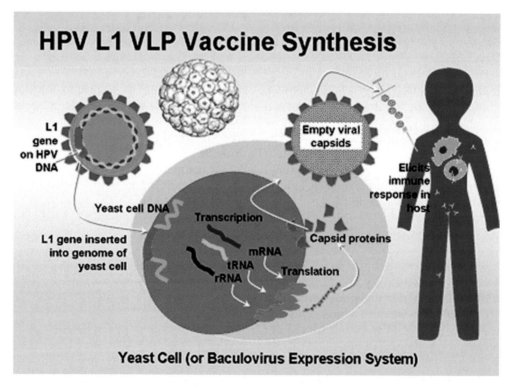

FIGURE 3-2   Human papillomavirus prophylactic vaccine. (From www.cancer.gov)

or vaginal intraepithelial neopaslia (VAIN); or cancer and the incidence of CIN, AIS, or cancer associated with HPV types 6, 11, 16, or 18. Vaccine efficacy was 100% for each of the coprimary end points. In an intention-to-treat analysis (which included those with prevalent infection or disease caused by vaccine-type and non–vaccine-type HPV) vaccination reduced the rate of any vulvar or vaginal perianal lesions regardless of the causal HPV type by 34% (95% CI, 15-49), and the rate of cervical lesions regardless of the causal HPV type by 20% (95% CI, 8-31).

The FUTURE I and II data, along with the immunogenicity trial led to FDA approval of GARDASIL in 2006. The latter study enrolled 506 girls and 510 boys (10-15 years of age) and 513 women age 16-23 years and demonstrated noninferior immunogenic responses to all four human HPV types in the quadrivalent vaccine, permitting the bridging of efficacy data that were generated in FUTURE I and II to girls. Current U.S. FDA approval for GARDASIL is for prevention of anogenital warts, CIN, AIS, cervical cancer, VIN, vulvar cancer, VAIN, and vaginal cancer in females ages 9 to 26 years, and prevention of anogenital warts in males ages 9 to 26 years. The Advisory Committee on Immunization Practices (ACIP) recommends routine vaccination of females aged 11 and 12 years, with catch-up vaccination for females ages 13 to 26 years who have not been previously vaccinated. Vaccination may be started as young as age 9.

With respect to males, phase III data presented at the 2008 European Research Organisation on Genital Infection and Neoplasia (EUROGIN) in Nice, France demonstrated that GARDASIL vaccine efficacy was 89.4% (95% CI 65.5, 97.9) in preventing genital warts in previously uninfected men ages 16 to 26 years. There were no cases of penile intraepithelial neoplasia in the vaccinated group, and three cases occurred in the placebo group. In October 2009 the ACIP supported the permissive use (i.e., at the discretion of the patient's health care provider) of GARDASIL for boys and young men ages 9 to 26 years to reduce the likelihood of acquiring genital warts. The ACIP also voted to recommend that funding be provided for the use of GARDASIL in males through the Vaccines for Children (VFC) program.

The generation of immune memory and long-term efficacy, safety, cross-protection, impact on vaccination on HPV transmission rates, vaccination in women beyond age 26 years, impact on repeat testing/procedures, cost containment, and disease recrudescence continue to be studied. In 2009 data from an extended follow-up study of a 1998 to 1999 randomized controlled trial to assess the longer term efficacy of a prophylactic monovalent HPV type 16 VLP in women suggested that the Merck platform for the monovalent VLP remained efficacious through 8.5 years after its

administration. In another study designed to evaluate the induction of immune memory with the quadrivalent VLP vaccine, stable anti-HPV levels were present for at least 5 years. Although anti–HPV-18 titers decline, there has been no breakthrough HPV-18 type-specific disease among patients who were seronegative to HPV-18 and did not have HPV-18 DNA on their cervix at the time of vaccine administration.

Brown and colleagues studied the impact of GARDASIL against disease endpoints (CIN I-III, AIS) and persistent infection caused by oncogenic HPV types in addition to HPV-16 and -18. The investigators found that the administration of the quadrivalent vaccine to a generally HPV-naïve population resulted in a 32.5% reduction in CIN II–III and AIS caused by 10 nonvaccine HPV types that cause more than 20% of cervical cancer worldwide. The cross protection of GARDASIL was most apparent for the A9 species of HPV, which causes most cases of CIN II–III and AIS.

In a double-blind, randomized trial of 3817 women aged 24 to 45 years, quadrivalent vaccine efficacy against the first coprimary endpoint (disease or infection related to HPV-6, -11, -16, and -18) was 90.5% (95% CI 73.7, 97.5) and 83.1% (95% CI 10.6, 95.8) against the second coprimary end point (disease or infection related to HPV-16 and HPV-18 alone). In 2008 Huh and colleagues from the University of Alabama showed that use of the quadrivalent vaccine results in reduction of high-grade squamous intraepithelial lesion (HSIL) by 43%, and in 2010 Huh and colleagues announced that among vaccinated patients who had previously undergone surgical treatment for CIN, the quadrivalent vaccine was associated with a 40% less likelihood of needing another procedure. At present, Merck is comparing the efficacy of a nanovalent HPV vaccine (6, 11, 16, 18, 31, 33, 45, 52, 58) to GARDASIL.

Bivalent Vaccine

In 2009 results from a phase III, randomized, double-blind, controlled trial called the PApilloma TRIal against Cancer In young Adults (PATRICIA) using the bivalent HPV-16 and -18 AS04-adjuvanted vaccine (CERVARIX, Glaxo-Smith-Kline) were published. For the study 18,644 women aged 15 to 25 years were vaccinated or received placebo at months 0, 1, and 6. At a mean follow-up of 34.9 months after the third dose, the vaccine efficacy against CIN II+ associated HPV-16 and -18 was 92.9% (96.1% CI 79.9, 98.3) in the primary analysis. Of importance, CERVARIX substantially reduced the overall burden of cervical precancerous lesions (CIN II+) by 70.2% in an HPV-naïve population approximating young girls before first sexual intercourse. Of interest, among women previously exposed to HPV types 16 or 18, once patients were unblinded it was noted that there was 91.5% efficacy against 12-month persistent infection in women who received three doses of CERVARIX and were seropositive at baseline and HPV DNA negative for HPV-16 or HPV-18 at baseline and month 6 (96.1% CI 54.0, 99.2).

Initial evidence of potential cross-protection efficacy conferred by the bivalent vaccine appeared in the analysis of those patients who were without current HPV-16 or HPV-18 infection at the time of vaccination and without prior exposure. In this group, the vaccine prevented 70.2% of CIN II–III and AIS and 87% of CIN III or AIS. The prevalence for CIN II and III associated with HPV-16 and -18 ranged from 32% to 64% in the control arm. To assess reductions in disease caused by nonvaccine HPV types, investigators analyzed the data combining 12 nonvaccine oncogenic HPV types (31, 33, 35, 39, 45, 51, 52, 56, 58, 59, 66, and 68) and reported that the bivalent vaccine reduced the incidence of CIN II and III. In analyses including lesions in which HPV-16 or -18 were also detected, bivalent vaccine efficacy in prevention of CIN II–III or AIS associated with HPV-31 was 92.0% (99.7% CI: 49.0, 99.8) and 100% (99.7% CI: 62.3, 100), respectively.

It should be noted that the duration of immunity following a complete schedule of immunization has not been established. In the randomized phase II CERVARIX trial, the bivalent vaccine has maintained 100% demonstrable efficacy against persistent infection at 12 months and CIN II and III and AIS for a mean of 5.9 years. The bivalent vaccine has also had a successful pediatric immunogenicity bridge and is available through the VFC program.

A direct head-to-head efficacy trial between the quadrivalent and bivalent vaccines has not been conducted. In a recent head-to-head immunogenicity trial, the bivalent vaccine (CERVARIX) induced significantly superior neutralizing antibody levels for HPV-16 and -18 in all age groups studied. Positivity rates for anti-HPV-16 and -18 neutralizing antibodies in cevicovaginal secretions and circulating HPV-16 and -18–specific memory B-cell frequencies were also higher after vaccination with bivalent compared with quadrivalent vaccines. Some explanations that have been proposed to account for the apparent higher immunogenicity seen in the head-to-head trial include the use of the proprietary-owned adjuvant system in CERVARIX, which confers additional immunogenicity through its bacterium-derived lipopolysaccharide backbone. In addition, others have proposed that higher valencies increase the potential for interference in antibody generation. It should be emphasized that it is unclear what clinical significant titers impart; as has been discussed earlier, in studies of GARDASIL in which anti–HPV-18 titers decline, there has not been any breakthrough disease.

MICROINVASIVE CARCINOMA OF THE CERVIX

The diagnosis and management of microinvasive carcinoma of the cervix remains controversial. The evolution and sometimes revolution concerning the diagnosis and management have occurred since Mestwerdt, in 1947, observed that invasive cervical cancer diagnosed only microscopically could be cured by nonradical surgery. During the last three decades definitions and treatment plans have changed dramatically. It is hoped that most of these changes had occurred as new data became available and that changes were therefore logical. Much of the confusion can be related to the fact that the Federation of International Gynecologists and Obstetricians (FIGO) has changed the criteria for early-stage invasive carcinoma of the cervix since 1960. These changes were made as additional information in regard to this disease process became available. Other influences, however, also contributed to the confusion. Over the years as many as 20 different definitions have been proposed and as many as 27 terms have been applied to this entity. The recommended therapy has also changed, going from radical surgery with any invasion to being more conservative with various depths of invasion.

In 1971 FIGO designated stage Ia carcinoma of the cervix as those cases of preclinical carcinoma. In 1973 the Society of Gynecologic Oncologists (SGO) accepted the following statement concerning the definition of microinvasive carcinoma of the cervix:

1. Cases of intraepithelial carcinoma with questionable invasion should be regarded as intraepithelial carcinoma; and
2. A microinvasive lesion should be defined as one in which a neoplastic epithelium invaded the stroma in one or more places to the depth of <3 mm below the base of the epithelium and in which lymphatic or vascular involvement is not demonstrated.

In 1985, for the first time, FIGO attempted to quantify the histologic definition of stage Ia carcinoma of the cervix. Stage Ia was defined as the earliest form of invasion in which minute foci of invasion are visible only microscopically. Stage Ia2 is a macroscopically measurable microcarcinoma that should not exceed 5 mm in depth and 7 mm in width. Vascular space involvement, either venous or lymphatic, should not alter staging. This definition has been criticized for several reasons. Although the upper limits of invasion for depth and width were stated, upper limits for measurement for stage Ia1 were not defined. It was therefore difficult to quantify patients in the two subgroups. Other areas of criticism were aimed at the fact that the FIGO definition could not be used as a guide for treatment, and the definition covered patients with vascular lymphatic channel involvement. These variations illustrate the problem with a specific definition.

In 1994 FIGO, in an attempt to better qualify the definition of microinvasive carcinoma of the cervix, adopted the following definition for microinvasive carcinoma of the cervix (Table 3-3). Stage Ia1 cancers would be those with stromal invasion up to 3 mm in depth and no greater than 7 mm. Stage Ia2 would be when invasion is present at 3 to 5 mm in depth and no greater than 7 mm. Lymphatic vascular space involvement would not exclude a patient from this definition. The recurrence rate of patients in these two substages would probably be no more than 1% to 2%. Survival of stage Ia1 would approach 99%, and stage Ia2 survival would approach 97% to 98%. This new definition allows further evaluation of what might be appropriate therapy for the different substages, particularly stage Ia2 cancers.

Vascular space involvement was not excluded from the FIGO definition for several reasons. Pathologists disagree with regard to the reproducibility of this entity. At least in one study, the number of slides prepared from the cervix depended on the incidence of capillary-like space involvement. Shrinkage artifact can lead to an overdiagnosis, and verification has been suggested with special staining to verify true capillary-like space involvement. In one study in which immunoperoxidase staining with Ulex Europaeus agglutinin 1 lectin (UEAI) was used, 10 of 32 cases of vascular space involvement were excluded in which involvement was initially thought to exist. In a combined study of 1004 patients at three reference centers, Burghardt and colleagues observed that the frequency with which angiolymphatic space involvement was detected ranged from 9% in Munich to 23% in Erlangen and finally up to 43% in Graz.

CLINICAL PROFILE OF INVASIVE CANCER

A substantial and well-publicized screening program is needed to make the public and the profession more aware of cervical cancer as the possible cause of even minimal gynecologic symptoms. All public education should emphasize the prevention and cure of cancer, and a more optimistic attitude would help motivate patients and physicians to seek appropriate action. The need for early diagnosis rests on the incontrovertible fact that definite cure, in actuarial terms, is readily achieved when cervical cancer is minimal—but almost impossible if the tumor is given time to grow and spread to the pelvic wall or into adjacent structures such as the bladder and rectum. The gradient of percentage curability from early invasive cancer to late, grossly invasive disease is such a steep one that even a moderate reduction in tumor size could not fail to create a substantial improvement in curability. It is true, of course, as with other cancers, that some carcinomas of the cervix grow more rapidly than others. The basis for this difference in growth rate is still beyond our knowledge, but it is not beyond our capability to prevent unnecessary growing time. Even the relatively slow-growing malignancy, if given enough time, will become incurable, and the most rapid-growing tumor, if diagnosed while of still moderate dimension, is definitely curable. The earlier that most tumors are detected and treated, the better will be the chance of cure. A Pap smear from a patient with early invasive squamous cell carcinoma illustrates a typical multinucleated "tadpole" cell (Figure 3-3). Cytology and colposcopy are valuable tools in the eradication of cervical cancer. Every opportunity should be taken to disseminate modern concepts of cancer control to schools of nursing and other paramedical organizations because

TABLE 3-3   Stage Ia Cancer of the Cervix

Stage Ia	Cancer invasion identified only microscopically. All gross lesions, even with superficial invasion, are stage Ib cancers. Measured stromal invasion with maximum depth of 5 mm and no wider than 7 mm*
Stage IaI	Measured invasion of stroma up to 3 mm
Stage Ia2	Measured invasion of stroma of 3-5 mm and no wider than 7 mm

The depth of invasion should not be >5 mm taken from the base of the epithelium, either surface or glandular, from which it originates. Vascular space involvement, either venous or lymphatic, should not alter the staging.

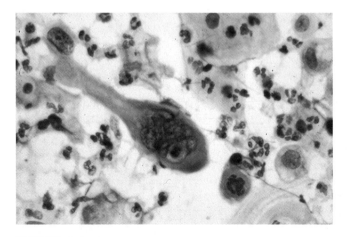

FIGURE 3-3   Multinucleated "tadpole" cell–early invasive squamous cell carcinoma.

there is still a need for more coordinated effort in these fields. The burden should not be left with the physician alone. The frequency with which invasive cervical cancer occurs in the United States is unknown, but the best incidence data indicate a rate of approximately 8 to 10/100,000/year (Figure 3-4). The incidence and mortality rates in the United States have been slowly declining (Figure 3-5). The occurrence of cervical cancer is apparently less frequent in Norway and Sweden than in the United States. However, in the underdeveloped areas of the world, the frequency of cervical cancer is more noteworthy, relative to the overall cancer problem, especially compared with that in the United States (see Table 3-3) and Western Europe.

In many South American and Asian countries, cervical cancer accounts for the largest percentage of cancer

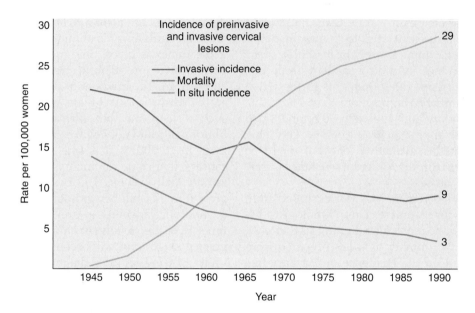

FIGURE 3-4   American Cancer Society data for 1991. Cervical cancer incidence and mortality.

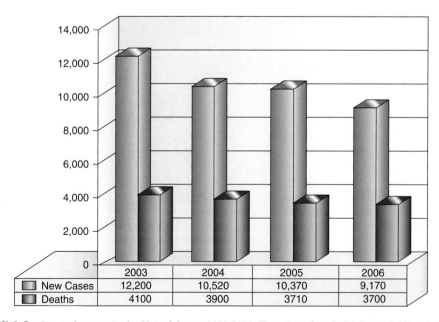

FIGURE 3-5   Cervical cancer in the United States: 2003-2006. *(From Jermal et al: CA Cancer J Clin 56:106, 2006.)*

deaths in women. One wonders whether nutritional deficiencies in these underdeveloped nations play a role in the etiology of cervical cancer. Orr and colleagues reported that abnormal vitamin levels were more commonly present in patients with cervical cancer. When compared with control values, levels of plasma folate, beta-carotene, and vitamin C were significantly lower in patients with cervical cancer. Personal cigarette smoking and exposure to passive smoke as risk factors for cervical carcinoma have been examined in case-control studies. Personal cigarette smoking increases the risk of cervical cancer after adjustment for age, educational level, church attendance, and sexual activity. The adjusted risk estimate associated with being a current smoker was 3.42; for having smoked for 5 or more pack-years, it was 2.81; and for having smoked at least 100 lifetime cigarettes, it was 2.21. The adjusted risk estimate associated with passive smoke exposure for 3 hours or more per day was 2.96. This study, reported by Slattery and colleagues in 1989, has been reinforced by others, confirming a strong association of smoking and increased risk of squamous cell carcinoma of the cervix.

Some studies suggest that cancer of the cervix is more frequent among oral contraceptive users; however, these studies may be influenced by confounding factors such as early onset of sexual activity after puberty, multiple sexual partners, and previous history of sexually transmitted diseases. Ursin and colleagues reported a twofold greater risk of adenocarcinoma of the cervix, especially among those who used oral contraceptives for 12 years or more.

Because of the cervix's sensitivity to hormonal influences, it may be considered biologically plausible that oral contraceptives could induce or promote cervical carcinoma. Piver reviewed a large number of early investigations of this issue and failed to show a consistent association. Moreover, these data are based on exposure to oral contraceptive preparations that contained high doses of estrogen and progestin and are no longer available.

In most large series, approximately 85% to 90% of malignant lesions of the cervix are squamous cell, but other lesions are possible (Table 3-4). Most information regarding etiology and epidemiology is pertinent only to the more common squamous cell lesions.

The greatest risk for cervical cancer is not ever having a Pap test or obtaining one infrequently. Everywhere in the world where the incidence of cervical cancer and its death rates have decreased, an active screening program is present. The older patients have a higher incidence of cervical cancer, at least in the United States, and these women have the most infrequent Pap smear screening.

TABLE 3-4   Histologic Classification of Cervical Cancer

Epithelial Tumors		
Nonglandular	Glandular	Other, Including Mixed
Squamous cell carcinoma	Adenocarcinoma, usual endocervical type	Adenosquamous
Verrucous carcinoma	Mucinous adenocarcinoma	Glassy cell carcinoma
Warty (condylomatous) carcinoma	Endometrioid adenocarcinoma	Mucoepidermoid carcinoma
Papillary squamotransitional carcinoma	Well-differentiated villoglandular adenocarcinoma	Adenoid cystic carcinoma
Lymphoepithelial-like carcinoma	Adenoma malignum (minimal deviation)	Adenoid basal carcinoma
Sarcomatoid carcinoma	Intestinal-like adenocarcinoma	Small cell carcinoma
	Signet ring cell adenocarcinoma	Classical carcinoid tumor
	Colloid adenocarcinoma	Gestational choriocarcinoma
	Clear cell adenocarcinoma	
	Serous papillary adenocarcinoma	
	Mesonephric adenocarcinoma	
Nonepithelial Tumors		
Mesenchymal Tumors	Germ Cell Tumors	Miscellaneous
Carcinosarcoma	Mature teratoma	Melanoma
Leiomyosarcoma	Immature teratoma	Lymphoma
Epithelioid leiomyosarcoma	Yolk sac tumor	Primitive neuroectodermal
Extrauterine endometrial stromal sarcoma	Nongestational choriocarcinoma	tumor
Adenosarcoma		
Embyronal rhabdomyosarcoma		
Granulocytic sarcoma (chloroma)		

From Tewari KS, Monk BJ: Tumors of the cervix. In: Raghavan et al, eds. Textbook of Uncommon Cancer. Ed 3. Hoboken, NJ, 2006, John Wiley & Sons, Ltd.

Symptoms

A typical patient with clinically obvious cervical cancer is a multiparous woman between 45 and 55 years who married and delivered her first child at an early age, usually before age 20. Probably the first symptom of early cancer of the cervix is a thin, watery, blood-tinged vaginal discharge that frequently goes unrecognized by the patient. The classic symptom is intermittent, painless metrorrhagia or spotting only postcoitally or after douching, although not the most common symptom. As the malignancy enlarges, the bleeding episodes become heavier and more frequent, and they last longer. The patient may also describe what seems to her to be an increase in the amount and duration of her regular menstrual flow; ultimately, the bleeding becomes continuous. In the postmenopausal woman, the bleeding is more likely to prompt early medical attention.

Late symptoms or indicators of more advanced disease include the development of pain referred to the flank, or leg, which is usually secondary to the involvement of the ureters, pelvic wall, or sciatic nerve routes. Many patients complain of dysuria, hematuria, rectal bleeding, or obstipation resulting from bladder or rectal invasion. Distant metastasis and persistent edema of one or both lower extremities as a result of lymphatic and venous blockage by extensive pelvic wall disease are late manifestations of primary disease and frequent manifestations of recurrent disease. Massive hemorrhage and development of uremia with profound inanition may also occur and occasionally be the initial presenting symptom.

Gross Appearance

The gross clinical appearance of carcinoma of the cervix varies considerably and depends on the regional mode of involvement and the nature of the particular lesion's growth pattern. Three categories of gross lesions have traditionally been described. The most common is the exophytic lesion, which usually arises on the ectocervix and often grows to form a large, friable, polypoid mass that can bleed profusely. These exophytic lesions sometimes arise within the endocervical canal and distend the cervix and the endocervical canal, creating the so-called barrel-shaped lesion. A second type of cervical carcinoma is created by an infiltrating tumor that tends to show little visible ulceration or exophytic mass but is initially seen as a stone-hard cervix that regresses slowly with radiation therapy. A third category of lesion is the ulcerative tumor (Figure 3-6), which usually erodes a portion of the cervix, often replacing the cervix and a portion of the upper vaginal vault with a large crater associated with local infection and seropurulent discharge.

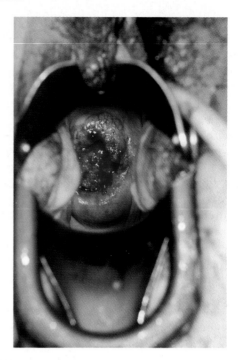

FIGURE 3-6 Ulcerative squamous cell carcinoma of the cervix.

Routes of Spread

The main routes of spread of carcinoma of the cervix are as follows:

1. Into the vaginal mucosa, extending microscopically down beyond visible or palpable disease.
2. Into the myometrium of the lower uterine segment and corpus, particularly with lesions originating in the endocervix.
3. Into the paracervical lymphatics and from there to the most commonly involved lymph nodes (i.e., the obturator, hypogastric, and external iliac nodes).
4. Direct extension into adjacent structures or parametria, which may reach to the obturator fascia and the wall of the true pelvis. Extension of the disease to involve the bladder or rectum can result, with or without the occurrence of a vesicovaginal or rectovaginal fistula.

The prevalence of lymph node disease correlated well with the stage of the malignancy in several anatomic studies. Lymph node involvement in stage I is between 15% and 20%; in stage II it is between 25% and 40%; and in stage III, it is assumed that at least 50% have positive nodes. Variations are sometimes seen with different material. The best study of lymph node involvement in cervical cancer was done by Henriksen (Figure 3-7). The nodal groups described by Henriksen follow.

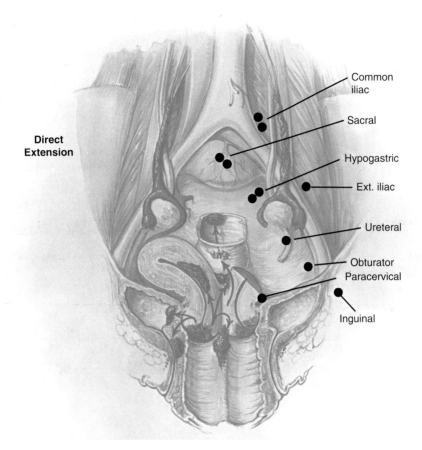

Direct Extension

Common iliac

Sacral

Hypogastric

Ext. iliac

Ureteral

Obturator
Paracervical

Inguinal

FIGURE 3-7   Lymph node chains draining the cervix. *(From: Henriksen E: Am J Obstet Gynecol 58:924, 1949.)*

Primary Group

1. The parametrial nodes, which are the small lymph nodes traversing the parametria
2. The paracervical or ureteral nodes, located above the uterine artery where it crosses the ureter
3. The obturator or hypogastric nodes surrounding the obturator vessels and nerves
4. The hypogastric nodes, which course along the hypogastric vein near its junction with the external iliac vein
5. The external iliac nodes, which are a group of six to eight nodes that tend to be uniformly larger than the nodes of the other iliac groups
6. The sacral nodes, which were originally included in the secondary group

Secondary Group

1. The common iliac nodes
2. The inguinal nodes, which consist of the deep and superficial femoral lymph nodes
3. The periaortic nodes

In his autopsy studies, Henriksen plotted the percentage of nodal involvement for treated and untreated patients (Figures 3-8 and 3-9). Distribution is, as one would expect, with a greater number of involved nodes found in the region of the cervix than in distant metastases. Although the series was an autopsy study, Henriksen found that only 27% had metastasis above the aortic chain. Cervical cancer kills by local extension, with ureteral obstruction in a high percentage of patients.

In 1980 the Gynecologic Oncology Group (GOG) reported the results of a series of 545 patients with cancer of the cervix who were surgically staged within their institutions. This study was prompted because traditional ports of radiation therapy were destined to treatment failure when the disease extended to the periaortic nodes (Figure 3-10). They found periaortic node involvement in 18.2% of patients with stage IIa disease and up to 33.3% in patients with stage IVa disease. Piver correlated the size of the cervical lesion with the incidence of lymph node metastasis in stage I disease (Table 3-5).

When clinical staging was compared with surgical staging, inaccuracies were found of the magnitude of a 22.9% misstaged occurrence in stage IIb disease and a 64.4% misstaged occurrence in stage IIIb disease. These data raise the question of whether knowing that disease has spread to the periaortic area enables the clinician to

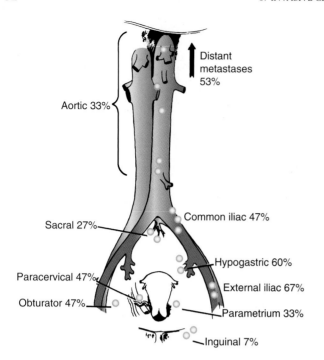

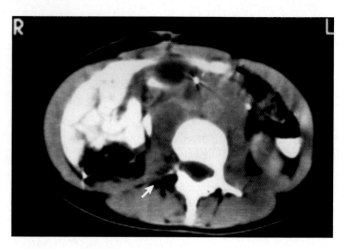

FIGURE 3-8   Percentage involvement of draining lymph nodes in treated patients with cervical cancer. *(From: Henriksen E: Am J Obstet Gynecol 58:924, 1949.)*

FIGURE 3-10   A computed tomography scan of the abdomen illustrating very enlarged periaortic nodes that have eroded a portion of the vertebral bone on the right.

TABLE 3-5   Size of Cervical Lesion and Lymph Node Metastasis in Stage Ib Cervical Cancer

Site (cm)	Patients	Patients with Metastasis	%	
≤1	22	4	18.1	21.1
2-3	72	16	22.1	
4-5	45	16	35.5	35.2
≥6	6	3	50	
Total	145	39	26.9	

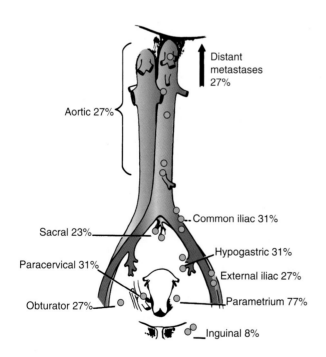

FIGURE 3-9   Percentage involvement of draining lymph nodes in untreated patients with cervical cancer. *(From Henriksen E: Am J Obstet Gynecol 58:924, 1949.)*

TABLE 3-6   Percentage Increase of Pelvic and Periaortic Node Metastasis by Clinical Stage

Clinical Stage	Positive Pelvic Nodes	Positive Periaortic Nodes
I	15.4	6.3
II	28.6	16.5
III	47.0	8.6

institute therapeutic modalities that can result in increased salvage. In other words, does the treatment of patients with spread of disease beyond the pelvis result in more cures? Berman and colleagues, reporting the GOG experience with staging laparotomy, indicated that 20% of 436 patients (stages IIb-IVa) were found to have metastatic disease to periaortic nodes. He also reported that 25% of these patients, or 5% of those surgically staged, demonstrated a 3-year, disease-free survival. Most of the patients with known periaortic node involvement received extended postoperative field irradiation.

Cumulative results from many studies utilizing lymphadenectomy in the surgical staging of cervix cancer have shown increased frequency of positive pelvic nodes, as shown in Table 3-6.

GLANDULAR TUMORS OF THE CERVIX

Approximately 75% to 80% of cervical cancers are squamous cell, and most of the remaining cases are adenocarcinomas. There appears to be an increase in the frequency of cervical adenocarcinomas, but this may be a result of the decrease in the incidence of invasive squamous cell lesions. With respect to histopathology, a SEER population study conducted on cases registered from 1973 to 2002 noted increasing numbers of adenocarcinomas despite a general decline, suggesting the inefficiency of conventional screening for these tumors. Adenocarcinoma arises from the endocervical mucous-producing gland cells, and because of its origin within the cervix, it may be present for a considerable time before it becomes clinically evident. These lesions are characteristically bulky neoplasms that expand the cervical canal and create the so-called barrel-shaped lesions of the cervix. The spread pattern of these lesions is similar to that of squamous cell cancer, with direct extension accompanied by metastases to regional pelvic nodes as the primary routes of dissemination. Local recurrence is more common in these lesions, and this has resulted in the commonly held belief that they are more radioresistant than are their squamous counterpart. It seems more likely, however, that the bulky, expansive nature of these endocervical lesions, rather than a differential in radiosensitivity, accounts for the local recurrence. Two controversial issues continue with regard to management of adenocarcinoma of the cervix. First, does this cell type carry a worse prognosis than squamous or adenosquamous cell types? Second, for early-stage disease, which therapy (radical surgery, radiation, or combined treatment) is superior?

Most studies suggest no difference in survival when adenocarcinomas are compared to squamous carcinomas after correction for stage. The 1998 FIGO Annual Report, which reported more than 10,000 squamous carcinomas and 1138 adenocarcinomas using multivariant analysis, noted no difference in survival in stage I cancers. In a study by Chen and associates of 302 adenocarcinomas, it was noted that in early stages, multivariant analysis noted better survival in patients treated with radical surgery compared with those treated with radiation therapy.

Kjorstad and Bond investigated the metastatic potential and patterns of dissemination in 150 patients with stage Ib adenocarcinoma of the cervix treated from 1956 to 1977. All cases were treated with a combination of intracavitary radium followed by radical hysterectomy with pelvic lymph node dissection. The incidence of pelvic metastases and distant recurrences and the survival rates were the same as those given in previously published reports for squamous cell carcinoma treated in the same manner. In one respect, the adenocarcinomas showed a significant difference from the squamous cell cancers. The incidence of residual tumor in the hysterectomy specimens after intracavitary treatment was much higher (30% vs 11%). Kjorstad and Bond considered this a strong argument for surgical treatment of patients with early stages of adenocarcinoma of the cervix.

Moberg and colleagues reported on 251 patients at Radiumhemmet in Stockholm with adenocarcinoma of the uterine cervix. The 5-year survival rate was compared with that in the total of cervical epithelial malignancies, and the rate was lower in the adenocarcinoma cases, with respective crude 5-year survival rates of 84%, 50%, and 9% in stages I, II, and III, respectively. Combined treatment consisting of two intracavitary radium treatments with an interval of 3 weeks followed by a radical hysterectomy with pelvic lymphadenectomy done within 3 months gave improved 5-year survival in a nonrandomized series. Prempree and colleagues also suggested combined therapy for stage II lesions or for those greater than 4 cm.

A large series of 367 cases of adenocarcinoma of the cervix was reported by Eifel and associates. Their conclusions were that the central control of adenocarcinomas with radiation therapy is comparable to that achieved for squamous cell carcinomas of comparable bulk. They found no evidence that combined treatment (radiation therapy plus hysterectomy) improved local regional control or survival. In their study, radiation therapy alone was as effective a treatment for most patients with stage I disease. They noted, as others have, that patients with bulky stage I (>6 cm), stage II, or stage III disease, particularly with poorly differentiated lesions or evidence of nodal spread, had a very high rate of extrapelvic disease spread.

Eifel reported the results of 160 patients with adenocarcinoma of the cervix. Of those patients, 84 were treated with radiation therapy alone; 20 were treated with external and intracavitary radiation followed by hysterectomy; and 56 were treated with radical hysterectomy. Survival was strongly correlated with tumor size and grade. There was a 90% survival rate for lesions smaller than 3 cm. After 5 years, 45% of the patients treated with radical hysterectomy had a recurrence. These recurrences were strongly correlated with lymph/vascular space invasion, poorly differentiated lesions, and larger tumor size.

Chen and associates from Taiwan reviewed 3678 cases of cervical cancer treated between 1977 and 1994, of which 302 (8.5%) were adenocarcinoma. A higher proportion of cases with adenocarcinoma were of the lower stages and in the younger patient even within a given stage. Survival was better in all stages in patients with squamous compared with adenocarcinoma (81% vs 76% in stage I, $P = 0.0039$). When surgery was primary therapy, there was no difference in survival in stage I (83% vs 80.3% survival of squamous and adenocarcinoma, respectively). Survival with radiation therapy noted 71% vs 49%, respectively ($P = 0.0039$), in stage I. Survival decreased as age increased within a given stage.

The MD Anderson Hospital group compared 1538 patients with squamous cell carcinoma with 229 patients with adenocarcinoma, all stage Ib and treated with radiation. In patients with tumors larger than 4 cm, multivariate analysis confirmed that those patients with adenocarcinoma had a significantly poorer survival than did those with squamous carcinoma (59% vs 73%). In a study by the GOG, 813 stage Ia2 and Ib cancers were evaluated. All were treated with radical hysterectomy. There were 645 squamous, 104 adenocarcinoma, and 64 adenosquamous cancers. Radiation was given postoperatively to 16% squamous, 13% adenocarcinomas, and 20% of adenosquamous patients. After adjusting for multiple risk factors, survival was worst for adenosquamous cancer compared with squamous and adenocarcinoma (71.8%, 82.1%, and 88%, respectively). A similar finding was noted in a study from Taiwan in which 134 stage Ib or II cervical adenocarcinomas or adenosquamous cancers were compared with 757 similarly staged squamous carcinomas treated with radical hysterectomy. The overall survival was 72.2% for the former compared with 81.2% for the squamous cancers. The histology was an independent prognostic factor for recurrence-free survival and overall survival.

STAGING

The staging of cancer of the cervix is a clinical appraisal, preferably confirmed with the patient under anesthesia; it cannot be changed later if findings at operation or subsequent treatment reveal further advancement of the disease.

International Federation of Gynecology and Obstetrics

International classification of cancer of the cervix according to the International Federation of Gynecology and Obstetrics (FIGO) was recently revised in 2009 (Figure 3-11, A through J):

Stage 0   Carcinoma in situ, intraepithelial carcinoma

Stage I   The carcinoma is strictly confined to the cervix (extension to the corpus should be disregarded)

Stage Ia   Invasive cancer identified only microscopically; all gross lesions even with superficial invasion are stage Ib cancers. Invasion is limited to measured stromal invasion with maximum depth of 5 mm and no wider than 7 mm

Stage Ia1   Measured invasion of stroma no greater than 3 mm in depth and no wider than 7 mm

Stage Ia2   Measured invasion of stroma greater than 3 mm and no greater than 5 mm and no wider than 7 mm

The depth of invasion should not be more than 5 mm taken from the base of the epithelium, surface or glandular, from which it originates. Vascular space involvement, venous or lymphatic, should not alter the staging.

Stage Ib   Clinical lesions confined to the cervix or preclinical lesions greater than stage Ia

Stage Ib1   Clinical lesions no greater than 4 cm

Stage Ib2   Clinical lesions greater than 4 cm

Stage II   Involvement of the vagina but not the lower third, or infiltration of the parametria but not out to the sidewall

Stage IIa   Involvement of the vagina but no evidence of parametrial involvement

Stage IIa1   Clinically visible lesion no greater than 4 cm in greatest dimension

Stage IIa2   Clinically visible lesion greater than 4 cm in greatest dimension

Stage IIb   Infiltration of the parametria but not out to the sidewall

Stage III   Involvement of the lower third of the vagina or extension to the pelvic sidewall; all cases with a hydronephrosis or nonfunctioning kidney should be included, unless they are known to be attributable to other causes

Stage IIIa   Involvement of the lower third of the vagina but not out to the pelvic sidewall if the parametria are involved

Stage IIIb   Extension onto the pelvic sidewall or hydronephrosis or nonfunctional kidney

Stage IV   Extension outside the reproductive tract

Stage IVa   Involvement of the mucosa of the bladder or rectum

Stage IVb   Distant metastasis or disease outside the true pelvis

The clinical evaluation of patients with cervical cancer is outlined in Table 3-7. The following diagnostic aids are acceptable for determining a staging classification: physical examination, routine radiographs, colposcopy, cystoscopy, proctosigmoidoscopy, IVP, and barium studies of the lower colon and rectum. Other examinations, such as lymphography, CT scans, magnetic resonance imaging (MRI) examinations, arteriography, venography, laparoscopy, and hysteroscopy, are not recommended for staging because they are not uniformly available from institution to institution. It is important to emphasize that staging is a method of communicating between one institution and another. Probably more important, however, is that staging is a means of evaluating the treatment plans used within one institution. For these reasons, the method of staging should remain fairly constant. Staging does not define the treatment plan, and therapy can be tailored to the architecture of the malignancy in each patient.

Positron Emission Tomography

In 2005 the Centers for Medicare and Medicaid Services implemented coverage for 18-fluorodeoxyglucose positron emission tomography (FDG-PET) for patients with

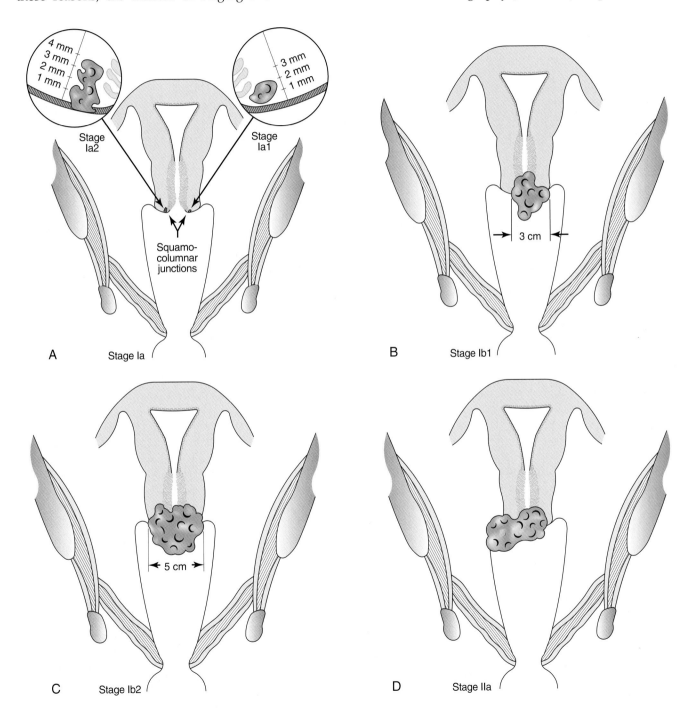

FIGURE 3-11   **A through J,** FIGO stagings and classification of cancer of the cervix. *(From DiSaia PJ: Adv Oncol 8:15, 1992.)*

Continued

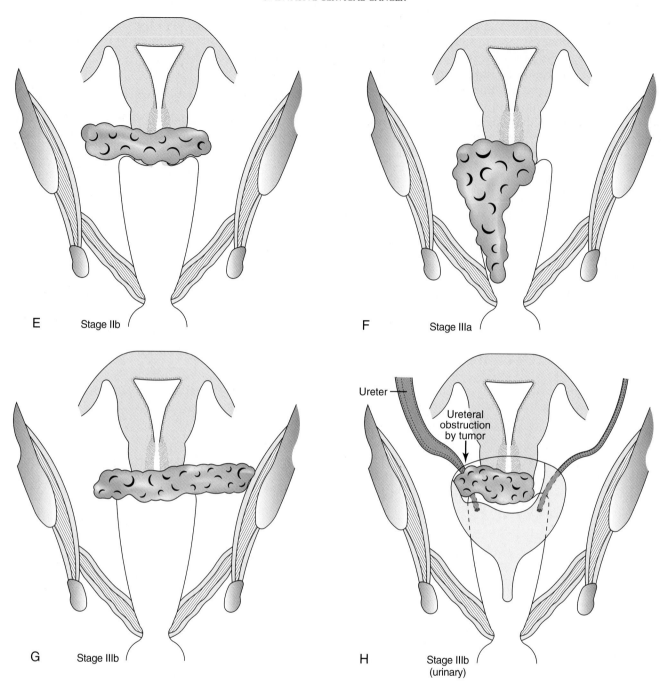

E   Stage IIb

F   Stage IIIa

G   Stage IIIb

H   Stage IIIb
     (urinary)

Ureter

Ureteral
obstruction
by tumor

FIGURE 3-11, cont'd

newly diagnosed and locally advanced cervical cancer undergoing pretreatment staging who have no extrapelvic metastases on conventional imaging studies (Figure 3-12). It should be noted that all imaging modalities are more specific than sensitive in detecting nodal metastases. The pooled sensitivity of PET in detecting pelvic nodal metastases in patients with untreated cervical cancer approaches 80% compared with MRI (approximately 70%) or CT (approximately 48%). It is important to recognize that the available studies are limited by low numbers of patients and wide confidence intervals.

Grosu and colleagues from Munich analyzed the results of clinical studies on the integration of PET in target volume definition for lung, head and neck, genitourinary, and brain tumors. FDG-PET had a significant impact on gross tumor volume and planning target volume delineation in lung cancer and was able to detect

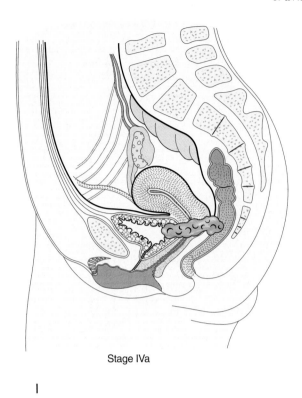

Stage IVa

I

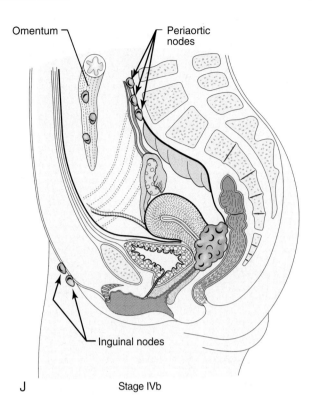

Omentum

Periaortic nodes

Inguinal nodes

J   Stage IVb

FIGURE 3-11, cont'd

TABLE 3-7   Clinical Evaluation of Patients with Newly Diagnosed Cervical Cancer

History	Review of Systems	General Physical Examination
Risk factors (STDs, smoking, OCPs, HIV), prior abnormal Pap tests, previous dysplasia and treatment	Abnormal vaginal bleeding or discharge; pelvic pain, flank pain, sciatica, hematuria, rectal bleeding, anorexia, weight loss, bone pain	Peripheral lymphadenopathy
Evaluation	Common procedures (FIGO)	Alternative procedures
Invasive cancer	Cervical biopsy	Histologic diagnosis required
	Endocervical curettage	
	Cervical conization	
Tumor size; involvement of the vagina, bladder, rectum and parametria	Pelvic examination under anesthesia	MRI pelvis preferred over CT
Anemia	Complete blood count	—
Renal failure	Serum chemistries	—
Hematuria	Urinalysis	—
Bladder involvement	Cystoscopy with biopsy and urine cytology	CT, MRI pelvis
Rectal infiltration	Proctoscopy with biopsy	CT, MRI pelvis; barium enema
Hydronephrosis	Intravenous pyelogram	Renal ultrasound; CT abdomen
Pulmonary metastases	Chest radiograph	CT chest; PET scan
Retroperitoneal lymphadenopathy	—	Lymphangiogram, CT, MRI, PET scan

CT, Computed tomography; HIV, human immunodeficiency virus; MRI, magnetic resonance imaging; OCP, oral contraceptive pill; PET, positron emission tomography; STDs, sexually transmitted diseases.

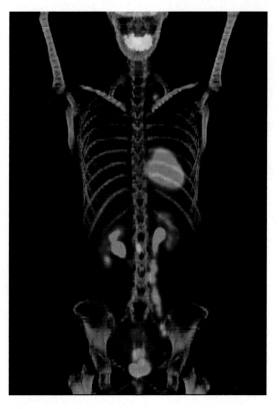

FIGURE 3-12 Positron emission tomography. *(From www. radassociates.com)*

TABLE 3-8   Sensitivity of FDG-PET for Lymph Node Staging in Locally Advanced Disease

	n	FIGO Stages	Imaging Modality	Lymph Nodes	Sensitivity
Sugawara et al	21	IB-IVA	PET vs CT	Overall	0.86 (PET) 0.57 (CT)
Rose et al	32	IIB-IVA	PET	PALN	0.75
				PELN	1.00
Yildirim et al	16	IIB-IVA	PET	PALN	0.5
Grigsby et al	152	IB-IV	PET	Overall	0.67
Narayan et al	7	IB-IVB	PET	PELN	0.80
Yeh et al	42	IB-IVA	PET	PALN	0.83
Lin et al	50	IB-IVA	PET	PALN	0.86
Yen et al	135	IB2-IVB + recurrence	PET	PELN	0.88
				PALN	0.95
Choi et al	22	IB-IVA	PET-CT	PELN	0.77
Amit et al	75	I-IV	PET-CT	PELN	0.60
Loft et al	119	IB1-IVA	PET-CT	PELN	0.96
				PALN	1.00

Adapted from Magne N et al: Cancer Treat Rev: 34:671, 2008.
CT, Computed tomography; PALN, para-aortic lymph nodes; PELN, pelvic lymph nodes; PET, positron emission tomography.

lymph node involvement and differentiate malignant tissue from atelectasis. In high-grade gliomas and meningiomas, methionine PET helped to differentiate tumor from normal tissue. Furthermore, the investigators suggest that FDG-PET seems to be particularly valuable in lymph node status definition in cervical cancer. With limited experience, several commentators have noted that FDG-PET may be superior to CT and MRI not only in the detection of lymph node metastases but also in the detection of unknown primary cancer and in the differentiation of viable tumor tissue after treatment. The accurate delineation of gross tumor volume suggests the potential for sparing of normal tissue. The imaging of hypoxia, cell proliferation, angiogenesis, apoptosis, and gene expression by new PET tracers such as choline and acetate may lead to the identification of different areas of a biologically heterogeneous tumor mass that can be individually targeted using intensity modulated radiotherapy (IMRT). In addition, a biological dose distribution can be generated permitting dose painting.

A 2007 meta-analysis of 41 studies was undertaken to compare the diagnostic performances of CT, MRI, and PET or PET/CT in patients for detection of metastatic lymph nodes in patients with cervical cancer. PET or PET/CT showed the highest pooled sensitivity (82%) and specificity (95%), whereas CT showed 50% and 92%, and MRI showed 56% and 91%, respectively (Table 3–8). In a recent investigation of 83 women with FIGO stages IB1 to IIIB cervical cancer, F-18 fluorodeoxyglucose-avid pelvic lymph nodes (SUVPLN) was found to be a prognostic biomarker, predicting treatment response, pelvic recurrence risk, and disease-specific survival. Finally, a prospective validation study conducted between 2000 and 2009 enrolled 560 women who underwent pretreatment FDG-PET lymph node staging. Overall, 47% of patients had lymph node involvement by FDG-PET at diagnosis and within a stage, patients with PET-positive lymph nodes had significantly worse disease-specific survival than those with PET-negative lymph nodes (P<0.001). The hazard ratios for disease recurrence increased incrementally based on the most distant level of nodal disease: pelvic 2.4 (95% CI 1.63, 3.52), para-aortic 5.88 (95% CI 3.8, 9.90), and supraclavicular 30.27 (95% CI 16.56, 55.34).

Surgical Staging

Findings uncovered by fusion PET-CT or conventional MR and/or CT examinations can be used in the planning of therapy but should not influence the initial clinical staging of the lesion. Unfortunately, clinical staging is only a rough value in prognosis because disease distribution and extent are often included under one stage

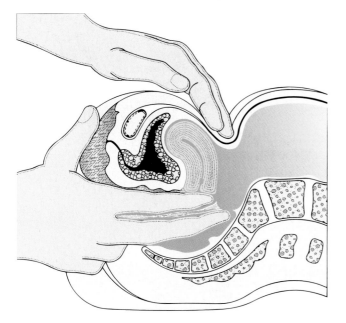

FIGURE 3-13   Technique of rectovaginal examination.

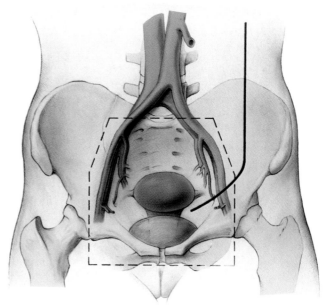

FIGURE 3-14   Pelvic diagram. The *dashed line* indicates the radiation field and the position of the uterus and cervix within the field. The *bold line* indicates the J incision path relative to the field and to the major vessels.

subheading. Clinical staging is enhanced with the liberal use of rectovaginal examinations (Figure 3-13) in that this type of pelvic examination allows more complete palpation of the parametria and cul-de-sac. The role of surgical assessment of lymph nodes with extraperitoneal, laparoscopic, or robotic lymphadenectomy is expanding. The ability to perform pelvic and paraaortic lymphadenectomy provides prognostic information, improves direction of radiation therapy (i.e., extended field radiation with positive paraaortic nodes), and may offer a therapeutic effect particularly in grossly involved lymph nodes. To date, no prospective data on surgical staging of cancers of the cervix exist to indicate a survival advantage to this approach.

Some gynecologic oncologists believe that limited staging procedures are warranted on patients with advanced-stage cervical cancer to place patients on institutional or national group protocols. The status of paraaortic nodes should be known before treatment is initiated in such cases to plan appropriate modalities, such as the extent of the radiation field or concomitant chemotherapy. An extraperitoneal approach for removal of the periaortic nodes is preferred by many clinicians in an effort to reduce morbidity from the procedure. More advanced lesions have been investigated with a retroperitoneal lymphadenectomy to determine the extent of disease before planning radiotherapy fields (Figure 3-14). Figure 3-15 illustrates one such approach. With the increased use of PET, it is expected that the indications for surgical staging in cervical cancer will decrease.

TREATMENT OF EARLY-STAGE DISEASE

After the diagnosis of invasive cervical cancer is established, the question is how to best treat the patient. Proposed management algorithms for early-stage disease, locally advanced malignancy, and disseminated tumors appear in Figure 3-16. Specific therapeutic measures are usually governed by the age and general health of the patient, by the extent of the cancer, and by the presence and nature of any complicating abnormalities. It is thus essential to carry out a complete and careful investigation of the patient (see Table 3–7), and then a joint decision regarding treatment should be made by the radiotherapist and gynecologic oncologist. The choice of treatment demands clinical judgment, but apart from the occasional patient for whom only symptomatic treatment may be best, this choice lies between surgery and radiotherapy (almost always given with cisplatin chemotherapy). In most institutions, the initial method of treatment for locally advanced disease is chemoradiation, both intracavitary and external radiographic therapy. The controversy between surgery and radiotherapy has existed for decades and essentially surrounds the treatment of stage I and stage IIa cervical cancer (Figure 3-16). For the most part, most patients with stages more advanced than stage I and stage IIa are treated with combination cisplatin and radiotherapy (see Figure 3-16). The 5-year survival figures from two

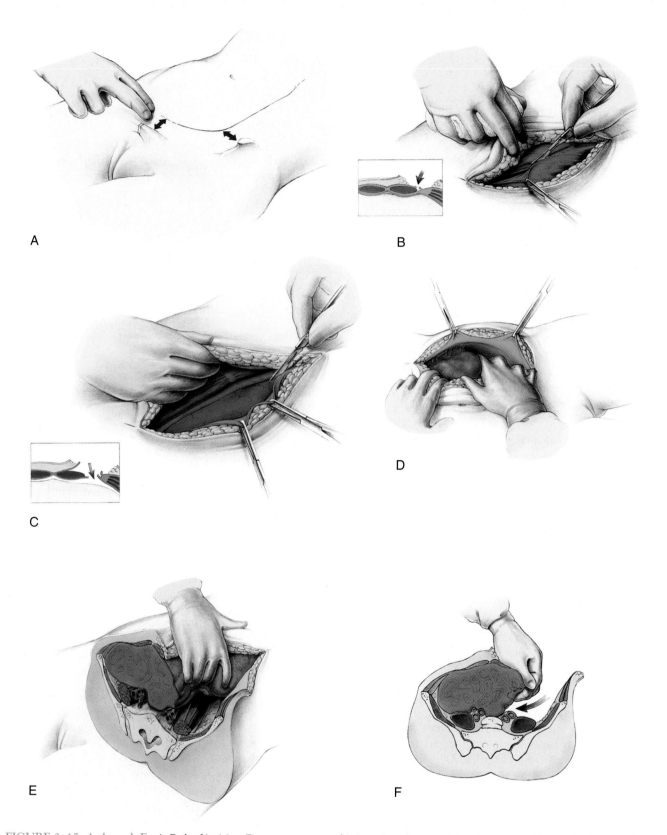

FIGURE 3–15, A through F   **A,** Path of incision. First measurement of 2–3 cm (two finger widths) above the pubic symphysis; second measurement 2–3 cm medial to the anterior superior iliac spine. A diagonal line connects these points. A vertical line is drawn superiorly to 3–4 cm above the level of the umbilicus. The incision begins at the lateral margin of the rectus muscle. **B,** Division of the external sheath of the rectus and a cross section. After the initial incision through the skin, the lateral margin of the sheath is divided with a bovie along the length of the muscle. On cross section, an *arrow* points to the ideal point of separation. **C,** Division of the internal sheath of the rectus and a cross section. The rectus muscle is mobilized medially. The internal sheath is divided carefully to preserve the underlying exposed peritoneum. **D,** Blunt dissection. Blunt dissection with a hand following the plane of the peritoneum and separating it from the transversalis fascia. **E,** Blunt dissection: perspective cross section. Dissection along the peritoneum until contact is made with the left ureter. The ureter is preserved with the peritoneum and is mobilized medially as dissection continues. The psoas muscle and the common iliac vessels are exposed. **F,** A cross section. Proper pathway of dissection along the peritoneum over the psoas.

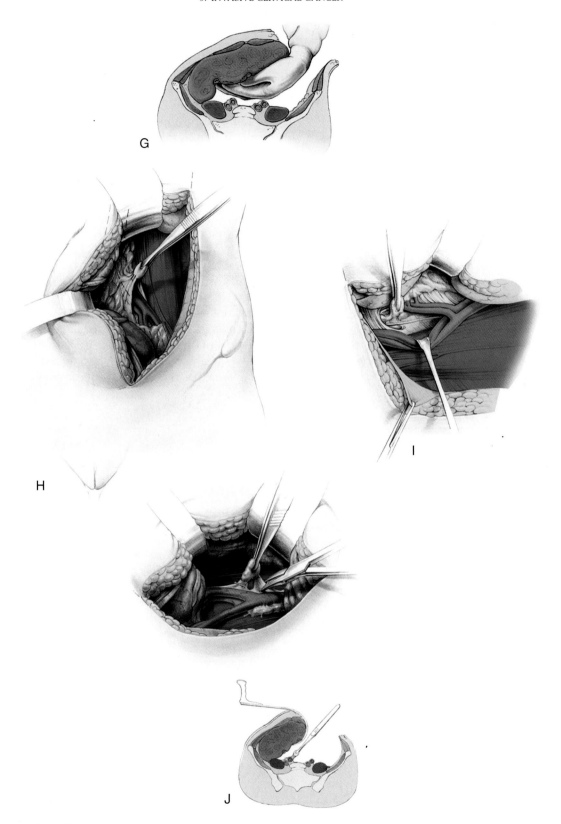

FIGURE 3-15 G through J, cont'd **G,** Cross section of deep dissection. Exposure of the left and right common iliac vessels underneath the peritoneum at about the level of L5-S1. Avoid damage to the inferior mesenteric artery. **H,** Lymphadenectomy begins along the left common iliac vessels. After medial and superior retraction of the mesentery and beginning about the bifurcation of internal and external iliac vessels, lymph nodes are removed along the length of the left common iliac to the junction with the aorta. **I,** Obturator nodes. Lateral mobilization of the external iliac vessels with a vein retractor. The obturator nerve is identified, and nodes are removed. **J,** The right common iliac. The right common and para-aortic lymph nodes are clipped and removed. The diagram shows deep access to the right common iliac nodes.

large series, one treated with radiotherapy alone and the other with surgery, are included here. Currie reported the results of 552 radical operations for cancer of the cervix:

Preinvasive carcinoma in situ	555 cases (99.9%)
Stage I	189 cases (86.3%)
Stage IIa	103 cases (75%)
Stage IIb	78 cases (58.9%)
Other stages	41 cases (34.1%)

Some of these patients with positive nodes received postoperative radiotherapy.

In 1981 Zander and colleagues reported results of a 20-year cooperative study from Germany of 1092 patients with stages Ib and II cancer of the cervix treated with radical hysterectomy of the Meigs type and bilateral pelvic lymphadenopathy. Of the 1092 patients, 50.6% had surgery only, with a 5-year survival rate of 84.5% in stage Ib and 71.1% in stage II (most were stage IIa). This correlates well with the figures reported by Currie and Falk. The rest of the patients reported by Zander received postoperative whole-pelvis irradiation therapy.

No significant difference could be observed in the survival rates of patients undergoing only surgery compared with those of patients undergoing adjuvant postoperative radiation. In fact, in 199 patients with lymph node involvement, the difference in survival rates of those undergoing only surgery and those undergoing additional postoperative radiation therapy was statistically insignificant.

Landoni and colleagues from the University of Milan conducted a prospective randomized trial in 243 patients comparing class II versus class III radical hysterectomy in stage IB to IIA cervical cancer. Although mean blood loss and transfusions were similar for both arms, mean operative time and late urologic morbidity were significantly lower in patients who underwent class II radical hysterectomy. The use of adjuvant radiotherapy was similar in both arms (54%, 55%). The recurrence rate (24%, 26%) and overall disease-free survival (75%, 73%) were not significantly different in either arm. Multivariate analysis confirmed that survival did not depend on the type of operation. This rare phase III surgical trial in early-stage cervical cancer has served as the platform from which our (non–phase III) experience in less radical

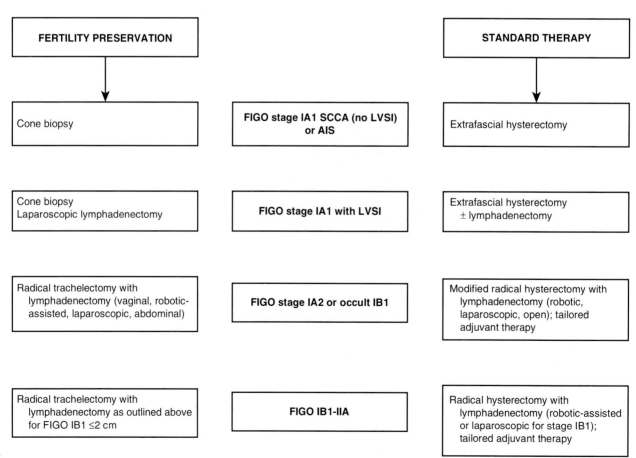

FIGURE 3-16 **A and B,** Algorithm for therapy.

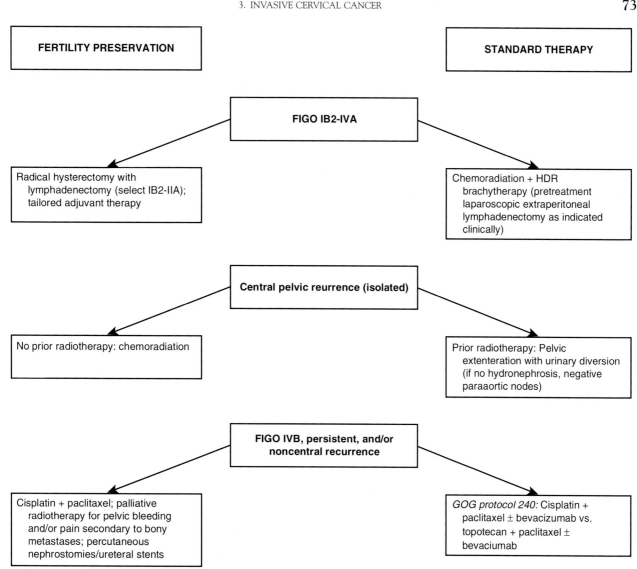

FIGURE 3-16, cont'd

surgery for early-stage disease is based (e.g., radical trachelectomy and cervical conizaton for fertility preservation in the setting of invasive disease).

In general, in early stages, comparable survival rates result from both treatment techniques. The advantage of radiotherapy is that it is applicable to almost all patients, whereas radical surgery of necessity excludes certain patients who are medically inoperable. The possible occurrence of immediate serious morbidity must be kept in mind when this treatment plan is selected. In many institutions, surgery for stage I and stage IIa disease is reserved for young patients in whom preservation of ovarian function is desired and improved vaginal preservation is expected. The modern operative mortality and the postoperative ureterovaginal fistula rate both have been reported to be less than 1%, making an objective decision for therapy even more difficult. Other

reasons given for the selection of radical surgery over radiation include cervical cancer in pregnancy, concomitant inflammatory disease of the bowel, previous irradiation therapy for other disease, presence of pelvic inflammatory disease or an adnexal neoplasm along with the malignancy, and patient preference. Among the disadvantages of radiation therapy, one must consider the permanent injury to the tissues of the normal organ bed of the neoplasm and the possibility of second malignancies developing in this bed.

Radical Abdominal Hysterectomy with Lymphadenectomy

The use of radical hysterectomy in the United States was initiated by Joe V. Meigs at Harvard University in 1944, and shortly thereafter the radical hysterectomy with pelvic lymphadenopathy was adopted by many clinics in the United States because of dissatisfaction with the limitations of radiotherapy. Some had found that many lesions were not radiosensitive, and some patients had metastatic disease in regional lymph nodes that were alleged to be radioresistant. Radiation injuries had been reported, and one of the overriding points in favor of surgery was that gynecologists were surgeons rather than radiotherapists and thus felt more comfortable with this treatment. At the time of the popularization of this procedure, modern techniques of surgery, anesthesia, antibiotics, and electrolyte balance had emerged, reducing the enormous morbidity that once attended major operative procedures in the abdomen.

Radical hysterectomy is a procedure that must be performed by a skilled technician with sufficient experience to make the morbidity acceptable (1%-5%). The procedure involves removal of the uterus, the upper 25% of the vagina, the entire uterosacral and uterovesical ligaments (Figure 3-17), and all of the parametrium on each side, along with pelvic node dissection encompassing the four major pelvic lymph node chains: ureteral, obturator, hypogastric, and iliac. Metastatic lesions to the ovaries are rare, and preservation of these structures is acceptable, especially in young women with small lesions. The procedure is complex because the tissues removed are in close proximity to many vital structures

such as the bowel, bladder, ureters (Figures 3-18 and 3-19), and great vessels of the pelvis. The object of the dissection is to preserve the bladder, rectum, and ureters without injury but to remove as much of the remaining tissue of the pelvis as is feasible.

There is no doubt that in stage I, and in the more restricted stage II cases, surgical removal of the disease is feasible. The addition of pelvic lymphadenectomy to the operative procedure caused considerable controversy in the early part of the century. Wertheim removed nodes only if they were enlarged and then not systematically. He believed that when accessible regional nodes were involved, the inaccessible distant nodes were also involved, and removal of suspicious nodes was more for prognostic than therapeutic value. He thought that node involvement was a measure of the lethal quality of the tumor and not merely a mechanical extension of the disease. The operative procedure popularized by Meigs included meticulous pelvic lymphadenectomy. Meigs demonstrated a 42% 5-year survival rate in another series of patients with positive nodes. Lymphadenectomy is now an established part of the operative procedure for any patient with disease greater than stage Ia1. There has been some interest in combining a radical vaginal operation with a retroperitoneal lymphadenectomy, and the results reported by Mitra, Navratil and Kastner, and McCall are surprisingly good. The survival

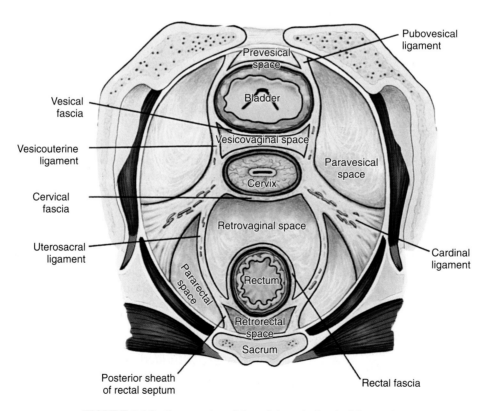

FIGURE 3-17   Cross section of the pelvis at the level of the cervix.

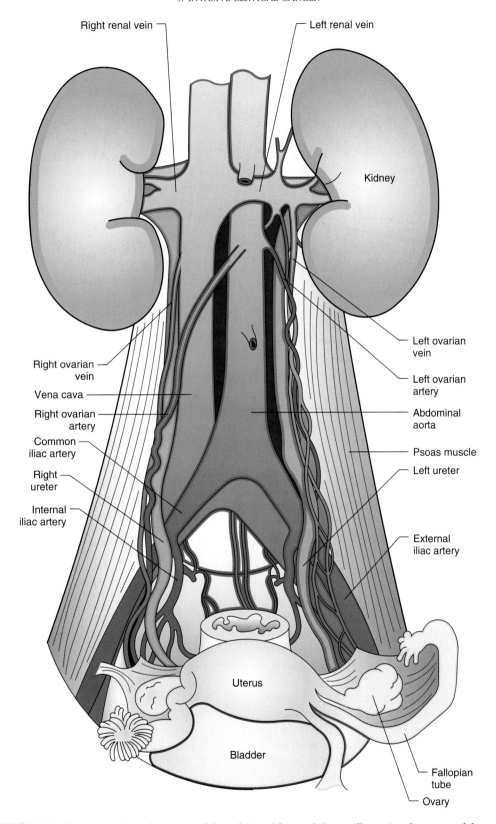

FIGURE 3-18   The retroperitoneal anatomy of the pelvis and lower abdomen illustrating the course of the ureters.

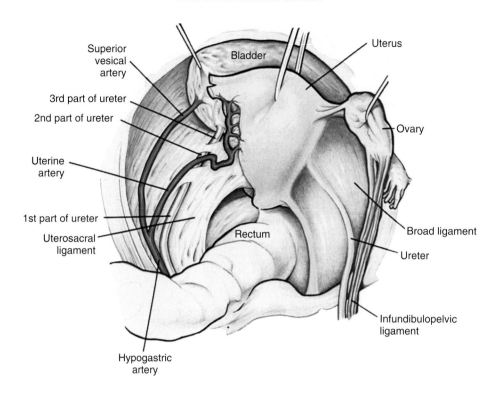

FIGURE 3-19   Relationship of the ureter to the uterosacral ligaments, uterine artery, infundibulopelvic ligament, and uterus.

rate in patients with negative nodes is usually in the range of 90% or more.

Rutledge and colleagues devised a system of rating radicality of hysterectomy (Table 3-9) used in treating women with cervical cancer at the MD Anderson Hospital. He suggested that the term "radical hysterectomy" is not adequate to record and communicate the different amounts of therapy attempted and the subsequent risk of complications when different surgeons report their results. These authors believed that describing the technical features of five operations enabled them to evaluate more accurately their results and provided a better understanding of the need to tailor each patient's treatment by using an operation that was adequate but not excessive.

The goal of the class I hysterectomy was to ensure removal of all cervical tissue. Reflection and retraction of the ureters laterally without actual dissection from the ureteral bed allows one to clamp the adjacent paracervical tissue without cutting into the side of the cervical tissue itself. Class I operations are advocated primarily for in situ and true microinvasive carcinomas of the cervix. A class I procedure is also performed after preoperative radiation in adenocarcinoma of the cervix or after preoperative radiation in the so-called barrel-shaped endocervical squamous cell carcinoma. The operation described is essentially the extrafascial hysterectomy used routinely at the MD Anderson Hospital.

TABLE 3-9   Rutledge's Classification of Extended Hysterectomy

Class	Description	Indication
I	Extrafascial hysterectomy; pubocervical ligament is incised, allowing lateral deflection of the ureter	CIN, early stromal invasion
II	Removal of the medial half of the cardinal and uterosacral ligaments; upper third of the vagina removed	Microcarcinoma postirradiation
III	Removal of the entire cardinal and uterosacral ligaments; upper third of the vagina removed	Stages Ib and IIa lesions
IV	Removal of all periureteral tissue, superior vesical artery, and three fourths of the vagina where preservation of the bladder is still possible	Anteriorly occurring central recurrences
V	Removal of portions of the distal ureter and bladder	Central recurrent cancer involving portions of the distal ureter or bladder

From Piver MS, Rutledge FN, Smith PJ: Obstet Gynecol 44:265, 1974. Reprinted with permission from The American College of Obstetricians and Gynecologists. CIN, Cervical intraepithelial neoplasia.

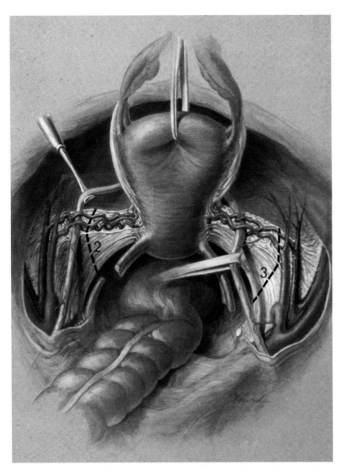

FIGURE 3-20 *Broken lines* identify the point of transection of the cardinal ligaments in class II and class III radical hysterectomy. *(Courtesy Gregorio Delgado, MD.)*

Class II extended hysterectomy is described as a modified radical hysterectomy. The purpose of the class II hysterectomy is to remove more paracervical tissue (Figure 3-20) while still preserving most of the blood supply to the distal ureters and bladder. The ureters are freed from their paracervical position but are not dissected out of the pubovesical ligament. The uterine artery is ligated just medial to the ureter as it lies in "the tunnel," ensuring preservation of the distal ureteral supply. The uterosacral ligaments are transected midway between the uterus and their sacral attachments (Figure 3-21). The medial halves of both cardinal ligaments are removed, as is the upper 25% of the vagina. A pelvic lymphadenectomy is usually performed with a class II hysterectomy. A class II operation is reported to be suitable for the following conditions:

1. Microinvasive carcinomas in which the depth of invasion is considered greater than early stromal invasion
2. Small postirradiation recurrences limited to the cervix

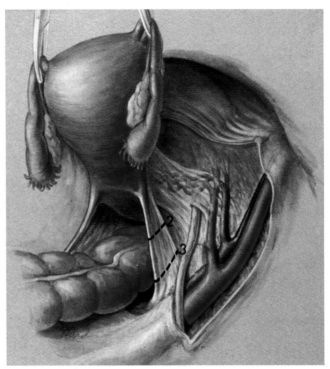

FIGURE 3-21 *Broken lines* identify the point of transection of the uterosacral ligaments in class II and class III radical hysterectomy. *(Courtesy Gregorio Delgado, MD.)*

The class III procedure is a wide radical excision of the parametrial and paravaginal tissues in addition to the removal of the pelvic lymphatic tissue. The uterine artery is ligated at its origin on the internal iliac artery. In the dissection of the ureter from the pubovesical ligament (between the lower end of the ureter and the superior vesical artery) care is taken to preserve the ligament, maintaining some additional blood supply to the distal ureter. The hazard of fistula formation is decreased by preservation of the superior vesical artery, along with a portion of the associated pubovesical ligament. The uterosacral ligaments are resected at the pelvic sidewall. The upper 25% of the vagina is removed (Figure 3-22), and a pelvic lymphadenectomy is routinely performed. This operation is primarily for the patient with stage I or IIa carcinoma of the cervix with or without preservation of ovarian function.

The aim of the class IV radical hysterectomy is complete removal of all periureteral tissue; a more extensive excision of the paravaginal tissues; and, when indicated, excision of the internal iliac vessels along an involved portion of the medial pelvic wall tissue. This differs from the class III operation in three respects:

1. The ureter is completely dissected from the pubovesical ligament
2. The superior vesical artery is sacrificed
3. 50% of the vagina is removed.

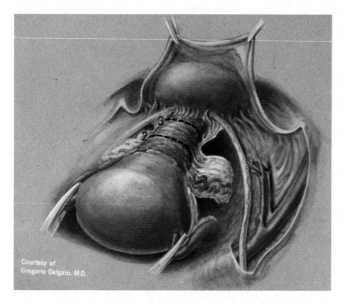

Courtesy of
Gregorio Delgato, M.D.

FIGURE 3-22   *Broken lines* illustrate the level of vaginal removal of class II and class III radical hysterectomy. *(Courtesy Gregorio Delgado, MD.)*

This procedure is used primarily for more extensive anteriorly occurring central recurrences when preservation of the bladder is seemingly still possible. Extension of the dissection laterally is needed when the disease has focally involved the medial parametrium. Sacrificing blood vessels to the bladder is unfavorable because the risk of fistula formation increases significantly. In most cases, these patients are more appropriately treated with an anterior exenteration.

The purpose of the class V hysterectomy is to remove a central recurrent cancer involving portions of the distal ureter or bladder. It differs from a class IV operation because the disease involves a portion of the distal ureter or bladder, or both, which is removed with the disease. A reimplantation of the ureter into the bladder, often as a utereroneocystostomy, is then performed. This procedure has a rare application to a small, specifically located recurrence when exenteration is considered unnecessary or has been refused by the patient.

The modified Rutledge classification of extended hysterectomies has considerable practical value. It once again underlines the necessity for the surgeon to tailor the operative procedure to the disease extent. A stage Ia2 lesion does not need an operative procedure that is as radical as the procedure for a large IIa lesion. This is particularly pertinent in the decision between a class II and class III radical hysterectomy. In many countries the class II radical hysterectomy (called a modified radical hysterectomy) is combined with a bilateral pelvic lymphadenectomy as standard therapy for early-stage cervical cancer. Indeed, the class III type of radical hysterectomy is a phenomenon of particular prevalence in

the Western hemisphere and Asia because of the dual influences of Meigs and Okabayashi. The class III, or Meigs–Okabayashi procedure, is a derivative of the Halstedian principle that a lesion should be removed en bloc with its draining lymphatics; thus, the class III radical hysterectomy calls for removal of all the parametria at the pelvic sidewall and transection of the uterosacral ligaments at the sacrum. Advocates of the modified radical hysterectomy or class II procedure with pelvic lymphadenectomy for stages I and IIa lesions suggest that the intervening lymphatics are not at risk in an early cancer of the cervix. Indeed, spread from the primary lesion to the draining pelvic wall nodes probably occurs as an embolic phenomenon. One virtually never finds a tumor in lymphatics except surrounding the primary lesions. However, it is prudent for the pathologist to take several sections of the most distal portion of the parametria following a class III radical hysterectomy for stage I or IIa cervical cancer in an effort to determine the presence or absence of malignant cells in lymphatics distant from the primary lesion. In the presence of a bulky central lesion, the need for an adequate surgical margin of resection often mandates a more extensive procedure than the typical class II radical hysterectomy. However, preservation of any portion of the lateral parametria appears to be associated with a greatly diminished incidence of bladder atony. Forney reported on 22 women extensively studied after undergoing radical hysterectomy; in 11 women, the cardinal ligaments had been divided completely, and in the other 11, the inferior 1 to 2 cm of these ligaments had been spared. Satisfactory voiding occurred significantly earlier (20 vs 51 days) in women who had undergone an incomplete transection. In a similar manner, preservation of a portion of the uterosacral ligaments appears to be associated with fewer complaints of postoperative obstipation. Undoubtedly, the preserved tissue contains intact nerve tracts, which avoid the extensive denervation associated with the typical class III type or radical hysterectomy.

Complications

Acute complications of radical hysterectomy include pelvic hemorrhage, urinary tract injury, injury to the genitofemoral or obturator nerves, deep venous thrombosis, and pulmonary embolism. Although hemorrhage requiring transfusion of blood products is a risk of any radical hysterectomy, this complication may occur more frequently when this procedure is performed in obese patients. Soisson and colleagues reported on 43 women undergoing radical hysterectomy for early-stage cervical cancer. All patients had a body weight at least 25% greater than their ideal weight. Survival was not compromised, and the incidence of serious complications was not increased in obese patients when compared

TABLE 3-10 Complications of Radical Hysterectomy with Approximate Incidences

Vesicovaginal fistula	1%
Ureterovaginal fistula	2%
Severe bladder atony	4%
Bowel obstruction (requiring surgery)	1%
Lymphocyst (requiring drainage)	3%
Thrombophlebitis	2%
Pulmonary embolus	1%

to a control group. The operative technique is more difficult; the procedure lasts longer, and surgery is associated with greater blood loss.

Pulmonary embolism is the one complication most likely to cause mortality in the period surrounding the operative therapy of cervical cancer. This must be kept in mind at all times, and particular care must be exercised during and after surgery to avoid this devastating complication. The operative period is the most dangerous period for the formation of a thrombus in the leg or pelvic veins. Care should be taken to ensure that a constriction of veins in the leg does not occur during the operative procedure, and careful dissection of the pelvic veins should lead to minimal thrombus formation in those structures. Because of the risk of pulmonary embolism and deep venous thrombosis, prophylactic heparin and/or pneumatic compression boots are strongly recommended.

Chronic complications following radical hysterectomy include urinary dysfunction, lymphocyst formation, lymphedema, extensive abdominal scarring, fistula formation (vesicovaginal and rectovaginal), compromised sexual function, and loss of fertility. All these complications are preventable, and the incidence is decreasing steadily (Table 3-10). With highly successful surgical treatment programs in place for early-stage disease, quality of life among survivors becomes important.

The major complication following radical surgery for invasive cancer of the cervix is postoperative bladder dysfunction. Reports in the literature by Seski and Carenza and Nobili and Giacobini suggest that bladder dysfunction is a direct result of injury to the sensory and motor nerve supply to the detrusor muscle of the bladder. The more radical the surgery, the greater will be the extent of damage and the more likely postoperative bladder dysfunction will result.

This dysfunction is usually manifested in the patient by a loss of the sense of urgency to void and an inability to empty the bladder completely without the Credé maneuver. Although most patients learn to compensate for the sensory and motor loss and return to near-normal function, patients occasionally need to be taught intermittent self-catheterization, or long periods of constant bladder drainage may be necessary postoperatively. Sophisticated urodynamic studies have shown that a residual hypertonicity in the bladder detrusor muscle and urethral sphincter mechanism sometimes produces dysuria and stress incontinence. Treatment is symptomatic, with near total recovery in most patients. Limitation of the extent and radicality of surgery, especially in patients with early lesions, can minimize this morbidity. Bandy and colleagues reported on the long-term effects on bladder function following radical hysterectomy (class III) with and without postoperative radiation. In his study, the necessity for bladder drainage of 30 or more days after surgery in 30% of patients was associated with significantly worse long-term residual and other bladder dysfunction. Adjunctive pelvic radiation was associated with significantly more contracted and unstable bladder. In a study reported from Greece of stage Ib cancers, 68 had a Rutledge type III and 50 had a type II radical hysterectomy. Age, grade, bulky tumor, and lymph node metastasis were similar in the two groups. Postoperative radiation was given to 31% of type III and 64% of type II hysterectomies. Major complications, mainly voiding problems, were significantly more common in those treated with type III hysterectomy; however, the disease-free survival was better in the class III hysterectomy (86.5% vs 76.5%, $P < 0.05$). This study would suggest type III surgery is better than type II plus radiation.

Ureteral fistulas are now infrequent (0%-3%), primarily as a result of the improvement in techniques, such as avoiding excessive damage to the structure itself and preserving alternate routes of blood supply. With respect to lymphocyst formation, two studies testing the hypothesis that avoiding reperitonealization of the pelvic peritoneum obviates the need for such drainage have been reported; both studies suggest that drainage is not necessary if the peritoneum is left open over the surgical site. Ligation of the lymphatics entering the obturator fossa under the external iliac vein helps reduce the flow of lymph into this area, where lymphocyst formation is prevalent. Lymphocysts, if present, rarely cause injury and are usually reabsorbed if given enough time. Choo and colleagues reported that cysts smaller than 4 to 5 cm usually resolve within 2 months and that only observation is necessary. Surgical intervention is necessary when there is some evidence of a significant ureteral obstruction. During laparotomy, the surgeon should unroof the lymphocyst and prevent re-formation by suturing a tongue of omentum into the cavity (internal marsupialization). Percutaneous aspiration of the cyst, which is often associated with subsequent infection, should be used cautiously.

Preservation of ovarian function is often desirable for patients who must undergo a surgical procedure for invasive cancer of the cervix. Often, after a careful histologic examination of the operative specimen, including the pelvic lymph nodes, a postoperative recommendation for pelvic radiation is indicated. Standard pelvic placement of preserved ovaries will result in postirradiation ovarian failure; therefore a procedure for transposition of the ovaries to an extrapelvic site (Figure 3-23) has been devised. Shielding during postoperative pelvic irradiation is possible with the ovaries so placed. The ovaries receive some radiation but not usually enough to prevent continued steroid production. A word of caution has been interjected by Mann and others regarding the rare occurrence of occult metastases to the ovary in patients with adenocarcinoma of the cervix. The two largest studies suggest that the incidence is between 0.6% and 1.3%, respectively. Most patients with metastatic disease in the ovary are postmenopausal or have had gross adnexal pathology or positive pelvic lymph nodes. These guidelines can be helpful in identifying patients for whom preservation of ovarian tissue is unwise. The incidence of occult metastasis to the ovary from squamous cell carcinoma of the cervix (stages I and IIa) is so rare that preservation of ovarian tissue does not carry the same concerns. Lateral ovarian transposition will be discussed further in the following section on fertility preservation.

Indications for Postoperative Adjuvant Therapy

Table 3-11 contains data sets from two randomized studies that have established the role for adjuvant therapy following radical surgery based on intermediate and high-risk surgicopathologic factors. In a GOG study

(protocol 92) of 277 patients with intermediate risk factors, stage Ib cancers were randomized to radical hysterectomy with or without postoperative irradiation. Of these patients, 137 were randomly assigned to radiation therapy and 140 were not given further treatment. Based on a previous GOG study, intermediate risk was defined as greater than one third of stromal invasion, lymph space involvement, and large clinical tumor diameter.

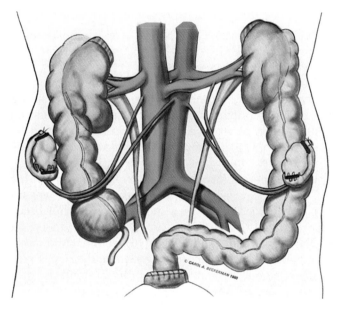

FIGURE 3-23 Diagram illustrating the location of transposed adnexae to a nonpelvic site where they can be spared from postoperative pelvic irradiation. *(From DiSaia PJ: Surgical aspects of cervical carcinoma. Cancer 48:548, 1981. Copyright 1981 American Cancer Society. Reprinted by permission of Wiley-Liss, Inc., a subsidiary of John Wiley.)*

TABLE 3-11   When to Use Adjuvant Therapy after Radical Hysterectomy

RANDOMIZED TRIAL OF ADJUVANT PELVIC RADIOTHERAPY FOR FIGO STAGE IB

GOG 92*	N	Recurrence (%)	RR[†]
Adjuvant pelvic RT	137	n = 21 (15)	0.53, P = 0.008
No further therapy	140	n = 39 (28)	

RANDOMIZED TRIAL OF SYNCHRONOUS ADJUVANT RADIATION THERAPY AND CHEMOTHERAPY FOR FIGO STAGE IA2-IIA

GOG 109/SWOG 8797/RTOG 91-12[‡]	N	Projected PFS (%)	Projected OS (%)
Adjuvant pelvic RT + CT	127	80 HR 2.01, P = 0.003	81 HR 1.96, P = 0.007
Adjuvant pelvic RT alone	116	63	71

GOG-92 data from Sedlis A, Bundy BN, Rotman MZ et al: Gynecol Oncol 73:177, 1999.
GOG 109/SWOG 8797/RTOG 91-12 data from Peters WA 3rd, Liu PY, Barrett RJ 2nd et al: J Clin Oncol 18:1606–1613, 2000.
RT, radiation therapy
*All patients underwent radical hysterectomy and lymphadenectomy, followed by randomization based on intermediate surgicopathologic risk factors (i.e., depth of stromal invasion, tumor size, presence of angiolymphatic space involvement).
†Reduction in the relative risk of recurrence.
‡All patients underwent radical hysterectomy and lymphadenectomy, followed by randomization based on high surgicopathologic risk factors (i.e., metastatic tumor to the lymph nodes, parametria and/or vaginal margin).

(Note that the term lymph space involvement is used interchangeably with vascular space involvement) All patients had negative lymph nodes. Four combinations of the risk factors were developed. Tumor size varied to greater than 4 cm. Although the two arms were equal with regard to the four combinations, in which group(s) the recurrences occurred is not stated. Using a one-tail test, there is a greater recurrence-free survival for the combined group (84.6% compared with 72.1%). Overall survival was not significant; 11% died of cancer compared with 18% of the radical hysterectomy only group. There was a 10% noncompliance rate in the radiation group. These authors are able to apply this information to clinical practice because greater than 90% of patients would be treated without benefit with regard to survival. Data were presented with an intent-to-treat evaluation (see Table 3-11).

Patients with positive pelvic nodes usually receive postoperative whole-pelvis irradiation and chemotherapy (see Table 3-11). Peters and colleagues randomized 268 patients with FIGO stage Ia2, Ib, and IIa carcinoma of the cervix, initially treated with radical hysterectomy and pelvic lymphadenectomy and found to have positive pelvic lymph nodes and/or positive margins and or microscopic involvement of the parametrium, to receive either pelvic radiation therapy alone or concurrent chemoirradiation. Among the 243 patients who were accessible, progression-free survival (PFS) and overall survival (OS) were significantly improved in the patients receiving chemotherapy. The projected PFS at 4 years was 63% with pelvic radiation therapy alone and 80% with concurrent chemoirradiation (hazard ratio 2.01, $P = 0.003$). The projected overall survival rate at 4 years was 71% with pelvic radiation therapy alone and 81% with concurrent chemoirradiation (hazard ratio 1.96, $P = 0.007$). The combined therapy arm had more frequent grade III and IV4 hematologic and gastrointestinal toxicity. This landmark intergroup study of the GOG (protocol 109), the Southwest Oncology Group (protocol 8797), and the Radiation Therapy Oncology Group (protocol 91–12) was one of five randomized trials to be published between 1999 and 2000 attesting to the value of radiosensitizing chemotherapy in the management of cervical cancer (discussed further later).

Prognostic factors have been evaluated by several authors in patients with early-stage disease who have been treated surgically. In a study by Francke and associates, 105 patients with stage Ib were treated with radical hysterectomy and had negative lymph nodes. Only LSI showed significant correlation with local failure. There were 32 patients with squamous carcinoma and positive LSI, 17 received postoperative radiation with 0 of 17 recurrences, and 4 of 15 (27%) treated with surgery only developed recurrence. The overall survival at 5 years was 96% in those treated with radiation and 93.3% in those with LSI not treated with radiation. Stockler and colleagues evaluated 194 patients with stage Ib and IIa who were treated with radical hysterectomy and had negative nodes. Nuclear grade 2 or 3 ($P = 0.02$) and small cell squamous histology ($P = 0.001$) were each associated with a fourfold increase in risk of recurrence, whereas LSI ($P = 0.02$), age younger than 36 years ($P = 0.03$), and either tumor size greater than 28 mm ($P = 0.03$) or surgical clearance less than 5 mm ($P = 0.02$) were associated with a 2.5-fold increase in risk of recurrence. Survival data were not given. Delgado, in reporting a GOG study of 645 women with stage Ib squamous carcinoma, including 100 patients with positive nodes, found depth of invasion, tumor size, and lymph space involvement to be important risk factors for recurrence in multivariate analysis. The group from Boston evaluated 171 patients with lymph node–negative stage Ib and IIa cervical cancer treated primarily with surgery. One hundred and sixteen (68%) were treated with surgery only and 55 (32%) received radiation. Overall, 28 patients (16%) developed recurrent disease with no difference in the two treatment groups. After correction for other factors, patients with LSI who received radiation were less likely to develop recurrence than similar patients treated with surgery only ($P = 0.04$); however, overall survival was similar in the two groups. In a study from Gateshead, United Kingdom, 527 patients with stage Ib to IIb cervical cancer treated with radical hysterectomy were evaluated. There were 102 (19.3%) with lymph node metastasis. In those with lymph node metastasis, histologic differentiation ($P = 0.009$) and metastatic extent ($P = 0.045$) were the only independent prognostic factors for risk of cervical cancer deaths.

Shibata and colleagues evaluated adjuvant chemoradiation in 37 patients who had undergone radical hysterectomy with pelvic lymphadenectomy. In addition to accepted high-risk surgicopathologic criteria (e.g., positive pelvic lymph nodes and/or positive surgical margins), the investigators also included the presence of lymphovascular space involvement (LVSI) as part of their inclusion criteria for protocol eligibility. Adjuvant chemotherapy consisted of cisplatin ($70 \, mg/m^2$ on day 1) and 5-FU ($700 \, mg/m^2$/per day on days 1-4) every 4 weeks for a total of three cycles. Pelvic radiotherapy was started concurrently with the first cycle of chemotherapy and administered to a dose of 45 Gy in 25 fractions. The incidence of grade III/IV toxicities included neutropenia (24.3%), nausea and vomiting (8.1%), and diarrhea (18.9%). The 5-year progression-free survival (PFS) was 89.2%. Both the GOG and the Korean GOG have emphasized the importance of further improvement of outcomes of women found to have high-intermediate surgicopathologic risk factors (e.g., large tumor diameter, deep stromal invasion, LVSI) following radical surgery for early-stage disease. A prospective, randomized trial involving adjuvant pelvic radiotherapy versus adjuvant single agent weekly cisplatin-based chemoradiation has recently been designed through collaboration of both cooperative groups.

The optimal adjuvant therapy for patients found to have high-risk surgicopathologic factors has not yet been determined. Specifically the role of adjuvant chemotherapy in place of or in addition to adjuvant chemoradiation has been the subject of much debate. Takeshima and colleagues treated 65 consecutive patients with FIGO stage IB to IIA cervical carcinoma with adjuvant chemotherapy following radical hysterectomy and pelvic lymphadenectomy. Patients with intermediate-risk factors (stromal invasion >50%, $n = 30$) and those with high-risk factors (positive surgical margin, parametrial invasion, and/or lymph node involvement, $n = 35$) were treated with bleomycin, vincristine, mitomycin, and cisplatin (three cycles for intermediate-risk cases and five cycles for high-risk cases). Chemotherapy was well tolerated with no significant adverse effects and no cases of severe bleomycin-related pulmonary toxicity. The 5-year disease-free survival was 93.3% for the intermediate-risk group and 85.7% for the high-risk group. All patients with squamous cell carcinomas in the intermediate-risk group and 89.3% of high-risk patients with squamous cell carcinoma remained disease free. Despite the absence of adjuvant pelvic radiotherapy, local-regional recurrence occurred in 3.3% of the intermediate-risk group and in 8.6% of the high-risk group. A randomized trial comparing adjuvant chemoradiation with and without continued systemic "consolidation" platinum-based and taxane-based chemotherapy is being considered by the GOG for patients found to have high-risk surgicopathologic factors following radical surgery.

To summarize, the recommendation for postoperative adjuvant therapy (pelvic radiotherapy with or without radiosensitizing chemotherapy) following radical hysterectomy is based on high–intermediate risk surgicopathologic factors (i.e., tumor diameter, depth of stromal invasion, and presence of lymphovascular space involvement) and high-risk surgicopatholgic factors (i.e., presence of tumor at the vaginal margin, in the parametria, and/or lymph nodes). The major research questions center around limiting the toxicity of chemoradiation, continued intravenous systemic therapy, and the triage of patients with locally advanced resectable lesions (i.e., IB2-IIA) to primary chemoradiation versus potentially trimodality therapy (i.e., radical surgery followed by adjuvant chemoradiation).

Sexual Function

The subject of sexual function after therapy for cervical cancer is often ignored. Many patients never regain pretreatment sexual function. Patients treated with full pelvic irradiation therapy (i.e., external-beam and vaginal brachytherapy) will experience decreased sexual function resulting from vaginal stricture formation with obliteration and premature ovarian failure (see forthcoming discussion). Andersen studied the sexual behavior, the level of sexual responsiveness, and the presence of sexual dysfunction of 41 women with uterine cancer compared with a matched group of healthy women. The two groups were similar until the onset of signs of disease, which sometimes occurred long before diagnosis, at which time the patients with cancer began experiencing significant sexual dysfunction. Sexual morbidity therefore begins actually in the prediagnosis period for many patients. Seibel reported on 46 patients who were interviewed more than 1 year after treatment for carcinoma of the cervix to establish the effects of radiation therapy and of surgical therapy on sexual feelings and performance. The patients who were irradiated experienced statistically significant decreases in sexual enjoyment, opportunity, and sexual dreams. The surgically treated group had no significant change in sexual function after treatment. Both groups experienced a change in self-image but did not feel that their partners or family viewed them differently. Myths about cancer and the actual effects of pelvic irradiation were found to have disrupted the sexual marital relationships of many women. Therapeutic programs with counseling and vaginal rehabilitation with the use of estrogen vaginal creams and possibly the use of dilators may be beneficial. Although radical hysterectomy offers an enhanced functional outcome, the procedure does not always leave sexual function undisturbed, with orgasmic problems and dyspareunia resulting from reduced vaginal size having been reported.

Nerve-Sparing Radical Hysterectomy

Lin and colleagues evaluated urodynamic function in 20 women with cervical cancer who underwent radical hysterectomy. Urodynamic parameters measured preoperatively and postoperatively included bladder voiding and bladder storage functions, both of which were found to be significantly impaired in all 20 cases following surgery. Surgical damage to the pelvic autonomic nerves is likely to be responsible for not only subsequent impaired bladder function but also in defecation problems and sexual dysfunction. The development of a nerve-sparing procedure that does not compromise the radicality of the operation is highly desirable.

Trimbos and colleagues introduced elements of the Japanese nerve-sparing technique in their Dutch population, citing that in various Japanese oncology centers it had been recognized that the anatomy of the pelvic autonomic nerve plexus permits a systematic surgical approach to preserve these structures. The investigators first identified and preserved the hypogastric nerve in a loose tissue sheath underneath the ureter and lateral to the uterosacral ligament; next, the inferior hypogastric plexus in the parametrium is lateralized and avoided during parametrial transection; finally, the most distal part of the inferior hypogastric plexus is preserved during the dissection of the posterior part of the vesicouterine ligament. Trimbos and colleagues concluded that the procedure is feasible and safe and deserves further consideration.

An updated series was presented by Maas and colleagues, who observed that the incidence of urinary dysfunction appears to be very low after nerve sparing. These findings have been supported by an Italian series of 23 patients reported by Raspagliesi and colleagues and by two recent Japanese papers for which urodynamic data were recorded for 27 patients. In the study by Sakuragi and colleagues, none of 22 patients for whom the nerve-sparing procedure was performed had urinary dysfunction, compared to 3 of the 5 patients for whom the procedure could not be performed.

Nerve-sparing radical hysterectomy is an attractive approach because of improved urogenital, anorectal, and sexual functions. The sympathetic fibers that innervate the uterus, vagina, urinary bladder, and rectum come from T11-L2 and form the superior hypogastric plexus. The parasympathetic fibers come from S2-4 at the pelvic wall as the pelvic splanchnic nerve. These fibers merge and form the inferior hypogastric plexus and branch to innervate the uterus and the urinary bladder. Professor Fujii from the Kyoto University Gynecology Group has gone to great lengths to provide a step-by-step anatomic identification of the nerve-sparing radical hysterectomy (Table 3-12). The first step in the nerve-sparing procedure involves isolation and separation of the deep uterine vein from the pelvic splanchnic nerve (Figure 3-24). This is then followed by isolation and separation of the hypogastric nerve. Ultimately, the bladder branch from the inferior hypogastric plexus is identified running parallel to the blood vessels in the paracolpium, and the uterine branch from the inferior hypogastric plexus is separated and divided (Figure 3-25). This procedure can be accomplished only through meticulous division of the posterior leaf of the vesicouterine ligament. Through separation of the inferior vesical vein in this ligament, the bladder branch from the inferior hypogastric plexus can be identified and preserved.

van den Tillaart and colleagues evaluated the feasibility, safety, and local recurrence rate in 122 patients with FIGO stage IA-IIA lesions, and compared them to 124

TABLE 3-12 Comparison of Nerve-Sparing Radical Hysterectomy (RH) to Traditional Radical Hysterectomy

	Nerve-Sparing RH	Traditional RH	P Value
FIGO stage IB1	10	8	ns
FIGO stage IB2	0	1	
FIGO stage IIA	0	1	
Mean operative time (min)	197	155.5	0.05
Median number lymph nodes removed	17.8	15.7	ns
Hospital stay (days)	7.6	8.4	ns
Postvoid residual urine volume >50 mL (days)	3.5	9.1	0.00078
Mean decrease in hgb concentration (g%)	1.7	2.5	ns
Complications	1 (blood transfusion)	0	ns

Modified from Skret-Magierlo J et al: Gynecol Oncol 116:502, 2010.
ns, Not specified.

patients who underwent non-nerve-sparing surgery. Unilateral or bilateral sparing of nerves was possible in 80% of cases in the nerve-sparing group. Operative time and blood loss were less in the nerve-sparing group, whereas postoperative courses were similar. The local recurrence rates were not significantly different at 2 years of follow-up. Nerve-sparing surgery was not a significant prognostic factor for local recurrence in univariate and multivariate regression analyses.

Neuronavigation systems and robotic-assisted nerve-sparing techniques are under investigation, as is the incorporation of the nerve-sparing procedure to radical trachelectomy for fertility preservation.

Sentinel Lymph Node Identification

Although the risk of nodal metastases is low in women with small, early cancers (i.e., FIGO Ia2 and Ib1 lesions), the need for bilateral pelvic lymphadenectomies must still be emphasized. Controversy has centered on the existence and ability to identify sentinel lymph nodes (SLN) in cervical cancer. The rationale for identifying an SLN in cervical cancer is to avoid full pelvic lymphadenectomies, which can result in lymphocyst formation and lower-extremity lymphedema, especially when adjuvant pelvic radiotherapy is given. Two techniques for sentinel node identification are available. An injection is performed around the tumor using either a blue dye or an isotopic colloid. Ideally the two techniques are used concomitantly in patients with early-stage lesions (Figure 3-26).

Dargent and Enria reported the results on 70 consecutive patients. Failure in identification of the SLN occurred in 14 of the 139 attempted dissections. One

FIGURE 3-24 Nerve-sparing.
(From Fujii S: Gynecol Oncol 111:S33, 2008).

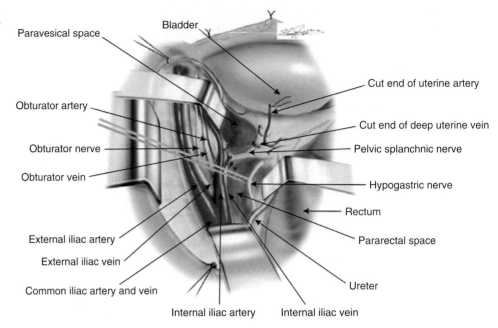

FIGURE 3-25 Nerve-sparing.
(From Fujii S: Gynecol Oncol 111:S33, 2008).

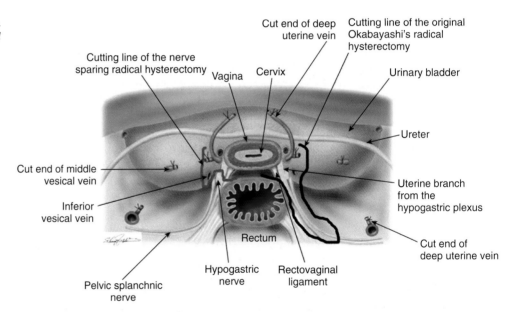

FIGURE 3-26 Sentinel node.
(A from Niikura H et al: Gynecol Oncol 2004;94:528. B from Gil-Moreno A et al. Gynecol Oncol 96:187, 2005.)

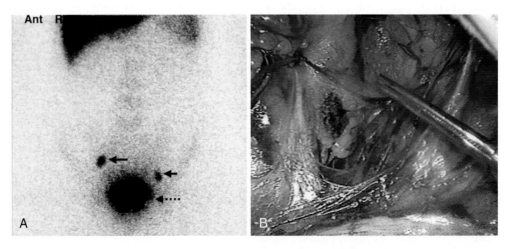

SLN was detected in 121 dissections, and two SLNs were detected in 4 dissections. The investigators carried out a systematic pelvic lymphadenectomy after removal of the SN. A metastatic involvement of the SLN was put in evidence in 19 of the 129 retrieved SLNs. The other regional lymph nodes were involved in 13 cases and not involved in 6 cases. In the 110 cases in which the SLN was not involved all the other regional nodes were free from metastasis.

Table 3-13 contains studies on sentinel node detection in cervical cancer from 2007 to 2010. Most studies were performed with a combination of blue dye and a radioactive tracer with detection rates ranging from 87.3% to 100%. False-negative rates have ranged from 0% to 22.6%. Darlin and colleagues noted that the technique appears to be an accurate method for identifying lymph node metastases in cervical cancer patients with tumors of 2 cm or smaller. The investigators recommend that in the case of a unilateral SLN only, a complete lymphadenectomy should be performed on the radionegative side. Although a randomized clinical trial to assess the equivalency of SLN mapping will not be feasible because a sample size of more than 1800 patients will be required to evaluate a decrease in recurrence rate from 15% to 10%, the GOG is prospectively studying the utility of lymphatic mapping and SLN identification in patients with early-stage cervical cancer (GOG protocol 206).

Laparoscopic Radical Hysterectomy with Lymphadenectomy

Advantages of minimally invasive surgery include magnification for improved visualization, decreased blood loss, shorter hospitalization, more rapid recovery to full function, less adhesion formation, improved cosmesis, and decreased wound complications (e.g., infection, hernia formation). A type III Wertheim–Meigs radical hysterectomy with bilateral pelvic and aortocaval lymphadenectomies can be accomplished via operative laparoscopy and has been reported by several centers (Table 3-14, Figure 3-27). Malzoni and colleagues published a series of 77 patients, 60 of whom underwent a class III operation and 17 who underwent a class II operation. The median body mass index was 27 kg/m^2 (range, 19-35 kg/m^2). Mean operative time was 186 minutes, median blood loss was 57 mL (range, 30-90 mL), and the median hospital stay was 4 days (range, 3-7 days). Chen and colleagues performed 290 laparoscopic radical hysterectomies with lymphadenectomy. The median blood loss was 230 mL (range, 50-1200 mL), and the mean operative time was 162 minutes (range, 110-350 minutes). Positive lymph nodes were detected in 27.1%, and surgical margins were clear in all patients. Postoperative complications occurred in 10.8% and included ureterovaginal fistula ($n = 5$), vesicovaginal fistula ($n = 4$), ureterostenosis ($n = 3$), deep venous thrombosis ($n = 9$), lymphocyst ($n = 4$), lymphedema ($n = 5$), and trocar insertion site metastasis ($n = 1$). Recurrent disease occurred in 16.3% ($n = 48$) at a median follow-up of 36.5 months.

TABLE 3-13 Studies on Sentinel Node Detection in Cervical Cancer

Reference	N	Technique	Detection Rate (%)	Metastases Sentinel Node (%)	False-Negative (%)
Frumovitz et al	831	R/B	89.8	20.5	8.2
Bats et al	71	R/B	87.3	25.8	11
Altgassen et al	590	R/B	88.6	15.7	22.6
Diaz-Feijoo et al	50	R/B	100	Unknown	0
Kara et al	32	R/B	100	28.1	0
Fader et al	38	R/B	92.1	15.7	16.7
Van de Lande et al	58	R/B	96.6	21.4	0
Pluta et al	60	R/B	100	8.3	0

Modified from Oonk MHM et al: Curr Opin Oncol 21:425, 2009.
B, Blue dye; R, radioactive tracer.

TABLE 3-14 Literature Review of Total Laparoscopic Radical Hysterectomy with Lymphadenectomy

Authors	N	BMI	OR Time (min)	EBL (ml)	Hospital Stay (days)	Transfusion	Pelvic Lymph Nodes
Spirtos et al	78	≤35	205	225	2.9	1	34
Ramirez et al	20	26	332.5	200	1	1	13
Gil Moreno et al	27	26	285	400	5	2	19.1
Abu-Rustum et al	19	23.1	371	301	4.5	1	25.5
Pomel et al	50	21.5	258	200	7.5	1	13.22
Nezhat et al	7	—	293	143	3.2	—	27.8
Puntambekar	248	—	92	165	3	—	18
Frumovitz	35	28.1	344	319	2	6	14
Malzoni et al	77	27	186	57	4	0	23

Modified from Malzoni M et al: Surg Oncol 18:289, 2009.

FIGURE 3-27 LSC radical hysterectomy. (**A** *from Frumovitz M and Ramirez PT: Gynecol Oncol 2007;104(1 Suppl):13–6.* **B** *from Abu-Rustum NR et al: Gynecol Oncol 91:402, 2003.)*

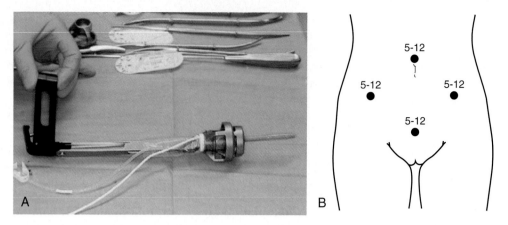

Single-site laparoscopic surgery platforms have been developed and are being evaluated in gynecologic oncology centers. Reports of this technique using the multi-channel single-incision laparoscopic surgery port for laparoscopic cases or a single channel Gelport for robotic-assisted cases on the da Vinci Surgical System in the performance of radical hysterectomy with lymphadenectomy using articulating endoscopes and articulating instrumentation are forthcoming.

Robotic-Assisted Laparoscopic Radical Hysterectomy with Lymphadenectomy

Worldwide adoption of a minimally invasive surgical approach for radical hysterectomy with lymphadenectomy using standard laparoscopic techniques has been slow because of technical difficulties, long surgeon learning curve, and long operative time in many cases. The counterintuitive hand movements, two-dimensional visualization, and limited degrees of instrument motion within the body in addition to ergonomic difficulty and tremor amplification constitute additional obstacles. The development of the robotic-assisted laparoscopic technique using the da Vinci surgical system has allowed for high-definition three-dimensional visualization, instruments that increase surgical accuracy by mimicking the complex movements of the human hand, enhanced dexterity with tremor abolition, and faster suturing (Figure 3-28). In both laboratory drills and in clinical settings, robotic-assisted laparoscopic techniques appear to require a shorter learning curve.

During the preceding 5 years, reports of robotic-assisted laparoscopic radical hysterectomy with lymphadenectomy has started appearing in the literature (Table 3-15). Maggioni and colleagues compared the surgical outcome of robotic radical hysterectomy ($n = 40$) with that of radical abdominal hysterectomy ($n = 40$ historic cases). The two groups did not differ significantly in body mass index, stage, histology, or intraoperative complications. The median age did differ

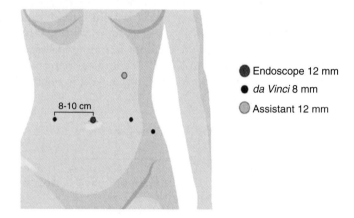

FIGURE 3-28 Robotic (Da Vinci). *(From Shafer A and Boggess JF: Gynecol Oncol 111(1 Suppl):S18, 2008.)*

significantly (44 years in the robotic cohort vs 49 years in the historic group, $P = 0.035$). The mean operative time was significantly shorter for the laparotomy group (mean, 200 minutes vs 272 minutes, $P = 0.0001$), whereas the mean blood loss was statistically significant in favor of the robotic group (78 mL vs 222 mL, $P < 0.0001$). A higher number of pelvic lymph nodes was removed via laparotomy (mean, 26 nodes vs 20 nodes, $P < 0.05$). The mean length of stay was significantly shorter for the robotic group. There were no significant differences in terms of postoperative complications between the two groups.

Finally, Cantrell and colleagues reported their 3-year experience involving 63 patients who underwent successful robotic-assisted laparoscopic type III radical hysterectomy. There was one intraoperative complication (asystole after induction) and two postoperative complications (intensive care unit admission for cardiac evaluation and reoperation for vaginal cuff dehiscence. Thirty-two percent of patients received adjuvant therapy. At a median follow-up of 12.2 months, there has been recurrence and death of one patient, resulting in a 94% PFS and OS. These survival outcomes did not differ

TABLE 3-15 Case-Matched Analysis of Robotic Radical Hysterectomy with Lymphadenectomy Compared with Laparoscopy and Laparotomy

	Robotic (n = 32)	Laparoscopic (n = 17)	Laparotomy (n = 14)	p-Value
IA2	—	2 (11.8%)	—	ns
IB1	29 (90.6%)	14 (82.4%)	13 (92.9%)	ns
IB2	3 (9.4%)	1 (5.9%)	1 (7.1%)	ns
BMI (mean)	29.7	28.1	29.5	ns
Operative time (mean)	2.4 hr	2.2 hr	1.9 hr	0.05 (robotic vs laparotomy)
EBL (mean)	130 cm^3	209.4 cm^3	621.4 cm^3	0.009 (robotic vs laparoscopy); <0.0001 (robotic vs laparotomy)
Total nodes (mean)	32.4	18.6	25.7	<0.001 (robotic vs laparoscopy); <0.05 (robotic vs laparotomy)
Positive margins	5 (15.6%)	3 (17.7%)	3 (21.4%)	ns

Modified from Estape R et al: Gynecol Oncol 113:357, 2009.
ns, Not specified.

TABLE 3-16 Conization for Microinvasive Adenocarcinoma of the Cervix

Author	Depth ≤3.0 mm	Recurrences	Depth 3.1-5.0 mm	Recurrences
Schorge	5	0	—	—
McHale	4	0	—	—
Webb	20	Not specified	18	Not specified
Smith	31	1	29	1
Ceballos	1	0	—	—
Poynor	2	0	1	0
Bisseling	16	0	2	0
Total	79	1	50	1

Modified from Bisseling KCHM et al: Gynecol Oncol 107:424, 2007.

lymphovascular space involvement, FIGO Ia2, and FIGO Ia adenocarcinoma) (see Figure 3-16). In addition, patients with FIGO stage Ib lesions less than 2 cm with limited endocervical involvement and no pathologic evidence of lymph node metastases may be candidates for radical trachelectomy. In patients who are selected for conservative therapy, there should be no clinical evidence of impaired fertility and a strong desire for future childbearing. In addition, close surveillance should be instituted with scheduled Pap testing, colposcopic evaluation, and endocervical curettage.

significantly from those of a historic cohort at the investigators' institution.

Robotic-assisted techniques for the management of early-stage cervical carcinoma appear to be feasible, but continued evaluation of oncologic outcomes and a cost–benefit analysis is still needed. Important complications that also require careful evaluation and scrutiny are those that may be specific to robotic techniques, including adverse effects associated with prolongation of steep Trendelenberg position, herniation at 8-mm port sites, vaginal cuff dehiscence, freezing of the robotic arms intraoperatively, and consequences of collisions. In addition, there has been a recent report of an 8-mm robotic port-site metastasis in a patient who underwent robotic-assisted laparoscopic radical hysterectomy and bilateral pelvic lymphadenectomy for a node-negative FIGO stage IB1 adenocarcinoma of the cervix.

Fertility-Preserving Surgery for Early-Stage Tumors

For patients with microinvasive cervical carcinoma, management depends on the depth of invasion and select patients may undergo conservative treatment with either cervical conization (FIGO Ia1) or radical trachelectomy with lymphadenectomy (FIGO Ia1 with

Cervical Conization for Adenocarcinoma In Situ and Microinvasive Carcinoma

There has been a movement during the past decade to seriously explore fertility-sparing surgery for patients with AIS and microinvasive carcinomas. For many patients with AIS, local excision appears to be sufficient treatment provided ectocervical and endocervical margins are clear and patient compliance with follow-up is demonstrable. It would appear that cold knife, CO_2 laser, and large loop excision of the transformation zone (LLETZ) conization procedures produce acceptable results; however, these approaches should be reserved for highly selected patients.

Cold knife conization is preferable in cases in which margin status is critical (e.g., glandular lesions and suspected microinvasion) (Table 3-16). Patients with margin involvement should be considered for repeat excisional biopsy. A 2009 meta-analysis composed of 33 studies indicated a recurrence rate for AIS of 2.6% for negative margins and 19.4% for positive margins (OR 2.48; 95% CI 1.05, 1.622, P <0.001). Invasive adenocarcinoma was more commonly associated with positive margins (5.2%) compared with negative margins (0.1%).

In a study of 85 patients with FIGO stage IA1 squamous cell carcinoma treated by electrosurgical conization and cold conization to preserve fertility, there was one recurrence (1.2%) at a median follow-up of 81 months. In a second report containing 75 patients with FIGO stage IA1 squamous cell carcinoma, there were no recurrences among the 53 women who underwent conization followed by hysterectomy nor in the 22 who underwent conization alone. As in the case with AIS and microinvasive squamous cell carcinoma, conservative fertility-preserving therapy may be considered for select cases of microinvasive adenocarcinoma, although this remains controversial. It would seem that for FIGO stage IA1 adenocarcinomas, conization is safe. When LVSI is present, laparoscopic pelvic lymphadenectomy seems advisable. In summary, for highly selected patients with early-stage disease seen in consultation with a gynecologic oncologist, cold knife cervical conization is a reasonable alternative to preserve fertility provided compliance with follow-up is not problematic and pathology review has excluded highly aggressive histologic subtypes (e.g., neuroendocrine tumors).

Vaginal Radical Trachelectomy with Laparoscopic Lymphadenectomy

Radical trachelectomy involves removing all or most of the cervix along with the bilateral parametria and upper vagina. This procedure allows for preservation of the uterus for childbearing and can be performed vaginally, abdominally, or through a minimally invasive approach (i.e., straight-stick laparoscopy or robotic-assisted laparoscopy). Of note, patients with stage Ia2 disease have a 6.3% risk of nodal metastases and therefore treatment must include a formal pelvic lymphadenectomy.

In 1987 Dargent designed a fertility-preserving operation for stage Ia2 and some Ib1 lesions. A variant of the classical Shauta operation of vaginal radical hysterectomy, the vaginal radical trachelectomy (VRT) is performed in conjunction with bilateral laparoscopic lymphadenectomies. The VRT is performed with division of the uterus underneath the isthmus, and at the completion of the procedure the uterus is sutured to the vagina. Oncologically, the technique is satisfying because a wide margin around the lesion is obtained containing the parametria and the upper vagina but leaving the body of the uterus in situ.

Plante and colleagues collected more than 600 reports of the vaginal technique from the past decade's literature, including 115 of her own. Oncologic outcomes have been satisfactory with an overall recurrence rate of 4.5% and death from disease of 2.5% (Table 3-17). Risk factors for recurrence include lesions 2 cm or larger (29% vs 1%) and the presence of LVSI (12% vs 2%). Adenocarcinomas and adenosquamous carcinomas are not clearly associated with an increased risk of recurrence. Patients with neuroendocrine tumors should probably not be offered fertility-sparing surgery. Approximately 10%-12% of patients selected for vaginal radical trachelectomy are found to have more extensive endocervical disease at the time of surgery or positive nodes on frozen section leading to abandoning the procedure in favor of adjuvant therapy or completion radical hysterectomy.

Plante and colleagues also tabulated obstetric outcomes for 256 patients (Table 3-18). Approximately 62% of pregnancies following vaginal radical trachelectomy

TABLE 3-17 Oncologic Outcomes After Vaginal Radical Trachelectomy

Author	N	Median f/u (mo)	Recurrence Rate (%)	Death (%)
Marchiole	118	95	7 (6)	5 (4)
Plante	115	74	4 (3)	2 (2)
Shepherd	112	45	3 (3)	2 (2)
Hertel	100	29	3 (3)	2 (2)
Covens	93	30	7 (7.5)	4 (4)
Sonoda	36	21	1 (3)	0
Burnett	19	21	2 (10.5)	?
Schlearth	10	48	0	0
TOTAL	**603**		**27 (4.5)**	**15 (2.5)**

From Plante M: Gynecol Oncol 111:S105, 2008.

TABLE 3-18 Obstetrical Outcomes After Vaginal Radical Trachelectomy

Author	Pregnancies	TAB, Ectopic (%)	1st-Trimester Loss (%)	2nd-Trimester Loss (%)	3rd-Trimester Deliveries (%)	Deliveries <32 wk (%)	Deliveries 33-36.6 wk (%)	Deliveries >37 wk (%)	Currently Pregnant
Plante	87	4 (5)	17 (20)	3 (4)	58 (66)	3 (5)	8 (14)	47 (81)	5 (5)
Mathevet	56	5 (9)	9 (16)	8 (14)	34 (61)	2 (6)	3 (9)	29 (85)	0
Shepherd	55	3 (5)	14 (25)	7 (13)	28 (51)	8 (29)	12 (43)	8 (29)	3 (5)
Bernardini	22	0	3 (14)	1 (4)	18 (82)	3 (17)	3 (17)	12 (67)	0
Hertel	18	2 (11)	1 (5)	0	12 (67)	—	—	—	3 (16)
Sonoda	11	0	3 (27)	0	4 (36)	0	0	4 (100)	4 (36)
Burnett	3	0	0	1	2	1	0	1	0
Schlearth	4	0	0	2	2	1	0	1	0
TOTAL	256	14 (5)	47 (18)	22 (8.6)	158 (62)	18 (12)	26 (16)	102 (65)	15 (6)

From Plante M: Gynecol Oncol 111:S105, 2008.

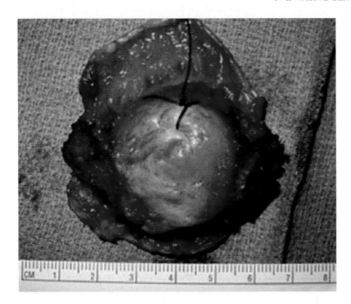

FIGURE 3-29 Vaginal radical trachelectomy. *(From Einstein MH et al: Gynecol Oncol 112:73, 2009.)*

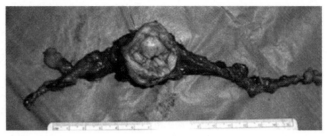

FIGURE 3-30 Abdominal radical trachelectomy. *(From Einstein MH et al: Gynecol Oncol 112:73, 2009.)*

TABLE 3-19 Pathologic Results of the Unfixed Trachelectomy Specimens with Bilateral Parametrial Measurements by the Pathologist

	VRT ($n = 28$)	ART ($n = 15$)	P Value
Median gross length (cm)	1.45 (0.73-1.63)	3.97 (2.7-5.36)	0.01
Median histologic length (cm)	1.07 (0.89-1.25)	1.51 (1.36-1.77)	≤0.0001
Patients with parametrial lymph nodes detected	0 (0%)	8 (57.3%)	0.0002

From Einstein MH et al: Gynecol Oncol 112:73, 2009.
ART, Abdominal radical trachelectomy; VRT, vaginal radical trachelectomy.

will reach the third trimester, of which 65% will reach term. The preterm delivery rate is in the range of 28%, but only 12% will end with significant prematurity (<32 weeks) in which most neonatal morbidity occurs. Overall, 40% of all pregnancies can be expected to culminate with the birth of a healthy newborn at term.

Abdominal approaches to radical trachelectomy may include nerve-sparing, laparoscopic, and/or robotic-assisted techniques. Potential benefits of the abdominal approach for radical trachetectomy include wider parametrial resection, possible lower intraoperative complication rates, and techniques familiar to most gynecologic oncologists (Figure 3-29). Cibula and colleagues reviewed the more than 100 reported cases of abdominal radical trachelectomy (ART) in 2008, and then updated their own experience with the abdominal approach in 2009. Specific indications for the abdominal approach have included clear cell carcinoma of the upper vagina, clear cell cervical carcinoma in pediatric patients, cervical cancer in patients with distorted vaginal anatomy, cancer in the cervical stump after subtotal hysterectomy, bulky exophytic cervical cancer, extent and location of cervical cancer that requires increased radicality of parametrial resection (type III), and cervical cancer in the first half of pregnancy. In total, a total of nine live births have been reported, of which at least two were premature deliveries.

Einstein and colleagues compared surgical and pathologic outcomes for 43 adult patients with FIGO stage IB1 lesions who underwent VRT ($n = 28$) or ART ($n = 15$) (Table 3-19). The median measured parametrial length in the VRT group was 1.45 cm compared to 3.97 cm in the ART group (P <0.0001). Parametrial nodes were only

detected in the ART specimens ($n = 8$, 57.3%). There was no difference in histologic subtypes, LVSI, or median total regional lymph nodes removed in the two groups. Median blood loss was greater but not clinically significant in the ART group, and median operating time was less in the ART group. The two groups did not differ significantly in the overall complication rate. The investigators concluded that the abdominal approach allows for wider parametrial resection, including contiguous parametrial nodes.

By allowing for the preservation of the body of the uterus and thereby the potential for reproductive function, the radical trachelectomy emerges as a true breakthrough in the management of young women with early-stage cervical cancer (Figure 3-30). It is currently the fertility-sparing procedure with the most available data supporting its use. Although these results are encouraging, there is lack of level I evidence (i.e., randomized controlled trials) comparing safety and survival rates between conservative and radical methods. Therefore these techniques should be used by fully trained operators. In our opinion, the technique can be considered in conjunction with laparoscopic transperitoneal lymphadenectomy in the patient who strongly desires future fertility and harbors a stage Ia1 lesion with LVSI, an Ia2 lesion, or an Ib1 tumor less than 2 cm in diameter.

Lateral Ovarian Transposition

As described previously, young patients with FIGO stage I to IIa cervical carcinoma who are considered to be at high risk for requiring adjuvant pelvic irradiation (with or without radiosensitizing chemotherapy) should have the ovaries transposed to the paracolic gutters at the time of radical abdominal hysterectomy. The infundibulopelvic ligament is mobilized and two large metallic clips should be placed in an "X" formation across the mesosalpinges to assist in radiographic localization during radiation treatment planning. Patients with locally advanced carcinomas (i.e., FIGO stage Ib2 to IVa) who will receive primary chemoirradiation can undergo lateral ovarian transposition via laparoscopy in anticipation of therapy.

The incidence of ovarian failure following transposition ranges from 28% to 50% when pelvic irradiation is used. There is a tendency to become postmenopausal if the scatter radiation dose at the transposed ovaries is greater than 300 cGy. This scatter radiation dose does not appear to depend on the distance the ovaries are placed from the linea innominata. The risk of premature ovarian failure when adjuvant radiation therapy is not required is approximately 5% in patients who have undergone lateral ovarian transposition. The risk of developing symptomatic ovarian cysts appears to be approximately 5%.

Husseinzadeh and colleagues performed lateral ovarian transposition in 22 patients with invasive cervical cancer, 15 of whom received whole pelvic external radiation therapy. Nine patients also received one or two intracavitary insertions. Ovarian function was measured by the serum gonadotropins, follicle-stimulating hormone (FSH), and luteinizing hormone (LH). Five patients developed postmenopausal symptoms. Ovarian function was preserved in seven patients, all of whom received an average dose of 250 cGy to the ovaries via external radiation and intracavitary insertion(s). FSH values ranged from 3.3 to 38.8 mIU mL-1 (mean = 17.7 mIU mL-1).

TREATMENT OF LOCALLY ADVANCED DISEASE

Radiotherapy

Over the past century radiotherapy has emerged as a notable alternative to radical surgery, primarily because of improvements in technique. The number of radiation-resistant lesions was discovered to be small, and skilled radiologists limit radiation injury, especially with the moderate dosages used for early disease. Much evidence has been presented that proves that radiotherapy can

destroy disease in lymph nodes and in the primary lesion. Over the past two decades, radical hysterectomy has been reserved in many institutions for patients who are relatively young, lean, and in otherwise good health. In other areas of the United States, radiotherapy or surgery is used alone when the alternative modality is not available. The relative safety of both treatment modalities and the high curability for stages I and IIa lesions give physician and patient a true option for therapy.

Radiotherapy for cancer of the cervix was begun in 1903 in New York by Margaret Cleaves. In 1913 Abbe was able to report an 8-year cure. The Stockholm method was established in 1914, the Paris method in 1919, and the Manchester method in 1938. Radium was the first element used; it has always been the most important element in radiotherapy of this lesion. External irradiation was used to treat the lymphatic drainage areas in the pelvis lateral to the cervix and the paracervical tissues.

Successful radiation therapy depends on the following:

1. Greater sensitivity of the cancer cell, compared with the cells of the normal tissue bed, to ionizing radiation
2. Greater ability of normal tissue to recuperate after irradiation
3. A patient in reasonably good physical condition

The maximal effect of ionizing radiation on cancer is obtained in the presence of a good and intact circulation and adequate cellular oxygenation. Preparation of the patient for a radical course of irradiation therapy should be as careful as the preparation for radical surgery. The patient's general condition should be as well maintained as possible with a diet high in proteins, vitamins, and calories. Excessive blood loss should be controlled and hemoglobin should be maintained well above 10 grams.

Some consideration must be given to the tolerance of normal tissues of the pelvis, which are likely to receive relatively high doses during the course of treatment of cervical malignancy. The vaginal mucosa in the area of the vault tolerates between 20,000 and 25,000 cGy. The rectovaginal septum is said to tolerate approximately 6000 cGy over 4 to 6 weeks without difficulty. The bladder mucosa can accept a maximal dose of 7000 cGy. The colon and rectum will tolerate approximately 5000 to 6000 cGy, but small bowel loops are less tolerant and are said to accept a maximal dose of between 4000 and 4200 cGy. This pertains to small bowel loops within the pelvis; the tolerance of the small bowel when the entire abdomen is irradiated is limited to 2500 cGy. One of the basic principles of radiotherapy is implied here: The normal tissue tolerance of any organ is inversely

TABLE 3-20   Suggested Therapy for Cervical Cancer

	Whole Pelvis		
Stage	(cGy)	Brachytherapy (mg/hr)	Surgery
Ial true microinvasive			Extrafascial hysterectomy
Ia2	2000 (2000 parametrial)	8000 (2 applications)	Radical hysterectomy with bilateral pelvic lymphadenectomy as an option
Ib	4000	6000 (2 applications)	
IIb	4000-5000*	5000-6000 (2 applications)	Consider pelvic exenteration for tumor persistence
IIIa	5000-6000*	2000-3000 or interstitial implant	
IIIb	5000-6000*	4000 (1 application), 5000 (2 applications)†	
IVa	6000	4000 (1 application), 5000 (2 applications)†	
IVb	500-1000 pulse 2-4 times 1 week apart	Palliative	

*Patients with larger lesions or poor vaginal geometry merit the higher dose of external radiation.
†Two applications are suggested following whole-pelvis radiation with larger lesions or when the first application has less than optimum dosimetry.

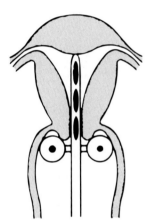
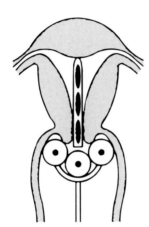
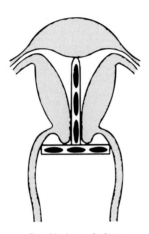
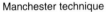

Manchester technique   Paris technique   Stockholm technique

FIGURE 3-31   Three techniques of intracavitary brachytherapy.

related to the volume of the organ receiving irradiation. External irradiation and intracavitary radium therapy must be used in various combinations (Table 3-20). Treatment plans must be tailored to each patient and her particular lesion. The size and distribution of the cancer, not the stage, should be treated. Success in curing cancer of the cervix depends on the ability of the therapy team to evaluate the lesion (and the geometry of the pelvis) during treatment and then make indicated changes in therapy as necessary. Intracavitary radium therapy is ideally suited to the treatment of early tumors because of the accessibility of the portio of the cervix and the cervical canal. It is possible to place radium or cesium in close proximity to the lesion and thus deliver surface doses that approximate 15,000 to 20,000 cGy. In addition, normal cervical and vaginal tissue has a particularly high tolerance to irradiation. One therefore has an ideal situation for the treatment of cancer because there are accessible lesions that lie in a bed of normal tissue (cervix and vagina) that is highly radioresistant.

Radium and Cesium Therapy

Radium is the isotope that has been used traditionally in the treatment of cancer of the cervix. Its greatest value is that its half-life is approximately 1620 years; therefore it provides a very stable, durable element for therapy. In recent years, both cesium and cobalt have been used for intracavitary therapy. Cesium has a half-life of 30 years; with the current technology, cesium provides an adequate substitute for radium. Four major technologies for the application of radium in the treatment of cervical cancer continue to be favored among gynecologists. Of these technologies, three are intracavitary techniques using specially designed applicators, and the fourth technique involves the application of radium in the form of needles directly into the tumor. The variations among the three techniques of intracavitary brachytherapy are found in the Stockholm, Paris, and Manchester schools of treatment (Figure 3-31). The differences are mainly found in the number and length of time of applications,

FIGURE 3-32 Fletcher-Suit radium applicators: Ovoids and tandem with inserts.

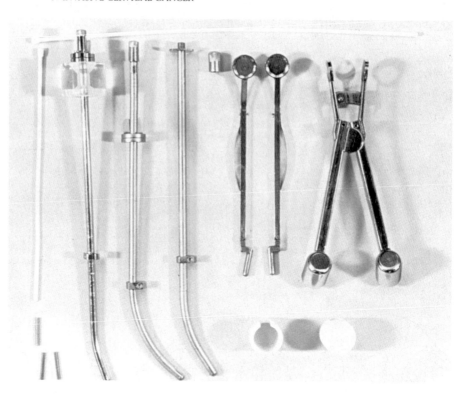

the size and placement of the vaginal colpostats, and radium loading. In the United States, the tendency has been to use fixed radium applicators with the intrauterine tandem and vaginal colpostats originally attached to each other. Over the last three decades, a flexible afterloading system, Fletcher-Suit, has gained increasing popularity because it provides flexibility and the safety of afterloading techniques.

The Paris method originally used a daily insertion of 66.66 mg of radium divided equally between the uterus and the vagina. The radium remained in place for 12 to 14 hours, and the period of treatment varied from 5 to 7 days. An essential feature of the Paris method, and a part of the modification of this technique, is the vaginal colpostat, which consists of two hollow corks that serve as radium containers joined together by a steel spring that separates them into the lateral vaginal wall.

The Stockholm technique uses a tandem in the uterine cavity surrounded by a square radium plaque applied to the vaginal wall and portio vaginalis of the cervix. No radium is placed in the lower cervical canal, and vaginal sources are used to cover the cervical lesion. The uterine tandem and vaginal plaque are immobilized by packing and left in place for 12 to 36 hours. Two or three identical applications are made at weekly intervals.

The Manchester system is designed to yield constant isodose patterns regardless of the size of the uterus and vagina. The source placed in the neighborhood of the cervical canal is considered the unit strength. The remaining sources in the corpus and vagina are applied as multiples of this unit and are selected and arranged to produce equivalent isodose curves in each case and an optimal dose at preselected points in the pelvis. The applicator is shaped to allow an isodose curve that delivers radiation to the cervix in a uniform amount. The Fletcher-Suit system (Figure 3-32) previously mentioned is a variation of the Manchester technique.

An effort is made in the two radium insertions to administer approximately 7000 cGy to the paracervical tissues as the total of the dose from both external and intracavitary irradiation. The isodose distribution around a Manchester system is pear-shaped (Figure 3-33). The maximal total dose delivered by the two radium insertions is a function of the total dose to the bladder and rectum. The total dose received by the rectal mucosa from both radium applications usually ranges between 4000 and 6000 cGy. The nearest bladder mucosa may receive between 5000 and 7000 cGy. When whole-pelvis irradiation is used, the radium dose must be reduced to keep the total dose to the bladder and rectum within acceptable limits.

In conjunction with the development of a system of radium distribution, British workers have defined two anatomic areas of the parametria (see Figure 3-33) where dose designation can be correlated with clinical effect. These are situated in the proximal parametria adjacent to the cervix at the level of the internal os and in the distal parametria in the area of the iliac lymph nodes and

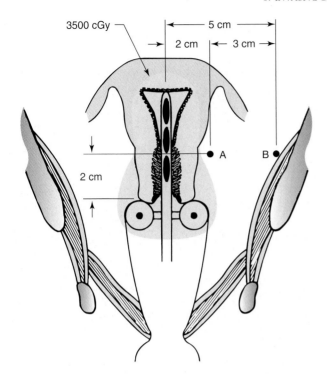

FIGURE 3-33 Pear-shaped distribution of radiation delivered to tissues surrounding a typical radium application with the Manchester type of applicators. Points *A* and *B* are noted as reference points.

are designated point A and point B. The description states that point A is located 2 cm from the midline of the cervical canal and 2 cm superior to the lateral vaginal fornix. The dose at point A is representative of the dose to the paracervical triangle, which correlates well with the incidence of sequelae and with the 5-year control rate in many studies. Point B is 3 cm lateral to point A. This point, together with the tissue superior to it, is significant when considering the dose to the node-bearing tissue. It is clear from what has been said relative to points A and B that they can represent important points on a curve describing the dose gradient from the radium sources to the lateral pelvic wall. This gradient is different for the various techniques. In a comparison of the physical characteristics of radio techniques, the ratio of the dose at point A to the dose at point B should help define physical differences. In addition, determining the dose at point A relative to the calculated dose at points identified as bladder trigone and rectal mucosa provides a means of assessing the relative safety of one application over another. The concepts of points A and B have been questioned by many authors, including Fletcher and Rutledge. They remain as imaginary points but seem to provide a framework in which therapy is planned. Again, the distribution of the disease must be the primary guide in planning therapy, and the total dose to either point A or point B is relative only to their position with regard to the disease distribution.

Whole-pelvis irradiation is usually administered in conjunction with brachytherapy (e.g., intracavitary radium or cesium) in a dose range of 4000 to 5000 cGy. Megavoltage machines such as cobalt, linear accelerators, and the betatron have the distinct advantage of giving greater homogeneity of dose to the pelvis. In addition, the hard, short rays of megavoltage pass through the skin without much absorption and cause very little injury, allowing almost unlimited amounts of radiation to be delivered to pelvic depths with little if any skin irritation. Orthovoltage, because of its relatively long wavelength and low energy, has the disadvantage that doses to the skin are particularly high and, in delivering the required amount of radiation to the pelvis, may cause temporary and permanent skin changes. Thus, for pelvis irradiation, high-energy megavoltage equipment has definite advantages over orthovoltage and even low-energy megavoltage equipment.

Interstitial Therapy

In advanced carcinoma of the cervix, the associated obliteration of the fornices or contracture of the vagina may interfere with accurate placement of conventional intracavitary applicators. Poorly placed applicators fail to irradiate the lesion and the pelvis homogeneously. Syed and Feder have revived a solution to this problem by advocating transvaginal and transperineal implants. The technique uses a template to guide the insertion of a group of 18-gauge hollow steel needles into the parametria transperineally (Figure 3-34). These hollow needles are subsequently "afterloaded" with iridium wires when the patient returns to her hospital room. Theoretically, this technique locates a pair of paravaginal interstitial colpostats in both parametria. This approach appears promising, but long-term studies illustrating improved survival rate and reasonable morbidity are not available. Also, there is no report reflecting, prospectively, the effectiveness, in comparable groups of patients, of the interstitial technique versus the standard intracavitary approach.

Interstitial therapy may have particular value in the treatment of carcinoma of the cervical stump. Although carcinoma of the cervical stump has become a relatively rare disease, accounting for less than 1% of all gynecologic malignancies, it does create difficult problems in terms of optimal geometry for delivery of effective irradiation therapy. In some series of cervical cancer, the incidence of carcinoma of the cervical stump is approximately 10%. Prempree, Patanaphan, and Scott reported excellent results with absolute survival rates of 83.3% for stage I, 75% for stage IIa, and 62.5% for stage IIb using radiation therapy with an emphasis on parametrial interstitial implants in the more advanced diseases. Similar results have been obtained by Puthawala and associates.

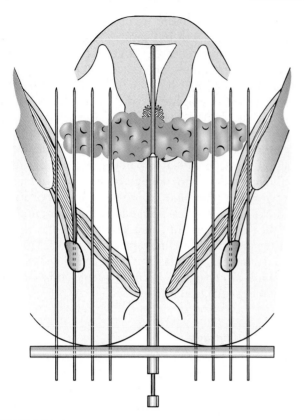

FIGURE 3-34 Diagram of the technique of interstitial therapy for advanced cervical cancer using a Syed–Noblett template.

Extended Field Irradiation Therapy

Over the past two decades, attempts have been made to improve survival for more patients with advanced cervical cancer by identifying the presence of paraaortic lymph node metastases and applying extended field irradiation to the area (Figure 3-35). The en bloc pelvic and periaortic portals extend superiorly as far as the level of the dome of the diaphragm and inferiorly to the obturator foramen. The width of the periaortic portion of the field is usually 8 to 10 cm, and the usual dose delivered is between 4000 and 5000 cGy in 4 to 6 weeks. A booster dose of 1000 cGy is often given to the pelvic field alone. Identification of paraaortic lymph node involvement was initially attempted by use of lymphangiography, but this technique did not find general acceptance because of varied accuracy from institution to institution and from radiologist to radiologist. Surgical localization of periaortic involvement has been more satisfactory.

Several reports have discussed survival and complications in patients with carcinoma of the cervix and periaortic metastases who received extended field irradiation (Table 3-21). Piver and Barlow of Roswell Park Memorial Institute, Buffalo, reported on 20 women with previously untreated cervical cancer who received

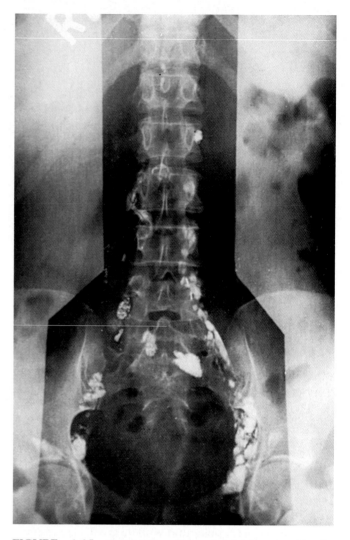

FIGURE 3-35 Abdominal radiograph showing portals for extended-field irradiation in cervical cancer.

TABLE 3-21 Late Complications of Radiation Therapy with Approximate Incidence

Sigmoiditis	3%
Rectovaginal fistula	1%
Rectal stricture	1%
Small bowel obstruction	1%
(with extended field)	20%
Vesicovaginal fistula	1%
Ureteral stricture	1%

radical irradiation to the periaortic lymph nodes and pelvis after the diagnosis of periaortic lymph node metastases had been established by surgical staging. They noted that 90% of these patients received 6000 cGy to the periaortic nodes and pelvis in 8 weeks using a split-course technique. A later report shows that 30% died of complications of this therapy and 45% died of recurrent disease. Only 25% of patients survived disease free for 16, 18, 24, and 36 months. The criticism may be that the dose is too high, yet a lesser dose might be ineffective, and 4 patients did survive. It is obvious that a safe yet effective dosage level for extended field irradiation therapy has not yet been established.

Wharton and colleagues of the MD Anderson Hospital reported on 120 women treated with preirradiation celiotomy. Of these patients, 32 had severe bowel complications and 20 (16.6%) eventually died as a result of the surgery or of the surgery and irradiation. Four of these patients died immediately as a result of the surgical procedure. Of 64 patients with positive nodes who were irradiated, 17% lived for 13 to 38 months after treatment. No patient had survived for 5 years. Wharton and associates further reported that in 36 women with positive nodes it was possible to accurately determine the failure sites after completion of the full course of irradiation therapy. In 25 of these patients, distant metastases were the first evidence of treatment failure; 11 had disease or developed recurrence within the treatment fields; and disease of the pelvic wall was found in only 2 patients.

The role of surgical staging in removal of paraaortic or pelvic nodes in cervical cancer remains controversial. The results of the aforementioned experience would question significant benefit in view of the complications and survival. Retroperitoneal lymphadenectomy, compared with the intraperitoneal approach, has decreased complications mainly as a result of adhesions and possible bowel complications. More recently, patients with advanced disease have had the paraaortic nodes reevaluated so that extended fields could be added if necessary. The laparoscopic approach is currently being evaluated. Less invasive approaches such as lymphangiogram, CT, and MRI studies have also been evaluated. The sensitivity is less, and false-negative results may be as high as 24% in patients with stage IIIB disease. Many gynecologic oncologists will obtain a CT scan and, if positive, do a fine-needle aspiration. If the result is negative, then surgical removal may be done. An alternative is to radiate the paraaortic areas prophylactically. This has been done with little or no survival benefit. All the studies note that the severe complication rate essentially doubles (5%-10%) when radiation was given to the paraaortic area.

Experience has shown that doses of about 4500 cGy, particularly when administered in daily fractions of 150 to 180 cGy, are safely tolerated by the organs in the periaortic treatment volume, and a complication rate of 5% should be expected. Extraperitoneal surgery appears to be associated with less postradiation morbidity, probably because of reduced bowel adhesions. The issues of the utility of periaortic radiation and surgical staging in the management of cervical carcinoma are closely intertwined. Although many hypotheses have been raised to support or reject the use of surgical staging, it is clear that some patients with biopsy-proven periaortic node metastases can be cured with radiotherapy using extended fields. Approximately 20% of patients who receive extended-field radiotherapy survive cervical cancer metastatic to the periaortic lymph nodes. Rubin and colleagues had a 50% survival in a group of patients with stage Ib disease with documented periaortic lymph node involvement. In many reports, the true value of extended field radiation is clouded because patients with periaortic node involvement often have advanced disease in which any node or regional therapy may have little effect on long-term survival.

The incidence of pelvic recurrence following irradiation alone for stages Ib, IIa, and IIb carcinomas of the cervix increases with the diameter of the tumor. Data from the MD Anderson Hospital showed an improved pelvic control rate, and a small increase in survival, when patients with the bulky, so-called barrel-shaped lesions were treated with preoperative irradiation followed by extrafascial hysterectomy. The subject continues to be controversial, with conflicting studies in the literature. Gallion and colleagues reported on 75 patients with "bulky, barrel-shaped" stage Ib cervical cancer; 32 patients received radiation alone and 43 patients were treated with radiation followed by extrafascial hysterectomy. The incidence of pelvic recurrence was reduced from 19% to 2% and extrapelvic recurrence was reduced from 16% to 7% in patients treated by combination therapy, which produced no increase in treatment-related complications. However, Weems and colleagues described 123 such patients treated from two different eras at his institution. Examination of pelvic control rates, and disease-free survival, showed no significant advantage in pelvic control, disease-free survival, or absolute survival for either treatment group when compared by stage and tumor size. Unfortunately, no large prospective randomized study has been done that could clarify this issue.

Radiation and Chemotherapy

Radiation therapy alone fails to control the progression of cervical cancer in 35% to 90% of women with locally advanced disease. Concurrent chemoirradiation has been used in the treatment of many cancers in an attempt to improve local control and eradicate distant metastases and has been successfully integrated into the therapeutic program of not only cervical carcinomas but also those of the head and neck and anal canal. The rationale for chemoradiation is based on the finding that tumor radiosensitivity can be enhanced through the formation of DNA-platinum adducts. There is a correlation of radiosensitivity with platinum sensitivity. Specifically, the therapeutic index may be improved by loading the tumor with platinum salts containing fast atomic ions. Mechanisms of drug–radiation interaction leading to enhanced radiation kill may include modification of the slope of the dose-response curve, inhibition of sublethal damage repair, inhibition of recovery from potentially lethal damage, alterations in cellular kinetics, decrements in tumor volume leading to improved blood supply and tissue oxygenation, and increased radiosensitivity.

Five phase III trials of concurrent chemoirradiation performed by the Gynecologic Oncology Group, the Radiation Therapy Oncology Group (RTOG), and the Southwestern Oncology Group (SWOG) have demonstrated a reduction in the risk of recurrence by up to 50% in patients with locally confined bulky or advanced-stage cervical cancer, regional spread, or high-risk features after hysterectomy (Tables 3-22). Three studies compared radiotherapy alone with radiotherapy plus cisplatin-based chemotherapy, one of which addressed the prescription of adjuvant therapy following radical

surgery for early-stage tumors (Intergroup Trial, discussed previously). Excluding patients with nodal involvement by CT scan, GOG protocol 123 evaluated the benefit of preoperative chemoiradiation therapy (weekly cisplatin 40 mg/m^2, maximal weekly dose of 70 mg) compared to radiation therapy alone in patients with locally advanced disease confined to the cervix (i.e., stage IB2). All patients underwent adjuvant hysterectomy. In this landmark study, the rates of both progression-free survival ($P <0.001$) and overall survival ($P = 0.008$) were significantly higher in the combined therapy group at 4 years. Patients receiving radiosensitizing chemotherapy experienced higher frequencies of grade III and grade IV adverse hematologic effects and adverse gastrointestinal effects. An update of GOG 123 was provided by Stehman and colleagues in which chemoradiation was found to significantly improve long-term PFS and overall survival (OS) without significantly increasing serious late effects.

Morris and colleagues reported the results from RTOG protocol 90-01. In this study the effects of pelvic radiation plus concurrent cisplatin and 5-FU were compared

TABLE 3-22 Five Pivotal Trials of Chemoradiation in Locally Advanced Cervical Cancer

Trial	Author	Year	Eligibility	Arms	N	Complete Response		Median Survival	
GOG 85	Whitney et al	1999	IIB-IVA§	Pelvic RT + cisplatin 50 mg/m^2 + 5-FU 4 g/m^2/96 hr (2 cycles)	177	60%	$P = 0.033$	65%	$P = 0.018$
				Pelvic RT + hydroxyurea 3 g/m^2 (2×/wk)	191	48%		50%	
						PFS at 4 yr		**OS at 4 yr**	
GOG 109*	Peters et al	2000	IA2-IIA	Adj pelvic RT + cisplatin 70 mg/m^2 + 5-FU	127	80%	$P = 0.003$	81%	$P = 0.007$
				Adj pelvic RT	116	63%		71%	
						PFS at 4 yr		**OS at 4 yr**	
GOG 120	Rose et al	1999	IIB-IVA§	Pelvic RT + cisplatin 40 mg/m^2/wk	176	60%	$P = <0.001$‖	60%	$P = 0.002$-0.004‖
				Pelvic RT + cisplatin 50 mg/m^2 + 5-FU 4 g/m^2/96 hr + hydroxyurea 2 g/m^2	173	60%		58%	
				Pelvic RT + hydroxyurea 3 g/m^2 (2×/wk)	177	45%		34%	
						PFS at 4 yr		**OS at 4 yr**	
GOG 123	Keys et al	1999	IB2†	Preoperative pelvic RT + cisplatin 40 mg/m^2/wk	183	80%	$P <0.001$	86%	$P = 0.008$
				Preoperative pelvic RT	186	64%		72%	
						DFS at 5 yr		**OS at 5 yr**	
RTOG 90-01	Morris et al	1999	IB‡-IIA tumor ≥5 cm IIB-IVA or positive pelvic nodes	Pelvic RT + cisplatin 75 mg/m^2 + 5-FU 4 g/m^2/96 hr (3 cycles	193	67%	$P <0.01$	73%	$P = 0.004$
				Pelvic RT + extended field RT	193	40%		58%	

*Intergroup: GOG 109/SWOG 8797/RTOG 91-12; no randomization.
†Negative nodes.
‡IB lesions included bulky tumors and those with positive pelvic lymph nodes.
§Negative paraaortic nodes.
‖Platinum-based regimens compared to hydroxurea.
PFS, Progression-free survival; OS = overall survival; RT, radiation therapy.

with pelvic radiation plus extended field radiation therapy. This was the only trial to include chemotherapy during low-dose-rate brachytherapy. Eligibility requirements for this study differed from the previous GOG studies with the inclusion of patients with FIGO stage IB2 to IIA tumors. The estimated 5-year survival rates were 73% versus 58%, respectively, for patients treated with chemoirradiation therapy vs radiation therapy alone. A significant difference in disease-free survival was also seen in favor of the chemotherapy arm. The addition of chemotherapy to radiation therapy was effective in reducing both the frequency of local recurrences and distant metastases, with the latter observation refuting those detractors who claim that the benefit conferred by radiosensitizing chemotherapy is strictly a function of increasing the relative dose intensity of the radiation that can be delivered to the pelvis. These results have been sustained in an update of RTOG protocol 90-01 with 8 years of follow-up provided by Eifel and colleagues.

Two additional phase III trials have confirmed the superiority of cisplatin-based chemoirradiation for the treatment of locally advanced cervical cancer. Whitney and colleagues published the results of concurrent cisplatin plus 5-FU and pelvic radiation therapy versus hydroxyurea plus pelvic radiation therapy in women with FIGO stage IIB to IVA disease who had undergone surgical staging and were found to have negative common iliac and aortocaval lymph nodes (GOG protocol 85). Among 368 eligible patients, the median follow-up time among survivors was 8.7 years. Disease progression occurred in 43% of patients randomly assigned to cisplatin plus 5-FU versus 53% of patients randomized to hydroxyurea. Progression-free survival was significantly better among patients treated with the combined chemotherapy regimen ($P = 0.033$), with 3-year survival rates of 67% (cisplatin–5-FU arm) versus 57% (hydroxyurea).

Rose and colleagues reported the results from the three-arm GOG trial of pelvic radiation therapy plus concurrent single-agent cisplatin versus cisplatin plus 5-FU plus hydroxyurea vs hydroxyurea alone (protocol 120). All patients had FIGO stage IIB to IVA cervical cancer with surgically confirmed negative common iliac and aortocaval lymph nodes. The median duration of follow-up was 35 months for 526 women included in the final analysis. Significant improvements in progression-free and overall survival were observed in patients randomly assigned to either cisplatin-containing arm. Effectively, the results from GOG protocol 85 and GOG protocol 120 were critical in supplanting hydroxyurea as the radiosensitizer of choice. In 2007 Rose and colleagues provided their own update of GOG 120 in which once again it was found that the improvement in PFS and OS observed with cisplatin-based

TABLE 3-23 Updates and Ad Hoc Analysis of Pivotal Chemoradiation Trials in Cervical Cancer

Study	Description	Update
Intergroup trial	Adjuvant RT Adjuvant CRT	Absolute 5YS benefit for CRT: tumors >2 cm, ≥2 positive nodes
GOG 123	RT plus adjuvant hysterectomy CRT plus adjuvant hysterectomy	CRT significantly improves long-term PFS and OS; serious late effects not increased significantly
RTOG 9001	RT plus EFRT CRT	CRT: superior OS and DFS (IB-IIB); superior DFS (III-IVA); serious late effects not increased significantly
GOG 120	CDDP-RT CDDP/HU/5FU-RT RT-HU	CDDP-based CRT improves long-term PFS and OS; no significant increase in late toxicity

chemoradiation was sustained without significant increases in late toxicity (Table 3-23).

Because the combination of cisplatin plus 5-FU results in added toxicity, weekly single-agent cisplatin dosed at 40 mg/m^2 has emerged as the standard radiosensitizer in locally advanced cervical cancer. At present, radiosensitizing chemotherapy is recommended during that part of the treatment program when external-beam pelvic radiotherapy is administered.

These pivotal phase III trials not only identified a significant survival advantage associated with the addition of concurrent chemotherapy but also were noteworthy in that the degree of benefit achieved with chemotherapy was remarkably similar for each of the four trials that studied chemoirradiation for primary therapy (Figure 3-36). The results changed the standard of care for the treatment of locally advanced cervical cancer and formed the basis for the 1999 NCI Clinical Announcement (Practice Alert) in cervical cancer. At that time, NCI Director, Richard D. Klausner, MD, stated the following: "The findings of these five trials are remarkably consistent. They are likely to change the standard of care for invasive cervical cancer."

A meta-analysis of 19 randomized controlled trials of chemoradiation versus radiation therapy alone containing a 4580 patients treated from 1981 to 2000 was published in 2001 by Green and colleagues. In their report the hazard ratios for both PFS and OS favored chemoradiation (HR 0.61, P <0.0001 and HR 0.71, P <0.0001, respectively). The Cochrane Review from 2005 analyzed 24 randomized controlled trials of 4921 patients. Chemoradiation was associated with a 10% absolute benefit in OS, a 13% absolute benefit in PFS, and a significant benefit was noted for local control. Acute hematologic

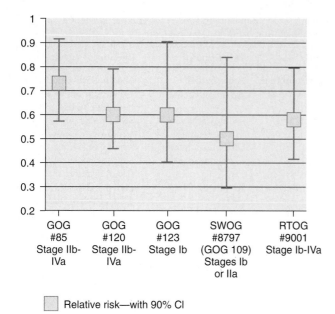

Relative risk—with 90% CI

FIGURE 3-36   Relative risk estimate of survival from five phase-III, randomized controlled clinical trials of chemoradiation in women with cervical cancer. (*GOG*, *Gynecologic Oncology Group; RTOG, Radiation Therapy Oncology Group; SWOG, Southwestern Oncology Group.*)

and gastrointestinal toxicity were reported more frequently with chemoradation, but treatment-related deaths attributable to multimodality therapy were rare. Late effects were not able to be adequately determined in the Cochrane Review. Most recently, a meta-analysis of 18 randomized trials containing 3517 patients again reported superiority of chemoradiation to radiation therapy alone in terms of relative risk, 3-year survival, and 5-year survival. In this third meta-analysis, although gastrointestinal toxicity, myelosuppression, and leukopenia occurred more frequently with the use of chemoradation, there were no significant differences noted between the two modalities in terms of proctitis, cystitis, and nausea/vomiting.

The most recent phase III experience comes from the Ion Chiricuta Cancer Institute in Romania, where 566 patients with FIGO IIB-IIIB lesions were randomly assigned to pelvic radiation therapy (46 Gy) plus high-dose rate brachytherapy (10 Gy) with or without cisplatin (20 mg/m^2 × 5 days). The 5-year survival rate was significantly improved with the use of chemoradation (74% vs 64%, P <0.05), as was the local control rate (78% vs 67%, P = 0.01).

In a 2007 study of practice patterns within the Gynecologic Cancer Intergroup, a global consortium of 14 cooperative groups, the mean external-beam radiation therapy dose was 47 Gy (3.5 Gy SD). The mean total dose to point A was 79.1 Gy (7.9 Gy SD), and the upper border for extended-field radiation therapy among 63% of respondents was T12-L1. Approximately 85% used

high-dose rate systems for vaginal brachytherapy. Of note, all groups reported using concurrent chemotherapy, with weekly cisplatin being the agent of choice for 83%.

The National Comprehensive Cancer Network (NCCN) Clinical Practice Guidelines in Oncology were updated in 2010 for cervical cancer. For patients with selected bulky tumors, those with FIGO stage IB2 and IIA lesions (>4 cm), and those patients with FIGO stage IIB to IVA disease, Category 1 treatment constitutes pelvic radiotherapy plus concurrent cisplatin-containing chemotherapy plus brachytherapy.

Although multimodality therapy has emerged as the standard of care of patients with locally advanced disease, chemoradiation has some shortcomings related to access, efficacy, and tolerability in certain populations. Neoadjuvant chemotherapy is the most studied alternative treatment modality for FIGO stage IB2 to IVA and is discussed in detail later in this chapter. Other modalities under investigation include proton beam therapy, cyberknife radiosurgery, intensity modulated radiation therapy (IMRT), radiosurgery, radiohyperthermia, and the incorporation of antiangiogenesis and other targeted agents into chemoradiation protocols.

Kagei and colleagues treated 25 patients with FIGO stage IIB to IVA disease with external-beam radiation therapy plus proton beam irradiation. The median total tumor dose was 86 Gy. At a median follow-up of 139 months (range, 11-184 months), the 10-year OS was 89% for stage IIB, and 40% for stages IIIB/IVA. Grade IV gastrointestinal and genitourinary toxicities were reported in 4% of patients. Choi and colleagues treated 30 women with isolated paraaortic nodal metastases with the cyberknife. Grade III to IV toxicity requiring hospitalization occurred in 1 patient. The 4-year OS and 4-year locol control rates were 50.1% and 67.4%, respectively. A nonrandomized trial comparing 135 women with locally advanced disease treated with IMRT using FDG-PET/CT simulation to 317 non-IMRT patients was reported to have had no significant impact on recurrence-free survival, although the grade III to IV bowel and bladder toxicities were reportedly higher in the non-IMRT cohort (P = 0.0351). Although the radiobiologic rationale for these three investigational modalities is promising, there have been no randomized trials for the population under discussion.

A recent Cochrane Collaboration Review identified six randomized controlled trials of radiotherapy versus radiohyperthermia for patients with locally advanced cervical carcinoma during the period from 1987 to 2009. Seventy-four percent of patients treated had FIGO stage IIIB tumors. The hazard ratios for 3-year local recurrence and 3-year survival favored the 43°C hyperthermia arms (HR 0.48, 95% CI 0.37-0.63, P <0.001, and HR 0.6, 95% CI 0.45-0.99, P = 0.05, respectively). There were no significant differences in acute or late-grade III to IV toxicity. The review did indicate that these studies were limited by small numbers and important methodologic flaws.

Two studies are ongoing studying targeted therapy in chemoradiation protocols. The RTOG protocol 0417 is a phase II trial investigating the response rate (RR), efficacy, and tolerability of pelvic irradiation with concurrent cisplatin plus the antiangiogenesis agent bevacizumab. The GOG is studying antiepidermal growth factor (EGF) therapy in GOG protocol 9918, a phase I trial designed to evaluate pelvic irradiation with concurrent cisplatin plus cetuximab.

Neoadjuvant Chemotherapy

As a result of limited access to sophisticated radiotherapy centers in resource-poor areas of the world, neoadjuvant chemotherapy has emerged as a viable alternative for treatment of women with locally advanced lesions. This approach was popularized by Sardi and colleagues in their "Buenos Aires Protocol." In one of the first prospective randomized studies of neoadjuvant chemotherapy in early-stage cervical cancer, Sardi and colleagues reported their final results in 205 cases of stage Ib carcinoma of the cervix. Patients were treated with radical hysterectomy followed by 50-Gy radiotherapy to the pelvis with or without neoadjuvant chemotherapy. In patients with stage Ib1, neoadjuvant chemotherapy did not improve overall resectability or survival compared with those not receiving chemotherapy. In patients with stage Ib2, there was 83.6% (51 of 61) partial or complete response to chemotherapy. Overall survival after 9 years of follow-up was 61% for the control group (no chemotherapy) and 80% for the neoadjuvant group (P <0.01). Resection was possible in 85% of the control group and 100% in the neoadjuvant group. Patients who responded to neoadjuvant therapy had an overall survival of 88% compared with 23% for nonresponders. Of interest, the stage Ib1, neoadjuvant groups had an 82% overall survival compared with 80% for stage Ib2. The control groups' survival was 77% and 61%, respectively. Neoadjuvant chemotherapy improved resectability and survival in the patients with stage Ib2. All patients received postoperative radiation.

The Cochrane Collaboration visited this subject originally in 2004 and returned to it recently. In their 2010 report the authors identified 1072 patients from six trials (Table 3-24). Although PFS was significantly improved with neoadjuvant chemotherapy (HR = 0.76, 95% CI 0.62-0.94, P = 0.01), no OS benefit was observed (HR = 0.85, 95% CI 0.67-1.07, P = 0.17). Neoadjvuant chemotherapy was associated with a significant decrease in

TABLE 3-24 Neoadjuvant Chemotherapy Plus Surgery Versus Surgery Alone: Hazard Ratios And Confidence Intervals for Overall Survival

Study	N^*	HR	95% CI
Sardi 1997	210	0.53	0.31, 0.92
Katsumata 2006	134	1.12	0.56, 2.22
Cai 2006	106	0.74	0.33, 1.65
Napolitano, 2003	288	0.84	0.51, 1.40
TOTAL	930	0.85	0.67, 1.07

Modified from Rydzewska L et al: Cochrane Database Syst Rev 1:CD007406, 2010.
*Number of participants analyzed.

adverse pathologic findings, including lymph node status and parametrial infiltration. Total cisplatin dose and schedule did not influence the findings, nor did stage of disease. The authors concluded that it remains unclear whether neoadjuvant chemotherapy consistently offers a benefit over surgery alone for patients with early-stage or locally advanced cancer.

Suboptimal Treatment Situations

Several clinical situations pose unique challenges in the management of cervical cancer, causing some patients with invasive cancer of the cervix to receive suboptimal treatment.

1. Cancer in a cervical stump
2. Simple hysterectomy in the setting of invasive cervical cancer
3. Poor vaginal geometry for intracavitary radiation

Cancer that occurs in a cervical stump is fortunately a diminishing problem because supracervical hysterectomies are performed less frequently. Carcinoma occurring in a cervical stump presents a special problem because often an optimal dose of intracavitary radium cannot be applied as a result of the insufficient place to insert the central tandem, which contributes significantly to the radiation dose to the central tumor and to the pelvic sidewall. Radical surgery is also more difficult; the bladder and rectum firmly adhere to the stump and may adhere to each other. Also, the ureters are more difficult to dissect cleanly from the parametrial tissue because of fibrosis from the previous surgery. The net result is an increase in the risk of significant surgical complications involving the ureters, bladder, and rectum. In modern gynecologic surgery, supracervical hysterectomy is rarely indicated, although in recent years concerns regarding pelvic support and even sexual function have prompted some surgeons to consider the procedure.

In a report of the MD Anderson Hospital experience with 263 patients with carcinoma of the cervical stump,

Miller and colleagues noted a 30% complication rate after full therapy with radiation. Urinary and bowel complications result from postsurgical adhesions; the absence of the uterus, which acts as a shield; and a tendency to emphasize external radiation therapy. We have had a similar experience, resulting in a preference for radical trachelectomy in patients with cancer of the cervical stump in whom stage and medical conditions allow. The increased technical difficulty of performing such a procedure seems to be outweighed by the low complication rate and comparable survival of patients.

A simple hysterectomy performed for invasive cervical cancer is not adequate therapy for most patients. This situation may occur because of poor preoperative evaluation or because the surgery was performed under emergency conditions without an adequate preoperative cervical evaluation. Such a situation may occur in a patient presenting with acute abdomen from ruptured tuboovarian abscesses. In any event, if an extensive cancer is found in the cervix, the prognosis is poor because optimal irradiation cannot be given with the cervix and uterus absent. An even more ominous situation occurs when a hysterectomy is performed with a "cut through" of the cancer—that is, the hysterectomy dissection passes through the cancer. The prognosis is uniformly poor in this event. In the examples just given, surgical cures are not obtained, and the probability of curative radiotherapy is greatly diminished.

In 1968 Durrance reported survival rates of 92% to 100% using postoperative radiation therapy in selected patients with presumed stage I or II disease after suboptimal surgery. Excellent survival rates were also reported by Andras and colleagues in 148 patients who had invasive cervical carcinoma found incidentally in the hysterectomy specimen. Of these patients, 126 were treated with postoperative radiation therapy. Patients with microscopic disease confined to the cervix had a 96% 5-year survival rate. Those with gross tumor confined to the cervix had an 84% 5-year survival. Patients with tumor cut through at the margins of surgical resection, but with no obvious residual cancer, had a 5-year survival rate of 87%. Patients with obvious residual pelvic tumor had a 47% 5-year survival rate. In 1986 Heller and colleagues reviewed the literature and reported equivalent survival rates in 35 patients who were also treated mainly with radiation.

Orr and colleagues have preferred radical parametrectomy, upper vaginectomy, and lymphadenectomy as the treatment of choice following a simple hysterectomy. We also prefer this approach, particularly because many of these patients are young and desirous of preserving optimal sexual function. We are also concerned about postoperative small bowel adhesions and the difficulty of delivering effective irradiation to the medial parametria in the absence of a uterus. Survival rates with either approach appear to be exceptionally good; undoubtedly, this clinical situation creates a bias for smaller lesions that may be easier to eradicate.

Adequate radiotherapy is also compromised in patients who have a vagina or cervix that cannot accommodate a complete intravcavitary radiation application. This situation is encountered with atrophic stenotic pelvic structures. These patients are treated by inserting the tandem and ovoids in a compromised manner, such as insertion of the ovoids singly or independently of the central tandem. In any event, standard optimal doses are usually not obtained, and the possibility of sustaining a radiation injury is increased.

NEUROENDOCRINE AND OTHER UNCOMMON TUMORS OF THE CERVIX

Neuroendocrine (small cell) cervical cancer (Figure 3-37) is a rare malignancy, representing less than 5% of all cases of cervical cancer. These tumors provide a therapeutic challenge for the clinician because they are characterized by frequent and early nodal and distant metastases. The pathologist's dilemma results from the large number of pathologic entities all described as "small cell cancers," including fully differentiated small cell nonkeratinizing squamous cell carcinoma, reserved cell carcinoma, and neuroendocrine (oat cell) carcinoma. Neuroendocrine carcinomas, which can be identified by characteristic light and electron microscopic criteria, are indistinguishable from oat cell cancers of the lung. In addition, they appear to have the poorest prognosis of the various small cell cancers. Therefore, it is important to distinguish this particular subtype of cancer from the rest and to consider innovative approaches to treatment. Neuroendocrine markers are commonly used to assist in classification, with up to 80% of tumors staining for

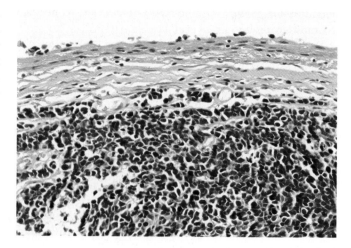

FIGURE 3-37 Small cell carcinoma. (*Courtesy Ibrahim Ramzy, MD, UCI, College of Medicine.*)

synaptophysin, chromogranin, and/or CD56 (neural cell adhesion molecule). At least in one series, Pap smear results were abnormal in only one of seven patients.

Abeler and colleagues reported on 26 cases of true neuroendocrine cervical carcinoma. The 5-year survival was 14% despite aggressive therapy including surgery, radiation, and chemotherapy. Viswanathan and colleagues observed a 66% relapse rate, with a course frequently characterized by the development of widespread hematogenous metastases. Locoregional recurrence outside irradiated fields was also frequently observed. In the group studied, the overall survival rate at 5 years was only 29%, with none of the patients who had disease more extensive than FIGO stage Ib1 or clinical evidence of lymph node metastases surviving their disease.

In our experience in the 1980s with 14 patients in stage Ib or IIa treated by radical hysterectomy with postoperative radiation therapy, all 14 have experienced recurrence, 12 before the 31st month after therapy. Innovative approaches to treating this subset of unfortunate patients are under study. Recently Chan and colleagues updated our series and performed a multivariate analysis of different prognostic factors among 34 patients. His group documented that only those with early lesions amenable to extirpation were curable. The role of primary or postoperative radiation with or without chemotherapy is unclear and yields uniformly poor results, particularly in patients with advanced lesions.

Hoskins and colleagues treated 31 patients with small cell neuroendocrine carcinoma (SCNEC) using protocols containing etoposide, cisplatin, and radiation therapy with concurrent chemotherapy with and without the addition of carboplatin and paclitaxel. The reported 3-year failure-free rate for patients with early-stage disease (stage I and II) was 80%. Chang and colleagues have reported that regimens containing a combination of vincristine, doxorubicin, and cyclophosphamide or cisplatin and etoposide constitute active adjuvant therapies following radical hysterectomy. Zivanovic and colleagues examined the outcomes of 17 patients with SCNEC. The estimated 3-year PFS and OS rates were 22% and 30%, respectively. Median OS for early-stage disease (IA1-IB2) was 31.2 months and 6.4 months for those with advanced-stage disease (IIB-IV, $P = 0.034$). In the early-stage disease group, the 3-year distant recurrence-free survival rate was 83% for patients who received platinum-based combination chemotherapy and 0% for those who did not receive chemotherapy as part of their initial treatment ($P = 0.025$). These data support the role of chemotherapy for distant control as an addition to radiation therapy for local control. Of interest, combined modality treatment with definitive chemotherapy and radiotherapy are used in the current management of small cell lung cancer, with surgical resection playing a limited role in patients with stage I

and stage II disease. It is unclear which patients, if any, should undergo radical hysterectomy for SCNEC of the cervix. Zivanovic and colleagues advise proceeding with combined modality therapy when the diagnosis is established by cervical biopsy, holding surgery in reserve to be used in the adjuvant setting if necessary. It should be recognized that there are advocates of primary radical hysterectomy for patients with early-stage tumors.

GLASSY CELL CARCINOMA, CARCINOSARCOMA, LYMPHOMA, AND MELANOMA

Glassy cell carcinoma of the cervix has also been classically regarded as a poorly differentiated adenosquamous carcinoma, which is infrequently diagnosed and associated with a poor outcome regardless of the modality of therapy. Many recurrences occur in the first year after therapy, and most have occurred by 24 months. Reported survival rates are more encouraging than are those associated with neuroendocrine carcinomas; rates have been seen to be as high as 50% for stage I disease in some series.

In the SEER report of 6549 cases of cervical carcinoma from 1973 to 1977, there were only 36 cases of cervical sarcoma, which is an incidence of 0.55%. Ninety-six cases of cervical sarcoma were reviewed by Rotmensch and colleagues, and no clear statement could be made regarding management, although surgery was consistently utilized for early-stage lesions. Laterza and colleagues reviewed the literature and described the outcomes of 33 patients with carcinosarcoma of the cervix including two of their own (Figure 3-38). Of 16

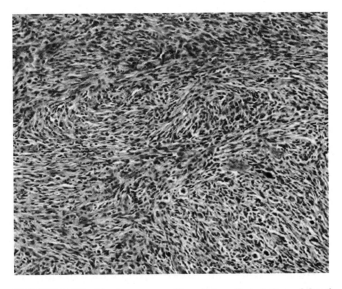

FIGURE 3-38 Carcinosarcoma. *(From Laterza R et al: Gynecol Oncol 107(1 Suppl):S98–100, 2007.)*

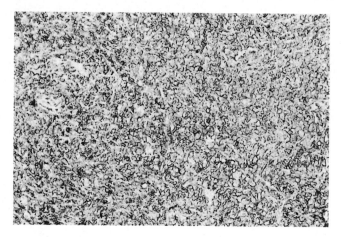

FIGURE 3-39 Lymphoma. *(From Szantho A et al: Gynecol Oncol 89:171, 2003.)*

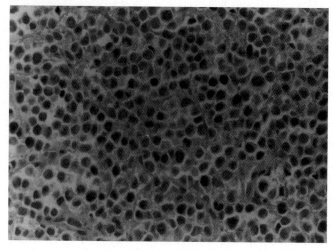

FIGURE 3-40 Melanoma. *(From Kristiansen SB et al: Gynecol Oncol 47:398, 1992.)*

patients with stage I disease, 8 were reported to be NED following a variety of treatment modalities including surgery, radiation, or chemotherapy, alone or in combination. The impact of radiotherapy on survival is uncertain. Given the propensity for distinct histologic subtypes to respond to systemic regimens irrespective of organ site of origin (e.g., small cell neuroendocrine carcinomas of the cervix and lung, malignant germ cell tumors of the ovary and testis), ifosfamide-based regimens, particularly ifosfamide plus paclitaxel, may be expected to exhibit some activity in this disease, similar to what has been reported in carcinosarcoma of the uterine corpus.

In contrast to systemic lymphomas, fever, night sweats, and weight loss rarely have been reported in cervical lymphoma (Figure 3-39). Most present with abnormal vaginal bleeding or discharge, but pelvic pain and dyspareunia may also be present. The differential diagnosis of cervical lymphomas should include benign chronic inflammations, poorly differentiated and small cell cervical carcinomas, sarcomas, and lymphoma-like lesions. Immunophenotyping can be used to make the diagnosis.

The prognosis of extranodal lymphomas is usually poorer than that of nodal lymphomas as a result of inaccurate or delayed diagnosis. Early-stage diagnosis of cervical lymphoma has been associated with favorable outcomes. Some authors have suggested that surgical resection in localized lymphoma may improve survival, although this is unclear. The CHOP regimen (cyclophosphamide, doxorubicin, vincristine, prednisone) is the most commonly used regimen.

Malignant melanoma of the uterine cervix is a rare manifestation (Figure 3-40). A careful survey should be done of the patient's skin and mucous membranes for a possible primary site. Almost 90% of the patients are asymptomatic, and vaginal bleeding is the main complaint among 10%. Most lesions present as an exophytic polypoid cervical mass with obvious coloring. Immunohistochemistry can be used to identify melanin granules, and positive staining for S100, HMB 45, and/or melan-A can help in establishing the diagnosis. Although there is little consensus on the best approach for therapeutic management, the majority of patients have undergone radical hysterectomy with or without pelvic lymphadenectomy and upper vaginectomy. The efficacy of radiation therapy has not been established, although it has been used in the adjunctive and palliative settings. Likewise, the use of adjuvant chemotherapy is under debate. To date there have been no reports of immunotherapy, including the use of interferon, for this disease. The 5-year survival rate is very poor, not exceeding 40% of stage I and 14% of stage II.

SURVIVAL RESULTS AND PROGNOSTIC FACTORS FOR EARLY-STAGE AND LOCALLY ADVANCED DISEASE

For early-stage tumors, results may imply that one form of therapy (i.e., radical surgery vs radiotherapy) has advantages over the other, but considering the rather wide dispersion that, in fact, may be unrelated to treatment, we must maintain collective openmindedness about the efficacy of individual therapeutic regimens. The best available figures for the two methods give results that are almost identical, and because the presence of other factors affect the samples being compared, large differences would be necessary to be significant. Individual physicians will probably continue to decide on the basis of personal preferences and comparison of complications and later disabilities.

The recovery rates of patients with operative squamous cell carcinoma of the cervix depend on many factors, including the histologically documented extent of the carcinoma. Baltzer and associates studied 718 surgical specimens of patients with squamous cell carcinoma of the cervix. Lymphatic and blood vessel invasion significantly influenced survival, blood vessel invasion being much more ominous. In their study, 70% of the patients who demonstrated blood vessel invasion succumbed to the disease, whereas 31% of the patients demonstrating only lymphatic invasion succumbed to the disease process. Other studies have not found prognostic significance for vascular invasion. A definite linkage was noted between the size of the carcinomas and the frequency of metastases. Fuller and colleagues drew similar conclusions. In their study of 431 patients who underwent radical hysterectomy for stages Ib or IIa carcinoma of the cervix at Memorial Sloan-Kettering Cancer Center, they found 71 patients who had nodal spread that correlated closely with increased primary tumor size, extracervical extension of tumor, and the presence of adenocarcinoma. Although these factors were recognized as having prognostic significance, the authors were unable to demonstrate that these detrimental effects could be overcome by postoperative pelvic radiation. Patients receiving postoperative irradiation therapy seemed to have some better local control, but the problem of systemic spread of disease resulted in little overall improvement in survival. In a similar study, Abdulhayogu and associates reported on a series of patients with negative lymph nodes at the time of radical hysterectomy who subsequently developed recurrent disease. They too pointed out the histologic architecture of invasion as an important prognostic indicator. Recurrence was more likely in patients who had deep invasion of the cervical stroma, especially when it extended to the serosal surface (even when the parametria were not involved). Once again the volume of tumor correlated with the eventual prognosis for the patient. They suggested that these patients were in need of postoperative therapy, and radiation therapy for local control was recommended in the absence of any other demonstrated effective adjuvant modality for this set of circumstances. Gauthier and colleagues had similar results and, in a multifactorial analysis of clinical and pathologic factors, demonstrated that the depth of stromal invasion is the single most important determinant of survival.

The role of intraperitoneal tumor spread was evaluated by an Italian group. They evaluated 208 patients with advanced local disease who received neoadjuvant chemotherapy. There were 183 clinically responsive patients who underwent radical surgery; 7 (4%) and 13 (7%) showed macroscopic and microscopic peritoneal tumor, respectively. Multivariant analysis showed that the peritoneal tumor involvement, stage, pathologic parametrial involvement, and lymph node metastasis were independent factors associated with survival.

About one quarter of those with pelvic lymph node metastasis had intraperitoneal involvement compared with only 6% of node-negative patients. If intraperitoneal disease was present, survival was similar, irrespective of stage (Ib-IIb compared with III-IVa).

A study from Austria evaluated 166 patients with stage Ib cancers treated with radical hysterectomy. In a multivariant analysis, microvessel density, lymph node involvement, tumor size, and postoperative radiation remained independent prognostic factors for survival. LSI failed to be a prognostic factor. Of interest, patients with negative lymph nodes but increased microvessel density had similar survival to patients who were node positive but with low microvessel density. A study from Norway evaluated HPV DNA in 97 patients with squamous carcinoma (all stages). When corrected for stage and age, prognosis was significantly poorer for HPV-18– and -33–positive tumors; however, overall when all HPV-positive tumors were compared with HPV-negative tumors, no survival difference was noted.

When age was evaluated in the Annual Report, overall survival in stage I decreased with age. Patients between 15 and 39 years of age in stage II had a worse survival rate compared with older patients. This was true for patients 30 to 49 years of age with stage IV cancers compared with patients of other ages. Mitchell and colleagues reviewed 398 patients with stages I to III cervical cancer of whom 338 patients were 35 to 69 years of age and 60 patients were 70 years of age or older. Although elderly patients had a higher rate of comorbidity resulting in more frequent treatment breaks and less ability to receive definitive therapy with intracavity radiation, the 5-year actuarial disease-free and cause-specific survival rates were comparable between the two groups.

RECURRENT AND ADVANCED CARCINOMA OF THE CERVIX

It is estimated that approximately 35% of patients with invasive cervical cancer will have recurrent or persistent disease after therapy. The diagnosis of recurrent cervical cancer is often difficult to establish (Table 3–25). The optimal radiation therapy most patients receive makes

TABLE 3-25 MD Anderson Hospital Central Recurrence Rate for Carcinoma of the Cervix Following Treatment with Radiation Therapy

Stage I	1.5%
Stage IIb	5%
Stage IIIa	7.5%
Stage IIIb	17%

cervical cytologic findings difficult to evaluate. This is especially true immediately following completion of radiation therapy. Suit, using mammary carcinomas in C3H mice, demonstrated that persistence of histologically intact cancer cells in irradiated tissue was not indicative of the regrowth of a tumor. Radiobiologically, a viable cell is one with the capacity for sustained proliferation. A cell would be classified as nonviable if it had lost its reproductive integrity, although it could carry out diverse metabolic activities. This reproductive integrity was demonstrated by the transplantation "take" rate when histologically viable tumor cells were transplanted into a suitable recipient. It was evident from these experiments in mice that relatively normal-appearing cancer cells can persist for several months following radiation therapy but that these cells are "biologically doomed." Thus cytologic evaluation of a patient immediately after radiation therapy may erroneously lead to the supposition that persistent disease exists. In addition, subsequent evaluation of the irradiated cervix is difficult because of the distortion produced in the exfoliated cells, often called radiation effect. Thus histologic confirmation of recurrent cancer is essential. This can be accomplished by punch or needle biopsy of suspected areas of malignancy when they are accessible. An interval of at least 3 months should elapse following completion of radiation therapy. The clinical presentation of recurrent cervical cancer is varied and often insidious. Many patients develop a wasting syndrome with severe loss of appetite and gradual weight loss over a period of weeks to months. This is often preceded by a period of general good health following completion of radiation therapy. Because most recurrences of cancer occur within 2 years after therapy, the period of good health rarely lasts more than 1 year before the symptoms of cachexia become evident. Diagnostic evaluation at this time of suspected recurrence may include a chest radiograph and CT scan and complete blood count, blood urea nitrogen, creatinine clearance, and liver function tests.

Autopsy studies of the location of advanced recurrent and persistent disease have been reported (Figures 3-41 and 3-42). After radical hysterectomy, about one fourth of recurrences occur locally in the upper part of the vagina or the area previously occupied by the cervix. The location of recurrence after radiation therapy showed a 27% occurrence in the cervix, uterus, or upper vagina; 6% in the lower two thirds of the vagina; 43% in the parametrial area, including the pelvic wall; 16% distant; and 8% unknown. Often one notes the development of ureteral obstruction in a patient who had a normal urinary tract before therapy. Although ureteral obstruction can be caused by radiation fibrosis, this is relatively rare, and 95% of the obstructions are caused by progressive tumor. Central disease may not be evident, and in the absence of other findings, a patient with ureteral obstruction and a negative evaluation for metastatic disease following therapy should undergo exploratory laparotomy and selected biopsies to confirm the diagnosis of recurrence. Patients with ureteral obstruction in the absence of recurrent malignancy should be considered for urinary diversion or internal antegrade ureteral stents.

The definition of primary healing after radiation therapy is a cervix covered with normal epithelium or an obliteration of the vaginal vault without evidence of ulceration or discharge. On rectovaginal examination, the residual induration is smooth with no nodularity. The cervix is greater than 2.5 cm in width, and there is no evidence of distant metastasis. The definition of persistent disease after radiation therapy is as follows:

1. Evidence of a portion of the tumor that was clinically present before treatment, or
2. Development of a new demonstrable tumor in the pelvis within the treatment period.

The definition of recurrence after radiation therapy is a regrowth of tumor in the pelvis or distally, which is noted after complete healing of the cervix and vagina.

Recurrence after surgery is defined as evidence of a tumor mass after all gross tumor was removed and the margins of the specimen were free of disease. Persistent disease after surgery is defined as persistence of gross tumor in the operative field or local recurrence of tumor within 1 year of initial surgery. A new cancer of the cervix would be a lesion that occurs locally at least 10 years after primary therapy.

The triad of weight loss accompanied by leg edema and pelvic pain is ominous. Leg edema is usually the result of progressive lymphatic obstruction, occlusion of the iliofemoral vein system, or both. The clinician should consider the possibility of thrombophlebitis, but recurrent cancer is more likely. Patients characteristically describe pain that radiates into the upper thigh either to the anterior medial aspect of the thigh or posteriorly into the buttock. Other patients describe pain in the groin or deep-seated central pelvic pain. The appearance of vaginal bleeding or watery, foul vaginal discharge strongly suggests a central recurrence. These lesions are among the more readily detectable recurrent cervical cancers, and histologic confirmation is easily obtained.

Less than 15% of patients with recurrent cervical cancer will develop pulmonary metastasis. When this does occur, patients will complain of cough, hemoptysis, and occasionally chest pain. In many cases, there will be enlargement of supraclavicular lymph nodes, especially on the left side. Needle aspiration of enlarged lymph nodes can be accomplished easily and avoids the necessity for an open biopsy of the area.

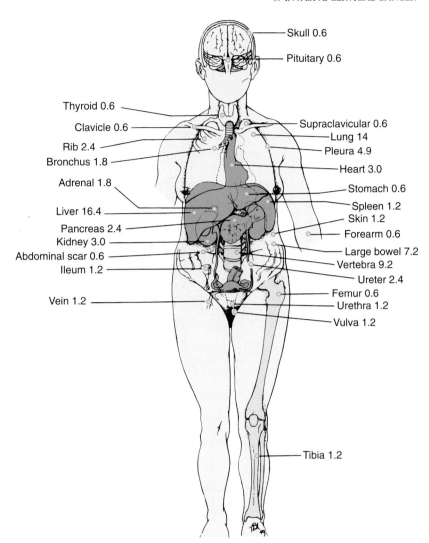

Skull 0.6
Pituitary 0.6
Thyroid 0.6
Clavicle 0.6
Rib 2.4
Bronchus 1.8
Adrenal 1.8
Liver 16.4
Pancreas 2.4
Kidney 3.0
Abdominal scar 0.6
Ileum 1.2
Vein 1.2
Supraclavicular 0.6
Lung 14
Pleura 4.9
Heart 3.0
Stomach 0.6
Spleen 1.2
Skin 1.2
Forearm 0.6
Large bowel 7.2
Vertebra 9.2
Ureter 2.4
Femur 0.6
Urethra 1.2
Vulva 1.2
Tibia 1.2

FIGURE 3-41 Metastatic sites of treated patients with cervical cancer and the percentage of involvement. *(From Henriksen E: Am J Obstet Gynecol 58:924, 1949.)*

In almost every case, the diagnosis of recurrent cervical cancer must be confirmed histologically. CT-directed needle biopsies have provided us with a tool that avoids the necessity of more elaborate operative procedures. In addition to the standard radiographic evaluations, such as IVP and chest radiograph, the clinician may find more sophisticated studies such as lymphangiography and MRI helpful in localizing deep-seated areas of recurrent cervical cancer.

Bony metastases presenting clinically are particularly rare. In a study of 644 patients with invasive cervical carcinoma, Peeples and colleagues were able to find only 29 cases of remote metastases. Of these, 15 were to the lungs and only 12 were to the bone, which is an incidence of 1.8%. No bony metastases were found at initial staging and diagnosis. The earliest discovery of bone metastasis came 8 months after diagnosis. Therefore a bone survey was not recommended as part of the staging examination for cervical cancer.

Blythe and associates reported on 55 patients who were treated for cervical carcinoma and who developed bony metastases. Radiographs were diagnostic in all except 2 of the patients. In 15 patients, a combination of radioactive scans and radiographs was used to establish the diagnosis. The most common mechanism of bony involvement from carcinoma of the cervix was extension of the neoplasia from periaortic nodes, with involvement of the adjacent vertebral bodies. The longest interval from the primary diagnosis until the discovery of bony metastases was 13 years. Of the patients, 69% were diagnosed within 30 months of initial therapy and 96% died within 18 months. Of the 36 patients treated with radiation therapy, 4 received complete relief of symptoms, 24 gained some relief, and 8 received no relief.

Van Herik and colleagues examined the records of 2107 cases of cervical cancer for recurrence after 10 years. Sixteen (0.7%) patients had a recurrence 10 to

FIGURE 3-42   Metastatic sites of untreated patients with cervical cancer and the percentage of involvement. *(From Henriksen E: Am J Obstet Gynecol 58:924, 1949.)*

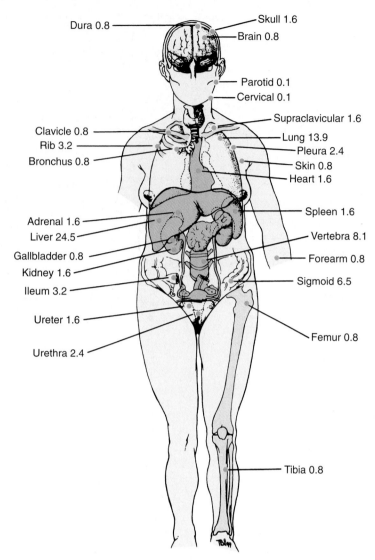

Dura 0.8

Skull 1.6
Brain 0.8

Parotid 0.1
Cervical 0.1

Supraclavicular 1.6

Clavicle 0.8
Rib 3.2
Bronchus 0.8

Lung 13.9
Pleura 2.4
Skin 0.8
Heart 1.6

Spleen 1.6

Adrenal 1.6
Liver 24.5
Gallbladder 0.8
Kidney 1.6
Ileum 3.2

Vertebra 8.1

Forearm 0.8

Sigmoid 6.5

Ureter 1.6

Femur 0.8

Urethra 2.4

Tibia 0.8

26 years after the initial therapy. Of these patients, 25% had bony metastasis or extension of the recurrence into bone. The finding of metastasis after 10 years correlates with the findings of Paunier and associates, who indicated that 92.5% of deaths resulting from carcinoma of the cervix occur in the first 5 years after diagnosis. In addition, their cumulative death rate curve was flat after 10 years.

Deaths resulting from cancer of the cervix occur most frequently in the first year of observation and decrease thereafter. About half of all the deaths occur in the first year after therapy, 25% in the second year, and 15% in the third year, for a total of 85% by the end of the third year. Because more than three-fourths of the recurrences are clinically evident in the first 2 years after initial therapy, post-treatment evaluation done at frequent intervals during this critical period is mandatory. The patient should be examined every 3 to 4

months, and cervical cytologic testing should be done at these visits. In addition, particular attention should be paid to the parametria on rectovaginal examination to detect evidence of progressive disease. For several months after the completion of radiation therapy, the examiner may observe a progressive fibrosis in the parametria, creating the so-called horseshoe fibrosis. The amount of fibrosis may sometimes be alarming, but smoothness of the induration should be reassuring when compared with the nodular presentation of recurrent parametrial malignancy. Parametrial needle biopsies, with the patient under anesthesia, may be helpful when the palpatory findings are equivocal. Generous use of endocervical curettage at these follow-up visits is recommended, especially when central failure is suspected following radiation therapy. Every follow-up examination should include careful palpation of the abdomen for evidence of periaortic enlargement, hepatomegaly, and unexplained masses. Every follow-up examination should begin with a careful palpation of the supraclavicular areas for evidence of nodal enlargement. This frequently omitted portion of the examination will sometimes reveal the only evidence of recurrent disease.

The prognosis for the patient with recurrent or advanced cervical cancer depends on the location of the disease. Of those patients with recurrent cervical cancer, the most favorable for therapy after primary irradiation are those with a central recurrence. These patients are candidates for curative radical pelvic surgery, including pelvic exenteration. There will be further discussion of this group of patients later in this chapter. With the advent of sophisticated methods of radiation therapy, including improved methods of brachytherapy and supervoltage external irradiation therapy, patients with pure central recurrence have become a rarity.

Isolated lung metastases from pelvic malignancies have responded in very selected cases to lobectomy. Gallousis reported metastases to the lung from cervical cancer in 1.5% of 5614 cases reviewed, with solitary nodules present in 25% of the cases. A surgical attack for isolated pulmonary recurrence should be considered, especially if the latent period has been longer than 3 years.

Other patients who deserve serious consideration are those with radiation bowel injury. Over the past decade, the limits of human tolerance to radiation therapy have been reached, with treatment techniques for advanced disease that include large extended fields to the periaortic area. Many patients with advanced-stage primary lesions have been treated with large doses of pelvic radiation (6000-7000 cGy), often following intraabdominal surgery. These techniques, standard radiation therapy can lead to a small but significant number of patients with chronic radiation injury to the large or small bowel. These patients often develop cachexia, which is indistinguishable from the clinical presentation of recurrent and progressive malignancy. These patients are often quickly and superficially diagnosed as having recurrent disease, and no further investigation is initiated. Careful investigation of these patients reveals a history of postprandial crampy abdominal pain causing anorexia and weight loss. The diagnostic evaluations discussed previously reveal no conclusive evidence of persistent malignancy. In most cases, these patients can be returned to health with appropriate bowel surgery, including internal bypass procedures. In every patient suspected of recurrent malignancy, an effort should be made to confirm this suspicion by biopsy (histologic confirmation), and patients who do not have a recurrence and who have radiation bowel injury should be identified.

Management and Prognosis

Persistent or recurrent carcinoma of the cervix is a discouraging clinical entity for the clinician, with a 1-year survival rate between 10% and 15%. Treatment failures are, as expected, much more common in patients with more advanced stages of the disease; therefore, most patients are unlikely candidates for a second curative approach with radical pelvic surgery. Cases of curative therapy applied to isolated lung metastases or lower vaginal recurrences are reported but occur rarely. Unfortunately, most recurrences are suitable for palliative management only.

Surgical Therapy: Radical Hysterectomy

Radical hysterectomy has been reported as therapy for patients with a small recurrent cervical carcinoma following radiation. Coleman's series of 50 patients from the MD Anderson Hospital were treated with radical hysterectomy (type II or III). Severe postoperative complications occurred in 42% of these patients. Of these patients, 28% developed urinary tract injury. Survival was 90% at 5 years for patients with lesions less than 2 cm as opposed to 64% in patients with larger lesions. Excessive morbidity can be limited if an omental pedicle is placed at the operative site at the end of the procedure, bringing in a new blood supply to the operative field that has undergone previous radiation therapy.

Pelvic Exenteration

In 1948 Brunschwig introduced the operation of pelvic exenteration for cancer of the cervix (Figure 3-43). Since then, extensive experience with pelvic exenteration has been accumulated, and the techniques and patient selection have steadily improved so that now, 50 years later, this procedure has attained an important role in the treatment of gynecologic malignancies for a selected group of patients. It is now accepted as a respectable procedure that can offer life to selected patients when no other possibility of cure exists. The criticism of this procedure has been lessened by steadily improving mortality and morbidity and a gratifying 5-year survival record. Most important, however, is that patients who survive this procedure can be rehabilitated to a useful and healthful existence.

Although pelvic exenteration has been used for various pelvic malignancies, its greatest and most important role is in the treatment of advanced or recurrent carcinoma of the cervix. Total exenteration (Figure 3-44) with removal of the pelvic viscera, including the bladder and rectosigmoid, is the procedure of choice for carcinoma of the cervix recurrent or persistent within the pelvis after irradiation. In select cases, the procedure may be limited to anterior exenteration (Figure 3-45)

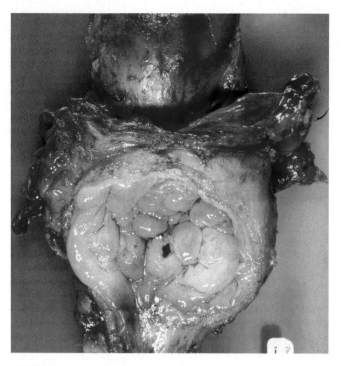

FIGURE 3-43 Specimen from an anterior exenteration done for recurrent cervical carcinoma; the specimen consists of the uterus, vagina, and bladder (the anterior wall has been opened to expose bullous edema of the trigone).

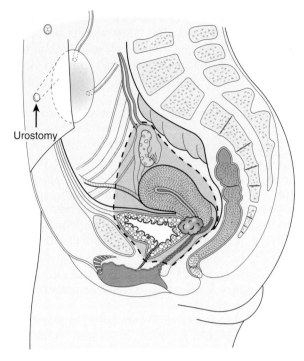

Shaded tissue within the *dashed outline* is permanently removed.

FIGURE 3-45 Anterior exenteration with removal of all pelvic viscera except the rectosigmoid. The urinary stream is diverted into an ileal or sigmoid conduit or a continent pouch. *(Redrawn from DiSaia PJ et al: Calif Med 118:13, 1973.)*

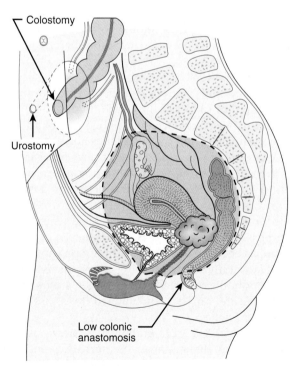

Shaded tissue within the dashed outline is permanently removed. Unshaded tissue within the dashed outline is first removed and then reconstructed.

FIGURE 3-44 Total exenteration with removal of all pelvic viscera. Fecal stream is diverted via a colostomy, and urinary diversion is via an ileal or sigmoid conduit or a continent pouch. *(Redrawn from DiSaia PJ et al: Calif Med 118:13, 1973.)*

with removal of the bladder and preservation of the rectosigmoid or posterior exenteration (Figure 3-46) with removal of the rectosigmoid and preservation of the bladder. Cogent objections have been raised regarding these limited operations, especially in patients with carcinoma of the cervix recurrent after irradiation, because of the increased risk of an incomplete resection. In addition, those patients in whom the bladder or rectum is preserved often have multiple complications and malfunctioning of the preserved organ. Consequently, some surgeons have completely abandoned subtotal exenterations, and most oncologists use them very selectively.

One of the greatest technical advances in the evolution of pelvic exenteration is the intestinal conduit for diversion of the urinary stream. Originally, Brunschwig transplanted the ureters into the left colon just proximal to the colostomy, thus creating the so-called wet colostomy. The complication rate from this procedure, especially electrolyte imbalance and severe urinary tract infections, was unacceptable. Bricker popularized the use of an ileal segment conduit for urinary diversion. The incidence of both postoperative pyelonephritis and hypochloremic acidosis has been greatly reduced. Furthermore, the patients are dry and comfortable and

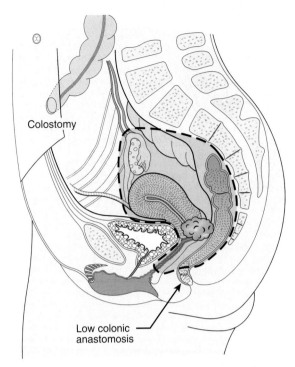

Colostomy

Low colonic
anastomosis

Shaded tissue within the *dashed outline* is permanently
removed. Unshaded tissue within the *dashed outline* is first
removed and then reconstructed.

FIGURE 3-46 Posterior exenteration with removal of all pelvic
viscera except the bladder. The fecal stream is diverted via a colostomy.
(*Redrawn from DiSaia PJ et al: Calif Med 118:13, 1973.*)

therefore more easily rehabilitated. More recent developments have resulted in several techniques for creation of a continent reservoir, again utilizing a segment of bowel (Figure 3-47). Another significant advancement in surgical technique of these patients is the use of the intestinal stapling device. Whereas a permanent colostomy was a standard part of the exenterative procedure, today, it is rare. In many, if not most, cases, reanastomosis with the end-to-end anastomosis stapler can be performed and the fecal stream continues through the anus.

Patient Selection

Only a few patients with recurrent cancer of the cervix are suitable for this operation (Table 3-26). Metastases outside the pelvis, whether manifested preoperatively or discovered at laparotomy, are an absolute contraindication to pelvic exenteration. The triad of unilateral leg edema, sciatic pain, and ureteral obstruction is pathognomonic of recurrent and unresectable disease in the pelvis. The triad must be complete, however, to be entirely reliable. Weight loss, cough, anemia, and other aberrations suggestive of advanced disease are not sufficient justification by themselves to discontinue efforts toward surgical management. Obesity, advanced age, and systemic disease may interdict extensive surgery in direct relation to the severity of these factors. Some patients are unsuitable because of psychological reasons, and a number of women who are otherwise candidates

TABLE 3-26   Survival Following Pelvic Exenteration

Author	Institution	Patients Treated	Operative Deaths (%)	No. Surviving 5 Years* (%)
Douglas and Sweeney (1975)	New York Hospital	23	1 (4.3)	5 (22)
Parsons and Friedell (1964)	Harvard University	112	24 (21.4)	24 (21.4)
Brunschwig (1965)	Memorial Hospital	535	86 (16)	108 (20.1)
Bricker (1967)	Washington University	153	15 (10)	53 (34.6)
Krieger and Embree (1969)	Cleveland Clinics	35	4 (11)	13 (37)
Ketcham et al (1975)	National Cancer Institute	162	12 (7.4)	62 (38.2)
Symmonds et al (1975)	Mayo Clinic	198	16 (8)	64 (32.3)
Morley and Lindenauer (1976)	University of Michigan	34	1 (2.9)	21 (62)
Rutledge et al (1977)	MD Anderson Hospital	296	40 (13.5)	99 (33.4)
Averette et al (1984)	University of Miami			
1966-1971		14	4 (28.5)	5 (36)
1971-1976		45	15 (33.3)	10 (22)
1976-1981		33	4 (12.1)	19 (58)
		65	6 (9.2)	15 (23)
Lawhead (1989)	Memorial Hospital	65	6 (9.2)	15 (23)
	1972-1981			
Soper et al (1989)	Duke University	69	5 (7.2)	28 (4.5)
Shingleton et al (1989)	University of Alabama	143	9 (6.3)	71 (50)
Sharma et al (2005)	Roswell Park Cancer Institute	48	2 (4.2)	16 (33)
Fotopoulou et al (2010)	Virchow University Hospital Berlin	47†	4 (8.5)	25 (53.2)‡
Total		2012	248 (12.3)	663 (33.7)

*In almost every series, the operative death rate and the 5-year survival rate improved dramatically in the later years of each series.
†Includes eight vaginal cancers.
‡Five-year survival not reached and therefore not included in the total.

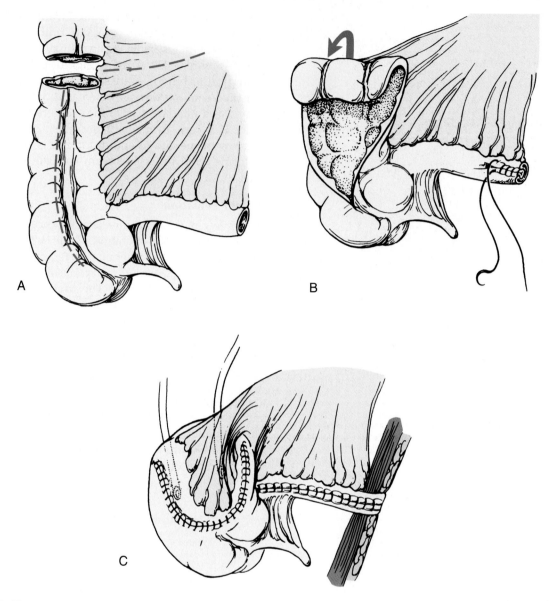

FIGURE 3-47   A–C, Construction of an Indiana pouch from the colon and the terminal ileum. *(From: Amis ES et al: Radiology 168:395, 1988.)*

for pelvic exenteration elect to accept the fate of unresected recurrence. If the time from primary treatment to recurrence is short (<2 years), this usually indicates aggressive biologic activity of the tumor and resectability is usually limited.

Evaluation studies before surgery include chest film, CT scan of the abdomen and pelvis with intravenous contrast, creatinine clearance, liver function tests, and assessment of the patient's hemostatic mechanism. Any suspected disease outside the pelvis noted on any of the diagnostic studies should prompt an attempt at confirmation using a fine needle biopsy technique. Bone survey and liver scan are not part of the "routine" evaluation.

Preparation for pelvic exenteration is often traumatic to patients with recurrent cervical cancer, especially when the procedure is aborted. The increased use of CT-directed fine-needle aspirants has contributed greatly to lowering the fraction of patients explored who are found to be unexenterable. At laparotomy, the entire abdomen and pelvis are explored for evidence of metastatic and intraperitoneal cancer (Figure 3-48). The liver should be carefully inspected visually and by palpation. The lymph nodes surrounding the lower aorta are the first to be sampled if the exploration of the abdomen has revealed no evidence of disease. If the lower aortic area findings are negative, a bilateral pelvic lymphadenectomy is performed.

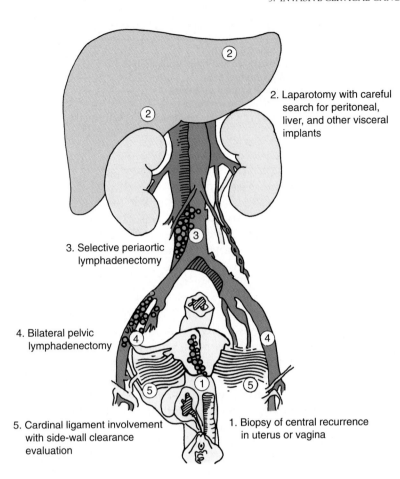

FIGURE 3-48 Steps in evaluation of a patient for an exenterative procedure. *(Courtesy A. Robert Kagan, MD, Los Angeles, California.)*

2. Laparotomy with careful search for peritoneal, liver, and other visceral implants

3. Selective periaortic lymphadenectomy

4. Bilateral pelvic lymphadenectomy

5. Cardinal ligament involvement with side-wall clearance evaluation

1. Biopsy of central recurrence in uterus or vagina

Morbidity and Mortality

Most of the morbidity and mortality directly related to exenteration occur within the first 18 months following the procedure. Many of the complications can be sequelae to any major surgery. These include cardiopulmonary catastrophes such as pulmonary embolism, pulmonary edema, myocardial infarction, and cerebrovascular accidents. The length of these surgical procedures and the magnitude of blood loss definitely increase the incidence of cardiovascular complications. This category of complications usually occurs within the first week after the procedure. Thezn there is a period when sepsis is the greatest threat to the patient's health and life. This sepsis usually originates in the pelvic cavity with occurrence of a pelvic abscess or, more commonly, diffuse pelvic cellulitis.

One of the most serious postoperative complications of exenteration is small-bowel obstruction related to the denuded pelvic floor. In the past decade, several techniques have been used in an effort to avoid the adherence of small bowel to this large raw surface, including mobilization of omentum (Figure 3-49) or abdominal wall peritoneum to cover the pelvic floor (Figure 3-50). When small-bowel obstruction does occur,

it is appropriately treated with conservative therapy. However, half these patients come to reoperation, and the mortality of this group is approximately 50% in some series. The risk of bowel obstruction is increased by the presence of pelvic infection. Both conditions predispose to the development of small-bowel fistulas, which always require reoperation and frequently are fatal. In general, complications are more common in patients who have recurrence after radiation therapy. Irradiated tissue is less likely to produce good wound healing, and the formation of granulation tissue is severely retarded.

The long-term morbidity from exenteration is predominantly related to urinary diversion. Once the period of susceptibility to sepsis has passed, urinary obstruction and infection become the major non-neoplastic life-threatening complications. Pyelonephritis is common and should be treated promptly and vigorously. Periodic IVPs can be obtained to assess the collecting system for hydronephrosis. A mild degree of obstruction is frequently retained following construction of an ileal conduit, but progressive hydronephrosis will require correction to salvage renal function. The incidence of complications appeared to be less in patients in whom

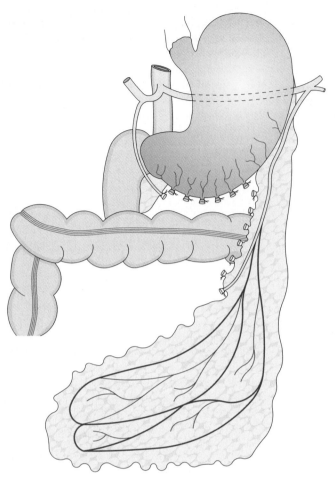

FIGURE 3-49 The omentum has been detached from the right transverse colon and the greater curvature of the stomach, keeping the left gastroepiploic vessels intact and creating a large "tongue of omentum" to cover the pelvic floor.

TABLE 3-27 Signs and Symptoms of Recurrent Cervical Cancer

Weight loss (unexplained)
Leg edema (excessive and often unilateral)
Pelvic or thigh–buttock pain
Serosanguineous vaginal discharge
Progressive ureteral obstruction
Supraclavicular lymph node enlargement (usually on the left side)
Cough
Hemoptysis
Chest pain

in the twenty-first century was comparable in both countries, with centrally recurrent cervical cancer or persistent tumor after chemoradiation being the main indication. PET-CT is more commonly used in the United States, whereas MRI is the preferred tool in Germany. Surgical staging is more commonly performed in the United States (61% vs 32%). Exenteration for FIGO stage IVA disease was more commonly recommended in Germany (43% vs 0%), as was the operation in the setting of fistulae involving the bladder or rectum (61% vs 29%). In Germany, interdisciplinarity with general surgeons, urologists, plastic surgeons, and radiation oncologists is more common. Although there is a consensus to administer adjuvant therapy after exenteration for patients with positive margins and/or positive lymph nodes, adjuvant therapy is more frequently recommended in Germany (93%) than in the United States (74%).

In 2010 Spahn and colleagues reported the results of 37 anterior pelvic exenterations and 6 total pelvic exenterations performed at the University of Wurzburg in Germany. A continent urinary diversion was constructed in 16 and an ileal conduit was constructed in 27. Continent urinary diversion was not associated with higher complication rates than ileal conduit formation. The overall disease-specific 5-year survival rate was 36.5%. Survival correlated significantly with surgical margin status.

For vaginal reconstruction, vascularized muscle flaps are preferred to fill the empty pelvis, and developments in bioengineering tissue are likely to have applications in neovaginal creation. De la Garza and colleagues reported the successful performance of a total pelvic exenteration with a split-thickness skin graft neovagina, continent orthotopic neobladder, and rectal anastomosis, resulting in no external ostomies and adequate sexual function.

Radiation

With recurrent disease outside the initial treatment field, irradiation is frequently successful in providing local control and symptomatic relief. External irradiation in

an unirradiated portion of bowel had been used for construction of the conduit.

Survival Results

The 5-year cumulative survival rate after pelvic exenteration varies in the literature from 20% to 62% (Table 3-27). Reported survival rates depend greatly on the circumstances of patient selection for exenteration. Cumulative survival rates are always improved when no patient is exenterated who has a positive pelvic node following pelvic irradiation. In general, however, both morbidity and mortality and the 5-year survival rate have improved steadily over the past two decades. Mortality in most centers is now well below 5%, and morbidity has been similarly lowered.

In 2009, 60 years following the first description of pelvic exenteration, Marnitz and colleagues surveyed and compared practice patterns in the United States and Germany. The number of exenterations performed

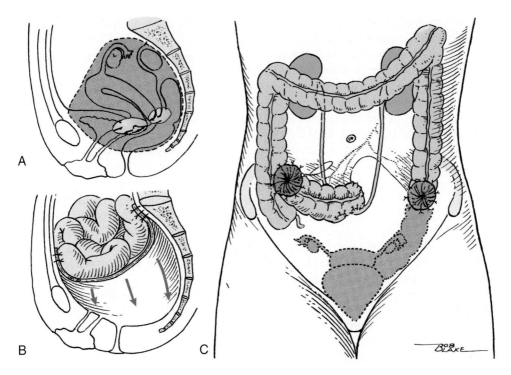

FIGURE 3-50 **A,** Lateral view of recurrent cancer involving the cervix and upper vagina with extension into the bladder and rectum. The stippled area indicates tissue to be removed by exenteration. **B,** A lateral view after pelvic viscera have been removed. The omental "carpet" is used to keep the intestines out of the pelvis during immediate postoperative period. With time, the omental "carpet" will descend into the pelvis and the "carpet" will adhere to the pelvic floor. **C,** Urinary conduit and colostomy diversion after exenteration. *Dotted areas* of the sigmoid, bladder, and internal genitalia have been removed.

moderate and easily delivered doses is usually effective in relieving pain from bone metastases. A dose of 3000 cGy delivered over 2 to 3 weeks is often sufficient to relieve pain from vertebral column or long-bone metastases.

Höckel and associates reported their experience with a combined operative and radiotherapy (CORT) for recurrent tumors infiltrating the pelvic wall. Although the combination therapy is not new, these authors surgically remove the recurrence more radically than previously reported. The bony pelvis and neurovascular support of the leg is preserved. Implantation of guide tubes, which exit from the skin for brachytherapy, is done after resection of the tumor. Considerable pelvic reconstruction is usually done. Although the indications and procedure are evolving, in the first 48 patients treated, survival probabilities are 50% and 44% after 3 and 5 years, respectively.

Reirradiation of pelvic recurrences of cervical cancer occurring within the previously treated field is a subject of some controversy. The results following reirradiation of patients with recurrent cervical malignancy have varied considerably. Truelsen reported a 3-year cure rate of 1.7%. Murphy and Schmitz reported a 9% salvage rate in 1956, and Nolan and associates reported on the use of 60Co teleradiation with a 25% salvage rate. At the Roswell Park Memorial Institute, Murphy and Schmitz adopted the policy of reirradiating patients with recurrence, delivering a full or almost full course for a second time. Among the highly selected series of 46 patients, 9% to 10% were living and well at the end of 5 years. Only 7 patients had biopsy-proven recurrences before treatment. Others have shown that the results of reirradiation depend on many factors, including the site of recurrence, initial clinical stage, and initial dose of radiation therapy.

Careful perusal of these reports suggests that most patients who benefited from reirradiation were those who received less than optimal radiation during initial therapy. This set of circumstances has become rare in recent times, when more sophisticated radiotherapy is being delivered in many areas of the United States. Therefore, reirradiation for recurrent disease is usually not a worthwhile consideration. The potential for necrosis and fistula formation with even moderate doses of reirradiation in the pelvis by external or interstitial sources can give very unfavorable results.

Recurrence after radical hysterectomy has been treated with radiation. In a study from Holland, 271 patients were treated with radical hysterectomy and 27 recurred with 14 limited to the pelvis. Of note, adjuvant radiotherapy had been administered in 14 (52%)

of the 27. In the 4 patients with isolated pelvic recurrence, only 1 died of disease, whereas all of the other patients with recurrences died of disease. The survivors were treated with radiation. In a study from the MD Anderson Cancer Center, 50 patients had recurrence after radical hysterectomy and were treated with radiation. Overall survival was 33%. In the 16 patients with central disease, 12 (69%) remained disease free. Survival of 29 patients with squamous carcinoma was 51% compared with 14% for the 14 patients with adenocarcinoma ($P = 0.05$).

Chemotherapy

The management of disseminated cervical cancer has improved with the development of modern chemotherapy. Figure 3-16 reviews the treatment of advanced or recurrent disease. Because concurrent platinum-based chemoradiation has become the standard of care for locally advanced disease, many recurrent tumors may therefore be platinum resistant. The GOG has completed eight multicenter, phase III randomized trials to study platinum-based therapies for recurrent and/or metastatic disease (Table 3-28). Drug discovery for the most part has fed into these phase III trial designs through the GOG's phase II series dedicated to exploring the activity and tolerability of cytotoxic compounds in cervical cancer.

The early trials of the GOG for recurrent and metastatic cervical carcinoma were designed to evaluate cisplatin dosing, schedules, and analogs. The next two trials evaluated the addition of ifosfamide, bleomycin, and mitolactol to cisplatin-based therapies. Among some of the lessons learned during the 1980s and 1990s governing chemotherapy for recurrent cervical cancer were that platinum-based therapies were most effective and that cisplatin was more active than carboplatin (19% vs 15%, respectively). Two ways through which the RR could be increased without prolongation in survival included increasing the platinum dose and/or adding ifosfamide to cisplatin. As a consequence of these first five phase III randomized clinical trials, single-agent cisplatin at 50 mg/m² emerged as the standard for recurrent disease, with a documented 19% RR on a 21-day schedule.

The combined regimen of cisplatin in combination with paclitaxel in GOG 169 yielded an impressive 36% RR, improvement in PFS, but no significant impact on OS when compared to single-agent cisplatin. The next trial, GOG 179, compared single agent cisplatin to cisplatin plus topotecan. The improvements observed in RR, PFS, and OS all favored the combined regimen, leading to FDA approval of the cisplatin 50 mg/m² plus topotecan 1.75 mg/m² days 1 to 3 in this population. In both GOG 169 and GOG 179, RRs were decreased in patients who had received prior platinum (Table 3-29). Because

TABLE 3-28 GOG Trials ×8

GOG protocol	Study Chair	Year	Arms	N	Objective Response			Median Duration of Response (mo)	Median PFS (mo)
					PR %	CR %	Overall %		
43	Bonomi et al	1985	Cisplatin 50 mg/m² IV q21d	150	10.7	10	20.7	4.9	7.1
			Cisplatin 100 mg/m² IV q21d	166	18.7	12.7	31.4	4.1	7
			Cisplatin 20 mg/m² IV × 5d q21d	128	16.4	8.6	25	4.8	6.1

GOG protocol	Study Chair	Year	Arms	N	PR %	CR %	Overall %	)	Median Survival (mo)
64	Thigpen et al	1989	Cisplatin 50 mg/m² 24 h cont inf	156	12	6	18	5.5	6.4
			Cisplatin 1 mg/min rapid inf	164	11	6	17	4.5	6.2

GOG protocol	Study Chair	Year	Arms	N	PR %	CR %	Overall %	Median PFI (mo)	Median Survival (mo)
77	McGuire et al	1989	Carboplatin 340-400 mg/m² IV q28d	175	9.7	5.7	15.4	2.7	6.2
			Iproplatin 230-270 mg/m² IV q28d	177	6.8	4	10.8	3	5.5

Continued

TABLE 3-28 GOG Trials ×8—cont'd

GOG protocol	Study Chair	Year	Arms	N	Objective Response			Median Duration of Response (mo)	Median PFS (mo)
					PR %	CR %	Overall %		
								Median PFS (mo)	Median Survival (mo)
110	Omura et al	1997	Cisplatin 50 mg/m² IV q21d	140	11.4	6.4	17.8	3.2	8
				147	11.6	9.5	21.1	3.3	7.3
			Cisplatin 50 mg/m² IV + mitolactol180 mg/m² po days 2, 6 q21d	151	18.5	12.6	31.1 *P* = 0.004	4.6 *P* = 0.003	8.3
			Cisplatin 50 mg/m² IV + ifosfamide 5 g/m² 24 h inf + MESNA 6 g/m² q21d						
									Median Survival (mo)
149	Bloss et al	2002	Cisplatin 50 mg/m² IV + ifosfamide 5 g/m² 24 hr inf + MESNA 6 g/m² q21d	146	NS	NS	32.2	4.6	8.5
				141	NS	NS	32.1	5.1	8.4
			Bleomycin 30 units 24-h inf followed by cisplatin 50 mg/m² IV + ifosfamide 5 g/m² 24 h inf + MESNA 6 g/m² q21d						
									Median Survival (mo)
169	Moore et al	2004	Cisplatin 50 mg/m² IV q21d	134	13	6	19	2.8	8.8
			Paclitaxel 135 mg/m² 24 h inf + cisplatin 50 mg/m² IV q21d	130	21	15	36 *P* = 0.002	4.8 *P* <0.001	9.7
									Median Survival (mo)
179	Long et al	2005	Cisplatin 50 mg/m² IV q21d	145	10	13	13	2.9	6.5
			Topotecan 0.75 mg/m² days 1-3 + cisplatin 50 mg/m² IV q21d	148	16	10	26 *P* = 0.004	4.6 *P* = 0.014	9.4 *P* = 0.017
			MVAC q4 wk	63	9	13	22	4.4	9.4
									Median OS (mo)
204	Monk et al	2009	Paclitaxel 135 mg/m² 24 h inf + cisplatin 50 mg/m² q21d	103	26.2	2.9	29.1	5.82	12.87
			Vinorelbine 30 mg/m² days 1 and 8 + cisplatin 50 mg/m² q21d	108	18.5	7.4	25.9	3.98	9.99
			Gemcitabine 1000 mg/m² days 1 and 8 + cisplatin 50 mg/m² q21d	112	21.4	0.9	22.3	4.7	10.28
			Topotecan 0.75 mg/m² days 1-3 + cisplatin 50 mg/m² q21d	111	21.6	1.8	23.4	4.57	10.25

GOG 179 was conducted during the era of chemoradiation and GOG 169 was under way before the adoption of multimodality therapy, 57% of patients on GOG 179 received radiosensitizing platinum compared to 27% on GOG 169.

GOG 204 compared four platinum-based doublets using paclitaxel, topotecan, gemcitabine, and vinorelbine. Because this study was activated before the data from GOG 179 were mature, cisplatin plus paclitaxel was selected as the control arm, primarily because of the 36% RR observed in GOG 169. None of the experimental arms outperformed the reference arm (Table 3-30 and Figure 3-51). For this reason, cisplatin plus paclitaxel has been selected as the control arm for the succeeding trial, which was activated in April 2009 (GOG 240).

In GOG 240 the experimental arms are designed to answer two critical questions. The first is a chemotherapy question and concerns whether nonplatinum agents would have greater activity in the recurrent setting given the increased usage of platinum-based chemoradiation initially for locally advanced cancers. Two phase II

experiences using nonplatinum doublets have been described. In the United Kingdom the Scotcerv trial piloted gemcitabine plus taxotere, which, when presented at ASCO, was not deemed to be suitable for further development. Tiersten and colleagues reported on their experience with the nonplatinum doublet topotecan plus paclitaxel. It is important to note that the regimen was active in previously irradiated patients (RR 26%) with acceptable toxicities. The laboratory work by Bahadori and colleagues demonstrating synergy between paclitaxel and microtubule-inhibiting agents (e.g., topotecan or vinorelbine) underscored this regimen's potential.[12] This nonplatinum doublet is being studied by the Arbeitsgemeinschaft Gynakologische Onkologie (AGO).

The second question to be addressed by GOG 240 involves targeted therapy. Tumor angiogenesis as measured by microvessel quantification has been shown to be a prognostic factor in cervical cancer. A small case series by Wright and colleagues described the

TABLE 3-29 Association of Prior Platinum Exposure with Response Rates in GOG 169 and GOG 179

GOG 179	No Prior Cisplatin (%)	Prior Cisplatin (57% of Patients) (%)
Cisplatin	20	8
Cisplatin + topotecan	39	15

GOG 169	No Prior Cisplatin	Prior Cisplatin (27% of Patients)
Cisplatin	26	5
Cisplatin + topotecan	37	32

TABLE 3-30 Objective Response by Treatment Regimen in GOG 204

Tumor Response	Cis + Pac (%)	Cis + Vin (%)	Cis + Gem (%)	Cis + Topo (%)	Total
CR	3 (2.9)	8 (7.4)	1 (0.9)	2 (1.8)	14
PR	27 (26.2)	20 (18.5)	24 (21.4)	24 (21.6)	95
SD	50 (48.4)	46 (42.6)	54 (48.2)	53 (47.8)	203
PD	23 (22.3)	34 (31.5)	33 (29.5)	32 (28.8)	122
Odds ratio*	—	1.17	1.43	1.34	
95% CI	—	0.54, 2.58	0.65, 3.19	0.61, 2.98	

Modified from Monk BJ et al: J Clin Oncol 27:4649, 2009.
*Odds ratios for response are provided for the reference arm, Cis + Pac, to the experimental therapies.
Cis + Pac, Cisplatin plus paclitaxel; Cis + Vin, cisplatin plus vinorelbine; Cis + Gem, cisplatin plus gemcitabine; Cis + Top, cisplatin plus topotecan.

FIGURE 3-51 GOG 204 survival curve. (*From Monk BJ et al: J Clin Oncol 27:4649, 2009.*)

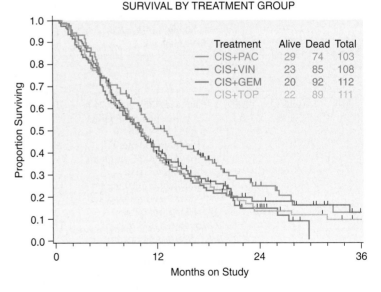

SURVIVAL BY TREATMENT GROUP

Treatment	Alive	Dead	Total
CIS+PAC	29	74	103
CIS+VIN	23	85	108
CIS+GEM	20	92	112
CIS+TOP	22	89	111

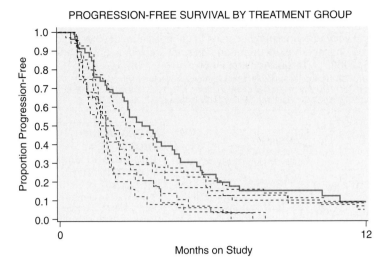

PROGRESSION-FREE SURVIVAL BY TREATMENT GROUP

Months on Study

FIGURE 3-52 GOG 227C Bevacizumab RRs. *(From Monk BJ et al: J Clin Oncol 27:1069, 2009.)*

successful combination of bevacizumab with cytotoxic agents in the recurrent and metastatic setting among previously irradiated patients. Of note, the antiangiogenesis agent bevacuzmab in combination with chemotherapy has been FDA approved for locally advanced and recurrent breast cancer, first-line and second-line therapy for metastatic colorectal cancer, and untreated non–small cell lung cancer (NSCLC). The drug is currently being studied by the GOG in primary advanced and platinum-sensitive recurrent ovarian carcinoma. A phase II evaluation of bevacizumab at 15 mg/kg q21 days was undertaken within the GOG (protocol 227C). The 26% RR of bevacizumab among previously irradiated patients was among the highest RRs noted within the GOG's phase II experience for recurrent cervical cancer (Figure 3-52).

Given the potential shared tumor biology between NSCLC and cervical cancer, the activity of platinum plus paclitaxel with bevacizumab in NSCLC supports the inclusion of this regimen as one of the experimental arms in GOG 240. Assuming no interaction between the nonplatinum doublet and bevacizumab, a 2 × 2 factorial design has been selected to answer both the chemotherapy question and the biologic/antivascular question. The schema for GOG 240 appears in Figure 3-53. This study will also prospectively validate important prognostic factors—including African-American race, performance status greater than 0, pelvic disease, prior radiosensitizer, and time interval from diagnosis to first recurrence less than 1 year—that have been recently reported by Moore and colleagues in a multivariate pooled analysis of three prior phase III studies in this population (Table 3-31).

We are seeing increasing evidence that therapy for metastatic cervical carcinoma does not need to be solely palliative. Qui and colleagues reported in 2007 on long-term survivors who presented with supraclavicular

TABLE 3-31 Multivariate Analysis of Prognostic Factors of Treatment Response in Recurrent, Persistent, and Metastatic Cervical Carcinoma

	OR	95% CI	P Value
Race: Black vs nonblack	0.49	0.28-0.83	0.008
GOG performance 1 or 2 vs 0	0.60	0.38-0.94	0.027
Site of disease: Pelvic vs nonpelvic	0.58	0.38-0.90	0.015
Radiosensitizer: Yes vs no	0.52	0.32-0.85	0.009
First recurrence within 1 year of diagnosis: Yes vs no	0.61	0.39-0.95	0.027

From Moore DH et al: Gynecol Oncol 116:44, 2010.
Odds ratio (OR) in favor of treatment response estimated from logistic regression model, adjusted for covariates.

metastases. Additionally, in 2009 Takano and colleagues reported complete remissions in two patients with metastatic and recurrent cervical cancer. Before recurrence, one patient had received chemoradiation for locally advanced disease and the other had been treated with adjuvant pelvic radiation following hysterectomy. Of note, both of these patients were treated with weekly paclitaxel (80 mg/m^2) plus carboplatin (AUC 2.0) (days 1, 8, 15) and weekly bevacizumab (days 1, 8, 15, 21). Notwithstanding significant unanticipated toxicities, the ongoing trials of the AGO, JCOG, and GOG have been positioned to further refine therapeutic options for this disease.

Targeted Therapies

Angiogenesis Inhibitors

As discussed earlier, biologic therapy in the form of angiogenesis inhibitors may be useful in retarding tumor growth and progression and even eliminating small-volume residual disease. Evidence that angiogenesis plays an important role in locally advanced cervical cancer has accumulated in recent years. In one study of 111 patients, Cooper and colleagues identified tumor

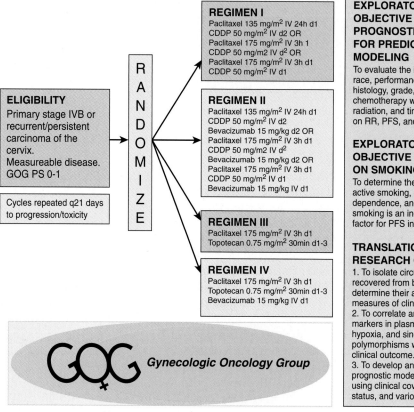

GYNECOLOGIC ONCOLOGY GROUP PROTOCOL 240

A randomized phase III trial of cisplatin plus paclitaxel with and without bevacizumab versus the nonplatinum doublet, topotecan plus paclitaxel, with and without NCI-supplied bevacizumab, in stage IVb, recurrent or persistent carcinoma of the cervix.

Activation Date – April 6, 2009   Target Accrual = 450

Study Chair: Krishnansu S. Tewari, MD (ktewari@uci.edu) Statistician: Michael Sill, PhD Pathologist: Helen Michael, MD
Co-Chairs: Harry J. Long, MD (Medical Oncology), Richard T. Penson, MD (Quality of Life), Michael J. Birrer, MD, PhD (Translational Research)
Scientific Collaborations: Steven Waggoner, MD. David H. Moore, MD. Kathleen M. Darcy, PhD, Bradley J. Monk, MD

PRIMARY OBJECTIVES
1. To determine whether the addition of bevacizumab to chemotherapy improves overall survival.
2. To determine whether the non-platinum chemotherapy doublet consisting of topotecan plus paclitaxel improves overall survival in comparison to the regimen involving cisplatin plus paclitaxel.
3. To determine the frequency and severity of adverse events as assessed by CTCAE version 3.0 for the regimens administered.

SECONDARY OBJECTIVES
1. To estimate and compare the progression-free survival of patients treated by the regimens investigated on this study.
2. To estimate and compare the proportion of patients with tumor responses by the regimens investigated on this study.

HEALTH-RELATED QUALITY OF LIFE OBJECTIVES
To determine whether the addition of bevacizumab to chemotherapy, or the substitution of cisplatin with topotecan improves the health-related QOL as measured by the FACT-Cx TOI and produces favorable toxicity profiles.

ELIGIBILITY
Primary stage IVB or recurrent/persistent carcinoma of the cervix. Measureable disease. GOG PS 0-1

Cycles repeated q21 days to progression/toxicity

R A N D O M I Z E

REGIMEN I
Paclitaxel 135 mg/m² IV 24h d1
CDDP 50 mg/m² IV d2 OR
Paclitaxel 175 mg/m² IV 3h 1
CDDP 50 mg/m2 IV d² OR
Paclitaxel 175 mg/m² IV 3h d1
CDDP 50 mg/m² IV d1

REGIMEN II
Paclitaxel 135 mg/m² IV 24h d1
CDDP 50 mg/m² IV d2
Bevacizumab 15 mg/kg d2 OR
Paclitaxel 175 mg/m² IV 3h d1
CDDP 50 mg/m2 IV d²
Bevacizumab 15 mg/kg d2 OR
Paclitaxel 175 mg/m² IV 3h d1
CDDP 50 mg/m² IV d1
Bevacizumab 15 mg/kg IV d1

REGIMEN III
Paclitaxel 175 mg/m² IV 3h d1
Topotecan 0.75 mg/m² 30min d1-3

REGIMEN IV
Paclitaxel 175 mg/m² IV 3h d1
Topotecan 0.75 mg/m² 30min d1-3
Bevacizumab 15 mg/kg IV d1

GOG *Gynecologic Oncology Group*

EXPLORATORY OBJECTIVE A: PROGNOSTIC MARKERS FOR PREDICTIVE MODELING
To evaluate the impact of age, race, performance status, stage, histology, grade, disease site, prior chemotherapy with primary radiation, and time to recurrence on RR, PFS, and OS.

EXPLORATORY OBJECTIVE B: IMPACT ON SMOKING
To determine the prevalence of active smoking, extent of nicotine dependence, and to determine if smoking is an independent risk factor for PFS in this cohort.

TRANSLATIONAL RESEARCH OBJECTIVES
1. To isolate circulating tumor cells recovered from blood and determine their association to measures of clinical outcome.
2. To correlate angiogenesis markers in plasma, biomarkers of hypoxia, and single nucleotide polymorphisms with measures of clinical outcome.
3. To develop an optimal prognostic model for PFS and OS using clinical covaniates, smoking status, and various biomarkers.

US NIH, 2010.

FIGURE 3-53   GOG 240 schema.

angiogenesis (as reflected by the tumor microvessel density, MVD) as a significant prognostic factor within a Cox multivariate analysis, where it was associated with poor locoregional control and overall survival. Conversely, among 166 women who underwent radical hysterectomy for stage Ib tumors, Obermair and colleagues demonstrated enhanced 5-year survivorship when the MVD was <20 per high power field (HPF) (90% vs 63% with MVD >20 HPF). The vascular endothelial growth factor (VEGF) receptor expression has also been shown to correlate with MVD in cervical carcinomas.

Several small-molecule inhibitors are actively being studied in cervical cancer, although none of these agents is currently approved in cervical cancer. Pazopanib is an oral tyrosine kinase inhibitor with antiangiogenic activity. It targets VEGFR, PDGFR, and c-Kit. Another oral tyrosine kinase inhibitor, lapatinib, targets EGFR

and HER2. Given existing evidence supporting a role for angiogenesis in cervical cancer and the observation that overexpression of EGFR correlates with poor outcome in this disease, Monk and colleagues studied these drugs in 230 patients with measurable stage IVB persistent/recurrent cervical carcinoma not amenable to curative therapy and at least one prior regimen. The randomization scheme included pazopanib 800 mg daily ($n = 74$) vs lapatinib 1500 mg daily ($n = 78$) vs pazopanib 400 mg daily plus lapatinib 1000 mg daily ($n = 78$). The futility boundary was crossed for the combined regimen at the planned interim analysis and this arm was discontinued, leaving a total of 152 patients in the monotherapy arms. Pazopanib improved PFS (HR = 0.66; 90% CI 0.48, 0.91 $P = 0.013$) and OS (HR = 0.67; 90% CI 0.46, 0.99 $P = 0.045$; median OS for P is 50.7 weeks; L is 39.1 weeks) with RR for pazopanib of 9% and that of lapatinib of 5%. Pazopanib was generally well tolerated, with the most common grade III adverse effect reported being diarrhea.

Therapeutic HPV Vaccine

Therapeutic vaccines target virus-infected cells using epitopes of major histocompatibility complex (MHC)-processed peptides. Through interaction with CD8+ lymphocytes and MHC I pathways, they engage the cellular machinery, resulting in production of cytotoxic T lymphocytes. The HPV oncoproteins E6 and E7 can be targeted for the development of antigen-specific vaccination. Molecular strategies to design a therapeutic vaccine can be based on bacterial or viral vectors, peptides, proteins, DNA, and even dendritic cells. They may be useful in inducing regression and/or halting progression of preinvasive disease and/or eradicating subclinical residual neoplastic disease following therapy.

With respect to prophylactic HPV vaccines, in 2003 the WHO convened a gathering of experts from both developing and developed countries to identify the appropriate end point measurements for HPV vaccine efficacy. The general consensus was that it would be desirable to have a globally agreed, measurable efficacy end point for considering deployment of HPV vaccines in public health settings. Because of the temporal lag between infection and the manifestation of invasive carcinoma, it was determined that a surrogate end point would be used to define the efficacy of HPV vaccines. Because persistent infection with the same high-risk HPV subtypes is considered a predictor for both moderate or high-grade cervical dysplasias and invasive cervical cancer, it was determined that CIN, rather than invasive cancer, would serve as the end point following HPV vaccine introduction.

Garcia and colleagues from the University of Arizona conducted a randomized, multicenter, double-blind, placebo-controlled trial in 161 women with biopsy-confirmed CIN II to III. Subjects received three intramuscular doses of placebo or ZYC101a, a vaccine containing plasmid DNA-encoding fragments derived from HPV-16 and -18 E6 and E7 oncoproteins. The vaccine was well tolerated and had demonstrable efficacy in promoting resolution of CIN II to III in women younger than age 25 years. Recently, Einstein and colleagues presented data from their phase II trial using the novel therapeutic vaccine HspE7. The fusion protein consists of an *Mycobacterium bovis* BCG heat shock protein (Hsp65) covalently linked at its C terminus to the entire sequence of HPV-16 E7. With an excellent safety profile on record, 32 HIV-negative women with CIN III were vaccinated. The investigators observed a 48% resolution of CIN III, 19% partial responses, and 33% of subjects with stable disease over a 4-month follow-up period.

For full reference list, log onto www.expertconsult.com ⟨http://www.expertconsult.com⟩

Endometrial Hyperplasia, Estrogen Therapy, and the Prevention of Endometrial Cancer

Lisa M. Landrum, MD, PhD, Rosemary E. Zuna, MD, and Joan L. Walker, MD

The endometrium is a very dynamic tissue in the reproductive-age woman. It is continuously changing in response to hormonal, stromal, and vascular influences, with the intended goal of implanting an embryo and supporting the nutritional needs of the developing pregnancy. Estrogen stimulation is associated with the growth and proliferation of the endometrium (Figure 4-1), whereas progesterone produced by the corpus luteum after ovulation inhibits proliferation and stimulates secretion in the glands and predecidual change in the stroma (Figure 4-2). Without conception and human chorionic gonadotropin (hCG) production, the corpus luteum fails to produce progesterone and hormonal withdrawal allows menses to occur. Continuous estrogen stimulation of the endometrium bypasses the normal recycling of the endometrium. Women have transitions in their lives—such as menopause or anovulation—during which the absence of ovulation predisposes them to unopposed estrogen stimulation because no corpus

luteum forms to secrete progesterone. Menarche and perimenopause are transitions of varying lengths of time, and some women (approximately 5%) have polycystic ovarian disease, which is a prolonged anovulatory condition. Obesity during menopause also produces a state of excess estrogen production. This results from the peripheral conversion, in the adipose tissues, of androgens secreted from the adrenal glands and ovaries into an estrogen, estrone, by the enzyme aromatase.

Unopposed estrogen stimulation will yield a continuous spectrum of change from proliferative endometrium (Figure 4-3) through many variations of endometrial hyperplasia until a malignant neoplasm develops. Endometrial cancer is defined by the ability to invade local tissue and metastasize (Figure 4-4). The fact that endometrial lesions are represented by glandular and stromal variations in continuous change explains the challenge of classifying endometrial hyperplasia into distinct categories, which are reproducible and predict neoplastic

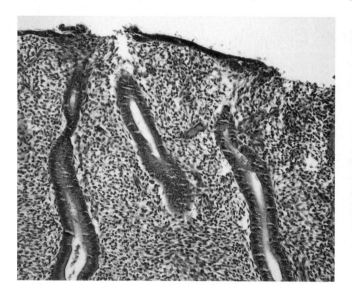

FIGURE 4-1   Proliferative endometrium: Simple tubular endometrial glands are set in a prominent stroma. This pattern is associated with normal estrogen stimulation in a cycling woman. (Hematoxylin and eosin, 10× original magnification.)

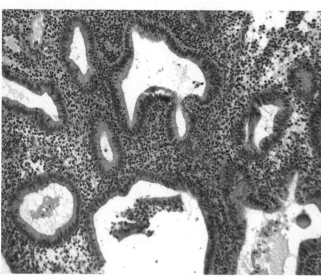

FIGURE 4-3   Simple hyperplasia without atypia: The endometrium shows an increase in the glandular epithelium usually as a result of unopposed estrogen stimulation. This results in irregular and unpredictable gland outlines that are often cystic. There is abundant stroma, so that the gland to stromal ratio is little altered from normal. (Hematoxylin and eosin, 10× original magnification.)

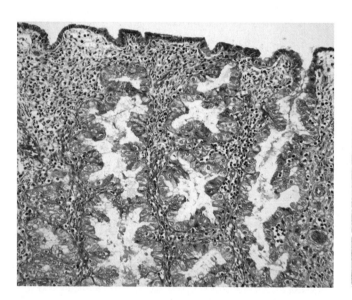

FIGURE 4-2   Secretory endometrium: Endometrial glands are present with a saw-tooth pattern. Each gland is an individual unit set in endometrial stroma. The epithelium has intracytoplasmic glycogen secretion that is eventually extruded into the gland lumen. (Hematoxylin and eosin, 10× original magnification.)

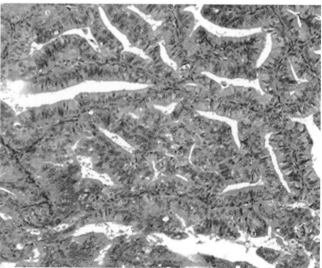

FIGURE 4-4   Endometrioid adenocarcinoma: Well-differentiated (FIGO G1) endometrioid adenocarcinomas typically show a "back to back" glandular arrangement with little intervening stroma. The glands are lined by tall columnar tumor cells. (Hematoxylin and eosin, 20× original magnification.)

risk and response to progesterone therapy. Histopathologic classification of endometrial lesions provides a stratification of risk for progression to cancer by defined endometrial changes.

Understanding the pathophysiology of excess unopposed estrogen production helps the clinician better predict which women are at risk for endometrial cancer and provides windows of opportunity for implementation of prevention strategies. These principles have also been used to treat hormonally active cancers, especially breast cancer. Selective estrogen receptor modulators (SERMs), such as tamoxifen and raloxifene, and, more recently, aromatase inhibitors are widely used as both treatment and chemoprevention of breast cancer. These drugs have toxicities that the obstetrician/gynecologist will be required to manage. Although tamoxifen is an antiestrogen in breast tissue, it paradoxically has estrogen-like properties in the endometrium and increases the risk of endometrial cancer. It is also associated with thromboembolism and stroke. Although tamoxifen provides protection against bone loss, osteoporosis, and fractures, it does not appear to carry increased risk of myocardial infarction. There does appear to be an association with cataracts. Unfortunately, tamoxifen accentuates menopausal symptoms. Aromatase inhibitors block the cytochrome p450 CYP-19 enzyme responsible for the peripheral conversion of androgens to estrogens and result in estrogen deficiency. This accelerates menopausal bone loss, which could lead to osteoporosis and fractures; therefore, prevention of these toxicities is important when they are prescribed. Other side effects include hot flashes, sweats, edema, myalgias, and fatigue.

Preventative health maintenance must balance all risks and benefits while maintaining quality of life and symptom control, and this is the central theme in this chapter. Many women want active control over these very important choices, and may value quality of life and their sexual relationship more than cancer prevention and cardiovascular risk reduction.

CLINICAL PRESENTATION

The scientific explanation for the low incidence rates for endometrial hyperplasia is that it is a lesion that is usually unrecognized and asymptomatic until cancer develops. Until endometrial cancer screening becomes routine and cost effective, the true prevalence of the precursor lesions will remain unknown. Women with endometrial hyperplasias are identified by endometrial biopsy performed because of abnormal vaginal bleeding (menorrhagia, or postmenopausal bleeding) or because a thickened endometrial stripe is found on transvaginal ultrasound when ordered for another reason such as the identification of endometrial cells in the Pap test of a woman older than age 40.

There is evidence of exogenous or endogenous unopposed estrogen stimulation of the endometrium in most women with endometrial hyperplasia. Some women will have an ovarian neoplasm producing the estrogen stimulation, which is the classic presentation of a granulosa cell tumor. The most common causes of excess estrogen are obesity, polycystic ovarian disease, or a prolonged perimenopause with anovulatory bleeding patterns. The development of hyperplasia secondary to anovulation at menarche is uncommon and should be easily reversible

with normalization of cyclic menses with oral contraceptive pills. The age at presentation depends on the source of the excess estrogen. Endometrial hyperplasias and cancers that are associated with estrogen stimulation have a good prognosis. Endometrial cancers in women without evidence of excess estrogen are usually not associated with hyperplasia and can be associated with a tumor suppressor gene abnormality such as p53-associated uterine serous carcinomas (Figures 4-5 and 4-6). These are aggressive tumors, behaving similarly to ovarian cancer with higher mortality rates.

Office endometrial biopsy has in general replaced the dilation and curettage procedure for the diagnosis of endometrial hyperplasia or carcinoma. There is interest in the potential benefit of curettage as therapy and providing more tissue for accurate histologic diagnosis. Others advocate the use of "hormonal curettage" in which medical therapy with progesterone is followed by the withdrawal bleed. This provides the same effect without the surgical cost or risk. Repeat office endometrial biopsy at 3-month intervals can reassure the patient and the clinician of the therapeutic effect of the hormonal therapy. There is little to no evidence of increasing a woman's mortality risk by potentially delaying a diagnosis of cancer by 3 months. It is expected that an underlying cancerous tumor will be identified periodically by this technique, but there is no evidence that dilation and curettage reduces a women's mortality risk. Outpatient office evaluation and management have become the usual and safest way to manage these patients until there is evidence that a hysterectomy is required. These

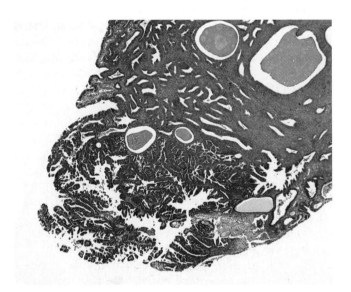

FIGURE 4-5 Endometrial serous carcinoma in a polyp: There is an irregular, complex pattern of papillary epithelium arising in the tip of an endometrial polyp. (Hematoxylin and eosin, 2× original magnification.)

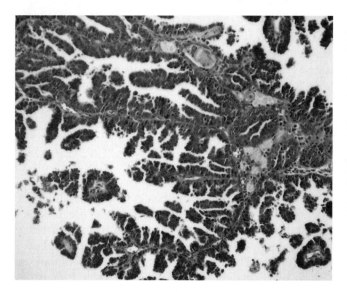

FIGURE 4-6   Endometrial serous carcinoma: This tumor shows a complex pattern of highly atypical cells with large irregular nuclei and prominent nucleoli. Typically, the tumor shows a papillary configuration, with abnormal epithelium covering a thin connective tissue core. (Hematoxylin and eosin, 10× original magnification.)

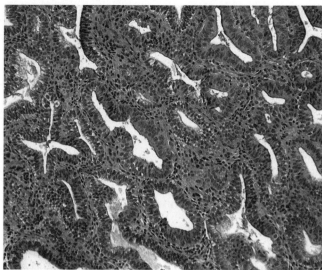

FIGURE 4-7   Complex hyperplasia without atypia: The gland to stromal ratio is increased with complex, closely set, irregular gland outlines. However, there is little nuclear atypia. (Hematoxylin and eosin, 20× original magnification.)

management decisions will be discussed further in later sections of this chapter.

ENDOMETRIAL HYPERPLASIA: PATHOLOGIC DIAGNOSTIC CRITERIA

The International Society of Gynecological Pathologists (ISGYP), International Federation of Gynecology and Obstetrics (FIGO), and the World Health Organization (WHO) currently classify endometrial hyperplasia based on a 1994 classification system into four categories based on architectural structure and cytologic features. The architecture is either simple or complex, and the cytologic features are described as with or without atypia. This yields four separate diagnoses (Table 4-1): simple hyperplasia without atypia (Figure 4-3), complex hyperplasia without atypia (Figure 4-7), simple hyperplasia with atypia (Figure 4-8), and complex hyperplasia with atypia (AEH) (Figure 4-9).

The terms adenomatous and cystic-glandular hyperplasia have been discarded, and when the abbreviation AEH is used, it refers to atypical endometrial hyperplasia, which reflects the two categories of hyperplasia with cytologic atypia (simple hyperplasia or complex hyperplasia with atypia). The presence of atypia appears to be the most important criteria for progression to adenocarcinoma or the coexistence of endometrioid adenocarcinoma. The rates of coexisting endometrioid adenocarcinoma with atypical endometrial hyperplasia are reported to be as low as 13% and as high as 43%.

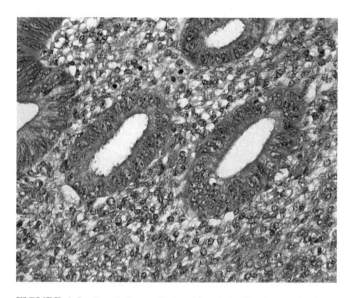

FIGURE 4-8   Simple hyperplasia with atypia: Uncommonly recognized form of hyperplasia in which the epithelium shows an increased gland to stromal ratio with simple glands. However, the glands are lined by epithelium with atypical nuclei. (Hematoxylin and eosin, 40× original magnification.)

TABLE 4-1   Classification of Endometrial Hyperplasia

Simple hyperplasia
Complex hyperplasia (adenomatous)
Simple atypical hyperplasia
Complex atypical hyperplasia (adenomatous with atypia)

From World Health Organization and Kurman RJ (ed.). Blaustein's Pathology of the Female Genital Tract, ed. 4., 1994.

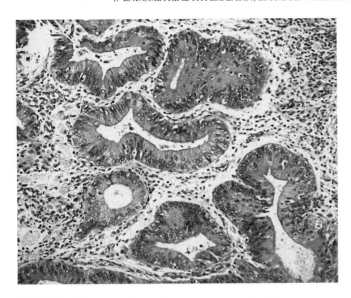

FIGURE 4-9 Atypical complex hyperplasia: The tissue shows a marked increase in the gland to stromal ratio with complex glandular outlines and nuclear atypia in the lining epithelium. (Hematoxylin and eosin, 10× original magnification.)

The pathologic diagnosis of these lesions is usually made with a small sampling of the endometrium in the office using a device called a pipelle. This small tissue sample then has to be categorized by the pathologist. A prospective study of the reproducibility of the diagnosis of atypical endometrial hyperplasia (both simple and complex) was undertaken by the Gynecologic Oncology Group (GOG). Women with the diagnosis of atypical endometrial hyperplasia who agreed to have a hysterectomy within 12 weeks of diagnosis of AEH were enrolled. The study population was 302 eligible cases with a median age of 57 years, and 31% were 50 years of age or younger. The endometrial biopsy specimens were rereviewed by three gynecologic pathologists independently (study panel diagnosis) in a blinded protocol. They agreed to categorize the endometrium as normal (cycling, menstrual, or atrophic), nonatypical hyperplasia (disordered proliferative, simple or complex hyperplasia), atypical hyperplasia (simple or complex), adenocarcinoma , or inadequate for evaluation. Two of three study pathologists had to agree on one of the aforementioned five diagnoses for a study panel diagnosis to be established. Correct diagnosis was determined by consensus agreement on the hysterectomy specimen during a panel review simultaneously with a multi-headed scope. The results found 40% of the cases had all three pathologists in agreement. The reproducibility was lowest for the diagnosis of AEH (kappa 0.28) and was better for adenocarcinoma (kappa 0.51). Reproducibility was best for dilation and curettage (kappa 0.47; CI 0.41:0.53) compared to small sampling devices (kappa 0.26-0.36). Two of three study panel members agreed

with the referring institution diagnosis of AEH in 38% of cases. The study panel diagnosis was less severe in 25% of cases and was adenocarcinoma in 29% of cases. The most important outcome for this study was the finding that 43% of the enrolled participants were found to have adenocarcinoma in their uterus at the time of hysterectomy. The second most important finding was the rate of adenocarcinoma in each study panel majority diagnosis category: normal or nonatypical hyperplasia 14/74 (18.9%), AEH 45/115 (39.1%), and adenocarcinoma 54/84 (64.3%). The uterine examination revealed the presence of some risk factors for metastatic disease present in 43 cases, including myometrial invasion, grade II or III lesions.

The natural history of simple hyperplasia without atypia is likely to follow a benign course. It is often seen in women near menopause, when anovulatory cycles are common. The removal of the estrogenic stimulation or treatment with progestogens influences the outcome. The majority of lesions will regress (60%) without treatment, and 84% will regress with progestin therapy. Only 3% are believed to progress to cancer. Complex hyperplasia is also expected to regress (56%) when atypia is not present. Atypical hyperplasia has a 36% progression rate, and even with progestins, 27% have been reported to progress, but it is unclear whether this is coexistent cancer that is eventually identified. Fifty-five percent of atypical hyperplasia is expected to regress with progestin therapy. The duration of treatment and the best agent for progestin therapy have not yet been identified; however, a recent study among Finnish women notes that a treatment regimen including continuous progestin rather than cyclical (10-14 days/month) progestin appears to reduce the risk of endometrial cancer in a postmenopausal population. It is assumed that unless the estrogen stimulation ceases, the progestin therapy may need to be lifelong. Alternatively, a hysterectomy is necessary to prevent the development of the most common endometrioid adenocarcinoma (Figure 4-4) or type I cancer (estrogen dependent). This estrogen-induced cancer is the most common histologic type and the least aggressive form of uterine malignancy and should be preventable and able to be successfully treated when detected.

Recent research involving molecular studies of endometrial lesions and objective computerized morphometrics has shown promise to increase the accuracy and reproducibility of the diagnosis of endometrial lesions. A new classification system was proposed as the 2003 WHO classification, which defines endometrial intraepithelial neoplasia (EIN) as the precancerous lesion. Early evidence suggests that it may be more predictive of progression to cancer, but it is not clinically used or accepted at this time.

Endometrial carcinomas of the serous papillary variety arise in a background of atrophic endometrium.

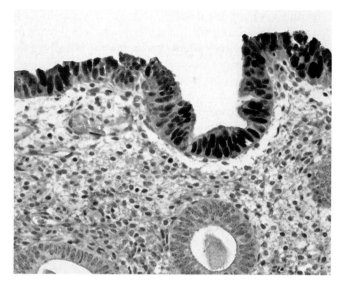

FIGURE 4-10   p53 immunostain of endometrial intraepithelial car-cinoma (EIC): Endometrial serous carcinoma is typically accompanied by p53 mutations that allow accumulation of p53 protein in the cells that can be identified by immunostaining. Normal cells do not stain positively for p53 because the amount of normal protein is below the threshold of the staining test. (Immunoperoxidase stain for p53 with DAB chromogen, 20× original magnification).

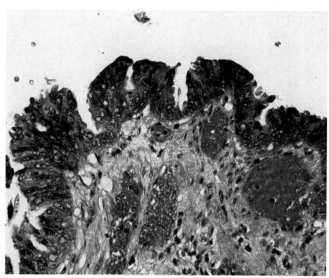

FIGURE 4-11   Endometrial intraepithelial carcinoma (EIC): Precur-sor lesion for serous carcinoma of the endometrium with markedly atypical, crowded epithelium with little architectural abnormality. This lesion is often observed on the surface of otherwise benign endometrial polyps. (Hematoxylin and eosin, 10× original magnification.)

These cancers are not associated with excess estrogen and have been classified as type II (estrogen indepen-dent) endometrial cancers. Serous papillary adenocarci-noma is less likely to be identified at an early stage compared with endometrioid histologic types. These lesions are often associated with abnormalities in p53 tumor suppressor gene that results in accumulation of p53 protein in the cell (Figure 4-10). Unlike normal cells or most endometrioid cancers, immunostaining with antibodies to p53 will be positive in the majority of serous cancers. Endometrial hyperplasia is not a precur-sor to serous carcinoma. Rather, the precursor has been identified as EIC. Serous EIC (Figure 4-11) can even be multifocal with disease found in the ovaries and omentum when no invasive component is found in the uterus. Comprehensive surgical staging is recommended as a result of the difficulty in establishing the diagnosis of invasive cancer intraoperatively. Postoperative therapy can be recommended after adequate histologic evaluation.

MANAGEMENT DECISIONS FOR ATYPICAL ENDOMETRIAL HYPERPLASIA

The patient's age, fertility plans and need for contra-ception, comorbidities, and personal preferences play a dramatic role in the management of these lesions.

Hysterectomy is indicated when fertility is not desired and AEH is identified. Atypical endometrial hyperplasia is commonly found with coexisting undiagnosed cancer already present in the uterus or progressing to endome-trial cancer in untreated women. As previously dis-cussed, the GOG reported that 43% of 306 women who had a community-based diagnosis of AEH on endome-trial biopsy and proceeded without medical treatment to hysterectomy had endometrial cancer on final pathol-ogy. Although 63% (77/123) of the cancers identified were grade I lesions confined to the endometrium, 31% were myoinvasive and 11% had deep myometrial inva-sion into the outer 50% of the myometrium. It is possible that future validation of a new EIN scoring system or another molecular marker will allow more precise pre-dictability for the neoplastic potential and the coexis-tence of cancer before hysterectomy.

The complexity of the surgical management of atypical endometrial hyperplasia is underappreciated. Intraoperative decision-making, using frozen section to determine the operative interventions, is never ideal, considering difficulty of the diagnosis and the variety of skill and expertise of the pathologist and gynecologists. It is to be expected that the postoperative diagnosis of cancer will be obtained in a substantial number of these cases. The recommendation is that the patient should be informed of the 20% to 45% risk of underlying malig-nancy, and hysterectomy is required for final diagnosis. She should be counseled about the desire to keep her ovaries or have them removed, based on her age, family history, and other medical conditions or comorbidities.

Vaginal hysterectomy may be all that is required, or laparoscopically assisted hysterectomy with bilateral salpingo-oophorectomy can be considered. In the event that high-grade cancer or deep myometrial invasion is found, another surgery may be necessary for comprehensive surgical staging and removal of retained ovaries. Staging can usually be accomplished laparoscopically if a previous laparotomy was not performed. This should be necessary in approximately 10% of the cases in which cancer is identified and will depend on the entire health history of the individual. Increased cost and more errors are likely if all hyperplasia cases are subjected to laparotomy, intraoperative frozen section, and staging based on intraoperative assessment of myometrial invasion. It should be noted that pelvic radiation is no longer a substitute for accurate and thorough surgical staging in endometrial cancer, so consultation with a gynecologic oncologist is appropriate for these difficult decisions when unexpected cancer is found in the hysterectomy specimen.

Women who desire childbearing, refuse hysterectomy, or have medical conditions that make hysterectomy an undesirable first choice can be treated hormonally. Megestrol, 160 mg/day in divided doses, has been the drug of choice with acceptable results even in the face of complex endometrial hyperplasia with atypia. It is unclear whether the treatment should be continuous or cyclic, but there are theoretical advantages to the endometrial shedding provided by the progesterone withdrawal bleed. The endometrium needs to be re-evaluated histologically, by office biopsy or dilation and curettage, at 3-month intervals for at least a year. Lifelong prevention strategies must be emphasized with the patient. The pathologist finds the evaluation of the endometrial sampling more straightforward if it is not complicated by exogenous hormonal influences. For this reason, it is best to withdraw the patient from the progestogen for 7 to 14 days to allow withdrawal bleeding before endometrial biopsies. Schedule the biopsy or dilation and curettage after the withdrawal bleeding ceases.

Ramirez reported in 2004 on successful pregnancies after treatment of grade I endometrial cancer with progestin. Eighty-one patients with a median age of 30 years were treated for approximately 6 months. Forty-seven were able to reverse the lesion, and 20 patients were able to become pregnant. Half of the patients required assisted reproductive technologies. The ACOG Practice Bulletin on endometrial cancer includes this general guideline: Women with atypical endometrial hyperplasia (AEH) and endometrial cancer who desire to maintain their fertility may be treated with progestin therapy. After therapy they should undergo serial complete intrauterine evaluation approximately every 3 months to document response. Hysterectomy should be recommended for women who do not desire fertility.

Local therapy of the endometrium with a progestin-containing intrauterine device (IUD; Mirena) is encouraging. Wildemeersch reported on 12 women with hyperplasia from 46 to 67 years of age. Their lesions were diagnosed as simple hyperplasia without atypia in 7 women and as atypical hyperplasia in 5 women. All women were without hyperplasia at 12 months. Montz and colleagues demonstrated the successful treatment of well-differentiated endometrial adenocarcinoma with the intrauterine progestin-secreting device. Hysteroscopic removal of all hyperplastic tissue was performed and the IUD was inserted in 13 women with grade I endometrioid adenocarcinoma. Endometrial biopsies were performed every 3 months, and 6 of the 12 evaluable cases were negative for carcinoma at 6 months. A total of 8 women completed 12 months of therapy, 6 of whom were negative for carcinoma at that time. Those 6 women have been maintained on this therapy and undergo annual endometrial biopsies. A recent systematic review indicates that the levonorgestrel-releasing intrauterine device prevents the development of benign endometrial polyps in patients with breast cancer who are taking tamoxifen; however, there is no clear evidence from randomized, prospective studies that local therapy prevents endometrial hyperplasia or malignancy.

In conclusion, management decisions in women with atypical endometrial hyperplasia are complex and require an understanding of the risk of invasive endometrial adenocarcinoma, the reproductive desires of the patient, her comorbidities, and risks for surgical management. Ideally, laparoscopic-assisted vaginal hysterectomy with bilateral salpingo-oophorectomy can be performed. The finding of adenocarcinoma in the uterus requires consultation with a gynecologic oncologist to determine whether observation or reoperation for surgical staging should be considered.

MANAGEMENT OF ENDOMETRIAL HYPERPLASIA WITHOUT ATYPIA

The diagnosis of simple or complex hyperplasia without atypia requires hormonal management and is not an indication for hysterectomy. These lesions are generally reversible with progestogen (synthetic progestin or progesterone). The initial approach is generally to treat in a cyclic fashion with the progestogen given for 14 days of the month to deliver predictable cyclic withdrawal menses. Women, including teenagers, who are premenopausal and sexually active are usually best treated with a regimen that provides contraception such as Depo-Provera or oral contraceptives. Women who want to conceive are likely to be anovulatory and require ovulation-induction agents after withdrawal bleeding is produced with a progestogen. Reassurance can be obtained from a reduction of menstrual flow and a bleeding pattern that is appropriately timed with the cyclic therapy. It is extremely important to counsel anovulatory women about the lifelong risk of endometrial cancer and methods for surveillance and prevention. Twenty-five percent of endometrial cancers occur in the premenopausal age range, and 5% occur in women 40 years of age and younger. These cancers may be part of the polycystic ovarian syndrome or the anovulatory transition before menopause and are all theoretically preventable with proper counseling and active management. Premenopausal patients with endometrial cancer should also be counseled about the possibility of Lynch syndrome. A family history should be taken, and if endometrial and colon cancers are frequent in the family, the patient should be referred to genetic counseling. Colonoscopy is often recommended to patients with endometrial cancer because of the association with colon cancer. There is a dramatic rise in the incidence rate of endometrial hyperplasia and endometrial cancer at 45 years of age and peaking at 65 years of age. This is likely a result of the combined effects of estrone (estrogen) production in the peripheral adipose tissue, particularly in obese women, and to the absence of progesterone that results from loss of ovulatory function in menopause.

PREVENTION OF ENDOMETRIAL CANCER

Endometrial stimulation by estrogens unopposed by progestins leads to endometrial hyperplastic conditions in a dose- and time-dependent manner. Experimental evidence has been obtained from prospective clinical trials conducted to identify the appropriate doses and schedules of hormone replacement therapies (HRT). Kurman reported a randomized trial of 1176 postmenopausal women receiving 1 mg of estradiol orally and either placebo or various doses of norethindrone acetate. Women treated with estradiol alone (247 evaluable participants) for 12 months had a 12.2% rate of simple hyperplasia without atypia, 1.6% had complex hyperplasia without atypia, and 0.8% had complex atypical hyperplasia. Norethindrone acetate at all doses used in this trial nearly eliminated that risk. The North American Menopause Society supports the addition of a progestogen whenever estrogen is prescribed for menopausal symptoms in women with an intact uterus for the prevention of estrogen-induced hyperplasia and adenocarcinoma. Unfortunately, the progestogen has undesirable side effects, and women have been known to discontinue this component of their prescribed hormone replacement.

The prevention of endometrial cancer has been complicated by the publication and early closure of the estrogen plus progestin (E+P) component of the Women's Health Initiative (WHI). This randomized, placebo-controlled clinical trial evaluated conjugated equine estrogens (CEE), 0.625 mg, plus medroxyprogesterone acetate (MPA), 2.5 mg orally per day (hormone replacement therapy [HRT]). This trial enrolled 16,608 women with a range of 50 to 79 years of age for an average of 5.2 years to determine the primary outcomes of coronary heart disease (CHD), invasive breast cancer, and a global index (including stroke, pulmonary embolism, endometrial cancer, colorectal cancer, hip fracture, and death from other causes). In May 2002 the data safety monitoring committee recommended premature closure of the trial as a result of the adverse outcomes of breast cancer and cardiovascular complications including coronary heart disease, stroke, and pulmonary embolus. Of note, overall mortality was not affected. The absolute excess risk per 10,000 person-years attributable to HRT was seven coronary heart disease events, eight strokes, eight pulmonary emboli, eight invasive breast cancers and a reduction of five hip fractures. These risks need to be reviewed with women choosing HRT.

The WHI trial with conjugated equine estrogen alone versus placebo had a very different outcome. There was a nonsignificant reduction in breast cancer risk (P = 0.06), and coronary heart disease risk was unaffected (HR = 0.91; CI 0.75-1.12), strokes were increased (HR = 1.39; CI 1.10-1.77), and hip fractures were reduced (HR = 0.61; 0.41-0.91). This places women with an intact uterus, and their physicians, in a difficult situation of balancing risks. A woman with a uterus can decide to accept the potential risks of the addition of a progestin, or she may choose to take unopposed estrogen and follow the endometrium yearly with transvaginal ultrasound or endometrial biopsy. Unopposed estrogen use gives a woman a relative risk (RR) for endometrial cancer of three times the general population for less than 5 years of use and an RR of 10 after 10 years of use. The risk decreases but remains elevated after discontinuing the drug. Alternatively, other progestins and progesterone formulations are available that may carry a different, but as yet unknown, risk of breast cancer. Micronized progesterone is available as oral 100-mg or 200-mg capsules (Prometrium) and has been approved by the U.S. Food and Drug Administration (FDA) for use in combination with estrogen for relief of menopausal symptoms. The dose of 200 mg for 12 days per month in a cyclic fashion causes withdrawal bleeding in a predictable manner. The regimen of conjugated equine estrogen, 0.625 mg/day with oral micronized progesterone at a dose of 200 mg/day for 12 days per month, failed to see any increase in endometrial hyperplasia with 3 years of follow-up. There is available vaginal progesterone gel, which is FDA approved only for infertility use but has been studied in small numbers of menopausal women.

An additional provocative alternative is to use the progestin-containing intrauterine system (Mirena is FDA approved for contraceptive use only) and unopposed estrogen, which has been studied prospectively in menopausal women. These women were followed only 1 year, and they were able to convert proliferative endometrium to atrophic endometrium while using continuous estradiol 50 mcg per day via the transdermal route.

The official position statement of the North American Menopause Society is that a progestogen should be added to estrogen therapy for all postmenopausal women with an intact uterus. The type, route, or regimen can be individualized to minimize side effects while providing adequate endometrial protection.

BENEFITS AND RISKS OF ESTROGEN REPLACEMENT THERAPY

Quality of Life, Vasomotor Symptoms, and Sexual Function

The World Health Organization and the Stages of Reproductive Aging Workshop (STRAW) working group define menopause as the permanent cessation of menstrual periods that occurs naturally or is induced by surgery, chemotherapy, or radiation. Menopausal transition is the time of an increase in follicle-stimulating hormone and increased variability in cycle length. Postmenopause begins at the time of the final menstrual period but is not recognized until 12 months of amenorrhea have occurred. The National Institutes of Health, in the "State of the Science Conference Statement: Management of Menopause-Related Symptoms," defines menopausal symptoms as vasomotor symptoms, vaginal dryness and painful intercourse, and sleep disturbance. Estrogen is the most consistently effective therapy for vasomotor symptoms, vaginal dryness, and sleep disturbances and for improved quality of life, and a subset of women may find an improved mood with estrogen therapy. Testosterone has been demonstrated to improve libido, especially in women who have undergone oophorectomy; however, long-term risks have not been studied. Antidepressants, clonidine, and gabapentin have been studied in treatment of hot flashes; some efficacy has been seen.

Symptom control is the most common reason for initiating estrogen therapy and remains undisputed as the most appropriate indication for prescribing estrogen at the time of natural or surgical menopause. The epidemiology community recommendations are that the patient should be told that hormone replacement should be for symptom control only, is prescribed at the lowest effective dose, and is for the shortest duration of use possible. Women should consider tapering off after 5 years of use to avoid the adverse events of thromboembolic disorders, breast cancer, stroke, and cardiovascular events (myocardial infarction, death). Women must be active participants in the decision-making regarding estrogen use or estrogen plus progestogen use. They must experience the symptoms, recognize the reasons they are choosing to use these agents, and actively make the decision that the benefit is worth the small risk. Their own social situation or individual risk profile may influence their personal decisions.

The WHI reported the symptoms manifested by 8405 women between 8 and 12 months from the date the HRT participants were asked to discontinue conjugated equine estrogen plus medroxyprogesterone acetate. These women were mailed a survey, and 21.2% had moderate to severe vasomotor symptoms, which was significantly different (CI 4.92-6.89) compared to placebo. They also reported pain and stiffness (adjusted odds ratio 2.16), and these symptoms were reported by more than 10% of respondents. Other withdrawal effects were feeling tired, having difficulty sleeping, and a feeling of bloating or gas. Depression was also significantly increased after withdrawal of hormone replacement ($P < 0.001$).

The WHI documented the beneficial effects experienced from hormone replacement therapy in women with a uterus. Relief of hot flashes (85.7%), night sweats (77.6%), vaginal or genital dryness (74.1%), and joint pain or stiffness (49.1%) was seen, compared to placebo effects ranging from 57.7% to 38.4%, respectively. Women taking HRT were more likely to complain of breast tenderness (9.3%) and vaginal bleeding (51%) than those on placebo 2.4% and 5%, respectively.

In conclusion, the data summarized in the WHI is not generalizable to the 45 to 55 year old suffering from menopausal symptoms. These women must prioritize their own situation, health risks, and quality-of-life benefits. Most will find the best symptom relief from estrogen use. Alternatives to estrogen include progestogens, antidepressants (venlafaxine, paroxetine, fluoxetine), clonidine, and the anticonvulsant gabapentin. Over-the-counter remedies include isoflavones, black cohosh, and vitamin E. None of the alternatives resolve the entire menopausal syndrome including sexual dysfunction.

Estradiol may also be delivered by a silicone ring placed in the vagina (Estring, Femring). The Estring (Pfizer US Pharmaceuticals) contains 2 mg of estradiol, and on average 0.02 mg/day is released over a 90-day period. Studies have demonstrated a median plasma estradiol increase from 4.5 pmol/L before insertion to 12.5 pmol/L at steady state. The comparison with a 0.05-mg estraderm patch was tenfold greater serum concentrations of estradiol. A study of endometrial thickness in 60 postmenopausal women over a 12-month period showed a thickness of 2.8 mm before Estring and 2.6-mm thickness after 12 months of use. This is reassuring to women unable to tolerate progestins. Another randomized controlled study demonstrated a decrease in urinary tract infections with the use of Estring. The use of Estring may be preferred for women wanting local therapy for vaginal dryness symptoms with an inability to take progestins or a history of breast cancer. Femring is available when an increase in vaginal dose is desired.

Estrogen alone does not always resolve the sexual dysfunction complaints following bilateral salpingo-oophorectomy. Testosterone is currently undergoing FDA review for the use in female sexual dysfunction. Testosterone has been demonstrated in clinical trials to help with decreased sexual desire, arousal, and orgasmic response. A recent study evaluated the efficacy and safety of testosterone treatment in 814 postmenopausal women with hypoactive sexual desire not receiving estrogen therapy. Patients were randomized to receive testosterone by patch (150 or 300 mcg/day) or placebo. At 24 weeks, efficacy was measured and the group of women receiving 300 mcg/day of testosterone reported significantly greater sexual satisfaction compared to the placebo group and the group treated with 150 mcg/day of testosterone. The rate of adverse events related to androgens, specifically unwanted hair growth, was also highest in this group. Furthermore, breast cancer was diagnosed in 4 women treated with testosterone, compared to none of the women who received placebo. The long-term effects of testosterone, including effects on the breast, remain unclear.

Breast Cancer

Probably the greatest concern of women who do take HRT is the concern regarding a possible breast cancer relationship. It should be remembered that breast cancer as a generalization takes a long time to become clinically apparent. From the time the initial cell is determined to be malignant, it may be up to 10 years before it is clinically detected based on 100-day doubling time. Obviously, the use of mammography will allow detection earlier and that is the window of opportunity for making an early breast cancer diagnosis. Bush and associates in 2001 reviewed the studies of HRT and breast cancer that had been published from 1975 to 2000. In 45 studies in which estrogen alone was used, 82% showed no increased or decreased risk for breast cancer. In the 20 studies that evaluated E+P, 80% found no increase or decrease, with an equal number having a significant decrease or a significant increase. Several meta-analyses were carried out during the latter portion of the twentieth century, and all showed no significant increase in breast cancer with ever use of estrogen alone or E+P.

The WHI in 2002 published their preliminary unadjudicated report indicating that the study was being terminated because of the increased risk of developing breast cancer. In the E+P category, the HR was 1.26 (1.00-1.59), which was not statistically significant. They did estimate 8/10,000 excess breast cancers per woman-years in the E+P arm. The annualized deaths were equal between the two arms, and there was no difference in the in situ cancers. To date, to our knowledge, the pathology has never been centrally reviewed in these breast cancer patients. The data have been further evaluated in regard to the time from menopause when E+P was begun. In the women who were less than 10 years since menopause, the HR was 1.19 (CI 0.84-1.70). The HR in the estrogen-only arm was 0.77 (CI 0.59-1.01). When only women 50 to 59 years of age were evaluated, the HR was 0.72 (CI 0.43-1.21). With more than 7 years of follow-up in the estrogen-only arm, in those individuals who had had no prior estrogen therapy the HR was 0.76 (CI 0.58-0.99). The incidence of ductal cancers in the estrogen-only arm noted an HR of 0.71 (CI 0.52-0.99), and in those patients who were adherent with more than 80% compliance, the HR was 0.67 (CI 0.47-0.97). It appears that, even though the initial report suggested that the rate of breast cancer was significantly increased in women who were receiving HRT, subsequent data revealed that even in those who are on E+P, the increase was not statistically significant. In those taking estrogen-only HRT, it would appear that particularly in those who were adherent, there was actually a statistically significant decrease in the risk of breast cancer.

Osteoporosis

Osteoporosis is a disease characterized by low bone mass and microarchitectural deterioration of bone tissue, which leads to increased bone fragility and increased fracture risk. Low bone mass is related to a low peak bone mass (mainly under genetic influence) and to a decrease in bone mass, which occurs after menopause and with aging. Menopause induces an accelerated bone loss within 5 to 8 years followed by a linear rate of bone loss.

Bone density readings are standardized to healthy women of similar age. Osteopenia is defined as bone loss of greater than one standard deviation from the mean, and osteoporosis is bone loss greater than two standard deviations from the mean.

Osteoporosis prevention strategies should begin before 40 years of age as a result of a decline in peak bone mass. An even more dramatic loss of bone occurs at menopause with the loss of estrogen support of osteoblastic activity. Women should take active measures to protect their bones by doing regular weightbearing exercise (at least 30 minutes three times a week), taking calcium supplementation (1500 mg elemental calcium for the postmenopausal woman), and ensuring adequate vitamin D supplementation (800–1200 IU per day). At menopause a baseline bone density is recommended and then repeated every other year unless osteopenia or osteoporosis is detected. Estrogen replacement therapy has been the traditional main prevention strategy to prevent this deterioration in bone strength. A number of medications are approved by the FDA for the prevention and/or treatment of osteoporosis. Bisphosphonates such as alendronate (Fosamax), risedronate (Actonel), and ibandronate (Boniva) act by preventing bone resorption by blocking the action of osteoclasts. Gastrointestinal side effects (reflex, esophagitis, esophageal ulcers) have been a primary concern for patients taking oral biphosphonates. These drugs should be taken first thing in the morning on an empty stomach with an 8-ounce glass of water. The patient should then wait a full hour before eating or taking any other medications. Lying down or eating before the recommended time increases risk for gastrointestinal distress. There are also theoretical concerns that prolonged therapy with bisphosphonates leads to oversuppression of bone remodeling, which allows microdamage to accumulate and increase skeletal fragility. Microscopic crack frequency is increased in animals treated with high doses of bisphosphonates, although this has yet to be demonstrated in biopsies taken from postmenopausal women treated with long-term use. Selective estrogen receptor modulators (SERMs) such as raloxifene (Evista) bind with high affinity to estrogen receptors and promote estrogen-like activity on bone. Unfortunately, raloxifene has the same thromboembolic risk of estrogen without the benefit of menopausal symptom relief. Drugs approved for treatment only include calcitonin (Miacalin), which is administered by nasal spray, and teriparatide (Forteo), which is administered through daily subcutaneous injections. Both of these pharmacologic agents serve to increase bone formation.

Two anatomic areas are of interest in the bone remodeling process. The first is the axial skeleton, composed primarily of trabecular bone. The second is the appendicular skeleton, composed primarily of cortical bone. The remodeling cycle is the same in both types of bone. However, because of the greater surface area, approximately 40% of trabecular bone, as opposed to 10% of the cortical bone, is in "turn over" each year. The osteoclast is responsible for the resorption of old bone, which results in the formation of a resorption cavity. Osteoblasts are then attracted to the cavity, where they secrete osteoid, which is primarily type I collagen. The collagen is mineralized mainly with calcium, thus producing new bone with an appropriate mechanical strength. Under normal circumstances, the amount of bone removed is replaced with fresh bone; however, this process can become uncoupled if osteoclasts remove more bone than can normally be replaced by osteoblasts, resulting in net loss of bone mass. In menopausal women, accelerated bone loss is associated with a high bone turnover rate and increased osteoclast activity. Estrogen may inhibit osteoclast activity and increase proliferation of osteoblasts and collagen production.

The beneficial effects of estrogen in preventing or treating postmenopausal osteoporosis are well recognized. At the same time, there is growing recognition that osteoporosis is a major public health problem in the United States. It is estimated that approximately 8 million women in the United States have osteoporosis and another 14 million are at risk because they have low bone mass. Osteoporosis causes more than 1.5 million fractures each year, including 300,000 hip, 700,000 vertebral, and 200,000 wrist fractures. These fractures are seen mainly in women. For a 50-year-old woman the lifetime risk of fracture of any of the three is 40%. Traditional risk factors for osteoporosis include estrogen deficiency, fair complexion, high caffeine intake, low calcium intake, small and thin build, smoking, inadequate physical activities, and multiple disease processes and medications. The cost of osteoporosis in the United States is estimated to be $14 billion per year, of which 70% of cases are associated with hip fractures. Excess mortality associated with hip fracture is 12% to 20% during the first year after the injury. Less than one half of patients with hip fractures ever return to their prefracture activity. Many require assistance, have lost their independence, and require long-term domiciliary care. Vertebral fractures may be asymptomatic in 50%, but successive fractures can lead to loss of height, kyphotic distortion of posture, and chronic back pain. Approximately 10% of patients with hip fractures die of surgical complications within 6 months of fracture. Approximately 25% of all white women older than 60 years of age have spinal compression fractures resulting from osteoporosis. The risk of hip fracture is 20% by the age of 90, and hip fractures are about 2.5 times more common in women than in men. An increased rate of loss of both cortical and cancellous bone is associated with menopause. In a follow-up study of 82 postmenopausal women 5 to 10 years after their first examination, Meema and colleagues concluded that (1) as a group, menopausal women lost bone, and the beginning of this loss is less related to age than to loss of ovarian function; (2) the rate of loss was not significantly correlated with age; and (3) the bone loss was prevented by estrogen administration (i.e., 0.625 mg of conjugated estrogens).

Nachtigall and associates conducted a 10-year, double-blind prospective study to evaluate the effects of estrogen replacement therapy (ERT). They took a sample population of 84 pairs of randomly chosen postmenopausal patients who were matched for age and diagnosis. Half of the patients received conjugated estrogens and cyclic progesterone, whereas the other half received a placebo. The estrogen-treated patients whose

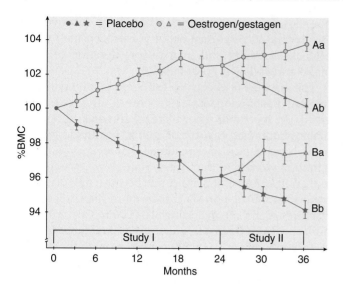

FIGURE 4-12   Bone mineral content as a function of time and treatment in 94 (study I) and 72 (study II) women soon after menopause. (*From Christensen C et al: Bone mass in postmenopausal women after withdrawal of estrogen/progestin replacement therapy. Lancet 1:459, 1981.*)

TABLE 4-2   Case Control Studies of Hormone Replacement Therapy in the Prevention of Hip Fracture

Authors	Relative Risk
Hutchinson et al	0.70
Weiss et al	0.43-0.77
Paganini-Hill et al	0.42
Kreiger et al	0.50
Kiel et al	0.34-0.65
Naesser et al	0.79
Kanis et al	0.55

therapy was started within 3 years of menopause showed improvement or no increase in osteoporosis. The patients in the control group demonstrated an increase in osteoporosis. A subsequent report by the same authors showed that there was no statistically significant difference in the incidence of thrombophlebitis, myocardial infarction, or uterine cancer in the two groups. Indeed, there was a lower incidence of breast cancer in the treated group. Estrogen-treated patients did show a higher incidence of cholelithiasis. The low number of cases precludes drawing any real conclusions from the data on diseases of low frequency. The study excludes a high incidence of complications from estrogens.

In another crossover study comparing the effects of estrogen–progestin therapy with those of placebo, bone mineral content increased during the 3 years of combination hormone therapy but continued to decrease in the placebo-treated group (Figure 4-12). When the placebo was given to some of the estrogen–progestin group, bone density decreased, whereas the women treated with placebo had an increase in bone mineral content after being given estrogen–progestin therapy. Other factors are also important in preventing osteoporosis, such as adequate dietary calcium, exercise, and vitamin D intake. Many case-control studies have noted considerable protection from hip fracture with HRT (Table 4-2).

Colorectal Cancer

Colorectal cancer is the third most common cancer and the third leading cause of cancer deaths in women in the United States. Several epidemiologic studies have noted

that HRT may reduce the risk of colorectal cancers. WHI demonstrated a HR of 0.63, demonstrating slight protection from colorectal cancer in their E+P arm but not in the estrogen-alone study (HR = 1.08). There appear to be some biologic reasons why estrogen may be protective. Bile acids are thought to initiate or promote malignant changes in the epithelium of the colon. Exogenous estrogen decreases secondary bile-acid production. Estrogen also decreases serum levels of insulin-like growth factor-1, which is an important mitogen associated with colorectal cancer.

Both case-control and prospective studies have been reported. Kampman and associates reported the largest case controlled study with 815 postmenopausal women with colon cancer and 1019 population base controls. After adjusting for multiple risk factors, they noted an 18% decrease in risk of colon cancer in HRT users compared with the nonusers (RR = 0.82, CI 0.67-0.99). In a large study by the American Cancer Society, 897 deaths from colon cancer were identified during 7 years of follow-up of 422,373 postmenopausal women. The authors reported a 29% decrease in risk of colon cancer deaths in hormone users compared with nonusers (R = 0.71, CI 0.61-0.83). In the review and meta-analysis by Grodstein and colleagues, 18 studies were evaluated. They found a 20% decrease of colon cancer in ERT users compared with the nonusers (RR = 0.8, CI 0.72-0.92) and a 19% decrease in rectal cancer (RR = 0.79, CI 0.72-0.92). Ten studies provided data on timing of hormone use. Current users had an RR of 0.66 (CI 0.59-0.74) compared with that of the nonusers. In the Nurses' Health Study, current users noted an RR of 0.65; in past users the RR was 0.84 (nonsignificant). Among past users, the decreased risk continued during the first 4 years after quitting ERT; however, 5 years or more after stopping ERT, the risk was similar to that of nonusers (RR = 0.92, CI 0.70-1.21). Recently, the effect of ERT on colon cancer risk was evaluated in the California Teachers Study among 56,864 postmenopausal women. A significantly lower risk for colon cancer was noted in women who had used ERT within the past 15 years than in women who had never taken hormones (RR = 0.64, CI 0.51-0.80). Five studies evaluated the duration of current use and found similar apparent protection for all women currently taking ERT, regardless of duration. Four studies evaluated ERT and colorectal adenoma. Most studies noted a significantly decreased risk of development of adenomas in women on ERT. This decrease did not appear to be caused by increased surveillance (sigmoidoscopy) in the ERT users. In several, but not all, studies there was a suggestion that colorectal cancers increased in women who were taking tamoxifen.

Cardiovascular Disease

Cardiovascular morbidity (i.e., heart disease and stroke) constitutes the most frequent cause of death among women in the United States. It is estimated to account for approximately 432,709 deaths in the United States in 2006. The second leading cause of death in women is cancer (269,819) followed by chronic respiratory diseases (65,323) in 2006. Cardiovascular risks factors can be found, and potentially modulated, in women; for instance, high cholesterol levels are present in 50% of women, high blood pressure is observed in 32% of all women, and 45% of black women have high blood pressure. The prevalence of cardiovascular diseases increases dramatically with age, starting at a low level of 17.6% for women age 35 to 44, 36.6% for women age 45 to 55, 56.5% for women age 55 to 64, and 75% for women age 65 to 74. The possible effects of estrogen and progestin on the incidence of cardiovascular disease in women is the subject of ongoing research. Most of the cohort studies suggest that ERT effectively diminishes the risk of cardiovascular disease in women who are 50 to 60 years of age, but protection decreases with age (Table 4-3). Unfortunately, recent studies (WHI, HERS) reveal that initiating estrogen therapy in women with established vascular disease (mean ages of 63-67) will not prevent cardiovascular events or deaths. These studies are unable to be generalized to estrogen use in the younger perimenopausal age groups, and the cohort and epidemiologic studies reveal some benefit, but use of progestin consistently decreases benefit.

Prevention of cardiovascular disease includes smoking cessation, blood pressure control, weight control, exercise, and blood sugar and cholesterol control. Blood cholesterol level is the main risk factor for cardiovascular disease in postmenopausal women. A high positive correlation has been found between levels of low-density lipoprotein (LDL) and coronary morbidity. Conversely, the level of high-density lipoprotein (HDL) shows a high negative correlation with the probability of coronary disease and with the extent of damage to the coronary vessels. Matthews has shown the beneficial effects of ERT on LDL and HDL levels. In a prospective study, he showed clearly a corresponding rise in HDLs and a decrease in LDLs in postmenopausal patients treated with ERT. The association of increased HDL and decreased LDL levels with reduced risk of cardiovascular disease is well documented for both men and women.

Lobo reported on the impact of different dosages of MPA on metabolism and hemostasis in postmenopausal women treated with conjugated estrogens. In this prospective, double-blind study, 525 women were randomly assigned to five treatment regimens at 26 sites in the United States and Europe. All participants received 0.625 mg of conjugated estrogens daily for up to 13 cycles; four groups also received MPA, either 2.5 or 5 mg/day continuously or 5 or 10 mg/day for the last 14 days of each cycle. Effects on lipid and carbohydrate metabolism and coagulation were evaluated.

All of the treatment groups experienced increases in HDL-cholesterol (HDL-C), the HDL2-C subfraction, and apolipoprotein A-1 compared with baseline; however, at each time point the increases from baseline in the conjugated estrogens-only group were significantly greater than were those for the conjugated estrogens-MPA groups. Additionally, all treatment groups had significant decreases in LDL-cholesterol (LDL-C) and apolipoprotein B. Decreases from baseline in total cholesterol (TC) levels were significantly greater than were those in the conjugated estrogens-only group. HDL3-C levels increased significantly from baseline in the conjugated estrogens-only group but not in the other treatment groups. Triglyceride levels increased significantly in all groups. The mean increase in the MPA-treated groups was less than that in the conjugated estrogens-only treatment group. Although MPA modified some of the effects of conjugated estrogens on lipid metabolism, the direction of changes in lipid parameters was unaltered.

Additional data on the conjugated estrogens regimen were reported in the results of the Postmenopausal Estrogen/Progestin Intervention (PEPI) trial. In this 3-year, randomized, double-blind, placebo-controlled trial, the investigators evaluated differences in selected heart disease risk factors among 875 postmenopausal women who received placebo, conjugated estrogens, or one of three conjugated estrogens/progestin regimens.

TABLE 4-3 Effect of Estrogen Treatment on Cardiovascular Morbidity in Menopausal Women

Authors	Year	Relative Risk
Bush et al	1983	0.4
Bush et al	1987	0.3
Wilson et al	1985	1.3-32*
Stampfer et al	1985	0.3
Colditz et al	1987	0.42

*Smokers.

One of the regimens used in this study was identical to that present in conjugated estrogens.

The investigators reported that after 3 years of therapy, women taking the conjugated estrogens regimen experienced significant increases in HDL-C levels compared with the placebo. However, the increases were significantly less than those experienced by women taking conjugated estrogens alone. Compared with the placebo, LDL-C values were significantly decreased in women taking the conjugated estrogens, with no significant difference between groups. TC levels decreased significantly among women taking the conjugated estrogens regimen compared with the placebo. Significant increases in serum triglyceride levels occurred in all treatment groups compared with the placebo group. There were no significant changes in blood pressure, fasting insulin levels, or 2-hour insulin levels among treatment groups. Treatment groups had significant increases in 2-hour glucose levels and significant decreases in fasting glucose levels compared with the placebo group. In paired comparisons, women in the placebo group had greater increases in fibrinogen than did women in the active treatment groups; no significant differences were present among active treatment groups. Among their findings, the investigators concluded that, ". . . oral estrogen taken alone or with MPA . . . is associated with improved lipoprotein and lower fibrinogen levels compared with placebo and the magnitude of these differences is likely to be clinically significant."

Multiple studies have evaluated HRT and CHD. In 1998 an overview by Barrett-Connor and Grady included 25 studies. Overall, the RR of CHD for women who took ERT compared with those who never took ERT was 0.70 (CI 0.65-0.75). When HRT was evaluated, the RR was 0.66 (0.53-0.84) compared with the nonusers. This analysis evaluated cohort case-control and angiographic studies. The apparent benefit is limited mainly to current or recent use. These findings are consistent across diverse populations and various study designs.

The U.S. National Health and Nutritional Examination Survey (NHANES-1) evaluated HRT and death from all cardiovascular disease in 1944 white women 55 years of age or older who were monitored for up to 16 years. After adjusting for risk factors of CHD, the risk of death from CHD was 0.66 (0.48-0.90) in the HRT users. The study by Ettinger and associates noted similar findings. In their patient population followed for 25 years, the death from any cause in HRT users compared with nonusers was 0.54, which was mainly the result of a reduction in CHD (RR 0.40) and other cardiovascular diseases (RR 0.27).

Many studies, including the PEPI randomized control trial, have noted that estrogen therapy in postmenopausal women decreased serum TC, LDL, and Lp(a) lipoproteins. HDL and triglyceride concentrations increase. The route of administration does affect the serum lipids. Transdermal application has less effect on the serum lipid concentrations than the oral route. The type of progestins can also affect the serum lipids. Synthetic progestins tend to blunt the beneficial effects on the HDL but do not decrease it below the baseline. Micronized progesterone does not decrease HDL compared with estrogen alone. Estrogen tends to decrease plasma fibrinogen concentrations, as do anticoagulant proteins, antithrombin III, and protein S. There also appears to be a decrease in the antifibronolytic protein plasminogen B activator inhibitor type I with an overall increased potential for fibrinolysis. In some reports, factor VII was also lowered with estrogen. The net effect on coagulation depends on the type of estrogen, dose, and duration of treatment.

As mentioned earlier, the 2002 Women's Health Initiative was a study looking at the role of HRT in regard to several disease entities, which included coronary artery disease, stroke, pulmonary embolus, and deep venous thrombosis; three cancers (breast, colorectal, and endometrial); and hip fractures. They also looked at total deaths. This intent-to-treat study was evaluated using a nominal and adjusted statistical methodology and included women ages 50 to 79 with a mean age of 63.3 years who received either estrogen plus progesterone (E+P) or a placebo. Of particular interest is that only 10% of the women in this study were age 50 to 54 years. There was a very large dropout rate—42% in the E+P group and 38% in the placebo group. As noted, this was a preliminary report that had not been adjudicated before publication. The overall hazard ratio was statistically significantly increased in those women who were taking E+P for congestive heart disease, stroke, and venous thrombolic phenomenon at the nominal level. Interestingly enough, the incidence of breast cancer was the reason that the study was stopped and, although the hazard ratio was elevated, it was not statistically significant. There was a statistically significant decrease in colorectal cancer, hip fractures, and total fractures. When the adjusted methodology was applied (not multivariant analysis) the only item that remained statistically significant was the venous thrombolic phenomenon—and only the venous thrombosis in that category. The authors noted that the congestive heart disease rates were low; however, they stated there were 7 more per 10,000 women years of CHD in those taking E+P versus the placebo. When the data were further analyzed, it was noted that there was an increase in events the first 4 months of the trial; however, the rate then decreased and at 6+ years there was a higher incidence of CHD in the placebo arm than in those taking E+P. Subsequent publications noted that the hazard ratio for CHD after adjudication had dropped from 1.29 to 1.24 (CI 1.00-1.54), and after multivariant analysis the confidence interval was 0.97 to 1.60.

In 2005 the WHI reported cardiovascular disease incidence in their observational arm compared with the clinical study. The WHI initially had about 160,000 women enrolled, for which there were three prospective randomized studies, and those who did not qualify or did not wish to participate in the randomized studies became the observational arm. In the clinical study, the risk ratio of those women taking HRT for CHD was 1.21, but in more than 53,000 women in the observational arm, it was only 0.71. In addition, stroke was 1.33 versus 0.77 and DVT was 2.1 versus 1.06. The big difference between the two is that in the clinical study the median age was 63.3 years where it is assumed that in the observational arm women who went on HRT did so at the time of menopause, which would be on average a decade or more earlier than in the clinical study.

The data from the observational arm also were confirmed in the large observational study from the Nurses' Health Study in which HRT was started near menopause. Those taking estrogen only had a risk ratio of 0.66 (CI 0.54-0.80), and in those taking E+P the RR was 0.72 (CI 0.56-0.92). Both of these figures were based on multivariant analysis. In 2004 the WHI published their data on estrogen only in which more than 10,000 women who had previously had a hysterectomy were randomly assigned to receive estrogen only or placebo. When the total group was analyzed for CHD, the HR was 0.91 (CI 0.75-1.12); however, in those women 50 to 59 years of age, the HR was 0.56 (CI 0.30-1.03). When the estrogen-only arm was further evaluated in the 50 to 59-year-old group, the outcome for cardiovascular disease, which included myocardial infarction, coronary death, coronary revascularization, and confirmed angina, the HR was 0.55 (CI 0.45-0.96) favoring the estrogen arm. On further evaluation in the E+P arm at commencement of HRT in the 50- to 59-year old, the HR was 1.29, which was not statistically significant, however, if it was started less than 10 years postmenopause, the HR was 0.88 but not statistically significant.

Further evaluation was carried out in a subset in the estrogen-only study of women 50 to 59 years of age. Coronary artery calcium scores were determined by computed tomography (CT) scans and measured on an average of 8.7 years after the start of the study. In more than 1000 women so evaluated, the mean score in the estrogen-only arm was 83.1 compared with the no-estrogen arm of 123.1 ($P = 0.02$). When the intent-to-treat evaluation was performed, the P value was 0.03; however, when 80% adherence to the medication was evaluated, the P value was 0.002. This evaluation used multivariant analysis. Test score at each level was better in the adherence compared to the intent-to-treat group. In 2007 the American Association of Clinical Endocrinology published a position statement on HRT

and cardiovascular risk that said, "It seems clear from statistical analysis of previous large observational studies and randomized control clinical trials that young women in early menopause not only have no excess cardiovascular risk but the benefit many indeed be shown in the future."

Cardiovascular risk reduction recommendations are smoking cessation, exercise, weight control, and blood pressure and cholesterol management. Aspirin has been shown to reduce the risk of stroke without affecting the risk of myocardial infarction or death from cardiovascular causes in most women. In this randomized trial of 39,876 healthy women 45 years of age or older, patients received 100 mg of aspirin or placebo on alternate days for 10 years and were monitored for cardiovascular events. There was a 17% reduction of strokes for the entire study population randomly assigned to aspirin (RR = 0.83, CI 0.69; 0.99, $P = 0.04$). There was benefit for prevention of myocardial infarction only in women 65 years of age and older at enrollment (RR = 0.66, CI 0.44; 0.97, $P = 0.04$). The conclusion of this study is that physicians should perform a careful risk assessment to determine who is likely to benefit from aspirin and who is likely to be harmed by the increase of gastrointestinal hemorrhage requiring transfusion ($P = 0.05$)

A 2008 ACOG Committee Opinion recommended that HRT should not be used for the primary or secondary prevention of CHD; instead, women should be prescribed estrogen or estrogen plus a progestogen (when a uterus is present) at the onset of moderate or severe menopausal symptoms. The dose should be the lowest necessary to achieve the symptom control desired, and the duration of therapy should be 5 years or less. Discontinuation of this medication is not without side effects, and withdrawal symptoms may be minimized by a tapering schedule over a long period. It is accepted, however, that once a woman is on therapy, the risk of continuing such treatment is low; risk is greatest during the first year or two after initiating treatment, especially when preexisting vascular disease may already be present.

ESTROGEN REPLACEMENT THERAPY FOR ENDOMETRIAL AND BREAST CANCER SURVIVORS

Estrogen Replacement Therapy for the Endometrial Cancer Survivor

Historically, hormone replacement therapy has been contraindicated for the patient who has been treated for cancer of the uterus. Although estrogen administration has not been shown to have adverse effects on patients who have been treated for endometrial cancer, many physicians continue to be reluctant to administer this medication to these women. No data in the literature substantiate the detrimental effects of estrogen in these patients. It is not unusual for women with endometrial cancer to have severe symptoms as a result of withdrawal of estrogen at the time of their diagnosis and surgical treatment.

The GOG conducted a prospective trial to evaluate the potential risk of estrogen replacement in women after treatment of endometrial adenocarcinoma. This randomized clinical trial of estrogen replacement therapy (CEE 0.625 mg orally per day, Premarin) compared to placebo in women treated for stage I and II endometrial cancer closed after the WHI was halted prematurely in 2002 because of a decrease in accrual and lack of feasibility. For the trial, 1236 eligible women were randomly assigned and the median follow-up was 35.7 months. The median age at endometrial cancer diagnosis was 57 years (range, 26-91 years). Compliance with medication for the entire treatment period was 41%, and for those on the ERT arm, 71% knew to which arm they had been randomly assigned. A summary of the results on the ERT arm demonstrated endometrial cancer recurrence in 14 patients (2.3%) and 8 patients (1.3%) developed a new malignancy, one of which was breast cancer. There were 26 deaths (4.2%) on the estrogen arm; 5 were from endometrial cancer. An important finding is that women with stage I and II endometrial cancer are more likely to die of causes unrelated to the cancer diagnosis; therefore other health issues must take priority when planning for preventive health maintenance (Table 4-4). Women on the placebo arm of this study suffered 19 deaths (3.1%; not statistically different), and 4 were from endometrial cancer. Ten patients receiving placebo developed a new malignancy (1.6%), 3 of which were breast cancer. Although there were no significant differences in recurrence between the ERT and placebo arms for all comers,

further investigation suggested that racial disparities in outcome may exist. With a median follow-up of 3 years, recurrent disease was noted in 5 of 56 black patients on the ERT arm compared with only 8 of 521 white patients. The RR of recurrence among blacks in the ERT group was 11.2 (95% CI, 2.86-43.59, $P = 0.0005$) after adjustment for age, body mass index, and tumor grade.

This study was admittedly underpowered for the endpoints of new breast cancer or endometrial cancer recurrence, but at least women can be informed that the rate of recurrence of endometrial cancer was equally low on each arm of this study. The exception to this may lie with ERT for specific subgroups. Although the number of outcome events was limited in this study, these findings suggest that the use of ERT in black women should be judicious and given only after appropriate patient education. The decision to prescribe estrogen must be individualized based on symptom control and quality-of-life concerns, which only the patient can assess.

Many physicians do not hesitate to give ERT in patients with well-differentiated or superficially invasive cancers because recurrences are generally very low in these patients. There is greater hesitancy to treat poorly differentiated or deeply invasive cancers with ERT. This is also true for patients with extrauterine disease. The belief is that because recurrence is more frequent, ERT may increase the risk. The data would suggest the opposite. Those patients with high-risk factors and taking ERT have a lower recurrence rate than do those who are not taking ERT. Although theoretically a possible advantage, it does not appear that the addition of a progestin to estrogen is beneficial. We initially followed this routine of a combination of E+P; however, for several years now we have not done so, and we have noticed no difference in outcomes.

The optimal time to begin ERT post treatment has not been determined. Some would suggest waiting for at least 2 years because most patients who will develop recurrences will have done so. The data currently would suggest no benefit in waiting. Within a few days of surgical treatment, many patients will develop disturbing vasomotor symptoms. These symptoms can be prolonged with subsequent adverse symptomatology, such as vaginal thinness and dryness that can lead to unpleasant intercourse. As a result, symptoms can be treated as soon as they become troublesome.

In 1993 the American College of Obstetricians and Gynecologists released the following statement: "In women with a history of endometrial cancer, estrogens could be used for the same indications as for any other woman, except that the selection of appropriate candidates should be based on prognostic indicators and the risk the patient is willing to assume." In the absence of good prospective studies, this statement appropriately leaves the issue with the patient and the physician.

TABLE 4-4   GOG Randomized Trial of Estrogen in Endometrial Cancer Recurrence and Survival

	Treatment Group			
	Placebo*	%	ERT*	%
Alive, NED	591	(95.6)	583	(94.3)
Alive with disease recurrence	8	(1.3)	9	(1.5)
Total deaths	19	(3.1)	26	(4.2)
Endometrial cancer	4	(0.6)	5	(0.8)
MI/CHD	4	(0.6)	3	(0.5)
Pulmonary embolism	0	(0.0)	2	(0.3)
Other	6	(1.0)	9	(1.5)
Unknown	5	(0.8)	7	(1.1)

From JCO 2006 Barakat et al 24:587.
*618 evaluable patients in each treatment group
CHD, coronary heart disease; ERT, estrogen replacement therapy; MI, myocardial infarction; NED, no evidence of disease.

Fear of medico–legal liability, as a result of the contraindication of estrogen in breast and endometrial cancer in the package insert, requires that physicians document a lengthy discussion of the risks/benefits and have the patient actively participate in the decision and understand the process of informed consent needed for this therapy.

Hormonal Therapy for the Breast Cancer Survivor

Women diagnosed with breast cancer are faced with many challenging decisions, especially if they are premenopausal. They are asked to review their family history to determine if they may have developed breast cancer because of a genetic predisposition (BRCA 1 or 2 gene), which transmits risk of familial breast and ovarian cancer. Genetic counseling and testing may then be recommended in order to properly counsel the patient, and her family members, about the benefits and risks of prophylactic mastectomy and bilateral salpingo-oophorectomy. This places premenopausal breast cancer patients in the unique position of being asked to undergo surgery to remove their ovaries to prevent ovarian cancer when they may be told they cannot take estrogen replacement for the menopausal symptoms, which will occur postoperatively. Appropriate estrogen and/or testosterone replacement after premenopausal oophorectomy is not condoned in this population by oncologists. The challenges to her emotional well-being, while simultaneously facing a life-threatening illness, menopausal symptoms, sexual dysfunction, and potential problems with her marriage, are overwhelming.

The benefits to bilateral salpingo-oophorectomy in a BRCA 1 or 2 carrier are the potential reduction in risk of breast cancer recurrence and the 90% risk reduction from ovarian cancer. If symptom control from the surgery was feasible, this would be a great benefit. The risk of estrogen and androgen withdrawal can be decreased libido, lubrication, hot flashes, insomnia, and depression; some women conclude that the benefit is not worth the risk. For this reason the age at which prophylactic oophorectomy should be planned is not known in genetic carriers and must be individualized. Some allow patients a reversible trial period of Depo-Lupron® to simulate menopause and help them with this decision-making process.

The treatment of breast cancer may consist of tamoxifen, aromatase inhibitors, local radiation, and chemotherapy. Some would argue that the purpose of the chemotherapy is to destroy ovarian function. Oophorectomy may be able to replace the benefit of chemotherapy, but this has not yet been adequately scientifically compared. Women are also eligible for treatment with aromatase inhibitors if they are menopausal, which has demonstrated a 43% reduction in breast cancer recurrence after completion of 5 years of tamoxifen.

There is increasing concern for the long-term morbidity of the standard breast cancer therapies, which are poorly captured in research trials. Women report cognitive function impairment from chemotherapy, in addition to fatigue, weight gain, osteoporosis, and sexual dysfunction. Further study is required in this area to determine prevention strategies: bone density testing frequency, calcium and vitamin supplementations, benefits of biphosphonates, bone density monitoring, and prevention of cognitive dysfunction and sexual dysfunction.

The use of tamoxifen for the treatment or prevention of breast cancer has many known consequences including thromboembolic disease, strokes, and endometrial cancer. The expected annual rate of endometrial cancer in the breast cancer patient is 1 per 1000. The patient taking tamoxifen has an excess risk of 2 per 1000 or a total risk of 3 per 1000 per year. Studies on the appropriate monitoring of women taking tamoxifen have demonstrated that transvaginal ultrasound and routine annual endometrial biopsies increase a woman's risk. The current recommendation is to "do no harm" by conducting a routine annual gynecologic examination with cervical cytology and inquire about symptoms such as bleeding or discharge.

For many years it has been stated that ERT in patients who have had breast cancer is absolutely contraindicated, yet the data are inconsistent in substantiating this admonition. During the last couple of decades there has been increasing evidence that ERT can protect against osteoporosis and colon cancer, and recent data suggest benefits in prevention of Alzheimer's disease, macular degeneration, and tooth loss. Because the benefits of ERT are substantial and no data are available to note detrimental effect in patients with breast disease, these authors firmly believe that a reappraisal of the admonition against ERT in patients with breast cancer is needed. Historically, it has been the dictum that women who have had breast cancer should not, under any circumstances, receive ERT. When one looks in the literature for data to support that recommendation, there is a huge void. In 1989 Wile and DiSaia suggested that in the absence of a prospective study of ERT in breast cancer survivors, one could analyze situations in which these patients were exposed to high levels of estrogens at a time when they may have been harboring breast cancer cells. These situations were defined as pregnancy coexistent with breast cancer, pregnancy subsequent to breast cancer, breast cancer in previous and current users of oral contraceptives, and breast cancer in women receiving ERT. After extensive evaluation of these situations, there appears to be very little, if any, relationship. Currently, approximately 192,000 cases of breast cancer

TABLE 4-5 Hormone Replacement Therapy in Women with Breast Cancer

Author	Recurrence (%)	Deaths (%)
Stoll	0/65 (0)	0
Powles	2/35 (8)	0
Sellin	1/49 (2)	0
Bluming	12/189 (6)	1 (1)
Brewster	13/145 (9)	3 (2)
Natrajan	2/50 (4)	3 (6)
	30/533 (6)	7 (1)

TABLE 4-6 Hormone Replacement Therapy Following Breast Cancer

	Recurrence		Deaths	
	ERT (%)	Controls (%)	ERT (%)	Controls (%)
CASE-CONTROLLED				
Wile et al	1/25 (4)	2/50 (4)	1 (4)	2 (4)
DiSaia et al	6/41 (14)	7/82 (8)	2 (5)	6 (7)
Eden et al	6/90 (7)	30/108 (17)	0	11
Cohort				
Dew et al	?/167	/1472	2 (1)	167 (13)
Espie et al	5/120	/240	*	*

*No difference in disease-free survival.
ERT, Estrogen replacement therapy.

occur in the United States annually. More and more of these individuals are surviving their cancer; in many, long-term survival of greater than 90% can be expected. Because many will survive their cancer, they will experience old age. We must address the advisability of HRT in this setting.

In fact, some data suggest that ERT in the patient with breast cancer is not deleterious. Historically, we must remember that before cytotoxic agents, postmenopausal women with metastatic or recurrent cancer received estrogen as a first line of therapy. We now understand that its effectiveness depended to a certain extent on the receptor status of the cancer. At least seven prospective, randomized, double-blind studies have compared estrogen with tamoxifen in patients with recurrent or metastatic breast cancer. The response rate of estrogen and tamoxifen is essentially the same. In prospective randomized studies comparing estrogen and tamoxifen as adjuvant therapy, the recurrence rate was essentially the same. It would appear that we have a very short medical history memory.

At least six retrospective studies have evaluated HRT in women with breast cancer. These patients were recurrence free at the time, and they were given estrogen to combat vasomotor symptoms or to prevent the chronic illness of cardiovascular disease, osteoporosis, and colon cancer. In this select group of more than 500 patients, there have been 30 (6%) recurrences and only 7 (1%) deaths. In the authors' study of 145 patients in which patients with in situ, stage I to IV cancer were treated, there have been 13 (9%) recurrences. Patients with both node-positive and node-negative disease were treated. Of the 96 node-negative patients, 11 recurred, whereas only 1 of 34 node-positive patients to date has had a recurrence. There was 1 of 15 recurrences in individuals in whom the lymph nodes were not pathologically evaluated. It appears that evaluation of the receptor status in patients who had this performed did not have an impact one way or the other with regard to recurrences (Table 4-5).

In addition, there have been three case-controlled studies and three cohort-type studies (Table 4-6) in which recurrences and deaths were similar in both the patients on ERT and the controls. A cohort study of 125 patients with breast cancer who received HRT post cancer therapy were compared with 362 patients with breast cancer who did not receive HRT. Patients were matched for stage, age, and year of diagnosis. All stages were included, although 78% had carcinoma in situ (14%) or stage I and II cancers. There was a survival advantage for HRT users compared with non-HRT users, with an odds ratio of 0.28 (CI 0.11-0.71). Six endometrial cancers were subsequently diagnosed in the patients who took HRT.

The HABITS trial was a prospective randomized, open, nonblinded study of HRT in women who had postmenopausal symptoms and had been previously treated for breast cancer. The study lasted 2 years and primarily looked at recurrence and breast cancer death rates and quality of life. Eligibility included patients with in situ, stage I or stage II breast cancers with up to four positive lymph nodes, and they should be recurrence free at the time of randomization. It was recommended that a recent (within 3 months) mammography be obtained. Receptor status was not taken into consideration, and the patient may be taking tamoxifen. Hormone therapy (HT) was "what was commonly given in an environment where the patient lived" and the control was "best symptomatic treatment without hormones." In their initial report it was noted that there were 18% recurrences in the HT group vs 8% in the no-hormone group. Cancer deaths were equal (3% vs 2%, respectively). This gave an HR of 3.3 (CI 1.5-7.4). Subsequently, a follow-up at 4 years was reported and a non-adjusted HR had dropped to 2.4 (CI 1.3-4.2); when adjusted using multivariant analysis, the HR was 2.2 (CI 1.0-5.1). When the two reporting times were evaluated, it was apparent that the largest number of recurrences/new cancers in the HT group occurred during the first 2 years of the study, suggesting that the cancer was probably present at the time the patients were randomized for the study. Between 2 and 4 years of follow-up, the incidence of the new recurrences/new cancers were equal in the two groups; 13 in the HT group and 10 in the no-HT group. The authors did state that there were limitations to their study, and items that could affect results were patient characteristics, the type of the HR used, and the fact that the placebo was not controlled. They stated "some judgments about disease recurrence can be subjective."

At the same time, the Stockholm trial was a prospective, randomized, open study. Postmenopausal women who had surgery for primary operable breast cancer were eligible for this study. Stratification was carried out for tamoxifen use, the type of hormone therapy (cyclic, spacing, estrogen-only), and the time since primary surgery (more or less than 2 years). There were 175 patients randomized to the HT compared with 184 in the no-HT. The compliance for more than 2 years was very good (77% and 90%, respectively). The recurrence rate was 6% in the HT group and 7% in the no-HT group. There were 2 deaths from breast cancer in the HT group compared with 4 in the no-HT group. Total mortality was 4 and 9, respectively.

Some differences were seen between the HABITS and the Stockholm study. Of the patients in the HABITS study, 27% had positive lymph nodes compared with 19% in the Stockholm group, and tamoxifen was being used in 21% vs 52%, respectively. The hormone therapy was described in the Stockholm study but not in the HABITS study. Although the median follow-up was equal in the two studies, the length of therapy was 2 years in the HABITS study but 5 years in the Stockholm study.

In conclusion, the risk of recurrent breast cancer in postmenopausal women receiving ERT is unclear. In postmenopausal women with previously treated breast cancer, consideration of ERT is an option but must be reviewed with caution. In other words, there must be informed consent. Women are interested in information for which they can make informed decisions. To not even discuss replacement therapy with these individuals is not in their best interest. In the United States today >36,000 women who are younger than 50 years of age will develop breast cancer. Most, if not all, will begin cytotoxic chemotherapy, and a significant number will become amenorrheic even though they are younger than 35 years of age. Unfortunately, if amenorrhea occurs while receiving chemotherapy, permanent ovarian failure occurs in the vast majority. Even in the very young (less than 40 years of age), 86% will have ovarian failure. We therefore are seeing an increasing number of young women who are going through a chemotherapeutic-induced premature menopause. A significant number of these women will be cured of their breast cancer; however, because of the premature menopause, they may have significant vasomotor symptoms that are much greater than those expected with a natural menopause. Long-term benefits of replacement therapy may even be greater because of the premature menopause. These patients should be made aware of the rationale for replacement (i.e., the benefits and risks) so that intelligent decisions can be made. The patient with breast cancer may be the ideal candidate for the vaginal, slow-release forms of estradiol rings. Estring contains a very low dose of estradiol, which can successfully treat vaginal atrophy symptoms and only increase plasma estradiol levels to one-tenth the amount of a 0.05 Estraderm patch. If menopausal symptoms remain intolerable, Femring has a higher estradiol dose of 0.05 mg/day and may provide some relief of symptoms also.

For full reference list, log onto www.expertconsult.com
⟨http://www.expertconsult.com⟩

Adenocarcinoma of the Uterine Corpus

William T. Creasman, MD, and David Scott Miller, MD

INCIDENCE

In the United States, cancer of the uterine corpus is the most common malignancy unique to women. It was estimated by the American Cancer Society that uterine cancer will develop in approximately 42,160 women in 2009 in the United States, making it the fourth most common cancer in women. The increased incidence of carcinoma of the endometrium has been apparent only during the last three decades. In reviewing the predicted incidence for the 1970s, the American Cancer Society noted a one and a half-fold increase in the number of patients with endometrial cancer; however, there was a decline in incidence during the late 1980s. In the past several years, the incidence has remained constant. During the period of increased incidence, predicted deaths from this malignant neoplasm actually decreased slightly. More recently, deaths from uterine cancer have increased. In 1990 the American Cancer Society estimated 4000 deaths from this cancer, increasing to 7780 in 2009. An estimation of the most common new cancers and the percentage of female deaths for 2009 in the United States is shown in Figure 5-1. The increased use of estrogen has been implicated in the apparent increased incidence during the 1970s and early 1980s; however, Norway and Czechoslovakia report a 50% to 60% increase in endometrial cancer, despite the fact that estrogens are rarely prescribed or are not generally available there. However, the increasing prevalence of overweight and obesity in women, especially in developed countries, may account for this apparent increase. Regardless of the reason for the increased number of women with corpus cancer, this malignant neoplasm has become an important factor in the care of the female patient.

EPIDEMIOLOGY

Endometrial adenocarcinoma occurs during the reproductive and menopausal years. The mean age for patients with adenocarcinoma of the uterine corpus is 63 years; most patients are between the ages of 50 and 59 years (Figure 5-2). Approximately 5% of women will have adenocarcinoma before the age of 40 years, and 20% to 25% will be diagnosed before menopause. Bokhman

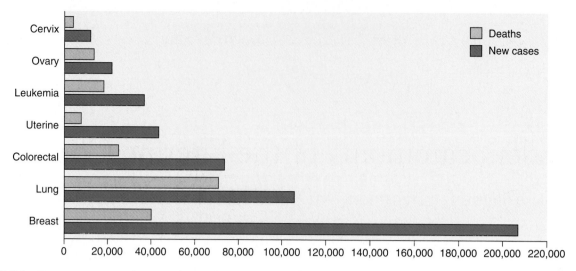

FIGURE 5-1   Common new cancer cases and deaths in women for 2010 in the United States. *(Modified from American Cancer Society. Cancer Facts and Figures 2010. Atlanta. American Cancer Society, 2010.)*

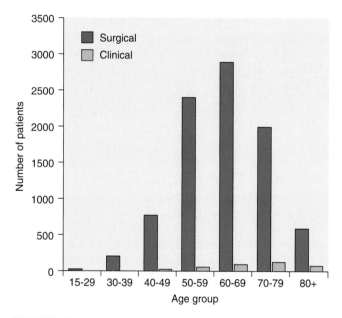

FIGURE 5-2   Carcinoma of the corpus uteri; patients treated in 1999–2001. Age distribution by mode of staging. *(Modified from Creasman WT et al: Int J Gynecol Obstet 95(1):S105-143, 2006)*

suggested that there are two pathogenic types of endometrial cancer. The first type arises in women with obesity, hyperlipidemia, and signs of hyperestrogenism, such as anovulatory uterine bleeding, infertility, late onset of menopause, and hyperplasia of the stroma of the ovaries and endometrium. The second pathogenic type of disease arises in women who have none of these disease states or in whom the disease states are not clearly defined. Bokhman's data suggest that patients with the first pathogenic type mainly have well-differentiated or moderately differentiated tumor, superficial invasion of the myometrium, high sensitivity to progestins, and favorable prognosis (85% 5-year survival in his material). The patients who fall into the second pathogenic group tend to have poorly differentiated tumors, deep myometrial invasion, high frequency of metastatic disease in the lymph nodes, decreased sensitivity to progestin, and poor prognosis (58% 5-year survival rate).

Multiple risk factors for endometrial cancer have been identified, and MacMahon divides these into three categories:

- Variants of normal anatomy or physiology
- Frank abnormality or disease
- Exposure to external carcinogens

Obesity, nulliparity, and late menopause are variants of normal anatomy or physiology classically associated with endometrial carcinoma. These three factors are evaluated in regard to the possible risk of developing endometrial cancer in Table 5-1. If a patient is nulliparous and obese and reaches menopause at age 52 years or older, she appears to have a fivefold increase in the risk of endometrial cancer above that of the patient who does not satisfy these criteria (Table 5-2).

The type of obesity in patients with endometrial cancer has been evaluated. In a study from the University of South Florida, it was noted that women with endometrial cancer had greater waist-to-hip circumference ratios, abdomen-to-thigh skin ratios, and suprailiac-to-thigh skin ratios than those of matched-control

TABLE 5-1 Endometrial Cancer Risk Factors

Risk Factors	Risk
Obesity	2.5-4.5×
Nulliparity	
Compared with 1 child	2×
Compared with 5 or more children	3×
Late menopause	2.4×

TABLE 5-2 Multiple Risk Factors

	Risk	
Nulliparous		Parous
Top 15% in weight	5× more than	Lower two thirds in weight
Menopause at 52 years		Menopause at <49 years

women. As these ratios increased, the relative risk (RR) of endometrial cancer increased. The researchers concluded that upper-body fat localization is a significant risk factor for endometrial cancer. In a large multicenter case-control study of 403 endometrial cancer cases and 297 control cases, Swanson and associates confirmed and amplified these findings. Women whose weight exceeded 78 kg had a risk 2.3 times that of women weighing less than 58 kg. For women weighing more than 96 kg, the RR increased to 4.3. Upper-body obesity (waist-to-height ratio) was a risk factor independent of body weight. Patients in the highest quartile of both weight and waist-to-thigh circumference had a risk of 5.8 times. The amount of body fat has been associated with decreased circulating levels of both progesterone and sex hormone-binding proteins. There was a strong inverse association between sitting height and risk of endometrial cancer. This may be related to sex hormone-bound globulin (SHBG), which appears to be depressed in women with endometrial cancer. The level of SHBG is progressively depressed with increasing upper-body fat localization. With lower SHBG, there is a higher endogenous production of non–protein-bound estradiol. Because endometrial cancer is related to obesity, dietary habits appear to be important. Data suggest that the levels of estriol, total estrogens, and prolactin were lower and those of SHBG were higher in postmenopausal women who were vegetarians. In a case-control study, Levi and colleagues evaluated dietary factors in 274 patients with endometrial cancer and 572 control subjects from two areas in Switzerland and northern Italy. Extensive dietary history was obtained. Their data confirmed the relationship between obesity and endometrial cancer. In relation to diet, they noted an increased association with total energy intake. After correction for total energy intake, a risk was present with the frequency of consumption of most types of meats, eggs, beans, added fats, and sugar. Conversely, significant protection was noted with an elevated intake of most vegetables, fresh fruits, whole grain bread, and pasta. This reflected a low risk with increased intake of ascorbic acid and beta-carotene. Of dietary interest is that the intake of olive oil seemed beneficial in Switzerland but resembled other added fats in the Italian women. It has been previously noted that the amount and type of dietary fat influence estrogen metabolism because estrogen reabsorption from the bowel seems to be increased by diets rich in beef or fats.

Diabetes mellitus and hypertension are frequently associated with endometrial cancer. Elwood and colleagues reported a RR of 2.8 associated with a history of diabetes after controlling for age, body weight, and socioeconomic status. High levels of insulin-like growth factor I, coupled with elevated estrogen levels, are thought to have neoplastic potential that accounts for the observed increased risk of endometrial cancer. High blood pressure is prevalent in elderly obese patients but does not appear to be a significant factor by itself, even though 25% of patients with endometrial cancer have hypertension or arteriosclerotic heart disease.

As extensively detailed in Chapter 4, the relationship of unopposed estrogen and endometrial cancer is well documented. Fortunately, the addition of a progestin appears to be protective. Adequacy of progesterone is important in prevention of endometrial cancer. In a study from Sweden, at the end of 5 years excess risk of endometrial cancer was 6.6 but with combined estrogen progestin (E + P), RR was 1.6 for 11 to 15 days of progestin, 2.9 for 10 days of use, and 0.2 if continuous E + P was given. The Million Women study from the United Kingdom has recently reported their findings of endometrial cancer and hormone replacement therapy (HRT). This study, which first reported on HRT and breast cancer, has been severely criticized mainly on methodology factors. They had an average follow-up of 3.4 years, during which 1320 incident endometrial cancers were diagnosed. At time of recruitment 22% of HRT users (total number was 320,953 women) last used continuous combined therapy, 45% last used cyclic combined therapy with progestogen usually added for 10 to 14 days per month, 19% last used tibolone, and 4% used estrogen alone. Compared with nonusers, RR of endometrial cancer was 0.71%, CI 0.56 to 0.90, P = 0.005; 1.05, CI 0.91 to 1.22; 1.79, CI 1.43 to 2.25, P <0.001; and 1.45, CI 1.02 to 2.06, P = 0.04, respectively. Of note, the adverse effects of tibolone and estrogen only were greatest in the nonobese woman and the beneficial effects of combined HRT were greatest in obese women. Although the risk of unopposed estrogen is present, women taking estrogen who develop endometrial cancer appear to have favorable prognostic factors. Several but not all studies suggest that risk factors such as multiparity and obesity are lower in the estrogen users. Stage of disease and histologic grade appear to be lower in estrogen users. With correction for stage and grade, estrogen users still have less myometrial invasion than nonestrogen users do. The poor prognostic subtypes, such as clear cell carcinoma and adenosquamous cancer, appear less frequently in estrogen users. As a result, survival rates with estrogen-related endometrial cancer are much better than those of nonestrogen cancers. In fact, some studies note just as good if not better survival in estrogen users than in women with nonestrogen, nonendometrial cancers.

Data indicate that the use of combination oral contraceptives decreases the risk for development of endometrial cancer. The Centers for Disease Control and Prevention evaluated endometrial cancer cases of all women aged 20 to 54 years from eight population-based cancer registries and compared them with control patients selected at random from the same centers. A comparison of the first 187 cases with 1320 control cases showed that women who used oral contraceptives at some time had a 0.5 RR of developing endometrial cancer compared with women who had never used oral contraceptives. This protection occurred in women who used oral contraceptives for at least 12 months, and protection continued for at least 10 years after oral contraceptive use. Protection was most notable for nulliparous women. These investigators estimated that about 2000 cases of endometrial cancer are prevented each year in the United States by past or current use of oral contraceptives. Of interest, cigarette smoking appears to decrease the risk for developing endometrial cancer. In a population-based case-control study of women aged 40 to 60 years, Lawrence and associates found a significant decline in RR of endometrial carcinoma with increased smoking (P >0.05). The RR decreased by about 30% when one pack of cigarettes was smoked per day and by another 30% when more than one pack was smoked per day. The effects of smoking did not appear to vary with menstrual status or exogenous estrogen. There was a fourfold increase in smoking-related odds ratio with body weight; the greatest reduction in risk by smoking was in the heaviest women. However, the estimated risk increased twelvefold in overweight women who were nonsmokers and whose primary source of estrogen was peripheral conversion of androgen to estrogen. Although smoking apparently reduces the risk for development of early-stage endometrial cancer, this advantage is strongly outweighed by the increased risk of lung cancer and other major health hazards associated with cigarette smoking.

Incidence and survival are higher in white women compared with black women. Reasons for these differences are unexplained. An analysis of the Gynecologic Oncology Group (GOG) database evaluated this factor in 600 white and 91 black women with clinical stage I or stage II endometrial cancer. A larger number of the African American women were diagnosed after age 70 years, and they had a higher proportion of papillary serous (PS) and clear cell histologic types; the black women also had more advanced disease, grade, vascular space involvement, depth of invasion, and lymph node metastases than the white women did. Survival (5-year) was 77% for white women and 60% for black women. Survival difference remained even in high-risk groups such as grade III tumors (59% vs 37%, respectively). The unadjusted hazard rate was 2.0, which was statistically significant. With adjustment for age, cell type, and extent of disease, the RR dropped to 1.2. The adjusted risk rate suggests that race is not a significant factor; nevertheless, race does denote an increased risk for poor prognostic factors, which clinically may be important.

Tamoxifen is used to prevent or treat breast cancer. Tamoxifen was first introduced in clinical trials in the early 1970s and was approved in 1978 by the U.S. Food and Drug Administration (FDA) for treatment of advanced breast carcinoma in postmenopausal woman. Tamoxifen, although labeled an antiestrogen, is known to have estrogenic properties and truly is a weak estrogen. Women receiving tamoxifen also appear to have some protection from osteoporosis and heart disease (decreased lactate dehydrogenase and cholesterol), much like women receiving estrogen replacement therapy. Extensive experience with this drug has been reported. It is estimated that more than 4 million women in the United States have taken tamoxifen for almost 8 million women-years of use. One of its major benefits is that in women taking tamoxifen, there has been a substantial decrease in the incidence of a second cancer in the opposite breast compared with similar women who were taking a placebo.

The Early Breast Cancer Trialists Collaborative Group (EBCTCG) has produced an important meta-analysis of 194 randomized trials of adjuvant chemotherapy or endocrine therapy with at least 15 years of follow-up. The analysis evaluated the effects of adjuvant tamoxifen on breast cancer recurrence and survival. It was shown that 5 years of tamoxifen therapy, compared to no adjuvant therapy, reduced the 15-year probability of breast cancer recurrence (from 45% to 33%) and breast cancer mortality (from 35% to 26%). In addition, tamoxifen has been shown to provide a preventive benefit in women at risk for developing breast cancer.

There has been a considerable amount of discussion in the literature in regard to the association of tamoxifen with endometrial cancer. At least three studies (Fisher and colleagues, Powels and colleagues, and Veronesi and colleagues) evaluating the prophylactic use of tamoxifen in women without breast cancer have reported an association between tamoxifen use and endometrial cancer. In addition, several cases of endometrial cancer have been described in women receiving tamoxifen. In a prospective, randomized study of the National Surgical Adjuvant Breast and Bowel Project (NSABP), 2843 patients with node-negative estrogen receptor–positive invasive breast cancer were randomly assigned to receive a placebo or 20 mg/day of tamoxifen. An additional 1220 tamoxifen-treated patients were registered and given the drug. The average time in the study was 8 years for the randomly assigned patients and 5 years for the registered patients. Of the 1419 patients randomly assigned to tamoxifen, 15 developed uterine cancer, of which two were sarcomas. One patient randomly assigned to receive tamoxifen did not take the drug and developed endometrial cancer 78 months after randomization. In the placebo group, two developed endometrial cancer; however, both were receiving tamoxifen at the time of their uterine malignant disease. One patient had a breast recurrence and was prescribed tamoxifen, and the other was given tamoxifen after colon cancer. Two of the patients with endometrial cancer had been taking tamoxifen for only 5 and 8 months before their diagnosis of uterine disease was made. Five patients in the tamoxifen group developed endometrial cancer after the drug had been discontinued for 7 to 73 months. In the registered patients who received tamoxifen, eight uterine tumors (seven endometrial) were subsequently diagnosed. Three of these patients had been taking tamoxifen for less than a year (2 months, 2 months, and 9 months). The authors determined the average annual hazard rate of endometrial cancer per 1000 women in their population of patients. This was 0.2 per 1000 in the placebo group and 1.6 per 1000 for the randomized tamoxifen-treated patients. In the registered patients receiving tamoxifen, the average annual hazard rate was 1.4 per 1000, similar to that of the randomized tamoxifen-treated group. The hazard rate of endometrial cancer in the placebo group was low compared with the Surveillance, Epidemiology, and End Results (SEER) data and with previous NSABP randomized tamoxifen–placebo studies; these data suggest that the average annual hazard rate is 0.7 per 1000.

These data, based on a limited number of patients with endometrial cancer while receiving tamoxifen, suggest that there may be a RR of 2.3 for development of endometrial cancer while receiving tamoxifen. This does not take into account the well-known fact that women who develop breast cancer are at an increased risk for development of endometrial cancer irrespective of subsequent treatment. The RR of 1.72 to more than 3 has been reported. The risks and benefits of

the prevention of recurrences and new breast cancer in comparison to new endometrial cancers were evaluated in the NSABP study. The benefits suggest that 121 fewer breast-related events per 1000 women treated with tamoxifen were seen compared with 6.3 endometrial cancers per 1000 women. Therefore the benefit from tamoxifen is apparent.

It was initially suggested that the rate of endometrial cancers associated with tamoxifen might be equal to that associated with unopposed estrogen replacement therapy. Because tamoxifen is a weak estrogen, similar characteristics of endometrial cancer were also implied (i.e., well-differentiated superficially invasive cancers). Barakat and associates reviewed five studies, including the study by Magriples, the NSABP, their own data from Memorial Sloan-Kettering Hospital, and two studies from overseas. A total of 103 patients were evaluated in regard to histologic features, grade of tumor, International Federation of Gynecology and Obstetrics (FIGO) staging, and deaths from uterine cancer; an increase was not found in poor prognostic histologic findings, tumor differentiation, or stage compared with what would be expected in a similar group of non–tamoxifen-treated patients with uterine cancer. Jordan, in an evaluation of the SEER data and of tamoxifen-associated endometrial cancer in the literature, reported similar findings.

It is suggested that all women, irrespective of whether they are taking tamoxifen, should have yearly gynecologic examinations. The endometrium should be evaluated if the patient is symptomatic. We do not currently recommend endometrial sampling or ultrasound evaluation of the endometrium just because an individual is taking tamoxifen. This possible concern of tamoxifen and endometrial cancer may lessen in the near future because the aromatase inhibitors (AIs) may appear to be better than tamoxifen in the prevention of recurrent or contralateral breast cancer. Several clinical trials have demonstrated the comparable if not greater efficacy of AIs compared to tamoxifen. Although tamoxifen remains an option for adjuvant therapy for postmenopausal women, AIs are thought to be more effective in preventing breast cancer recurrence in the first 2 years after surgery. AIs reduce estrogen levels in postmenopausal women by inhibiting or inactivating aromatase, the enzyme that synthesize estrogens from circulating androgens. AIs should be avoided in premenopausal women, including those who have experienced chemotherapy-induced amenorrhea. Whereas tamoxifen is a partial agonist, AIs are not agonists and are not associated with estrogenic-related thromboembolic events and uterine cancers. The activity of third-generation agents anastrozole, letrozole, and exemestane is generally considered comparable. Although AIs are associated with a significant risk of osteoporosis, they do not increase the risk of gynecologic problems. In one large adjuvant therapy trial (the Anastrozole, Tamoxifen Alone or in Combination Trial [ATAC]), anastrozole was associated with fewer cerebrovascular events (2.0% vs 2.8%), endometrial cancers (0.2% vs 0.8%) thromboembolism (2.8% vs 4.5%), hot flashes (41% vs 36%), and vaginal bleeding (5.4% vs 10.2%) compared with tamoxifen. The role of AIs as prophylaxis is being investigated, but data are lacking at the present time.

Although most cases of endometrial cancer are sporadic, hereditary endometrial cancer has been identified in association with hereditary nonpolyposis colon cancer (HNPCC), also known as Lynch II syndrome. This is an autosomal-dominant inherited cancer that involves a germline mutation in one of the genes in the DNA mismatch repair gene family, which includes MSH2, MLM1, and MSH6. Fortunately, HNPCC accounts for only 1% to 5% of all colorectal cancers, but it is associated with a 39% to 54% lifetime risk of developing colon cancer. There is a lifetime risk of 30% to 61% of developing endometrial cancer. There is also an increased risk of ovarian cancers and other nongynecologic cancers. In a study by Lu and associates, they noted that about half the time, the endometrial or ovarian cancer appeared before the colon cancer. In both instances, the age at diagnosis was in the early 40s. There was a median of 11 years between the gynecologic cancer and the colon cancer. About 14% of the time the gynecologic and colon cancers were diagnosed simultaneously. Several "red flags" should prompt an evaluation for HNPCC. These include any individual with a personal or family history of colon cancer at an early age of onset (usually before age 50) or endometrial cancer at an early age of onset (premenopausal or before age 50) and two or more HNPCC-related cancers in an individual or family. Assessing a patient's risk for hereditary cancer is an important process, beginning with screening for the "red flags" of hereditary colon (and endometrial) cancer. Individuals with any of the "red flags" should enter into a discussion about genetic testing to determine if this is appropriate for them. Medical management strategies can be tailored depending on the genetic testing results and may include increased surveillance, chemoprevention, and prophylactic surgery. The Cancer Study Consortium suggests colonoscopy every 1 to 3 years beginning at age 25 in individuals with this hereditary disorder. The data suggest that if surveillance is done, survival is improved. Women should be offered surveillance with ultrasound and endometrial sampling from age 25 to 35, although there are no data to suggest this will improve survival if endometrial cancer is diagnosed by these means. As reported by Schmeler and colleagues, risk-reducing surgery consisting of removal of the uterus and bilateral ovaries has been shown to decrease the risk of uterine and ovarian cancer in these high-risk patients.

DIAGNOSIS

Routine screening for uterine adenocarcinoma and its precursors is not recommended. Women receiving HRT (estrogen and progesterone) do not need endometrial biopsy before institution of therapy or during replacement therapy unless abnormal bleeding occurs. Monthly withdrawal bleeding after progestin is not considered abnormal bleeding. However, breakthrough bleeding should be evaluated. The use of continuous estrogen alone increases the risk of adenocarcinoma. Estrogen plus progesterone appears to decrease the risk of adenocarcinoma and therefore is the preferred treatment. In asymptomatic high-risk patients, periodic screening may be advisable. All postmenopausal women with uterine bleeding must be evaluated for endometrial cancer, although only 20% of these patients will have a malignant genital neoplasm. As the patient's age increases after menopause, there is a progressively increasing probability that her uterine bleeding is caused by endometrial cancer. Feldman and associates found that age was the greatest independent risk factor associated with endometrial cancer or complex hyperplasia. In women aged 70 years or older, the odds ratio was 9.1. If complex hyperplasia was present, the odds ratio increased to 16. When a woman was older than 70 years, her chance of having cancer when vaginal bleeding was present was about 50%. If she was also nulliparous and had diabetes, the risk was 87%. A perimenopausal patient who may have abnormal uterine bleeding indicative of endometrial cancer is frequently not evaluated because the patient or her physician interprets her new bleeding pattern as resulting from menopause. During this time in a woman's life, the menstrual periods should become lighter and lighter and farther and farther apart. Any other bleeding pattern should be evaluated with carcinoma of the endometrium in mind. A high index of suspicion must be maintained if the diagnosis of endometrial cancer is to be made in the young patient. Prolonged and heavy menstrual periods and intermenstrual spotting may indicate cancer, and endometrial sampling is advised. Most young patients who develop endometrial cancer are obese, in many instances massively overweight, often with anovulatory menstrual cycles.

Historically, fractional dilation and curettage (D&C) has been the definitive diagnostic procedure used in ruling out endometrial cancer. Today, most advocate the routine use of the endometrial biopsy as an office procedure to make a definitive diagnosis and spare the patient hospitalization and an anesthetic. Several studies have indicated that the accuracy of the endometrial biopsy in detecting endometrial cancer is approximately 90%. Cytologic detection of endometrial cancer by routine cervical Papanicolaou (Pap) smear has generally been poor in comparison with the efficacy of the Pap smear in diagnosing early cervical disease. Several studies in the literature indicate that only one third to half of the patients with adenocarcinoma of the endometrium have abnormal Pap smears on routine cervical screening. The main reason for the poor detection with the cervical Pap smear is that cells are not removed directly from the lesion as they are on the cervix. When a cytologic preparation is obtained directly from the endometrial cavity, malignant cells are present in higher numbers than those found if routine cervical or vaginal smears are obtained. Techniques that obtain only a cytologic preparation are generally inadequate if they are used alone.

Several commercial apparatuses are available for sampling the endometrial cavity on an outpatient basis. If diagnosis of endometrial cancer can be made on an outpatient basis, the patient can avoid hospitalization and a minor surgical procedure. Devices that remove tissue for histologic evaluation have generally been good if tissue is obtained from the endometrial cavity. Stovall and colleagues evaluated 40 patients known to have endometrial cancer with the Pipelle instrument. Ninety percent of the women were postmenopausal. Only in one patient was cancer not identified with the Pipelle. This patient had a prior D&C that revealed a grade I lesion. The Pipelle diagnosis was atypical adenomatous hyperplasia, and the hysterectomy specimen revealed a focus of adenocarcinoma in situ. The pathologist noted that the obtainable tissue was acceptable for analysis in 100% of patients. Discomfort was recorded as mild in 80%, and only two patients (5%) reported severe pain. Goldchmit and coworkers reported similar accuracy with the Pipelle in 176 consecutive patients undergoing D&C. Whereas endometrial biopsy and D&C appear to be equivalent in terms of diagnosing cancer, the accuracy of endometrial biopsy appears to be inferior to D&C in predicting final posthysterectomy tumor grade. In a recent study by Leitao and colleagues, 18% of endometrial biopsy specimens were upgraded on final hysterectomy specimen, whereas only 9% of D&C specimens were upgraded. In the symptomatic patient in whom inadequate tissue (or no tissue at all) is obtained for pathologic evaluation, a D&C must be considered.

Hysteroscopy has been suggested as adjuvant in making the diagnosis of endometrial cancer and in establishing the extent of disease. Hysteroscopy has been used frequently in the evaluation of patients with abnormal uterine bleeding and has the advantages of allowing the physician to see the pathologic lesion and direct biopsy, identify other competing diagnoses (fibroids, polyps), and perform the procedure on an outpatient basis. Clark and colleagues analyzed data from 65 primary studies on the use of hysteroscopy to diagnose endometrial cancer and endometrial disease (cancer, hyperplasia, or both), including more than 26,000 women. All of the patients had abnormal premenopausal or postmenopausal uterine bleeding. Using endometrial histologic findings as a reference, a positive hysteroscopy result was associated with a 72% probability of endometrial cancer, whereas a negative result reduced this probability to 0.6%. The corresponding probabilities for endometrial disease were 55% with a positive result and 3% with a negative result. The accuracy of hysteroscopy tended to be higher among postmenopausal women and in an outpatient setting. They concluded that hysteroscopy is highly accurate and thereby clinically useful in diagnosing endometrial cancer in women with abnormal uterine bleeding and is moderately useful in diagnosing endometrial disease. Because many patients with endometrial cancer can be diagnosed with office biopsy, that is our preferred first diagnostic step. If the biopsy result is negative and further evaluation is needed, we proceed to hysteroscopy. With its use, surgeons can direct biopsies of focal lesions that might be missed by D&C. Hysteroscopy can also be used to evaluate the endocervical canal.

Ultrasonography (US) has been suggested as a diagnostic tool in evaluating women with irregular bleeding, particularly the postmenopausal patient (Figure 5-3). The endometrial stripe as seen with transvaginal US appears to be indicative of endometrial thickness. Several studies suggest that if a thin endometrial stripe is present, a histologic diagnosis is not necessary because atrophic endometrium would be present. Granberg and associates evaluated 205 women with postmenopausal bleeding, 30 postmenopausal asymptomatic women, and 30 postmenopausal patients with known endometrial cancer. In the two groups of 60 patients, the endometrial thickness was 3.2 (mean) versus 17.7, respectively. In the group of 205 women, 18 were found to have endometrial cancer. No cancers were present in the endometrium that had an endometrial thickness of 8 mm or less. There was considerable overlap of endometrial thickness by all histologic groups. The authors noted that if a cutoff of 5 mm was used, no false-negative findings were present. With this measurement, the positive predictive value was 87%, with specificity of 96% and sensitivity of 100% for identifying endometrial abnormalities. It has been suggested that if US could save a large number of endometrial biopsies, there would be a large cost savings with less discomfort to the patient. As previously noted, significant pain with the newer disposable endometrial biopsy techniques affects only a small number of patients; and a certain number of patients, because of considerable endometrial thickness, will require endometrial sampling anyway. Clark and colleagues investigated the cost-effectiveness of initial diagnostic strategies for

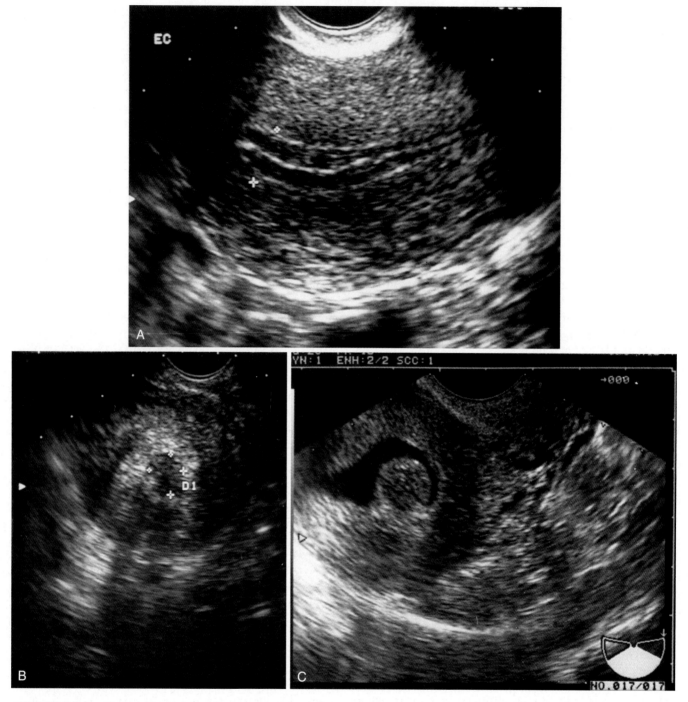

FIGURE 5-3 **A,** Ultrasound of the uterus showing the "triple line" indicating the thickness of the endometrium. **B,** Ultrasound of the uterus showing a "thickened endometrium" of more than 10 mm. **C,** Saline instillation of the endometrial cavity notes a well-defined submucous fibroid and not thickened endometrium.

postmenopausal bleeding. A decision analytic model was constructed to reflect current service provision, which evaluated 12 diagnostic strategies using endometrial biopsy, ultrasonography (4- and 5-mm endometrial thickness cutoff), and hysteroscopy. Diagnostic probability estimates were derived from systematic quantitative reviews, clinical outcomes from published literature and cost estimates from local and National Health Service sources. The main outcome measure was the cost per additional life year gained (£/LYG). Compared with carrying out no initial investigation, a strategy based on initial diagnosis with US using a 5-mm cutoff was the least expensive (£11 470/LYG). Initial investigation with endometrial biopsy or US using a 4-mm cutoff was comparably cost-effective (<£30 000/LYG vs US with a 5-mm cutoff). The strategies involving initial evaluation with test combinations or hysteroscopy alone were not cost-effective. They concluded that women presenting for the first time with postmenopausal bleeding should undergo initial evaluation with US or endometrial biopsy.

Unfortunately, endometrial cancer has been identified when the endometrial thickness is less than 5 mm. Although studies may evaluate several hundred patients, most do not have many cancer patients included. Wang and associates reviewed the ultrasound of 52 women who were diagnosed with papillary serous clear cell and other high-grade carcinomas. Of the 52, 34 (65%) had thickened endometrium measuring 5 mm or more; in 9 (17%) the endometrium was less tham 5 mm, and in an additional 9 women (17%) the endometrium was indistinct. In the women with nonthickened endometrium, other ultrasound abnormalities were noted: intracavitary fluid or lesion, myometrial mass, enlarged uterus, or adnexal mass. Multiple factors can affect endometrial thickness. These include estrogen, estrogen plus progestin, body mass index (BMI), diabetes, poor histotype, race, and postmenopausal status. The Committee on Gynecologic Practice of the American College of Obstetricians and Gynecologists issued an opinion on the role of transvaginal ultrasonography in the evaluation of postmenopausal bleeding. They concluded that women with postmenopausal bleeding may be assessed initially with either endometrial biopsy or transvaginal ultrasonography. This initial evaluation does not require performance of both tests. Transvaginal ultrasonography can be useful in the triage of patients in whom endometrial sampling was performed but tissue was insufficient for diagnosis. When transvaginal ultrasonography is performed for patients with postmenopausal bleeding and an endometrial thickness of less than or equal to 4 mm is found, endometrial sampling is not required. Meaningful assessment of the endometrium by ultrasonography is not possible in all patients. In such cases, alternative assessment should be completed. When bleeding persists despite negative initial evaluations, additional assessment is indicated.

The reliability determining endometrial thickness in the postmenopausal patient does not appear to be applicable to women taking tamoxifen. In all studies, the endometrium in the tamoxifen-treated patient is considerably thicker than in the non–tamoxifen-treated patient. Histologic evaluation revealed atrophic endometrium in a large number of these tamoxifen-treated patients. Lahti and colleagues evaluated 103 asymptomatic postmenopausal patients (51 receiving tamoxifen and 52 control subjects) with US, hysteroscopy, and endometrial histologic examination. In the tamoxifen group, 84% had endometrial thickness on US of 5 mm or more versus 19% in the non-tamoxifen group (51% vs 8% more than 10 mm, respectively). Hysteroscopy findings noted that 28% of uterine mucosa was atrophic versus 87% in the non-tamoxifen control group. Histopathologic examination noted atrophic endometrium in 60% of tamoxifen-treated patients versus 79% of control subjects. The biggest difference between the two groups was the finding of polyps in 18% of the tamoxifen group versus 0% of the control group; this appears to be a frequent finding in the tamoxifen-treated patient. So-called megapolyps measuring up to 12 cm have been described. Other uterine disease has been attributed to tamoxifen, including increased uterine volume, lower impedance to blood flow in uterine arteries, endometriosis, focal periglandular condensation of stromal cells, and epithelial metaplasia. Data now suggest that the markedly thickened endometrium (up to 40 mm) in patients receiving tamoxifen is not thickened endometrium but proximal myometrium.

US has also been evaluated as a means for determining depth of myometrial invasion. Gordon and associates studied 15 known patients with endometrial cancer by US and magnetic resonance imaging (MRI). By use of criteria of greater than 50% myometrial wall involvement as deep invasion and less than 50% as superficial invasion, US was judged to be more accurate than MRI in five studies; MRI was better in three, both were equally accurate in four, and neither was accurate in three. It has been suggested by some that US can accurately predict myometrial invasion in about 75% of cases. Although knowing the depth of invasion preoperatively would be important information to the clinician, the data from studies as noted before would currently appear to be too premature or too costly to use routinely. We prefer to evaluate depth of myometrial invasion intraoperatively with gross examination or frozen section.

Pathology

Careful evaluation of the uterus by the pathologist is essential for proper diagnosis and treatment of corpus cancer (Figure 5-4). Gross inspection of a bivalved uterus at the time of hysterectomy can offer an impression of the size of the lesion, its location (involvement of fundus, lower uterine segment, or cervix), and depth of tumor penetration into the myometrium (depth of invasion). A clinically enlarged uterus may be caused by increasing tumor volume, but this should not be the only gauge for significant local disease. Obviously, many patients can have enlarged uteri because of factors other than adenocarcinoma. Carcinoma of the endometrium may start as a focal discrete lesion, as in an endometrial polyp. It may also be diffuse in several different areas, in some situations involving the entire endometrial surface. As the

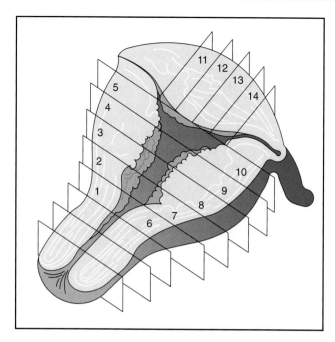

FIGURE 5-4   Pathologic evaluation of endometrial cancer. *(Courtesy Paul Underwood, MD.)*

TABLE 5-3   Endometrial Carcinoma Subtypes

Type	Number (%)
Endometrioid	6231 (84)
Adenosquamous	317 (4.2)
Mucinous	74 (0.9)
Papillary serous	335 (4.5)
Clear cell	185 (2.5)
Squamous cell	28 (0.04)
Other	285 (3.8)

From Pecorelli S (ed): Int J Gynecol Obstet 83:79, 2003.

tumor grows, it can become larger and/or spread within the endometrium or myometrium. Endometrial cancer may disseminate to regional lymph nodes, by embolization or direct extension into the pelvis or vagina, or hematogenously to distant organs (Figure 5-5). The risk of spread is related to several factors, including depth of invasion into the myometrium, tumor grade, and histologic type.

Adenocarcinoma, the most common histologic type, is usually preceded by a predisposing lesion, atypical endometrial hyperplasia (Table 5-3). Only those hyperplasias with cellular atypia are considered to be precursors of adenocarcinoma of the endometrium. For most patients with endometrioid-type tumors, particularly grade I-II lesions, and hyperplasia, hyperestrogenism is the etiologic basis. Pathologically, endometrial cancer is characterized by the presence of glands in an abnormal relationship to each other, with the hallmark of little if any intervening stroma between the glands. There can be variations in the size of the glands, and infolding is common. The cells are usually enlarged, as are the nuclei, along with nuclear chromatin clumping and nucleolar enlargement. Mitosis may be frequent. Differentiation of adenocarcinoma (mild, moderate, and severe, or grades I-III) is important prognostically and is incorporated into FIGO surgical staging (Figure 5-6). Most studies suggest that 60% to 65% of all endometrial cancers are of this subtype.

For almost a century, it has been recognized that a squamous component may be associated with an adenocarcinoma of the endometrium. This occurs in about 25%

of patients. Historically, patients with a squamous component were further stratified according to whether the squamous component appeared benign (designated adenoacanthoma, AA) or malignant (designated adenosquamous carcinoma, AS). It was suggested that AA indicated a good prognosis, and those with AS had a poor survival. Today, this distinction has been questioned in regard to its prognostic importance. Zaino and co-workers, in reporting data from the GOG, suggest that the notation of squamous component irrespective of differentiation does not affect survival. Patients with clinical stage I and stage II cancers were evaluated, and 456 with typical adenocarcinoma (AC) and 175 with squamous differentiation (AC + SQ) were identified. The latter were subdivided into 99 with AA and 69 with AS. Multiple known prognostic factors were compared with differentiation of glandular and squamous component of the tumor. Age, depth of myometrial invasion, architecture, nuclear grade, and combined grade were similar for AC and AC + SQ, although patients with AA were better differentiated than those with AS and had less myometrial invasion. Both glandular and squamous differentiation correlated with frequency of pelvic and para-aortic node metastasis. Nodal metastasis, when it was stratified for grade and depth of invasion, was similar in AC and AC + SQ patients. The differentiation of squamous component is closely correlated with the differentiation of the glandular element, and the glandular element is a better predictor of outcome. It would therefore appear that the previous designation of AA and AS has no added predictive property than differentiation of glandular component and probably should be dropped as a diagnostic term. The authors suggest the term squamous differentiation instead, with differentiation of the glandular component noted as the important prognostic factor. Subsequently, Abeler and Kjorstad reviewed 255 cases and made the same recommendations.

Secretory adenocarcinoma (Figure 5-7) is an uncommon type of endometrial cancer. It usually represents well-differentiated carcinoma with progestational changes. It is difficult to differentiate it from secretory

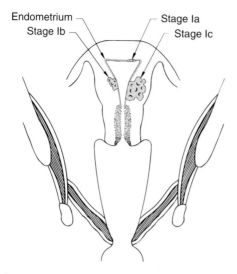

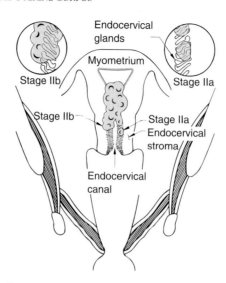

Stage Ia: Tumor limited to endometrium
Stage Ib: Invasion to less than half the myometrium
Stage Ic: Invasion to more than half the myometrium

Stage I

Stage IIa: Endocervical glandular involvement only
Stage IIb: Cervical stroma invasion

Stage II

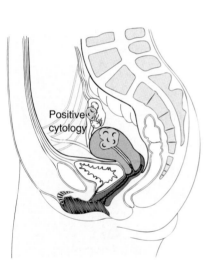

Stage IIIA

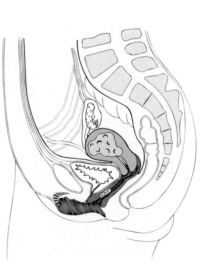

Stage IIIB

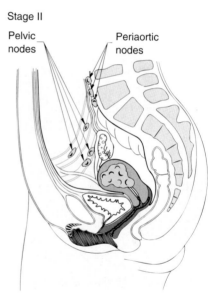

Stage IIIC

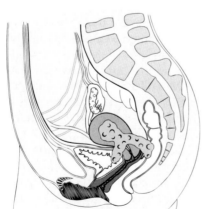

Stage IVa

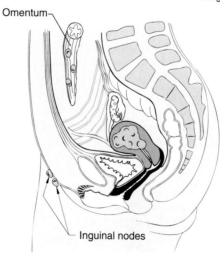

Stage IVb

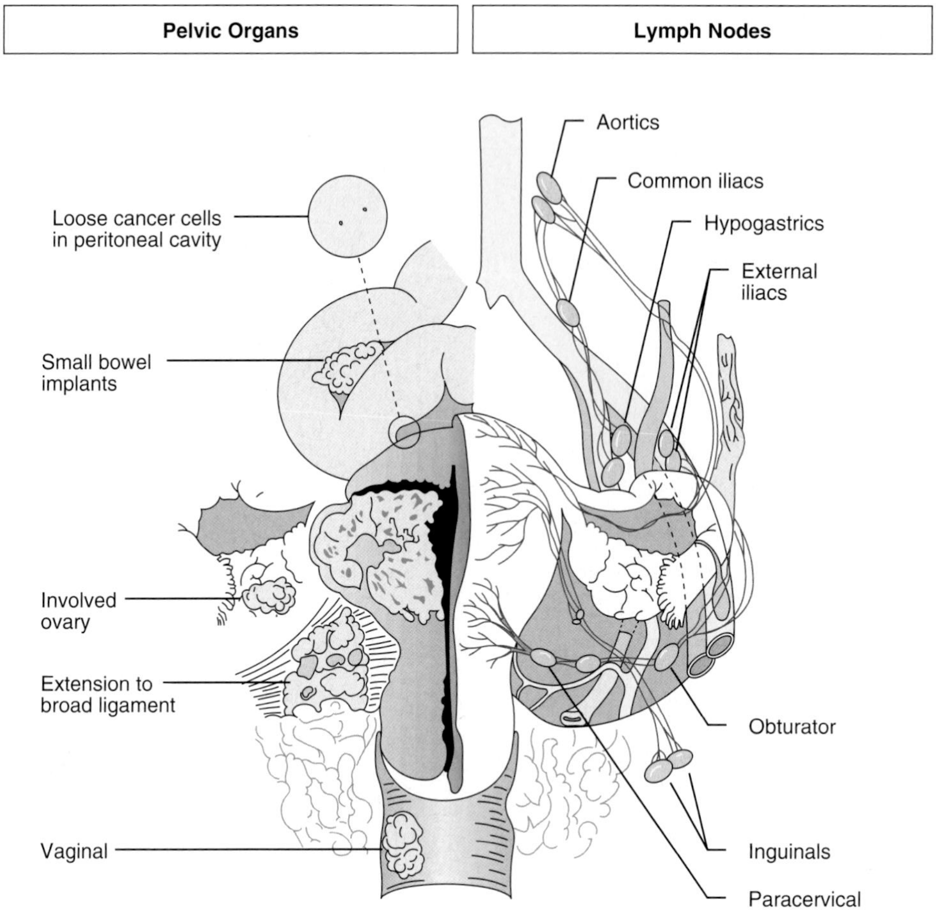

FIGURE 5-5   Spread pattern of endometrial cancer with particular emphasis on potential lymph node spread. Pelvic and periaortic nodes are at risk, even in stage I disease.

endometrium. Survival is good and comparable to that associated with the pure adenocarcinoma. Although it is an interesting histologic variant, the separation of the entity as it relates to treatment and survival is probably not warranted.

Increasing emphasis has been placed on the importance of the histologic subtype serous adenocarcinoma (SC) of the uterus (also called uterine papillary serous carcinoma, UPSC). This subtype represents less than 10% of all adenocarcinomas but is a highly aggressive carcinoma of the uterus. Unlike the more common variants, PS is not associated with hyperestrogenism and frequently develops in the setting of atrophic endometrium. It is more commonly seen in older and nonwhite patients. Hendrickson, in the early 1980s, noted that in more than 250 endometrial cancers, only 10% had histologic features of SC, but these accounted for 50% of all treatment failures. The histopathologic appearance resembles a high-grade serous carcinoma of the ovary

that has a propensity for vascular or lymphatic vascular space involvement (LVSI). Well-formed papillae are lined by neoplastic cells with grade III cytologic features (Figure 5-8). Differentiation between papillary architecture and syncytial metaplasia with benign endometrial alterations must be made because the papillary architecture alone does not designate PS. The uterus may appear grossly normal but can have extensive myometrial invasion. Most UPSC tumors are aneuploid and have a high S-phase. Serous cancers can be pure or admixed with other histologic types (endometrioid, clear cell, carcinosarcoma).

Clear cell carcinomas (Figure 5-9) are also infrequent in number but have distinct histologic criteria. Clear cell tumors are characterized by large polyhedral epithelial cells that may be admixed with typical non–clear cell adenocarcinomas. Some authorities accept the mesonephritic-type hobnail cells as part of this pattern, whereas others believe that this histologic type should

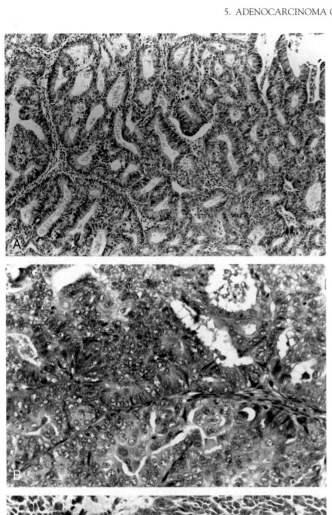

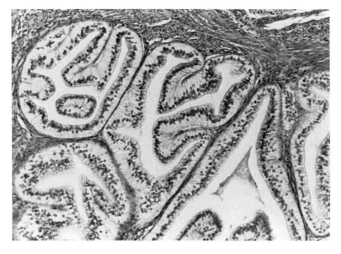

FIGURE 5-7 High-power view of well-differentiated secretory carcinoma invading inner one-third of the myometrium. *(Courtesy William M. Christopherson, MD, Louisville, Kentucky.)*

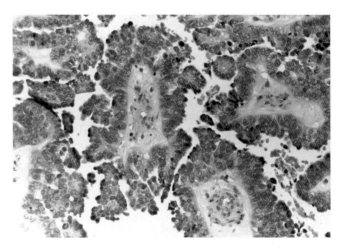

FIGURE 5-8 Serous adenocarcinoma. Similarity to ovarian carcinoma is apparent. *(Courtesy Gregory Spiegel, MD.)*

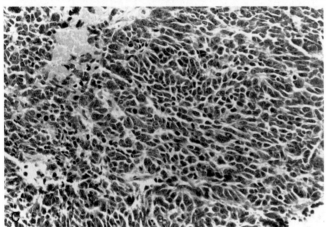

FIGURE 5-6 Histologic patterns of differentiation in endometrial carcinoma. **A,** Well-differentiated (G1). **B,** Moderately differentiated (G2). **C,** Poorly differentiated (G3). *(Courtesy Gregory Spiegel, MD.)*

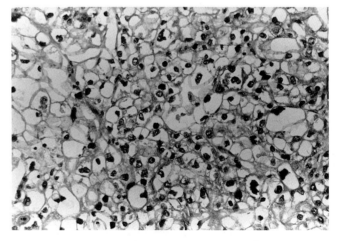

FIGURE 5-9 Clear cell carcinoma of the endometrium. Clear cell component is quite evident. *(Courtesy Gregory Spiegel, MD.)*

be excluded from the clear cell category. Silverberg and DeGiorgi and Kurman and Scully suggested a worse prognosis for clear cell adenocarcinoma than for pure adenocarcinoma. This was confirmed in studies by Christopherson and co-workers. Even in stage I disease, only 44% of patients with clear cell carcinomas survive 5 years. Neither the FIGO classification nor nuclear grade correlates with survival. Photopulos and associates, in a review of their material, noted that their patients with this entity were older and tended to have a worse prognosis. They did note that patients with stage I clear cell carcinomas had a 5-year survival similar to that of patients with stage I pure adenocarcinoma of the endometrium.

Tumor Grade

In addition to histologic type, pathologists assign a measure of tumor differentiation, known as grade, to endometrial cancers. Grade I lesions are well differentiated, are frequently associated with estrogen excess, closely resemble hyperplastic endometrium, and are generally associated with a favorable prognosis. Grade III lesions are poorly differentiated, do not resemble normal endometrium, and frequently have a poorer prognosis. Grade II tumors are moderately well differentiated and have an intermediate prognosis. Both architectural criteria and nuclear grade are used to classify. Architectural grade is related to the proportion of solid tumor growth, with grade I having an adenocarcinoma in which less than 5% of the tumor growth is in solid sheets, grade II has 6% to 50% of the neoplasm arranged in solid sheets of neoplastic cells, and grade III has greater than 50% of the neoplastic cells in solid masses. Regions of squamous differentiation are excluded from this assessment. The FIGO rules for grading state that notable nuclear atypia, inappropriate for architectural grade, raises the grade of a grade I or grade II tumor by one. By convention, serous and clear tumors are considered grade III/high-grade tumors.

PROGNOSTIC FACTORS

Following hysterectomy and lymph node dissection, clinical-pathologic characteristics are commonly used to predict risk of recurrence and to optimize therapy. Multiple factors have been identified for endometrial carcinoma that have prognostic value (Table 5-4). Essentially all reports in the literature agree stage (extent of disease spread), grade of tumor, and depth of invasion are important prognostic considerations. Before 1988 endometrial cancer was clinically staged with stage assignments based on uterine size and clinical extent of disease. Because of the considerable discrepancy between the clinical extent of disease spread and pathologic spread noted after surgical staging, FIGO adopted a surgical-pathologic staging classification in 1988. In 2009 FIGO updated the staging system (Table 5-5). FIGO staging classification attempts to categorize patients into prognostic groups based on extent of disease and tumor grade.

TABLE 5-4   Prognostic Factors in Endometrial Adenocarcinoma

Histologic type (pathology)
Histologic differentiation
Stage of disease
Myometrial invasion
Peritoneal cytology
Lymph node metastasis
Adnexal metastasis

TABLE 5-5   2009 FIGO Staging System for Carcinoma of the Endometrium

Stage I*		Tumor contained to the corpus uteri
	IA	No or less than half myometrial invasion
	IB	Invasion equal to or more than half of the myometrium
Stage II		Tumor invades the cervical stroma but does not extend beyond the uterus[†]
Stage III*		Local and/or regional spread of tumor[‡]
	IIIA	Tumor invades the serosa of the corpus uteri and/or adnexas
	IIIB	Vaginal and/or parametrial involvement
	IIIC	Metastases to pelvis and/or para-aortic lymph nodes
		IIIC1 Positive pelvic nodes
		IIIC2 Positive para-aortic lymph nodes with or without positive pelvic lymph nodes
Stage IV*		Tumor invades bladder and/or bowel mucosa and/or distant metastases
	IVA	Tumor invasion of bladder and/or bowel mucosa
	IVB	Disant metastases, including intra-abdominal metastases and/or inguinal lymph nodes

*Includes grades 1, 2, or 3.
[†]Endocervical glandular involvement only should be considered as stage I and no longer as stage II.
[‡]Positive cytology has to be reported separately without changing the stage.

Stage of Disease: Depth of Invasion, Cervical Involvement, Adnexal Involvement, and Nodal Metastasis

Staging of patients with malignancies is designed to have prognostic value by classifying the size and extent of tumor. The survival rate in regard to stage of disease has been consistent, and Table 5-6 and Figure 5-10 show the 5-year survival rate reported by FIGO (FIGO 1988 staging). The patterns of disease spread in endometrial cancer was evaluated in a prospective study performed by the GOG (GOG protocol 33) and reported by Creasman. This study is required reading for physicians who

care for patients with endometrial cancer. GOG protocol 33 was a surgical-pathologic study of 621 patients with clinical stage I endometrial cancer who were uniformly treated with total abdominal hysterectomy, bilateral salpingo-oophorectomy, peritoneal cytologic evaluation, and selective pelvic and para-aortic selected lymphadenectomy. Before this study, it was presumed most patients with endometrial cancer were at risk for nodal metastases and nearly all patients required some form of pelvic radiation therapy (either preoperatively or postoperatively). The study demonstrated important relationships between pathologic factors and risk of nodal disease. For example, factors associated with nodal disease included higher tumor grade, deeper myometrial invasion, cervical involvement, (+) cytology, and LVSI. As a result of this study FIGO accepted a surgical-based staging system of endometrial cancer in 1988.

For endometrial cancer, FIGO staging reflects the progression of disease within the uterus and at extrauterine sites. Approximately 75% of patients with endometrial cancer present with disease limited to the uterus (Table 5-7). For stage I disease, depth of tumor invasion into the myometrium is an important prognostic factor. The degree of myometrial invasion is a consistent indicator of tumor virulence (Figure 5-11). DiSaia and associates noted that recurrences were directly related to depth of myometrial invasion in patients with stage I cancer treated primarily with surgery (Table 5-8). The Annual

TABLE 5-6   Five-Year Survival in Endometrial Cancer: Surgical Stage

Stage	No. of Patients	Five-Year Survival (%)
Ia	1063	91
Ib	2735	90
Ic	1219	81
IIa	364	79
IIb	426	71
IIIa	484	60
IIIb	73	30
IIIc	293	52
IVa	47	15
IVb	160	17

From Pecorelli S (ed): Int J Gynecol Obstet 83:95, 2003.

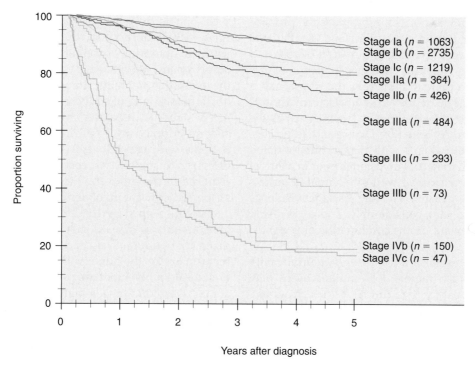

FIGURE 5-10   Carcinoma of the corpus uteri; patients treated in 1990–1992 (FIGO). Survival by surgical stage (*n* = 5694). *[From Pecorelli S (ed): Int J Gynecol Obstet 83:95, 2003. © International Federation of Gynecology and Obstetrics.]*

TABLE 5-7   Distribution of Endometrial Carcinoma by Stage (Surgical)

Stage	Patients (%)
I	3839 (73)
II	574 (11)
III	694 (13)
IV	166 (3)

From Pecorelli S (ed): J Epidemiol Biostat 3:41, 1998.

TABLE 5-8   Relationship between Depth of Myometrial Invasion and Recurrence in Patients with Stage I Endometrial Carcinoma

Endometrial only	7/92 (8%)
Superficial myometrium	10/80 (13%)
Medium myometrium	2/17 (12%)
Deep myometrium	15/33 (46%)

Modified from DiSaia PJ et al: Am J Obstet Gynecol 151:1009, 1985.

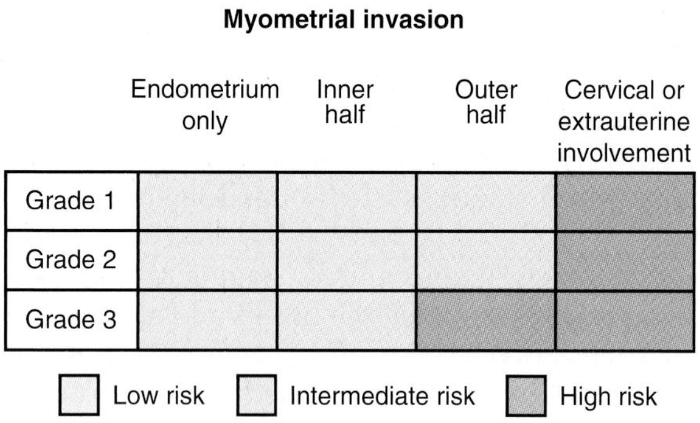

Myometrial invasion

FIGURE 5-11   Risk assignment based on surgical staging/extent of disease in patients with endometrial cancer.

TABLE 5-9   Relationship between Depth of Myometrial Invasion and Five-Year Survival Rate (Stage I)

Stage	Patients	5-Year Survival (%)
IaG1	698	93
IbG1	1030	88
IcG1	442	87
IaG2	229	91
IbG2	1307	93
IcG2	485	84
IaG3	66	75
IbG3	280	82
IcG3	247	66

From Pecorelli S (ed): Int J Gynecol Obstet 83:95, 2003.

Report of FIGO demonstrated a decrease in the survival rate as myometrial penetration increased (Table 5-9). Lutz and co-workers determined that the depth of myometrial penetration was not as important as the proximity of the invading tumor to the uterine serosa. Patients whose tumors invaded to within 5 mm of the serosa had a 65% 5-year survival rate, whereas patients whose tumors were more than 10 mm from the serosa had a 97% survival rate. The depth of myometrial invasion is associated with the other prognostic factors, such as the grade of the tumor. As noted by DiSaia and associates, the survival rate of patients with poorly differentiated lesions and deep myometrial invasion is poor in contrast to that of patients who have well-differentiated lesions but no myometrial invasion. This suggests that virulence of the tumor may vary considerably, and as a result, therapy should depend on the combination of prognostic factors.

Location of the tumor within the endometrial cavity is important because tumors low in the cavity may involve the cervix earlier than fundal lesions. Prognosis for women with cervical involvement (stage II) is worse than with stage I disease. Cervical involvement is often a surrogate marker for extrauterine disease spread or for risk of local recurrence. Data from GOG 33 showed that those with disease of the lower uterine segment had a higher incidence of pelvic lymph node metastases (16%) than do those with only fundal disease (8%). There is a similar frequency of para-aortic nodal metastases: a 16% incidence from disease of the lower uterine segment and a 4% incidence when only fundal disease is present. Previously, endocervical curettage (ECC) was commonly used to determine whether the patient had cervical involvement. Many false-positive results occur through the use of this technique, however. In addition, the prognostic significance of endocervical glandular spread (formerly stage IIa) has been challenged. The new surgical staging adopted by FIGO in 2009 includes only those patients with cervical stromal invasion in the stage II category. In some cases, cervical biopsy and/or ECC is required in the pretreatment planning of a patient with suspected cervical involvement.

Patients with stage III-IV disease may have a heterogeneous mix of disease characteristics. It is well recognized that endometrial cancer can and frequently does metastasize to the adnexa. Patients with adnexal and/or serosal involvement are categorized as stage IIIA and are considered to have a higher risk of peritoneal recurrence. In GOG 33, 5% of patients had adnexal involvement. Adnexal metastasis was significantly associated with involved pelvic (32%) and para-aortic (20%) lymph nodes. In a large surgical trial comparing laparoscopy to open staging (GOG Lap 2 trial), 5% of 2616 patients enrolled were found to have stage IIIA disease (FIGO

TABLE 5-10   Grade vs Positive Pelvic and Aortic Nodes

Grade (n)	Pelvic Nodes (%)	Aortic Nodes (%)
G1 (180)	5 (3)	3 (2)
G2 (288)	25 (9)	14 (5)
G3 (153)	28 (18)	17 (11)

Modified from Creasman WT et al: Cancer 60:2035, 1987.

TABLE 5-11   Maximal Invasion and Node Metastasis

Maximal invasion (n)	Pelvic Nodes (%)	Aortic Nodes (%)
Endometrium only (87)	1 (1)	1 (1)
Superficial muscle (279)	15 (5)	8 (3)
Intermediate muscle (116)	7 (6)	1 (1)
Deep muscle (139)	35 (25)	24 (17)

Modified from Creasman WT et al: Cancer 60:2035, 1987.

TABLE 5-12   Frequency of Pelvic and Para-Aortic Nodal Disease

Depth of Invasion	Grade		
	Grade I (n = 180)	Grade II (n = 288)	Grade III (n = 153)
Endometrial only (n = 86)	0%/0%	3%/3%	0%/0%
Inner one-third (n = 281)	3%/1%	5%/4%	9%/4%
Middle one-third (n = 115)	0%/5%	9%/0%	4%/0%
Outer one-third (n = 139)	11%/6%	19%/14%	34%/23%

(Pelvic Nodal Positivity/Para-aortic Nodal Positivity)
Modified from Creasman WT et al: Cancer 60:2035, 1987.

1988 staging). In an analysis of 222 patients with clinical stage I carcinoma of the endometrium reported by DiSaia and colleagues, 16 (7%) were found to have metastasis in the adnexa. This finding correlated with many but not all of the other prognostic factors. Spread to the adnexa did not seem to be related to the size of the uterus. The grade of the disease did not appear prognostically important in regard to this in that 6% of patients with grade I tumors had adnexal disease compared with only 10% if poorly differentiated carcinoma was present. The depth of invasion did appear to be significant, however, in that only 4% of patients with only the endometrium involved had adnexal spread, compared with 24% who had adnexal metastases if deep muscle was involved. If tumor was limited to the fundus of the uterus, only 5% of patients had disease in the adnexa; however, if the lower uterine segment or the endocervix was involved, one-third had spread to the adnexa. When metastasis was present in the adnexa, 60% of patients had malignant cells in the peritoneal cytologic fluid, compared with only 11% if the adnexa were not involved. Recurrences appeared in only 14% of these individuals who did not have metastasis to the adnexa, compared with recurrences in 38% of patients with adnexal metastasis.

Metastatic spread to lymph nodes (stage IIIC) has prognostic and therapeutic implications. It is clear that lymphadenectomy is the most sensitive way to identify nodal disease. The GOG 33 study demonstrated that as the depth of tumor invasion or tumor grade increased, the frequency of pelvic and para-aortic nodal metastases also increased (Tables 5-10 and 5-11). For all 621 patients, 58 (9%) had positive pelvic nodes and 34 (6%) had positive para-aortic nodes. Patients with grade 1, 2, and 3 tumors had pelvic nodal metastases of 3%, 9%, and 18% respectively. Similarly, patients with no myometrial invasion, inner one third, middle one third, and outer one third invasion had 1%, 5%, 6%, and 25% pelvic nodal disease, respectively. The highest risk group included patients with grade III tumors and outer one third invasion who had pelvic nodal involvement in 34% of cases (Table 5-12). Without a lymphadenectomy, one may grossly estimate the probability of nodal involvement based on these data to select for or against the use of adjuvant therapy. This strategy potentially results in undertreatment or overtreatment of patients, however. In two large prospective randomized trials, routine lymphadenectomy resulted in the identification of more patients with nodal disease (9% to 13%), compared to when only clinically suspicious nodes were removed (1% to 3%). It is clear that patients with nodal disease have poorer prognosis (3- to 5-year survival of 50% to 75%) and different patterns of failure (nodal, distant) than patients with negative nodes (3- to 5-year survival of 80% to 95%, vaginal cuff failures predominate). Patients with nodal involvement include those with pelvic nodal disease (IIIC1) or any para-aortic involvement (IIIC2). The substaging was created in 2009 given the belief of different outcomes associated with different levels of nodal involvement. The number of involved nodes and the extent of resection of grossly involved nodes also affect outcome. In addition Mariani and McMeekin have suggested that patients with (+) nodal disease plus other stage III defining features (positive cytology, adnexal or serosal involvement) have a much poorer prognosis than those with nodal disease only. Patients with stage IV/distant disease spread (intraperitoneal, lung, liver) have a particularly poor prognosis, with 5-year survival of less than 20%. The extent of surgical resection has been suggested to alter prognosis in patients with advanced-stage disease. As with ovarian cancer, the extent of resection of disease reflects biology of the tumor, aggressiveness of the surgery, and response to postoperative therapies.

Tumor Grade

The degree of histologic differentiation (tumor grade) of endometrial cancer is a sensitive indicator of prognosis and is included in FIGO stage assignment. The Annual Report on the Results of Treatment in Gynecological Cancer has evaluated survival in regard to grade in patients with clinical stage I adenocarcinoma of the endometrium (Table 5-13). Tumor grade is inversely related to survival decreases; as grade increases, survival is poorer. In their review of 244 patients with stage I disease, Genest and colleagues noted that patients with grade I disease had a 5-year survival rate of 96%. This dropped to 79% and 70% for grade II and grade III, respectively. Data presented by Morrow for outcomes in patients enrolled on GOG 33 show that recurrence-free survival markedly diminishes with increasing grade, with progression-free survival (PFS) at 48 months being approximately 95%, 85%, and 68% for grade I, II, and III tumors, respectively. Grade of tumor also correlates with other factors of prognosis. Table 5-14 shows the relationship between differentiation of the tumor and depth of myometrial invasion as reported by Creasman from the GOG 33 study. As the tumor becomes less differentiated, the chances of deep myometrial involvement increase. However, exceptions can occur: Patients with a well-differentiated lesion can have deep myometrial

invasion, whereas patients with a poorly differentiated malignant neoplasm might have only endometrial or superficial myometrial involvement.

Lymphovascular Space Involvement

Hanson and colleagues described 111 patients with stage I endometrial cancer and found capillary-like space (CLS) involvement in 16. This was most frequently found in patients with poorly differentiated tumors with deep invasion. These patients had a 44% recurrence rate, compared with 2% if the CLS was not involved. This was an independently significant prognostic factor. In the GOG study of 621 patients, it was shown that 93 (15%) had CLS involvement. The incidences of pelvic and para-aortic node metastases were 27% and 19%, respectively. This compares with a 7% occurrence of pelvic node metastasis and a 3% occurrence of para-aortic node metastasis when there is no CLS involvement. In risk models predicting risk of recurrence in node-negative/early-stage endometrial cancer, the GOG has suggested that LVSI is an important risk factor. In the Post Operative Radiation Therapy in Endometrial Cancer (PORTEC) trial, LVSI was considered to be a factor associated with distant site of failure.

Tumor Size

Schink and co-workers evaluated tumor size in 91 patients with stage I disease. The incidence of lymph node metastases in patients with tumor size less than 2 cm was only 6%. If tumor was greater than 2 cm in diameter, there were nodal metastases of 21% and up to 40% if the entire endometrium was involved. Patients with lesions greater than 2 cm in size and less than half myometrial invasion had no nodal metastasis. Using multivariate analysis, the authors showed that tumor size was an independently significant prognostic factor. Watanabe and associates did not find cancer size was predictive of lymph node metastasis. Gynecologic oncologists from the Mayo Clinic have developed a risk model predicting nodal metastases and have suggested that grade I-II tumors that are less than 2 cm are particularly low risk for nodal disease.

Peritoneal Cytology

The importance of peritoneal cytology in endometrial cancer is controversial. In GOG 33, 76 (12%) had malignant cells identified by cytologic examination of peritoneal washings. Of these patients, 25% had positive pelvic nodes, compared with 7% of patients in whom no malignant cells were found in peritoneal cytologic specimens ($P > 0.0001$). It is true that peritoneal cytology, to a certain degree, mimics other known prognostic factors—that is, if peritoneal cytologic specimens are positive, other known poor prognostic factors may also be identified. In addition, data from GOG 33 also suggested that the

TABLE 5-13   Relationship between Tumor Differentiation and Five-Year Survival Rate, Stage I (Surgical)

Grade	Survival ($n = 5017$) (%)
1	91
2	90
3	81

From Pecorelli S (ed): FIGO Annual Report, years 1996–98, Int J Gynecol Obstet 83:95, 2003.

TABLE 5-14   Correlation of Differentiation and Myometrial Invasion in Stage I Cancer

Myometrial Invasion	Grade		
	1 (%)	2 (%)	3 (%)
None	24	11	11
Superficial	53	45	35
Mid	12	24	16
Deep	10	20	42

Modified from Creasman WT et al: Cancer 60:2035, 1987.

RR for recurrence with positive cytology was 2.4 (*P* = 0.02).

Given the relationship of positive cytology with other known risk factors, it is important to evaluate data sets coming from patients who undergo complete surgical staging. Saga and colleagues reported on a series of 307 (32 with positive cytology, 275 with negative cytology) patients with endometrioid-type cancer, all who underwent complete staging and had negative lymph nodes. The authors reported that 5-year survival was 87% with (+) cytology compared to 97 with negative cytology. Most patients with positive cytology received chemotherapy postoperatively. Havrilesky reported on experience from Duke University. Patients with positive cytology alone (*n* = 37) were compared to patients with adnexal/serosal involvement (*n* = 20). Five-year survival was similar between the groups (62% positive cytology, 68% adnexal/serosal disease), but in a multivariable analysis cytology was an independent predictor of recurrence and poorer survival. This study included patients with nonendometrioid histologies, and lymphadenectomy was not routinely performed. In another review of the literature, Wethington demonstrated that in endometrioid-type tumors with low risk factors (superficial invasion, grade I-II), the recurrence rate was only 4%. By comparison, 32% patients with higher grade tumors or deeper invasion and positive cytology had a recurrence. These results suggest that for at least a subset of cytology patients, the risk of recurrence approximates that driven by other uterine factors (depth of invasion, tumor grade). In 2009 FIGO dropped cytology as a stage IIIA defining characteristic.

Milosevic and colleagues reviewed 17 studies. In 3820 patients, the prevalence of positive cytologic findings was 11%. The three largest studies totaling more than 1700 patients (Haroung and associates, Turner and colleagues, Morrow and co-workers) using multivariate analysis noted that the finding of malignant cells on cytologic examination was independently significantly associated with either recurrence or reduced survival. Pooled odds ratio for the entire series was 4.7 (confidence interval 3.5 to 6.3) for disease recurrence. All studies note the highest correlation of malignant cytologic specimens with extrauterine disease. It does appear that with multivariate analysis, the presence of malignant cells is an important prognostic factor even when disease is limited to the uterus.

Optimal therapy has not been determined to date. Historically, intraperitoneal ^{32}P or oral progestins have been used to manage disease in patients with positive cytology. Today, uterine risk factors are largely used to define postoperative adjuvant therapy independent of cytology status and, increasingly, in otherwise low-risk patients (endometrioid-type tumors, negative nodes), observation is often considered. Chemotherapy has also been used in the adjuvant setting for patients with positive-cytology.

Molecular Indices

Hormone Receptors

Historically, estrogen and progesterone receptors were the first "targets" describing the molecular biology of endometrial cancer. Using multivariate analysis to analyze hormone receptor status, Creasman and associates noted that in stage I and stage II cancers, progesterone receptor–positive status was a highly significant, independently prognostic factor in endometrial cancer. Without progesterone receptor status in the model and with the evaluation of estrogen receptor status in its stead, estrogen receptor–positive status was an independent prognostic factor but not to the degree of progesterone receptor–positive status. Hormone receptor status may closely mirror grade, however.

Today there is an explosion of research into the molecular makeup of endometrial cancer. Cytogenetic studies have described gross chromosomal alterations, including changes in the number of copies of specific chromosome. The extent of abnormalities in a given tumor is relatively low. About 80% have normal diploid DNA content. Aneuploidy in 20% is usually associated with high-grade, extrauterine disease, high-risk histotypes, and poor prognosis. So-called loss of heterozygosity occurs at a relatively low frequency in comparison to other solid tumors. When chromosomal loss of heterozygosity does occur, underlying molecular genetic defects have been observed on 17p and 10q that correlates with mutational inactivation of *TP53* and *PTEN*, respectively. Individual tumors with a greater number of gains and losses are associated with a poorer prognosis, and some changes seen in cancer are also present in atypical hyperplasia but not simple hyperplasia lesions.

Mutational activation or aberrant expression of some oncogenes has been described but to a lesser degree than tumor suppressor genes. The *RAS* gene family is the most commonly identified oncogene aberration in human cancers and is present in 10% to 30% of endometrial cancers. This mutation appears to occur early in the neoplastic process, and the incidence is the same in endometrial hyperplasia. Correlation of *RAS* mutation to survival has produced conflicting results. About 10% to 15% of endometrial cancer has overexpression of ERBB-2 (HER2/neu) protein. Overexpression appears to be confined to high-grade or advanced-stage tumors.

The *FMS* oncogene encodes a tryosine kinase, which serves as a receptor for macrophage colony-stimulating factor (m-CSF). Expression of *FMS* correlates with advanced stage, high grade, and deep myometrial invasion. Expression of *C-MTC*, which has been observed in normal endometrium and endometriosis, has a higher expression in secretory endometrium. Several studies suggest amplification is present in a fraction of endometrial cancers.

Mutation of TP53 tumor suppressor gene, the most common genetic abnormality currently recognized in human cancers, is present in 10% to 30% of endometrial cancers. Overexpression and/or mutation are associated with prognostic factors. In a study of more than 100 endometrial hyperplasia specimens, TP53 mutation was not present. PTEN mutation analysis in endometrial cancer indicates that this gene is somatically inactivated in 30% to 50% of all tumors, the most frequent molecular genetic alteration defined in endometrial cancer. There does appear to be a correlation between microsatellite instability and PTEN mutation. PTEN mutation is observed in 20% of endometrial hyperplasias, suggesting that this is an early event in the development of some type I endometrial cancers.

Inherited mutations in gene encoding DNA mismatched repair proteins, primarily MSH2 and MLM1, are responsible for HNPCC, for which endometrial cancer is the second most common cancer in women with these mutations. Cancers in these individuals are characterized by frame shift mutations in multiple microsatellite repeat sequences throughout the genome. This instability is also seen in 20% of sporadic endometrial cancers. In these sporadic cancers, acquired mutation in mismatched repair genes is rare. Endometrial cancers that exhibit microsatellite instability tend to be type I, which has a more favorable prognosis. This microsatellite instability is present in some cases of complex hyperplasia associated with endometrial cancer but is not seen in papillary serous cancers.

Type I endometrial cancers are commonly described to include tumors seen in obese and nulliparous women, are well-differentiated, are superficially invasive, and frequently carry a good prognosis. These tumors also share several common molecular changes and tend to have the following genetic features: diploid, low allelic imbalance, K-RAS, MLH1 methylation, and PTEN. In contrast, type II with poor prognostic pathologic features have aneuploid, high allelic imbalance, K-RAS, TP53, and HER2/neu changes.

Recently, array-based technology has allowed a more comprehensive characterization of endometrial cancers. It should be noted that these new technologies are in their infancy, although multiple papers using these techniques have been reported, many with DNA microassay. The effects of exogenous PTEN expression in endometrial carcinoma cell lines lacking PTEN function has been studied by Matsushima-Nishiu and associates. They observed increased expression in 99 genes and repression of 72 genes, many of which are known to be involved in cell proliferation, differentiation, and apoptosis, suggesting the potential power of expression profiling identifying molecular pathways affected by critical cancer-related genes. Proteomic profiling, which is the study of intact and fragmented proteins and their function, is being evaluated. Newer technologies allow the creating of proteomic fingerprints that reflect in serum what is happening in the end organs. The biochip is playing a major role in this evaluation. As little as a microliter of serum can be evaluated, and this technology is very sensitive to low molecular weight protein regions. The GOG is currently collecting material (tissue, serum, urine) on a large number of endometrial cancer patients to be stored in its tumor bank for in-depth research using these newer technologies, which will hopefully allow us to understand the malignant process.

Correlation of Multiple Prognostic Factors

The GOG 33 protocol identified the extent of disease spread identified at surgery correlated with outcomes. Although single factors were associated with recurrence, the combination of factors could also establish risk. For example, Morrow showed that patients with no risk factors (LVSI, cervical involvement, adnexal involvement, nodal disease) had a very low risk of recurrence, whereas 20% with one, 43% with two, and 63% with three or more factors recurred. In multivariate analysis, those patients with disease limited to the uterus were at increased risk for recurrence if there were deep myometrial invasion, vascular space involvement, or positive washings. Figure 5–11 is the author's attempt to compartmentalize these risk factors into risk categories for predicting prognosis and guiding decisions for adjuvant therapy. The lines between categories are somewhat porous, consistent with most clinical situations.

Data from three randomized trials evaluating the use of postoperative pelvic radiation therapy have been useful in shaping models predicting risk of recurrence after surgery. Aalders identified a subset of the 95/540 (18%) patients enrolled in a randomized trial of vaginal cuff brachytherapy with or without pelvic radiation therapy with grade III tumors and greater than 0% myometrial invasion to be particularly notable for risk of recurrence. Patients with these factors had a pelvic recurrence rate of 20% with vaginal brachytherapy alone compared to 5% with the combination of pelvic and vaginal radiation. It is interesting that approximately 15% of patients with these tumor characteristics failed at a distant site, regardless of radiation technique. The PORTEC trial compared pelvic radiation therapy to observation following hysterectomy without lymph node dissection in patients with endometrial cancer. In this trial of 714 patients, a subset of patients with grade III tumors (10%), age greater than 60 (72%), or greater than 50% depth of invasion (59%) was identified in which having two of three factors defined a high-risk

TABLE 5-15 High-Intermediate Risk Model: Early-Stage
Endometrial Cancer

Age	Risk Factor
Any age + 3 factors	LVSI
≥50 years + 2 factors	Grade II-III tumor
≥70 years + 1 factor	Outer one-third invasion

Modified from Keys: Gynecol Oncol 2004;92:744–751.
LVSI, Lymphovascular space invasion.

group. The locoregional failure rate was 23% in this group who underwent surgery followed by observation compared to 5% after pelvic radiation therapy. There was no difference in distant sites of recurrence (~5% each group) or in cancer-related deaths (8% observation, 11% radiation). The GOG conducted a randomized trial (GOG 99) of observation versus pelvic radiation in a group of patients with surgically documented negative nodes and any amount of myometrial invasion. Depending on patient age and number of risk factors (LVSI, grade I-II tumor, outer one-third myometrial invasion) (Table 5-15), a high-intermediate (H-IR) risk group could be identified. The H-IR group accounted for one third of all patients enrolled but two thirds of recurrences. Perhaps equally important was the identification that two thirds of the patients enrolled who did not have H-IR features had an incredibly low risk of recurrence (2.1% to 2.9%), suggesting that in addition to defining high-risk groups, low-risk groups who may avoid postoperative adjuvant therapy may also be identified.

The value of risk models is that they can be applied to an individual patient incorporating all of the information (age, uterine characteristics) so as to provide a reasonable estimate of risk of recurrence and probability of benefit of selected adjuvant therapy. Research is under way to identify molecular markers that may augment clinical-pathologic information in establishing risk. Other cancer types (breast, prostate, bladder) have well-validated disease-specific nomograms predicting risk and benefit to adjuvant therapy. Similarly developed and validated models for endometrial cancer are needed.

TREATMENT

Surgical Management of Endometrial Cancer

We prefer to sample the endometrium in symptomatic postmenopausal patients as the first diagnostic technique. If histologic findings are "negative," the patient is observed. A D&C is done only if the patient continues to be symptomatic after the negative biopsy result. Once a tissue diagnosis of endometrial cancer is established, the patient should be assessed for surgical options of therapy. Most patients require routine blood counts

(CBC), metabolic profile, and a metastatic evaluation with chest radiograph. Routine use of computed tomography (CT) or MRI scans has not shown to be useful and should be reserved for unusual situations (high-risk tumor types, evidence of intraperitoneal disease, positive chest radiograph). Most patients with endometrial cancer are candidates for definitive surgery, including surgical staging (lymphadenectomy). Routes of hysterectomy include vaginal, abdominal, laparoscopic (total or assisted), and robotic and have broadened the surgical options for patients.

The surgical evaluation of most patients with endometrial cancer requires a thorough inspection of the peritoneal cavity, collection of cytologic washings, and pelvic and para-aortic lymphadenectomy in addition to hysterectomy. Cytologic evaluation of peritoneal fluids, or washings, has been a common surgical step in staging endometrial cancer because of associations with extra-uterine disease and prognosis. Once the peritoneal cavity is opened, an assessment of the amount of peritoneal fluid in the pelvis is made. If none is present, 100 to 125 mL of normal saline solution is injected into the pelvis. This can be done easily with a bulb syringe. The saline solution is admixed in the pelvis, withdrawn with the syringe, and sent for cytologic evaluation. We continue to recommend that peritoneal cytologic evaluation be performed in all patients undergoing surgery for endometrial cancer, although FIGO no longer uses cytology as a stage-defining characteristic. Omental biopsy may be considered in patients with gross spread to the omentum or adnexa or in cases with high-risk histologies such as serous or clear cell tumors. Approximately 10% of all patients will be found with nodal metastasis when surgically staged, whereas only 1% to 3% will be found to have nodal disease if nodes are evaluated only when clinically suspicious. In a large GOG study of 621 staged patients, 6% of patients with clinical stage I disease were noted to have intraperitoneal disease.

The definitive treatment for patients with endometrial cancer is hysterectomy. The hysterectomy should be extrafascial, and removal of the upper vagina does not appear to decrease vault recurrences (Figure 5-12). Removal of the uterus removes the primary tumor and can provide important information that can be used to estimate risk of spread to lymph nodes or risk of recurrence. Removal of the adnexa is thought to be important given that approximately 5% of endometrial cancers have metastatic disease to the ovaries and/or fallopian tubes. In addition, synchronous ovarian and endometrial cancers are not infrequent, particularly in younger patients. Historically, total abdominal hysterectomy (TAH) and bilateral salpingo-oophorectomy (BSO) have been the hallmarks of therapy for endometrial cancer. There are no data to suggest that the route of hysterectomy influences recurrence-free or overall survival

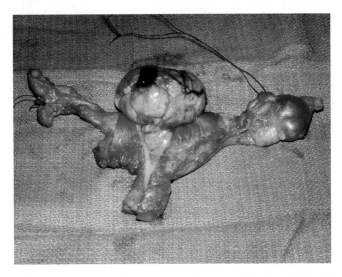

FIGURE 5-12 Total abdominal hysterectomy (TAH) and bilateral salpingo-oophorectomy (BSO) showing large polypoid adenocarcinoma of the endometrium with deep myometrial invasion.

outcomes for patients; as such, the hysterectomy (abdominal, laparoscopic, robotic) is the safest and facilitates rapid recovery and thus is suggested.

Several studies note the role of vaginal hysterectomy in highly selected patients with endometrial cancer for whom surgical staging cannot be performed safely (morbid obesity, significant cardiopulmonary medical comorbidities, advanced age). Because factors associated with the choice of vaginal hysterectomy (morbid obesity, medical comorbidities) are often associated with favorable uterine characteristics (low-grade lesions, smaller uterus), it is not surprising that survival rates are comparable to those of the abdominal approach. Chan reviewed 51 medically compromised patients treated with vaginal hysterectomy and reported 3- and 5-year disease-specific survival of 91% and 88%, respectively. Of note, approximately 50% of women could not have the ovaries removed at the time of vaginal hysterectomy. Smith evaluated 63 patients with obesity or medical comorbidities and found that vaginal hysterectomy was safe and well tolerated in this patient population. Vaginal hysterectomy may represent a reasonable tradeoff for patients who may not tolerate other approaches or for whom surgical staging is not being considered (atypical hyperplasia, some patients with grade I cancers).

Over time there has been a more widespread use of lymphadenectomy in the management of patients with endometrial cancer. Lymph node dissection provides the best estimate of spread of disease (vs palpation or use of imaging studies), the lymph node status is prognostically important (as evident by different survival rates seen with different stages of disease), and patients who are found to have positive or negative nodes receive different postoperative therapy vs patients with unknown status of lymph nodes. In a joint statement by ACOG and the SGO in 2005, both organizations suggested that most women with endometrial cancer should undergo systematic surgical staging including bilateral pelvic and para-aortic lymphadenectomy. Today, debate continues as to which patients (all, none, some) benefit most from lymphadenectomy and the technique (pelvic, pelvic and para-aortic, level of para-aortic dissection) that should be performed.

The technique of the lymph node dissection is thought to be important. Early studies were conducted with selective lymphadenopathy or lymph node sampling (only visibly enlarged lymph nodes are selectively removed). Some data suggest a true lymphadenectomy (complete skeletonization of vessels) should be performed. It seems intuitive that a sufficient number/distribution of nodes needs to be removed to represent an adequate sampling. When lymphadenectomy is done, the retroperitoneal spaces in the pelvis are opened in routine fashion. The vessels are outlined, and the lymph node–bearing tissue along the external iliacs from the bifurcation to the inguinal ligament is removed. The obturator fossa anterior to the obturator nerve is cleaned of lymphoid tissue. Lymph nodes along the common iliacs are also removed. The left and right para-aortic nodes are approached by retracting the small intestine into the upper abdomen and incising the peritoneum over the upper common iliac artery and lower aorta. The main vessels are outlined, and the ureter is retracted laterally. On the right, the tissue overlying the vena cava and the aorta is removed en bloc, beginning at the bifurcation of the aorta and extending caudad. On the left, the left common nodes are frequently quite lateral. Using this technique, one should have a total of 20 to 30 pelvic and para-aortic lymph nodes available for histologic evaluation. The upper limit of the dissection (unless enlarged nodes are noted above this area) is usually the inferior mesenteric artery (IMA), but some surgeons suggest that the dissection should extend to the level of the renal vessels.

The extent of nodal dissection to include para-aortic nodes is also thought to be important in endometrial cancer. There appear to be two nodal drainage basins—pelvic and para-aortic. Studies indicate that when lymph nodes are positive, approximately 50% to 60% of the time para-aortic nodes are involved. In a retrospective study from the Mayo Clinic, 137 patients at high risk for nodal involvement who underwent para-aortic lymphadenectomy (PAL+) were compared with those who did not undergo surgical evaluation of the para-aortic nodes (PAL–). The 5-year survival was 85% for PAL+ patients compared to 77% for PAL– patients. In 51 patients with pelvic or para-aortic node metastasis, survival was 77% for PAL+ patients compared to 42% in the PAL– group. It is generally thought that the rate of isolated

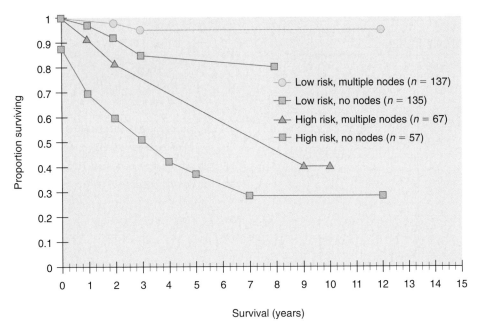

FIGURE 5-13　Survival by nodes sampled and risk groups: multiple-site pelvic node sampling versus no nodes. Low-risk group, $P = 0.026$; high-risk group, $P = 0.0006$. *(From Kilgore LC et al: Gynecol Oncol 56:29, 1995.)*

para-aortic lymph node metastasis is less than 5%; metastasis isolated to the para-aortic lymph node and metastasis above the IMA are seen. Mariani and colleagues reported on a study of 482 patients with endometrial cancer at the Mayo Clinic. A total of 281 underwent lymphadenectomy to the renal vessels, and 22% had positive lymph nodes; of these, 51% had both positive pelvic and para-aortic nodes, 33% had positive pelvic nodes only, and 16% had isolated involvement of the para-aortic nodes. Of note, 46% of those with isolated para-aortic lymph nodes were only positive above the IMA and 77% had at least one metastatic node located above the level of the IMA. However, the authors do report that there were no positive lymph nodes detected in those with grade I or II tumors with a tumor size of less than 2 cm with less than 50% invasion, raising the question of the benefit of lymphadenectomy in the truly low-risk group. Abu-Rustum and colleagues demonstrated a 1% risk of isolated para-aortic lymph node metastasis in both the low- and high-grade tumors. Based on these and other reports, para-aortic lymphadenectomy does have an important role in comprehensive staging. For high-risk patients, the data suggest even a therapeutic role for para-aortic lymph node dissection. However, prospective trials are needed to confirm this concept for patients with early-stage endometrial cancer with high-risk features.

Since 1988 when FIGO changed endometrial staging from clinical to surgical, there have been questions raised as to whether the lymphadenectomy is only diagnostic, which is an important determinate, or whether it also could be therapeutic. Kilgore and associates, in evaluating 649 patients, noted that those who underwent multiple-site lymph node removal had significantly better survival than those patients who had no lymph nodes removed (Figures 5-13 and 5-14). Lymph node removal resulted in a better survival than those without lymph node removal plus postoperative radiation. Cragun and colleagues reported that patients with grade III or poorly differentiated cancers with more than 11 lymph nodes removed had an improved survival (hazard ratio [HR], 0.25) and progression-free survival (HR, 0.26) when compared to those with fewer than 11 lymph nodes removed. However, the number of lymph nodes removed was not predictive of survival outcome in those with grade I and II tumors. This association between lymphadenectomy and improved survival remained when controlling for adjuvant radiation treatment, emphasizing the impact of extensive lymph node dissection. A retrospective review by Chan and colleagues of more than 12,000 patients showed an increased 5-year survival for the intermediate- and high-risk group who underwent an extensive lymph node dissection. However, there was no benefit of nodal dissection seen in the low-risk group.

Removal of nodes involved by tumor has been supported as a therapeutic option. In a study reported by Havrilesky, 91 patients were identified with stage IIIc

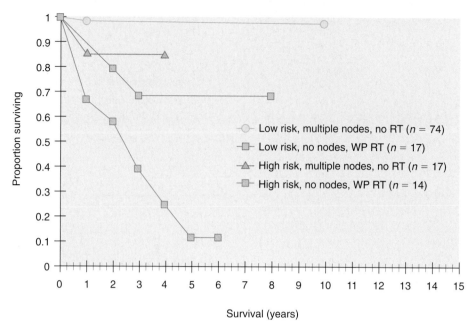

FIGURE 5-14 Survival comparisons of multiple-site pelvic node sampling to whole pelvic radiation therapy: Multiple nodes without RT vs no nodes plus whole pelvic RT. Low-risk group, *P* = 0.003; high-risk group, *P* = 0.041. (*RT,* Radiation therapy; *WP,* whole pelvic.) (*From Kilgore LC et al: Gynecol Oncol 56:29, 1995.*)

disease. There were 39 with microscopic involvement of the lymph nodes (LN) and 52 with grossly enlarged nodes. After surgery, 92% received some type of adjuvant therapy with 85% receiving radiation therapy. Survival (5 years) was 58% in the 39 with microscopic LN, 48% in 41 patients with grossly positive LN completely resected, and only 22% in the 11 with unresected LN. The authors felt that these data suggested a therapeutic benefit for lymphadenectomy. Similarly, in a small study of 41 patients, Bristow and co-workers noted disease-free survival was improved if patients with bulky adenopathy underwent complete resection of involved nodes compared with patients who had gross residual disease in lymph nodes remaining after surgery (37.5 vs 8.8 months; P = 0.006). Onda and colleagues carried out thorough pelvic and para-aortic lymphadenectomies on 173 patients with Stage I-III endometrial cancer. The average number of lymph nodes removed was 38 pelvic and 29 para-aortic. There were 30 patients (17%) with positive nodes; 10 to pelvis only, 2 para-aortic only, and 18 with metastasis to both pelvic and para-aortic nodes. Selected patients received radiation therapy with extended fields and/or combination chemotherapy. In the 10 patients with only pelvic metastasis, 5-year survival was 100%; it was 75% in those with para-aortic involvement. The authors suggest that although postoperative treatment may attribute to these excellent results, systematic pelvic and para-aortic lymphadenectomy was a contributing factor.

One of the important effects of lymph node dissection is that it identifies that most patients with negative lymph nodes are at very low risk for recurrence. As such, lymph node dissection has allowed for modifications of postoperative therapy away from pelvic radiation therapy. In one study, Mohan and associates evaluated 159 Stage I patients who had full pelvic lymphadenectomy and received vaginal brachytherapy rather than the more traditional pelvic radiation. In general vaginal brachytherapy is a quicker therapy (1-3 days vs 5-6 weeks for pelvic radiation) and is associated with fewer side effects. In the Mohan study, the 15-year overall survival was 92% and the recurrence rate was 4%, all at distant sites. Podratz and associates reviewed four studies that used thorough lymphadenectomies in moderate- and high-risk patients who did not receive postoperative radiation therapy. There were 20 recurrences (7%) in 305 patients; only 5 recurrences were local/regional, with 4 being in the vagina. Those 4 did not receive postoperative brachytherapy but were salvaged with subsequent radiation.

The disadvantages of a lymph node dissection include that the performance of lymph node dissection requires a specially trained surgeon, has the potential to increase complications (postoperative ileus, lymphedema), and has not been prospectively validated to improve outcomes. Two recent phase III trials compared the use of lymph node dissection or not in patients with endometrial cancer. In a large multicentric study (ASTEC study), 1408 patients were randomly assigned to abdominal hysterectomy or bilateral salpingo-oophorectomy with or without pelvic lymphadenectomy (PLA). A median follow-up of 37 months was obtained. There was no difference in survival between the two groups. This was an intent-to-treat study and has been criticized as having a relatively large noncompliance in regard to lymphadenectomy (LA) and subsequent therapy. In the LA arm, almost a half had no nodes or a small number (≤ 9) removed. This study was further complicated by the fact that many of these patients were secondarily randomly assigned into a postoperative radiation study not taking into consideration surgical findings. Para-aortic lymphadenectomy (PALA) was not the standard management, although some patients had these nodes removed.

The second study was presented by Pierluigi Benedetti Panici. The Italian study randomly assigned 514 stage I patients to systematic PLA or no LA. Although 13.3% of patients in the LA arm had known metastasis versus 3.2% in the no-LA arm, there was no difference in recurrence or overall survival. The protocol required a minimum of 20 lymph nodes to be removed; however, the LA was limited to the pelvis, although PALA could be removed at the discretion of the surgeon. Postoperative radiation was left to the discretion of the treating physician. Adjuvant therapy was similar in the two groups. Whether or not this had an effect on survival is unknown because this was not standardized.

A study from Japan (SEPAC study) was published in early 2010. This was a study of PLA ($n = 325$ patients) versus PALA ($n = 346$ patients) in endometrial cancer. It was not a randomized study; however, one hospital did only pelvic nodes and the other pelvic and para-aortic. LA was certainly adequate for using the number of lymph nodes removed as a parameter. Survival was significantly better ($P > 0.001$) in those women receiving the PLA and PALA. This was associated in intermediate- and high-risk patients but not in low-risk patients. In a multivariant analysis, the PLA plus PALA reduced the risk of death compared with PLA only. In the high-risk group, patients receiving chemotherapy plus PLA plus PALA had a better survival than patients receiving chemotherapy plus PLA only. PLA plus PALA and adjuvant chemotherapy were independently associated with improved survival.

The Cochrane Database recently concluded that there was no overall statistical difference between progression-free and overall survival in those patients who had a lymphadenectomy versus those who did not but did report more morbidity for those patients who had a lymphadenectomy. Cochrane only considered the ASTEC and the Italian study in reaching their conclusion. The extent of the lymphadenectomy appears to be critical in evaluating studies in determining an appropriate surgical procedure for patients with endometrial cancer. Multiple studies confirm that both pelvic and para-aortic lymph nodes are at risk for metastasis. Our practice is to discuss the data on lymph node dissection and the potential downstream effects (possible increased use of adjuvant therapy in unknown nodal status, possible increased complications with node dissection) with patients in an effort to make an informed choice.

Patients with stage II carcinoma of the endometrium, because of extension of disease into the endocervix, will have a greater propensity for lymph node metastasis. For example, in the GOG 33 protocol, 16% of patients with cervical involvement had positive pelvic lymph nodes versus 8% with a fundal location of tumor. In addition, parametrial and vaginal involvement are thought to be more common when the cervix is involved. As such, surgery in the form of radical hysterectomy and lymphadenectomy has been advocated when there is gross cervical involvement with tumor. Because many cases of cervical involvement are occult, and only recognized after surgery, simple hysterectomy with lymphadenectomy appears to be adequate surgery in most cases. Postoperative radiation therapy can be planned, depending on surgical-pathologic findings, including use of pelvic radiation or vaginal cuff brachytherapy, both, or neither.

In 1993 Childers and others pioneered laparoscopic lymph node removal in conjunction with vaginal hysterectomy and bilateral salpingo-oophorectomy. In the hands of those who acquired those surgical skills, the outcomes appeared comparable and some advantages were gained, such as short hospitalization and rapid postoperative recovery. A large GOG study comparing laparoscopic approach versus laparotomy has been completed. Walker and colleagues recently reported the results of GOGLAP2, which randomly assigned patients between laparoscopic versus open laparotomy surgical staging. Laparoscopy was initiated and completed without conversion in 74%. Conversion from laparoscopy to laparotomy was secondary to poor visibility in 15%, metastatic cancer in 4%, and bleeding in 3%. Patients randomly assigned to undergo laparoscopy had significantly fewer moderate to severe postoperative (14% vs 21%) complications and similar rates of intraoperative complications. Length of hospital stay was significantly shorter for those randomized to undergo laparoscopy (median 3 days vs 4 days), but operative time was significantly longer (median 204 minutes vs 130 minutes). Pelvic and para-aortic nodes were removed in 92% of patients undergoing laparoscopy and 96% of patients undergoing laparotomy, and cytology was performed in 96% vs 98%. Neither treatment arm demonstrated an improved ability to detect metastatic disease. Quality-of-life evaluation found a better body image and return to normal activities for the patients undergoing laparoscopy. Laparoscopic surgical staging is feasible and safe for patients with uterine cancer and results in fewer complications and a shorter hospital stay. A reduction in para-aortic node evaluation is a potential risk of laparoscopic staging. Data also have suggested that there is no difference in survival or recurrence between the surgical modalities. Today, advancements of laparoscopic surgery including use of a robotic surgical platform have been suggested as the next step. Robotic surgery offers three-dimensional graphics, improved ergonomics, and greater dexterity of surgical instruments. Robotic surgery may extend the applications of laparoscopy especially in obese patients or patients in whom a vaginal component are more difficult.

Surgical staging has now been accepted as standard therapy in patients with endometrial cancer unless clinical conditions suggest otherwise. Of the 6260 patients with endometrial cancer reported to the last Annual Report of FIGO, 94% were surgically staged. It is appreciated that those institutions reporting to the Annual Report are academic ones and that most endometrial cancers, at least in the United States, have their primary surgery at academic hospitals. Because endometrial cancer staging has been determined by surgical staging, it has been suggested by some that these are patients who are at low risk (i.e., grade I) for lymph node metastasis and lymphadenectomy is not worthwhile. Increasing data suggest that even in grade I, as noted on endometrial biopsy, a significant number of patients have on full surgical staging findings that would have an impact on further therapy. Ben-Shachar and colleagues in evaluating 181 grades I endometrial cancers found 19% had grade change on hysterectomy specimen, 11% had extrauterine disease, 4% had lymph node metastasis, and 26% on final evaluation had high-risk intrauterine factors. Of note, the authors felt because of full surgical staging that 12% needed and received adjuvant therapy and 17% who may have received postoperative treatment did not based on full surgical findings. Geisler and associates found in 349 patients that of those with grade I lesions, 16% had positive nodes and 3% had positive para-aortic nodes only. Of all positive nodes, 31% occurred in grade I lesions. As a result of these and other studies, many feel that all endometrial cancer patients should have the benefit of full surgical staging, which includes peritoneal cytology, bilateral pelvic and para-aortic lymphadenectomy, and total abdominal hysterectomy and bilateral salpingo-oophorectomy. Obviously, complete evaluation of the entire peritoneal cavity and its contents should be performed and any suspicious areas should be pathologically evaluated.

Straight and associates reported on a large number of patients who were surgically staged. Low-risk factors, stage IaG1 and 2 were present in 103 patients. None received postoperative therapy and none had recurred. Intermediate risk was defined as stage IaG3 and all stage

I and Ic cancers. There were 440 patients of which 93% received no further therapy. Twenty-eight patients received postoperative therapy and one (4%) had a recurrence compared with 5% of those not radiated. The latter patients received therapy at time of recurrence, and 62% were successful. The Annual Report (2003) noted 5-year survival with surgery only of 93%, 91%, 73%, 79%, and 73%, respectively, for stages Ia, b, c, and IIa and b. This compares with 89%, 91%, 83%, 83%, and 75%, respectively, if surgery plus postoperative radiation is used. There is a suggestion that in stage Ic, survival is somewhat better when postoperative radiation is added than surgery alone. What factors went into decision-making regarding postoperative therapy is unknown. In a multi-institutional study, 220 surgically staged Ic patients were identified. High-risk histotypes were excluded. Adjuvant radiation was used in 99 (45%), 56 brachytherapy only, 19 whole-pelvis radiation, and 24 received both. Overall survival between those treated with surgery and surgery plus radiation was similar (92% vs 90%).

Radiation Therapy

Radiation therapy has been the mainstay of adjuvant therapy for endometrial cancer. Historically, nearly all patients received some form of preoperative or postoperative radiation therapy given the perception of risk for recurrence was high. Whereas GOG 33 defined relationships between depth of invasion and tumor grade and extrauterine spread following surgical staging, it also showed that most patients were not at risk for extrauterine disease spread. As such, the routine use of pelvic radiation therapy became increasing questioned. To date, there have been four large prospective randomized studies comparing external pelvic radiation to observation or vaginal brachytherapy in women with endometrial cancer (Table 5-16). Aalders and colleagues compared vaginal cuff brachytherapy with or without pelvic radiation in 540 patients with early-stage endometrial cancer. Patients did not undergo lymph node dissection. The addition of pelvic radiation therapy reduced local failures (2% vs 7%), but there was no difference in 5-year survival between the groups (89% pelvic, 91% brachytherapy).

In the Dutch PORTEC trial, Creutzberg enrolled 714 patients with grade I lesions with greater than 50% myometrial invasion, grade II lesions with any amount of invasion, or grade III with less than 50% invasion. Patients were randomly assigned postoperatively to receive either external radiation or observation. None of the patients were surgically staged, and all histologies were eligible. In the 654 eligible for follow-up, local and regional recurrences were less frequent in the radiation therapy group (4% vs 14%) than in the observational

TABLE 5-16 Radiation in Early-Stage Carcinoma of the Endometrium

	Local Recurrence (%)	Survival (%)
Aalder		
Surgery + VCB (n = 277)	7*	91
Surgery VCB + RT (n = 263)	2†	89
Creutzberg (PORTEC)		
Surgery (n = 300)	14†	85
Surgery + RT (n = 354)	4†	81
Keyes (GOG 99)		
Surgery (n = 202)	4	86
Surgery + RT (n = 190)	2	92
ASTEC/ NCIC CTG EN.5		
Surgery ‡(n = 454)	6§	84
Surgery + RT (n = 452)	3§	84

*P <0.01
†P <0.001
‡50% received vaginal brachytherapy
§P = 0.038
RT, Pelvic radiation therapy; VCB, vaginal cuff brachytherapy.

TABLE 5-17 Survival Rate in Stage I Carcinoma of the Endometrium with Regard to Grade and Treatment

	Survival	
Grade	Surgery Only (%)	Combined Therapy (%)
1	1295/1375 (94)	2284/2389 (96)
2	488/510 (96)	1490/1721 (87)
3	100/135 (74)	398/498 (80)

From Pettersson F (ed): Annual Report on the Results of Treatment in Gynecological Cancer, Vol 21. Stockholm, International Federation of Gynecology and Obstetrics, 1991.

TABLE 5-18 Recurrences in Stage I Carcinoma of the Endometrium with Regard to Depth of Invasion and Treatment

Recurrence	Surgery and Radium	Surgery and External Radiation
Endometrium only	6/88 (7%)	0/4 (0%)
Inner and mid thirds	3/68 (4%)	9/29 (31%)
Outer third	3/9 (33%)	11/24 (46%)

Modified from DiSaia PJ et al: Am J Obstet Gynecol 151:1009, 1985.

group, but 5-year survival was similar, 81% versus 85%, respectively.

The GOG performed a phase III trial of surgery with or without adjunctive external pelvic radiation in intermediate-risk endometrial adenocarcinomas. These included all women with any degree of myometrial invasion, any grade, and no evidence of lymph node metastasis (stage Ib, IC, IIA occult, and IIB occult). All patients were required to have surgical staging with histologic evaluation of the lymph nodes. There were 202 who received no radiation (NAT) and 190 who received pelvic radiation (RT). Median follow-up was 69 months. There were 15% total recurrences in the NAT group compared to 6% to 8% in the RT (P = 0.007). Local recurrences were 9% versus 2%, respectively. The overall survival at 48 months was 86% for NAT and 92% for RT, with intercurrent diseases accounting for half or more of the deaths in both groups. Deaths from disease were 8% in both the NRT versus RT group. Grade III and IV toxicity by treatment was 5% versus 14% in the NRT and RT, groups, respectively. In 12 of the 13 women who had isolated vaginal recurrences, the NAT arm were treated with radiation and 5 have died of disease. An H-IR subgroup appeared to derive the best benefit from pelvic radiation, with 27% of H-IR patients followed with observation compared to 13% after pelvic radiation, recurring. All other eligible patients were considered low-intermediate risk and had recurrence rates less than 1% to 3% regardless of the use of radiation therapy. The most recent data from a pooled trial of the MRC ASTEC and NCIC CTG EN.5 randomized trials also showed no survival advantage for adjuvant external-beam radiotherapy in the treatment of endometrial cancer (5-year survival ~84% both groups). In this study including 906 patients randomly assigned to pelvic radiation or observation, 30% of patients underwent lymphadenectomy and 50% received vaginal brachytherapy. Pelvic radiation reduced local failures (6% with observation vs 3% after pelvic radiation). In a subsequent Cochrane Review on the use of adjuvant radiation therapy for stage I endometrial cancer, the authors concluded that there is no survival advantage with routine use of pelvic radiation therapy and that benefits must be balanced against the toxicity/morbidity of therapy. In addition, risk factors within stage I groups (grade III, outer 50% invasion) should be considered in an effort to better select populations who may get the best benefit.

Essentially all studies evaluating pelvic radiation therapy show improved local control rates compared to observation. The local control, however, is largely a result of reduction in vaginal cuff recurrences. A considerable amount of data have been collected to evaluate vaginal recurrence and survival rate with surgery alone or combined therapy when mainly preoperative application of brachytherapy and surgery were used. Data have also been evaluated in regard to the grade of the tumor (Table 5-17) and, in some instances, the depth of myometrial involvement (Table 5-18). In patients who had postoperative irradiation, there appeared to be a lower incidence of vaginal vault recurrences, although there does not appear to be much difference in the grade I and grade II lesions. Vaginal vault recurrence did not appear to affect survival. Recently, results of a randomized prospective trial comparing adjuvant external-beam radiotherapy versus vaginal brachytherapy in 427 patients with intermediate-risk early-stage endometrial cancer have been reported (PORTEC-2). No differences in recurrence rate (vaginal failure 2% with pelvic radiation, 0.9% with vaginal brachytherapy) or overall survival (3-year survival ~90% both groups) were observed between the two treatment arms, suggesting that patients with intermediate-risk early-stage endometrial cancer can be treated with adjuvant vaginal brachytherapy alone. Although these findings have led many clinicians in the United States to move away from the routine use of external-beam radiation therapy in early-stage endometrial cancer, it is important to note that in the patients who did not undergo a lymph node dissection, pelvic failure rates were higher in vaginal brachytherapy group (3.5% vs 0.7%), and the study excluded higher-risk patients such as those with grade III/deeper invasion tumors.

Chemotherapy

The role of chemotherapy in endometrial cancer is evolving. Traditionally reserved for patients with recurrent or disseminated cancer, chemotherapy has become increasingly used in the first-line management of advanced-stage and high-risk early-stage patients. Historically, radiation therapy has been the adjuvant of choice for patients at risk of recurrence. Although the overall prognosis of patients in adjuvant radiation trials has been favorable, 3% to 23% of patients have a recurrence at distant sites, demonstrating the need for effective systemic therapy.

Drug Development

Progestins have been an important systemic therapy given response rates in up to one third of patients and low toxicity. The identification of active cytotoxic chemotherapy regimens has led to a re-evaluation of chemotherapy. Phase II studies have identified several single agents with activity in advanced or recurrent endometrial cancer. In a report of the GOG experience, Thigpen and colleagues noted that 37% with advanced or recurrent cancer experienced an objective response with use of doxorubicin alone. Unfortunately, response lasted only 7 months. The Eastern Cooperative Oncology Group achieved only a 19% response rate in its doxorubicin trial; however, a dosage lower than the GOG dosage was used. When one evaluates the doxorubicin data, one notes that only about 10% of patients who received this drug had a complete response rate. Patients designated as giving a partial response had survival rates no greater than those of patients who had no response to this cytotoxic agent. Likewise, phase II studies have identified platinum agents (cisplatin, carboplatin) and taxanes (paclitaxel) to have significant activity.

Combining two or more active agents in combination has been an important strategy. Phase III studies have shown better response rates when the agents were combined compared to used alone. Several chemotherapy combinations have been used in recurrent or advanced endometrial cancer. The GOG, in a randomized trial, compared doxorubicin with or without cisplatin. The combination produced tumor response in 66% versus 35% for the single agent, with a median progression-free interval of 6.2 and 3.9 months, respectively. The GOG reported a 45% response rate (22% complete response) for the combination of doxorubicin and cisplatin in advanced or recurrent endometrial cancer compared to 17% response for doxorubicin alone. The European Organization for Research and Treatment of Cancer Gynecological Cancer Cooperative Group (EORTC-GCCG) compared doxorubicin alone with doxorubicin and cisplatin. Response rate was 17% and 57%, respectively. The GOG (GOG 163) has compared doxorubicin and cisplatin to doxorubicin and paclitaxel (24-hour infusion) with filgrastim in advanced/recurrent endometrial cancer. There were 317 patients randomly assigned to the two regimens. Response rates were similar (40% vs 43%). PFS was median 7.2 versus 6 months, and overall survival was median 12.6 vs 13.6 months). Toxicities were also similar. A phase III study by the GOG (GOG 177) compared doxorubicin plus cisplatin with or without paclitaxel plus filgrastim in advanced endometrial cancer. There were 273 women registered and objective response was 57% versus 34% (P <0.01); PFS (median 8.3 vs 5.3 months, P <0.01) and overall survival (median 15.3 vs 12.3 months, P = 0.037) were improved with the triple combination (TAP regimen). This study marked for the first time a statistically significant improvement in response rate, PFS, and survival with a combination regimen in endometrial cancer. However, the three-drug regimen required a 2-day treatment and the use of growth factors on day 3 and was associated with moderate peripheral neuropathy. The GOG has recently concluded a randomized trial comparing the three-drug TAP regimen to carboplatin plus paclitaxel.

Advanced Disease

Drug development trials are largely designed to assess the efficacy of new drugs or combinations in patients with incurable disease (recurrent, disseminated). The concept of using chemotherapy in patients with advanced but potentially curable disease was once considered controversial. Treatment of patients with stage III or stage IV disease depends largely on the extent of surgical resection. Patients with stage III-IV disease and resection to less than 1 to 2 cm residual may be treated with curative intent with chemotherapy, radiation, or a combination of the two. The GOG studied patients (GOG 122) with stage III/IV endometrial cancer with 2 cm or less residual disease (distant metastases were excluded). After surgery, patients were randomly assigned to receive doxorubicin and cisplatin every 3 weeks for eight courses or whole abdominal radiation with 3000 cGy to the whole abdomen. A boost to the pelvic and para-aortic lymph node region (1500 cGy) could be given for positive nodes. Two years after therapy, overall survival was improved by 11% and cancer-free survival was improved by 13% with chemotherapy compared to those treated with radiation therapy. Side effects were more common in the chemotherapy-treated patients.

In an effort to build on improvements noted with the first-line chemotherapy into the management of patients with advanced endometrial cancer, the GOG performed a randomized trial (GOG 184) comparing volume-directed radiation (pelvic radiation with or without extended field to cover para-aortic lymph nodes) followed by six cycles of doxorubicin/cisplatin with or without paclitaxel chemotherapy. The results showed no improvement in PFS with the addition of paclitaxel to pelvic radiation plus cisplatin and doxorubicin except in patients with gross residual disease. Although the results of GOG 184 may seem to conflict with the results of GOG 177, several important observations can be made. First, the addition of pelvic radiation therapy may supplant the benefit of adding paclitaxel the two-drug regimen seen in GOG 177. Second, this trial demonstrates the feasibility of combining multi-agent cytotoxic chemotherapy with adjuvant radiation. This study has finished the accrual phase and results are awaited.

Factors associated with response to chemotherapy have been studied. Behbakht and colleagues evaluated prognostic factors in 137 patients with advanced disease (stage III and stage IV). Multivariate analysis noted age, parametrial involvement, and abdominal metastasis as significant prognostic indicators. An increased frequency of advanced stage was also noted with papillary serous histology. Unfortunately, multiple therapies were used and conclusions concerning treatment cannot be made. Kadar and associates evaluated 58 patients with surgical stage III and stage IV disease. Extrapelvic peritoneal metastasis and positive peritoneal cytologic findings affected survival. If either of these factors was present, 2-year survival was only 25% compared with 83% if they were not present. Postoperative therapy varied, but it did not appear to have any effect on survival.

Adjuvant Therapy: High-Risk Disease

Given the results of GOG 122, new considerations for chemotherapy in a variety of settings have been considered. Today, the role of adjuvant chemotherapy in intermediate- and high-risk early-stage endometrial cancers is increasingly considered. Several trials have assessed the role of chemotherapy in high-risk endometrial cancer. The Japanese GOG group performed a randomized trial of chemotherapy (at least three cycles of cyclophosphamide, doxorubicin, cisplatin [CAP regimen]) versus pelvic radiation in patients with endometrial cancer. Most patients had stage IC/II disease (75%), but patients with IIIA and IIIC disease were included. For all patients, there was no difference in PFS or OS between the regimens. The study did identify a group of patients with higher-risk features (IC/grade III, stage II-III with depth of invasion >50%) for whom PFS and OS were significantly improved in the chemotherapy arm. Maggi and colleagues performed a similar study comparing five cycles of CAP chemotherapy to pelvic radiation in 340 patients with endometrial cancer. In this trial 62% of patients had stage IIIA-C disease. The 5-year PFS and OS were not statistically different between the groups. Neither of these studies used paclitaxel, an agent that in phase II and III studies appears to offer improved efficacy.

The role of adjunctive chemotherapy in addition to surgery and radiation therapy has been addressed by the GOG in patients with high-risk stage I and occult stage II endometrial cancers. One hundred and eighty-one patients were treated with TAH and BSO, peritoneal cytologic evaluation, and selective pelvic and para-aortic lymphadenectomy, followed by external irradiation (pelvic, with or without extended field) and were then randomly assigned to receive doxorubicin 60 mg/m^2 every 3 weeks for eight doses. Patients participating in the doxorubicin arm of the protocol had a higher incidence of metastases to pelvic nodes (20% vs 10%) than did those in the nondoxorubicin arm; otherwise, the risk factors were equal between the two groups. There were recurrences in 22 of 92 (23%) in the doxorubicin arm versus recurrences in 23 of 89 (26%) in the nondoxorubicin arm. Of those patients with recurrence, those who received doxorubicin had a greater chance of metastasis to the abdomen than did those not receiving it (40% vs 17%). However, distant metastases occurred more frequently without the use of doxorubicin than with it (56% vs 18%). The small sample size (and reduced power), the heterogeneous population, and the use of single-agent doxorubicin (as opposed to combination therapy) are weaknesses of the study. The Radiation Oncology Group (RTOG) and the European Organization for Research and Treatment of Cancer (EORTC) have both published data on patients with high-risk early-stage endometrial cancers treated with adjuvant radiation therapy ± adjuvant platinum-based chemotherapy. Both trials suggest that adjuvant radiation combined with adjuvant chemotherapy in high-risk early-stage endometrial cancers is feasible and may result in better overall survival.

Based on the experience with current studies, two important trials assessing the role of chemotherapy have been developed. The PORTEC-3 trial is an ongoing randomized phase III trial comparing concurrent chemoradiation followed by adjuvant paclitaxel/carboplatin chemotherapy versus pelvic radiation alone. The GOG is currently accruing patients for a randomized phase III trial (GOG 249) comparing vaginal brachytherapy plus adjuvant carboplatin and paclitaxel versus pelvic radiation. Neither the PORTEC-3 trial nor GOG 249 will require lymph node dissection as part of the inclusion criteria. However, full surgical staging is encouraged in the GOG trial. It is hoped that the results of these trials will elucidate the role of adjuvant chemotherapy combined with adjuvant radiation in high-risk early-stage endometrial cancer.

Hormones

Progestins have been used for more than 30 years, and the objective responsiveness of recurrent carcinoma of the endometrium to these hormones has been substantiated (Figure 5-15). Historically, approximately one third of all patients with recurrent carcinoma of the endometrium are said to respond to the hormone, although patients with well-differentiated tumors have a response rate much higher than that of patients with moderately or poorly differentiated lesions. The GOG described 420 patients with advanced or recurrent endometrial

carcinoma treated with medroxyprogesterone acetate (MPA) 50 mg three times a day. Of the 219 patients with objective measurable disease, there were only 17 complete responders (8%) and 13 partial responders (6%). More than half of the patients remained stable and one third progressed. Median survival was 10.5 months. Grade I lesions responded more frequently than poorly differentiated carcinomas did. The GOG evaluated, in a randomized phase III trial, MPA at 1000 mg/day compared with 200 mg/day. In almost 300 patients there was no difference in response rate or survival between the two groups. Lentz reported another GOG trial of high-dose megestrol acetate (800 mg/day) in patients with advanced or recurrent endometrial carcinoma. Of 58 patients, 13 (24%) responded; 6 (11%) had a partial response. Four of the responses lasted more than 18 months and were primarily between the grade I and grade II lesions.

More recently, considerable interest has been shown in the presence of specific estrogen and progesterone receptors in neoplastic human uterine tissue. These receptors are definitely present and vary from tumor to tumor. It has been shown that there is a greater number of both estrogen and progesterone receptors in well-differentiated lesions than in poorly differentiated ones (Table 5-19). In a small group of patients, it was noted that about one third of those with recurrent cancer had a positive receptor site analysis to both estrogen and progesterone. The receptor data may therefore correlate with clinical findings of responsiveness to progesterones in patients with recurrent cancer. Preliminary data suggest an excellent correlation (Table 5-20). Obviously, considerable additional data are needed to verify these findings; however, the prospects are excellent. If direct correlation can be substantiated, the receptor site

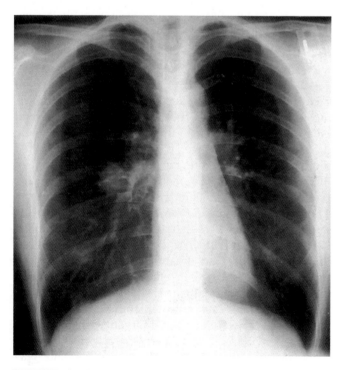

FIGURE 5-15 Patient with right hilar metastases that resolved completely on progestin therapy.

TABLE 5-19 Correlation of Tumor Differentiation with Receptor Content

Differentiation	ER and PR Positive (%)
Well	28/40 (70)
Moderate	21/38 (55)
Poor	11/27 (41)

From Creasman WT et al: Am J Obstet Gynecol 151:922, 1985.
ER, Estrogen receptor; PR, progesterone receptor.

TABLE 5-20 Response to Progestin Therapy in Regard to Receptor Content

Receptor Content	Progestin Response (%)
Positive	44/55 (80)
Negative	4/76 (5)

Based on papers by Ehrlich, Benraad, Creasman, Kauppila, Pollow, and Quinn.

analysis can guide the type of progestin therapy or chemotherapy given for recurrent endometrial cancer. If receptor site analysis is positive for both estrogen and progesterone, a patient's chances of responding to progestins are extremely good, even if she has a poorly differentiated lesion. However, if the receptor site analysis is negative, the data suggest that the patient's response to progestins may be extremely low, making it more advisable to go directly to cytotoxic agents without wasting time on progestin therapy. Kauppila noted from five studies in the literature that 89% of progesterone receptor-positive tumors were hormonally responsive, compared with only 17% of progesterone receptor-negative tumors. The GOG noted that 4 of 10 (40%) estrogen receptor-positive, progesterone receptor-positive tumors responded to progestins, compared with 5 of 41 (12%) progesterone receptor-negative tumors.

Progestin therapy may be administered in several different ways; MPA (Depo-Provera), 400 mg intramuscularly at weekly intervals, oral MPA (Provera) in the range of 150 mg/day, and megestrol acetate (Megace) 160 mg/day are recommended progestins. Progestins are continued indefinitely if an objective response is obtained. If progression of disease is noted, progestins should be discontinued and chemotherapy should be considered.

Progestins have been evaluated as adjunctive therapy in the hope of preventing recurrences. Lewis and coworkers, in a randomized study, treated endometrial cancer patients postoperatively with MPA or placebo. The 4-year survival was similar in the two groups. Kauppila and associates, in describing more than 1100 patients who received adjunctive progestin therapy for 2 years after surgery and radiation therapy, found that even in stage I low-grade tumors, recurrences did appear; it was their belief that prophylactic progestins were not of benefit to these patients. In a prospective study of 363 patients with stage I disease who received adjuvant MPA for 12 months, DePalo and colleagues compared survival with that of 383 patients with stage I disease who did not receive MPA postoperatively; there was no difference in survival between the two groups. In a British study in which 429 patients with stage I or stage II cancers were randomized between postoperative MPA and observation, no difference in survival was seen after 5 years. A Cochrane Database review concluded that current evidence did not support the use of adjuvant progestin therapy in the primary treatment of endometrial cancer

With only modest response to progestins, other hormonal agents have been evaluated. Tamoxifen has been shown to bind estrogen receptors and thereby block access of the estrogen into the nucleus. It has also been suggested that tamoxifen can increase the number of progesterone receptors in vivo. Combined results of several small studies noted a response rate of 22% (complete response rate of 8%) in 257 patients. These studies suggest that grade I lesions are more responsive than other grades of tumors. Progestins plus tamoxifen have been evaluated in combination in recurrent carcinoma of the endometrium. Tamoxifen, 40 mg daily, with intermittent Provera, 200 mg daily on alternate weeks, had a 33% response rate with a median progression-free survival of 3 months and median survival of 13 months (GOG 0119). A Phase II trial of megestrol acetate, 160 mg orally for 3 weeks, alternating with tamoxifen, 40 mg daily for 3 weeks, until disease progression showed an overall response rate of 27% with a median progression-free survival of 2.7 months and median overall survival of 14 months (GOG 0153). The response rate was 38% in patients with histologic grade I tumors, 24% in those with grade II, and 22% among patients with grade III. Although tamoxifen is theoretically attractive (it causes an increase in progesterone receptors for better progestin effect), studies of small groups of patients have not produced favorable results. The use of tamoxifen is interesting in view of the reports of endometrial cancer in patients taking tamoxifen. This is in contrast to in vitro data suggesting that tamoxifen does not stimulate and in fact may inhibit established endometrial cell line growth.

Gonadotropin-releasing hormone (GnRH) analogues have been evaluated in the treatment of endometrial cancer in a small number of patients. These analogues suppress gonadotropins with a reduction in estrogen but not cortisol levels. Gallagher and associates treated 17 patients with recurrent endometrial cancer who had received previous progesterone therapy; 6 (35%) had a response that continued for a median of 20 months. Further study is needed, but it appears that GnRH analogues may have a direct inhibitory effect on cancer cells.

Special Circumstances

Multiple Malignant Neoplasms

Simultaneous or subsequent primary cancers involving the breast, ovary, and large intestines occur more frequently in patients with endometrial cancer than might be expected. The reverse also appears true, in that women with breast or ovarian cancer have a higher than expected risk for development of subsequent primary cancers of the endometrium. As a result, the recommendation in a patient with one of these malignant neoplasms is to evaluate the other organ sites at the time of diagnosis or during follow-up visits. Appropriate screening, such as mammography, should be emphasized.

Simultaneous malignant neoplasms of the ovary and endometrium are noted in about 8% of patients with carcinoma of the uterus, and twice that rate is noted in patients with ovarian carcinoma. Ovarian involvement in cases in which endometrial cancer is present has been reported to be as high as 40% of autopsy specimens and 15% of specimens obtained at the time of hysterectomy and bilateral salpingo-oophorectomy. In approximately one third of cases of endometrioid carcinoma of the ovary, endometrial carcinoma has also been noted. When the occurrence is simultaneous, the question arises whether these are simultaneous multiple malignant neoplasms or one is metastatic from the other. It appears that if metastasis is present, it is more common for it to go from the endometrium to the ovary than from the ovary to the endometrium. Metastasis to the ovary is suspected if the endometrial carcinoma involves significant myometrium, particularly with lymphatic or vascular channel invasion, or if the tumor is on the ovarian surface. If, however, the corpus carcinoma is small and limited to the endometrium or superficial myometrium, with associated atypical hyperplasia, and the ovarian tumor is centrally located, the tumors are probably independent of each other. Most common tumors are the endometrioid type, but they can occasionally be of different histologic types in the two organs. Most studies suggest that most of the synchronous ovarian and corpus carcinomas are independent primary tumors. The survival of patients with what is believed to be multiple primaries mimics the excellent prognosis of the individual cancer, suggesting that the two tumors are probably each stage I and not stage III. This has certainly been true when the simultaneous endometrial and ovarian carcinomas are of the endometrioid type. In one study, the survival was 100% of the 16 patients described. It appears that when such a situation is encountered (i.e., when there is no evidence of direct extension of either tumor), myometrial invasion is usually absent or superficial, there is no lymphatic or blood vessel invasion, there is atypical hyperplasia of the endometrium frequently associated with the cancer, both tumors are usually confined to the primary sites and have minimal spread, and tumor is predominantly within the ovary or the endometrium. Whether the histologic type is uniform or dissimilar, therapy should be appropriate for stage I disease, which in many instances may be treated adequately with surgery only (hysterectomy and bilateral salpingo-oophorectomy with appropriate surgical staging).

Serous Carcinoma

Much debate has surrounded the biology and clinical behavior of PS tumors. There is a common perception that PS tumors behave differently than similarly staged patients with endometrioid tumors. Given the relative rarity of PS tumors, most series reported in the literature have been small, retrospective series covering a long time period, using variable levels of surgical staging, and a variety of postoperative therapies. Older studies

TABLE 5-21   Upstaging of Serous Carcinoma of the Uterus

Author	n	Patients Upstaged (%)
Mallipeddi	9	8
Lee	10	10
Carcangiu	64	32
Cirisano	53	26
Gehrig	16	10
Kato	28	19
Sutton	10	4
Gallion	13	6
Chen	13	5
Goff	50	36
Sherman	41	19
Frank	9	7
Ward	20	8
Total	339	190 = 56%

that did not include comprehensive surgical staging suggest that nearly 50% of "early staged" cases of PS recurred. One explanation for this finding is that for PS tumors, extrauterine disease spread is common at diagnosis, even in clinically stage I disease. One of the larger series by Goff and associates identified 50 patients with UPSC, 33 pure UPSC and 17 admixed with other histologic types. Unlike endometrioid tumors, PS tumors have a greater frequency of disease spread at presentation. In the Goff series, 72% had extrauterine disease; lymph node metastasis was found in 36% with no myometrial invasion, 50% with less than half invasion, and in 40% with outer half invasion. Of particular significance was the fact that 14 patients (28%) had disease limited to the endometrium, yet 36% had lymph node metastasis, 43% had intraperitoneal disease, and 50% had positive peritoneal cytologic findings, essentially equal to the findings in patients with outer-half myometrial invasion. In this study, the only significant predictor of extrauterine disease was LVSI. The propensity for extrauterine spread even in the absence of invasion is not an unusual feature in PS tumors. Chan evaluated 100 patients with PS tumors and identified 12 without myometrial invasion who had complete staging. Of these patients, 6 were found to have extrauterine disease spread. A pooled analysis of several studies (Table 5-21) show that approximately 50% of cases will be upstaged with comprehensive staging. It is not surprising that if patients with PS tumors do not undergo surgical staging, unrecognized disease spread will be a common occurrence, and survival for "early-stage" patients will be poorer.

Some suggest that in appropriately staged patients, outcomes of PS/CC tumors are comparable to patients with high-risk endometrioid tumors. Creasman and colleagues using the FIGO Annual Report database compared patients with surgically staged I PS and CC carcinomas to those with endometrioid G3 cancers. Of

3996 surgically stage I cancers, there were 148 PS, 59 CC (5% of all stage I), and 325 G3 (8%) cancers. These were more IA cancers (no myometrial invasion) with PS and CC than G3. Five-year survival for PS and CC was 72% and 81% respectively, compared to 76% for G3 lesions. Postoperative radiation therapy improved survival somewhat (6% to 8%), but the difference was not significant. The role of chemotherapy was not defined in this study because few patients had this treatment. Huh reported on 60 patients with comprehensively staged stage I PS cases and showed that 5-year OS for patients treated by surgery alone was 66%, and it was 59% by radiation alone. Of interest, there was no recurrences in a small group (n = 7) treated with chemotherapy. Nickels Fader evaluated data from a pooled multi-institutional dataset of 206 surgically staged, stage I-II PS patients. A variety of postoperative therapies were used, including observation following surgery, chemotherapy, radiation, and combinations of chemotherapy and radiation. Of all patients 21% recurred, including 11% of patients with no myometrial invasion.

The peritoneal cavity and distant sites (lung, liver) are common sites of failure in PS tumors. In an effort to improve peritoneal coverage whole abdominal radiation (WAR) has been studied extensively in this disease. In a small phase II study of WAR, Sutton reported 5-year PFS of only 38% in stage I-II disease. In GOG 122 (WAR vs chemotherapy), chemotherapy was superior for all patients, including the subset with PS/CC tumors. Given the histologic similarity and propensity for intraperitoneal disease spread like ovarian cancer, several investigators have advocated use of systemic chemotherapies active in ovarian cancer for PS tumors. Levenback and colleagues from MD Anderson treated 20 patients with UPSC using cisplatin, doxorubicin, and cyclophosphamide. This included patients with measurable disease (advanced and recurrent disease) and adjuvant therapy. Only 2 of 11 patients with measurable disease had an objective response. The 5-year survival for all patients was 23%. Paclitaxel and carboplatin have been increasingly used, and several series suggest improvements in outcomes with this regimen. For example, Huh demonstrated no recurrences in 12 patients with stage I disease treated with platinum-based therapy, and Kelly showed that 0 of 15 patients had a recurrence with IB PS tumors treated with platinum chemotherapy compared to 10 of 13 who did not receive chemotherapy. In a review of the GOG phase III experience of advanced/recurrent endometrial cancers, there was no difference noted in response rate to chemotherapy based on histologic type (endometrioid vs PS/CC).

The optimal therapy for PS/CC tumors remains to be determined. Chemotherapy alone or in combination with radiation is being investigated. Given unique molecular findings in PS and CC tumors, it is also hoped that targeted therapies may offer a unique option in this disease.

Follow-Up

Following surgery, with or without adjuvant therapy, patients with endometrial cancer should enter a routine surveillance program. We advocate for patients to be seen every 3 to 4 months for the first 2 years, then yearly. Most recurrences manifest within 2 years, making closer surveillance during this time reasonable. Surveillance visits should include a focused review of systems (questions related to pelvic, leg, or back pain; vaginal bleeding urinary changes; changes in bowel habits) and physical examination including pelvic examination. Routine Pap smear collection of the vaginal cuff is controversial. We tend to perform Pap smears as a sampling of the vaginal cuff in an effort to afford early detection of vaginal cuff recurrences. Some have suggested that routine Pap smears are not cost-effective and that most recurrences are clinically palpable or associated with patient symptoms. In addition, following radiation (vaginal or pelvic) vaginal cuff recurrences are uncommon, and radiation may produce cytologic changes occasionally difficult to classify. Most low- and intermediate-risk patients do not require routine, scheduled imaging studies to evaluate for recurrence. Patients with new complaints or worsening of abdominal/pelvic complaints may be considered for additional studies (CT scans, colonoscopy). It has been suggested by some that CA-125 can be used to monitor therapy in patients with advanced or recurrent adenocarcinoma of the endometrium, much as is done in ovarian cancer. Niloff and colleagues and others have noted that CA-125 is elevated in as many as three-fourths of these patients. Data are limited in regard to monitoring. Fanning and Piver did note in 21 women that clinical response, in addition to subsequent relapse, correlated with CA-125 levels of patients with advanced or recurrent disease. Monitoring with CA-125 is helpful, primarily in patients with high risk for recurrent disease, as in patients with recurrent disease receiving therapy who have a proven elevation of their serum value.

Even though the most patients with endometrial carcinoma do not experience recurrence or die of disease, the number of endometrial cancer deaths has risen over the past several years. Patients identified with recurrence are assessed for treatment options. Long-term disease control of recurrent disease is a function of site of recurrence. Patients with recurrence at a distant site or with multiple sites of recurrence are best treated with hormonal or chemotherapy, as discussed earlier in a palliative setting. Isolated vaginal cuff recurrences may occur, particularly in cases where postoperative radiation was not used. Provided no other disease spread is noted, 60% to 80% of patients with vaginal cuff recurrences can achieve long-term disease control with the use of surgery and/or radiation therapy. Patients with pelvic side wall or isolated para-aortic recurrences may have long-term disease control, but overall prognosis is poorer than with vaginal recurrence. Rarely, patients with vaginal/pelvic recurrence after radiation therapy may be offered pelvic exenteration with the hopes of cure.

For full reference list, log onto www.expertconsult.com ⟨http://www.expertconsult.com⟩.

Sarcoma of the Uterus

D. Scott McMeekin, MD

CLASSIFICATION

Sarcomas are uncommon tumors arising from mesenchymal elements and are distinguished from carcinomas that arise from epithelial elements. Uterine sarcomas are thought to arise primarily from two tissues: endometrial stroma and the uterine muscle itself. When endometrial mesenchymal tissue undergoes malignant transformation, it may be accompanied by a malignant epithelial component (carcinosarcoma, formerly referred to as malignant mixed müllerian tumor), it may be associated with a benign-appearing epithelial component (adeno-sarcoma), or it may have no recognizable epithelial component (endometrial stromal sarcoma). Tumors arising from malignant transformation of uterine smooth muscle are known as uterine leiomyosarcomas. Other sarcomas, such as angiosarcoma and fibrosarcoma, arise in supporting tissues and are rare.

Several classification schemas have been advanced over time for uterine sarcomas. The Gynecologic Oncology Group (GOG) has developed a histologic classification that reflects current trends (Table 6-1). The classification of tumors known as mixed müllerian sarcomas or malignant mixed müllerian tumors (MMMTs)

has undergone considerable evolution. These tumors must contain malignant epithelial (carcinoma) and mesenchymal (sarcoma) elements. Kempson and Hendrickson note that the carcinoma is usually endometrioid in type, but mucinous, squamous, papillary serous, and clear cell histologies alone or in mixtures are noted. When the malignant sarcomata's component has features that are unique to uterine tissue (spindle cell sarcoma, stromal sarcoma, leiomyosarcoma, fibrosarcoma), the tumors are called homologous types. When the stromal component produces tissue not normally found in the uterus, such as bone, cartilage, or skeletal muscle (osteosarcoma, chondrosarcoma, rhabdomyosarcoma), the tumors are designated as heterologous. There has been controversy as to the clinical importance of the presence of homologous versus heterologous elements in the sarcomatous component of these tumors.

Currently, most authorities make no distinction in terms of behavior or prognosis based on this factor, and MMMT tumors have been reclassified by most authorities under the heading of carcinosarcoma. As our understanding of these tumors at a cellular level has increased, there is now evidence that challenges whether cases of carcinosarcoma are actually sarcomas or if they represent an extreme manifestation of undifferentiated

TABLE 6-1   Gynecologic Oncology Group Classification
of Uterine Sarcomas

I. Nonepithelial neoplasms
   A. Endometrial stromal tumors
      1. Stromal nodule
      2. Low-grade stromal sarcoma
      3. High-grade stromal sarcoma
   B. Smooth muscle tumor of uncertain malignant potential
   C. Leiomyosarcoma
      1. Epithelioid
      2. Myxoid
   D. Mixed endometrial stromal and smooth muscle tumor
   E. Poorly differentiated (undifferentiated) endometrial sarcoma
   F. Other soft tissue tumors
      1. Homologous
      2. Heterologous
II. Mixed epithelial-nonepithelial tumors
   A. Adenosarcoma
      1. Homologous
      2. Heterologous
      3. With high-grade stromal overgrowth (see notes)
   B. Carcinosarcoma (malignant mixed mesodermal tumor or
      malignant mixed müllerian tumor)
      1. Homologous
      2. Heterologous

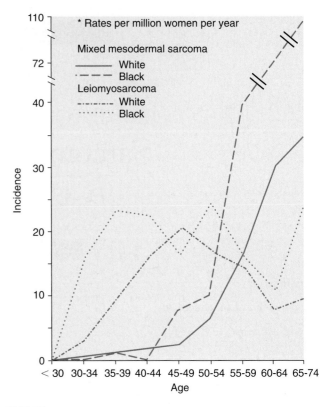

FIGURE 6-1   Incidence of uterine sarcoma among females by age, race, and histology: Surveillance, epidemiology, and end results (SEER) areas, 1973-1981. *(From Harlow BL, Weiss NS, Lofton S: J Natl Cancer Inst 76:399, 1986.)*

endometrial cancers. Clinical evidence to support classification of these tumors as "endometrial cancers" include tumor spread patterns similar to endometrial cancer, patterns of failure comparable (albeit at different frequency) to endometrial cancer, and the fact that carcinosarcoma metastases are usually with a carcinoma component and this component reflects biologic behavior. In addition, pathologically, monoclonal origin of tumor is suggested by the findings that p53 expression is concordant and X chromosome inactivation patterns are identical between carcinoma and sarcoma components. Debate has centered on the differences in outcomes between endometrial cancers and uterine carcinosarcoma, and research organizations continue to separate carcinosarcomas from endometrial cancers in clinical trials.

INCIDENCE AND EPIDEMIOLOGY

Sarcomas arising within the uterus are relatively rare and account for 3% to 8% of uterine cancers. According to the Surveillance, Epidemiology, and End Results (SEER) data reported by Brooks and colleagues covering 2677 cases from 1989 to 1999, the age-adjusted incidence for all sarcomas (per 100,000 women age 35 and older) in U.S. women was 2.68 for Native American/Asian/Hispanic, 3.58 for white, and 7.02 for black women. By comparison, the incidence for epithelial uterine cancers, per 100,000 women, is roughly 9 for black women and

20 for white women. Uterine sarcomas represented 8% of primary uterine malignancies in the most recent analysis of the SEER database. Harlow and co-workers had previously reported from SEER databases covering 1973-1981 that suggested an annual incidence of only 1.7 cases per 100,000 women. Sarcomas have been traditionally thought to represent only 3% to 5% of all uterine tumors. The increasing incidence of uterine sarcomas noted in the SEER studies may reflect better diagnosis and perhaps a true increase in an aging population. Of the sarcomas, the most common, in order of decreasing incidence, are carcinosarcoma, leiomyosarcoma, endometrial stromal sarcoma, and adenosarcoma. Of the 1452 uterine sarcomas in Harlow's study, 86% were classified as carcinosarcoma (MMMT) or leimyosarcoma. Sherman reporting on SEER data from 1992 to 1998 found that 53% of all sarcomas were carcinosarcomas.

The type and frequency of uterine sarcomas are related to both age and race. As Figure 6-1 demonstrates, carcinosarcoma is unusual before 40 years of age and begins to increase steadily thereafter. Leiomyosarcoma can occur at an early age, has an incidence plateau in middle age, and declines thereafter. In a large prospective surgical-pathologic study conducted by the GOG evaluating patients with all types of sarcomas, the median age of patients with leiomyosarcoma was 55 compared to 65 for those with carcinosarcoma. Brooks suggested that white women were older at the time of diagnosis of their sarcomas compared to black women.

Using SEER data (1992-1998), Sherman and colleagues reported on racial differences in uterine malignancies. They found that for all histopathologic categories the age-adjusted incidence of uterine cancers (per 100,000 women) was 23 for non-Hispanic white, 14 for white Hispanic, and 15 for black women. In contrast, carcinosarcomas and leiomyosarcomas are more common in black women. For carcinosarcomas, the incidence was 0.78, 0.63, and 1.82 for non-Hispanic white, white Hispanic, and black women, respectively. Similarly, for leiomyosarcomas, endometrial stromal sarcomas, and adenosarcomas combined, the incidence was 1.24 for black versus 0.79 for non-Hispanic white women. Harlow found the same trend reporting on an earlier SEER data set. It has also been suggested that blacks present with stage I disease less commonly than whites.

Given that uterine sarcomas are rare and form a heterogeneous group, little is known about other risk factors favoring development of these tumors. For carcinosarcomas, there is some evidence that exposure to radiation may increase risk. A history of pelvic irradiation is noted in 5% to 10% of patients with sarcoma. Sarcomas have been reported to develop from 1 to 37 years from radiation exposure. Meredith and colleagues reported on 1208 women with uterine malignancies and identified 30 who had a history of prior pelvic irradiation. The authors estimated that frequency of carcinosarcomas after radiation (17%) exceeded the 5% baseline rate expected. Postradiation sarcomas are predominantly carcinosarcomas.

Given the molecular evidence that carcinosarcomas are biologically related to epithelial endometrial cancers, some investigators have attempted to determine whether the two tumor types share similar risk factors. Zelmanowicz and co-workers performed a multicenter case-control study comparing risk factors associated with women diagnosed with endometrial carcinomas and those with carcinosarcomas. They found that the two tumor types share similar risk factors related to estrogen exposure (obesity, exogenous estrogen exposure, nulliparity) and suggested that the pathogenesis was similar between the two tumors. Larger studies will need to be performed to confirm these findings. Tamoxifen exposure has also been suggested to increase the risk of endometrial cancer, including carcinosarcoma. For women with leiomyosarcoma, a preoperative diagnosis of uterine leiomyoma is common. However, it has not been established that leiomyosarcoma arises in benign leiomyomas; in nearly all cases the sarcoma arises independently of the benign neoplasm.

CARCINOSARCOMA

Clinical Profile

Most patients with uterine carcinosarcoma present with postmenopausal bleeding. As in other cases of postmenopausal bleeding, histologic evaluation by endometrial biopsy or curettage is mandatory and will establish the diagnosis. Not infrequently, a large polypoid mass may extend from the endometrial cavity protruding through the cervical os, which can be easily biopsied (Figure 6-2). Carcinosarcomas have both malignant epithelial and mesenchymal elements, but on small biopsies, the epithelial component may be the only one recognized preoperatively (Figures 6-3 and 6-4). Some patients may present without bleeding but with an enlarging pelvic mass as a result of tumor and hematometrium. Patients with advanced-stage disease may present similarly to patients with ovarian cancer with pleural effusions, ascites, adnexal masses, and evidence of intraperitoneal disease spread.

Preoperative assessment with imaging studies is controversial. At a minimum, a chest radiograph is recommended given the potential for distant disease spread. For common endometrial cancers, routine preoperative computed tomography (CT) scans have not been shown to alter clinical management, but data are limited for patients with carcinosarcoma. Consultation with a gynecologic oncologist should strongly be considered in cases with a preoperative diagnosis of carcinosarcoma.

Surgical Management

The surgical management for patients with uterine carcinosarcoma should include collection of cytologic washings, hysterectomy with bilateral salpingo-oophorectomy, and pelvic and para-aortic lymph node dissection. Patients with carcinosarcoma of the uterus should be staged according to the 2009 FIGO staging system for endometrial cancer. Extrauterine disease spread in carcinosarcoma is not uncommon. In one analysis of the SEER data from 1988 to 2004, 40% of cases were classified as having stage III-IV disease. In cases where gross extrauterine disease is encountered, many advocate a debulking surgery akin to what is used to manage ovarian cancer.

The GOG prospectively evaluated disease distribution in 530 patients with clinical stage I-II uterine sarcomas. All patients underwent collection of pelvic washings, hysterectomy, and pelvic and para-aortic lymph node dissection. In the subgroup of 301 patients with carcinosarcoma, extrauterine disease was found commonly; 21% were identified with positive cytologic washing, 37% had myometrial invasion into the outer half of the myometrium, 12% had adnexal metastases,

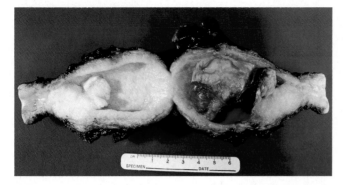

FIGURE 6-2 Uterine carcinosarcoma with polypoid mass filling uterine cavity and with deep myometrial invasion. (*Courtesy Dr. Pablo Souza, University of Oklahoma.*)

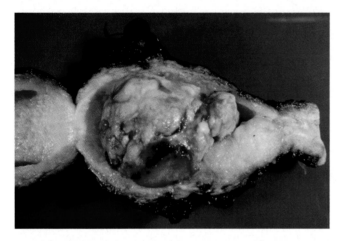

FIGURE 6-3 Close-up view of specimen in Figure 6-2 showing carcinosarcoma with tumor filling the endometrial cavity. (*Courtesy Dr. Pablo Souza, University of Oklahoma.*)

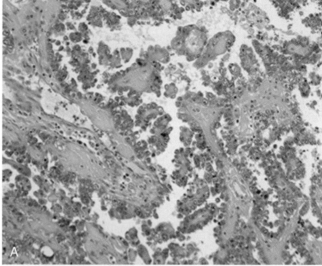

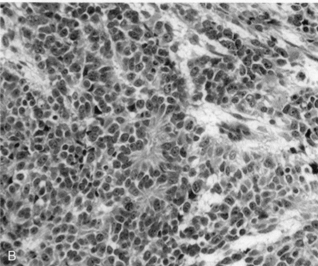

FIGURE 6-4 Photomicrograph of carcinosarcoma of the uterus. Within the tumor are two discrete malignant populations: a high-grade epithelial component (A) and a stromal component (B). (*Courtesy Dr. Pablo Souza, University of Oklahoma.*)

and 17% had nodal involvement. Compared to a similar surgical staging study conducted by the GOG evaluating endometrial cancer patients, positive cytology was found in only 12%, deep myometrial invasion in 22%, adnexal involvement in 5%, and nodal metastases in 9% of cases (Table 6-2). For carcinosarcoma, following surgical staging 59% were stage I, 21% were stage II, 9% were stage III, and 11% were stage IV. In almost every case, when extrauterine metastases are encountered, only the epithelial component of the tumor was present.

Carcinosarcomas frequently carry a poor prognosis. In some cases managed without complete surgical staging, unrecognized disease spread may account for poorer outcomes. For example, in the 1988-2004 SEER database, of 3962 cases of carcinosarcoma, only 53% underwent lymph node dissection. For patients with apparent uterine confined disease, 5-year cancer-specific survival was 59% for stage IA (no myometrial invasion), 54% for stage IB, and 38% for stage IC. Even in series with uniform use of staging recurrences are common, indicating that unrecognized disease spread occurs

frequently. In the GOG series, 53% of all patients with carcinosarcoma and 40% with stage I disease had a recurrence within 3 years of diagnosis. As in endometrial cancer, survival was related to the presence nodal metastases, to the depth of myometrial invasion, and to whether the lower uterine segment or cervix was involved. Patients with adnexal involvement also had a poor prognosis. Ferguson reported a series of 42 patients in stage I who all underwent pelvic nodal dissection and found 3-year disease-free and overall survival were 42% and 62%, respectively, even though nearly all patients received some form of postoperative adjuvant therapy.

Although many believe carcinosarcoma to actually represent a metaplastic high-grade/undifferentiated endometrial cancer (and not a true sarcoma), some data

TABLE 6-2   Frequency and Distribution of Disease Spread in Patients with Uterine Malignancies

	Carcinosarcoma (%) (n = 301)	Leiomyosarcoma (%) (n = 59)	Endometrial Adenocarcinoma (%) (n = 621)
Deep myometrial invasion	37	—	22
Positive peritoneal cytology	21	5	12
Adnexal involvement	12	3	5
Nodal metastases	17	3.5	9

(From Major FJ et al: Cancer 71:1702, 1993; Creasman WT et al: Cancer 60:2035, 1987.)

indicate a different clinical behavior between uterine carcinosarcoma and high-grade (grade III, serous, or clear cell) endometrial cancers. Amant and colleagues compared 104 patients with grade III, papillary serous, or clear cell endometrial cancers to 33 patients with carcinosarcoma. Among patients with stage I-II disease, those patients with carcinosarcoma had a poorer survival rate and a higher incidence of pulmonary metastases. Carcinosarcoma was also an independent predictor of survival with a hazard ratio of 3.2 for recurrence compared to the other histologies. In a population-based comparison between carcinosarcoma and grade III endometrioid cancers, patients with carcinosarcoma had poorer survival compared to endometrioid cancers when compared stage by stage. For example, 5-year survival was 38% versus 68% for patients with stage IC disease. Some have argued that based on the differences in clinical behavior carcinosarcoma should be studied separately from high-risk endometrial cancers.

Patterns of failure following surgery alone or after adjuvant therapies can help to inform how to best direct therapies for patients with cancers. For example, local therapies such as pelvic radiation may reduce local (vaginal/pelvic) failures but have no/minimal effect on the frequency that cancers recur at distant sites (lung, liver, abdominal cavity). In the GOG study, 40% of patients received postoperative pelvic radiation therapy, with 17% of these patients having a recurrence in the pelvis, 16% at an extrapelvic location, and 19% in the lung (Table 6-3). In the 60% of patients who received no radiation, 24% had a pelvic recurrence, 24% had an extrapelvic recurrence, and 10% recurred in the lung. In the GOG trial, therapy was not randomized but was selected by the physician. Pelvic recurrences usually develop within the first 12 to 18 months after diagnosis and surgery. In a series of 23 carcinosarcoma patients with surgically staged, stage I disease who received no postoperative therapy, 11 patients were noted to have recurrence. The median time to recurrence in these patients was 13 months, and patterns of failure showed that 3 patients had an isolated pelvic recurrence, 3 had an isolated distant recurrence, and 5 had both local and distant failures.

TABLE 6-3   Patterns of Failure in Uterine Sarcomas

Site of first failure	Carcinosarcoma (n = 301)		Leiomyosarcoma (n = 59)	
	No Radiation (n = 182)	Radiation (n = 119)	No Radiation (n = 46)	Radiation (n = 13)
Pelvis	24%	17%	17%	0
Extrapelvic	24%	16%	29%	8%
Lung	10%	19%	37%	54%
Other	11%	7%	4%	15%

(Adapted from Major FJ et al: Cancer 71:1702, 1993.)

Adjuvant Therapy

Postoperative radiation therapy or chemotherapy has been used to reduce the risk of recurrence in patients with uterine sarcoma. In older studies, all types of uterine sarcomas were commonly grouped together so that the effect of therapy on a particular histologic type of sarcoma was largely unknown. Historically, radiation therapy has been most commonly used in an effort to reduce pelvic failures. When radiation therapy is given, 4500 to 6000 cGy to the pelvis has been advocated, with some also recommending intravaginal brachytherapy to deliver a boost to the vaginal cuff or entire vagina. Preoperative radiation is infrequently used and typically reserved for cases with bulky cervical involvement or parametrial extension.

Several series have shown improved rates of local control with the use of radiation without necessarily improving survival compared to patients managed without radiation. In a prospective GOG study that included patients with stage I-II uterine sarcomas of all types, 156 patients were randomly assigned to postoperative treatment with doxorubicin or not. Pelvic radiation was permitted at the physician's discretion. In this study, which included 93 patients with carcinosarcoma, 47% of patients' disease recurred with or without the use of pelvic radiation therapy (Table 6-4). Pelvic radiation did appear to reduce local recurrences. Similarly, there was not a statistically significant difference in recurrence

TABLE 6-4 Gynecologic Oncology Group Randomized Trial of Doxorubicin versus No Further Therapy in Completely Resected Stage I and Stage II Uterine Sarcoma: Rates of Recurrence

	Adjuvant Doxorubicin ($n = 75$)		No Chemotherapy ($n = 53$)	
CS ($n = 90$)	39%		51%	
LMS ($n = 52$)	44%		61%	
	Adjuvant Doxorubicin ($n = 75$)		No Chemotherapy ($n = 53$)	
	Radiation ($n = 31$)	No Radiation ($n = 44$)	Radiation ($n = 28$)	No Radiation ($n = 53$)
All sarcoma types ($n = 156$)	39%	43%	57%	51%
	Radiation ± Chemotherapy ($n = 59$)		No Radiation ± Chemotherapy ($n = 97$)	
All sarcoma types ($n = 156$)	47%		47%	

(Modified from Omura GA et al: J Clin Oncol 3:1240, 1985.)
CS, Carcinosarcoma; LMS, leiomyosarcoma.

rates, progression-free survival (PFS), or survival in patients who did or did not receive doxorubicin. More recently, the European Organization for Research and Treatment of Cancer (EORTC) enrolled 224 patients with stage I-II uterine sarcomas (including 91 with carcinosarcoma) and randomly assigned patients to observation versus pelvic radiation therapy following surgery. For the group as a whole, there was no difference in disease-free or overall survival between the two treatment groups. For patients with carcinosarcoma, improved local control was noted with pelvic radiation therapy. The study found that following observation 47% of carcinosarcoma patients developed a local recurrence versus 24% after pelvic radiation. Distant sites of failure remained a significant problem regardless of treatment (35% following radiation, 29% with observation).

Because a common site of failure is at a distant site from the pelvis, the use of adjuvant local irradiation, although improving local control, may ultimately have no effect in increasing the overall survival rate. Systemic therapy using chemotherapy with or without radiation has been evaluated in adjuvant settings. The selection of drugs/regimens likely to be beneficial is based on information from studies performed with patient populations with advanced or recurrent disease. To date, ifosfamide, cisplatin, and paclitaxel have shown the most promise for development for carcinosarcomas. Kanjeekal and colleagues reviewed the literature on the chemotherapy for uterine sarcomas and noted that for carcinosarcoma the most promising regimens would likely include platinum-based combinations. Drawing on experience from patients with advanced and recurrent carcinosarcoma, which found that the combination regimen of ifosfamide and cisplatin produced nearly a doubling in response rate and a modestly prolonged progression-free survival

compared to ifosfamide alone, the GOG initiated a randomized trial comparing three cycles of ifosfamide and cisplatin to whole abdominal radiation therapy (WART). Eligible patients could have had stage I-IV disease provided no residual disease greater than 1 cm remained following surgery. For the group as a whole, stage was one of the most important prognostic factors, with 37% of patients with stage I disease versus 80% with stage IV disease having a recurrence by 5 years. The crude 5-year rate of recurrence was 58% for patients treated by WART versus 52% for chemotherapy. After adjusting for stage and age, the recurrence rate was 29% lower for chemotherapy; however, the results did not achieve statistical significance (relative hazard, 0.789, CI 0.48-1.04, $P = 0.245$). Despite this, the authors concluded the results supported further evaluation of combination chemotherapy in future research trials. A retrospective review by Makker and colleagues of 49 patients with stage I-IV disease treated by radiation alone versus chemotherapy ± radiation suggested that the inclusion of chemotherapy into an adjuvant regimen improved PFS and OS compared to chemotherapy alone.

Management of Recurrent Disease

Not unlike with surgical development, the development of chemotherapy in uterine sarcomas began with studies combining all uterine sarcoma types. This strategy appeared justified because, regardless of tumor type, about half the patients with early-stage uterine sarcoma developed a recurrence. Given its importance in patients with soft tissue sarcomas, doxorubicin has been used extensively in patients with uterine sarcomas. The GOG performed a randomized trial comparing doxorubicin with or without DTIC (dimethyl triazenoimidazole carboxamide) in 226 patients with stage III, stage IV, and recurrent sarcomas of the uterus. There was no difference in response rate, PFS, or survival between doxorubicin and doxorubicin plus DTIC-treated groups. Response rate for leiomyosarcoma was 25% versus 15% for carcinosarcoma, and survival time of patients with leiomyosarcoma was significantly longer than that of patients with other cell types. This study was important because it suggested that there was a difference between sarcomas types and response to different agents. With the recognition that there are differences in prognosis and response between the histologic types, carcinosarcoma and leiomyosarcoma are now studied in separate chemotherapy trials.

The first GOG trial to evaluate carcinosarcomas as a separate group was reported by Thigpen. This phase II study evaluated cisplatin in 28 patients with advanced or recurrent disease who had received prior chemotherapy and had measurable disease. The response rate was 18%, with two patients obtaining a complete response. A subsequent phase II study used cisplatin in a similar group of 63 patients who had not received prior chemotherapy and noted a response rate of 19% (8% complete response).

As a result of activity seen in soft tissue sarcomas, ifosfamide was selected for evaluation in uterine sarcomas. Using ifosfamide with the uroprotective agent mesna (2-mercaptoethane sodium sulfate), Sutton reported for the GOG on 28 patients with advanced or recurrent carcinosarcoma who had not received prior chemotherapy. He described a 32% response rate, including 18% of patients with a complete response. Given these promising results, interest in studying combination regimens in this disease resurfaced. The GOG evaluated ifosfamide and mesna with and without cisplatin in patients with advanced, persistent, or recurrent carcinosarcomas in a phase III study. The study evaluated 194 patients and found that response rate for ifosfamide alone was 36% compared to 54% for the combination. Patients treated with cisplatin had a modest improvement in median PFS (6 months vs 4 months), but there was no statistically significant improvement in survival (ifosphamide, 9 months vs ifosphamide plus cisplatin, 10 months, median survival). The combination regimen produced greater incidences of neutropenia, anemia, and peripheral neuropathy.

Paclitaxel has been evaluated in 44 patients with advanced or recurrent disease who all had received one prior chemotherapy regimen. Curtin for the GOG reported an 18% response rate with acceptable toxicity. The GOG has subsequently conducted a phase III trial comparing ifosfamide with and without paclitaxel. This trial enrolled 179 eligible patients with stage III, IV, or recurrent carcinosarcoma who had not received prior chemotherapy. The combination regimen produced

higher response rates (45% vs 29%), longer PFS (median, 5.8 months vs 3.6 months), and longer survival (median, 13.5 months vs 8.4 months). There was a 31% decrease in the hazard ratio of death ([HR] 0.69, 95% CI 0.49-0.97, $P = 0.03$). The combination regimen produced more neuropathy and thrombocytopenia and required 3 days for infusion. Because there is interest in improving convenience and cost and reducing toxicity, other regimens have been evaluated in patients with carcinosarcoma. Powell reported on a phase II study evaluating the combination of paclitaxel with carboplatin in 46 patients with advanced or recurrent carcinosarcoma. The response rate was 54% (13% complete response), and 59% of patients completed six or more cycles of therapy. The GOG is currently conducting a phase III trial comparing ifosfamide/paclitaxel to paclitaxel/carboplatin in untreated patients.

LEIOMYOSARCOMA

Clinical Profile

As opposed to patients with carcinosarcoma who present with postmenopausal bleeding, patients with leiomyosarcoma have a median age of diagnosis of only 55 years. Many of these patients experience perimenopausal bleeding, are found to have a pelvic mass on examination, and will be thought to have uterine leiomyomas. Giuntoli, reporting on the Mayo Clinic experience of 208 patients with uterine leiomyosarcoma collected over a 23-year period, found that vaginal bleeding was the most common symptom (56%), followed by a palpable pelvic mass (54%) and pelvic pain (22%). A commonly described "clinical pearl" has been the relationship of a rapidly enlarging uterus to leiomyosarcoma. The data to support such an observation are mixed, however. Parker evaluated 1332 patients who underwent surgery for presumed leiomyoma. In the group of 371 patients who had rapid uterine growth, only one case (0.2%) of leiomyosarcoma was identified. Similarly, in a subgroup of 198 patients who had carefully documented rapid uterine growth, no cases of leiomyosarcoma or carcinosarcoma were found. Leibsohn reported on 1432 patients undergoing hysterectomy for bleeding related to uterine leiomyomas and identified 7 (0.49%) patients with leiomyosarcoma.

Because leiomyosarcoma arises within the uterine smooth muscle, biopsy of the malignant tissue is difficult and many lesions are found only at final pathology. In Leibsohn's series none of the seven patients with leiomyosarcoma were identified on preoperative biopsy and in only three cases was there an intraoperative suspicion of sarcoma. Various authors have reported that leiomyosarcoma may be present in the submucosa of the uterus in 30% to 50% of patients, but even at that, biopsy diagnosis is not easily accomplished. Schwartz described the tumors to be both broad based and pedunculated and that in 19 of 20 cases the leiomyosarcoma was confined to one mass.

Because of the difficulty in establishing a preoperative diagnosis and the high frequency of uterine leiomyoma in the population, it is not unexpected that several case reports have detailed the finding of leiomyosarcomas in patients who have undergone conservative management of symptomatic leiomyomas by myomectomy, following lupron treatment before myomectomy, and following vascular embolization of presumed leiomyomas. These cases speak to the importance of pretreatment counseling of patients who undergo such therapies.

There is considerable discussion about the histologic criteria necessary for the diagnosis of leiomyosarcoma (Figure 6-5). Leiomyosarcomas must be distinguished from a variety of benign smooth muscle tumors (Table 6-5). The predominant differentiating features between benign and malignant tumors include mitotic activity (as gauged by the number of mitotic figures per 10 high power fields [hpf]), cellular atypia, and necrosis. Leiomyoma, cellular leiomyoma, and bizarre leiomyoma (also called atypical or symblastic leiomyoma) are considered to be benign. These entities are distinguished from leiomyosarcoma mainly by the mitotic count of the tumor. Although cellular leiomyomas and bizarre leiomyomas may appear at first sight to be malignant, they contain fewer than 5 mitoses/10 high power fields on histologic evaluation, and the prognosis is excellent with surgery only. Smooth muscle tumors of uncertain malignant potential (STUMP) include a group of smooth muscle tumors with 5 to 9 mitoses/10 hpf that can exhibit a variable behavior.

Intravenous leiomyomatosis is a rare smooth muscle tumor characterized by nodular masses of histologically benign smooth muscle cells growing within venous channels that are lined by epithelium; arteries are not involved. Treatment involves surgical removal, and the prognosis is good. Recurrences are unusual and are usually managed successfully with further surgical excision.

Benign metastasizing leiomyoma is another rare condition in which smooth muscle tumor deposits are found in the lung, lymph nodes, or abdomen and appear histologically like a benign leiomyoma. Most women have a history of pelvic surgery for benign leiomyomas years before these metastatic sites are recognized. Surgical excision has been the primary treatment.

Taylor and Norris believed that mitotic count was extremely important in that if fewer than 10 mitoses/10 hpf were identified, the lesion was benign regardless of the degree of cellular atypia; if more than 10 mitoses/10 hpf were present, the prognosis was grave. More recently, Norris stated that tumors with fewer than 5 mitoses/10 hpf can rarely metastasize. In a follow-up study from the Armed Forces Institute of Pathology, O'Connor and Norris evaluated 73 smooth muscle tumors of the uterus with 5 to 9 mitotic figures/10 hpf but lacking cytologic atypia. They concluded that the metastatic rate was too low to consider these as being sarcoma. Several of their patients were treated only with myomectomies with excellent results. Lissoni and colleagues have suggested extending this philosophy to additional patients.

Kempson and Bari believe that the mitotic count is important but state that prognosis is poor if more than 5 mitoses/10 hpf are identified. Their experience with tumors containing 5 to 9 mitoses/10 hpf indicates that the tumors usually behave aggressively and will metastasize. These authors believe that the degree of cellular atypia is of limited value by itself in determining the malignancy of smooth muscle tumors. In tumors with higher mitotic counts, there were usually a greater

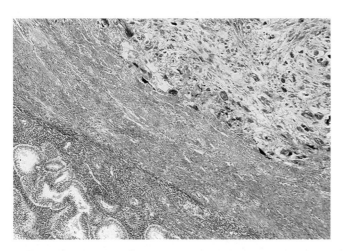

FIGURE 6-5 Photomicrograph of uterine leiomyosarcoma demonstrating the malignant lesion at the top right, normal endometrium at the bottom left, and normal myometrium between them.

TABLE 6-5 Metastatic Potential of Smooth Muscle Tumors of the Uterus

Mitotic Figures/10 hpf	Atypia*	Diagnosis	Metastatic Potential
1-4	Any degree	Leiomyoma	Very low
5-9	None	Leiomyoma with high mitotic activity	Very low
5-9	Grade 1	Smooth muscle tumor of uncertain malignant potential	Low
5-9	Grade 2 or 3	Leiomyosarcoma	Moderate
≥10	Grade 1	Leiomyosarcoma	High
≥10	Grade 2 or 3	Leiomyosarcoma	Very high

(From O'Connor DM, Norris HJ: Hum Pathol 21:223, 1990.)
*Grade based on a scale of 3.

number of very atypical cells. This atypia was also seen in tumors with 5 to 9 mitoses/10 hpf. Tumors with fewer than 5 mitoses/10 hpf were thought to be benign regardless of the atypia of the cells. None of Kempson and Bari's patients with fewer than 5 mitoses/10 hpf had disease outside the uterus, whereas distant disease was a common finding if more than 5 mitoses/10 hpf were noted. The presence of coagulative necrosis, especially with diffuse significant atypia, suggests strongly that the lesion is a leiomyosarcoma regardless of the mitotic count.

However, Silverberg believes that the mitotic count alone cannot be used as a strict histologic criterion because he had patients with fewer than 10 mitoses/10 hpf who succumbed to their disease. He emphasized that the grade of the tumor, which reflects the cytologic atypia, is a better criterion than mitotic count alone. Toledo and Oliva point out that mitotic rate alone is not sufficient to predict prognosis. Although mitotic rate and nuclear atypia are important features, tumor cell necrosis is a unique feature of leiomyosarcoma. Most uterine leiomyosarcoma with necrosis will also show high mitotic rate and atypia. Essentially all investigators note the gravity of the situation if intravascular invasion or disease outside the uterus is found. Silverberg believes that the single most important prognostic indicator is the menopausal status of the patient. Women who are premenopausal when the diagnosis is made tend to have a much better prognosis than that of women who are postmenopausal, even when criteria such as blood vessel invasion, growth pattern, grade, and mitotic counts are considered. Leiomyosarcomas occur in young patients and tend to be more localized when they are first diagnosed, and they probably exhibit a slower growth pattern than carcinosarcomas or endometrial stromal sarcomas do.

Surgical Management

Planning the surgical management of leiomyosarcoma is difficult because many cases go unrecognized preoperatively. Patients commonly undergo myomectomy or hysterectomy for presumptive leiomyomas, which are subsequently identified as a sarcoma. In cases where a preoperative diagnosis is known, hysterectomy should be performed. Retention of the ovaries in premenopausal patients has not shown to worsen outcome in several retrospective series and may be considered. Surgical staging with lymph node dissection is controversial, but most authorities tend to recommend biopsy of suspicious nodes only. In cases where leiomyosarcoma is recognized postoperatively, re-exploration for the purposes of completing surgical staging is not recommended. Following diagnosis, evaluation of the chest with chest radiograph or CT scan is reasonable given the propensity of spread to the lungs. Goff found that 10% of

TABLE 6-6 Figo 2009 Staging Classification for Uterine Sarcomas

Stage I (tumor limited to uterus)
IA: <5 cm tumor size
IB: ≧5 cm tumor size

For Leiomyosarcoma
IA: tumor limited to endometrium/endocervix without myometrial invasion
IB: tumor invades <50% myometrium
IC: tumor invades ≧50% myometrium

For Endometrial Stromal Sarcoma and Adenosarcoma
Stage II (tumor extension into the pelvis)
   IIA: adnexal involvement
   IIB: other extrauterine pelvic disease
Stage III (tumor invades abdominal tissues)
   IIIA: one site involvement
   IIIB: >1 site involvement
   IIIC: metastasis to pelvic and/or para-aortic lymph nodes
Stage IV (tumor invades bladder and/or rectum, and/or distant metastasis)
   IVA: involvement of bladder and/or rectum
   IVB: distant metastasis

Note: For stage I disease, two substages are used based on tumor type (Modified from Mutch DG: Gynecol Oncol 2009;115:325-328 and FIGO staging for uterine sarcomas. Int J Gynecol Obstet 2009;104:179.)

patients with leiomyosarcoma had lung metastases at presentation.

Data on patterns of spread for leiomyosarcoma are limited given the rarity of the tumor. Goff found that 16 of 21 patients had stage I disease at surgery, and only those patients with disseminated intra-abdominal disease had nodal involvement. Giuntoli reported that only 34 of 208 patients in the Mayo Clinic series had pelvic nodal dissections performed, and of the 4 with positive nodes, extrauterine disease was reported in 3. The GOG sarcoma study on patterns of spread found that in 59 surgically staged patients, 5% had positive extrauterine spread to peritoneal cytology, 3% had adnexal involvement, and 3.5% had nodal metastases (see Table 6-2). Following surgical staging 83% were stage I, and only 13% of patients were upstaged based on biopsies. In 2009 FIGO introduced a new staging system for leiomyosarcoma, endometrial stromal sarcoma, and adenosarcoma. For LMS, stage reflects tumor size and extrauterine spread (Table 6-6).

Leiomyosarcomas most commonly spread hematogenously. Corscaden and Singh reported the results of autopsies of 15 patients who died of leiomyosarcoma of the uterus. Of these patients, 100% had intra-abdominal visceral involvement, 80% had lung or pleural metastases, 40% had para-aortic nodal involvement, 33% had renal metastases, and 20% had liver metastases. In the GOG study the most common first site of recurrence was the lung (41%) and only 13% had a pelvic failure (see Table 6-3).

The prognosis for leiomyosarcoma is poor, even for early-stage disease. Vardi found that of the total group of 32 patients, 44% died of disease within the first 3 years after diagnosis. There was a 63.6% 5-year survival in women in whom diagnosis was made while they were premenopausal, compared with a 5.5% 5-year survival in postmenopausal women. The GOG found that only 31% of patients remained disease free at 3 years. Gadducci found that 39% of patients with stage I-II disease had a recurrence, with a median time to recurrence of 18 months. Berchuck reported that only 29% of patients with stage I-II disease remained free of disease, with a median follow-up of 7.5 years. Although almost all deaths and recurrences are during the 4 years after diagnosis, Gallup and co-workers reported a recurrence 25 years after initial therapy. Contrary to an older perception, these data would indicate that leiomyosarcomas have a poorer prognosis than carcinosarcomas.

Predictors of outcome have been assessed by several groups. The GOG found that patients with greater numbers of mitoses were associated with increased risk of recurrence such that 79% of patients with more than 20 mitoses/hpf recurred compared to 61% with 10 to 20 mitoses/hpf. Patients who present with extrauterine disease also have a very poor prognosis. Berchuck found no survivors beyond 2 years in this group of patients. Gadducci assessed 126 patients collected from a multi-institutional study and identified stage, mitotic count, and age as independent prognostic factors predicting recurrence. Giuntoli found that high grade, advanced stage, and having had ovaries removed at surgery were independent predictors of poorer survival.

Adjuvant Therapy

For patients with leiomyosarcoma, no adjuvant therapy has been shown to be effective in prolonging survival. As with other high-risk uterine cancers, leiomyosarcomas have been managed postoperatively by radiation therapy or chemotherapy. Berchuck found that among patients receiving any form of adjuvant therapy, 83% recurred compared to 68% who underwent surgery alone. Given the propensity for hematogenous spread, radiation does not adequately address the high frequency of distant sites of failure (lung, liver, abdominal cavity). Supporters of radiation note that pelvic control may be obtained, which can prevent bulky pelvic recurrences and improve patient comfort and quality of life. The GOG reported that only 3 of 13 patients who received radiation remained without recurrence, but no pelvic failures were seen. Giuntoli performed a subset analysis within his large series of patients, identifying 31 patients who received adjuvant radiation therapy. In a comparison to 31 well-matched patients who did not receive radiation, there was not a statistically significant

difference in survival between the groups, although 5-year survival for those receiving radiation was 60% compared to 40% without radiation therapy. In the only prospective randomized trial, the EORTC showed in the subgroup of 103 patients with leiomyosarcoma, there was no improvement of local control with radiation (local recurrence; 20% after radiation versus 24% after surgery alone). Of note, most patients developed distant sites of failure.

Given the importance of distant failures in this disease, chemotherapy has been used to manage early-stage leiomyosarcomas. As discussed with carcinosarcomas, early chemotherapy trial included patients with all types of uterine sarcomas. In the GOG adjuvant trial evaluating the role of doxorubicin with or without radiation, 61% of patients with leiomyosarcoma treated without doxorubicin compared to 44% who received chemotherapy had a recurrence (see Table 6-4). This study was too small to specifically evaluate the importance that histology played in response to therapy. With the identification of an active combination regimen of docetaxel plus gemcitabine for patients with advanced/recurrent disease, early data suggest this regimen may hold promise in an adjuvant setting. In one series of 18 patients with stage I-II LMS, 59% remain progression free at 3 years.

Management of Recurrent Disease

Data from randomized phase III trials conducted by the GOG, which included advanced and recurrent uterine sarcomas of all types, helped to identify the differential sensitivity of leiomyosarcomas compared to carcinosarcomas to different agents. In the trial comparing doxorubicin with and without DTIC, leiomyosarcomas were found to have a longer survival compared to other types when treated with a doxorubicin-containing regimen. In a subsequent study using doxorubicin with or without cyclophosphamide, histologic type was not found to be a prognostic indicator, however. Given that 80% of all patients died of disease within 2 years, the GOG adopted a strategy of performing phase II trials with the hope of identifying active agents that could later be tested in randomized studies. The rarity of leiomyosarcomas, however, has made randomized study of this tumor more difficult.

Historically, doxorubicin and ifosfamide have demonstrated the most activity in patients with recurrent disease with responses ranging from 25% to 33% for doxorubicin and 18% for ifosphamide when used as single agents. Sutton and the GOG published the results of a phase II study combining ifosfamide and mesna and doxorubicin, showing an overall response rate of 30%. The duration response was 4 months, and the regimen produced substantial toxicity. Paclitaxel has been studied in leiomyosarcomas, with an 8% response seen in patients who had received prior chemotherapy and a 9% response in those who were chemotherapy naïve. A novel combination of gemcitabine with docetaxel has shown a 53% response rate in a small phase II trial of patients that included 29 patients with uterine leiomyosarcoma. This regimen was subsequently evaluated in two phase II trials. In one trial of 39 patients with advanced/recurrent leiomyosarcoma who had received no prior chemotherapy, the regimen produced a 36% response rate and a median PFS of 4.4 mos. In a similar population of 48 patients who had received one prior chemotherapy regimen, a 27% response rate was noted. In both studies, myelosuppression was the most common toxicity. Targeted biologic agents are also being explored, although no agent has yet to demonstrate activity in this tumor type. A randomized trial comparing the docetaxel plus gemcitabine regimen with or without the antivascular endothelial growth factor antibody bevacizumab is currently ongoing. Patients with late recurrences of leiomyosarcoma in the form of isolated pulmonary metastases are candidates for thoracotomy and sequential resection of the lesions. Five-year survival of 30% to 50% has been reported after such therapy.

ENDOMETRIAL STROMAL SARCOMA

Clinical Profile

Endometrial stromal tumors are rare mesenchymal tumors composed of cells that resemble endometrial stromal cells of the proliferative endometrium. The most common symptom of endometrial stromal sarcoma (ESS) is irregular vaginal bleeding. Asymptomatic uterine enlargement, pelvic pain, or palpable mass are also common symptoms. The tumors are generally soft, fleshy, smooth, polypoid masses that may protrude into the endometrial cavity. The multiple-polyp form of the neoplasm has also been described, as has the characteristic yellow color of many of these lesions. On occasion, the uterine wall is diffusely enlarged by tumor without the presence of an obvious tumor mass. Preoperative diagnosis remains challenging because endometrial biopsy may not identify the lesion in many cases.

In the past endometrial stromal tumors were largely grouped as either endolymphatic stromal myosis or endometrial stromal sarcoma. Endolymphatic stromal myosis was distinguished from stromal sarcomas by the minimal extent of tumor infiltration into the myometrium, the lack of metastases, and an indolent clinical behavior. There was significant histologic overlap between the two entities that made diagnosis difficult, however. Currently, endometrial stromal tumors are classified into two groups based on their metastatic potential. Stromal nodules are benign proliferations with the appearance indistinguishable from endometrial stroma of proliferative endometrium. They tend to be well-circumscribed lesions less than 15 cm and do not demonstrate infiltrating margins or vascular space invasion. They behave like benign lesions without reported recurrences or metastases. Stromal sarcomas represent the second type of stromal neoplasm. Stromal sarcomas demonstrate local invasiveness or vascular and lymphatic space involvement, and infiltrate and separate the muscle fibers of the uterus. Stromal sarcomas have traditionally been divided into low- and high-grade endometrial stromal sarcomas, largely based on the mitotic activity. Today there is a greater recognition that most high-grade tumors should be classified as undifferentiated endometrial sarcomas.

Low-grade endometrial stromal sarcoma (LGESS), previously described as endolymphatic stromal myosis, can have an infiltrating growth pattern that on gross examination can project out in a wormlike fashion into the myometrium or into pelvic blood vessels. On microscopic examination, there is little or no cellular atypia, and there are few if any mitoses (Figures 6-6 and 6-7). Although metastasis can occur, the clinical course is usually indolent, and surgery only is usually adequate treatment. Low-grade sarcomas may recur, but their clinical course is marked by late recurrences, typically greater than 5 years from diagnosis, with recurrences up to 25 years having been reported. In a review of 72 cases of low-grade ESS, 88% of patients remained alive at 80 months.

High-grade ESS traditionally has been distinguished from low-grade ESS by having 10 or greater mitoses per 10 hpf based on work by Norris and Taylor. From a review of 17 stromal sarcomas, Kempson and Bari noted that 10 tumors contained more than 20 mitoses/10 hpf, and 9 of 10 patients died of disease. Seven patients had

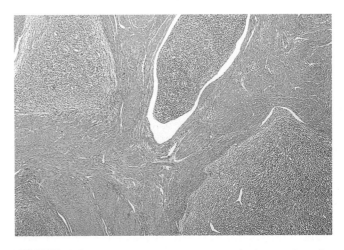

FIGURE 6-6 Low-power photomicrograph of a low-grade endometrial stromal sarcoma with invasion into myometrium.

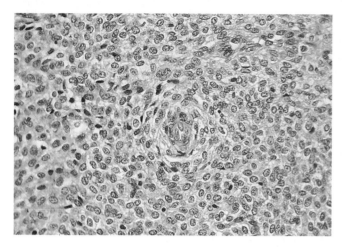

FIGURE 6-7   High power view of low-grade endometrial stromal sarcoma shown in Figure 6-6.

tumors that contained 5 mitoses or fewer/10 hpf, and none have developed a recurrence. Kempson and colleagues subsequently reviewed 109 cases of endometrial stromal sarcoma and found that stage was the predominant predictor of behavior, even more so than the number of mitoses. For example, disease in 45% of stage I patients with rare mitosis and minimal atypia recurred. In this series, as long as the stromal cells appeared bland (similar to normal proliferative endometrial stromal cells), the 10 mitoses/10 hpf cutoff was not predictive of recurrence or survival. Leath and colleagues demonstrated that the clinical behavior of HGESS is frequently aggressive, with more patients presenting with advanced stage (extrauterine disease 61% vs 32%) and poorer survival compared to LGESS. Today there is a belief that many HGESS tumors are in fact undifferentiated endometrial sarcomas. These tumors show myometrial invasion and nuclear pleomorphism and have a high mitotic rate and extensive necrosis but lack smooth muscle or endometrial stromal differentiation.

Surgical Management

The standard management for patients with stromal sarcoma is hysterectomy and bilateral salpingo-oophorectomy. The role of nodal dissections is unresolved, largely because there is a scarcity of data where complete surgical staging has been performed. Goff found no nodal disease, but only seven patients were evaluated. In the GOG surgical staging series, 52 stromal sarcomas were included, but the frequency of nodal disease was not reported. Data suggest that bilateral salpingo-oophorectomy should be performed. Several investigators have suggested that recurrences were higher in patients who had ovaries preserved. In 2009 FIGO introduced a new staging classification for endometrial stromal sarcomas (see Table 6-6).

Patients with LGESS tend to present with disease confined to the uterus, with stage I-II disease being reported in approximately 70% of series. In contrast, patients with HGESS had stage I-II disease in 40% to 50% of cases. In a retrospective review of 52 cases of LGESS by Piver and colleagues, 47% of stage I patients developed recurrence following surgery. Despite this, 5-year survival was 88% for stage I and 100% for stage II patients. Gadducci evaluated 66 patients with stromal sarcomas, including 26 with LGESS and 40 with HGESS. For 20 patients with stage I-II low-grade tumors, 25% recurred (median follow-up 86 months), all in the pelvis. The median time to recurrence was 36 months, with a range of 4 to 108 months. For LGESS, 5-year survivals have ranged from 80% to 100%, despite the fact that 20% to 40% of patients eventually have a recurrence. Piver reported on patterns of failure in stage I patients whose disease recurred, with 12 of 19 recurrences being in the pelvis, 3 of 19 being at distant sites, and 4 of 19 with combined pelvic and distant failures.

The prognosis for HGESS is comparable to carcinosarcoma and leiomyosarcomas. Gadducci reported 5-year disease-free survival of only about 20% for this group of patients. The median time to recurrence is shorter than with LGESS, with a median time of 7 months. Mitotic count was an independent predictor of survival with patients with 10 to 20 mitoses/10 hpf having a 2-year DFS of approximately 60% compared to approximately 10% if there were 20 mitoses or more/10 hpf. Other investigators have suggested 5-year survival between 20% and 55% for HGESS. Recurrences in the pelvis, abdomen, and lung are commonly seen, with the majority including at least some distant site of failure. A study of 24 patients with HGESS from the Mayo Clinic found that prognosis was related to the extent of disease, size of primary tumor, and grade. Mitotic count was not a prognostic factor, nor was DNA pattern.

Adjuvant Therapy

As with other uterine sarcomas, adjuvant therapy has been evaluated to reduce recurrences. Gadducci had no recurrences in five low-grade patients who received adjuvant therapy versus 5 of 15 (33%) who did not. In the Piver study, five low-grade patients received postoperative pelvic radiation, and no recurrences were seen. Piver, noting the sensitivity of advanced or recurrent disease to progestins, suggested that adjuvant progestin therapy may be an effective strategy. In the large multi-institutional series by Leath, 30 of 72 patients received adjuvant hormonal therapy and survival curves suggested a possible benefit associated with its use.

Berchuck reported recurrence rates of 57% with adjuvant chemotherapy or radiation therapy vs 56% who did not receive adjuvant therapy in 25 patients with stage I

ESS (high and low grade). Gadducci noted no benefit to adjuvant therapy in stage I-II high-grade tumors. Given the rarity of ESS, no prospective study has been performed to identify active agents to be used in adjuvant treatment. As with other sarcoma types, radiation therapy may have a role in reducing pelvic recurrences but with an unknown effect on survival.

Management of Recurrent Disease

Although initial studies did allow for patients with ESS, the small numbers of such patients included does not allow for interpretation of results. Low-grade endometrial sarcomas have a high frequency of progestin receptors, making progestational agents reasonable. Piver found that progestins produced a 46% response rate in a small number of patients with LGESS treated at recurrence. Responses lasted from 2 to 104 months. Recurrences of LGESS should be considered for local resection when they develop in the pelvis. For high-grade ESS, limited success has been reported with drugs commonly used for uterine sarcomas including ifosphamide and doxorubicin.

OTHER SARCOMAS

Clement and Scully described 100 cases of adenosarcoma of the uterus. This is an unusual tumor with low malignant potential. Like other endometrial lesions, adenosarcoma usually presents with abnormal vaginal bleeding. On gross evaluation, the tumor is usually a polypoid mass that can fill the endometrial cavity. Involvement of the cervix and myometrium is less commonly seen. In 2009 FIGO introduced a new staging classification for adenosarcomas (see Table 6-6). Histologic evaluation notes benign or atypical neoplastic glands with a sarcomatous stroma. In 78% of patients, the sarcomatous stroma was homologous. Stromal mitotic rate was 1 to 40/10 hpf. Extensive stromal fibrosis was common. Myometrial invasion was present in only 15, and it was deeply invasive in only 4. Recurrence became apparent in 23 patients and in one third appeared 5 years after diagnosis. Recurrence was confined to the vagina, pelvis, or abdomen, with two exceptions. Of those with recurrence, only 11 died with tumor. Only the presence of myometrial invasion was associated with an increased risk of recurrence. A variant of adenocarcinoma is a pattern that has been called adenosarcoma with sarcomatous overgrowth. This is characterized by overgrowth of the neoplasm by a pure sarcomatous component occupying at least 25% of the lesion. It is an ominous feature with reported recurrence rates exceeding 50% compared with the usual adenosarcoma.

Pure heterologous uterine sarcomas are rare. Of these, rhabdomyosarcoma is the most common, followed by chondrosarcoma and osteosarcoma. Rhabdomyosarcoma is derived from primitive myogenic precursors and is the most common soft tissue tumor in children and adolescents; 21% occur in genitourinary sites, and 20% of these in the uterus. Therapy has evolved from radical surgery and radiation therapy to more reliance on chemotherapy. Some authors have reported successful preservation of reproductive functions.

For full reference list, log onto www.expertconsult.com ⟨http://www.expertconsult.com⟩.

Gestational Trophoblastic Disease

Emily M. Ko, MD, and John T. Soper, MD

Gestational trophoblastic disease (GTD) comprises a spectrum of neoplastic conditions derived from the placenta. Hydatidiform moles, gestational choriocarcinoma, and placental site trophoblastic tumor (PSTT) are histologic diagnoses, whereas postmolar gestational trophoblastic neoplasia (GTN) is defined by clinical and laboratory criteria. The disease entities included in GTD have a wide variation in behavior, whereas GTN specifically refers to those with the potential for tissue invasion and metastases.

Gestational trophoblastic disease has been recognized since antiquity. Individual hydropic molar villi (Figure 7-1) were sometimes identified as separate fetuses. In the early nineteenth century Velpeau and Boivin recognized hydatidiform mole as a cystic dilation of the chorionic villi. In 1895 Marchand demonstrated that hydatidiform mole and less frequently normal pregnancy preceded the development of choriocarcinoma. In the early twentieth century Fels and associates identified elevated chorionic gonadotropic hormones in the urine of women with hydatidiform moles.

Before the mid-1950s the prognosis for women with GTN was dismal. In the 1940s Hertz demonstrated that fetal tissues required large amounts of folic acid and could be inhibited by methotrexate, but it was not until 1956 that Li and associates reported the first sustained remission in a patient with choriocarcinoma who was treated with methotrexate.

Since that report, GTN has been recognized as the most curable gynecologic malignancy. Reasons for this include the following: (1) identification and development of quantitative assays for human chorionic gonadotropin (hCG) in serum and urine allowed hCG to become the prototype of tumor markers; (2) sensitivity of GTN to various chemotherapeutic agents; and (3) identification of risk factors allowing individualization

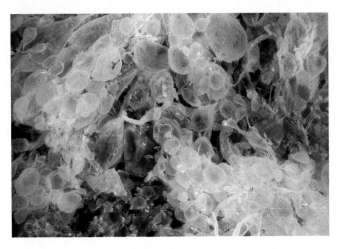

FIGURE 7-1 Complete hydatidiform mole, gross specimen. Note the diffuse hydropic placental villi, which make up almost the entire specimen. *(Courtesy John Soper, MD.)*

TABLE 7-1   Features of Partial and Complete Hydatidiform Moles

Feature	Partial Mole	Complete Mole
KARYOTYPE	**Most Commonly 69, XXX or –,XXY**	**Most Commonly 46, XX or –,XY**
PATHOLOGY		
Fetus	Often present	Absent
Amnion, fetal RBC	Usually present	Absent
Villous edema	Variable, focal	Diffuse
Trophoblastic proliferation	Focal, slight-moderate	Diffuse, slight-severe
CLINICAL PRESENTATION		
Diagnosis	Missed abortion	Molar gestation
Uterine size	Small for dates	50% large for dates
Theca-lutein cysts	Rare	25%-30%
Medical complications	Rare	10%-25%
Postmolar GTN	2.5%-7.5%	6.8%-20%

GTN, Gestational trophoblastic neoplasia; RBC, red blood cells.

of treatment, often using multimodality treatment with chemotherapy combined with surgery and/or radiation therapy in selected cases.

In general, GTD represents a derangement in the development of the conceptus, associated with unregulated trophoblastic proliferation and invasion, with the propensity for hematogenous metastasis in GTN. The diseases are characterized by paraneoplastic disorders from secretion of gestational hormones, most notably hCG. GTD is the only group of female reproductive neoplasms derived from paternal genetic material (androgenic origin).

Although largely unclear, the etiology of GTD likely involves genetic abnormalities involved in fertilization, but it likely also involves abnormalities in differentiation and pronuclear cleavage, decidual implantation, myometrial invasion, and host immunologic tolerance. Several candidate tumor suppressor genes (e.g., DOC-2/hDab2), chromosomal loci (e.g., 7qp12-7q11,23 and 9q13,3-13,4), and oncogenes (e.g., CD9) have been implicated in the pathogenesis of GTD.

HYDATIDIFORM MOLE

Two distinct forms of molar pregnancies, complete (CM) and partial (PM) moles, are currently recognized (Table 7-1). Cytogenetic studies have conclusively demonstrated that they are completely separate but related entities. Despite the cytogenetic, pathologic, and clinical differences outlined in Table 7-1, the clinical management of patients with complete and partial moles is similar.

Epidemiology

The incidence of molar pregnancies in the United States is approximately 1 in 1500 pregnancies. Race or ethnicity, age, socioeconomic status, diet, and prior reproductive history all influence the risk. The most reliable studies suggest that the incidence of hydatidiform mole is slightly less than 1 in 1000 pregnancies in most of the world, 1.2 in 1000 in South Africa, as high as 2 in 1000 in Japan, 7 in 1000 deliveries in Malaysia and the Philippines, and possibly higher in Saudi Arabia. The reported incidence of molar pregnancies among various ethnicities and races may be biased as a result of dependence on hospital records, particularly from tertiary centers, rather than population-based studies. Historically, GTD was thought to occur more frequently in the Asian population; however, recent population-based studies in Japan have shown a decreasing incidence of GTD in Japan, even with a relatively homogeneous population.

Extremes of reproductive age are associated with increased risk of molar pregnancy. Based on an analysis of 2202 patients with hydatidiform moles compared to a contemporary control group including all types of pregnancy events, a Duke study found a significantly higher incidence of molar pregnancy in women younger than 15 years and older than 40 years of age. Other studies have confirmed the peak incidence of molar pregnancies at the extremes of women's reproductive age in the teens and advanced maternal ages. Some of these studies noted an increased risk associated with increasing paternal age for CM but not for PM.

Dietary factors associated with an increased risk of hydatidiform mole may include a low-protein diet and vitamin A deficiency, although these factors are difficult to extrapolate from lower socioeconomic class alone. Berkowitz and co-workers have suggested that a deficiency of animal fat and fat-soluble vitamin carotene is associated with increased risk of molar pregnancies. Areas with high prevalence of vitamin A deficiency have been associated with higher incidences of hydatidiform mole. Although carotene-rich vegetables are available in these countries, the lack of dietary fat needed for carotene absorption may result in an overall carotene-deficient condition.

Prior molar pregnancy also increases the risk of recurrent molar pregnancy. Women with a single previous molar pregnancy have more than 10 times the risk of having another molar pregnancy compared to those who have never had one. Based on data by Bagshawe and colleagues, after having had one molar pregnancy, the risk for a second was 1 in 76; after two molar pregnancies, the risk for a third was 1 in 6.5. Sand reported that the risk of a third mole was 28%. Goldstein and associates noted that 9 of 1339 patients (1 in 150) had at least two consecutive molar pregnancies. Other centers have reported the incidence of a second mole as high as 1 in 50 women with a prior mole.

With recurrent molar pregnancies, there is also an increased risk of developing malignant GTN, although patients with consecutive molar pregnancies may have subsequent normal pregnancies. Berkowitz and associates noted that four of their patients with repeated moles later had full-term pregnancies. Lurain noted that five of eight patients with consecutive moles had normal full-term pregnancies. In a case-controlled study from Baltimore, factors found to be associated with GTN included professional occupation, history of prior spontaneous abortions, and the mean number of months from last pregnancy to the index pregnancy. Contraceptive history, irradiation, ABO blood groups, and smoking factors of the male partner were not relevant. Following partial moles, no clinical factor such as gravidity, parity, age, uterine size, gestational age at diagnosis, or hCG levels at presentation were associated with development of GTN.

Cytogenetics and Pathology

Molar pregnancies consist of complete moles and partial moles. In most series, CM and PM consist of approximately 70% and 30% of molar pregnancies, respectively.

Complete hydatidiform moles are completely derived from the paternal genome (Table 7-1). Most frequently, CMs have a diploid 46, XX genome with exclusively androgenetic markers on the chromosomes, implying duplication of a haploid sperm chromosomal complement in the fertilized ovum. Approximately 5% of CMs have a 46, XY androgenetic genome, however, indicating

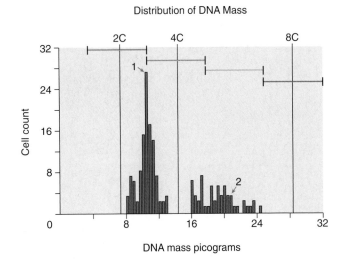

FIGURE 7-2   Flow cytometry of a partial mole. Note the peak at 3C, indicating triploidy. *(Courtesy Dr. Rex Bentley, Duke University Medical Center.)*

that dispermic fertilization occurs in some. The mechanism for exclusion of the maternal polar body from the nucleus of the fertilized ovum is unknown. No 46, YY moles have been reported, but aneuploid karyotypes, such as tetraploidy, have been associated with CM. The fetus fails to develop in CM; fetal red blood cells are not observed in sections of the villi.

In contrast, partial moles are composed of both paternal and maternal genomes (Table 7-1). Usually, two paternal haploid sets of chromosomes are combined with one maternal set, resulting in complete triploidy (Figure 7-2); 69, XXX karyotype is most common, but some PM, have a 69, XXY karyotype, implying dispermic fertilization. Sometimes other aneuploid karyotypes are observed in PM, but none with duplication of the Y chromosome. All karyotypes reported for PM feature a maternal haploid set and multiples of the paternal chromosomal complement. Gross or histologic evidence of fetal development such as fetal red blood cells is a prominent feature of PM.

Histopathology features of CM and PM differ. Complete moles have diffuse villous edema, often with central cisterna formation (Figure 7-3). Trophoblastic proliferation is usually diffuse (Figure 7-4) but may vary in extent. Histologic evidence of a fetus is lacking. Histologic features of PM can be subtle; PMs are probably underdiagnosed in the context of spontaneous abortions. A PM exhibits focal, varying degrees of hydropic villi with scalloping and trophoblastic inclusions within the villi (Figure 7-5). Focal trophoblastic proliferation is usually subtle compared to CM. Fetal red blood cells are observed within vessels of the villi (Figure 7-6) or a fetus can be grossly identified, although the fetus is usually nonviable and rarely survives beyond 20 weeks

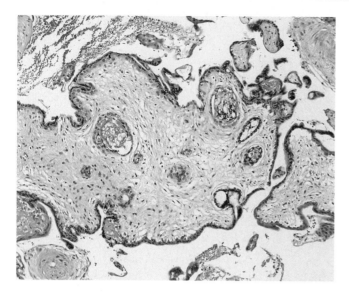

FIGURE 7-3   Low-power photomicrograph of a complete mole illustrating diffuse hydropic change of the villi, which have marked paucity of stroma in the central zone of each villus (cisternae formation). Sheets of trophoblast cell are adjacent to the villi. *(Courtesy Dr. Rex Bentley, Duke University Medical Center.)*

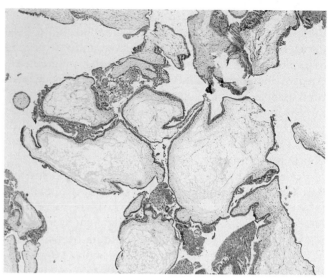

FIGURE 7-5   This low-power photomicrograph of a partial hydatidiform mole contains enlarged placental villi with stromal edema, scalloping at the edge of the villi, and trophoblastic inclusions within the stroma of the villi. Minimal trophoblastic proliferation is present. *(Courtesy Dr. Rex Bentley, Duke University Medical Center.)*

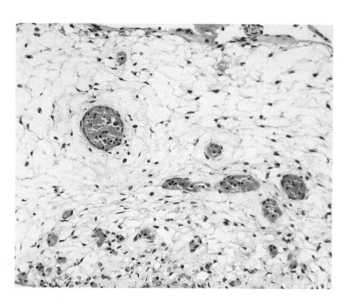

FIGURE 7-4   High-power photomicrograph of a complete mole. The villus *(upper left)* is associated with sheets of trophoblast cells, containing the multinucleated syncytiotrophoblasts and the small, polygonal cytotrophoblast cells. Production of hCG occurs mainly in the syncytiotrophoblast cells. *(Courtesy Dr. Rex Bentley, Duke University Medical Center.)*

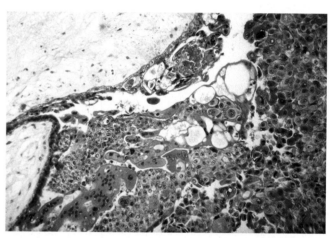

FIGURE 7-6   In this high-power photomicrograph of a villus from a partial mole, small vessels within the stroma are seen containing nucleated fetal red blood cells. *(Courtesy Dr. Rex Bentley, Duke University Medical Center.)*

of gestation. The difference in amount of trophoblastic proliferation between CM and PM is related to their different clinical presentations. Malignant GTN occurs in 2.5% to 7.5% of patients with PM compared to approximately 6.8% to more than 20% after evacuation of a CM mole (see Table 7-1).

Other techniques have been developed to differentiate CM from PM. These include karyotyping and flow cytometry, fluorescence in situ hybridization, and amplification of short tandem repeat loci. Additionally, p57 immunohistochemistry is absent in CM but present in PM because it is paternally imprinted but maternally expressed. Although most cases of mole can be classified as CM or PM using histopathology alone, histologic differences may not be apparent if diagnosis is made early in gestation. Here, these molecular genetic techniques may be critical for accurate diagnosis.

Presentation and Symptoms

Irregular bleeding is the hallmark symptom for hydatidiform moles. Nearly all patients with moles have delayed or irregular menses for varying time periods, with patients considered pregnant. Vaginal bleeding usually occurs during the first trimester. The bleeding may vary from dark-brown spotting to hemorrhage requiring blood transfusion. In earlier series, bleeding occurred in 73% to 100% of molar pregnancies including CM and PM. Expulsion of recognizable molar vesicles may accompany vaginal bleeding when the gestation approaches the second trimester.

There is increasing information that the presentation of moles may be changing as a result of earlier and improved diagnostic tests, including early ultrasound and hCG serum assays. The New England Trophoblastic Disease Center group compared symptoms in CM treated at their institution from 1988 to 1993 to those treated from 1965 to 1976. Vaginal bleeding was still the most common symptom but occurred in 84% compared to 97% in the earlier interval. Even more recently, a cohort of CM was compared to the NETDC cohort from 1988 to 1993; only 52% (56/108) of patients presented with vaginal bleeding compared to 84% in the earlier study. In the later study 38% were entirely asymptomatic and diagnosed by first-trimester ultrasound.

Other symptoms include nausea and vomiting. Nausea and vomiting were reported in almost one-third of patients with hydatidiform mole in older studies, although Curry and co-workers noted only 14% of 347 patients with this symptom. Berkowitz and colleagues found 8% of molar patients to have hyperemesis in their more recent cohort.

Preeclampsia-like symptoms in the first trimester of pregnancy are nearly pathognomonic of a hydatidiform mole. Symptoms of headache with hypertension, hyperreflexia, and proteinuria define preeclampsia. Preeclampsia was present in 28% of patients in the Boston cohort and in 12% of the patients in the study by Curry and colleagues. Fortunately, eclampsia in the setting of hydatidiform mole is rare.

Additionally, other medical comorbidities associated with mole—such as tachycardia and hypertension from hyperthyroidism or shortness of breath and chest pain from acute respiratory distress syndrome—may result. Hyperthyroidism occurs rarely but can be very severe. Laboratory evidence of hyperthyroidism can occur in as many as 10% of patients; however, clinical manifestations occur less frequently. Hyperthyroidism is caused by the production of elevated levels of normal hCG by molar tissue, which acts as a thyrotrophic substance. The hCG molecule binds to the TSH receptor site, resulting in thyroid hyperfunction. Furthermore, Yoshimura and colleagues demonstrated that isoforms of hCG with higher thyrotrophic activity are more frequently produced by trophoblastic tissues in hydatidiform mole compared with normal pregnancies. Clinical manifestations of hyperthyroidism disappear once the molar pregnancy is evacuated. Antithyroid therapy may be indicated for a short period to control hyperthyroidism during molar evacuation.

Acute respiratory distress caused by trophoblastic pulmonary embolization may also be a presenting symptom of GTN. Other factors that may alter cardiac or pulmonary function such as preeclampsia, hyperthyroidism, and anemia are often present and more frequently contribute to acute cardiopulmonary decompensation. Respiratory distress is most often associated with a large volume of molar tissue and uterine enlargement at greater than 16 weeks gestational size.

Theca-lutein cysts of the ovary are caused by hyperstimulation of the ovaries by excessive hCG production. Approximately 15% to 25% of patients with unevacuated moles have theca-lutein cysts larger than 6 cm. Although theca-lutein cysts will resolve after molar evacuation, there may be considerable lag behind the decline of hCG levels. Surgical intervention is rarely required for acute torsion or bleeding. Patients who develop theca-lutein cysts have a higher incidence of postmolar GTN. Furthermore, the combination of enlarged ovaries with a uterus that is large for gestational age results in an extremely high risk for malignant GTN. Up to 57% of patients with this combination require subsequent therapy for postmolar GTN.

Classically, a patient with a hydatidiform mole was said to have a uterine size excessive for gestational age. Historically this was found in more than 50% of patients with CM; however, approximately one-third of patients have uteri smaller than expected for gestational age. In the recent Boston study, uterine size was excessive for dates in only 28%, equal to dates in 58%, and less than dates in 14%.

Similar to the comparative study performed by NETDC, Mangili and colleagues from Italy compared clinical features of molar pregnancies between two historical cohorts, 1970 to 1982 versus 1992 to 2004. The later cohort had significantly less vaginal bleeding on presentation (51% vs 74%, $P < 0.0001$), fewer with increased uterine volume (29% vs 51%, $P < 0.0001$), and fewer with theca-lutein cysts (13% vs 21%, $P = 0.03$). There was no difference in rates of hyperemesis or preeclampsia. Because molar pregnancies are diagnosed at an increasingly early gestational age, clinical symptoms are less frequent. As a result, there is increasing reliance on histopathologic analysis to identify cases of molar pregnancies.

The previously outlined conditions are seen mainly in patients with CM. Patients with PM usually do not exhibit excessive uterine size, theca-lutein cysts, preeclampsia, hyperthyroidism, or respiratory problems. In most patients with PM, the clinical and ultrasound diagnosis is usually a missed or incomplete abortion. Partial moles are often underdiagnosed because of the clinical lack of suspicion and the often subtle or focal nature of the pathologic changes in the placental tissues. Therefore, products of conception from missed or incomplete abortions should be thoroughly examined by pathologists to prevent a missed diagnosis of PM; cytogenetic testing may be required to accurately diagnose GTD.

Diagnosis

The majority of patients with CM are clinically diagnosed by characteristic ultrasound features and markedly elevated hCG. In contrast, the majority of patients with PM and an increasing proportion of patients with CM are clinically diagnosed as missed abortion. A quantitative hCG of greater than 100,000 IU/L, an enlarged uterus with absent fetal heart sounds, and vaginal bleeding suggest a diagnosis of hydatidiform mole. However, a single hCG determination is not diagnostic. A single high hCG value may be seen with a normal single or multiple pregnancy, especially if there has been bleeding or disruption of the placenta. Therefore, an isolated hCG value alone should not be used as the sole determining factor in diagnosing hydatidiform mole. Conversely, a "normal" hCG level for an anticipated gestational age does not exclude the possibility of a molar pregnancy.

Ultrasound has replaced all other radiographic means (e.g., amniography or uterine angiography) for establishing the diagnosis of hydatidiform mole. Molar tissue typically is identified as a diffuse mixed echogenic, vesicular pattern replacing the placenta (Figure 7-7), traditionally labeled a "snowstorm appearance." More recently, with increasing use of ultrasonography earlier in pregnancy, classic features may be subtle or lacking in cases of early CM or PM. In a recent series based on histopathologic identification of molar pregnancies, 52% of patients were diagnosed on ultrasound examination before evacuation of the uterus. In another series, the abundant vesicular pattern that constructed the "snowstorm appearance" was absent in 10% of CM pregnancies and only subtly present in 63% of CM, based on ultrasounds performed at mean gestational age of 7.6 weeks.

The largest study to date, from Charing Cross in the United Kingdom, assessed more than 1000 cases of GTD from 2002 to 2005 and found an overall 44% detection rate by ultrasound of molar pregnancies before evacuation. The overall detection rate was 35% to 40% before 14 weeks of gestation and 60% after. The sensitivity was 44%, specificity 74%, positive predictive value 88%, and

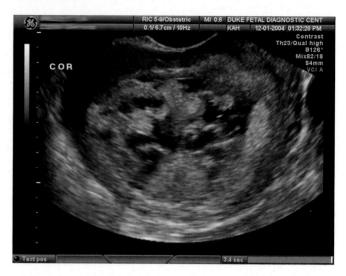

FIGURE 7-7 Transabdominal ultrasound of an unevacuated complete mole, illustrating the characteristic mixed echogenic pattern in the uterus. *(Courtesy John Soper, MD.)*

negative predictive value 23% for detecting molar pregnancy of any type. Detection rates were higher for CM versus PM and for later gestations. Nonetheless, less than 50% of molar pregnancies were diagnosed by ultrasound in first-trimester scans.

In a smaller series from St. George's in London, out of 90 cases the sensitivity of ultrasound diagnosis for mole was 44%: 95% for CM and 20% for PM. The group at Yale evaluated the combined use of both ultrasound and hCG values to determine the diagnosis of hydatidiform mole. When ultrasound was used alone, 15 (42%) of 36 patients with moles did not have a definite diagnosis on first examination. When hCG value above a threshold of 82,350 mIU/mL was used along with the initial ultrasound findings, 32 patients (89%) were correctly identified as having hydatidiform moles (Figure 7-8). A combined algorithm using hCG, clinical history, examination, and imaging is required to make the diagnosis of hydatidiform mole.

With improving ultrasound and serum testing technology, CMs have been diagnosed at an earlier mean gestational age of 11.7 weeks (95% CI, 11.1-12.4) versus 13.8 weeks (95% CI, 13.0-14.6) when comparing a cohort from 1994-2006 to 1977-1989 based on a large database in the Netherlands. Likewise the pre-evacuation median hCG was 4100 (ng/mL) compared to 8600, respectively. Of note, the median weeks to normalization of hCG was 7.4 versus 10.0, respectively.

Several reports have been made of a hydatidiform mole arising in ectopic sites, such as the fallopian tube. These patients tend to present with classic symptoms and signs of ectopic pregnancy, occasionally with hemorrhagic shock resulting from tubal rupture. Tubal GTD was diagnosed in 16 (0.8%) of 2100 women with GTD

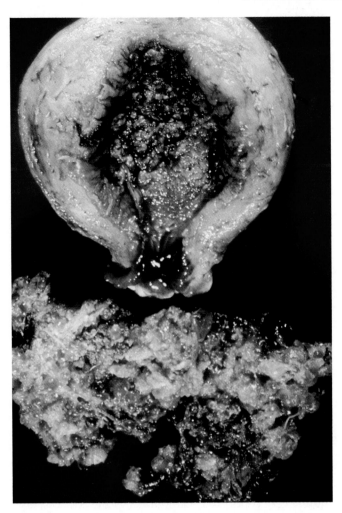

FIGURE 7-8 Gross specimen in a patient treated for complete hydatidiform mole with primary hysterectomy. *(Courtesy John Soper, MD.)*

TABLE 7-2   Management of Hydatidiform Mole

Evacuation: suction D&E (or hysterectomy in selected patients)
Postevacuation quantitative hCG level and chest radiograph
Monitor quantitative hCG levels every 1-2 weeks until normal value or criteria for GTN
Examination every 2-4 weeks while hCG elevated
Confirm normal hCG level, then monitor hCG levels every 1-2 months for 6-12 months
Initiate chemotherapy for GTN using indications listed in Table 7-4:
   1. Plateaued or rising hCG values
   2. Histologic diagnosis of choriocarcinoma, invasive mole or placental site trophoblastic tumor
   3. Persistent hCG >6 months after evacuation
   4. Metastatic disease

D&E, Suction dilation and evacuation; GTN, gestational trophoblastic neoplasia; hCG, human chorionic gonadotropin.

following laboratory evaluation is recommended (see Table 7-2): complete blood count with platelet determination, clotting function studies, renal and liver function studies, blood type with antibody screen, and determination of hCG level. A pre-evacuation chest radiograph should also be obtained.

Evacuation of molar pregnancies should be performed expeditiously. Medical complications are observed in approximately 25% of patients with uterine enlargement at more than 14 to 16 weeks gestational size with molar pregnancy. The mole should be evacuated as soon as possible after stabilization of any medical complications. The choice of facilities for molar evacuation should be based on the expertise of the physician, uterine size, and ability of the facility to manage existing medical complications. In most patients, the preferred method of evacuation is suction dilation and evacuation (D&E) (see Table 7-2).

Medical induction of labor with oxytocin or prostaglandin and hysterotomy are not recommended for evacuation because they increase blood loss and may increase the risk for malignant sequelae compared with suction D&E. The Charing Cross Group reported a significant trend toward more frequent evacuation by suction curettage compared with sharp curettage or medical induction for molar evacuation during their study interval. Postmolar GTN developed in 5.9%, 3.8%, and 9.1% of their patients evacuated with suction curettage, sharp curettage, and medical induction, respectively (*P* <0.05, for increased postmolar GTN in the medical induction group). Furthermore, many patients require D&E to complete the evacuation of the mole after medical induction of labor.

Evacuation is usually performed under general anesthesia, but local or regional anesthesia may be used for a cooperative patient with a small uterus. After serial dilatation of the cervix, uterine evacuation is accomplished with the largest cannula that can be introduced through the cervix. Evacuation may be accompanied

who were managed at the New England Trophoblastic Disease Center in the series reported by Muto. Usually tubal rupture occurs before the diagnostic features, suggesting molar gestation can be identified by ultrasound. Various authors have warned that the current trend of treating ectopic pregnancies with conservative surgery or single-dose methotrexate necessitates close monitoring of serum hCG levels to avoid missing the diagnosis of ectopic GTN.

Evacuation

With increasing frequency, the diagnosis of mole will be made only after histologic evaluation of uterine curettings. Curettage is often performed for a suspected incomplete spontaneous abortion. When GTD is diagnosed, patients should be monitored with serial hCG measurements. A baseline postevacuation chest radiograph should be considered. For patients in whom hydatidiform mole is suspected prior to evacuation, the by significant blood loss and evacuation of tissue, particularly with increasing gestational age. Intravenous oxytocin is begun after the cervix is dilated and continued for several hours postoperatively. Other uterotonics such as methylergonovine or misoprostol may be used if needed. After completion of suction D&E, gentle sharp curettage may be performed. Repeat uterine evacuation by D&E has been performed for persistent GTD, defined in the United Kingdom as failure of hCG to normalize within 4 to 6 weeks or a rise of hCG any time after primary dilation and curettage (D&C). The utility of repeat second D&C is controversial; it may subject patients to surgical complications, when hCG may normalize given more time, and it does not comply with current International Federation of Gynecology and Obstetrics (FIGO) guidelines for treatment of GTN.

Hysterectomy is an alternative to suction D&E for molar evacuation in selected patients who do not wish to preserve childbearing (Figure 7-9). Usually the adnexa may be preserved; theca-lutein cysts should be left in situ unless they are torsed or ruptured and actively bleeding. Hysterectomy reduces but does not eliminate the risk of malignant postmolar sequelae compared to evacuation by D&C. The risk of postmolar GTN after hysterectomy remains approximately 3% to 5%;

therefore these patients should be monitored postoperatively with serial hCG levels.

Risk Factors for Postmolar Gestational Trophoblastic Neoplasia

Many of the risk factors for development of postmolar GTN indirectly reflect the amount of trophoblastic proliferation at the time of evacuation. High pre-evacuation hCG levels, uterine size larger than expected by dates, theca-lutein cysts (see Figure 7-9), and increasing maternal age increase the risk. However, a recent study evaluating all GTD cases for 20 years revealed that maternal age was not a risk factor for developing GTN. Many of these factors interact; the combination of theca-lutein cysts and uterus larger than expected for dates increases the risk of postmolar GTN to 57%. In other series using multivariate analysis, age, parity, initial uterine size, presence of theca-lutein cysts, and initial hCG concentration were not found to be independent prognostic factors for postmolar GTN. Efforts to correlate outcome with the histopathologic features of uterine curettings have been inconsistent, possibly because of incomplete sampling.

Multiple risk factors have been incorporated into scoring systems that might identify high-, medium-, and low-risk subsets of patients. Unfortunately, Parazzini and associates found that, although 15% of their patients could be classified as high risk, these patients accounted for a minority of the cases of postmolar GTN. Of note, despite a lower incidence of clinical risk factors in the more recent cohort of CM reported by the NETDC, 23% of their contemporary patients required treatment for postmolar GTN, compared to 18% in the older cohort, a nonsignificant difference. More recently, analysis of PM at the NETDC did not reveal any clinical factors significantly associated with GTN. Other studies report up to 29% of patients requiring treatment for GTN after CM, despite earlier evacuation. This implies that other molecular biologic mechanisms may be responsible for the development of postmolar GTN, rather than the amount of trophoblastic proliferation at the time of evacuation. Most centers do not base treatment on risk factors; rather they rely on surveillance with serial hCG levels.

Postmolar Surveillance

After molar evacuation, it is important to monitor all patients carefully to diagnose and treat postmolar GTN promptly. Serial quantitative serum hCG measurements should be performed using one of several commercially available assays capable of detecting beta hCG to baseline values (<5 mIU/mL). Ideally, serum hCG levels should be obtained within 7 days of evacuation, every 1 to 2 weeks while elevated, and then at 1- to 2-month intervals for an additional 6 to 12 months (see Table 7-2).

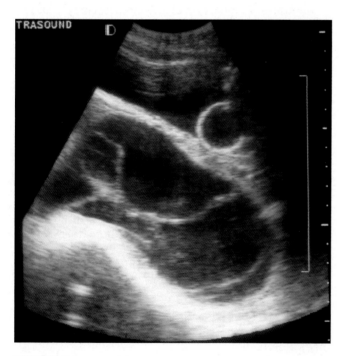

FIGURE 7-9   Ultrasound demonstrating a large theca-lutein ovarian cyst associated with a complete hydatidiform mole. These usually contain multiple thin septations and have an appearance similar to iatrogenic ovarian hyperstimulation during ovulation induction. Theca-lutein cysts regress spontaneously after evacuation of the molar pregnancy, but regression often lags behind hCG level decline. (*Courtesy John Soper, MD.*)

Reliable contraception is recommended during monitoring of hCG values. A chest radiograph is indicated if the hCG level rises. Patients with a histologic diagnosis of malignant GTN (choriocarcinoma, invasive mole, or PSTT), the development of metastatic disease, a rising hCG value, or a plateauing of the hCG values over several weeks' time are diagnosed with postmolar GTN, as discussed later. Approximately 6.8% to 30% of patients develop postmolar GTN after evacuation of CM, whereas 2.5% to 7.5% of patients develop postmolar GTN after PM.

Postmolar surveillance by serial hCG monitoring after achieving normal values allows identification of patients who develop late GTN. Although rare instances of long latent periods between molar evacuation and postmolar GTN have been reported, the vast majority of episodes of GTN after hydatidiform moles occur within approximately 6 months of evacuation. The New England Trophoblastic Disease Center analyzed 1029 patients followed with hCG assays after CM evacuation at their institution. Postmolar GTN occurred in 153 (15%) patients. Only 2 women developed postmolar GTN following normalization of hCG levels; both were followed by an older assay with a sensitivity of 10 mIU/mL.

None of their 82 (95% CI, 0%-4.5%) patients who were followed with an hCG assay having a sensitivity of 5 mIU/mL developed postmolar GTN after normalizing hCG levels. However, a substantial number of their patients were excluded from analysis because of incomplete follow-up, including 817 lost to follow-up after normalization of hCG and 60 patients lost to follow-up before hCG values normalized. The same group of investigators reported that patients with PM had spontaneous normalization of hCG, with a median time of 46 days, and suggested that surveillance in this group may also be abbreviated.

Kerkmeijer and colleagues reported from the Netherlands that 265 of 355 patients with molar pregnancies attained spontaneous normalization of hCG following evacuation. Only 1 case of GTN occurred out of 265 patients who obtained two normal hCG levels. Of note, 144 patients were followed for less than 6 months, and another 100 were followed for up to 12 months. They conclude that hCG surveillance can also be curtailed following normalization of values. Within the same database, they found that no GTN occurred in patients with CM who obtained spontaneous normalization of weekly hCG levels within 2 months after evacuation in a series of 414 patients, although they did report only 56% compliance for 6 months after normalization and 20% lost to follow-up before normalization. Because this total experience is relatively small, it is prudent to recommend continued surveillance after molar evacuation with hCG monitoring for several months following normalization of hCG values.

Although early pregnancies after molar evacuation are usually normal gestations, an early pregnancy obscures detection of an elevated hCG due to GTN. Oral contraceptives do not increase the incidence of postmolar GTN or alter the pattern of regression of hCG values. In a randomized study conducted by the Gynecologic Oncology Group (GOG), patients treated with oral contraceptives had half as many intercurrent pregnancies during hCG surveillance as those using barrier methods. Furthermore, the incidence of postmolar GTN was lower in patients using oral contraceptives. After completion of surveillance documenting remission for 6 to 12 months, pregnancy can be encouraged and hCG monitoring discontinued.

Prophylactic Chemotherapy after Molar Evacuation

Two randomized studies have evaluated prophylactic chemotherapy after molar evacuation. Kim and associates reported that a single course of methotrexate/folinic acid reduced the incidence of postmolar GTN from 47.4% to 14.3% (P <0.05) in patients with high-risk moles, but the incidence was not reduced in patients with low-risk moles. Patients who had received prophylactic chemotherapy but developed GTN required more chemotherapy than those who had not been exposed to prophylactic chemotherapy. In the study reported by Limpongsanurak, a single course of actinomycin-D was compared to observation in patients following evacuation of high-risk moles. Postmolar GTN was 50% in the control group, compared to 13.8% in the treatment group (P <0.05). In both studies there were no deaths in the treatment or control groups caused by GTN or treatment toxicity.

However, there are anecdotal cases of fatalities caused by prophylactic chemotherapy, and prophylactic chemotherapy does not eliminate the need for postevacuation follow-up. Furthermore, patients are exposed to drugs most frequently used to treat postmolar GTN, which could lead to relative chemoresistance. In compliant patients the low morbidity and mortality achieved by monitoring patients and instituting chemotherapy only in patients with postmolar GTN appears to outweigh the potential risk and small benefit of routine prophylactic chemotherapy.

Coexistent Molar Pregnancy with a Normal Fetus

Coexistence of a fetus with molar change of the placenta is relatively rare (Figure 7-10), occurring in 1 in 22,000 to 1 in 100,000 pregnancies. The majority of the literature covering this relatively rare entity consists of case reports, small case series, and review of cases reported

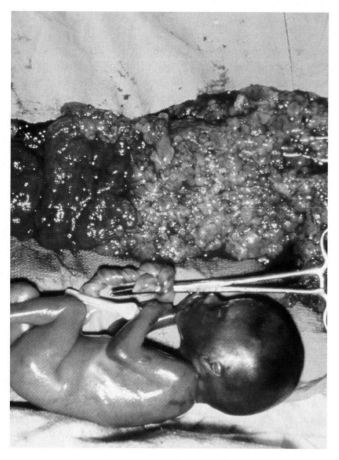

FIGURE 7-10   Gross photo of fetus and mole.

in the literature. Both CM and PM with a coexistent normal fetus have been reported. A variety of criteria have been used to evaluate these pregnancies. Many of the reports that antedated the histologic and cytogenetic distinction between CM and PM likely included twin gestations with coexistent fetus and molar gestation in addition to singleton PM. Although there might be an increased incidence of coexisting mole and fetus related to an increase in multifetal pregnancies caused by ovulation induction for infertility, this may only reflect reporting bias.

Most of these are diagnosed antepartum by ultrasound findings of a complex, cystic placental component distinct from the fetoplacental unit. However, in a few cases the diagnosis is not suspected until examination of the placenta following delivery. Medical complications of hydatidiform mole appear to be increased, including hyperthyroidism, hemorrhage, and pregnancy-induced hypertension.

Compared to singleton hydatidiform moles, twin pregnancy with fetus and mole has an increased risk for postmolar GTN, with a higher proportion of patients having metastatic disease and requiring multiagent chemotherapy. In patients with a coexistent mole and fetus

who continue pregnancy beyond 12 weeks, the subset that develops early complications leading to termination of the pregnancy before fetal viability has a markedly increased risk of postmolar GTN compared to patients whose pregnancy continues into the third trimester.

Among 72 patients collected by a national survey of physicians in Japan during 1997, 24 patients underwent first-trimester evacuation with 20.8% subsequently developing postmolar GTN. In comparison, 45.2% of 31 patients who required evacuation during the second trimester and 17.6% of the 17 who delivered in the third trimester developed postmolar GTN (P <0.05). Nine (50%) of the 18 patients with proven androgenic mole in association with a fetus subsequently were treated for postmolar GTN, but it is not certain that this apparent increased risk was a result of selection bias. Major congenital abnormalities have not been reported in surviving infants.

For patients with coexistent hydatidiform mole and fetus suspected by ultrasound, there are no clear guidelines for management. The ultrasound should be repeated to exclude retroplacental hematoma, other placental abnormalities, or degenerating myoma and to fully evaluate the fetoplacental unit for evidence of a PM or gross fetal malformations. If the diagnosis is still suspected and continuation of pregnancy is desired, fetal karyotype should be obtained, a chest radiograph should be performed to screen for metastases, and serial serum hCG values should be followed.

Patients are at an increased risk for medical complications of pregnancy requiring evacuation, including bleeding, premature labor, and pregnancy-induced hypertension. They should be counseled about these risks and the increased risk of postmolar GTN after evacuation or second-trimester delivery. If fetal karyotype is normal, major fetal malformations are excluded by ultrasound, and there is no evidence of metastatic disease, it is reasonable to allow the pregnancy to continue unless pregnancy-related complications force delivery. After delivery, the placenta should be histologically evaluated and the patient should be followed closely with serial hCG values, similar to a singleton hydatidiform mole.

GESTATIONAL TROPHOBLASTIC NEOPLASIA

GTN is defined by a plateaued, rising, or prolonged persistence of elevated hCG values after molar evacuation, histologic diagnosis of choriocarcinoma, invasive mole or PSTT, or identification of metastasis. The prompt diagnosis of malignant GTN is important because delay in the diagnosis may increase the patient's risk and adversely affect response to treatment. All patients with

TABLE 7-3 Distribution of Metastatic Sites from GTN

Metastatic Site	Number	(%)	(% Metastatic)
Nonmetastatic	195	54	
Metastatic	136	46	
Lung only	110		81
Vagina only	7		5
Central nervous system*	9		7
Gastrointestinal*	5	—	4
Liver*	2	—	1.5
Kidney*	1	—	0.7
Unknown†	4	—	3

Modified from Soper JT, Clarke-Pearson DL, Hammond CB: Obstet Gynecol 71:338, 1988.

*Concurrent lung metastases, highest-risk site recorded.

†Rising hCG after hysterectomy for hydatidiform mole, no identifiable metastases.

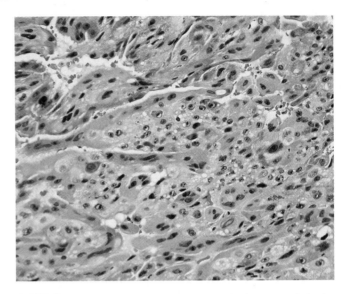

FIGURE 7-11   High-power photomicrograph of gestational choriocarcinoma, illustrating the dimorphic population of the polygonal cytotrophoblast and the multinucleated syncytiotrophoblast cells. *(Courtesy Dr. Rex Bentley, Duke University Medical Center.)*

malignant GTN should undergo a complete evaluation aimed at identifying metastatic sites (Table 7-3) and other clinically important prognostic factors. Several classification systems have been used to determine prognostic groups and assist in the triage of management for individual patients. FIGO revised its staging system for patients with malignant GTN in 2000 to reflect prognostic factors other than simple anatomic distribution of disease.

Diagnosis

Between half and two thirds of cases of GTN that require treatment follow evacuation of CM or PM. Because these patients are treated on the basis of hCG levels rather than hysterectomy, the distribution of histologic lesions is not known. Approximately 50% to 70% of patients with postmolar GTN have persistent or invasive moles, whereas 30% to 50% have postmolar gestational choriocarcinoma.

Gestational choriocarcinoma (Figure 7-11) derived from term pregnancies, spontaneous abortions, and ectopic pregnancies account for the vast majority of the other cases of malignant GTN. PSTT (Figure 7-12) is a rare form of GTN that can follow any pregnancy event.

Invasive moles are characterized by presence of edematous chorionic villi with trophoblastic proliferation that invade directly into the myometrium. Metastasis of molar vesicles may occur, and usually invasive moles will undergo spontaneous resolution after many months, but they are treated with chemotherapy to prevent morbidity and mortality caused by uterine perforation, hemorrhage, or infection. Gestational choriocarcinoma is a pure epithelial malignancy, comprising both neoplastic syncytiotrophoblast and cytotrophoblast elements without chorionic villi (see Figure 7-11). Gestational choriocarcinomas are highly malignant, and chemotherapy is clearly indicated when diagnosed.

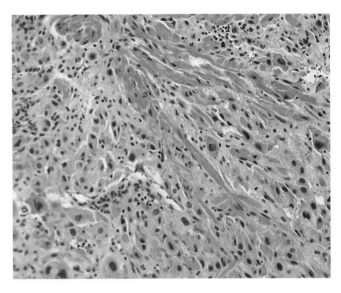

FIGURE 7-12   High-power photomicrograph of placental site trophoblastic tumor treated with hysterectomy. Sheets of anaplastic polygonal cells with frequent mitoses infiltrate the smooth muscle of the uterine wall. *(Courtesy Dr. Rex Bentley, Duke University Medical Center.)*

Placental site trophoblastic tumors are relatively rare. These tumors are characterized by absence of villi with proliferation of intermediate trophoblast cells (see Figure 7-12). The syncytiotrophoblast population observed in choriocarcinoma is lacking in PSTT, with relatively lower levels of intact hCG secreted by these tumors. In general, PSTTs are not as sensitive to simple chemotherapy as other forms of malignant GTN; therefore it is important to identify these tumors. Fortunately, most patients present with disease confined to the uterus and can be treated with hysterectomy.

Women with postmolar GTN are usually diagnosed early in the course of disease by serial hCG monitoring. In contrast, patients with malignant GTN after nonmolar gestations often present with predominantly nongynecologic symptoms and signs including hemoptysis or pulmonary embolism, cerebral hemorrhage, gastrointestinal or urologic hemorrhage, or metastatic malignancy of an unknown primary site. The index pregnancy event may have occurred years before presentation or may have been a subclinical spontaneous abortion. The possibility of malignant GTN should be suspected in any woman of reproductive age who presents with metastatic disease from an unknown primary site or undiagnosed cerebral hemorrhage. Under these circumstances the diagnosis is facilitated by a high index of suspicion coupled with serum hCG testing and exclusion of a concurrent pregnancy, most often without the need for tissue biopsy.

Before the development of effective chemotherapy, Delfs reported that of 119 patients followed after mole, 5 (4%) and 6 (5%) required hysterectomy for invasive mole or choriocarcinoma, respectively. Other prechemotherapy reports indicated a mortality rate of more than 20% among patients with invasive mole. Since the development of chemotherapy, between 15% and 36% of patients in the United States are treated after molar evacuation based on inclusive hCG level criteria for initiating chemotherapy in an attempt to limit the morbidity and mortality caused by postmolar GTN. In contrast, Bagshawe and colleagues used very conservative hCG criteria to initiate chemotherapy and reported treating only approximately 8% of their patients after molar evacuation.

The pattern of hCG regression after evacuation of hydatidiform mole is most often used to make a diagnosis of postmolar GTN. After evacuation, most patients will have an initial fall in hCG levels and should be followed with serial hCG values every 1 to 2 weeks. Almost every series has treated patients on the basis of a confirmed hCG rise. In many studies, however, chemotherapy was initiated on the basis of an hCG level plateau of relatively short (<3 weeks) duration. Kohorn noted that 15% of his patients had hCG plateaus after molar evacuation that lasted at least 2 weeks, followed by spontaneous regression without intervention. In a chemotherapy trial of actinomycin-D, Schlaerth and colleagues observed that 25% of their patients had a substantial spontaneous fall in hCG levels on the day that chemotherapy was initiated. Based on the correlation between hCG level and tumor burden, Kohorn has suggested an approach using shorter observation for patients with high hCG level plateaus but allowing

longer periods of observation for those who have hCG plateaus at levels under 1000 mIU/mL.

In some studies an additional criterion for initiating chemotherapy after molar evacuation has been persistence of hCG for an arbitrary length of time, ranging between 6 weeks and 6 months after evacuation. The initial reports of chemotherapy from the National Institutes of Health used persistence of detectable hCG for more than 60 days after molar evacuation as an indication for chemotherapy treatment. Many series have documented that persistence of hCG for more than 60 days after evacuation increases the risk for developing postmolar GTN. However, 60% to 64% of patients with delayed regression of hCG beyond 60 days will ultimately undergo spontaneous hCG regression, with no deaths in those who began therapy more than 60 days from molar evacuation. Furthermore, groups reporting from the United Kingdom, where care for GTD patients is centralized, follow patients with elevated hCG levels for up to 6 months without an increase in morbidity or mortality among those treated after this prolonged follow-up.

Lurain and associates from the John I. Brewer Trophoblastic Disease Center reported their experience with 738 patients with complete hydatidiform moles. In their study, 596 patients had spontaneous remission to normal of hCG values, although only 390 (65%) had done so by 60 days. An additional 206 patients reached normal values during the next 110 days. Overall, 142 (19%) were treated with chemotherapy because of rising or plateauing hCG levels. Of these, 125 had invasive moles and 17 had choriocarcinomas. Only 15% of the 142 treated patients, or 3% of the total, developed metastases outside of the uterus. Morrow and Kohorn treated a higher proportion of their patients (36% and 27%, respectively) using hCG criteria derived from regression curves, compared with studies that use the individual patient's hCG regression pattern. It appears that use of hCG regression curves may result in treatment of more patients than necessary, and it did not prevent metastatic disease.

In an effort to provide uniformity to the diagnosis of postmolar GTN, FIGO conducted workshops among members of the Society of Gynecologic Oncologists, International Society for the Study of Trophoblastic Disease, and International Gynecologic Cancer Society to formulate its current recommendations for evaluation and staging this disease. The current FIGO requirements for making a diagnosis of postmolar GTN are as follows (Table 7-4):

1. Four values or more of plateaued hCG (±10%) over at least 3 weeks: days 1, 7, 14, and 21.
2. A rise of hCG of 10% or greater for 3 values or more over at least 2 weeks: days 1, 7, and 14.
3. The histologic diagnosis of choriocarcinoma.

TABLE 7-4   Diagnosis and Evaluation of GTN

DIAGNOSIS OF GTN

After molar evacuation: 4 values or more of plateaued hCG (±10%) over at least 3 weeks: days 1, 7, 14, and 21
After molar evacuation: a rise of hCG of 10% or greater for 3 values or more over at least 2 weeks: days 1, 7, and 14
After molar evacuation: Persistence of hCG beyond 6 months
The histologic diagnosis of choriocarcinoma, invasive mole, or PSTT
Metastatic disease without established primary site with elevated hCG; pregnancy has been excluded

EVALUATION OF GTN

Complete physical and pelvic examination; baseline hematologic, renal, and hepatic functions
Baseline quantitative hCG level
Chest radiograph or CT scan of chest
Brain MRI or CT scan
CT or MRI scan of abdomen and pelvis

CT, Computed tomography; hCG, human chorionic gonadotropin; MRI, magnetic resonance imaging; PSTT, placental site trophoblastic tumor.

4. Persistence of hCG beyond 6 months after mole evacuation.

The level and duration for observation of the hCG plateau beyond 3 weeks would be determined at the discretion of the treating physician. Observation of hCG level plateau for longer than 3 weeks was permitted because this does not appear to have an adverse effect on survival.

Recently, laboratory assays for hyperglycosylated hCG have been found to be highly sensitive for differentiating active GTN or choriocarcinoma from inactive or "quiescent" GTD in patients with hCG level plateaus. These newer assays, developed by Cole and associates at the U.S. hCG Reference Service at the University of New Mexico, may allow earlier diagnosis of postmolar GTN in the future.

The majority of centers in the United States will also treat patients if metastases are identified. In contrast, Bagshawe and colleagues, reporting the results from monitoring patients after hydatidiform mole in the United Kingdom, stated that patients with pulmonary nodules were followed conservatively and treatment decisions based on hCG regression patterns. Although the overall results from this policy were excellent, outcome for patients with pulmonary metastases was not detailed. In the United States, where care is decentralized, identification of metastases is included as an indication for initiation of therapy.

"Phantom" Human Chorionic Gonadotropin

Rarely, women present with persistently elevated hCG levels but are subsequently found to have a false-positive hCG assay result, sometimes after receiving chemotherapy or surgery for presumed malignant GTN. Most patients with "phantom" hCG present with low-level hCG elevations, but occasionally values as high as 200 to 300 mIU/mL have been recorded. The false-positive hCG values result from interference with the hCG immunometric sandwich assays caused by nonspecific heterophile antibodies in the patients' sera. Many of these patients have an undefined previous pregnancy event and do not have radiographic evidence of metastatic disease. Serial hCG values usually do not substantially vary, despite often prolonged observation, and usually do not substantially change with therapeutic interventions such as surgery or chemotherapy.

"Phantom" hCG may also present after evacuation of a hydatidiform mole or following a clearly defined pregnancy event, such as an ectopic pregnancy. It should be suspected if hCG values plateau at relatively low levels and do not respond to therapeutic maneuvers such as methotrexate given for a presumed persistent mole or ectopic pregnancy. Evaluation should include study of serum hCG using a variety of assay techniques at different dilutions of patient serum combined with a urinary hCG level if the serum level is above threshold for the urinary assay. False-positive hCG assays will not be affected by serial dilution of patient sera and will have markedly different values using different assay techniques, with the majority of assays reflecting undetectable hCG. Heterophile antibodies are not excreted in the urine. Therefore, if they are the cause of serum hCG level elevation, urinary hCG values will not be detectable. Other techniques are available to inactivate or strip the patient's serum of heterophile antibodies. It is important to exclude the possibility of "phantom" hCG before subjecting these patients to hysterectomy or chemotherapy for GTN.

Pretherapy Evaluation

In contrast to epithelial endometrial cancer, GTN usually spreads by hematogenous dissemination. Venous metastasis can occur in the subvaginal venous plexus, resulting in vaginal metastases (Figure 7-13), or in the main uterine venous system with metastases to the parametrium and lungs. Although direct shunting into the systemic circulation rarely occurs, the majority of disseminated metastases develop only after pulmonary metastases have become established. The brain, liver, gastrointestinal tract, and kidneys are the distant organs most often affected, but metastases to virtually every organ have been reported. Although lymphatic spread can occur, it is relatively uncommon among patients with choriocarcinoma and invasive mole. The hematogenous pattern of metastatic involvement is important when considering the radiographic evaluation of patients with GTN (see Table 7-3).

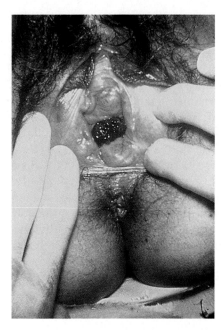

FIGURE 7-13   Vaginal metastasis of malignant GTN, presenting as vaginal bleeding with a discolored submucosal mass underlying the urethra. Vaginal metastases of GTN are highly vascular and should not be biopsied. *(Courtesy John Soper, MD.)*

Pretherapy evaluation of the patient with GTN (see Table 7-4) includes assessment of history for clinical risk factors, examination, laboratory evaluation, and radiographic survey for potential sites of metastatic disease and number of lesions. Clinical risk factors important for assigning staging and treatment include duration of disease as determined by interval from antecedent pregnancy, type of antecedent pregnancy, and previous treatment. Because of different clinical characteristics, patients with histologically proven PSTT are classified separately from patients with gestational choriocarcinoma or postmolar GTN. The laboratory evaluation should include a pretherapy hCG value. It should be emphasized that the hCG level obtained immediately before instituting treatment for malignant GTN is important for staging—not the hCG level obtained at the time of molar evacuation.

Vaginal metastases of GTN are diagnosed by physical examination. These lesions usually involve the mucosa of the anterior vagina and present as dark, often blue, soft nodules (see Figure 7-13). Ulceration or active bleeding may be present. Because of the highly vascular nature of these lesions, biopsy is not recommended. If the vagina is the only site of metastasis, the majority of these lesions will respond to chemotherapy. A few patients will require vaginal packing or selective embolization using interventional radiology to control active hemorrhage early in the course of treatment.

The recommended radiographic staging evaluation for patients with GTN includes chest radiograph or computed tomography (CT) scan, evaluation of the abdomen and pelvis with CT or magnetic resonance imaging (MRI) scan, and contrasted CT or MRI of the brain. An ultrasound of the pelvis should also be obtained to exclude the possibility of intrauterine pregnancy before instituting chemotherapy. Both ultrasound and MRI studies of the uterus can be used to identify intrauterine tumors and foci of myometrial invasion by GTN, but they are not sensitive or specific enough to replace serum hCG level monitoring for establishing the diagnosis of GTN or for following patients during treatment.

Approximately 45% of patients have metastatic disease when GTN is diagnosed. As indicated by the anatomic sites of metastatic disease encountered among patients initially treated for malignant GTN (see Table 7-3), the lung is the most frequent site of extrauterine metastasis (Figure 7-14). Although the majority of patients with high-risk metastatic sites have pulmonary metastases on chest radiograph or symptoms referable to metastatic involvement, a full metastatic evaluation is recommended, rather than relying on a negative chest radiograph alone to make a determination of nonmetastatic GTN.

Between 29% and 41% of patients treated for nonmetastatic GTN have pulmonary metastases identified on CT scans of the lungs that are not detected by chest radiograph. The clinical importance of occult pulmonary metastases is debated when they are the only sites of extrauterine metastases. However, many series of patients treated for high-risk metastases include patients who initially presented with normal chest radiographs. It would be a tragedy to miss the diagnosis of a high-risk metastasis in a patient and delay appropriate aggressive initial therapy.

Although operative procedures may be integrated into the treatment of patients with malignant GTN, they are rarely indicated for establishing the diagnosis or staging. Performing a secondary D&E before beginning chemotherapy in a patient with postmolar GTN is controversial. The experience at the University of Southern California indicated that it had an effect on the treatment in only 20% and was complicated by uterine perforation requiring hysterectomy in 8% of their patients. In contrast, Pezeshki and associates analyzed 544 women undergoing a second uterine evacuation for presumed postmolar GTN. After a second evacuation, 368 (68%) entered spontaneous remission. Of 251 patients with a histologic diagnosis of persistent GTD, 96 (38%) required chemotherapy compared to 39 (18%) of 219 with negative histology at the second D&C. Many clinicians in the United States treat patients with postmolar GTN without performing a second D&C because of the concern for preservation of fertility. Other operative procedures such as laparoscopy, thoracotomy, or craniotomy are only rarely justifiable to establish the primary diagnosis of GTN.

TABLE 7-5 Clinical Classification System for Patients with Malignant GTN

Category	Criteria
Nonmetastatic GTN	No evidence of metastases; not assigned to prognostic category
Metastatic GTN	Any entrauterine metastases
Good prognosis metastatic GTN	Short duration (<4 months)
	No brain or liver metastases
	Pretherapy hCG <40,000 mIU/mL
	No antecedent term pregnancy
	No prior chemotherapy
Poor prognosis metastatic GTN	Any one risk factor:
	Long duration (>4 months)
	Pretherapy hCG >40,000 mIU/mL
	Brain or liver metastases
	Antecedent term pregnancy
	Prior chemotherapy

GTN, Gestational trophoblastic neoplasia; hCG, human chorionic gonadotropin.

Classification and Staging

The classification and staging of malignant GTN has evolved over the past 50 years. The Clinical Classification System, based on risk factors, has been frequently used in the United States (Table 7-5). In this system patients with nonmetastatic disease are not assigned into a prognostic group because of uniformly good outcome using simple single-agent chemotherapy. The risk factors used in this system were derived by retrospective analysis to predict resistance to single-agent methotrexate and actinomycin-D regimens among women treated for metastatic GTN at the National Institutes of Health. Hammond and colleagues subsequently reported essentially 100% survival among women who presented with good-prognosis metastatic GTN treated with single-agent therapy. He noted survival of 70% among patients with metastatic poor prognosis disease initially treated with multiagent chemotherapy, compared to only 14% survival for patients in this category who initially received single-agent therapy. Poor tolerance of multiagent therapy was noted in the group of poor-prognosis patients receiving initial single-agent regimens, with toxicity causing death in half of these patients.

A more complicated system was adopted by the World Health Organization (WHO) in the early 1980s based on the experience at the Charing Cross Hospital in London between 1957 and 1973. Univariate analysis was used to identify prognostic factors among patients treated mainly with simple chemotherapy regimens. In the original study patient age, antecedent pregnancy, interval from antecedent pregnancy, hCG level, ABO blood type, size of the largest tumor, sites and number of metastases, and type of prior chemotherapy were each found to correlate with prognosis. The prognostic

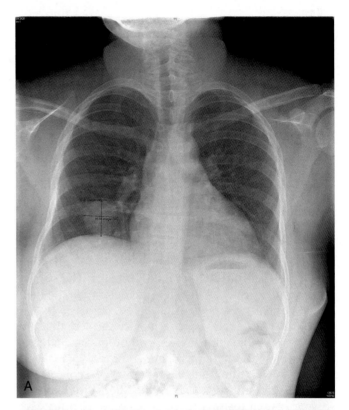

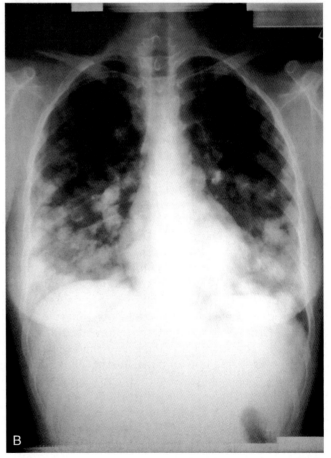

FIGURE 7-14 Pulmonary metastases of GTN can present as solitary (A) or diffuse (B) pulmonary nodules. *(Courtesy John Soper, MD.)*

TABLE 7-6　Prognostic Index Score Compared with Clinical Classification System

Clinical Classification	Low Risk (<5)	Medium Risk (5-7)	High Risk (>8)	Total Clinical Classification
Nonmetastatic GTN	99.5% (217)	100% (10)	—	99.7% (227)
Metastatic GTN				
Good prognosis	100% (86)	100% (5)	—	100% (91)
Poor prognosis	100% (8)	90.5% (21)	68.4% (38)	79.1% (67)
Total WHO	99.8% (311)	94.4% (36)	68.4% (38)	

Modified from Soper JT, Evans AC, Conaway MR, et al: Obstet Gynecol 84:969, 1994.
Data presented as life table survival percentage (number of patients).
GTN, Gestational trophoblastic neoplasia; WHO, World Health Organization.

index applied a weighted score to each of these factors, which were assumed to act independently. The sum of component scores was then used to determine the individual patient's risk category.

Multivariate analyses have not confirmed that the factors have independent effects on prognosis. Paternal blood-type information is not uniformly available and has been omitted in generating WHO score values by some investigators. Others modified the weighted scoring system using a highest risk score of 6 for each prognostic factor, while not changing the total score for assigning patients into risk categories. Furthermore, the WHO prognostic index score provided for reassignment of a score among patients who have previously received treatment for GTN, which might obscure the prognostic effects of some of the other clinical factors on primary treatment. Finally, there was no uniformity in assessing size of the largest tumor or assigning number of metastases. Despite these limitations, modifications of the WHO prognostic index score were useful for predicting risk groups of patients with malignant GTN.

In Table 7-6, the Clinical Classification System and WHO prognostic index score are compared among patients who presented for initial treatment of GTN at Duke University Medical Center. The Clinical Classification System had a greater sensitivity for identifying patients at risk for treatment failure and death (see Table 7-6). Although the WHO prognostic index score was able to provide slightly better discrimination of patients with poor prognosis metastatic disease in low-, intermediate-, and high-risk populations, stratification into three categories was considered less important than identifying patients at risk of failure for initial therapy. By multivariate analysis, both systems were roughly equivalent for stratifying patients into risk groups.

In the early 1980s FIGO proposed an anatomic staging system for malignant GTN (Table 7-7). Although this system recognized the stepwise development of metastatic disease, it did not incorporate any of the other prognostic factors into the FIGO stage. Although stage I

TABLE 7-7　Anatomic FIGO Staging System for GTN

Stage	Criteria
I	Disease confined to the uterus
II	Disease outside of uterus but is limited to the genital structures
III	Disease extends to the lungs with or without known genital tract involvement
IV	All other metastatic sites

Modified from Kohorn EI: Int J Gynecol Cancer 11:73, 2000.
FIGO, International Federation of Gynecology and Obstetrics; GTN, gestational trophoblastic neoplasia.

patients uniformly had low-risk disease and stage IV patients were uniformly high risk, there was considerable overlap of outcome within stages II and III. Revision of the FIGO staging in 1992 recognized hCG level and time from antecedent pregnancy as risk factors. These factors generated substages within each stage. Although this revised system did correlate with outcome, it resulted in a proliferation of substages of questionable importance.

In 2000 FIGO revised its staging system for GTN again. The original anatomic stages were retained, but the 1992 risk factors were replaced by a risk factor score that used a modification of the WHO prognostic index score (Table 7-8). Patients with histologically diagnosed PSTT were reported separately, reflecting the distinct tumor biology of these lesions. Changes to the WHO classification included elimination of ABO blood group risk factors and a change in the risk score for liver metastasis from 2 to 4, reflecting high risk for patients with liver metastasis. Radiographic staging studies were standardized. Finally, the three risk groups of the WHO prognostic index score were consolidated into two groups: Low Risk with a score of 6 or less and High Risk with a score of 7 or greater. Hancock and colleagues retrospectively compared the outcomes of patients

TABLE 7-8 The Revised FIGO 2000 Scoring System for GTN

FIGO score	0	1	2	4
Age (years)	<40	≥40		
Antecedent pregnancy	Hydatidiform mole	Abortion	Term pregnancy	
Interval from index pregnancy (months)	<4	4-6	7-12	≥13
Pretreatment hCG (mIU/mL)	<1000	1000 to <10,000	10,000 to 100,000	≥100,000
Largest tumor size including uterus (cm)		3-5	≥5	
Site of metastases	<3	Spleen Kidney	Gastrointestinal	Brain Liver
Number of metastases identified	0	1-4	5-8	>8
Previous failed chemotherapy			Single drug	≥2 drugs

From Kohorn EI: Int J Gynecol Cancer 11:73, 2000.
The total score for a patient is obtained by adding the individual scores for each prognostic factor. Total score 0-6 = low risk; >7 = high risk.

according to the risk score categories generated by the modified WHO prognostic index score and the proposed FIGO score. The consolidated risk categories generated by the FIGO score correlated better with outcome than the modified WHO prognostic index score did.

The current FIGO system counts and measures pulmonary metastases only if they are visible on chest radiograph. Other recommended studies include CT scan of the abdomen and pelvis, ultrasound of the uterus, and MRI or contrasted CT scan of the brain. It is important to realize that the hCG level used to generate the risk score refers to the level recorded at the time GTN is diagnosed, *rather than hCG at the time of molar evacuation.* Under the new FIGO system, reporting of patients includes both anatomic stage and FIGO risk score. For example, a 30-year-old patient with nonmetastatic GTN diagnosed 5 months after molar evacuation with an hCG level of 8000 mIU/mL would be recorded as a FIGO stage I: 2. Likewise, a 40-year-old with prior term pregnancy 7 months previously, hCG of 200,000 mIU/mL, 2 brain metastases, 10 lung lesions, and uterine tumor measuring 6 centimeters would be FIGO Stage IV: 17.

Adoption of the current revision of FIGO staging for GTN will allow uniformity for evaluation and reporting of outcomes. With accumulation of data through FIGO, it is hoped that multivariate analysis can confirm or refute the prognostic importance of individual factors used to generate the risk scores. Although these changes are important on an international scale and are the standard for reporting results of treatment, they are of lesser importance for the practicing general obstetrician/gynecologist initially encountering patients with malignant GTN. For these clinicians, the most important decisions revolve around identification of patients who should be referred out of the community to a specialist for treatment of high-risk disease. Because the clinical classification system (see Table 7-5) is relatively simple, it may be the best system for use by the generalist for the purpose of appropriate referral.

TABLE 7-9 Chemotherapy Regimens for Nonmetastatic and Low-Risk Metastatic GTN

Agent/Schedule	Dosage
METHOTREXATE*	
Weekly	30-50 mg/m² IM
5 day/every 2 weeks	0.4 mg/kg IM (maximum 25 mg/day total dose)
Methotrexate/folinic acid rescue	Methotrexate 1 mg/kg IM, days 1, 3, 5, 7; and
Every 2 weeks	Folinic acid 0.1 mg/kg IM, days 2, 4, 6, 8
Methotrexate infusion/folinic acid	Methotrexate 100 mg/m² IV bolus; and
Every 2 weeks	Folinic acid 200 mg/m² 12-hour infusion with 15 mg p.o. every 6 hours for four doses
DACTINOMYCIN†	
5 day/every 2 weeks	9-13 mcg/kg/d IV (maximum dose 500 mcg/day)
Bolus, every 2 weeks	1.25 mg/m² IV bolus
ETOPOSIDE‡	
5 day/every 2 weeks	200 mg/m²/day PO

Dose based on ideal body weight, maximum 2m²
†*Potential extravasation injury, gastrointestinal toxicity common*
‡*Alopecia, small leukemogenic risk*
IM, Intramuscular; IV, intravenous; PO, oral.

Treatment of Nonmetastatic and Low-Risk Metastatic Gestational Trophoblastic Neoplasia

Primary remission rates of patients treated for nonmetastatic or low-risk GTN are similar using a variety of chemotherapy regimens (see Table 7-9). Essentially all patients with low-risk GTN can be cured, usually without the need for hysterectomy. Randomized comparisons of the regimens detailed in Table 7-9 have not been completed, and comparison of the following results may not be valid because of slightly different criteria used to make the diagnosis of nonmetastatic GTN by different investigators. Patients with metastatic GTN who lack any of the clinical high-risk factors or have a total FIGO risk score of 6 or lower have low-risk disease and can be treated successfully with initial single-agent regimens similar to nonmetastatic GTN.

Methotrexate 0.4 mg/kg/day given by intramuscular (IM) injection for 5 days, with cycles repeated every 12 to 14 days, was the regimen originally used to treat GTN at the NIH. Hammond and colleagues reported the NIH experience treating 58 patients with nonmetastatic GTN. Only four (7%) patients had disease resistant to this regimen, and three of these were salvaged with single-agent actinomycin-D. In Lurain's series from the Brewer Trophoblastic Disease Center, all 337 patients with non-metastatic GTN were cured. Only 10.7% of 253 patients initially treated with 5-day IM methotrexate therapy required a second agent, only 1.2% needed multiagent chemotherapy, and only 0.8% required hysterectomy to achieve a complete remission. Factors significantly associated with the development of methotrexate resistance included pretreatment serum hCG in excess of 50,000 mIU/mL, nonmolar antecedent pregnancy, and histopathologic diagnosis of choriocarcinoma. Others have used 5-day IM methotrexate, reporting similar results. If patients have abnormal liver function, methotrexate should not be used because it is metabolized in the liver. Significant hematologic suppression, cutaneous toxicity, mucositis, alopecia, gastrointestinal toxicity, and serositis are frequently seen in patients receiving the 5-day methotrexate regimen.

Patients with low-risk metastatic GTN have higher failure rates. DuBeshter and associates used single-agent methotrexate or actinomycin-D to treat 48 patients with low-risk metastatic GTN at the New England Trophoblastic Disease Center. All patients achieved sustained remission but 51% required a second drug, 14% needed combination chemotherapy, and 12% required surgery to remove drug-resistant disease. Among 52 patients with low-risk metastatic GTN treated initially with the 5-day methotrexate regimen at Duke University Medical Center, 60% achieved primary remission within a median 3 cycles of methotrexate chemotherapy. Patients were treated with actinomycin-D for documented methotrexate resistance or toxicity with equal frequency. All patients achieved remission, with only 4% requiring multiagent regimens. Likewise, Roberts and Lurain treated 92 patients for low-risk metastatic GTN at the Brewer Trophoblastic Disease Center. Among their 70 patients who were initially treated with chemotherapy alone, 24.6% developed chemoresistant disease and 9.8% had therapy changed because of toxicity. Overall, 78% achieved remission using the primary regimen with or without hysterectomy; all eventually achieved remission, and only one (1.1%) required multiagent chemotherapy.

Bagshawe and Wilde first reported the use of alternating daily doses of IM methotrexate (1 mg/kg) and leukovorin factor or folinic acid (0.1 mg/kg) for four doses of each agent in an attempt to reduce the toxicity of daily methotrexate regimens. Whereas toxicity sparing may be true for high doses of methotrexate, Rotmensch and associates evaluated methotrexate levels in patients after daily methotrexate therapy compared to levels in patients receiving alternating daily doses of methotrexate and folinic acid, with a higher daily dose of methotrexate given in the methotrexate/folinic acid regimen. They noted that whereas patients on the methotrexate/folinic acid regimen had higher peak methotrexate levels after treatment with a higher methotrexate dose than those on single-agent methotrexate, trough levels were both subtoxic and subtherapeutic 24 hours after methotrexate administration. This finding alone might explain the therapeutic and toxicity benefit described for the low-dose methotrexate/folinic acid regimen used for treatment in GTN.

At Charing Cross Hospital in London, 347 of 348 (99.7%) low-risk patients treated with methotrexate and folinic acid survived; however, 69 (20%) had to change treatment because of drug resistance and 23 (6%) patients needed to change because of drug-induced toxicity. An analysis of the data from the Southeastern Trophoblastic Disease Center at Duke University indicated that 8 (27.5%) of 29 patients developed resistance to methotrexate with folinic acid given at 14-day intervals, compared to 3 (7.7%) of 39 treated with standard 5-day methotrexate for nonmetastatic disease. Although this difference was statistically significant, a similar proportion of patients were changed to a second agent in each group because a larger number of patients receiving 5-day methotrexate changed to another agent because of toxicity. Wong and associates also compared 5-day methotrexate to methotrexate with folinic acid, resulting in comparable sustained remission rates. In their series, however, patients who received methotrexate/folinic acid achieved remission earlier but experienced a higher incidence of hepatic toxicity compared with patients receiving the 5-day regimen.

McNeish and associates, reporting from the Charing Cross system, reviewed the results of 485 patients with low-risk GTN (prognostic index score <8, using their modification) treated with cyclical intramuscular methotrexate/folinic acid; overall survival was 100%. Two thirds achieved remission with primary chemotherapy, whereas150 patients were changed to an alternative agent because of chemoresistance. In patients with chemoresistant disease and hCG levels less than 100 mIU/mL, therapy was changed to single-agent actinomycin-D, with 89% responding to actinomycin-D and the remaining patients salvaged with multiagent regimens. If hCG levels were greater than 100 mIU/mL, patients were treated with a multiagent regimen containing etoposide, with 98.9% responding to the first salvage regimen and all patients entering sustained remission.

Berkowitz and associates, at the New England Tro-phoblastic Center, have used IM methotrexate with folinic acid rescue in 185 patients with GTN. Ninety percent of 163 patients with nonmetastatic disease and 68% of 22 patients with low-risk metastatic disease were placed into complete remission with this regimen. Rather than recycling treatment at fixed intervals, they treated patients based on hCG level response. More than 80% were placed into remission with only one course of che-motherapy. All patients with methotrexate resistance achieved remission with other agents. Other investiga-tors have used higher doses of intravenous (IV) metho-trexate (300-500 mg/m^2) followed by oral or intravenous folinic acid every 6 hours for 24 hours, resulting in primary remission rates of 45% to 86% in patients with nonmetastatic and/or low-risk metastatic GTN. Overall cure rates in these series were excellent and toxicity was minimal. A major disadvantage with these regimens is the need for a prolonged (up to 12-hour) IV infusion.

Oral methotrexate is readily absorbed via the gastro-intestinal tract. Barter reported a retrospective analysis of 15 patients treated solely with oral methotrexate 0.4 mg/kg for 5-day cycles that were repeated every 14 days. The primary remission rate was 87% with minimal toxicity. Concerns about patient compliance and the pos-sibility of unpredictable absorption in individual patients have led to infrequent use for this mode of treatment in GTN.

In a prospective phase II trial, the GOG reported an 82% primary remission rate for patients treated with weekly intramuscular methotrexate given at a dose of 30 to 50 mg/m^2. Remission was achieved within a median seven cycles of therapy. There was no apparent benefit for increasing the dose up to 50 mg/m^2. It was con-cluded that the weekly methotrexate regimen was most cost effective among several alternative methotrexate or actinomycin-D schedules when taking efficacy, toxicity, and cost into consideration. Hoffman and colleagues and Gleeson and associates confirmed the low toxicity and overall remission rates for patients treated with this regimen. In the experience reported by Gleeson and associates, weekly methotrexate was compared with methotrexate/folinic acid, producing equivalent primary remission rates. Total doses of methotrexate required to induce remission were lower in the weekly methotrexate group. They also concluded that weekly methotrexate was minimally toxic, equally effective, and their pre-ferred regimen for nonmetastatic GTN.

In contrast to IM methotrexate regimens used for treating ectopic pregnancies, chemotherapy for GTN is recycled every week until hCG values have achieved normal levels, and then an additional course is admin-istered after the first normal hCG value has been recorded. Hematologic indices must be monitored carefully during chemotherapy, but significant hematologic toxicity is infrequent among patients treated with the weekly methotrexate regimen.

Other investigators have used 5-day courses of IV actinomycin-D 9 to 13 mcg/kg/day as primary therapy for nonmetastatic or low-risk GTN with equally good results. They believe that toxicity from 5-day actinomycin-D is less than that from 5-day methotrexate regimens. However, alopecia, nausea, and significant myelotoxicity can result. Furthermore, extravasation of actinomycin-D during administration can result in severe local soft tissue damage.

Treatment of nonmetastatic and low-risk metastatic GTN with actinomycin-D 1.25 mg/m^2 given as a single IV bolus dose every 2 weeks had equal remission rates in retrospective comparisons to 5-day courses of IV actinomycin-D. The GOG reported a phase II study of this regimen. Of 31 patients who were treated, 29 (94%) achieved remission after an average of 4.4 (range of 2-15) courses of therapy. The two patients who failed to respond to pulse therapy were subsequently cured by alternative treatment. The frequency of toxicity was quite low. The advantages of pulse dactinomycin-D over other treatment schedules include ease of administra-tion, greater patient convenience, and improved cost effectiveness. Moreover, the single bolus administration appears to reduce the risk of extravasation injuries com-pared to 5-day IV administration.

Other investigators have alternated courses of 5-day IM methotrexate with 5-day IV actinomycin-D in an attempt to limit toxicity and improve primary remission rates. Rose and Piver combined their experience using this approach in 9 patients with a literature review of 40 patients treated in this manner. All patients were cured with primary therapy when the two regimens were alternated. However, given the relatively small numbers of patients and selectivity of reporting small series of patients in the literature, one cannot conclude that this strategy is superior to beginning therapy in patients with GTN using a single agent and changing to the alternative only if chemoresistance or toxicity is encountered.

5-fluorouracil (5-FU) and oral etoposide are frequently used in Asia for primary treatment of patients with non-metastatic and low-risk metastatic GTN, but they are not often used in the United States. Among patients treated with a 10-day continuous intravenous infusion of 5-FU, Sung and colleagues reported a 93% primary remission rate. Acute toxicity included diarrhea, nausea and vom-iting, hepatotoxicity, and stomatitis. Likewise, Wong and co-workers reported a 98% primary remission rate among patients treated with 5-day courses of oral eto-poside 100 mg/m^2, recycled at 14-day intervals. Toxicity included frequent alopecia, myelosuppression, and gas-trointestinal toxicity. Furthermore, patients exposed to etoposide have a low but significant risk of developing

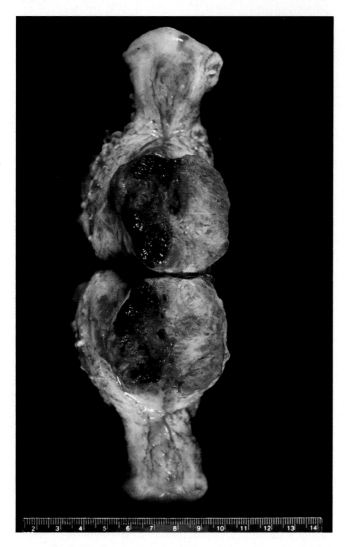

FIGURE 7-15 Hysterectomy specimen in a 39-year-old woman with nonmetastatic GTN who underwent surgery during her first course of methotrexate. She entered complete remission 4 weeks after initial therapy. *(Courtesy John Soper, MD.)*

TABLE 7-10 Management of Low-Risk Nonmetastatic or Low-Risk Metastatic GTN

Initiate single-agent methotrexate or dactinomycin regimen
  (Table 7-9)
Consider hysterectomy if fertility not desired
Monitor hematologic, renal, and hepatic indices before each cycle of
  chemotherapy
Monitor serum hCG levels weekly during therapy
Change to alternative single-agent if resistance or severe toxicity to
  first agent
If resistance to alternative agent:
  1. Repeat metastatic evaluation
  2. Consider hysterectomy if no extrauterine metastases
  3. Multiagent therapy (MAC or EMA/CO, see text)
Remission: three consecutive weekly hCG values in the normal
  range
1 or 2 cycles of maintenance/consolidation chemotherapy

EMA/CO, Etoposide, methotrexate, actinomycin-D, cyclophosphamide and vincristine; MAC, methotrexate, actinomycin-D, and cyclophosphamide.

acute myelogenous leukemia. Based on considerations of convenience, cost, and toxicity, these agents are not usually used as initial therapy for nonmetastatic GTN in the United States.

Few randomized trials have been conducted in patients with low-risk GTN. Lerkhachonsuk and colleagues randomly assigned 49 stage I low-risk patients to the 5-day IV actinomycin-D or IM alternating methotrexate/folinic acid. Six women in the methotrexate arm required cross-over to actinomycin-D because of rising liver function tests. All 20 women in the actinomycin-D arm achieved remission versus 14 (73.6%) in the methotrexate/folinic acid arm ($P = 0.02$). Mucositis and alopecia were more frequent in the actinomycin-D group, whereas elevations of liver function tests were more frequent in the methotrexate/folinic acid group.

Yarand and associates randomly assigned 131 women with FIGO low-risk GTN to pulsed weekly IM methotrexate 30 mg/m^2 versus biweekly IV bolus actinomycin-D 1.25 mg/m^2. Primary remission rates were 48% versus 90% ($P <0.01$) in the methotrexate and actinomycin-D groups, respectively. The mean number of treatment cycles needed to achieve remission was lower in the actinomycin-D group (4.8 vs 6.8). Toxicity was reported as low in each of the treatment arms. Likewise, a recently completed GOG study compared the same regimens in patients with low-risk GTN and reported similar results in an abstract. Further randomized trials are needed to confirm that actinomycin-D is superior to other methotrexate regimens at this time. Unfortunately, none of the trials reported to date have compared long-term effects on ovulation or reproductive function after treatment.

Among patients with nonmetastatic and low-risk GTN, early hysterectomy will shorten the duration and amount of chemotherapy required to produce remission. Therefore, each patient's desire for further childbearing should be evaluated at the onset of treatment. Hysterectomy may be performed during the first cycle of chemotherapy (Figure 7-15). However, further chemotherapy after hysterectomy is mandatory until hCG values are normal.

Treatment for nonmetastatic and low-risk metastatic GTN is outlined in Table 7-10. Most centers in the United States will begin therapy with the bolus actinomycin-D regimen or weekly IM methotrexate. Weekly hCG values should be monitored during treatment, along with hematologic and metabolic studies to monitor for toxicity. Chemotherapy is repeated until hCG levels normalize and at least one cycle of chemotherapy is given as maintenance chemotherapy to prevent recurrence. Reliable contraception should be used to prevent an intercurrent pregnancy during chemotherapy and monitoring after remission.

Patients in whom the rate of fall of hCG levels has plateaued or values are rising during therapy should be switched to an alternative single-agent regimen after radiographic restaging. If there are new metastases or failure of the alternative single-agent chemotherapy, the patient should be treated with multiagent regimens. Hysterectomy should be considered for the treatment of disease that is refractory to chemotherapy and confined to the uterus.

The overall cure rate for patients with nonmetastatic and low-risk GTN approaches 100%. The majority of women who wish to preserve fertility can be cured without hysterectomy. When chemotherapy is given for an additional 1 to 2 cycles after the first normal hCG value, recurrence rates are less than 5%.

High-Risk Metastatic Gestational Trophoblastic Neoplasia

Patients with metastatic disease and one or more of the Clinical Classification system risk factors or a FIGO risk score of 7 or greater have high-risk disease. They will require multiagent chemotherapy, often with additional surgery or radiation incorporated into treatment. It should be emphasized that patients with high-risk metastatic GTN should have their treatment directed by individuals who have experience in treating this relatively rare disease, preferably in a trophoblastic disease center. Survival ranges are up to 86%. In contrast to patients with nonmetastatic or low-risk metastatic GTN, early hysterectomy does not appear to improve the outcome in women with high-risk metastatic disease.

Aggressive treatment with multiagent chemotherapy is the major component for management of these patients. Triple therapy (Table 7-11) with methotrexate, actinomycin-D, and either chlorambucil or cyclophosphamide (MAC) was the standard regimen for many years in the United States, producing sustained remission rates of 63% to 73%. Studies from the Southeastern Regional and the Brewer Trophoblastic Disease Centers in the 1970s documented the importance of initial combination chemotherapy for these patients; single-agent

regimens followed by multiagent chemotherapy produced only 14% to 39% remissions, whereas patients with high-risk GTN treated initially with MAC chemotherapy had remission rates of 65% to 70%. Some studies indicated that patients with extremely high WHO prognostic index scores had poor survival following MAC chemotherapy.

In the late 1970s the Charing Cross group developed a complex, alternating regimen using cyclophosphamide, hydroxyurea, actinomycin-D, methotrexate/folinic acid, vincristine, and doxorubicin (CHAMOCA). Sustained remissions were reported for 56% to 83% of patients with high-risk GTN using modifications of this regimen, with an overall impression of reduced toxicity compared to previous experience with MAC. However, when the Gynecologic Oncology Group performed a randomized trial of MAC versus CHAMOCA, the primary remission rates were comparable at 73% and 65%, respectively. Of note, five of six patients who failed MAC were salvaged compared to only one of seven patients failing CHAMOCA. Perhaps initial exposure to marginally effective additional agents in CHAMOCA adversely affected the efficacy or tolerance of savage regimens. Furthermore, the CHAMOCA regimen had significantly more acute life-threatening toxicity, with a 45% incidence of grade 4 toxicity compared to only 9% with MAC ($P < 0.05$).

More recent regimens have incorporated etoposide into primary combination chemotherapy for GTN. Alternating weekly chemotherapy (Table 7-12) with etoposide, methotrexate/folinic acid rescue, actinomycin-D/cyclophosphamide, and vincristine (EMA/CO) was first developed by the Charing Cross group. Their initial report documented survival of 30 (86%) of 36 patients

TABLE 7-11 Triple Agent (MAC) Chemotherapy for High-Risk Gestational Trophoblastic Neoplasia

Day	Drug	Dose
1-5	Methotrexate	15 mg IM
	Actinomycin-D	500 mcg IV
	Chlorambucil	8-10 mg PO
	OR	
	Cyclophosphamide	3 mg/kg IV
15-22	Begin next cycle	

IM, Intramuscular; IV, intravenous; PO, oral.

TABLE 7-12 Alternating Weekly EMA/CO Chemotherapy for High-Risk Gestational Trophoblastic Neoplasia

Day	Drug	Dose
1	Etoposide	100 mg/m² IV
	Methotrexate*	100 mg/m² IV bolus
	Methotrexate	200 mg/m² IV infusion over 12 hours
	Actinomycin-D	350 mcg/m² IV
2	Etoposide	100 mg/m² IV
	Actinomycin-D	350 mcg/m² IV
	Folinic acid	15 mg PO, IM or IV every 12 hours × 4 doses, begin 24 hours after methotrexate bolus
8†	Cyclophosphamide	600 mg/m² IV
	Vincristine	1 mg/m² IV
15	Begin next cycle	

Methotrexate is sometimes given as a 12-hour IV infusion at a dose of 500-1000 mg/m² for treatment of brain metastases, with folinic acid rescue increased to 15 mg every 6 hours × 48 hours or 30 mg every 12 hours × 48 hours.
†*Some investigators give methotrexate 15 mg intrathecal injection for prophylaxis or treatment of brain metastases.*
IM, Intramuscular; IV, intravenous; PO, oral.

TABLE 7-13 Management of High-Risk GTN

Evaluate for high-risk metastases: brain, liver, kidney
Stabilize medical status of patient
Multiagent therapy with EMA/CO (Table 7-12) or MAC
- Aggressive recycling may require cytokine support
Management of brain metastases (see text):
- Consider early neurosurgical intervention if isolated brain lesion
- Consider stereotactic or whole brain irradiation if multiple brain lesions
Management of liver metastases (see text):
- Consider selective angiographic embolization or irradiation
Monitor hCG weekly during therapy
At least three cycles of maintenance chemotherapy after hCG values normalize

with high-risk GTN after primary treatment with EMA/CO. In their updated series, Bower and associates included 272 patients with high-risk GTN treated with EMA/CO. Complete remission was recorded in 213 (78%), whereas 33 patients who failed EMA/CO were salvaged with additional therapies, resulting in an overall 5-year survival of 86.2%. Other smaller retrospective series have reported complete response rates of 65% to 94% among patients with high-risk GTN treated initially with EMA/CO. As a result of these reports, EMA/CO has become the most widely used regimen for treatment of patients with high-risk GTN.

Patients receiving primary EMA/CO usually have limited toxicity; alopecia is almost universal, whereas stomatitis and emetogenic toxicities are frequently seen. Myelosuppression is the acute dose-limiting acute toxicity. Several investigators have used stem cell support with granulocyte colony-stimulating factor to avoid dose reductions or treatment delays during EMA/CO therapy. It is unclear whether the cyclophosphamide and vincristine are important components of the EMA/CO regimen; treatment with EMA alone has documented complete response rates of 71% to 78% in high-risk patients, whereas both cyclophosphamide and vincristine contribute to myelosuppression in this regimen.

Platin-containing regimens have also been found to be active in treating GTN. Cisplatin combined with etoposide and actinomycin-D (PEA) demonstrated complete responses in 57% to 100% of patients with high-risk GTN. A 1-day course of cisplatin and etoposide (EP) were originally substituted for CO and combined with EMA to treat patients with refractory GTN. Surwit and Childers successfully treated four high-risk patients initially with EMA/EP, but concerns about acute toxicity have kept it from becoming widely accepted as primary therapy. It should be emphasized that MAC and EMA/CO are the two regimens that have been most extensively evaluated for the treatment of high-risk GTN (Table 7-13), but these have never been compared in a

randomized trial. The majority of the literature for other regimens has been in the form of retrospective analyses of relatively small numbers of patients using slightly different definitions of "high-risk" GTN. Regardless of the regimen selected, aggressive recycling of multiagent therapy is the cornerstone for management of patients with high-risk disease (see Table 7-13). The need for randomized comparisons of EMA/CO or the newer combinations with MAC is obvious, but they are unlikely to be done given the relative rarity of this disease.

Management of cerebral metastases is controversial. Radiation therapy has been used concurrently with chemotherapy in an attempt to limit acute hemorrhagic complications from these metastases. Brain irradiation combined with systemic chemotherapy is successful in controlling brain metastases, with cure rates up to 75% in patients who initially present with brain metastases. However, a similar primary remission rate has also been reported among patients treated with combination regimens that incorporated high-dose systemic methotrexate combined with intrathecal methotrexate infusions without brain irradiation. The best treatment for liver or other high-risk sites of metastases has not been established. Even with intense chemotherapy, additional surgery may be necessary to control hemorrhage from metastases, remove chemoresistant disease, or treat other complications to stabilize high-risk patients during therapy.

Treatment of patients with high-risk GTN who have developed chemoresistant disease is extremely challenging and is largely determined by prior chemotherapy exposure and cumulative toxicity from prior treatment. Patients who have not been exposed to etoposide-containing regimens are usually treated with EMA/CO, with remission rates of 71% to 82% reported for this group in several studies. The Charing Cross group used EMA/EP to treat 34 high-risk patients previously exposed to EMA/CO, reporting remission rates of 95% in patients with hCG level plateau during EMA/CO compared to 75% for those with rising hCG levels. Myelosuppression is more severe in patients receiving regimens for salvage than when they are used as primary therapy.

Variations of combination regimens used in the treatment of testicular and ovarian germ cell tumors have been used as salvage therapy in patients with GTN. Etoposide-platin (± bleomycin ± doxorubicin) and vinblastine-bleomycin-cisplatin have remission rates reported between 50% and 86% in a small series of patients treated with these regimens, but they have long-term survival rates of usually less than 50% and considerable myelosuppression when these combinations are used in a salvage setting. Ifosfamide-containing chemotherapy produced responses in four of five patients reported by Sutton and colleagues, but only one patient

TABLE 7-14   Surveillance During and After Therapy of GTN

Monitor serum quantitative hCG levels every week during chemotherapy:
1. Response: >10% decline in hCG during one cycle
2. Plateau: ±10% change in hCG during one cycle
3. Resistance: >10% rise in hCG during one cycle or plateau for two cycles of chemotherapy
   • Evaluate for new metastases
   • Consider alternative chemotherapy (see text)
   • Consider extirpation of drug-resistant sites of disease
Remission: Three consecutive normal weekly hCG values
1. Maintenance chemotherapy (see text)
Surveillance of remission:
1. hCG values every 2 weeks × 3 months
2. hCG values every month to complete 1 year of follow-up
3. hCG values every 6-12 months indefinitely; at least 3-5 years

had a sustained remission. Anecdotal case reports and small series of patients also indicate activity of paclitaxel regimens, high-dose chemotherapy with autologous bone marrow or colony-stimulating factor support, and 5-FU/actinomycin-D in treating drug-resistant disease.

Chemotherapy is continued until hCG values have normalized, and this is followed by at least three courses of maintenance chemotherapy in the hope of eradicating all viable tumor (Table 7-14). Despite using sensitive hCG assays and maintenance chemotherapy, up to 13% of patients with high-risk disease will develop recurrence after achieving an initial remission.

Surgery

Brewer and associates reported that survival of patients treated with hysterectomy was only 40% for women with nonmetastatic choriocarcinoma and only 19% for those with metastatic choriocarcinoma before effective chemotherapy was developed. The majority of their patients died of progressive disease within 2 years of surgery. The emergence of effective chemotherapy has lessened the importance of surgical procedures for primary management of malignant GTN. However, many procedures remain useful adjuncts when integrated into the management of these patients.

Primary or delayed hysterectomy can be integrated into management to remove central disease, and surgical extirpation of metastases may cure highly selected patients with drug-resistant disease. At Duke University Medical Center, extirpative procedures such as hysterectomy were usually performed during a course of chemotherapy to minimize the possibility of inducing metastases by surgical manipulation of tissues. There did not appear to be an increase in surgical morbidity using this combined modality approach. Surgical procedures are often required during therapy of patients with high-risk disease to treat complications of the disease, such as hemorrhage or abscess, and allow stabilization during chemotherapy.

Percutaneous angiographic embolization can allow relatively noninvasive control of hemorrhagic complications of pelvic tumors or metastatic lesions. Finally, indwelling central venous catheters are useful for most patients with high-risk malignant GTN, who will often require prolonged courses of chemotherapy and intravenous support with blood products, crystalloid, antiemetics, and total parenteral nutrition during treatment.

Most patients with malignant GTN are in their peak reproductive years and do not wish sterilization. Furthermore, the majority can be cured with chemotherapy alone, especially women with nonmetastatic or low-risk metastatic disease. Hysterectomy, however, continues to have a role in the management of women with malignant GTN.

Hammond and colleagues reported an overall 100% sustained remission rate among 194 patients treated at Duke University Medical Center for nonmetastatic or low-risk metastatic GTN. Of these, 162 wished to retain childbearing capacity and 89% were able to avoid hysterectomy. All 32 women treated with primary hysterectomy combined with methotrexate or actinomycin-D single-agent chemotherapy regimens entered sustained remission. When compared to similar patients who had low-risk disease and were treated with chemotherapy alone, patients receiving primary hysterectomy had shorter duration of chemotherapy and lower total dosage of chemotherapy, roughly equivalent to one cycle of chemotherapy. Suzuka and associates also analyzed the total dosage of chemotherapy in women treated with etoposide for low-risk GTN. They found that the total dosage of etoposide was decreased in women with nonmetastatic disease treated with adjuvant hysterectomy compared to those who were treated with chemotherapy alone, again roughly equivalent to a single cycle of chemotherapy. This effect was not observed among their patients with low-risk metastatic disease, where similar total dosages of etoposide were given to patients treated with adjuvant hysterectomy or chemotherapy alone. In other series hysterectomy was incorporated into the primary therapy of approximately 25% of patients with low-risk GTN.

Primary adjuvant hysterectomy was not effective in reducing chemotherapy requirements or improving cure rates for women with high-risk GTN in the experience reported by Hammond and colleagues. These patients usually present with disseminated disease and hysterectomy would be expected to contribute much less to reduction of tumor burden compared to patients with low-risk GTN. Therefore, the major role of primary hysterectomy should be as part of primary treatment for women with nonmetastatic disease or with limited metastatic involvement if there is no wish to preserve fertility.

Delayed hysterectomy is often considered for patients who fail to respond to primary chemotherapy. In the Duke experience reported by Hammond and colleagues, almost all of the patients with low-risk GTN who were treated with a delayed hysterectomy because of resistance to primary chemotherapy achieved remission without requiring multiagent chemotherapy. Others have reported that salvage hysterectomy is effective in producing remissions in most patients with nonmetastatic or low-risk metastatic disease. Control of extrauterine disease is central in the success of salvage hysterectomy for these patients.

Salvage hysterectomy may be integrated into the treatment of selected patients with high-risk metastatic GTN who have a small extrauterine tumor burden, but results are not as beneficial as in patients with low-risk disease. Patients with recurrent GTN often present with limited extrauterine dissemination and may benefit from salvage hysterectomy. Among 28 women with recurrent GTN treated at Duke University Medical Center, 14 (50%) were selected to undergo salvage hysterectomy during their therapy. The majority of these patients had no radiographic evidence of extrauterine disease, and 10 (83%) had sustained remissions. However, salvage hysterectomy performed when there is disseminated metastasis is unlikely to have a significant impact on the survival of patients with high-risk or recurrent GTN.

PSTT is much rarer than invasive mole or gestational choriocarcinoma. In contrast to other forms of GTN, production of hCG is relatively lower and these tumors are usually resistant to conventional methotrexate- or actinomycin-D-based chemotherapy regimens. Papadopoulos and colleagues noted that two thirds of their patients were cured following surgery alone if PSTT was confined to the uterus, similar to the reported experience of others in smaller series. Hysterectomy should be integrated into the primary management of PSTT unless there are widespread metastases or in the rare case of localized disease that has been removed by D&C or localized myometrial resection in a woman who strongly desires childbearing.

The majority of women undergoing hysterectomy for malignant GTN have been treated with abdominal hysterectomy, with or without preservation of the adnexa. Ovarian removal is not required because GTN rarely metastasizes to the ovaries and these tumors are not hormonally influenced. Vaginal hysterectomy may be considered in women with nonmetastatic GTN who have a small uterus and low hCG levels, but it does not allow assessment of the upper abdomen for occult metastases. Laparoscopic assisted vaginal hysterectomy (LAVH) or total laparoscopic hysterectomy (TLH) has been used in a few patients with GTN. In contrast to vaginal hysterectomy, LAVH and TLH allow surveillance of the upper abdomen combined with a shorter acute convalescence than abdominal hysterectomy.

More conservative myometrial resections combined with uterine reconstruction can be considered in highly selected patients with nonmetastatic GTN who wish to avoid hysterectomy. Previous anecdotal reports of local myometrial resections of invasive moles have documented the use of resection and uterine repair for primary therapy of nonmetastatic GTN and PSTT. Kanazawa and colleagues evaluated this procedure in 22 patients with invasive moles diagnosed on the basis of abnormal hCG regression after molar evacuation. All patients had lesions localized in the myometrium and defined by pelvic angiography, ultrasound, and computerized tomography techniques. Seven (32%) of their patients required chemotherapy after surgery. Pregnancies have been documented after conservative resections of invasive moles; Kanazawa and colleagues observed that reproductive performance was similar to that of patients treated with chemotherapy alone. Because of the high cure rates reported following chemotherapy alone in similar patients, it is more rational to consider these as salvage procedures in women with localized chemoresistant disease. Each patient considered for this procedure should be carefully evaluated for systemic metastases and the uterine lesion should be localized using a combination of color-flow ultrasound, MRI, and hysteroscopy. Intraoperative frozen sections should be used to assess surgical margins. Small lesions associated with low hCG levels are more likely to be completely excised with a conservative myometrial resection than lesions greater than 2 to 3 cm in diameter.

The most frequently used surgical procedure for extirpation of extrauterine metastases of GTN is thoracotomy with pulmonary wedge resection, but there are few large series of patients reported recently because of the relative rarity for the need to perform extirpation of metastases. Although this can safely be performed in conjunction with chemotherapy, it is not necessary to resect lung metastases in the majority of patients. Radiographic evidence of tumor regression often lags behind hCG response to treatment and some patients will have persistent pulmonary nodules months after completion of therapy. In women with low-risk GTN the overall risk of recurrence is less than 5%. Even though women with persistent pulmonary nodules may be at an increased risk for recurrence, these patients can be safely followed with serial hCG levels without surgical resection.

Many series of patients with GTN treated with thoracotomy include patients whose disease was not suspected until after resection of a pulmonary nodule. As in the case of brain, liver, or renal metastases, any woman of reproductive age who presents with an apparent metastatic malignancy of unknown primary site should be screened for the possibility of GTN with a serum hCG level. Excisional biopsy is not indicated to histologically confirm the diagnosis of malignant GTN if the patient is not pregnant and has a high hCG value.

Resection of pulmonary nodules in highly selected patients with drug-resistant disease may successfully induce remission. Immediately before performing pulmonary resection, it is important to exclude the possibility of active disease elsewhere by performing a comprehensive metastatic survey. Patients with isolated, unilateral nodules associated with low hCG values are much more likely to benefit from thoracotomy with pulmonary resection than patients with bilateral or multiple unilateral lesions or those with disease in other locations. Tomoda and colleagues reported that 14 (93%) of their 15 patients with isolated nodules and low hCG values survived after pulmonary resection, compared to none of 4 patients with either hCG values greater than 1000 mIU/ml or evidence of active disease elsewhere. Others have reported that hCG level remission within 1 to 2 weeks of surgery portends a favorable outcome. Highly selected patients will require more than one pulmonary resection during the course of treatment in order to achieve a durable remission.

Brain metastases (Figure 7-16) occur in 8% to 15% of patients with metastatic GTN and are associated with a worse prognosis than vaginal or pulmonary metastases. Metastases from GTN tend to be highly vascular and have a tendency for central necrosis and hemorrhage. A significant portion of early deaths is caused by central nervous system metastases of GTN with acute neurologic deterioration before effective therapy is initiated or very early in the course of treatment. The major goals of treatment include early detection of brain metastases through complete radiologic metastatic survey, stabilization of the patient's neurologic status, and initiation of therapy. Craniotomy solely for the purpose of tissue confirmation is not justified if GTN is clinically diagnosed on the basis of metastatic disease associated with an elevated hCG level.

In series of patients with brain metastases of GTN reported from the United States, brain irradiation is usually integrated into treatment in an attempt to prevent hemorrhage and neurologic deterioration. Craniotomy is usually used only to prevent deterioration. However, Rustin and colleagues recommended an approach using early craniotomy with excision of isolated lesions combined with high-dose systemic and intrathecal chemotherapy to treat patients with brain metastases. In their experience, brain irradiation was not used routinely. Both primary radiation therapy combined with chemotherapy and the approach emphasizing early surgical intervention appear to have similar efficacy in previously untreated patients. In sharp contrast to the outlook for women with brain metastases from other solid

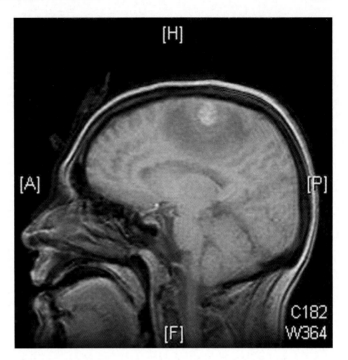

FIGURE 7-16 Brain magnetic resonance image of a patient presenting with high-risk metastatic GTN, pulmonary metastases, and seizures associated with a solitary brain metastasis. She is in remission following surgical resection of this brain lesion during her first cycle of chemotherapy followed by multiple cycles of chemotherapy with high-dose methotrexate combinations, platin-taxane, and hysterectomy. *(Courtesy John Soper, MD.)*

tumors, 75% to 80% of women with brain metastases presenting for primary therapy and 50% of patients overall with brain metastases from malignant GTN will be cured. Craniotomy for resection of drug-resistant brain lesions is only rarely performed. In these patients, it is important to exclude active disease elsewhere before attempting surgical resection. Sometimes craniotomy is required for women who require acute decompression of central nervous system hemorrhagic lesions to allow stabilization and institution of therapy.

Surgical extirpation of metastatic disease at other sites is occasionally beneficial for primary or salvage therapy of malignant GTN. Because PSTT is more often resistant to conventional chemotherapeutic agents, multiple surgical resections of metastatic sites may be required in highly selected patients in order to produce a cure. In general, resection of distant metastases is unlikely to be successful if there is evidence of disseminated disease resistant to chemotherapy.

Vaginal metastases of malignant GTN are highly vascular, originating via metastasis through the submucosal venous plexus of the vagina. These should not be biopsied or resected unless they represent the only site of drug-resistant disease. Biopsy of a metastatic vaginal lesion often results in massive hemorrhage. Packing or

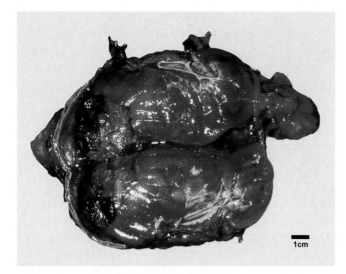

FIGURE 7-17   Nephrectomy specimen with a large hemorrhagic metastasis of choriocarcinoma involving the superior pole. (*Courtesy John Soper, MD.*)

angiographic localization with selective embolization is usually used in an attempt to control bleeding from vaginal metastases during initial therapy.

Renal metastases occur in 1% to 20% of patients treated for metastatic GTN. They are usually associated with other high-risk factors and disseminated disease. All three survivors with renal metastases treated at Duke University Medical Center had nephrectomy incorporated into initial therapy (Figure 7-17); however, three of the five fatalities also underwent nephrectomy. Survivors had limited metastatic involvement elsewhere when compared to patients with renal metastases who died. However, the role for this procedure appears limited because others have reported patients with high-risk metastatic GTN involving the kidneys who entered remission after treatment with etoposide-containing chemotherapy regimens without nephrectomy.

Less than 5% of patients with metastatic GTN have initial involvement of other intra-abdominal organs or the gastrointestinal tract. Most often these patients' illness can be managed with chemotherapy alone, but occasional patients will develop bleeding that requires resection for stabilization. Liver metastases, although prone to catastrophic intra-abdominal hemorrhage, are less likely to be successfully controlled with surgical resection. Selective angiographic embolization techniques should be considered as an option if possible. Only rarely will resection of isolated liver metastases be feasible for treatment of drug-resistant disease because most patients will have other sites of active disease or diffuse involvement of the liver.

Approximately 30% of patients with high-risk malignant GTN require other procedures, such as D&C or drainage of an abscess, for stabilization during therapy.

Another ancillary procedure that is often used is insertion of a tunneled catheter or subcutaneous infusion port to provide long-term venous access among patients with high-risk GTN. These patients often require prolonged courses of chemotherapy, transfusion of blood products, nutritional support, and antibiotics during the course of their treatment.

With the development of advanced interventional radiology techniques, selective angiographic localization and embolization techniques have been used to conservatively manage hemorrhage from active sites of metastatic GTN and to treat intrauterine arteriovenous malformations (AVM) that can occasionally develop after treatment of GTN. Vaginal metastases are the site of active disease most often treated with selective angiographic embolization, when simple packing or suturing techniques have failed to control hemorrhage. Grumbine and associates managed a patient with liver metastases of GTN with the prophylactic placement of a catheter in the hepatic artery for balloon occlusion or embolization in the event of rupture, and others have successfully used selective embolization to treat hemorrhage from hepatic metastases. Lang used selective catheter placement for chemoembolization in three patients with liver metastases and two with pelvic tumors from GTN. All had chemoresistant GTN and relatively localized persistent tumors. Two of the patients with liver metastases achieved long-term remissions, with minimal hematologic toxicity recorded during treatment.

Angiographic abnormalities in the uterus caused by GTD can persist for many months after evacuation of hydatidiform mole or treatment of malignant GTN. The occurrence of intractable bleeding from intrauterine AVM after successful treatment for GTD is a relatively rare complication. Lim and colleagues reported 14 patients treated over a 20-year interval with selective angiographic embolization for this indication. Hemorrhage was initially controlled with the first procedure in 11 (78%) and 6 (45%) patients required a second embolization for treatment of recurrent bleeding, while only 2 (15%) patients required hysterectomy. Successful term pregnancies have been reported after this procedure.

Radiation Therapy

With the continued evolution of chemotherapy regimens active in this disease, radiation therapy has a limited role in the management of patients with malignant GTD. Radiation is used most frequently to treat patients with brain or liver metastases in an effort to minimize hemorrhagic complications from disease at these sites.

Brace first reported control of brain metastases using 2000 cGy whole brain irradiation for patients with GTN treated at the NIH with single-agent regimens. He reported 5 (24%) survivors among 21 patients treated for brain metastases; 3 required re-treatment for recurrent symptoms of intracranial disease. Whole brain irradiation has been used in the majority of series of patients with brain metastases reported from the United States. Most series report administration of between 2000 and 4000 cGy in 10 to 20 equal fractions that are given concurrently with combination chemotherapy, with reduced field boosts given in selected patients. Total doses correlate with control of central nervous system metastases. Schecter and colleagues reported that the 5-year actuarial local control for patients given doses less than 2200 cGy was only 24%, significantly worse than 91% local control among patients given 2200 to 6000 cGy.

Survival rates of 50% to 75% are reported in series of patients who initially presented with brain metastases and received combined chemoradiation. Survival of these patients is influenced in part by the extent and subsequent control of extracranial disease, in addition to the extent of central nervous system involvement. Small and colleagues reported that women who were asymptomatic at presentation had a 100% survival rate compared to only 38% survival rate in those who presented with symptoms from brain metastases, a significant difference. Evans and associates reported that patients with new brain metastases diagnosed at the time of recurrence or who developed brain metastases during chemotherapy had survival rates of only 38% and 0%, respectively. These groups had significantly worse survival than the 75% survival rates of their patients, who presented with brain metastases for primary therapy.

Chronic central nervous system toxicity such as mental retardation has been reported among long-term survivors of leukemia and other tumors treated with a combination of whole brain irradiation and concurrent moderate-dose methotrexate regimens. These reports have diminished the enthusiasm for combining whole brain radiation with chemotherapy regimens that incorporate infusions of 300 to 1000 mg/m² of methotrexate used to treat GTN, such as EMA/CO. Stereotactic treatment of individual brain metastases could be considered in these circumstances, but concerns persist that therapeutic levels of chemotherapy might not cross the blood–brain barrier, allowing development of occult brain metastases outside of the radiated fields. However, 6- to 12-hour infusions of methotrexate greater than 500 mg/m² result in therapeutic cerebrospinal fluid levels of methotrexate, suggesting that doses of methotrexate in these ranges should be used when focal irradiation or surgical resection of individual brain metastases is performed. The group at Charing Cross Hospital reported 80% survival for patients who received primary therapy with this approach. They did not routinely administer radiotherapy to their patients and advocated early neurosurgical intervention. Although the number of patients available for randomization between concurrent

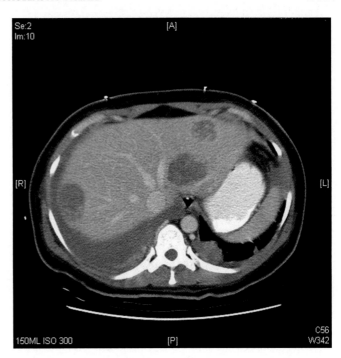

FIGURE 7-18 Multiple liver metastases in a woman presenting less than 4 weeks after term delivery with lung, brain, and liver metastases of GTN. Selective hepatic arterial embolization was required to control bleeding from the hepatic metastases; note fluid density around liver from intra-abdominal blood. This patient was treated aggressively with multimodality therapy and placed into remission. (*Courtesy John Soper, MD.*)

chemoradiation and combined systemic/intrathecal chemotherapy is small, the need for comparative studies is obvious.

Hepatic metastases are identified in 2% to 8% of patients presenting for primary therapy of malignant GTN (Figure 7-18). Involvement of the liver constitutes a poor prognostic factor, as evidenced by survival rates of 40% to 50% for women with primary liver involvement and dismal survival for those who develop new liver metastases during therapy. These are highly vascular and tend to produce catastrophic intra-abdominal hemorrhage. In an attempt to minimize this risk, patients treated at Duke University Medical Center for liver metastases received approximately 2000 cGy whole liver irradiation concurrently with MAC chemotherapy. Administration of chemotherapy was limited in only 1 of 15 patients because of hepatitis, but survival was very poor among these patients, with only 2 (13%) survivors overall and no survivors among patients who developed liver metastases during therapy. Bakri and colleagues reported survival in none of their patients who were treated with methotrexate-dactinomycin-cyclophosphamide combined with whole liver radiation, compared with survival in 5 of 8 patients who were treated with etoposide-based combination regimens. Others have

TABLE 7-15   Treatment Results for GTN

CLINICAL CLASSIFICATION	Survivors/Total	Life Table Survival
Nonmetastatic	226/227	99.7%
METASTATIC		
Good prognosis	91/91	100%
Poor prognosis	54/67	79.1%
WHO CLASSIFICATION (SCORE)		
Low risk (<5)	310/311	99.8%
Medium risk (5-7)	34/36	94.4%
High risk (>7)	27/38	68.4%

Modified from Soper JT, Evans AC, Conaway MR et al: Obstet Gynecol 84:969, 1994.

reported survival of approximately 27% among patients treated with etoposide-based regimens without hepatic irradiation.

Radiation therapy is occasionally administered to other sites of disease in an attempt to treat drug-resistant foci, with anecdotal responses to multimodality therapy. However, the overall efficacy of radiation therapy to sites other than the brain is unclear. Most of the successes probably reflect the summation of an aggressive multimodality approach to individual patients with high-risk metastatic GTN.

It must be emphasized that cure rates of 75% to 86% for patients with high-risk metastatic GTN are reported from centers that specialize in the treatment of women with this relatively rare malignancy. Patients with high-risk disease present multiple challenges for management. They often require a highly individualized approach to address the extent of their disease and treatment toxicity. All women with high-risk disease should be treated by physicians experienced in the management of patients with GTN who can coordinate all aspects of therapy. The overall treatment results for patients with malignant GTN at Duke University Medical Center are displayed in Table 7-15.

Placental Site Trophoblastic Tumor

This rare tumor has the potential to metastasize and cause death. Approximately 100 cases have been reported in the literature. It may be found after abortion, mole, or normal pregnancy. Bleeding, the most common symptom, can appear shortly after termination of pregnancy or years later. Bleeding is often accompanied by uterine enlargement and the diagnosis of pregnancy is often entertained. The result of a pregnancy test may be positive, but these tumors characteristically produce lower levels of intact hCG than other forms of GTD. Gross uterine findings may vary from a diffuse nodular enlargement of the myometrium, which is usually well circumscribed, to a large polypoid projection into the uterine cavity with involvement of the myometrium. Invasion may extend to the serosa or even with extension to the adnexae. Microscopically, it is difficult to differentiate from benign trophoblastic infiltration. It is characterized by mononuclear infiltration of the uterus and its blood vessels with occasional multinucleated giant cells. The predominant cell is an intermediate trophoblast with large polyhedral cells and pleomorphic nuclei. Occasionally, syncytial trophoblast giant cells are present. Mitotic counts have not been a reliable prognostic factor.

PSTTs must be distinguished from choriocarcinoma and can occasionally be interpreted as sarcomas. Histochemical stains for human placental lactogen are usually diffusely positive but only focally positive for hCG. The serum hCG, although elevated enough to give a positive pregnancy test result, is often low, even with metastasis; therefore, it is a poor predictor of prognosis. Most of these tumors behave in a locally aggressive fashion, although they may metastasize, with at least 20 deaths reported, indicating approximately a 15% to 20% mortality rate. Metastases have been reported at various sites. Some patients may be cured with a D&C only, but a hysterectomy is considered optimal therapy and is usually adequate in most situations. Swisher and Drescher reported a complete response to EMA/CO in a patient with metastasis to lung and vagina. In their review, 2 of 7 patients treated with EMA/CO had a complete response. In a review by Chang and associates of 88 patients with placental site tumor, 58 of 62 patients with FIGO stage I and II survived and were treated mainly with a hysterectomy with or without chemotherapy. Apparently, 9 of 10 patients survived after a D&C alone. Only 7 of 21 patients with stage III or IV disease survived. All received chemotherapy, and only 6 received a hysterectomy. Leiserowitz and Webb reported a patient whose tumor was localized with ultrasonography and MRI and treated with local excision and uterine reconstruction. Surgical-free margins were present, and the patient has had three subsequent pregnancies including two spontaneous abortions and one term delivery.

OTHER CONSIDERATIONS

Future Childbearing

After effective treatment for malignant GTN, molar pregnancies occur in only about 1% to 2% of subsequent pregnancies, and many patients have subsequently had normal gestations without difficulty (Table 7-16). Because of the increased risk for the development of a mole in subsequent pregnancies, it is reasonable to evaluate these pregnancies with first-trimester ultrasonography.

TABLE 7-16 Fertility after Treatment for GTN

Desired Fertility	109/122 (89%) Patients	
REPRODUCTIVE OUTCOME		
Infertility	62/109 (57%) patients	
Pregnancies	47/109 (43%) patients	57 pregnancies
Normal infants		45*/57 (79%)
Spontaneous abortion		7/57 (12%)
Therapeutic abortion		3/57 (5%)
Mole		2/57 (4%)

Modified from Hammond CB, Weed JC Jr, Currie JL: Am J Obstet Gynecol 136:844, 1980.
*Two sets of twins.

A particular dilemma has been noted in women undergoing ovulation induction after previous molar gestations. In such cases, patients have occasionally developed repeated hydatidiform moles or malignant GTN subsequent to the implementation of assisted reproductive technologies. In one such patient, in vitro fertilization (IVF) of oocytes retrieved showed a significantly high incidence of abnormal fertilization resulting in the development of triploid embryos. The authors suggested the possible association of an oocyte defect predisposing to abnormal fertilization resulting in the high incidence of triploid embryos. Investigators have proposed the use of intracytoplasmic sperm injection (ICSI) with preimplantation genetic diagnosis or donor oocyte IVF as therapeutic alternatives in these cases.

It appears that the pregnancy outcomes in women with history of molar gestations are no different from the outcomes in women who have no such history with respect to term live births, first- and second-trimester abortions, anomalies, stillbirths, prematurity, and primary cesarean section rate (see Table 7-16). For individuals with prior molar gestations, subsequent pregnancy outcome appears similar irrespective of whether the mole is complete or partial.

Treatment of malignant GTN with chemotherapy is compatible with the preservation of fertility and is not associated with an increased risk of congenital malformations. Ayhan and colleagues from Turkey reported on 49 women who had received chemotherapy for GTN and subsequently became pregnant a total of 65 times with 42 (64.7%) term births and 3 (4.6%) molar pregnancies. No congenital malformations or obstetric complications were observed. Of the 63 patients in the Southeastern Trophoblastic Center study of poor prognosis metastatic GTN, only 19 were able to preserve their reproductive capacity. Only 4 of these patients have had subsequent pregnancies that resulted in 1 spontaneous abortion and 4 normal deliveries.

In the Charing Cross experience of women treated with EMA/CO, 56% of women who were in remission for at least 2 years and had fertility-conserving therapy achieved pregnancy after completing EMA/CO. At the time of their report there were 112 live births including 3 babies with congenital abnormalities. Woolas and colleagues updated the outcome data of posttreatment reproductive intent and outcome from 1121 GTN survivors. Of 728 women who had tried to become pregnant, 607 reported at least 1 live birth, 73 conceived but had not registered a live birth, and 48 did not conceive. No differences were apparent among the 392 women who received methotrexate as single-agent chemotherapy and the 336 treated with multiple-agent chemotherapy. Women who had registered a live birth were significantly younger. They concluded that standard chemotherapy protocols in the treatment of malignant GTN have minimal impact on the subsequent ability to reproduce.

Coexistence of Normal Pregnancy and Gestational Trophoblastic Neoplasia

Rare cases of metastatic GTN coexisting with normal gestations have been reported; some have been treated successfully with delivery and subsequent chemotherapy. In one case, a patient with a normal intrauterine pregnancy of 27 weeks had a coexisting pulmonary metastatic choriocarcinoma. Treatment with single-agent methotrexate during pregnancy resulted in favorable outcomes for both the mother and the child.

Transplacental Fetal Metastases

Rare cases (only 15 to 20 cases have been reported, and only 5 since 1990) of maternal GTN metastatic to the fetus have been described. The diagnosis of widely metastatic disease in the delivered neonate may occur in the absence of metastatic GTN in the mother (found only in retrospective examination of the term placenta) or precede diagnosis of metastatic GTN in the mother.

Survivorship Issues after Successful Treatment of Gestational Trophoblastic Neoplasia

Survivors of nonmalignant and malignant GTN may be at risk for unique physical and psychosocial problems. This generally relates to the increased risk for the development of secondary malignancies after treatment with agents such as etoposide and to issues related to reproductive capacity.

Rustin conducted a population-based study in the United Kingdom analyzing the incidence of secondary malignancies after successful treatment of malignant GTN. Using a sophisticated epidemiologic design, an overall 50% excess of risk (RR = 1.5, 95% CI, 1.1-2.1; P <0.011) was observed. The risk was significantly increased for myeloid leukemia (RR = 16.6; 95% CI, 5.4-38.9), colon (RR = 4.6; 95% CI, 1.5-10.7), and breast cancer when the survival exceeded 25 years (RR = 5.8; 95% CI, 1.2-16.9). The risk was not significantly increased among the 554 women who received single-agent therapy (RR = 1.3; 95% CI, 0.6-2.1). Leukemias only developed in patients who received etoposide plus other cytotoxic drugs. Wenzel and colleagues reported on 76 women with GTN from the New England Trophoblastic Disease Center in regard to chronic psychosocial effects. Across all levels of disease, they found that patients with GTN experience clinically significant levels of anxiety, anger, fatigue, confusion, and sexual problems and are significantly affected by pregnancy concerns for protracted periods.

For full reference list, log onto www.expertconsult.com ⟨http://www.expertconsult.com⟩.

8

Invasive Cancer of the Vulva

Jeanne M. Schilder, MD, and Frederick B. Stehman, MD

The International Federation of Gynecology and Obstetrics (FIGO) 6th Annual Report published in 2006 noted that cancer of the vulva accounted for 4% of all female genital malignant neoplasms. With the exception of the rare sarcomas, the peak incidence is in women between 65 and 75 years old (Figure 8-1); in some series, almost half are 70 years of age or older. Classically, vulvar cancer has been a disease of elderly women, but the trend in recent years is an increasing prevalence among younger women, which cannot be accounted for by immunocompromised patients alone. Many authors have observed this shift in the demographics of women developing vulvar cancer and have proposed age-dependent risk factors. Younger women are more likely to have early-stage disease arising in a field of human papillomavirus (HPV)–related preinvasive disease and often have a history of tobacco use. HPV-related preinvasive lesions are rare in older women, and these malignancies may be found in association with chronic vulvar dystrophies, such as lichen sclerosis, although a direct association has not been proven. No race or culture is spared, and gravidity and parity are not involved in the pathogenesis of this neoplasm. Vulvar cancer is common in the poor and elderly in most parts of the world, and this has led to the hypothesis that inadequate personal hygiene and medical care are contributing factors in this disease.

Younger patients frequently have early stromal invasion associated with diffuse intraepithelial neoplasia of the vulvar skin. Choo found 17 patients younger than age 35 years with invasive carcinoma of the vulva. Of these, 8 had microinvasion. Al-Ghamdi evaluated 21 patients younger than age 40 years with invasive vulvar cancer and found that most, but not all, had associated HPV. Outcomes in these populations were excellent. Lanneau and colleagues have corroborated these results in a study that evaluated 56 women younger than age 45 with squamous cell carcinoma of the vulva. They concluded that vulvar cancer in this population is associated with early-stage disease, HPV, vulva intraepithelial neoplasia (VIN), and smoking.

The development of squamous cell carcinoma of the vulva may be similar to the process that occurs on the cervix. The association between HPV and both preinvasive and invasive urogenital lesions has been well described. Susceptibility of the cervical, vaginal, and

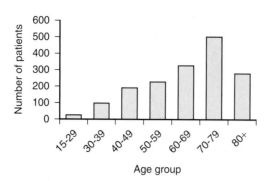

Age group	Patients (*n*)	Percentage (%)
15-29	22	1.3
30-39	97	5.9
40-49	188	11.4
50-59	227	13.7
60-69	332	20.1
70-79	505	30.6
80+	280	17.0
Total	1651	100.0

FIGURE 8-1   Carcinoma of the vulva: Patients treated in 1999-2001. *(Adapted from the 6th Annual Report on the Results of Treatment in Gynecological Cancer. Int J Gynaecol Obstet Vol 95, 2006.)*

vulvar epithelium is referred to as the "field effect." This effect is more pronounced in tobacco users and in patients who are immunocompromised, such as those with HIV/AIDS, or organ transplant recipients. The association of condyloma acuminatum with vulvar carcinoma is well known, but no cause and effect relationship has been confirmed as yet. HPV is suspected in the etiology of squamous neoplasia of the vulva, as it is in similar lesions of the cervix. Bloss and colleagues looked at the clinical and histologic features of vulvar carcinomas analyzed for HPV status. Of 21 invasive carcinomas of the vulva analyzed, 10 were found to contain HPV-16 DNA. Others have confirmed this observation, suggesting that HPV DNA associations with malignant changes of the vulva are similar to those observed elsewhere in the genital tract. The correlation is not as strong as in VIN. Andersen and colleagues, among others, noted a variable detection rate of HPV nucleic acids in vulvar cancer. Only 13% of the invasive lesions contained HPV on analysis by in situ hybridization.

Many previously reported associated features seen in patients with vulvar cancer, such as diabetes, obesity, hypertension, and arteriosclerosis, may just reflect the increased incidence of these diseases associated with aging.

INVASIVE SQUAMOUS CELL CARCINOMA

Histology

The overwhelming majority of all vulvar cancer is squamous in origin. The vulva is covered with skin, and any malignant change that appears elsewhere on the skin can occur in this region. Table 8-1 depicts the incidence of vulvar neoplasia from several collected studies in the literature. The following discussion focuses mainly on squamous cell carcinoma because of its preponderance,

TABLE 8-1   Incidence of Vulvar Neoplasms by Histologic Type*

Tumor Type	%
Epidermoid	86.2
Melanoma	4.8
Sarcoma	2.2
Basal cell	1.4
Bartholin gland	
Squamous	0.4
Adenocarcinoma	0.6 } 1.2
Adenocarcinoma	0.6
Undifferentiated	3.9

Modified from Plentl AA, Friedman EA: Lymphatic system of the female genitalia. Philadelphia, WB Saunders, 1971.
*Based on 1378 reported cases.

but as a generalization, the other lesions can be treated similarly, except as noted.

Clinical Presentation and Diagnosis

In many cases of squamous cell vulvar cancer, the initial lesion appears to arise from an area of intraepithelial neoplasia that subsequently develops into a small nodule that may break down and ulcerate (Figures 8-2 and 8-3). On other occasions, small, warty, or cauliflower-like growths evolve, and these may be confused with condyloma acuminatum. Long-term pruritus or a lump or mass on the vulva is present in more than 50% of patients with invasive vulvar cancer (Table 8-2). Biopsy must be done of all suspicious lesions of the vulva, including lumps, ulcers, and pigmented areas, even in the patient not complaining of burning or itching (Table 8-3).

Significant delay in diagnosis and appropriate treatment is not uncommon. Several series of carcinoma of the vulva report a delay of 2 to 16 months following onset of symptoms before medical attention is sought. Further delay can occur when medical treatment of vulvar lesions continues without biopsy for definitive diagnosis or referral.

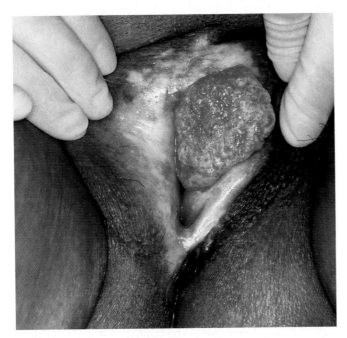

FIGURE 8-2 Squamous cell carcinoma arising in a bed of lichen sclerosis.

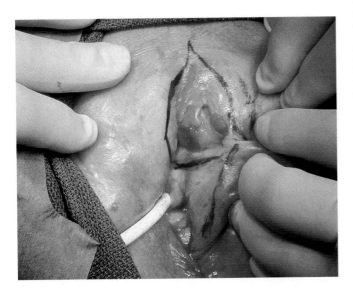

FIGURE 8-3 Small, well-localized lesion of the vulva.

Fortunately, vulvar cancer is commonly indolent, extends slowly, and metastasizes fairly late. Hence, we have a good opportunity for preventing the serious advanced stages of this disease through education of patients and physicians. Lawhead proposed a technique for routine vulvar self-examination and urges that this practice be incorporated into every woman's preventive health care regimen.

TABLE 8-2 Signs and Symptoms of Vulvar Cancer

Sign/Symptom	%
Pruritus	45.0
Mass	45.0
Pain	23.0
Bleeding	14.0
Ulceration	14.0
Dysuria	10.0
Discharge	8.0
Groin mass	2.5

TABLE 8-3 Indications for Excisional Biopsy of Vulvar Lesions

Change in surface area of nevus
Change in elevation of a lesion: raised, thickened, or nodular
Change in color: especially brown to black
Change in surface: smooth to scaly or ulcerated
Change in sensation: itching or tingling

Location and Spread Pattern

Primary disease can appear anywhere on the vulva. Approximately 70% arise primarily on the labia. Disease more commonly occurs on the labia majora; however, it may appear on the labia minora, clitoris, or perineum. The disease is usually localized and well demarcated, although it can occasionally be so extensive that the primary location cannot be determined (Figure 8-4). Multifocal growth pattern in invasive squamous cell carcinoma of the vulva is uncommon, except for the so-called kissing lesions that can occur as isolated lesions.

Verrucous carcinoma of the vulva (Figure 8-5) is a special and unusual variant of squamous cell carcinoma that is locally invasive but nonmetastasizing. The lesion, which may involve the cervix, vagina, and the vulva, presents as a warty, fungating, ulcerated mass with a bulky, elevated appearance reminiscent of a benign HPV lesion. Identification of this variant is important because the biologic behavior of the disease influences therapy. Condyloma may initially be diagnosed on microscopic examination, but distinction from ordinary condylomata is aided by the absence of fibrovascular cores within the proliferating papillary masses of tumor. There is usually a uniform lack of malignant features histologically. Adequate material, including underlying stroma for pathologic evaluation, is necessary to differentiate verrucous carcinoma from condyloma. The tumor may invade deeply into the underlying tissue, often requiring extensive surgery, and has a propensity to recur locally. Woodruff noted a lack of lymph node metastases in 27 patients (from the literature and his patients) who were treated with radical vulvectomy and inguinal lymphadenectomy. As a result, he advocated a more conservative approach, with wide local excision and tumor-free

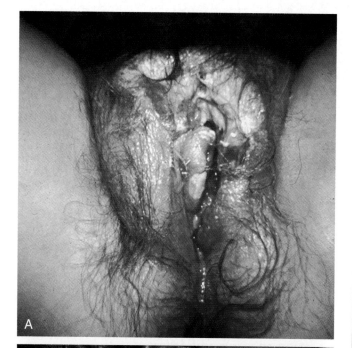

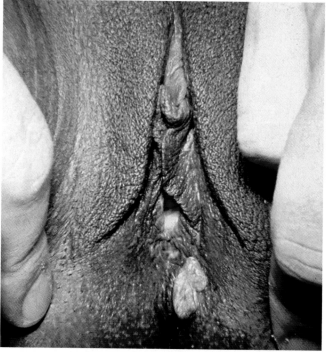

FIGURE 8-5   Verrucous carcinoma of the vulva.

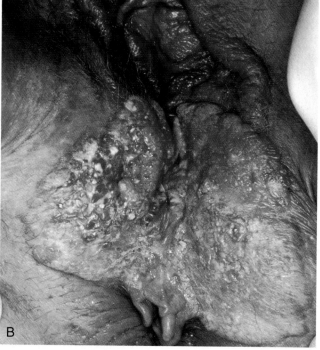

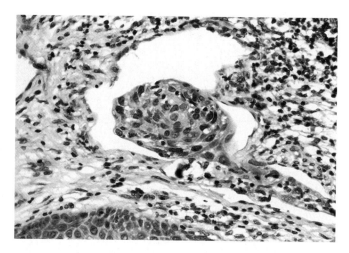

FIGURE 8-6   Photomicrograph of a tumor nodule invading a vulvar lymphatic.

FIGURE 8-4   **A,** Large ulcerating squamous cell malignancy of the vulva with destruction of the clitoris and the urethra. **B,** Large exophytic squamous cell carcinoma of the vulva.

margins as the therapeutic aim. Lymphadenectomy is of questionable value except when nodes are obviously involved. Historically, it was felt that radiotherapy is contraindicated because of its ineffectiveness, and reports indicate that it can be an instigator of more aggressive behavior by this tumor.

Fundamental to the understanding of therapy for invasive cancer of the vulva is thorough knowledge of the lymphatic drainage of this region. In general, the four histologic types of invasive cancer primarily use the lymphatic route for initial metastases (Figure 8-6). Lymphatic drainage of the external genitalia begins with minute papillae, and these are connected in turn to a multilayered meshwork of fine vessels. These fine vessels extend over the entire labium minus, the prepuce of the clitoris, the fourchette, and the vaginal mucosa up to the

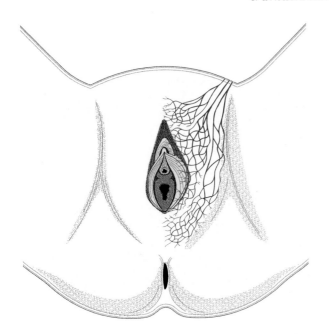

FIGURE 8-7 Lymphatic drainage of the external genitalia.

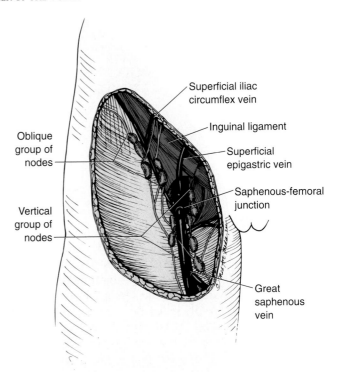

FIGURE 8-8 The superficial inguinal lymph nodes can be divided into the horizontal group and the perpendicular group.

level of the hymenal ring (Figure 8-7). Drainage of these lymphatics extends toward the anterior portion of the labium minus, where they emerge into three or four collecting trunks whose course is toward the mons veneris, bypassing the clitoris. Vessels from the prepuce anastomose with these lymphatics. Similarly, vessels from the labium majus proceed anteriorly to the upper part of the vulva and mons veneris, there joining the vessels of the prepuce and labium minus. These lymphatic vessels abruptly change direction, turning laterally, and terminate in ipsilateral or contralateral femoral nodes. Drainage is usually limited initially to the medial upper quadrant of the femoral node group. The nodes are medial to the great saphenous vein above the cribriform fascia and in turn may drain secondarily to the deep femoral group. The next echelon of nodes is the pelvic/iliac nodes.

The superficial inguinal lymph glands are located immediately beneath the integument and Camper fascia, with an average of 8 to 10 in number. Most authors agree that this is the primary node group for the vulva and can serve as the sentinel lymph nodes (SLNs) (Figure 8-8). The deep femoral nodes, which are by classic teaching located beneath the cribriform fascia, are the secondary node recipients and are involved before drainage into the deep pelvic nodes occurs. The Cloquet node, the last node of the deep femoral group, is located just beneath the Poupart ligament. The multilayered meshwork of lymphatics on the vulva itself is always limited to an area medial to the genitocrural fold (Figure 8-9). Lymphatic drainage of the vulva is a progressive systematic mechanism, and therapy can be

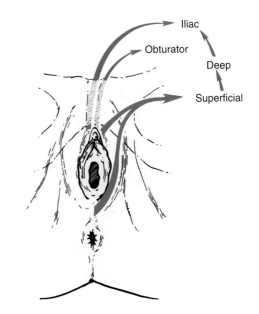

FIGURE 8-9 Lymphatic spread of a vulvar malignancy. See the text for details.

planned according to where in the lymphatic chain tumor is present.

Borgno and colleagues examined 100 inguinal lymphadenectomy specimens at autopsy and demonstrated that the deep femoral nodes are always situated within

TABLE 8-4 Incidence of Positive Nodes

Series	No. of Cases	Positive Groin or Pelvic Nodes (%)	Positive Pelvic Nodes (%)
Morley (1976)	374	37.0	—
Curry, Wharton, and Rutledge (1980)	191	30.0	4.7
Simonsen (1984)	122	50.0	10.0
Sutton et al (1991)	150	24.0	—
Homesley (1994)	277	29.2	—
Creasman et al (1997)	1553	31.0	—

TABLE 8-5 Groin Node vs Tumor Diameter

Feature	N	Positive Groin Nodes	%
TUMOR DIAMETER			
≤2.0 cm	190	36	19
>2.0 cm	390	163	43
INVASION			
≤5 mm	272	57	21
>5 mm	286	137	48
CLINICAL EXAMINATION			
N0-1	477	114	23
N2-3	111	89	80

From Homesley HD et al: Prognostic factors for groin node metastasis in squamous cell carcinoma of the vulva (a Gynecologic Oncology Group study). Gynecol Oncol 49:279, 1993.

the openings in the fascia at the fossa ovalis, and no lymph nodes are distal to the lower margin of the fossa ovalis, under the fascia cribrosa. The implication is that a carefully performed deep femoral lymphadenectomy does not require removal of the fascia lata (cribriform fascia) because no lymph nodes are to be found between the femoral vein and artery, lateral to the artery or distal to the lower margin of the fossa ovalis beneath the cribriform fascia. They also found that the node of Cloquet or Rosenmüller, which is the uppermost node among the deep femoral lymph nodes, was absent in 54% of the specimens dissected. Borgno and colleagues also demonstrated that during surgery, when traction is persistently applied to the lymphovascular fat tissue above the cribriform fascia, all inguinal nodes can be removed. No nodal tissue was found when the cribriform fascia and the fat beneath were submitted separately for pathologic review. Hudson and colleagues confirmed this finding in cadaver dissection, and Micheletti and coworkers found supporting evidence with careful embryologic study.

Although lymphatics draining from the clitoris directly to the deep pelvic lymph nodes are described, their clinical significance appears to be minimal. It is unusual to find a case in which metastasis is present in the pelvic lymph nodes without metastatic disease in the inguinal lymph nodes, even when the clitoris is involved. Curry and associates noted clitoral involvement in 58 patients of 191 studied; none had positive deep pelvic nodes without involvement of inguinal nodes also. Similar results were observed in a study of 38 patients with carcinomas of the clitoris by Ericksson and coworkers, who found also that the deep inguinal or femoral nodes were never positive in the absence of positive superficial inguinal nodes.

The incidence of positive inguinal and pelvic nodes varies considerably, as noted in Table 8-4. Unfortunately, most of these studies were unstaged, although, in general, the larger the tumor, the greater the propensity for inguinal and pelvic node metastases. Morley noted a 20.7% incidence of lymph node involvement if there was a T1 lesion (<2 cm in diameter. In T2 lesions (>2 cm

but limited to the vulva), the incidence of lymph node involvement more than doubled to 44.8%. Malfetano and colleagues reported the incidence of inguinal node metastases in patients with stage III and stage IV lesions to be 53% and 90%, respectively. Clinical evaluation of the groin is somewhat more accurate than tumor size. Homesley found that approximately 24% of patients with clinically nonsuspicious nodes had positive nodes when dissected and approximately 75% of patients with suspicious (palpable, fixed, or ulcerated) groins had positive nodes. Table 8-5 demonstrates the association between inguinal lymph node involvement and tumor size, depth of invasion, and clinical examination. Of note, these data did not evaluate laterality or unifocal versus multifocal lesions.

Staging

Many staging systems have been applied to invasive cancer of the vulva. Significant discrepancy exists between clinical and surgical-pathologic evaluation of lymph node status. This has been documented in a study by Iversen with 258 patients seen at the Norwegian Radium Hospital. Overdiagnosis (lymph node involvement suspected clinically but negative pathologically) was seen in 40 of 258 patients (15%). Of the 100 patients with metastasis to the inguinal lymph nodes, lymph node involvement was not suspected clinically in 36 patients. Patients with "micrometastasis" (lymph node involvement not suspected clinically but positive microscopically) had a significantly better survival rate than did those with gross metastasis. As a result of these repeated findings, it was suggested that staging be based on surgical-pathologic evaluation instead of clinical evaluation alone. FIGO agreed, and the original clinical staging system was replaced in 1988 by a

TABLE 8-6   Figo Staging of Invasive Cancer of the Vulva

Stage I	Tumor confined to the vulva
IA	Lesions ≦2 cm in size confined to the vulva or perineum and with stromal invasion ≦1.0 mm*, no nodal metastasis
IB	Lesions >2 cm in size confined to the vulva or perineum with stromal invasion greater than 1.0 mm*, no nodal metastasis
Stage II	Tumor of any size with extension to adjacent perineal structures (1/3 lower urethra, 1/3 lower vagina, anus), no nodal metastasis
Stage III	Tumor of any size with or without extension to adjacent perineal structures (1/3 lower urethra, 1/3 lower vagina, anus) with positive inguinofemoral lymph nodes
IIIA	(i) With 1 lymph node metastasis (≧5 mm), or (ii) 1-2 lymph node metastasis(es) (<5 mm)
IIIB	(i) With 2 or more lymph node metastases (≧5 mm), or (ii) 3 or more lymph node metastases (<5 mm)
IIIC	With positive nodes with extracapsular spread
Stage IV	Tumor invades other regional (2/3 upper urethra, 2/3 upper vagina), or distant structures
IVA	Tumor invades any of the following: (i) upper urethra and/or vaginal mucosa, bladder mucosa, rectal mucosa, or fixed to pelvic bone, or (ii) fixed or ulcerated inguinofemoral lymph nodes
IVB	Any distant metastasis, including pelvic lymph nodes

*The depth of invasion is defined as the measurement of the tumor from the epithelial-stromal junction of the adjacent most superficial dermal papilla to the deepest point of invasion.

surgical-pathologic, or tumor-node-metastasis (TNM), classification system. The most recent revised FIGO staging for carcinoma of the vulva was published in 2009 (Table 8-6) and further characterizes the number and type of lymph node metastases. Previous studies noted poorer survival among individuals with bilateral lymph node metastasis; thus laterality was incorporated into the staging system. However, recent studies have demonstrated that the number of lymph node metastases and extracapsular spread are predictive of survival regardless of laterality. It is important to remain aware that many reports in the literature use older staging systems depending on when data were compiled, and this must be considered when analyzing these publications.

Donaldson and colleagues thoroughly evaluated the prognostic parameters in 66 patients with squamous cell carcinomas of the vulva. The size of the lesion predicted the incidence of lymph node metastasis (19% metastasis if the lesion was <3 cm, and 72% metastasis if the lesion was >3 cm). Likewise, grade of tumor correlated with node metastasis (onethird of well-differentiated tumors had metastasis, compared with 75% of the poorly differentiated lesions). Of 38 patients, 11 (29%) had node involvement if invasion of the primary lesion was 5 mm or less, compared with 17 of 28 (61%) if invasion was greater than 5 mm. If the tumor did not involve lymphatic or vascular spaces, only 2 of 33 (6%) had positive nodes, whereas 26 of 33 patients (79%) with lymphatic or vascular space involvement had metastasis to the regional lymph nodes. None of 25 patients with lesions invading less than 5 mm and without lymphatic or vascular space involvement had lymph node metastasis.

The use of sentinel lymph node biopsy (SLNB) in the evaluation of vulvar cancer was first proposed in 1979,

with the original lymphatic mapping data being published by Levenbach and colleagues in 1994. When a sentinel node or nodes are identified, the tissue is resected and submitted for frozen section. If the frozen section is positive, then a complete inguinofemoral node dissection is performed. If the frozen section is negative, then there appears to be a low likelihood that other nodes in that groin would be positive. If this technique can be proven to be highly effective, it would offer the opportunity to reduce the morbidity of the groin dissection.

Despite several studies that appear promising, definitive conclusions have yet to be drawn, and significant limitations remain. The first mapping studies of SLNB in vulvar cancer evaluated 21 patients with isosulfan blue dye only, and an SLN was identified in only 86% of patients and 66% of groins. Addition of lymphoscintigraphy with radiolabeled technetium was used by subsequent investigators, improving the SLN detection rate. A collective review of the literature in 2002 noted a detection rate of 92% with the combined technique, and this was confirmed in a subsequent Gynecologic Oncology Group (GOG) study published in abstract in 2009. This GOG study evaluated the SLN procedure prospectively. Patients with primary lesions 2 to 6 cm and clinically nonsuspicious nodes underwent SLNB and then had a complete inguinofemoral node dissection. The combined procedure resulted in an SLN detection rate of 93%.

Van der Zee and colleagues reported a multicenter observational study using the combined technique in patients with vulvar squamous cell carcinoma. Eligible patients had T1 or T2 lesions less than 4 cm, invasion greater than 1 mm, and clinically nonsuspicious inguinofemoral lymph nodes. SLNB was performed, and if the

SLN was negative, then an inguinofemoral dissection was not performed; 623 groins in 403 patients were evaluated. The authors selected 259 selected patients with unifocal vulvar disease and a negative SLN to describe in detail. Among these, there were 6 groin recurrences (2.3%) and the 3-year survival rate was 97%, with a mean follow-up of 35 months. They concluded that recurrence was low and survival was excellent. Short-term morbidity (groin wound breakdown and cellulitis) and long-term morbidity (recurrent cellulitis and lower-extremity lymphedema) were significantly lower in the SLNB group compared to those from the node-positive group who underwent inguinofemoral lymphadenectomy. The largest North American experience to date with the longest follow-up was published by Frumovitz and colleagues at the MD Anderson Hospital. Fifty-two patients underwent the procedure between 1993 and 1999, and 14 suffered a recurrence. Eight of the recurrences (15.4%) were on the vulva, 3 (5.8%) in the groin, and 3 (5.8%) distant. The pattern of recurrence is similar to that seen with standard approaches, although the rate of relapse in the groin appears somewhat high.

Levenbach and coauthors have reported the results of a prospective GOG trial in abstract. There were 510 patients with T2 lesions between 2 and 6 cm and clinically nonsuspicious nodes who underwent SLNB followed by inguinofemoral node dissection. There were 129 patients who had positive groin nodes and the SLN procedure identified 116 of these as positive, for a sensitivity of 90%. Of the 13 patients with false-negative results, 8 had tumors greater than 4 cm. Although these results are encouraging, it should be noted that 13 of 394 patients with a negative SLN had positive nodes that were missed (3.3%, 95% CI 1.71-5.50). Without the inguinofemoral dissection, these patients would have been expected to relapse in the groin, and almost all patients who relapse in the groin will succumb to the disease. This false-negative predictive value is comparable to that observed in breast cancer, but salvage rates for this disease are more favorable.

Results to date suggest a low rate of false negativity, and the results compare favorably to SLNB performed for melanoma and breast cancer; however, questions remain. It is important to recall that the gold standard for the rate of groin relapse in a node-negative groin is 0.3% based on Homesley's GOG experience. Despite higher rates of recurrence with SNLB, some gynecologic oncologists have adopted SNLB as routine practice. Prior to implementing this procedure, strict criteria should be applied that can reduce the false-negative rate. Levenbach and colleagues noted a steep learning curve, both for the operating surgeon and for the institution. The rate of SLN detection improved from 84% to 93% in all patients and from 64% to 85% in all groins in the first 2 years of their experience. If a sentinel node cannot be identified and in any case in which the mapping procedure appears inadequate, SNLB should be abandoned in favor of complete lymphadenectomy. Levenbach suggests that it takes at least 10 cases of SNLB followed by complete lymphadenectomy to achieve competence. The University of Groningen in the Netherlands recently conducted a multicenter study evaluating the association between the size of metastasis within the sentinel node and the chance of non–sentinel node involvement. This study demonstrated a higher likelihood of non–sentinel node metastasis when sentinel node involvement was identified with routine pathologic evaluation (23/88, or 27%) versus those identified only with ultrastaging (3/56, or 5%.) The authors concluded that a size cutoff below which non–sentinel node involvement is near zero does not appear to exist. Given the high risk of mortality if such nodes are missed, additional groin treatment remains the current recommendation for all patients with sentinel node involvement.

In the GOG trial the false-negative predictive value was only 2% for lesions 2 to 4 cm in size increasing to 6% for those between 4 and 6 cm. Careful patient selection is crucial to success. Ideal candidates include those with unifocal T_1/T_2 primary tumors <4 cm in diameter and clinically nonsuspicious groin nodes. Preoperative imaging such as computed tomography (CT) or magnetic resonance imaging (MRI) may be useful to exclude patients with gross nodal disease, in whom lymphatic mapping is less accurate. Nodes that are totally replaced by tumor may not be identified by mapping because of blockage of lymphatic channels by tumor cells. If a positive sentinel node is found on one side, then a complete groin dissection should be done bilaterally. In addition, the pathologist should be aware of the consequences of false-negative results and should be familiar with ultrastaging of the sentinel node via step sectioning, which increases the yield (Puig-Tintore). This is problematic with frozen sections, and thus some patients initially noted to be negative will be identified with lymph node metastasis on final pathology, requiring a return to the operating room for completion inguinofemoral lymph node dissection.

Management

Way originally reported improved survival in carcinoma of the vulva by use of the en bloc dissection of radical vulvectomy plus inguinal and pelvic lymphadenectomy, which subsequently became the mainstay of treatment in vulvar cancer. Corrected 5-year survival rate for stage I and stage II disease has been reported by many authors to be approximately 90%. This so-called "longhorn" en bloc resection has evolved into a more tailored approach depending on size and laterality of the lesion, resulting in similar cure rates with lower morbidity. Modified

TABLE 8-7   Unilateral Lesions: Percentage of Positive Groin Nodes by Tumor Thickness

Tumor Thickness (mm)	Ipsilateral Positive Only	Contralateral Positive Only	Bilateral Positive	Total	n
<2	6.8	0.0	0.0	6.8	59
3-5	20.4	1.9	2.8	25.0	108
6-10	28.8	3.8	11.3	43.8	80
>11	36.7	6.7	6.7	50.0	30
Total	21.7	2.5	5.1	29.2	277

From Homesley HD et al: Prognostic factors for groin node metastasis in squamous cell carcinoma of the vulva (a Gynecologic Oncology Group study). Gynecol Oncol 49:279, 1993.

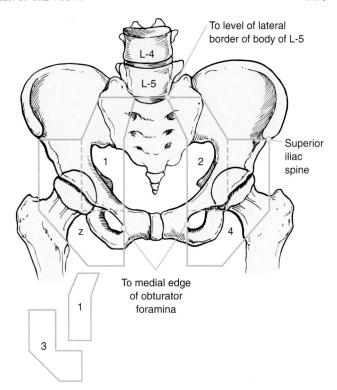

FIGURE 8-10   Radiation ports for inguinal and pelvic treatment. *1, 2,* anteroposterior pelvic and inguinal port; *3, 4,* anterior boost, or "wing." (*From Prolog: Gynecologic Oncology and Surgery, 2nd ed. The American College of Obstetricians and Gynecologists, 1991, p 51.*)

radical vulvectomy is the current approach to resect the primary lesion with a 2-cm margin, sparing a significant amount of normal tissue, especially with smaller lesions. The lymph nodes are resected via separate incisions. Well-lateralized lesions, defined as less than 1 cm from the midline, can be managed with modified radical vulvectomy and ipsilateral inguinofemoral lymph node dissection (LND). Homesley presented the GOG experience with such lesions (Table 8-7) and confirmed the low incidence of contralateral node involvement, making ipsilateral inguinal lymphadenectomy a rational initial approach. However, central lesions must be evaluated with bilateral LND. This is based on the lymphatic drainage of the vulva confirmed by anatomic studies demonstrating contralateral lymphatic drainage of lesions near the anus and clitoris, thus warranting the evaluation of both groins in central lesions.

Adjuvant therapy is based on surgicopathologic findings following radical vulvectomy and evaluation of appropriate lymph nodes. Historically, if metastasis was noted in the groin nodes, pelvic lymph node dissection was performed. This practice has now been largely abandoned in favor of pelvic radiation therapy to treat the next nodal chain when groin nodes are involved. The pelvic nodes are essentially never involved with metastatic disease when the inguinal nodes are uninvolved. A study by Curry and associates at the M.D. Anderson Hospital showed that of 191 patients, only 9 (4.7%) had positive pelvic nodes and all 9 patients also had metastatic disease in the groin nodes. In 1986 the GOG (Homesley) performed a prospective randomized study in patients with vulvar carcinoma who had positive groin nodes; 114 patients with positive inguinal nodes were randomly assigned to receive radiotherapy vs ipsilateral pelvic node dissection. The group treated with radiotherapy had a 68% relative 2-year survival rate, and the group undergoing pelvic node dissection had a 54% relative 2-year survival rate. The authors now recommend pelvic lymph node irradiation (Figure 8-10) for patients with positive inguinal nodes.

A randomized Gynecologic Oncology Group trial attempted to evaluate groin irradiation vs groin dissection for patients with N0/N1 nodes. (Stehman, 1992). This study was closed prematurely when interim monitoring demonstrated an excess groin failure rate in the radiation arm. Although this study's radiation prescription has been criticized, a Cochrane Database Systematic Review (van der Velden, 2005) concluded that follow-up studies do not support better disease control with radiation of the intact groin and that lymph node dissection continues to be the cornerstone of therapy. There may still be some role for radiation therapy, especially in patients who are not surgical candidates, although the risks of groin failure and hip fracture must be taken into account (Katz, 2003).

Boronow also emphasized the possible role of primary radiation therapy in vulvar and vaginal cancers. His report dealt mostly with advanced disease involving vaginal mucous membrane, necessitating an exenterative procedure if a primary surgical approach was used. As an alternative, he recommends surgical extirpation of the lymph nodes with a combination of external and interstitial irradiation for control of the central lesion. In a small, highly individualized series, this approach appeared promising. Similar reports by Fairey and associates and Hacker and colleagues substantiated this.

Although neoadjuvant radiation has gained acceptance in this setting, significant challenges remain. Low anterior and posterior fields must be used, resulting in intense exposure of the vulvar skin because the axis of the x-ray beam runs parallel to (and often within) the skin and mucous membrane. Vulvitis may result, and interruption of therapy is often necessary because of the patient's discomfort. Similarly, radiation therapy to enlarged, obviously positive inguinal nodes becomes technically difficult. Surgical removal of enlarged nodes with subsequent radiation therapy to the area has been our preference. Requisite preoperative doses of 45 to 50 Gy to either groin or vulvar areas produce a hazardous situation for any subsequent surgical approach. Delaying surgical intervention for 4 to 6 weeks following radiation therapy reduces the risk of wound complications.

Neoadjuvant concurrent chemoradiation therapy to provide optimal reduction in the size of the central lesion has also been evaluated. Russell and coworkers described 25 women with locoregionally advanced squamous cancer of the vulva. Eighteen patients were previously untreated, and all patients received external-beam radiation and synchronous radiopotentiating chemotherapy. Complete clinical response was obtained in 16 of 18 previously untreated patients and in 4 of 7 patients with recurrent disease. Concurrent chemoradiation with cisplatin and 5-fluorouracil has been prospectively evaluated by the GOG and found to be highly effective. Moore and colleagues reported on 73 patients with T3/T4 tumors who would have required ultraradical surgery to clear disease. Resection was accomplished after chemoradiation in 69/71, and only 3 patients required urinary or fecal diversion. Montana and colleagues reported the companion trial for patients with unresectable groin nodes. Many of these poor-prognosis patients suffered progression or intercurrent death during chemoradiation. Still, 38 of 40 who completed treatment had resectable disease and 15 of 37 had negative lymph nodes.

It has been suggested that in selected stage IV carcinomas of the vulva, ultraradical surgery may be applicable. Cavanagh and Shepherd, in a review of their data and the literature, identified 53 patients since 1973 who were treated with exenteration and radical vulvectomy and were eligible for a 5-year follow-up. Most of the patients were young, and 47% were alive without recurrence. In their series, Cavanagh and Shepherd found all survivors to have negative pelvic lymph nodes.

Technique of Radical Vulvectomy

The goal of radical vulvectomy is to remove the primary lesion to the depth of the perineal fascia with a 2-cm circumferential margin. Ipsilateral or bilateral inguinofemoral lymph nodes are harvested based on the size and laterality of the lesion, as discussed previously. The single incision technique is described in Figure 8-11 and can be modified to incorporate one or both groins. Another possibility is to limit the skin incision to the inguinal area, thereby preserving the bridge of skin between the inguinal and vulvar incisions (three-incision technique, Figure 8-12). All tissue is removed from the inguinal lymph node bundles. An 8-cm incision is made parallel to the inguinal ligament two fingerbreadths (4 cm) beneath the inguinal ligament and two fingerbreadths (4 cm) lateral to the pubic tubercle (Figure 8-13). The incision is carried down through the Camper fascia, and at this point skin flaps are bluntly and sharply dissected superiorly and inferiorly, allowing access to the fat pad containing the superficial nodes. The sentinel nodes are located in the fatty layer of tissue beneath the Camper fascia, in part anterior to the cribriform plate and also protruding from beneath the fascia lata (Figure 8-14). The dissection should be carried superiorly to the inguinal ligament and inferiorly to a point approximately 2 cm proximal to the opening of the Hunter canal. The dissection should be carried laterally to the sartorius muscle and medially to the adductor longus muscle fascia (Figure 8-15). Blunt dissection facilitates identification of the cribriform fascia, which is most easily identified just below the inguinal ligament or in the area of the saphenous opening. The cribriform fascia unites with the fascia lata and thus is contiguous with the fascia on the surface of the adductor longus and sartorius muscles; this may facilitate its identification. The portion of the fascia covering the femoral triangle is perforated by the saphenous vein, by lymph nodes of the vertical set, and by numerous blood and lymphatic vessels, hence the name cribriform fascia. If the dissection is carried out properly, the adventitia of the femoral vessels should not be clearly seen except through the vessel openings mentioned earlier.

Bell showed that a complete inguinal dissection could be achieved while leaving the fascia intact. He and his coinvestigators retrieved a mean of 10 nodes per groin without removing the cribriform fascia. Borgno and colleagues demonstrated that the deep inguinal or femoral nodes are exposed in the fossa ovalis and other openings of the cribriform fascia, allowing access to all inguinal nodes with this technique. The result is that a dissection that uses the boundaries of the femoral triangle and is carried out to the level of the cribriform fascia with optimal traction on the lymphovascular fat bundle of the inguinal area will produce a specimen that contains all of the inguinal and femoral nodes.

Frozen-section analysis can be obtained if the initial plan is to perform an ipsilateral LND and suspicious nodes are encountered during the dissection. If metastatic disease is confirmed, a contralateral LND is

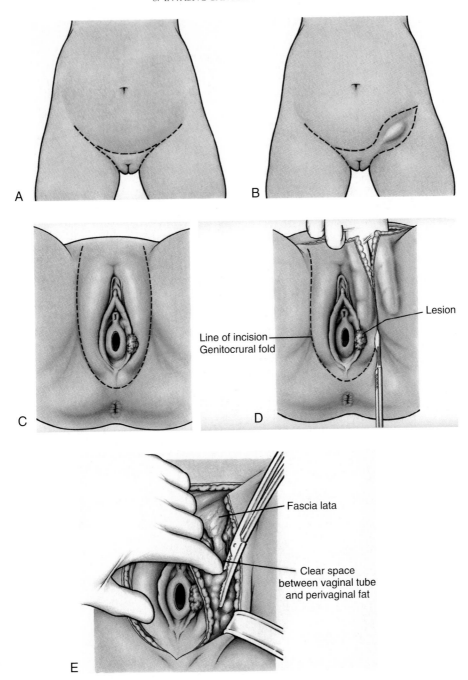

FIGURE 8-11 **A,** Groin incision for moderate-sized lesions. **B,** Groin incision for a patient with a matted left inguinal node. **C** and **D,** Vulvar incision along the genitocrural fold. **E,** Clamping the perivaginal tissue.

performed. Closed-suction drains are then placed in the groin dissection, and the skin incision is closed by means of a running delayed absorbable suture. The lymph node dissection is typically performed first (with two teams if bilateral node dissection is planned), and attention is then turned to the vulvectomy itself.

A complete radical vulvectomy is accomplished by defining the margin of dissection. The mons is incised anteriorly, extending medially to the genitocrural fold

and posteriorly midway between the anus and posterior fourchette. A bloodless space can be dissected between vulvar fat and the subcutaneous tissue of the thigh, using a finger dissection (Figure 8-11, C and D). The tissue is transected and ligated with 0 or 2-0 delayed absorbable suture at the level of the fascia of the thigh (Figure 8-11, E). The posterior dissection is performed sharply (Figure 8-11, F). Special attention is directed to the location of the anus and rectum. It is sometimes

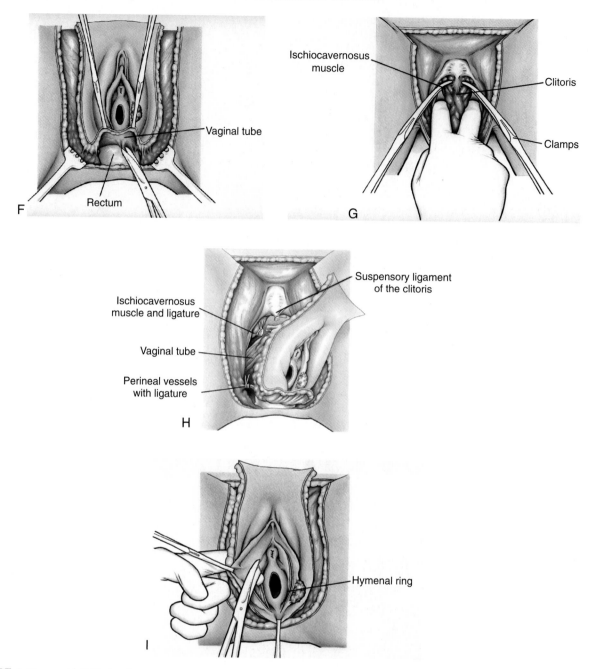

FIGURE 8-11, cont'd **F,** Vagina being separated from the rectum. **G,** Clamping the ischiocavernosus muscle and the crura of the clitoris. **H,** Mobilized specimen is prepared for excision. **I,** Excision along the inner margin of the specimen.

helpful for the operator to place a double-gloved finger in the rectum to ascertain its location and avoid damage during this part of the procedure. The clitoris is then isolated and its suspensory ligament is clamped, divided, and suture ligated at its inferior attachment to the pubic bone. It is often helpful at this point to attempt to isolate the ischiocavernosus muscle and divide this structure as laterally as possible (Figure 8-11, *G*). The pudendal artery and vein are ligated bilaterally. At this point of the procedure, only the vagina remains attached to the vulva

(Figure 8-11, *H*). A decision about the amount of vagina to be removed should be made relative to the location and size of cancer and based on knowledge of the lymphatic drainage of the vulva. Every effort should be made to avoid resection of the urethra unless it is close to the cancer. If it is indicated, the distal 1 to 2 cm of this organ can be removed without damage to the functional sphincter. The perineal defect is closed primarily with mattress sutures of 0 or 2-0 delayed absorbable suture. Tension on this closure can be prevented, if necessary, by

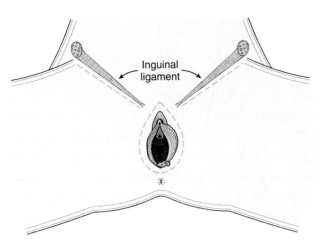

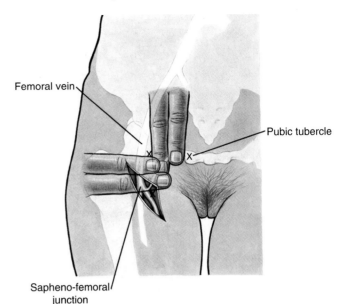

FIGURE 8-12 Three-incision technique for vulvar cancer.

FIGURE 8-13 Incision can be made as noted so that superficial inguinal nodes can be removed easily. (*Modified from Cabanas RM: An approach to the treatment of penile carcinoma. Cancer 39:456, 1977. Copyright © 1977 American Cancer Society. Reprinted by permission of Wiley-Liss, Inc., a subsidiary of John Wiley & Sons, Inc.*)

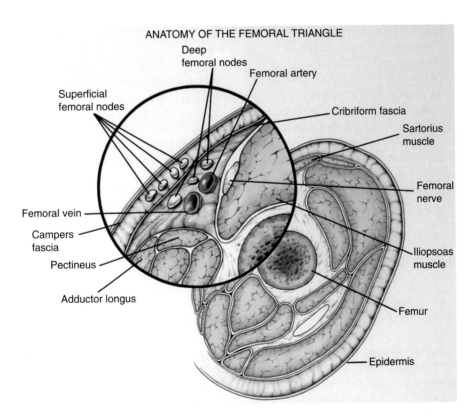

FIGURE 8-14 Many inguinal nodes are located between the Camper fascia and the cribriform fascia, as noted on cross section through the femoral triangle. Additional nodes are clustered in the foramen ovalis, in the part protruding from beneath the plane of the cribriform fascia. (*Modified from Cabanas RM: An approach to the treatment of penile carcinoma. Cancer 39:456, 1977. Copyright © 1977 American Cancer Society. Reprinted by permission of Wiley-Liss, Inc., a subsidiary of John Wiley & Sons, Inc.*)

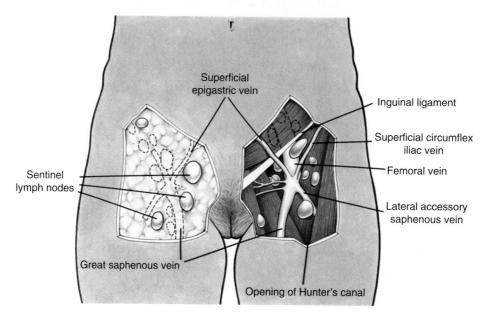

FIGURE 8-15 The right side demonstrates the two groups of lymph nodes making up the "sentinel" nodes. The left side notes the limits of the dissection with the cribriform fascia removed. The triangle that is dissected in a full inguinal lymphadenectomy is clearly identified on the patient's left side. The inguinal ligament forms the base of the triangle, and the opening of Hunter's canal becomes the apex. The triangle is bound laterally by the sartorius muscle and medially by the adductor muscles and fascia.

sharp and blunt mobilization of the vaginal barrel or subcutaneous tissue of the thigh. The most anterior extent of the dissection may be allowed to granulate secondarily for large defects if closure would result in significant tension. This prevents distortion of the urethra and alteration of the urinary stream. If the defect is too large for primary closure, intraposition of a split-thickness skin graft or rhomboid flaps can be used.

Several studies have demonstrated that the classical radical vulvectomy can be safely modified depending on the laterality and extent of the lesion without compromising outcomes if a 2-cm circumferential margin is maintained. If a unilateral lesion is present, hemivulvectomy can be done with preservation of the uninvolved side.

Morbidity Associated with Treatment of Vulvar Carcinoma

In the early series of Way, operative mortality approached 20%. In the last two decades, this has been reduced to 1% to 2%. This procedure is commonly carried out in the ninth and tenth decades of life with surprising safety. However, morbidity remains high and most commonly includes wound breakdown, lower-extremity lymphedema, lymphocyst formation, decreased pelvic support, and decreased sexual function.

Wound breakdown occurs in more than 50% of patients in most series. This aspect of morbidity is

usually limited to skin loss at the margin of the groin incision. Podratz and colleagues at the Mayo Clinic noted impaired primary wound healing in 148 of 175 patients (85%) who were treated with radical vulvectomy and inguinal lymphadenectomy. Removing lesser amounts of skin and decreasing the undermining of the skin flaps have reduced the incidence of wound breakdown. Routine prophylactic antibiotics and the use of closed suction drainage aid in wound healing and decrease the incidence of wound cellulitis and wound breakdown. Careful débridement and vigorous care to keep the wounds clean and dry almost always result in adequate healing. Bed rest is maintained for 1 to 3 days depending on the extent of resection. Vigorous local cleansing of the perineal and groin incisions is continued until these incisions are completely healed.

Lymphedema of the lower extremities is another major problem, especially in patients who have had inguinal and pelvic node dissection (see Figure 8-16). In the study reported by Podratz and colleagues, varying degrees of lymphedema of the lower extremities occurred in 69% of their patients. The incidence of this debilitating long-term complication can be reduced by routine use of custom-made elastic support hose during the first postoperative year while collateral pathways of lymph drainage are being developed. Streptococcal lymphangitis in the lower extremities dramatically increases the incidence of lymphedema; thus Rutledge and colleagues have for many years advised that patients also receive low-dose prophylactic antibiotic therapy (similar to that

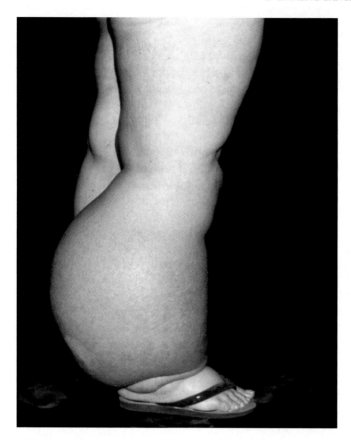

FIGURE 8-16 Marked lymphedema of the left leg after inguinal and pelvic lymphadenectomy.

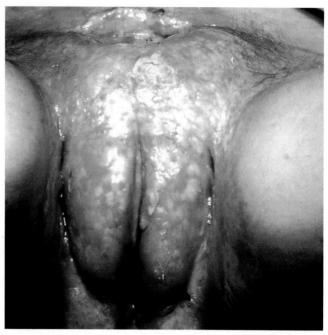

FIGURE 8-17 Severe edema of the vulva following radiation therapy with necrosis at the site of the primary lesion.

used to prevent subacute bacterial endocarditis) after lymphadenectomy. Established lymphedema can be kept under control in many patients with routine use of pneumatic hose devices that have become widely available. Zhang and colleagues confirmed Plaxe's observation that sparing of the saphenous vein reduces the incidence of chronic lymphedema, and does not compromise the outcome, with similar recurrence rates in patients undergoing complete resection versus preservation of the saphenous vein during inguinal lymphadenectomy.

The development of a lymphocyst in the groin area is an infrequent occurrence, and it usually resolves spontaneously. The incidence can be reduced by careful ligation of all the lymph-bearing tissue during the groin dissection and by maintaining closed suction drains in these spaces postoperatively until drainage is less than 30 cc per day. On occasion, intermittent aseptic aspiration of the fluid facilitates resolution of these collections.

The rate of complications has been reduced in this era of modified radical operation, although it continues to be high. Three contemporary series (Rouzier, 2003; Gaarenstroom, 2003; and Gould, 2001) have shown that wound cellulitis occurs in 25% to 39% of patients; wound

breakdown in 17% to 31% of patients; and lymphedema in 28% to 39% of patients. Although these results are encouraging, it is clear that further improvements are needed.

Morbidity is also associated with radiation therapy. The use of radiation therapy as a priori treatment, especially in patients with fixed inguinal nodes, can result in significant vulvar edema. This is especially true when low fields are used to include vulvar disease. Figure 8-17 illustrates severe edema in a patient treated primarily with radiation therapy. Necrosis is seen at 5 o'clock, which is residual from the large lesion occupying that area before irradiation. Pelvic radiation therapy also increases risk of pelvic fracture, especially in older women. This risk was quantified in a study reported in *JAMA* in 2005. Risk varied with primary site of disease, with more fractures noted in those treated for anal cancer, followed by rectal cancer and cervical cancer. Although risk in vulvar cancer was not specifically evaluated because of small numbers, all women undergoing pelvic radiation had a higher rate of pelvic fracture than women with pelvic malignancies who did not undergo irradiation, and the majority of fractures (90%) involved the hip.

Symptoms related to stress incontinence and the development of cystocele or rectocele are sometimes reported by patients undergoing surgery or radiation for the treatment of vulvar cancer. These conditions are secondary to the loss of the support of the lower end of the vagina and subsequent enlargement of the introitus.

The findings may also simply reflect the increased frequency of pelvic visceral prolapse among older women.

Removal of significant vulvar tissue, particularly the clitoris, can result in decreased sexual satisfaction. With small lesions in which the clitoris is not involved, hemivulvectomy with preservation of the clitoris can be performed. This allows sexual satisfaction to be achieved without a decrease in survival. Loss of the subcutaneous tissue prevents mobility of the external genitalia, which can also hinder sexual pleasure. Although this has been a detriment in many patients, others report that orgasm is still obtainable after vulvectomy.

Survival Results

Survival in cancer of the vulva, as with all other malignant neoplasms, is directly related to the extent of disease at the time diagnosis is made and treatment is undertaken. In addition, because this malignant neoplasm is initially diagnosed in the elderly woman, many patients succumb to intercurrent disease while they are tumor free. In stage I and stage II disease, the corrected 5-year survival rate should approach 90%. A 75% corrected 5-year survival rate for all stages of vulvar cancer is not unusual.

Regardless of stage, nodal status is of particular prognostic significance. In many series, if the lymph nodes are negative irrespective of stage, more than 90% of these patients will survive 5 years (corrected survival), whereas only 40% to 50% will survive if the lymph nodes are positive (Table 8-8). The large National Cancer Data Base (NCDB) study reported a 5-year survival of 93% for stage I and 87% for stage II. In those patients with negative nodes, irrespective of size or primary lesion, the 5-year survival rate was 90%. Survival was 55% with one positive node, 59% with two or three positive nodes, and 33% with four positive nodes. In those patients with positive nodes, survival was 62% if the primary lesion was 2 cm or less and 43% if the primary lesion was more than 2 cm. Overall survival results by stage are found in Figure 8-18.

Curry and associates noted that in patients with three or fewer unilateral groin nodes involved with metastasis, the 5-year survival rate was still fairly high (17 of 25, or 68%); however, of five patients in whom more than three nodes were involved, none survived. None of the patients with three or fewer unilateral involved nodes had pelvic node metastases. Boyce and associates and Shimm and coworkers reported similar results, with prognosis worsening not only with an increase in the number of positive nodes, but also to a lesser extent with bilateral inguinal node involvement. Of the patients with more than four unilateral nodes, 50% had pelvic node metastasis, and if bilateral groin nodes were involved, 26% had positive pelvic nodes. In patients with positive pelvic nodes, the survival rate is poor. Collected series indicate that only one fifth of patients with pelvic node metastasis survived 5 years (Table 8-9).

More recently, features of nodal metastasis have been noted by some investigators to carry prognostic significance. Raspagliesi and associates evaluated features including FIGO stage, depth of invasion, grade, lymph node status, lymphovascular space involvement (LVSI),

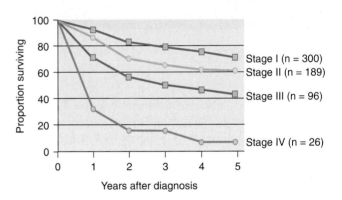

FIGURE 8-18 Carcinoma of the vulva: Patients treated in 1990-1992. (*From the Annual Report of Gynecological Cancer. FIGO, Vol 23, 1998.*)

TABLE 8-9   Survival Rates for Patients with Positive Pelvic Nodes

Series	5-Year Survival Rate (%)
Way (1957)	2/9 (22.2)
Green et al (1958)	2/16 (12.5)
Way (1960)	3/8 (37.5)
Merrill and Ross (1961)	1/3 (33.3)
Collins et al (1963)	1/6 (16.7)
Franklin and Rutledge (1971)	3/12 (25.0)
Morley (1976)	1/6 (16.7)
Curry, Wharton, and Rutledge (1980)	2/9 (22.2)
Boyce (1985)	0/6 (0)
Shimm et al (1986)	0/7 (0)
Total	15/82 (18.3)

TABLE 8-8   Survival Rates for Carcinoma of the Vulva

Series	Status of Nodes	No. of Patients	Percentage Surviving Positive	Percentage Surviving Negative
Boyce (1985)	Positive	30	50	
	Negative	49		82
Shimm et al (1986)	Positive	33	52	
	Negative	65		77
Cavanagh et al (1990)	Positive	77	39	
	Negative	126		85
Creasman (1997)	Positive	444	49	
	Negative	983		90

DNA ploidy, and patient age and found that lymph node status and LVSI were both significant independent prognostic factors. Pathologic analysis of metastatic lymph nodes determined that percentage of nodal replacement and extracapsular spread were both statistically significant also, whereas number of positive nodes and laterality were not significant. Similarly, Fons and colleagues confirmed that extracapsular spread was an important prognostic factor. In addition, the significance of bilateral lymph node involvement was lost once the total number of metastatic nodes was taken into account. In other words, the total number of metastatic nodes is more important than their location—either unilateral or bilateral. FIGO recently recommended modifications for vulvar cancer staging incorporating these findings. The new system now includes degree of tumor burden within metastatic lymph nodes, number of involved nodes, and presence of extracapsular lymph node spread (Table 8-6). Tumor size is now included in stage I substaging, rather than stage I and stage II, and laterality of lymph node metastasis is no longer included.

Tolerance of the Elderly Patient to Therapy

The rate of squamous cell carcinoma of the vulva increases with age, often affecting patients in the eighth, ninth, and tenth decades of life. As the average life span of women increases, gynecologic malignant neoplasms in geriatric patients have become more common. The reason for the increase in incidence of cancer in this population has not been clearly established, although a number of factors may be involved. These include the possibility of decreased immunosurveillance, the longer duration of carcinogenic exposure, and an increased susceptibility of aging cells to carcinogenesis.

Although elderly patients should not be categorically excluded from aggressive therapy because of their age, treatment may need modification to accommodate changes that occur with age. For example, it is clear that older patients who are treated with intensive chemotherapy have a much higher initial toxicity rate because of bone marrow suppression. Therefore, doses should be initiated at a reduced level and then increased as tolerated to avoid difficulty. However, surgical therapy such as radical vulvectomy with bilateral inguinal lymphadenectomy is well tolerated by elderly patients, even those in their 90s. Undoubtedly this is because body cavities are not violated. Much of the risk lies in the anesthesia required.

Recurrence

Recurrence may be local or distant, and more than 80% will occur in the first 2 years after therapy, demanding initial close follow-up. Oonk noted that 65% of

TABLE 8-10 Sites of Recurrence After Modified Radical Operation

Author	n	Local (%)	Bridge (%)	Groin (%)	Distant (%)
de Hullu (2002)	238	18 (8)	1 (0.4)	2 (0.8)	12 (5)
Gonzalez-Bosquet et al (2005)	330	64 (19)	—	8 (2.4)	37 (11)
Maggino et al (2000)	502	100 (20)	—	35 (6.9)	25 (5)
Oonk et al (2003)	238	49 (20)	2 (0.8)	6 (2.5)	8 (3)
Rouzier (2002)	215	26 (17)	7 (3.3)		

recurrences were found at scheduled follow-up visits and that half of those patients were asymptomatic. Recurrences found at scheduled follow-up tended to be smaller. Local recurrence is more common with larger tumors and positive capillary-lymphatic space involvement (Table 8-10). Is it surprising that more than half of the recurrences are local and near the site of the primary lesion. This is more common in patients with large primary tumors or metastatic disease in the lymph nodes at initial surgery. The margin of resection has long been recognized to be a significant prognostic factor also. Heaps and colleagues found that if the formalin-fixed margin was greater than 8 mm (equivalent to 1 cm in fresh tissue), the risk of local recurrence was very low. This finding has been confirmed by de Hullu and Rouzier. The high incidence of local recurrence demands careful attention to adequate margins in the removal of the primary lesion. Some recurrences on the vulva occur at a site remote from the primary excision, often manifesting later in follow-up. Rouzier and colleagues (2001) noted that these patients, who may actually have new primary lesions, had a better prognosis than those who recurred earlier and near the site of the prior excision.

Wide local excision and the triple incision technique may lead to a slightly increased risk for local recurrence (van der Velden, 2004). Care must be given to excising the entire lesion with at least a 1- to 2-cm margin. In many instances, local recurrences can be successfully treated by local excision or interstitial irradiation. Patients with recurrent local disease in the lymph node area or distant disease are difficult to treat, and the salvage rate is poor. Simonsen reported a 40% salvage rate with local recurrence and an 8% survival at 5 years with regional metastases. Both groups were treated with a combination of surgery and radiation therapy. Prempree and Amornmarn had similar results using radiation alone. Disease limited to the introitus gave the best prognosis: six of six patients survived. As expected, extensive recurrences have the poorest prognosis, especially when bone metastases occur. Patients with distant recurrences have been treated with cisplatin-based chemotherapy, and a 30% overall response rate has been achieved. Responses are more likely outside the radiation field.

EARLY VULVAR CARCINOMA

Andreasson and Nyboe constructed three different models of groups at low risk for metastasis in squamous cell carcinoma of the vulva region. They concluded that a definite, distinct profile of low-risk patients would require data from large accruals of patients and international collaboration. Based on such studies, the International Society for the Study of Vulvovaginal Disease (ISSVD) has proposed the following pathologic definition of microinvasive carcinoma of the vulva: "a squamous carcinoma having a diameter of less than 2 cm, as measured in the fresh state, with a depth of invasion of less than 1 mm, measured from the epithelial-stromal junction of the most superficial adjacent dermal papilla to the deepest point of invasion." Vascular space involvement by tumor excludes the lesion from this definition, and groin nodes should be clinically nonsuspicious. The current staging system classifies these lesions as stage Ia. Microinvasive, or stage Ia, lesions are managed with wide local excision and do not require inguinal lymphadenectomy. A review of the literature reveals only two cases of stage Ia vulvar squamous cell carcinoma with lymph node metastasis.

Assessing depth of invasion is obviously critical in obtaining this diagnosis, and unfortunately, there remains considerable inconsistency regarding pathologists' methods of measurement. In most current publications, a method is described that measures from the most superficial dermal–epidermal junction of the most superficial adjacent dermal papilla. This is the measurement required in the FIGO staging system. Others have used a method that measures from the surface of the lesion; although this method is simpler, it appears not to be as reflective of true invasion. The importance of vascular invasion adjacent to the vulvar carcinoma in predicting lymph node metastasis, or prognosis, remains controversial. However, data support the hypothesis that vascular space involvement by tumor at the site of the primary tumor is associated with increased frequency of lymph node metastasis. There does not appear to be a definitive correlation between tumor differentiation and lymph node metastasis and survival. There may be an association between depth of tumor invasion and tumor differentiation, with deeply invasive tumors being more undifferentiated. More study of this issue is needed.

Podratz and colleagues reported a 5-year survival rate of 90% if the primary lesion was less than 1 cm, 89% if the lesion was 1 to 2 cm, and 83% if the lesion was 2 to 3 cm. They found that the 5- and 10-year survival rates of patients with stage I disease were independent of the extent of the surgical procedure, suggesting that more selectivity of the treatment is feasible without sacrifice of curability. There continues to be a lack of unanimity concerning the proper surgical approach to the patient

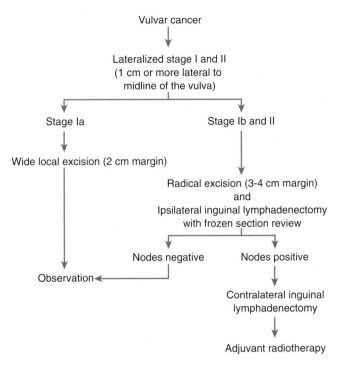

FIGURE 8-19   Algorithm for management of lateralized stage I or II vulvar cancer.

with an early invasive carcinoma of the vulva. The morbidity produced by radical vulvectomy, both to body image and with sexual function, makes this issue worthy of serious consideration.

Stehman and colleagues reported the GOG experience with 121 patients with stage I disease and invasion less than 5 mm treated with a modified radical vulvectomy and superficial inguinal lymphadenectomy. There were 19 recurrences including 5 groin-only recurrences and 7 deaths. Gordiner reported on the MD Anderson experience. They observed 9 groin recurrences in 104 patients treated with superficial dissection. In these 9 patients, the median number of nodes removed per groin was 7, but there were 4 groins with 0 to 2 nodes. In contrast, in Kirby's report, only an average of 2.7 nodes was retrieved per groin. The difference among all these reports is likely to be in the extent of the inguinal lymphadenectomy. Our suggestions for management are presented in Figures 8-19 to 8-21.

PAGET'S DISEASE

Paget's disease of the vulva is rare. Even among vulvar neoplasms, it is an unusual finding. It most often occurs in women in the seventh decade of life but can be seen in young patients. Pruritus and tenderness are the most common presenting symptoms. These symptoms may be present for years before the patient seeks medical

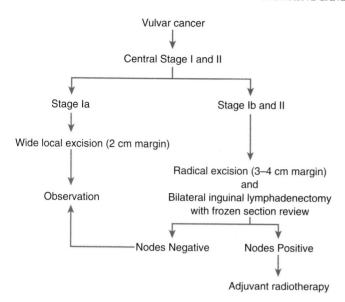

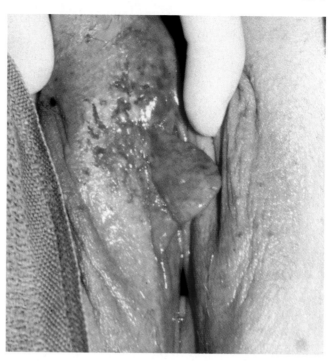

FIGURE 8-22   Paget's disease of the vulva involving the lower half of the left labium major and labium minor. The white medial portion is characteristic of "cake-icing effect." The red medial aspect is also commonly seen and called "violaceous coloring."

FIGURE 8-20   Algorithm for management of central stage I or II vulvar cancer.

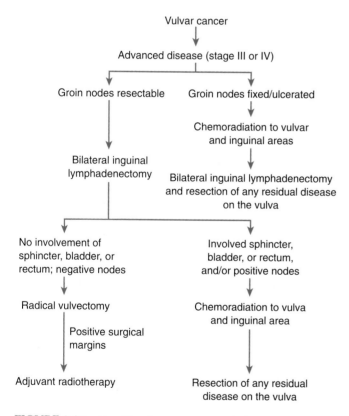

FIGURE 8-21   Algorithm for management of advanced (stage III or IV) vulvar cancer.

Clinical and Histologic Features

On examination, the vulvar lesions are usually hyperemic, sharply demarcated, and thickened, with foci of excoriation and induration. The vulvar skin is often thick and smooth, leading to the impression of leukoplakia. It is not unusual for the hyperemic areas associated with a superficial white coating to give the impression of "cake-icing effect." This finding is classic and, if present, is almost pathognomonic for Paget's disease (Figure 8-22). Typically, areas of leukoplakia are mixed with patches of redness where excoriation has occurred because of intense pruritus. Vulvar changes are usually superficial, but palpation may indicate thickness or a masslike effect under the epithelial changes raising concern of an underlying adenocarcinoma. If clinical findings are suspicious, adequate biopsy of the lesion relative to width and depth of tissue must be obtained to enable adequate histologic evaluation. One should perform a needle aspiration of any thickness or mass that is palpated beneath the skin involved with Paget's disease.

Historically, it appears that there are two separate lesions: intraepithelial extramammary Paget's disease and pagetoid changes within the skin associated with an underlying adenocarcinoma. More recently, invasive Paget's disease has been described based on depth of

attention. The vulvar lesion may be localized to one labium or involve the entire vulvar epithelium. It is not unusual for the disease process to extend to the perirectal area, buttocks, inguinal area, or mons. Extension into the vagina has been reported.

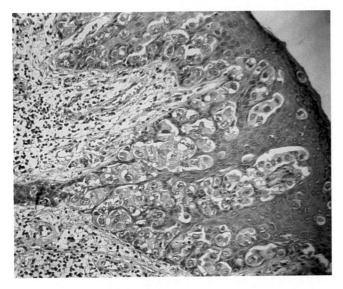

FIGURE 8-23   Histologic picture of Paget's disease of the vulva. Large cells with clear cytoplasm are apparent in the epidermis. Note the heavy lymphocytic infiltration in the dermis.

invasion. Minimally invasive Paget's disease is that in which the Paget cells have broken through the basement membrane into the underlying dermis to less than 1 mm. Invasive vulvar Paget's disease is a lesion in which the Paget cells break through the basement membrane into the underlying dermis greater than 1 mm. Therapy for these two lesions is considerably different, and a definitive diagnosis is therefore imperative.

A thickened, often acanthotic epidermis is the typical histologic finding. Characteristic large cells with clear granular cytoplasm are found within the epidermis (Figure 8-23). A single layer of squamous cells often separates the Paget cells from the epidermis, but neoplastic cells may be in immediate contact with the dermis. Intraepidermal formation of glands with true lumens may also be present. The hair follicles may also be involved with Paget cells. These cells contain intracytoplasmic mucin demonstrated by Mayer's mucicarmine or Alcian blue. A mixed inflammatory infiltrate of variable intensity composed usually of lymphocytes and plasma cells is present in the upper dermis.

Clinical Course and Management

If only intraepithelial Paget's disease is present, the clinical course may be prolonged and indolent, often associated with recurrence of intraepithelial disease. Rarely, the disease can have an invasive component or be associated with an underlying adenocarcinoma of underlying apocrine glands. The latter is not actually Paget's disease, but rather a secondary infiltration of the vulvar skin with pagetoid cells from the primary adenocarcinoma. Paget's disease with an underlying adenocarcinoma can

be aggressive, with metastasis to the regional lymph nodes and distant spread.

The literature has been confusing with regard to the association of invasive carcinoma and concomitant intraepithelial Paget's disease. Earlier reports suggested invasive underlying adenocarcinomas in up to 20% of patients with histologically confirmed pagetoid cells in the vulvar skin. Recent literature suggests a much lower incidence. Similarly, older studies suggest that up to 25% of patients have a concomitant carcinoma at another site, such as the breast, colon, anus, or cervix. Here, too, recent studies have not confirmed these numbers, with only a rare patient having a simultaneous lesion. In a review of 100 cases from eight institutions, Fanning and colleagues noted 12% of patients with invasive vulvar Paget's disease and 4% with an underlying primary vulvar adenocarcinoma. A review of the literature noted an underlying adenocarcinoma in 8% and 10% with invasive Paget's disease; 20 patients had a total of 26 nonvulvar malignant neoplasms. It was thought by the authors that the nonvulvar cancers were probably related to the older age of the patients and not necessarily related to Paget's disease.

Because Paget's disease without an underlying adenocarcinoma appears to be a true intraepithelial neoplasia, it can be treated as such. Wide local excision to include the entire lesion is usually sufficient. Even with apparently wide margins, it is not unusual to find Paget's disease extending to the edge of the surgical margin, and recurrences are common. In the Fanning study, 31 of 84 patients with intraepithelial disease developed a recurrence. Radical vulvectomy, hemivulvectomy, and wide excision were used as treatment. Recurrence was similar with all three treatments. Because of the high recurrence rate and challenges in evaluating the margin grossly, intraoperative examination of the surgical margins by cryostat frozen sectioning has been recommended in the past (Figure 8-24). Unfortunately, this approach is time- and personnel-intensive, adding considerable time to the operation without leading to an improved outcome. Fishman and colleagues evaluated 14 patients with Paget's disease who underwent a total of 25 operations. Margin status was determined by frozen section in 8, with an average of 5.5 biopsies per patient to achieve a negative margin. Visual inspection was used to determine the margin in the remaining 17 patients. Frozen section was incorrect in 3/8 (37.5%), whereas visual inspection was wrong in 6/17 (35%). Furthermore, outcome was not significantly different with respect to the margin status. Two of five (40%) with a positive margin and 3/9 (33%) with a negative margin experienced recurrent disease.

New lesions can be handled in the same manner as the primary disease—that is, by wide local excision. Studies show that removal of full-thickness skin plus a

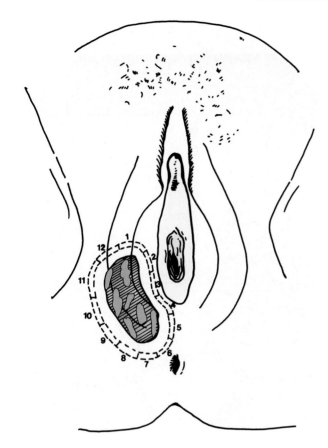

FIGURE 8-24 Diagram of the vulva with an area of Paget's disease involving the right labium majus. The two parallel lines lateral to the lesion represent the surgical margin sent intraoperatively for frozen section analysis. The margin is serially cut in a clockwise fashion, labeled, and analyzed. If any segment of the margin reveals Paget's disease, the resection is extended in that direction. *(From Bergen S et al: Conservative management of extramammary Paget's disease of the vulva. Gynecol Oncol 33:151, 1989.)*

TABLE 8-11 High-Risk Group for Development of Melanoma

Increased risk with one or more of the following:
Family history of melanoma
Poor or no tanning ability, often with a history of sunburn in adolescence
Unusual moles with any of the following characteristics:
  Dark (blue-black) look
  Speckled or splotchy color pattern
  Jagged or fuzzy border
  Recent change in size, shape, or color of a mole
  Any mole larger than a dime

TABLE 8-11 High-Risk Group for Development of Melanoma

Increased risk with one or more of the following:
Family history of melanoma
Poor or no tanning ability, often with a history of sunburn in adolescence
Unusual moles with any of the following characteristics:
  Dark (blue-black) look
  Speckled or splotchy color pattern
  Jagged or fuzzy border
  Recent change in size, shape, or color of a mole
  Any mole larger than a dime

TABLE 8-12 Clark's Staging Classification of Melanoma by Levels

Level	Definition
I	In situ melanoma: all demonstrable tumor is above the basement membrane in the epidermis
II	Melanoma extends through the basement membrane into the papillary dermis
III	The tumor fills the papillary dermis and extends to the reticular dermis but does not invade it
IV	The tumor extends into the reticular dermis
V	The tumor extends into the subcutaneous fat

microscopic amount of subcutaneous fat routinely results in an operative specimen that is 6 mm thick (Figure 8-25). Because the base of the hair follicles in vulvar skin is at a depth of 4 mm, one need not be concerned about the possibility of leaving neoplastic cells that may have involved hair shafts. Lesions can be extensive in the primary and recurrent stages, and treatment should be determined accordingly. A skin graft to cover the removed tissue may be warranted and should be used freely. DiSaia described two patients who developed recurrent Paget's disease in the middle of a split-thickness skin graft. A process labeled *retrodissemination* was given as an explanation for this curious phenomenon whereby pagetoid cells from peripheral occult sites of persistent disease are postulated to metastasize back into a skin graft site.

Besa and coworkers reported good results when radiotherapy was used in conjunction with surgery or for patients for whom surgery was not possible. A dose of 50 to 55 Gy appeared to be adequate. Voigt and colleagues reported a dramatic response of extramammary Paget's carcinoma in a man with chemotherapy using carboplatin and 5-fluorouracil with folinic acid, suggesting another possible approach when surgery is not appropriate.

Patients in whom an underlying adenocarcinoma is identified in association with Paget's disease of the vulva should be treated in the same manner as patients with other invasive malignant neoplasms of the vulva. This usually includes radical vulvectomy and inguinal lymphadenectomy. If the lymph nodes have no evidence of metastatic disease, the prognosis is good; however, if metastases are present in the lymph nodes, the prognosis is guarded.

MELANOMA

Melanoma of the vulva is rare but represents the second most common malignant neoplasm of the vulva. This malignant neoplasm probably arises from a lesion containing a junctional or a compound nevus. Tables 8-11, 8-12, and 8-13 define the high-risk group and describes the characteristics of pigmented lesions of the vulva or any skin that determine the need for excisional biopsy.

The clinical characteristics are as elsewhere on the body; melanomas are usually pigmented and raised, and they may be ulcerated (Figure 8-26). In a nationwide

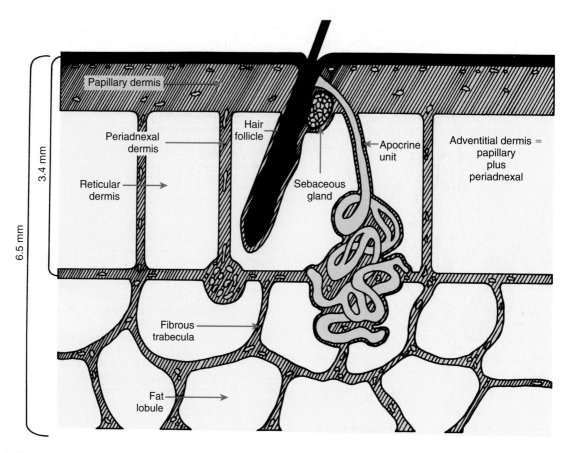

FIGURE 8-25 Schematic of vulvar skin anatomy showing the extension of skin appendages into the subdermal adipose tissue. *(From Bergen S et al: Gynecol Oncol 33:151, 1989.)*

TABLE 8-13 Lymph Node Metastasis and Clark's Level of Vulvar Melanoma

Clark's Level (*n*)	Nodes Examined (%)	Positive Nodes (%)
I (38)	3 (8)	0 (44)
II (80)	30 (60)	3 (10)
III (70)	38 (54)	6 (16)
IV (90)	55 (61)	13 (23)
V (45)	31 (69)	9 (29)

Modified from Creasman WT, Phillips JL, Mench HR: J Am Coll Surg 188:670, 1999.

study of 198 women from Sweden, vulvar melanoma was overrepresented by 2.5 times compared with cutaneous melanoma. Most vulvar melanomas are on the labia majora or clitoris. Of all melanomas, 46% of lesions were in glabrous (nonhairy) skin, 12% in hairy skin, and 35% in both areas. The median age of patients with these lesions is 65 years in a series reported by Tasseron and coworkers. In a large NCDB study of melanoma of the vulva, age ranged from 7 to 97 years with a median of 66 years; in this study, 50% were 70 years old or older and macroscopic amelanotic tumors were present in 27%

of patients. The patient may have experienced pruritus, bleeding, or enlargement of a pigmented area. Melanomas are often misdiagnosed as undifferentiated squamous cell cancers, especially when they are histologically amelanotic. The histologic diversity of melanoma can make the diagnosis challenging. In difficult cases, ultrastructural analysis with electron microscopy and immmunohistochemistry staining (especially with S-100 protein and HMB antibody) in conjunction with histologic evaluation can help confirm the diagnosis.

Prognosis is related to the size of the lesion and the depth of invasion. The Clark classification, commonly used for melanomas elsewhere on the skin, is of prognostic benefit for the vulva also. The Clark classification, which uses histologic levels, is outlined in Table 8-14. In 1970 Breslow recognized that survival was relative to the greatest thickness of the invasive portion of the melanoma by micrometer measure (Figure 8-27). The Breslow technique appeals to many because of its simplicity. In 1975 Chung and associates described a third system of reporting level of involvement of vulvar melanoma (Figure 8-28). Survival is influenced by histology as well. Five-year survival rates for superficial spreading and nodular melanomas were 71% and 38%, respectively; 10-year survival rates were 66% and 25%, respectively.

Although it has been suggested that all patients with melanoma of the vulva be treated with radical vulvectomy and inguinal and pelvic lymphadenectomy, there has been a tendency of late to be more conservative. In the 596 patients described by the NCDB, surgery was used in more than 90% of patients with stage 0 to stage III disease. Local excision was performed mainly in early stage (stage 0 and stage I) disease. Lymph node evaluation was performed in more than 50% of the patients, with greater frequency for patients with advanced disease. Radical local excision with a margin of 2 cm for thin lesions (up to 7 mm) and 3 to 4 cm for thicker lesions appears to be adequate for most well-circumscribed melanomas. Because prognosis is directly related to depth of invasion, therapy can be tailored accordingly. If the disease is intraepithelial, cure should be close to 100%. Clark level I or level II melanoma may be adequately treated with wide local excision. As the melanoma extends deeper, the chance of lymph node metastasis increases and the prognosis worsens considerably. Podratz and colleagues reported that 10-year survival rates associated with Clark's level II, III, IV, and V tumors were 100%, 83%, 65%, and 23%, respectively. In the 323 patients described by the NCDB who had a Clark

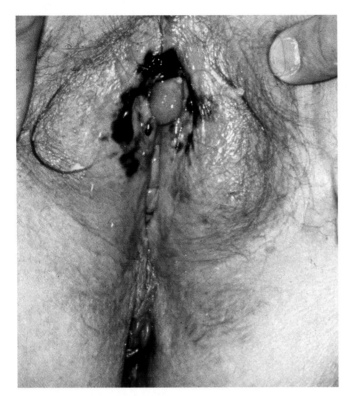

FIGURE 8-26   Melanoma of the vulva. A typical pigmented neoplasm is present.

TABLE 8-14   Correlation of Melanoma Thickness with Survival

Thickness	8-Year Survival Rates (%)
<0.85 mm	100
0.85-1.5 mm	99
1.5-4 mm	66
>4 mm	25-35

From Jaramillo BA et al: Malignant melanoma of the vulva. Obstet Gynecol 66:398, 1985; Day CL et al: The natural break points for primary tumor thickness in clinical stage I melanoma. N Engl J Med 305:1155, 1981.

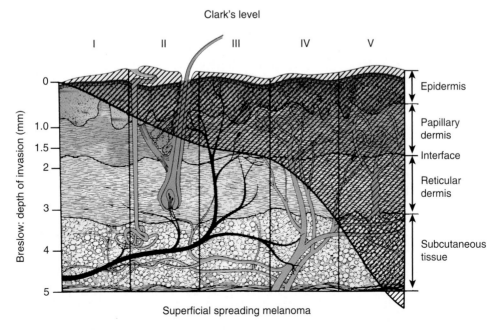

FIGURE 8-27   Comparison of Clark and Breslow classifications for skin melanomas.

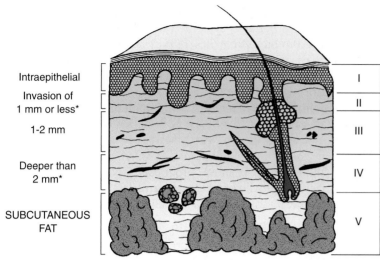

Intraepithelial

Invasion of
1 mm or less*

1-2 mm

Deeper than
2 mm*

SUBCUTANEOUS
FAT

I

II

III

IV

V

*As measured from the granular layer of surface epithelium

FIGURE 8-28   Chung system of reporting melanoma involvement.

level determination, 157 had lymph nodes evaluated. Most were in level II to level V, and as expected, metastasis increased as level of invasion increased (Table 8-15). In the patients with negative nodes, survival of level I to level IV was 88%, 77%, 88%, and 85%, respectively. Interestingly, 4 of 7 patients with positive nodes survived. Using the Breslow method, Jaramillo and coworkers and Day and coworkers reported nearly 100% survival in patients with lesions less than 1.5 mm in thickness, 65% to 70% survival in patients with lesions 1.5 to 4 mm, and 25% to 35% survival in patients with lesions greater than 4 mm (Table 8-16). Trimble and colleagues described 80 patients treated at Memorial Sloan-Kettering Cancer Center with a median follow-up of 193 months. By Chung level, 10-year survival for Chung level I to V was 100%, 81%, 87%, 11%, and 33% respectively.

Verschraegen and colleagues updated the experience from the MD Anderson hospital from 1970 to 1997. Thirty-two of 51 patients ultimately suffered a recurrence of their melanoma. Both Clark's and Breslow's assessments were predictive. The type of operation performed did not have an impact on recurrence. The role of lymphadenectomy in this disease is probably more prognostic than therapeutic and consideration can be given for SLN dissection as used for melanoma arising from other parts of the body. If disease is limited to the vulva, regardless of its extent, and the lymph nodes are negative, the survival rate is good. Most patients with positive inguinal or pelvic nodes eventually succumb to the disease.

Standard management of primary disease includes surgical resection, but there is a lack of consensus in the published literature regarding additional treatment options. Radiation, chemotherapy, biologic agents, and immunologic therapies have been implemented in

TABLE 8-15   Lymph Node Metastasis and Clark's Level of Vulvar Melanoma

Clark's Level	Nodes Examined	Positive Nodes
I ($n = 38$)	3 (8%)	0 (44%)
II ($n = 80$)	30 (60%)	3 (10%)
III ($n = 70$)	38 (54%)	6 (16%)
IV ($n = 90$)	55 (61%)	13 (23%)
V ($n = 45$)	31 (69%)	9 (29%)

Modified from Creasman WT, Phillips JL, Mench HR: J Am Coli Surg 188:670, 1999.

TABLE 8-16   Correlation of Melanoma Thickness with Survival of Patients

Thickness	Eight-year Survival Rates
<0.85 mm	100%
0.85-1.5 mm	99%
1.5-4 mm	66%
>4 mm	25% to 35%

From Jaramillo BA et al: Obstet Gynecol 66:398, 1985; and Day CL et al: N Engl J Med 305:1155, 1981.

high-risk and recurrent settings. Recommendations can be extrapolated from the experience in nongenital cutaneous melanomas. Therapy should be tailored to the individual patient.

SARCOMA

Sarcoma of the vulva is rare, and the experience is limited even in large referral institutions. The source of these tumors can be any of the supporting mesenchymal structures of the vulva. Symptoms and findings can be similar to those noted with squamous cell carcinoma, or patients can present with a well-circumscribed mass. In a review of 12 patients, DiSaia and colleagues noted that vulvar sarcoma occurred more often in younger patients (mean age 38 years) than other vulvar malignant neoplasms. A variety of histologic subtypes have been reported, all exceedingly rare, including leiomyosarcoma, rhabdomyosarcoma, malignant fibrous histiocytoma, epithelioid sarcoma, dermatofibrosarcoma protuberans, and even a few cases of Kaposi's sarcoma. The clinical course of these tumors tends to be similar to sarcomas occurring in other anatomic locations. The histologic grade appears to be the most important factor in prognosis. Undifferentiated tumors often grow rapidly, and metastasize early, whereas well-differentiated tumors may be cured with local resection or follow an indolent course. Primary therapy consists of radical vulvectomy and bilateral inguinal lymphadenectomy except in the low-grade lesions, in which node involvement is rare and wide local excision should be considered. Patients undergoing wide local excision are at risk for local recurrence and should be observed closely. Recurrences can be managed with re-resection, chemotherapy, radiation, or a combined modality approach, which should be tailored to the individual patient.

BARTHOLIN GLAND CARCINOMA

Adenocarcinoma of the Bartholin gland is a rare lesion occurring in only about 1% of all vulvar malignant neoplasms (Figure 8-29). The peak incidence is in women in their mid-60s, although it has been reported in a teenager. Because of its location, the tumor can be of

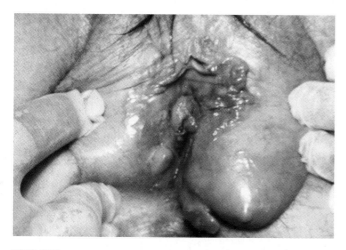

FIGURE 8-29 Adenocarcinoma of Bartholin's gland with local skin metastasis.

considerable size before the patient is aware of symptoms. Dyspareunia may be one of the first symptoms, although the finding of a mass or ulcerative lesion may be the first indication to the patient of her disease. An enlargement in the Bartholin gland area in a postmenopausal woman should be considered a malignant neoplasm until proved otherwise. The lesion can have a tendency to spread into the ischiorectal fossa and can have a propensity for lymphatic spread to the inguinal nodes by the common lymphatic spread pattern for vulvar cancer and for posterior spread to the pelvic nodes directly. Almost half of all carcinomas said to be of Bartholin gland origin are squamous cell carcinomas. Every attempt should be made to differentiate between a true Bartholin gland cancer and a primary squamous cell carcinoma of the vulva arising in proximity to the Bartholin gland. Prognosis is good if lymph node metastasis is not present.

Therapy includes radical vulvectomy with a large, wide, extensive dissection around the gland and inguinal lymphadenectomy. To have adequate margins, there may be a need to remove a considerable amount of vagina and, on occasion, part of the rectum. It appears that pelvic lymphadenectomy is not indicated A more conservative approach in selected patients with early disease may be appropriate. The largest series is that reported by Copeland and associates of 36 patients whose 5-year survival was 84%. Distribution of the tumors in FIGO stages included 9 stage I, 15 stage II, 10 stage III, and 2 stage IV. Cell types were squamous, 27; adenomatous, 6; adenoid cystic, 2; and adenosquamous, 1. Of 30 patients with lymph node dissections, 14 (47%) had nodal metastasis, and 11 remain free of disease. Disease recurred in 9 patients (6 local recurrences, 2 distant, 1 local and distant), and 4 were treated successfully. Less impressive results were reported by Wheelock and coworkers in a series of 10 patients. Radical vulvectomy with bilateral inguinal lymphadenectomy was performed in 9 patients; 5 of 9 had metastatic lymph node involvement, and 4 of the 5 died of disease.

Adenoid cystic carcinoma of the Bartholin gland is a rare entity manifested by frequent local painful recurrences and slowly progressive disease, including pulmonary metastasis, sometimes many years after initial therapy. The characteristic perineural and lymphatic invasion seen in these tumors are likely responsible for the pain and high rate of recurrence. Recommended primary treatment ranges from wide local excision to radical vulvectomy and inguinal lymphadenectomy followed by careful monitoring. Local recurrences are best treated by surgery. As with some other rare tumors, radiation and chemotherapy can be considered on an individual basis, especially in refractory cases and those with distant metastasis.

BASAL CELL CARCINOMA

Basal cell carcinoma usually presents in the eighth decade of life, comprising approximately 1.4% of all vulvar cancers. Clinical presentation often includes itching, irritation, or soreness and a lesion that bleeds and then seems to heal. The process repeats itself as the lesion slowly increases in size. No specific etiology or risk factors have been identified. Most lesions are small, and the most common location is the anterior hair-bearing aspect of the labia majora. A typical lesion has a rolled, pearly border showing fine telangiectatic vessels on the surface with central ulceration (Figure 8-30). These lesions typically behave like they do elsewhere on the body, with local invasion being the rule. Stromal infiltration is usually circumscribed and orderly with a slow and indolent growth rate. Lymphatics are rarely involved, and metastatic basal cell carcinoma of the vulva has been reported as a rare occurrence.

Primary treatment consists of wide local excision and primary closure without the need to surgically evaluate regional lymph nodes. Close follow-up is important. If a large lesion is present, a skin graft may be required following resection. In rare cases of very large lesions or clinically involved lymph nodes, successful response to preoperative radiation has been

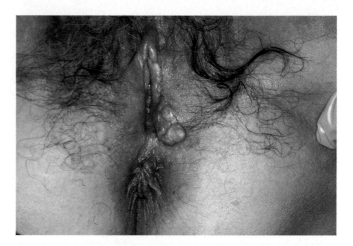

FIGURE 8-30   Basal cell carcinoma.

reported. Basal cell carcinoma must be differentiated pathologically from basosquamous cell carcinoma, which must be treated as one would treat a squamous cell carcinoma of the vulva.

For full reference list, log onto www.expertconsult.com ⟨http://www.expertconsult.com⟩.

Invasive Cancer of the Vagina

Brian M. Slomovitz, MD, and Robert L. Coleman, MD

The vaginal tissues, in sharp contrast to the uterine cervix and other gynecologic organs, rarely undergo malignant transformation. Primary cancer of the vagina is an uncommon malignancy, accounting for only 1% to 3% of gynecologic malignancies (Table 9-1). In 2011 there will be 2570 new cases of vaginal cancer and 780 women will die from this disease because the annual incidence of this disease is approximately 1 case in 100,000 women.

When primary cancer does occur in the vagina, it is usually in the upper third (Table 9-2) and it is most commonly an epithelial carcinoma. By convention, any primary malignant neoplasm involving both the cervix and vagina is classified as cervical cancer. The age incidence of this disease is between 35 and 90 years, with more than 50% of the cases occurring between the seventh and ninth decades of life (Figure 9-1).

Squamous cell carcinoma is the most frequent histologic subtype (78%). Adenocarcinoma (6%), melanoma (3%), and sarcoma (3%) have been described as primary vaginal cancers (Table 9-3). History of radiation therapy contributes to the development of vaginal sarcomas. The relationship of diethylstilbestrol (DES) intrauterine exposure to clear cell adenocarcinoma of the vagina has resulted in the reporting of significant numbers of cases

of adenocarcinoma of the vagina in both exposed and unexposed individuals.

The principal focus of this chapter is squamous cancers. Rare histologies will be discussed later in the chapter. However, the clinical evaluation and staging for vaginal tumors are the same for all types of vaginal cancers.

SQUAMOUS CELL CARCINOMA OF THE VAGINA

Epidemiology

Similar to cervical cancer, epidemiologic evidence suggests that vaginal cancer has a strong relationship with human papilloma virus (HPV) infection. HPV subtype 16 presence has been associated with up to two thirds of all new cases of vaginal cancer. In addition, approximately one-third of women who develop vaginal cancer have a history of cervical dysplasia or cervical cancer more than 5 years earlier. A study from the University of South Carolina found that the median interval between cervical disease and development of vaginal cancer was 14 years. In this study, 16% of patients had a history of

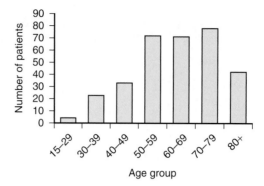

FIGURE 9-1 Carcinoma of the vagina: Patients treated in 1999-2001. Number of cases by age group. *(From IJGO Vol. 95, Suppl. 1 FIGO Annual Report, Vol. 26.)*

Age group	Patients (n)	Percentage (%)
15–29	4	1.2
30–39	23	7.1
40–49	33	10.2
50–59	72	22.2
60–69	71	21.9
70–79	78	24.1
80+	43	13.3
Total	324	100.0

TABLE 9-1 Incidence of Vaginal Cancer

Series	No. of Malignant Genital Neoplasms	Vaginal Cancer (%)
Smith (1955)	8199	1.5
Ries and Ludwig (1962)	14,785	2.1
Smith (1964)	6050	1.8
Wolff and Douyon (1964)	4665	1.8
Rutledge (1967)	5715	1.2
Palumbo et al (1969)	2305	1.9
Daw (1971)	564	1.9
Gallup et al (1987)	Not given	3.1
Manetta (1988)	2149	1.3
Eddy (1991)	2929	3.1

TABLE 9-2 Involvement of Vagina

Series	Upper Third	Middle Third	Lower Third
Livingstone (1950)	34	4	42
Bivens (1953)	22	3	14
Mobius (1956)	89	0	29
Arronet, Latour, and Tremblay (1960)	14	8	3
Whelton and Kottmeier (1962)	20	13	19
Blunt (1965)	13	15	10
Daw (1971)	24	14	13
Benedet (1983)	46	3	19
Manetta et al (1990)	22	8	16
Eddy et al (1991)	33	5	8
Total	317 (56%)	73 (13%)	173 (31%)

TABLE 9-3 Histologic Distribution of Primary Vaginal Cancer

Cell Type	Percentage %
Squamous	85
Adenocarcinoma	6
Melanoma	3
Sarcoma	3
Miscellaneous	3

Between 3% and 7% of patients with VAIN progress to invasive carcinoma despite treatment. Chronic vaginal irritation has also been suggested to contribute to the etiology of vaginal cancer; however, the mechanism by which this promotes carcinogenesis is not well understood and has not been extensively studied.

Screening

For women who have had a previous hysterectomy, the diagnosis of vaginal cancer may often be missed. It is particularly important that the lateral "horns" of the upper vaginal vault be thoroughly examined. For some patients, this may require use of an endocervical speculum to ensure a complete evaluation of the vaginal apices.

The Papanicolaou smear is effective in detecting vaginal cancer in an asymptomatic patient. For a screening test to be effective, however, the incidence of the disease must be sufficient to justify the cost. The American Cancer Society recommends that Papanicolaou screening for cervical cancer may be discontinued in women who have had a hysterectomy for conditions other than cervical dysplasia or cancer. However, women with a history of cervical dysplasia or cervical cancer are at increased risk and Pap testing should be continued whether or not they may have had a hysterectomy.

Because the incidence of vaginal cancer is so low, routine screening is not cost effective. However, development of vaginal cancer is possible even in women with a history of hysterectomy for benign disease. Bell and colleagues described 87 patients with primary

prior radiation. Proposed mechanisms for developing vaginal cancer with a remote history of cervical cancer include occult residual disease, radiation-induced tumorigenesis, and a new primary cancer in a high-risk individual. Regardless, a new vaginal lesion 5 years or more after treatment of cervical cancer constitutes a new primary vaginal cancer.

The natural course of vaginal intraepithelial neoplasia (VAIN) is not well understood because most patients are treated once diagnosed. Up to 99% of VAIN 1 and 93% of VAIN 2/3 result from HPV. HPV-16 is the most common type of HPV associated with vaginal dysplasia.

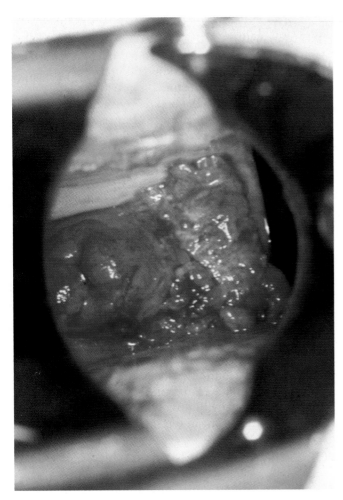

FIGURE 9-2   Lesion of the posterior fornix in squamous cell carcinoma.

cancer of the vagina, 31 of whom had undergone total hysterectomy for benign disease. Benedet and colleagues found that 19 of their 97 patients (20%) with vaginal cancer had surgery for benign diseases. Peters and associates reported that 38% (25 of 68) of the patients in their series had undergone prior hysterectomies for benign disease. Guidelines aside, these observations underscore the need to individualize vaginal cancer cytologic screening by careful consideration of estimated risks and benefits of such clinical activity.

Signs and Symptoms

The signs and symptoms of invasive vaginal cancer (Figure 9-2) are similar to those of cervical cancer. Painless vaginal discharge, often bloody, is the most frequent symptom in most series. Postcoital or postmenopausal vaginal bleeding is the initial symptom in many patients with invasive lesions, and a gross lesion is obvious on speculum examination. Urinary symptoms (pain and frequency) are more common than with cervical cancer

because neoplasms that are lower in the vagina are close to the vesicle neck, with resulting compression of the bladder at an earlier stage of the disease. Tenesmus is commonly associated with posterior vaginal lesions. Approximately 5% to 10% of women have no symptoms, and the disease is suspected on physical examination and confirmed by biopsy.

Diagnostic Considerations

All patients who present with a vaginal cancer need to have a full workup to rule out metastatic disease. Medical history should emphasize history of cancer, radiotherapy, and surgery. Physical examination, including an adequate pelvic examination (under anesthesia if necessary), should be performed. The diagnosis is often missed on first examination, especially if the lesion is small and covered by the blades of the speculum. Definitive diagnosis is made by biopsy.

In patients with an abnormal Pap smear and no gross abnormality, careful vaginal colposcopy is necessary. In order to differentiate between an early vaginal cancer and VAIN III, it is often necessary to perform a partial upper vaginectomy because the lesion may be buried by reapproximation of the vaginal vault at the time of hysterectomy. Hoffman and associates reported on 32 patients with VAIN III who underwent an upper vaginectomy. Invasive carcinoma was found in 28% of the patients.

Metastatic carcinoma to the vagina is seen much more often than primary disease. More than 80% of malignant vaginal lesions are the result of metastasis from other sites. In 269 patients with metastatic vaginal cancer, Mazur and colleagues found that 84% were from genital sites and the remaining 16% were most commonly metastatic from the gastrointestinal tract or breast. The cervix (32%) and endometrium (18%) are the most common primary sites of cancer. Endometrial carcinomas and choriocarcinomas often metastasize to the vagina, whereas rectal and bladder cancers invade the vagina directly.

When the primary site of growth is in the vagina and does not involve surrounding organs (e.g., vulva or cervix), the tumor is considered a vaginal primary cancer. Special consideration needs to be made for those patients with a remote (>5 years) or questionable history of a gynecologic malignancy (especially cervical cancer) who present with a vaginal lesion. By convention, these lesions are considered primary vaginal cancers. However, patients with a history of endometrial cancer and a vaginal lesion with a histologic diagnosis of adenocarcinoma consistent with recurrence are diagnosed with recurrent endometrial cancer.

Once diagnosed, patients with cancer of the vagina should be examined for evidence of local or distant spread in a manner analogous to that of cervical cancer. All patients should have at least the following diagnostic studies in addition to a thorough history and physical examination: chest radiograph, intravenous pyelography, cystoscopy, and proctosigmoidoscopy, the last two depending on the location of disease. A computed tomography (CT) scan or magnetic resonance imaging (MRI) can replace the pyelography, cystoscopy, and proctosigmoidoscopy. If bone pain is present, further radiographs are warranted. Although staging is clinical, not surgical, an imaging evaluation should be performed to evaluate lymph node metastasis, distant metastasis, and an evaluation of the genitourinary system.

PET/CT and Vaginal Cancer

CT imaging is only able to detect suspicious lymph nodes that are at least 1.5 cm in greatest dimension. Metabolic imaging with positron emission tomography (PET) has been shown to be more sensitive than CT and MRI, specifically for cancer of the head and neck, lung, esophagus, and cervix. In a study from Washington University, Lamoreaux and associates found that PET imaging detected primary and metastatic lesions more often than CT scans. We recommend that all patients with vaginal cancer have imaging, and the PET/CT is a reasonable option for these patients.

Sentinel Lymph Node Dissection

Patients with vaginal cancer rarely undergo lymph node dissections. Sentinel lymph node evaluation has been evaluated as a technique to determine if there is microscopic nodal metastasis. Frumovitz and colleagues evaluated the utility of radiocolloid and blue dye injection in 14 women with newly diagnosed vaginal cancer. These investigators found that the lymphatic drainage from the primary tumor does not always follow the lymphatic channels that would have been predicted. Pretreatment lymphoscintigraphy did improve treatment planning in this small study. Incorporation of sentinel lymph node dissection should be limited to research protocol.

Staging

Staging of vaginal cancer follows clinical parameters outlined by the International Federation of Gynecology and Obstetrics (FIGO) (Figure 9-3); a summary of the staging classification follows:

Stage 0   Carcinoma in situ, intraepithelial carcinoma
Stage I   Carcinoma is limited to the vaginal wall
Stage II   Carcinoma has involved the subvaginal tissue but has not extended onto the pelvic wall
Stage III Carcinoma has extended onto the pelvic wall
Stage IV   Carcinoma has extended beyond the true pelvis or has involved the mucosa of the bladder or rectum; bullous edema or tumor bulge into the bladder or rectum is not acceptable evidence of invasion of these organs
Stage IVa Spread of the growth to adjacent organs or direct extension beyond the true pelvis
Stage IVb Spread to distant organs

Perez and Camel have suggested modification of stage II. Stage IIa lesions would involve the submucosal area of the vagina but should not extend to the parametrium. Stage IIb lesions would significantly involve the parametrium but not extend to the pelvic wall. Although useful to stratify patients with stage II disease, this staging modification has not demonstrated prognostic significance. Although FIGO does not specify the stage of patients with inguinal lymph node involvement, the American Joint Committee on Cancer (AJCC) assigns patients with T1 to T3 tumors with positive inguinal lymph nodes to stage III. Involvement of the pubic symphysis places a patient in the stage III category.

Patterns of Spread

Vaginal cancer metastasizes by direct extension, lymphatic dissemination, and hematogenous spread. The pelvic soft tissues, pelvic bones, bladder, and rectum are commonly involved via direct extension in those patients with locally advanced disease. The lymphatic vasculature of the vagina begins as an extremely fine capillary meshwork in the mucosa and submucosa (Figure 9-4). In the deep layers of the submucosa and muscularis, there is a similar parallel but coarser network. Irregular anastomoses have been demonstrated between the two. Both systems drain into small trunks that coalesce at the lateral aspect of the vagina and form a number of collecting trunks. It is at this point that the efferent lymph drainage channels of the organ originate. The lymphatic trunks of the upper vagina drain into the iliac and eventually the para-aortic lymph nodes. The lower vagina is principally drained by a lymphatic network that anastomoses with the regional lymph nodes of the femoral triangle. All lymph nodes in the pelvis may at one time or another serve as primary sites or regional drainage nodes for vaginal lymph and its contents.

Because most patients with vaginal cancer are treated with radiation, the incidence of lymph node involvement is not well recorded. However, retrospective studies demonstrate that 30% to 35% of patients with

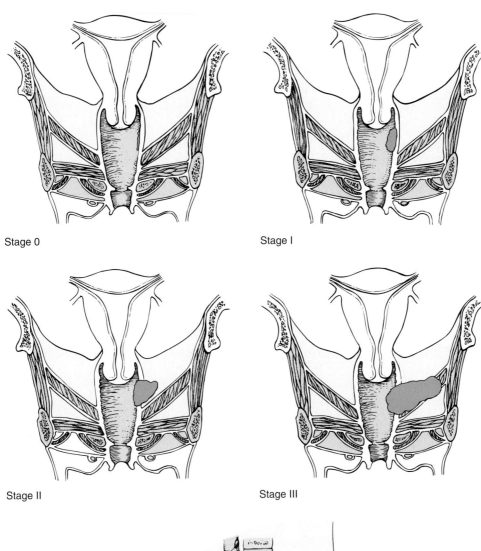

Stage 0

Stage I

Stage II

Stage III

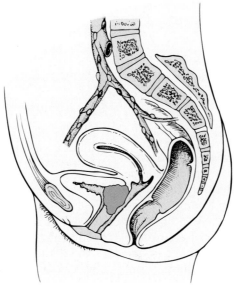

Stage IV

FIGURE 9-3   Staging diagrams for vaginal cancer.

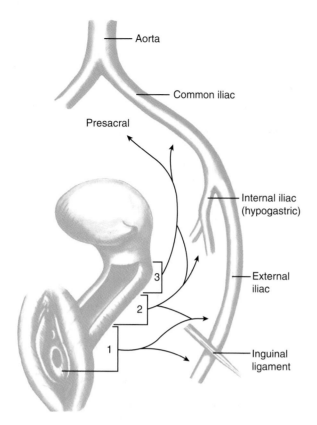

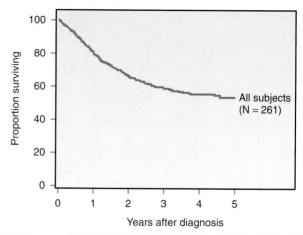

Patients (n)	Mean age (yr)	Overall survival (%) at				
		1 year	2 years	3 years	4 years	5 years
All subjects 261	62.7	80.1	66.7	59.0	55.6	53.6

FIGURE 9-5 Carcinoma of the vagina. Patients treated in 1990-1992. Five-year survival rates. *(From IJGO Vol. 95, Suppl. 1 FIGO Annual Report, Vol. 26.)*

FIGURE 9-4 Lymphatic drainage of the vagina: channels from the lower third drain into the femoral and external iliac nodes (*1*); the channels from the middle third drain into the hypogastric nodes (*2*); channels from the upper third drain into the common iliac, presacral, and hypogastric nodes (*3*). *(Modified from Plentl AA, Friedman EA: Lymphatic System of the Female Genitalia. Philadelphia, WB Saunders, 1971.)*

TABLE 9-4 Vaginal Cancer: Comparison of Survival

Authors	No. of Cases	Stage and Survival (%)				
		I	II	III	IV	All Stages
Krepart (1979)	14*	65	60	35	39	51.8
Nori et al. (1981)	36*	71	66	33	0	42.8
Perez and Camel (1982)	105*	81	42	30	9	50.8
Prempree (1982)	80*	78	57	39	0	8.8
Puthawala et al. (1983)	27*	100	75	22	0	56.8
Benedet et al. (1983)	75*	71	50	15	0	45.8
Reuben et al. (1985)	68*	79	52	54	0	49.8
Gallup et al. (1987)	28*	100	50	0	25	42.8
Eddy (1991)	84*	70	45	35	28	50.8
Stock et al. (1995)	100*	67	53	0	15	46.8
Creasman et al. (1998)	792*	73	58	58	58	

5-year survival.

vaginal cancer have lymph node metastasis. Para-aortic spread is almost exclusively seen in patients with concomitant pelvic node metastases.

Prognostic Features

The number of patients who survive vaginal cancer has increased, which reflects our better understanding of the disease and improved radiation techniques (Figure 9-5 and Table 9-4). Several investigators have remarked that age at time of diagnosis is one of the most important prognostic factors. Reflecting intolerance of aggressive multimodality therapy and attendant comorbidities, age acts as a surrogate of clinical outcome. Although not well described, performance status likely reflects a factor with greater precision in determining the impact of chronologic age. Tumor histology may also have prognostic relevance. It is clear that vaginal melanomas and sarcomas have the poorest prognosis when compared to squamous cell and adenocarcinomas. However, survival

differences among these histologies have not been well documented.

Stage, tumor location, and tumor size also appear to affect prognosis. In a review of 843 patients with vaginal cancer, patients with stage I disease had a 64% to 90% 5-year survival, 31% to 80% for stage II, 0% to 79% for stage III, and 0% to 62% for stage IV. In this study, lesions of the distal vagina had a poorer prognosis than those originating in the proximal vagina. In a review of 104 patients, Smith (1964) found 6.8% survivors among 29 patients with cancer of the lower third of the vagina, 25% of 48 patients with tumors of the middle third, and 37% of 27 patients with lesions of the upper third. In 1958 Merrill and Bender reported a 29% survival rate in 14 patients with upper third lesions and an 11% rate in 9 patients with distal third involvement. Recently, Tewari and colleagues reported that survival was better for patients with lesions smaller than 3 cm compared to those greater than 3 cm. Chyle and colleagues found that tumor size larger than 5 cm was associated with a higher local recurrence rate when compared to smaller tumors.

Frank and colleagues at MD Anderson Cancer Center reported their 30-year experience treating patients with vaginal cancer. In this series of 193 patients, disease-specific survival and pelvic disease control rates were correlated with stage (I, II, or III/IV) and tumor size (<4 cm or >4 cm).

Intuitively, lymph node status at the time of diagnosis would portend a worse prognosis; however, this has not been thoroughly evaluated. In one study by Pingley and colleagues, the 5-year survival for patients without lymph node involvement was 56% compared to 33% for those patients with lymph node involvement. Finally, as has been suggested in radiation treatment trials of patients with cervical cancer, time to treatment initiation and total treatment time affect survival. Lee and associates found that the pelvic control rate was 97% if the treatment was completed within 63 days compared to 54% if treatment lasted longer than this time.

In a review of the Surveillance, Epidemiology, and End Result (SEER) population-based cancer registry, 2149 women with vaginal cancer between 1990 and 2004 were identified. Advanced stage, tumor size greater than 4 cm, aggressive histologies (e.g., melanoma), and combined treatment modality (vs surgery alone) were associated with a worse prognosis.

Management

Until the 1930s, vaginal cancers were considered incurable. With advances in radiation oncology, cure rates for even advanced cancers approach those for cervical cancer. As mentioned, stage, tumor location, and size are the principle factors taken into consideration when planning treatment for patients with vaginal carcinoma. Other factors include history of surgery and/or radiation.

Prevention

Although the potential effect of HPV vaccines may not be as high for vaginal cancer as it may be for cervical cancer, vaccinating young women against HPV-16 and -18 should help to reduce the incidence of HPV-related vaginal disease.

TABLE 9-5   Radiotherapy for Vaginal Cancer

Stage	External Irradiation	Vaginal Therapy
0	Surgical excision preferred for localized disease	7000 cGy surface dose
I		
1-2 cm lesion		Brachytherapy irradiation, 6000-7000 cGy*
Larger lesions	4000-5000 cGy whole pelvis	Brachytherapy delivering 3000-4000 cGy
II	4000-5000 cGy whole pelvis	Same as for stage I
III	5000 cGy whole pelvis (optional 1000-2000 cGy through reduced fields)	Brachytherapy implant, 2000-3000 cGy (if tumor regression is satisfactory)
IV (pelvis only)	Same as for stage III	Same as for stage III

*Surgical excision for selected sites on 1- to 2-cm lesions may be used instead of brachytherapy.

Stage 0 and I

VAIN usually occurs at the vaginal apex. It is also a multifocal disease and is common in patients with a history of cervical dysplasia. Treatment options for patients with VAIN include surgery (i.e., wide local excision or vaginectomy), 5% fluorouracil cream, local ablation (Laser, cryotherapy, electrodiathermy, etc.), and intracavitary radiation (Table 9-5).

Creasman and associates reported the results of the National Cancer Data Base (NCDB), a large central registry of hospital data, for 10 years (1984-1994). There were 4885 cases reported, with 1242 carcinomas in situ (CIS) representing 26% of all vaginal lesions. CIS was almost exclusively treated with surgery; only 5% were treated with radiotherapy. Brown and colleagues reported no new cases of in situ or invasive carcinoma of the vagina developing after radiation therapy for CIS or early invasive carcinoma. Their report discouraged overly aggressive therapy for early-stage tumors because of the good prognosis for these lesions and the adverse effects of high-dose irradiation on the pliability of the vagina and on sexual function. Lee and Symmonds reported the results in 66 patients treated previously with wide local excisions or partial vaginectomies and in 7 patients with multicentric disease treated with total vaginectomies. Only 1 patient had recurrent carcinoma of the vagina, resulting in her death. In the young, sexually active patient with diffuse involvement of the vaginal epithelium, total or subtotal vaginectomy with split-thickness skin graft reconstruction of the vagina often allows excellent long-term results. When radiation therapy is chosen, patients who have CIS and superficial stage I tumors can be treated with intracavitary insertion alone.

TABLE 9-6   Primary Vaginal Carcinoma: Local Control and Disease-Free Survival By Stage

FIGO Stage	Local Control (%)	Five Years	
		Disease-Free Survival	No.
I	23	72	67
II	58	62	53
III	9	0	0
IV	10	21	15

From Stock RG et al: Gynecol Oncol 56:45, 1995.

Surgical management is an option for lesions 0.5 cm or less in patients with invasive carcinoma. For early lesions, particularly in the upper vagina (see Figure 9-2), surgery may be preferred in many patients. Peters and coworkers have described superficially invasive squamous cell carcinoma of the vagina as a lesion that invades less than 2.5 mm from the surface, is lacking involvement of lymphovascular spaces, and is developed in a field of CIS. Their experience with six patients suggests that local therapy was sufficient, and no attempt was made to treat pelvic nodes either surgically or with irradiation. This conservative approach might allow preservation of optimal sexual function in young patients who have these early invasive squamous and adenocarcinoma lesions.

For invasive carcinoma thicker than 0.5 cm, total vaginectomy and lymphadenectomy have been performed in the past. If the patient did not have a prior hysterectomy, a radical hysterectomy and upper vaginectomy would need to be performed. However, pelvic external-beam radiotherapy and interstitial implants are more commonly used. Patients with small stage I cancers (<2 cm) who are not good surgical candidates can adequately be treated with brachytherapy alone. For large vaginal tumors, options for radiating the primary lesion are tailored by physician preference and extent of disease. Bulky stage I cancers (>2 cm) of the upper portion of the vagina in patients with intact uteri are treated with techniques similar to those used for carcinoma of the cervix. External irradiation in a dose of 4000 to 5000 cGy is given initially in bulky stage I and stage II cancers (Table 9-6). For young patients who require radiation therapy, pretreatment laparotomy or laparoscopy with ovarian transposition and surgical staging is a rational approach.

Stage II to IVa

For patients who have stage II to IV vaginal cancer, treatment is tailored to the extent of the disease and the radiation therapy plan should reflect consideration of the depth of invasion of the lesion. Proper planning of radiation therapy and individualization of treatment plans are essential to minimize the more serious complications of acute and long-term radiation sequelae in these organs. The difficulty in applying radiation systems to vaginal cancer led some, like Wertheim and Brunschwig, to advocate radical exenterative surgery as primary therapy. However, the complications associated with these radical procedures, especially in older patients, have become a serious limiting factor to the surgical approach.

Patients with advanced-stage disease should be treated with external irradiation and brachytherapy. External irradiation to the pelvis is usually sufficient and para-aortic extension is not routinely administered. Groin radiation is often considered if the tumor involves the lower one third of the vagina or in the presence of metastatic groin disease. Perez and associates evaluated 149 patients with vaginal carcinoma and clinically negative lymph nodes who were not treated with groin radiation. In the group of patients with tumors confined to the upper vagina, there were no recurrences, compared with an 8% recurrence rate in those patients whose tumor involved the lower third of the vagina.

If the uterus is intact and the lesion is in the upper vagina, an intrauterine tandem and ovoids would be appropriate. If the patient has had a hysterectomy, interstitial radiation alone or in combination with intracavitary therapy optimizes dose distribution.

For those patients who can be treated with brachytherapy only, a minimum of 6000 to 7000 cGy is delivered to the neoplasm in 5 to 7 days. Pelvic and groin radiation consists of a total of 45 to 50.4 Gy given in 1.8-Gy fractions daily. Use of concomitant sensitizing radiotherapy is discussed in the following section.

If there is metastatic lymph node involvement to the pelvic or groin lymph nodes, external radiation is given to a dose of 60 to 66 Gy. In addition, adenopathy greater than 2 cm may be best controlled with excision. The deep nodes must be included in the treatment fields because large tumors have a high incidence of regional lymphatic metastasis. After receiving 5000 cGy, the patient with a large lesion should be re-evaluated for an additional 1000 to 2000 cGy external radiation to reduced field. Higher radiation doses, however, are associated with greater vaginal toxicity. Newer treatment planning protocols using intensity-modulated radiation therapy (IMRT) may lead to higher tumor control with less local normal tissue effects. Long-term morbidity outcomes with this technology are awaited.

Chemosensitizing radiation is standard for patients with carcinoma of the cervix. Because the natural history, the histology, and risk factors are similar for vaginal cancer, chemotherapy chemosensitization with weekly cisplatin has been recommended in patients receiving radiation for advanced-stage disease. Prospective studies will likely not be performed given the rarity of this disease.

Chemotherapy

Studies are limited regarding the experience with chemotherapy for patients with vaginal cancer. In a phase II Gynecologic Oncology Group (GOG) study, 26 patients with progressive or recurrent vaginal carcinoma were treated with cisplatin (50 mg/m^2 every 3 weeks). There was minimal, insignificant activity, particularly in the patients with squamous cell carcinoma. Other agents that have been used for the treatment of vaginal cancer include 5-fluorouracil (5-FU), mitomycin-C, epirubicin, and the combination of two of these agents.

A small series of patients with stage II vaginal carcinoma treated with neoadjuvant chemotherapy followed by radical surgery has been reported by Panici and colleagues. Eleven patients were treated with paclitaxel 175 mg/m^2 and cisplatin 75 mg/m^2 for three courses followed by surgery. There was a 27% complete response rate and 64% partial response rate. With a median of 75 months, 2 (18%) patients had a recurrence and 1 died of disease.

Special Considerations

Although one is often dealing with a radiosensitive neoplasm in a relatively radioresistant bed (the vagina), serious limitations may nonetheless exist. The proximity of relatively radiosensitive normal tissues, such as the bladder and rectum, provides a challenge to the therapist, especially in the treatment of tumors in the lower third of the vagina. Therapy must be individualized, and radical surgery should be reserved for treatment failures (Figure 9-6).

The incidence of complications after radiation therapy or surgery for vaginal cancer can be substantial. Serious complications consist primarily of rectal stenosis, rectovaginal fistulas, and severe rectal bleeding often requiring diversion. As many as 35% of patients experience cystitis or proctitis during or shortly after therapy, but symptoms usually resolve spontaneously. A few patients have extensive vaginal necrosis that usually resolves with prolonged conservative management.

Frank and associates found that the incidence of major complications associated with radiation were associated with FIGO stage. Four percent of stage I patients, 9% of stage II patients, and 21% of stage III/IVa patients suffered major complications.

Patients who are sexually active should be encouraged to continue regular intercourse. For others, vaginal dilators should be used to maintain vaginal patency during and after therapy.

Survival and Recurrence

A study by Rutledge in 1967 reported 3- and 5-year survival rates of 42% and 44%, respectively, for patients treated primarily with radiotherapy. Comparable survival results at 5 years were reported by Prempree and colleagues, who used radiotherapy for stage I (83%), stage II (63%), stage III (40%), and stage IV (0%) lesions; their absolute 5-year cure rate for all stages was 55.5%.

In 1982 Perez and Camel reported their long-term follow-up of patients treated with radiation therapy for invasive carcinoma of the vagina. The actuarial disease-free 5-year survival rate for stage I (39 patients) was 90%; stage IIa (39 patients), 58%; stage IIb (21 patients), 32%; stage III (12 patients), 40%; and stage IV (8 patients), 0%. Of 39 patients with stage I carcinoma, 37 (95%) showed no evidence of vaginal or pelvic recurrence. Most of them received interstitial or intracavitary therapy or both; the addition of external-beam irradiation did not

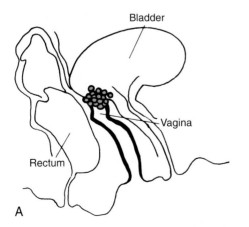
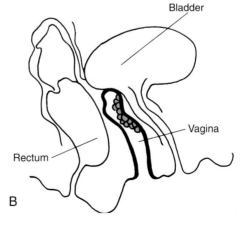

FIGURE 9-6 Diagrammatic representation of typical locations of vaginal cancer in a previously hysterectomized patient, illustrating the proximity of the bladder and urethra. **A,** Lesion at the vaginal apex. **B,** Lesion at the upper anterior vaginal wall. *(Courtesy A. Robert Kagan, MD, Los Angeles, California.)*

significantly increase survival or tumor control. In stage IIa (paravaginal extension), tumor was controlled in 22 of 34 patients (64.7%) with a combination of brachytherapy and external-beam irradiation; only 2 of 5 (40%) treated with brachytherapy alone exhibited tumor control in the pelvis. The incidence of complications was 9.7% for all stages.

In 1991 Eddy and coworkers published similar results for stage I and stage II lesions of the vagina treated with curative radiotherapy and reported a 5-year survival of 78% for patients assigned to stage I and 71% for patients assigned to stage II. In addition, Stock and colleagues (1995) reported local control rates of 72% for stage I and 62% for stage II disease (see Table 9-6). In the large database (NCDB) reported in 1998, the 5-year relative survival rate was 96% for stage 0, 73% for stage I, 58% for stage II, and 36% for stage III-IV. Women with stage I disease who were treated with surgery had a 5-year survival rate of 90% compared with 63% for patients treated with radiotherapy and 79% for patients treated with surgery and radiotherapy.

In the study from MD Anderson, the 5-year disease-specific survival rate was 85% for patients with stage I disease, 78% for stage II, and 58% for stage III/IVa. In this study, external-beam radiation fields and dose were determined by evaluating distribution of gross disease and possible sites of microscopic paravaginal and nodal disease.

Sinha and colleagues from Indiana University reviewed their experience with treating vaginal cancers. Overall survival rates were similar to the MD Anderson study (stage I, 92%; stage II, 82%; and stages III and IVA, 20%; $P = 0.0005$). Because of the poor prognosis associated with advanced stage disease, these investigators suggested routine use of combined chemotherapy and radiation as a treatment strategy for these patients.

Vaginal cancers appear to behave like cervical or vulvar cancer by first recurring locally. More than 80% of patients with recurrent disease have pelvic recurrence noted clinically, and most recurrences appear within 2 years of primary therapy. Distant sites of involvement occur later and much less frequently. Effective treatment for previously irradiated but locally recurrent or persistent vaginal cancer patients requires radical surgery (i.e., pelvic exenteration). However, for those with extrapelvic recurrence, the long-term prognosis is poor. Chyle and colleagues reported a 12% 5-year survival rate after first recurrence. Rubin and associates reported on 33 patients with recurrent vaginal cancer. Eighteen had recurrent disease in the pelvis; 15 were extrapelvic recurrences. At the time of the report, 30 patients had died of disease. The average length of survival from recurrence was 8 months. In the past, chemotherapy for recurrent squamous cell carcinoma of the vagina has been relatively ineffective. In the only GOG study of recurrent vaginal cancer, Thigpen and coworkers described 16 patients with squamous cell carcinoma of the vagina treated in a phase II study of cisplatin 50 mg/m^2 intravenously every 3 weeks. The results were disappointing. There was only 1 responder, and this was a complete responder who had extrapelvic disease and who had received no prior therapy. Most of the patients with recurrence in previously irradiated fields showed no response; 5 of the remaining 15 patients had stable disease.

In the SEER study, an apparent survival advantage was seen with the incorporation of chemoradiation (those patients treated since 2000) when compared to those patients treated with radiation alone (those patients treated between 1990 and 1994).

RARE HISTOLOGIES

Adenocarcinoma/Clear Cell Adenocarcinoma

Approximately 6% of vaginal cancers are adenocarcinomas. Before 1965 clear cell adenocarcinoma of the cervix in women younger than age 30 years was reported only rarely, and vaginal clear cell adenocarcinoma was unknown. In April 1970 Herbst and Scully reported seven cases of primary vaginal adenocarcinoma in patients between the ages of 15 and 22 years. These seven cases exceeded the number of cases in the world literature in adolescent girls born before 1945. Because of this case clustering, an epidemiologic study of the patients and their families was initiated to identify associative factors. With the addition of another patient to the study, it was discovered that the mothers of seven of the eight patients with vaginal adenocarcinoma had been treated with DES, a nonsteroidal synthetic estrogen, in the first trimester of the relevant pregnancy. Since that time, additional cases of vaginal and cervical adenocarcinoma have been reported in patients whose mothers ingested nonsteroidal estrogen during pregnancy. DES and related drugs were used to support high-risk pregnancy and reduce fetal wastage in the mid-1940s and 1950s, but their use then declined. The incidence of DES-induced clear cell carcinoma peaked in the mid-1970s.

As of 1992, 594 cases of vaginal and cervical (approximately 40% involve the cervix) adenocarcinoma have been accessioned by the registry established by Herbst and colleagues. Among the cases in which a maternal history was obtainable, the proportion that was positive for medication with DES or chemically related estrogens was approximately two thirds. Progestins had been administered in six of the cases, and a steroidal estrogen had been administered in another three cases. The risk for development of these carcinomas in the DES-exposed female patient through the age of 24 years has been estimated to be 0.14 to 1.4 per 1000. Of the cases, 90% have occurred in patients 14 years of age or older. About 68% of the individuals with clear cell adenocarcinoma of the cervix and 86% of those with primary vaginal tumors had a history of hormone exposure. In addition, there was a lower risk for cancer among women whose mothers began DES after the 12th week of pregnancy. It is not known how many exposed women are in the United States, but estimates place this population at 0.5 million to 2 million.

Patients 15 years of age and younger appeared to have more aggressive carcinomas than those of patients 19 years of age and older. Abnormal bleeding was the initial symptom in most of the patients, but 20% were asymptomatic and carcinomas were discovered on routine pelvic examinations. Cytologic testing has proved useful, but a false-negative rate of up to 20% has been reported, probably because of the heavy polymorphonuclear infiltration seen with these lesions. The carcinomas may occur anywhere on the vagina or cervix, but most have been in the upper part of the vagina, particularly on the anterior wall (Figure 9-7). Adenosis (the presence of glandular epithelium or its mucinous products in the vagina) has been found accompanying vaginal clear cell adenocarcinoma in virtually all cases. Adenosis is benign tissue, but it may be the non-neoplastic precursor of the clear cell adenocarcinoma in some cases, although direct transitions from adenosis to cancer have not been identified. The same observations apply to cervical eversion (ectropion, "congenital erosion") and clear cell adenocarcinoma of the cervix.

Both surgery and radiation have been effective in treating these tumors (Table 9-7), although follow-up for many of these patients is limited. Incidence of lymph node metastases is fairly high, with approximately 16% in stage I and 30% or more in stage II. The clear cell adenocarcinomas tend to remain superficial, suggesting the possibility that this disease can be treated locally, especially if the lesion is small.

The Registry for Research on Hormonal Transplacental Carcinogenesis has reported a study examining the effectiveness of various forms of therapy for early-stage vaginal clear cell adenocarcinomas. Of 219 patients with stage I vaginal clear cell adenocarcinomas, 20% received local therapy and 80% underwent conventional therapy. Actuarial survival rates at 5 and 10 years for patients treated with local therapy and conventional therapy were equivalent (92% and 88%, respectively). This study

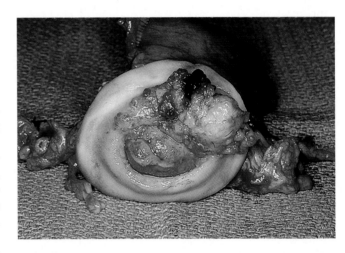

FIGURE 9-7   Clear cell adenocarcinoma (radical hysterectomy and upper vaginectomy specimen). Note the involvement of the cervix and the anterior wall of the upper vagina.

TABLE 9-7   Suggested Management of Clear Cell Adenocarcinoma of the Cervix and Vagina

Stage	Surgery	Radiation
CERVIX		
Ib	Radical hysterectomy with clear vaginal margins and bilateral pelvic lymphadenectomy	5000 cGy whole pelvis in patients with positive pelvic nodes
IIa	Radical hysterectomy with bilateral pelvic lymphadenectomy and upper vaginectomy	5000 cGy whole pelvis in patients with positive pelvic nodes
IIb	Consider exenteration for radiation failures	5000 cGy whole pelvis, tandem and ovoids
IIIa and IIIb	Consider exenteration for radiation failures	6000 cGy whole pelvis, tandem and ovoids
IV	Individualize	
VAGINA		
I (upper third of vagina)	Radical hysterectomy with bilateral pelvic lymphadenectomy and upper vaginectomy	5000 cGy whole pelvis in patients with positive nodes
I (lower two thirds of vagina)	Radical hysterectomy with bilateral pelvic lymphadenectomy and total vaginectomy with vaginal reconstruction	5000 cGy whole pelvis, vaginal application or interstitial implant
II	Consider exenteration for radiation failures	5000 cGy whole pelvis, interstitial implant
III	Consider exenteration for radiation failures	6000 cGy whole pelvis, interstitial implant
IV	Individualize	

indicated that for certain early cancers, local therapy, which can conserve reproductive function, is an effective mode. Another study showed that pregnancy does not appear to affect the prognosis or behavior of clear cell adenocarcinoma. However, one instance of pelvic node metastasis has been reported in a patient with invasion of less than 3 mm.

If the cancer is confined to the cervix or upper vagina, or both, radical hysterectomy with upper vaginectomy and pelvic lymphadenectomy with retention of the ovaries is the recommended therapy. In young patients, avoidance of pelvic irradiation is desirable in view of the increased risks of long-term morbidity (radiation-induced carcinogenesis and progressive vasculitis) in patients surviving many decades after full-dose pelvic irradiation and the possible decrease of optimal vaginal function.

More extensive tumors and lesions involving the lower two thirds of the vagina are more suitable for radiation, which would include the pelvic nodes and parametrial tissues. Although some experienced surgeons have used radical hysterectomy with total vaginectomy and split-thickness skin graft vaginal reconstruction in this group of patients, it is difficult to get negative surgical margins (especially on the bladder). Herbst and coworkers reported a discouraging 37% recurrence rate among 22 patients treated by conventional irradiation, but 21 of these 22 patients had large vaginal adenocarcinomas and probably would not have been good surgical candidates for vaginectomy. Pelvic exenterations are reserved for radiation failures in patients with central persistence of the neoplasm and involvement of the lower two-thirds of the vagina.

Transvaginal local excision of stage I vaginal adenocarcinoma, which is associated with higher recurrence rates than transabdominal approaches, appears to be an inferior treatment. Some institutions have attempted radiation treatment with transvaginal cone or implant, especially for small vaginal tumors after local excision. The identification of the risk for pelvic lymph node spread, even in cases of small stage I tumors, led to the recommendation that retroperitoneal node dissection be carried out before the local treatment. Follow-up of many of the cases is limited. Therefore, comparing the efficacy of various modes of therapy is difficult.

Survival percentages are highly correlated with tumor stage. The following percentages were found for patients at these stages:

Stage I	91%
Stage II vaginal	82%
Stage IIa cervical	80%
Stage IIb cervical	56%
Stage III	37%

TABLE 9-8   Five- and Ten-Year Survival Rates for 588 Patients with Clear Cell Adenocarcinoma of the Vagina and Cervix By Stage

Stage	5-Year Survival (%)	10-Year Survival (%)
I	91	85
IIa	80	67
IIb	56	47
II (vagina)	82	67
III	37	25
IV	0	0

From Herbst AL: Neoplastic diseases of the vagina. In Mishell DR Jr et al (eds): Comprehensive Gynecology, 3rd ed. St. Louis, Mosby Year Book, 1997.

The overall survival rate of 80% is somewhat better than the 65% crude survival rate reported for squamous cell carcinoma of the cervix and much higher than the 35% to 45% overall survival rate reported for squamous cell carcinoma of the vagina. The better prognosis might be the result of early detection because it is occurring mainly in young patients exposed to DES (Table 9-8).

Recurrent Adenocarcinoma

A higher proportion of clear cell adenocarcinomas metastasize to the lungs and supraclavicular area when compared to squamous cancers. In the study by Herbst and colleagues, 346 patients were analyzed for frequency, site, and treatment of recurrent disease. Of the 346 patients, 20 were never free of disease after initial therapy and 19 had died at the time of the report. Recurrence developed in 58 patients, and diagnosis was made in most of these within 3 years after primary tumor treatment: 60% had recurrence in the pelvis, almost half of these being in the vagina; 36% (21 patients) had recurrence in the lungs; and 20% (12 patients) had recurrence in the supraclavicular lymph nodes. Surgery and radiation have been effective in the control of pelvic recurrences in some cases.

The results of chemotherapy are disappointing. Objective responses (>50% reduction of tumor size for longer than 3 months) were observed in 8 of 34 cases in which chemotherapy regimens were analyzed. Two patients who received doxorubicin (Adriamycin) had objective remissions, but an alkylating agent was also given in one of these. Two patients who received combination chemotherapy (5-FU, methotrexate, vincristine, cyclophosphamide, and prednisolone; and 5-FU, dactinomycin, and cyclophosphamide) also had objective remissions. No total remissions were observed. There were no responses in 9 cases in which a progestational agent alone was used.

In a 1981 report by Herbst, follow-up data of 409 patients for periods up to 15 years were published. In this study, 55 patients had an initial recurrence in the pelvis (60% of the total group with recurrence) up to 7 years after initial therapy. This emphasizes the importance of prolonged follow-up. Of the 58 patients with recurrences, 12 survived 3 years or longer after treatment of their first recurrence. A second recurrence was observed in 17 of the patients, and 12 of them died within 1 year of the diagnosis. However, 3 patients had survived longer than 2 years after treatment of their second recurrence.

Primary adenocarcinoma of the vagina can occur unrelated to intrauterine DES exposure. Some cases that were thought to have arisen in association with vaginal adenosis or from foci of endometriosis generally resembled endocervical or endometrial carcinomas. Because of their content of clear cells, others were considered to be of mesonephric origin. A few exceptional cases may have arisen from Gartner's duct remnants and thus may have truly been mesonephric in origin. Therapy for these adenocarcinomas is presently analogous to that for their squamous counterpart.

Vaginal metastases from adenocarcinoma of other pelvic and abdominal organs are more common than primary vaginal cancers. Lesions of cervical and endometrial origin are most common. Ovary, tube, colon, rectum, and renal cell neoplasms can also be present with vaginal metastasis.

Malignant Melanoma

Malignant melanoma of the vagina is rare and represents less than 0.5% of all vaginal malignant neoplasms and 0.4% to 0.8% of all malignant melanomas in women. The main presenting symptoms are vaginal bleeding, vaginal discharge, and the feeling of a mass. The tumors are predominantly located in the lower third of the vagina, commonly on the anterior wall. It is primarily a disease of postmenopausal women. Lesions may be single or multiple, pigmented or nonpigmented, and arising from melanocytes present in the epithelium of the vagina (Figure 9-8).

Multiple therapies have been attempted during the past several decades, and surgery remains the treatment of choice. The surgical approach must be tailored to the location of the lesions. The NCDB report noted 192 patients with vaginal melanoma; 95 (49%) were 70 years of age or older. Surgery was used as the first course of treatment in 66%, and 40% received radiotherapy. External radiation was more frequently used to treat advanced melanoma cases. Neoplasms that involve the lower third of the vagina are usually treated similarly to vulvar melanoma, with radical vulvectomy, partial vaginectomy, and inguinal and deep node dissection. Neoplasms that involve the upper two thirds of the vagina require some form of exenteration for optimal results. Radiation therapy in general has not proved effective, and the

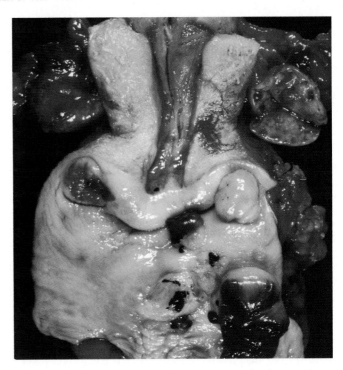

FIGURE 9-8 An exenteration specimen showing an open uterus, tubes, and ovaries with multifocal melanotic lesions of the vagina in a patient who underwent vaginectomy with her exenteration.

results of chemotherapy have been equally disappointing; thus the radical surgical approach remains the primary therapy when it is applicable.

Survival figures for this group of lesions are difficult to determine because of the infrequent occurrence of this disease. Patients with negative nodes who have disease involving the upper two thirds of the vagina and are treated by exenteration have about a 50% probability of surviving 5 years or longer. The overall survival rate for vaginal melanoma is about 15%. Lymph node metastases portend a poorer prognosis. Many patients have advanced disease at the time of diagnosis.

Treatment must be based on the extent of the disease, location, tolerance of the patient, and depth of invasion. Increasing emphasis is placed on the depth of invasion. Superficial lesions (Clark's level I and level II) can be managed with less than exenterative-type surgery, whereas more deeply invasive tumors must be managed with extended radical surgery with some expectation of a favorable outcome, as reported by Van Nostrand and associates. Survival appears to be more favorable with depths of invasion of less than 2 mm. In the NCDB report, the 5-year survival rate for 76 patients whose diagnosis was made between 1985 and 1989 was 14%. The number of diagnoses with Clark's level information was small (51 patients). The 3-year relative survival rate by Clark's level without regard to node status or presence of metastasis was as follows:

Level II	45% (11 patients)
Level III	36% (5 patients)
Level IV	27% (4 patients)
Level V	14% (9 patients)

No level I was reported.

The dissection of lymph nodes that are clinically negative for melanoma of the vagina, urethra, and vulva continues to be controversial. For level I and level II lesions, there appears to be little value in lymphadenectomy if nodes are clinically negative. Whether or not there is a role for selective sampling via lymphatic mapping and sentinel node localization is not known. However, in the few vulvovaginal primary lesions mapped, groin sentinel nodes have been isolated. Such dissections may provide prognostic information without extensive morbidity seen with inguinofemoral lymphadenectomy. Patients with level IV and level V lesions with positive nodes rarely survive, but local control may be achieved with lymphadenectomy. Recurrences develop primarily in the pelvis and lung. The interval to recurrence varies, but it is usually less than 1 year. Survival from point of recurrence averages 8 months.

Sarcoma

Spindle cell sarcomas of the vagina, such as leiomyosarcoma and fibrosarcoma, occur rarely. Tavassoli and Norris reported 60 smooth muscle tumors of the vagina. Only five neoplasms recurred, and these were all greater than 3 cm, with more than 5 mitotic figures per 10 high-power fields (hpf). Local excision was the treatment of choice when the tumor was well differentiated and well circumscribed and the margins were not infiltrated. In general, these lesions behave like their corresponding cell types on the vulva in that the well-differentiated lesions have a much better prognosis than the pleomorphic types, which tend to have poor prognosis regardless of therapy. The vagina, like the vulva, has a rich lymphatic and vascular network, possibly contributing to the early dissemination of these neoplasms (especially the pleomorphic types). In general, hematogenous dissemination occurs surprisingly late in the course of the disease, so that the importance of local therapy is underlined. However, after local excision of a circumscribed lesion and postoperative local radiation therapy, the value of pelvic radiation therapy is unclear. In most instances in which it has been successfully applied, the lesions were well differentiated and well circumscribed, suggesting that surgery itself was curative.

An unusual and tragic lesion that predominantly afflicts children is sarcoma botryoides (Figure 9-9). These lesions are usually multicentric and tend to arise in the anterior wall at the apex of the vagina. There is a tendency for this tumor to originate higher in the genital

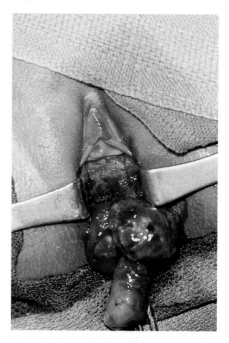

FIGURE 9-9   Sarcoma botryoides (rhabdomyosarcoma) in a 3-year-old child.

tract in older patients. In all patients, the tumor may be multifocal, but this is rare and should not be taken as a basis for extensive surgery.

Whereas these lesions were formerly treated by exenterative procedures, equal success has been obtained in recent years with less radical surgery and adjuvant chemotherapy, with or without radiotherapy. There were 30 sarcomas reported in children from the NCDB; 32 patients were between the ages of 20 and 49 years, 36 patients were between 50 and 69 years, and 37 patients were 70 years or older. The diagnosis was embryonal rhabdomyosarcoma in 70% of the children (21 patients), infantile embryonal carcinoma in 20% (4 patients), and rhabdomyosarcoma in 10% (3 patients). More than three quarters of the children received chemotherapy, including four fifths who were treated surgically. The 12 children whose diagnosis was made between 1985 and 1989 were younger than 5 years, and their 5-year survival rate was 90%.

A combination of vincristine, dactinomycin, and cyclophosphamide appears to be effective in this disease and results in a marked reduction in tumor size when the drug combination is used as initial therapy, permitting more conservative surgery. Although there is continued use of external radiation therapy in many centers, its role in managing sarcoma botryoides of the female genital tract remains unclear. Small lesions appear to be adequately treated with chemotherapy and surgery. A combination of chemotherapy and radiation therapy without surgery has been reported by Flamant and colleagues to be curative of localized vaginal lesions.

The tendency for genitourinary rhabdomyosarcoma to spread to regional lymph nodes is well established. The Intergroup Rhabdomyosarcoma Study reported a 26% incidence of known lymph node metastasis. The pelvis is the most common site for primary recurrences.

Leiomyosarcoma was the most frequent type of sarcoma for adults, accounting for 50% of the cases in patients aged 20 to 49 years and for 35% in those aged 70 years or older. Adjuvant chemotherapy was used less with increasing age, whereas radiotherapy was used most frequently for the older patient. Survival decreased with increasing age. Relative 5-year survival was 84% for those aged 20 to 49 years and 48% for those 50 to 69 years. Those older than 70 years had a 2-year relative survival of only 30%.

Endodermal Sinus Tumor

This rare carcinoma occurring in the vaginas of infants is most likely of germ cell origin. Norris and coworkers use the term mesonephroma or mesonephric carcinoma because of an alternative theory of their origin. The disease usually occurs in infants younger than 2 years, and survival rates have been poor, with less than 25% of patients alive at 2 years. Lesions most often occur on the posterior vaginal wall or fornices. Combination therapy (surgery and chemotherapy) appears appropriate. Patients who have vaginal endodermal sinus tumors are usually seen because of vaginal bleeding or discharge and have polypoid or sessile tumors. In the majority of cases, the differential diagnosis of endodermal sinus tumor is that of embryonal rhabdomyosarcoma (sarcoma botryoides). This is the most common vaginal tumor of children and almost always develops in patients younger than 5 years; the average age at the time of diagnosis is 3 years. The characteristic grapelike appearance of sarcoma botryoides differs from the usual endodermal sinus tumor. In addition, the edematous and cellular areas that are composed of immature skeletal muscle cells characteristic of embryonal rhabdomyosarcoma bear no resemblance to the histologic appearance of endodermal sinus tumor.

Young and Scully described 32 patients with endodermal sinus tumors. At the time of the report, 18 had died of their disease despite radical surgical therapy. Six patients were treated by surgery and then received vincristine, dactinomycin, and cyclophosphamide. Of these 6 patients, 2 also received radiation therapy. All were alive and free of disease 2 to 9 years after surgery. Copeland and associates have reported similar results with the same combination. Thus chemotherapy after conservative surgical excision can be effective in controlling this neoplasm.

Special Considerations

Pride and Buchler suggested that vaginal carcinoma might occur more frequently in patients who received pelvic irradiation 10 years or longer before the appearance of the new lesion. Of patients previously treated for cervical cancer, those who had received radiation therapy (>5 years previously) were more likely to develop vaginal cancer than were those whose cervical cancers had been treated surgically, according to Murad and colleagues. Abnormal vaginal cytologic findings are common after radiation, and many have ignored these dysplastic lesions as if they were routine results of irradiation therapy. However, a study from MD Anderson suggested that 30% of these "dysplastic" or "intraepithelial" lesions will progress to invasive cancer if they are left untreated. In this report, 28 patients with dysplasia or carcinoma in situ of the vagina after previous pelvic radiation therapy were observed for progression, and 9 developed invasive carcinoma. The median length of time from diagnosis of the intraepithelial lesion to invasion was 34 months. Therefore, treatment of these intraepithelial lesions by local excision is warranted. Laser vaporization or topical chemotherapy with 5-FU should be seriously considered.

For full reference list, log onto www.expertconsult.com ⟨http://www.expertconsult.com⟩.

The Adnexal Mass

D. Scott McMeekin, MD, Robert S. Mannel, MD, and Philip J. Di Saia, MD

THE ADNEXAL MASS

The adnexae consist of the fallopian tubes, broad ligament, ovaries, and structures within the broad ligament that are formed from embryologic rests. Detection of pelvic abnormalities is more frequent in women of reproductive age because these patients have serial examinations as part of periodic screening for cancer (i.e., Pap smears) and contraceptive counseling. Management of the adnexal mass is complex because of the scope of the disorders it encompasses and the numerous therapies that may be appropriate (Table 10-1). The risk of malignancy and the fundamental concept that early diagnosis and treatment in cancer are related to reduced mortality and morbidity propel the system. An adnexal mass often involves ovarian substance because of the propensity of the ovary for neoplasia. Fewer neoplasms occur in the fallopian tube, although that structure may commonly be involved in an inflammatory process that manifests as an adnexal mass. It is estimated that 5% to 10% of women in the United States will undergo a surgical procedure for a suspected ovarian neoplasm during their lifetime, and 13% to 21% of these women will be found to have an ovarian malignant neoplasm. The overwhelming majority of adnexal masses are benign, and it is important to determine preoperatively whether a patient is at high risk for ovarian malignant disease to minimize the number of operative procedures performed for self-limited processes.

Evaluative Approach

Patients may present with an adnexal mass in a variety of clinical settings. Some may be symptomatic (pelvic pain/pressure) as a result of the mass, others may have a mass identified as part of a workup for another condition (CT scan performed for back pain), and some have a mass incidentally identified as part of a normal well-woman examination. In addition, masses are occasionally identified during pregnancy as a result of the number of prenatal ultrasounds that are performed. The patient with a mass is approached differently depending

TABLE 10-1   Differential Diagnosis of Adnexal Mass

Organ	Cystic	Solid
Ovary	Functional cyst	Neoplasm
	Neoplastic cyst	Benign
	Benign	Malignant
	Malignant	
	Endometriosis	
Fallopian tube	Tubo-ovarian abscess	Tubo-ovarian abscess
	Hydrosalpinx	Ectopic pregnancy
	Paraovarian cyst	Neoplasm
Uterus	Intrauterine pregnancy in a bicornuate uterus	Pedunculated or interligamentous myoma
Bowel	Sigmoid or cecum distended with gas or feces	Diverticulitis
		Ileitis
		Appendicitis
		Colonic cancer
Miscellaneous	Distended bladder	Abdominal wall hematoma or abscess
	Pelvic kidney	Retroperitoneal neoplasm
	Urachal cyst	

TABLE 10-2   Pelvic Findings in Benign and Malignant Ovarian Tumors

Clinical findings	Benign	Malignant
Unilateral	+++	+++
Bilateral	+++	+++
Cystic	+++	+++
Solid	+++	+++
Mobile	+++	+++
Fixed	+++	+++
Irregular	+++	+++
Smooth	+++	+++
Ascites	+++	+++
Cul-de-sac nodules	−++	+++
Rapid growth rate	−++	+++

on the clinical scenario. The approach of what to do in the setting of adnexal mass can be broken down into two fundamental questions: (1) What is the suspicion that the mass is malignant? and (2) Is the patient symptomatic? Understanding these two issues helps focus treatment planning into a decision for surgery versus observation.

To determine the appropriate intervention for an adnexal mass, a thorough evaluation including complete history and physical examination, liberal use of transvaginal ultrasonography, and judicious use of serum tumor markers should be performed. Pelvic examination should always be performed under optimal circumstances. The patient's bladder should be empty. It is not unheard of for a patient with 10-cm midline mass to have the mass disappear with catheterization of the bladder. The rare pelvic kidney should always be kept in mind as a possible cause of a pelvic mass. Tragic reports of excision of such a mass in a patient with one kidney are found in the literature. Whenever possible, the rectum and rectosigmoid should also be empty when a pelvic examination is done. This avoids the misdiagnosis of fecal material as an adnexal mass. Detection of an adnexal mass is greatly facilitated by a rectovaginal examination (see Figure 3-13), which allows more complete access to the cul-de-sac and to the more superficial areas of the pelvic basin. Knowledge of the size, shape, contour, and general location of the mass within the pelvis helps the physician arrive at the most likely diagnosis. Benign tumors are commonly smooth walled, cystic, mobile, unilateral, and smaller than 8 cm

(7 cm is the exact diameter of a new tennis ball). Malignant tumors are usually solid or semisolid, bilateral, irregular, fixed, and associated with nodules in the cul-de-sac. Ascites usually is found with malignant neoplasms (Table 10-2). Koonings showed that the risk of malignant disease was 2.6-fold greater for women with bilateral neoplasms than for women with unilateral neoplasms.

Patient symptoms may derive from the physical nature of the mass by producing pressure against the bladder or rectum and increasing abdominal distention. Pain may be acute or chronic in nature. It may be a result of rapid size change and can be caused by torsion, hemorrhage into the mass, or rupture. Pain may also be a result of associated inflammatory processes from tubo-ovarian abscess or diverticular abscess. The nature and severity of the pain and other associated symptoms frequently lead to operative intervention, irrespective of the risk for malignancy.

Classifying the Mass

The complete evaluation of a patient with an adnexal mass requires that the physician assemble and analyze all of the available information from the history, examination, imaging studies, and tumor markers. One goal is to characterize the mass based on its malignant potential. Management then depends on a combination of many factors, including age and menopausal status of the patient, morphologic characteristics of the mass by ultrasound, clinical findings, and patient desires. Classically, features associated most commonly with benign masses include young age, absence of symptoms (nausea, vomiting, weight loss, changes in urinary frequency, pain), unilateral and unilocular cystic masses, and normal CA-125 level. Despite these factors, it is clear that no single characteristic guarantees that a mass will be benign. Increasingly models taking into account all available information have shown the best ability to predict benign vs malignant masses.

Of all variables, however, age is probably the most important factor for predicting the potential for malignancy. For example, Moore and colleagues showed in one large prospective series of 531 patients with adnexal mass for whom surgery was to be performed, 7% of premenopausal versus 39% of postmenopausal patients had a diagnosis of an epithelial ovarian malignancy on final pathology. The differential diagnosis of an adnexal mass varies with the age of the patient. In premenarchal girls and postmenopausal women, an adnexal mass should be considered highly abnormal and must be immediately investigated. In premenarchal patients, most neoplasms are germ cell in origin and require immediate surgical exploration. Stromal, germ cell, and epithelial tumors are seen in postmenopausal women. It was once dogma that a postmenopausal patient with any enlargement of the ovary be considered to have "cancer until proven otherwise." In an era before pelvic ultrasound, examining a patient with a "palpable postmenopausal ovary" was thought pathonomonic for ovarian cancer. Today, with common use of imaging studies, it has been shown that adnexal masses in postmenopausal women are more frequent than previously recognized, and many of these will be benign. Greenlee and colleagues demonstrated in a prevalence study of more than 15,000 women over 55 years of age who underwent pelvic ultrasound, 14% had an adnexal cyst at initial screening. As with patients in all age groups, a complete evaluation can better characterize risk of malignancy. (See section on postmenopausal ovary.)

One of the most common modalities used for characterizing an adnexal mass is pelvic ultrasound. Pelvic ultrasound may be performed transabdominally (better for larger masses extending out of the pelvis) or transvaginally (best for masses in the cul-de-sac or pelvis) to characterize masses. Many adnexal masses have characteristic appearances that define them as benign or suspicious for malignancy. The ultrasound shows size, mass morphology, unilateral or bilateral involvement, and associated findings such as ascites. Ultrasound is the most valuable initial tool and should be considered the first choice in assessing an adnexal mass by imaging. In some cases CT or MRI imaging may augment information on the mass and provide additional relevant anatomic information (e.g., description of upper abdominal findings and information on adenopathy and ureteral patency). Masses may be described as purely cystic (so-called simple cyst), solid, or mixed solid/cystic (so-called complex cyst). The risk of malignancy increases with increasing complexity. Large series have shown that simple cysts have a very low risk of malignancy. Cysts with septations and no solid component also have been shown to have low risk of malignancy. Malignancy is more commonly associated when a cyst wall or septation is thickened or has nodularity or the cyst contains solid components.

Much research has been devoted to developing accurate biomarkers that can detect malignancy and better characterize adnexal masses. To date, no single marker has been shown to be accurate in distinguishing a mass as benign or malignant. Information from tumor markers may be useful in characterizing the potential risk of malignancy so appropriate therapy may be offered (e.g., surgery vs observation) and patients may be appropriately triaged to specialists who are trained to perform complete surgical staging and debulking as needed.

One of the most widely used serum biomarkers for ovarian cancer is cancer antigen 125 (CA-125). CA-125 is used to monitor response of therapy and to assess for possible recurrence in patients with a known diagnosis of ovarian cancer. It is elevated in approximately 80% of patients with nonmucinous, epithelial ovarian cancers. It is elevated in only approximately 50% of stage I ovarian cancers, however. In combination with examination and serial pelvic ultrasounds, CA-125 has been evaluated in several large screening studies including asymptomatic women at risk for ovarian cancer to identify those with unrecognized disease. These studies show that CA-125 may augment the information from ultrasound alone. CA-125 testing has limited sensitivity and specificity, making routine CA-125 testing problematic. Conditions associated with peritoneal or serosal inflammation/irritation of any etiology may be associated with CA-125 level elevations. In addition to ovarian cancer, CA-125 levels may be elevated by a number of other malignancies and benign conditions including endometriosis, uterine leiomyomata, benign adnexal masses, tubal inflammation/infection, liver disease/hepatitis, congestive heart failure, menses, and pregnancy. Because most of these conditions are seen in younger women, CA-125 testing in premenopausal women is particularly difficult to interpret. A higher sensitivity has been reported in postmenopausal women, in whom CA-125 levels greater than 50 have been associated with a high risk of ovarian malignancy. In a prospective study comparing ultrasound to CA-125 levels to characterize patients with persistent adnexal masses ($N = 1066$), Van Calster reported ultrasound pattern classification correctly classified 93% of tumors as benign or malignant compared to 83% by CA-125 testing. Histologic diagnoses most commonly misclassified by CA-125 testing were fibromas, endometriosis, abscess, and borderline tumors. CA-125 information in the setting of an adnexal mass may provide information in conjunction with patient symptoms, examination, and imaging studies as to whether to offer observation or perform surgery, make referral to specialists, or perform additional testing.

OVA1 Test

A biomarker panel that measures five proteins (OVA1 test) was approved by the FDA in 2009 to better classify adnexal masses to assist physicians with making referral to gynecologic cancer specialists. The concept is that an abnormal test result should prompt referral to specialists trained in staging and debulking of ovarian cancer. The OVA1 test produces a score from 0 to 10, with a cutoff of 5 for premenopausal and 4.4 for postmenopausal women. In a pivotal trial of 516 patients, OVA1 testing augmented information from radiologic imaging and laboratory testing. The Society of Gynecologic Oncologists in September 2009 noted support for testing that resulted in appropriate referral of patients but also noted OVA1 testing has not been validated as a screening tool and should not be used in this manner.

HE4

Human epididymis protein 4 (HE4) is a novel tumor marker that is indicated for women with known ovarian cancer who have been treated as a marker for recurrence. HE4 is a glycoprotein produced in normal glandular epithelium of the reproductive tract, renal tubules, and respiratory epithelium. HE4 levels appear to be less susceptible to peritoneal irritation, perhaps reducing false-positive findings. For example, in one study, HE4 levels were not increased in patients with endometriosis. HE4 testing has been investigated in combination with CA-125 levels to increase sensitivity and specificity of biomarker testing. In combination with patient menopausal status and CA-125 and HE4 testing, Moore reported a sensitivity of 94% for all patients.

Multimodality Approach

Because no single test or finding in a vacuum is accurately predictive of a benign or malignant status of an adnexal mass, combining all information is our best option. Jacobs introduced the concept of the Risk of Malignancy Index (ROMI) in 1990 combining demographic, sonographic, and tumor marker data into the assessment of a patient with an adnexal mass. It was a simple, reproducible system that has been modified and studied in several large trials. In a systematic review of the literature of ROMI, Geomini suggested that all models have acceptable sensitivity and specificity, but the best predictors accounted for data from ultrasound findings, menopausal status, and CA-125 level. One modification proposed by Tingulstad created a formula of $U \times M \times CA-125$ level, where U = ultrasound score (higher-risk morphology = 3, low-risk morphology = 1), M = menopausal status (postmenopausal = 3, premenopausal = 1), and CA-125 level is the actual testing value. van den Akker reported a prospective observational study of 548 women with adnexal masses using this

TABLE 10-3   Benign Ovarian Tumors

Nonneoplastic tumors
Germinal inclusion cyst
Pregnancy luteoma
Endometrioma
Neoplastic tumors derived from coelomic epithelium
Cystic tumors
Serous cystoma
Mucinous cystoma
Mixed forms
Fibroma, adenofibroma
Brenner tumor
Tumors derived from germ cells
Dermoid (benign cystic teratoma)

modified ROMI with a threshold value of 200 and achieved a sensitivity of 81% and specificity of 85%. They found that using the ROMI they could accurately refer 80% of ovarian cancers to specialists using a threshold value of 200.

Differential Diagnosis

The differentiation between benign (Table 10-3) and malignant ovarian enlargements is often the exclusive decision of the pathologist, but a short discussion of these lesions is pertinent even in a textbook of oncology. Although functional ovarian cysts are usually asymptomatic, they can on occasion be accompanied by a minor degree of lower abdominal discomfort, pelvic pain, or dyspareunia. In addition, rupture of one of these fluid-filled structures can result in additional peritoneal irritation and possibly an accompanying hemoperitoneum; however, this is rarely serious. More intense lower abdominal discomfort results when these ovarian tumors undergo torsion or infarction. Similar to functional cysts of the ovary, benign ovarian neoplasms do not produce any symptoms that readily differentiate them from malignant tumors or from various other pelvic diseases. Although these tumors are more likely to twist, resulting in infarction, malignant neoplasms may have the same fate. Indeed, one of the most unfortunate features of benign ovarian neoplasms is that they are indistinguishable clinically from their malignant counterparts. Although it is not known whether malignant ovarian tumors arise de novo or develop from benign tumors, there is strong inferential evidence that at least some benign tumors will become malignant. All too often, the first symptom of cancer in an ovarian tumor is increasing abdominal distention, although benign ovarian neoplasms may become apparent because of increasing abdominal girth, and indeed the "giant tumors" of the ovary are often benign mucinous cystadenomas. Benign mucinous cystadenomas weighing up to 300 pounds have been reported.

EXTRAOVARIAN ADNEXAL MASSES

Given the proximity in the pelvis, a variety of nonovarian structures may be responsible for the appearance of an "adnexal mass." This category includes disorders of the uterus, fallopian tubes, intestines, and adjacent structures. The process that creates the mass can be congenital, functional, neoplastic, or inflammatory. It is important to keep a broad differential diagnosis of the adnexal mass and to use all of the information available based on the history, physical examination, and imaging studies. On occasion, extragenital lesions, which are often large and cystic, are found on pelvic examination; exploratory laparotomy is indicated because of the size alone. These extragenital lesions include peritoneal cysts, omental cysts, retroperitoneal lesions, and diseases of the gastrointestinal tract (cecum, appendix, sigmoid, and even small bowel, any of which can fall into the pelvis and become adherent). Retroperitoneal disorders may also be palpated on pelvic examination. Retroperitoneal sarcomas, lymphomas, and teratomas of the sacrococcygeal areas are commonly noted on rectovaginal examination and misdiagnosed as an adnexal mass.

Uterine Masses

Pregnancy should always be kept in mind as a cause of uterine enlargement. Most physicians are familiar with the unreliability of a menstrual history, and any patient of reproductive age with a pelvic mass should first have pregnancy ruled out by any of a variety of pregnancy tests or by detection of a fetus with ultrasound examination.

Myomas of the uterus are the most common uterine neoplasms (Figure 10-1). They are usually discrete, relatively round tumors that are firm to palpation and may be single or multiple. Myomas may be located within the myometrium (intramural), just beneath the endometrial lining (submucosal), or on the surface of the uterus (serosal). A myoma may frequently be found in the broad ligament attached to the lower uterine segment by a thin pedicle. This will often confuse the examiner and suggest that the mass originates in the ovary or tube. In the United States, myomas are found in at least 10% of white women and 30% to 40% of black women older than age 35 years. In the postmenopausal group, it is said that the incidence increases to 30% in white women and 50% in black women. Fortunately, these neoplasms usually shrink after menopause, especially in patients not receiving high doses of exogenous estrogen stimulation. It appears that most of these benign neoplasms are somewhat estrogen dependent. Growth is commonly seen during pregnancy, probably secondary to elevated hormone levels. Degeneration, infarction, and infection can occur in these lesions, and these complications are associated with considerable lower abdominal pain.

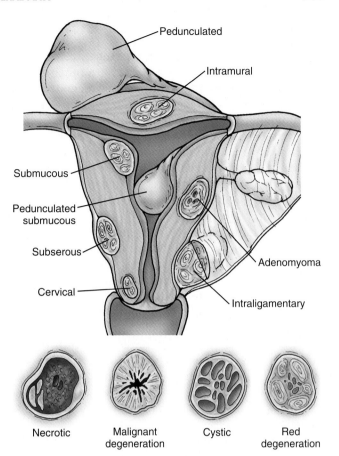

Pedunculated
Intramural
Submucous
Pedunculated submucous
Subserous
Adenomyoma
Cervical
Intraligamentary

Necrotic
Malignant degeneration
Cystic
Red degeneration

FIGURE 10-1 Myomas can be seen initially in multiple sizes and states of growth, disease, and degeneration. (*Courtesy Erle Henriksen, MD, Los Angeles, California.*)

Sarcomatous elements, associated with myomas less than 0.1% of the time, are most often recognized postoperatively. Symptoms of associated sarcomatous elements may include a rapidly enlarging pelvic mass, often accompanied by pain and tenderness. The mean age at diagnosis of these lesions is 50 to 55 years, with a range of 25 to 85 years.

A recent enlargement of the uterus in the postmenopausal patient is rarely caused by fibroids, particularly if the enlargement develops in a short time ("rapid" growth). The use of hormone replacement therapy in and of itself is not an explanation for such an enlargement. The most probable diagnosis is a malignant neoplasm, and physicians must prepare to do an appropriate surgical procedure even if the result of dilatation and curettage (D&C) is negative.

Other conditions that can cause enlargement of the uterus are adenomyosis and endometrial carcinoma or sarcoma. Endometrial carcinoma can enlarge the uterus to as much as four times normal size. Most patients with endometrial cancer will describe abnormal vaginal bleeding, and the diagnosis can be made appropriate endometrial sampling (office biopsy or D&C).

Tubal Masses

Neoplasms arising from the fallopian tube are rare. More commonly, adnexal masses secondary to tubal disease are inflammatory or represent an ectopic pregnancy. Distinction between tubal and ovarian masses on the basis of examination alone is often difficult. In the acute phase of salpingitis, the fallopian tube is distended by grossly purulent material. This infection may be secondary to gonorrhea or other organisms, including anaerobes. As the salpingitis process progresses, the adjacent ovary may become involved, creating a so-called tubo-ovarian abscess. Although this acute process may resolve, the patient is often subject to reinfection. As a result of repeated chronic infectious processes, the tubal ostia may close or firmly adhere to the adjacent ovary, and the fallopian tube fills with a clear fluid. As the structure distends, it creates a mass that can easily be mistaken for an ovarian cyst. Although the symptoms of acute pelvic inflammatory disease are distinct (pelvic pain, fever, increased vaginal discharge, and abnormal uterine bleeding), the symptoms of chronic pelvic infection may be subtle. Even the traditional elevation of the erythrocyte sedimentation rate or leukocyte count may be absent in as many as 30% of patients with chronic pelvic inflammatory disease and adnexal masses.

A cystic mass in the adnexal region may be neither ovarian nor tubal in origin but caused instead by remnants of embryologic structures. The paraovarium, located within the portion of the broad ligament containing the fallopian tube, consists of vestigial remnants of the Wolffian duct. Paraovarian cysts are found as distal remnants of the Wolffian duct system. They are characteristically located between the fallopian tube and the ovary; when large, they are often found with the fallopian tube stretched over the top of the cyst. These paraovarian cysts are most commonly unilocular and filled with clear yellow fluid. They often persist into the postmenopausal period and can appear as cystic structures in the adnexa on imaging studies done for other complaints.

Approximately 98% of ectopic pregnancies are tubal. Unfortunately, a pelvic mass can be found on examination in fewer than half the cases of tubal pregnancy, but sensitive testing (serum/urine) for beta human chorionic gonadotropin (BHCG) are positive. Rupture usually occurs when the distended fallopian tube reaches a diameter of 4 cm. Tubal pregnancy must be distinguished from pelvic inflammatory disease, torsion of the adnexa, and bleeding corpus luteum cysts because all produce pain or abnormal bleeding.

Carcinoma of the fallopian tube is rare and accounts for less than 0.5% of all female genital tract malignant neoplasms. Indeed, most of these neoplasms are discovered by serendipity, a preoperative diagnosis of ovarian neoplasm being most common. On gross evaluation, the fallopian tube is usually enlarged, smooth-walled, and sausage-shaped. On occasion, patients present with the symptom of several weeks of profuse watery vaginal discharge, the so-called hydrops tubae profluens.

Adnexal Masses of Nongynecologic Origin

Bowel

By far the most common entity of the gastrointestinal tract that initially appears to be an adnexal mass is fecal material in the sigmoid colon or cecum, which may on initial pelvic examination be palpated as a soft, mobile, tubular mass. Patients should be re-examined after appropriate cleansing enemas to confirm or rule out this possibility.

Inflammatory disorders of the large and small intestine can also be detected on pelvic examination. Diarrhea, nausea and vomiting, anorexia, or passage of blood or mucus per rectum should suggest these gastrointestinal tract disorders. Patients with diverticulitis, even with abscess formation, sometimes exhibit remarkably minor symptoms initially. Careful questioning to detect subtle changes in gastrointestinal symptoms is often rewarding. Periappendiceal abscesses may be formed as a result of rupture of the appendix and present as pelvic masses. Unfortunately, they vary in location, although they are generally found on the right side of the pelvis and are usually fixed, firm, and tender to palpation. Diverticulitis is a more common disorder with increasing age. Although it is usually located in the sigmoid colon, the mass may be midline or right sided. Inflammation of the ileum (regional ileitis) may occasionally present as a right-sided adnexal mass as the loops of thickened and inflamed ileum become fixed in the pelvis.

Gastrointestinal malignant disease is suggested by the presence of blood in the stool, anemia, and alterations in bowel habits. Neoplasms of the large intestine are particularly common with increasing age, and 60% to 70% occur on the left side within the reach of the palpating finger or flexible sigmoidoscope. However, carcinoma of the cecum often presents as a right-sided adnexal mass, and on examination, induration and irregularity may be found in the involved area. If one suspects gastrointestinal origin of the mass, appropriate endoscopic or radiographic studies usually help in the definitive diagnosis.

OVARIAN MASSES

Functional Cysts

The cyclic ovarian function of a reproductive-age women continually produces follicular growth and resorption. Among the most frequently found "masses" involving

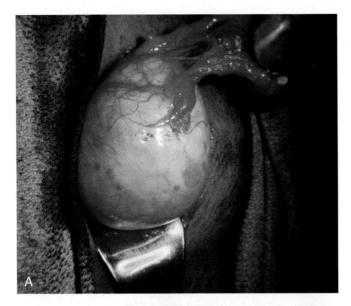

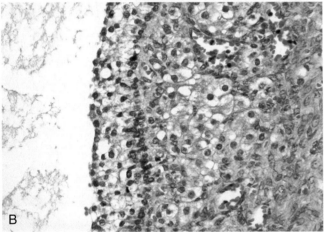

FIGURE 10-2 **A,** Follicular cyst (8 cm) with fimbria. **B,** Microscopic view of a follicular cyst as seen in **A**. *(Courtesy Ibrahim Ramzy, MD, UC, Irvine, California.)*

the adnexa are the non-neoplastic cysts related to the process of ovulation that are sometimes referred to as functional cysts. They are by far the most common clinically detectable enlargements of the ovary occurring during the reproductive years. If ovulation does not occur, a clear fluid-filled follicular cyst (Figure 10-2) lined by granulosa cells may result that can reach a size as large as 10 cm in diameter. These cysts usually resolve spontaneously within a few days to 2 weeks but can persist longer. When ovulation occurs, a corpus luteum is formed that may become abnormally enlarged through internal hemorrhage or cyst formation. The masses are of great significance because young women will have cysts on their ovaries at essentially all times (in varying sizes, numbers) during the reproductive years, and occasionally the cysts can produce pain and discomfort, and

a mass will be noted on examination or ultrasound. Clinical sequelae of these benign physiologic processes can also bring patients to the physician's attention as the masses may undergo torsion, acutely hemorrhage into the mass, or grow to sufficient size to produce pain/pressure/bloating symptoms. The clinical challenge is that these functional cysts cannot be readily distinguished from true neoplasms on clinical grounds alone. Ultrasound evaluation typically shows a thin-walled, simple-appearing, anechoic cyst without solid component or septations. A hemorrhagic cyst may also show more complexity on ultrasound given the presence of blood and fibrin stranding.

In addition, such cysts are often associated with variable delays in the onset of menses and confusion regarding the possibility of pregnancy. Theca-lutein cysts result from overstimulation of the ovary by human chorionic gonadotropin (hCG) and on histologic examination are characterized by extensive luteinization of the stroma surrounding the follicle. Although theca-lutein cysts do not commonly occur in a normal pregnancy, they are often associated with hydatidiform moles and choriocarcinoma. Gross examination of the ovary containing theca-lutein cysts shows a structure almost completely replaced by lobulated thin-walled cysts that vary in size and are smooth and yellow.

Corpus luteum, follicular, and theca-lutein cysts are benign and represent an exaggerated physiologic response of the ovary. In most instances, they involute over time, but they do present a problem requiring a differential diagnosis. Luteomas of pregnancy are often large, solid, but not neoplastic masses originating in the ovary during pregnancy. Most cases are discovered at cesarean section in the last 2 months of pregnancy. The exact cell of origin of luteoma has not been established. It is probably a chorionic hormone-dependent non-neoplastic hyperplasia and usually regresses after delivery. Therefore, surgical excision of these lesions at the time of cesarean section is not necessary.

Polycystic (sclerocystic) ovaries contain multiple follicle cysts with hyperplasia and luteinization of theca interna surrounding the cysts and atretic follicles. The ovaries are two to five times normal size with a thickened capsule. The condition is found most frequently in association with the Stein–Leventhal or polycystic ovarian syndrome.

Endometriotic Cysts

Endometriosis is a condition in which implants of normal-appearing endometrial glands and stroma are found outside their normal location in the uterine cavity. Presumptive evidence of endometriosis is also supported by significant scarring in the pelvis and the presence of hemosiderin-laden macrophages in the cyst wall or peritoneum. The most common sites for endometriosis are the ovaries, the supporting ligaments of the uterus, and the peritoneum of the cul-de-sac and bladder. Endometriosis is most common in women 35 to 45 years of age and is more common in white and nulliparous women. Endometrioitic cysts sometimes may be distinguished from ovarian neoplasms by patient history (history of endometriosis or symptoms suggestive of endometriosis including dysmenorrhea, pelvic pain, infertility) and examination findings (nodularity of the uterosacral ligaments). Pelvic pain is by far the most usual symptom of endometriosis. Although physical activity and sexual intercourse usually increase the discomfort, the amount of endometriosis present does not seem to correlate with the intensity of the symptoms. For some, pain produced from small peritoneal implants appears to be incapacitating. Ultrasound may show a homogenous echo, sometimes referred to as having a "ground glass appearance," and on occasion may be misinterpreted as a solid mass. Septations and wall nodularity are also seen commonly. Of note, CA-125 levels are frequently elevated in patients with endometriosis. The morphologic complexity on ultrasound coupled with CA-125 level elevations make endometriotic cysts among the most common masses incorrectly thought to be suspicious for malignancy on workup. At surgery the ovary may be enlarged and cystic. The lumen contains blood of varying color, depending on the amount and age of the hemorrhage. In most instances, it is dark brown (chocolate cyst). In at least 50% of cases, both ovaries are involved. These cysts rarely exceed a diameter of 12 cm. They are frequently adherent to surrounding structures.

Benign Ovarian Neoplasms

The ovary is composed of tissue derived from coelomic epithelium, germ cells, and mesenchyme, and any one of these components may undergo neoplastic change (benign or malignant). Morphologically, neoplasms can be divided into solid and cystic types based on ultrasound and gross appearances. The most common benign cystic neoplasms of the ovary are serous and mucinous cystadenomas and cystic teratomas (dermoids). Benign cystadenomas may vary in size from 5 to 50 cm and are thin-walled, ovoid, and frequently unilocular. Benign neoplasms do not spontaneously regress, nor do they have the potential to disseminate/ metastasize. Whether some begin neoplasms are premalignant is a source of controversy. Intraepithelial neoplasia has been reported in otherwise benign serous cystadenomas; in early-stage invasive epithelial cancer, several authors have described the presence of transitional changes from normal epithelium to intraepithelial neoplasia to invasive cancer.

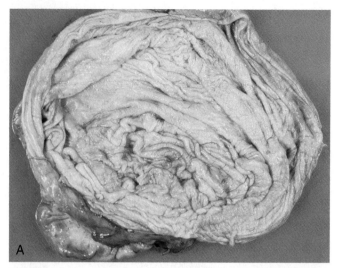

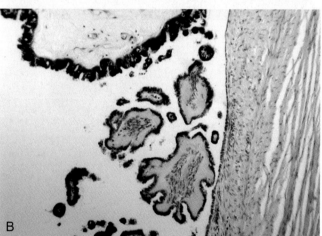

FIGURE 10-3 **A,** Gross photograph of an opened serous cyst adenoma that contained 500 mL of clear straw-colored fluid. Note the papillary projections on the inner surface, especially on the right. **B,** Microscopic view of a serous cystadenoma with a few papillary projections from the surface.

Serous Cystadenoma

Serous cystadenomas are more common than the mucinous type of tumor, but as a rule, they do not attain the large size characteristic of their mucinous counterparts. On gross evaluation, the cyst fluid is usually thin, watery, and yellow tinged. The surface of the cyst is usually smooth and frequently unilocular (Figure 10-3). Septations dividing the cyst can be seen, however. Some serous tumors may have small papillary projections on the surface of the cyst wall, which at times are so numerous that a cauliflower pattern is produced. Large, frond-like solid projections or nodules or areas of necrosis should raise the concern for malignancy. On microscopic examination, the epithelium is usually of the low columnar type with cilia. Particularly characteristic of this type

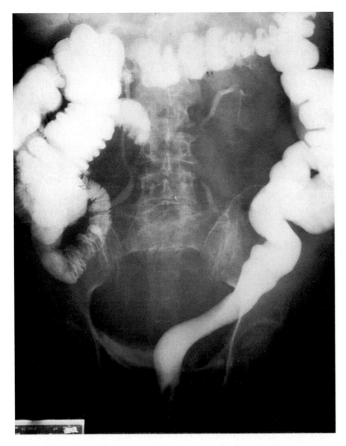

FIGURE 10-4 Barium enema film of a patient with a large mucinous cystadenoma of the right ovary filling the pelvis and lower abdomen.

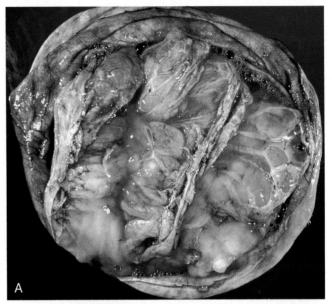

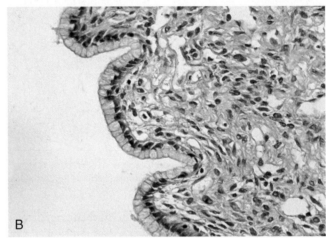

FIGURE 10-5 Mucinous cystadenoma. **A**, Gross appearance. **B**, Histologic section showing tall epithelial lining with pale-staining nuclei at basal pole. (*A, Courtesy of Ibrahim Ramzy, MD, UC, Irvine, California.*)

of cyst are small calcific granules, the so-called psammoma bodies, which are an end product of degeneration of the papillary implants. Associated fibrosis may lead to the so-called cystadenofibroma.

Many serous cystadenomas of the ovary are asymptomatic and are discovered as an incidental finding during routine pelvic examination or through imaging studies performed for another reason. Symptoms may develop because of the size of the mass (pain, pressure on bladder/rectum) or as a result of rupture or torsion. Ultrasound appearance is frequently similar to a large functional cyst, unilocular and simple.

Mucinous Cystadenoma

Mucinous cystadenomas (Figure 10-4) may become huge, with some (Figure 10-5) reported to weigh more than 300 pounds. On gross evaluation, the masses are round or ovoid with smooth capsules that are usually translucent or bluish to whitish gray. The interior is divided by a number of discrete septa into loculi containing in general a clear, viscid fluid. Papillae are rarely noted. However, on microscopic examination, the lining

of the epithelium is of a tall, pale-staining secretory type with nuclei at the basal pole; the presence of goblet cells is common. The cells will be found to be rich in mucin if suitable stains are obtained. It is believed that this type of cyst usually arises from simple metaplasia of the germinal epithelium. It may occasionally arise from a teratoma in which all the other elements have been lost. It rarely occurs from a Brenner tumor in which there has been mucinous transformation of the epithelium.

Bilaterality may be found in as many as 10% of patients with serous cystadenomas, in contrast with mucinous cystadenomas, for which there is essentially no significant incidence of bilaterality. This information is helpful when the surgeon needs to make a judgment about surgical inspection of the opposite ovary in a

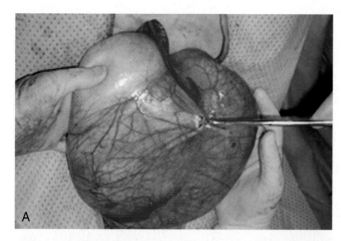

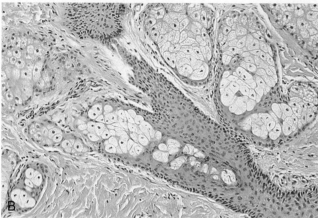

FIGURE 10-6 **A,** Ruptured dermoid cyst with sebaceous material seen. **B,** Photomicrograph of a mature teratoma (dermoid) of the ovary.

young woman desirous of further childbearing. If the other ovary is of normal size, shape, and configuration, surgical evaluation is not needed.

Dermoid Cyst (Benign Cystic Teratoma)

Dermoid cysts are rarely large (typically <10 cm), are often bilateral (15% to 25%), and occur with disproportionate frequency in younger patients. On gross evaluation, there is a thick, opaque, whitish wall; on opening of the cyst, one frequently finds hair, bone, cartilage, and a large amount of greasy fluid, which rapidly becomes sebaceous on cooling. On microscopic examination, all types of mature ectoderm, mesoderm, and endoderm may be present. Stratified squamous epithelium, hair follicles, sebaceous and sudoriferous glands, cartilage, neural and respiratory elements, and indeed all elements normally seen in fetal life may be present. Sequelae include growth of the mass, rupture (Figure 10-6), and malignant degeneration. Malignant degeneration occurs in benign cystic teratomas in 1% to 3% of these tumors, and it is usually of a squamous type. These neoplasms are thought to arise from early ova that have been

triggered by some type of parthenogenetic process. Imaging evaluation of teratomas can be useful. For example, abdominal radiographs may demonstrate calcifications (teeth, bone), and CT imaging is excellent at showing fat densities commonly seen with dermoids. Ultrasound appearance is variable and complex morphology with hyperechoic areas is common.

Removal of the ovary or cyst is recommended, and given the young age of many patients with mature teratoma, cystectomy (open or laparoscopically) in a patient desirous of further childbearing is standard. In most instances, a significant portion of normal ovary can be preserved and reconstituted. Care must be taken to remove the entire capsule of the neoplasm to avoid recurrence. In our experience, bilaterality is relatively rare when the opposite ovary is normal in appearance and is usually identified by preoperative ultrasound. We do not recommend bivalving/opening a normal-appearing contralateral ovary in these circumstances. Care should be taken to prevent spillage of the contents of the dermoid cyst because this material can cause a chemical peritonitis. Because many of the masses are found in pregnant patients undergoing routine prenatal ultrasound, conservative management until delivery is reasonable. Caspi reported on 49 women with ultrasonographically diagnosed ovarian cystic teratoma less than 6 cm in pregnancy who were followed for change in size. A total of 68 pregnancies resulted. None of the classic complications of dermoid cysts such as torsion, dystocia, or rupture occurred. The authors concluded that such small lesions are safe to just follow, especially in pregnancy.

Fibroma

Benign solid tumors of the ovary are usually of connective tissue origin (fibromas, thecomas, or Brenner tumors). They vary in size from small nodules found on the surface of the ovary to large neoplasms weighing several thousand grams. On physical examination, these neoplasms are usually firm, slightly irregular in contour, and mobile. The occurrence of fibromas (Figure 10-7) is not at all infrequent. Sometimes they are first noted as small nodules on the ovarian cortex. In other instances, they can be extremely large, filling the entire pelvis and lower abdomen. The tumors are characterized by their firmness and resemblance to myomas, and they are frequently misdiagnosed as such. The cut surface has a homogeneous grayish-white and firm appearance, although areas of cystic degeneration are common in larger tumors. On microscopic examination, one finds stellate or spindle-shaped cells arranged in fusiform fashion. The cells are uniformly well differentiated with nothing to suggest malignancy. Hyalinization is frequent, particularly in the larger tumors, and if fat stains

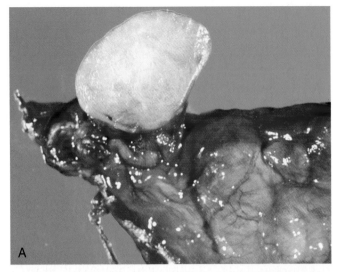

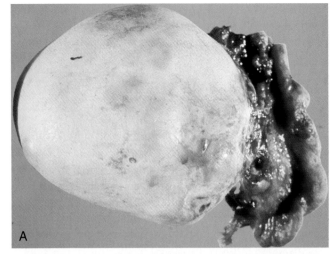

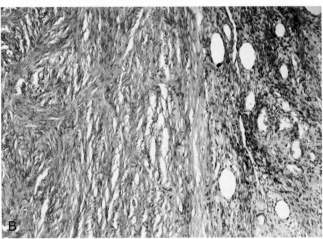

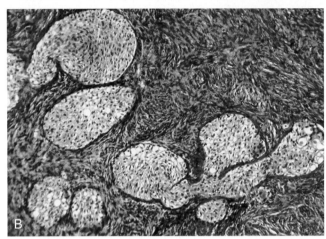

FIGURE 10-7   Ovarian fibroma. **A,** Gross appearance-solid white lesion with a firm cut surface and fallopian tube. **B,** Histologic section-whorls of fibromatous matrix. *(Courtesy Ibrahim Ramzy, MD, UC, Irvine, California.)*

FIGURE 10-8   Brenner tumor. **A,** Gross appearance-solid, firm, white cut surface. **B,** Histologic section-hyperplastic fibromatous matrix interspersed with nests of epithelioid cells. *(Courtesy Ibrahim Ramzy, MD, UC, Irvine, California.)*

are done, admixtures of theca cells may be seen. Meigs' syndrome is characterized by ascites, hydrothorax, and an ovarian tumor that was originally believed to be specifically a fibroma; however, many other types of ovarian tumors are now known to be associated with this syndrome, such as Brenner tumors and Krukenberg tumors. The cause of Meigs' syndrome is not completely understood, but it seems that the hydrothorax occurs by certain lymphatics through the diaphragm. After removal of the ovarian neoplasm, there is a prompt resolution of both abdominal and pleural fluid.

Brenner Tumor

Brenner tumor (Figure 10-8), an uncommon type of ovarian neoplasm, is grossly identical to a fibroma. Frequently, the tumor is an incidental finding in an otherwise unremarkable ovary. On microscopic examination, one finds a markedly hyperplastic fibromatous matrix interspersed with nests of epithelioid cells. The epithelioid cells under high magnification show a "coffee bean" pattern caused by the longitudinal grooving of the nuclei. The cell nests show a frequent tendency toward central cystic degeneration, producing a superficial resemblance to a follicle. Although it was originally believed that Brenner tumors arise from simple Walthard cell rests, it has been conclusively demonstrated that Brenner tumors can arise from diverse sources, including the surface epithelium, rete ovarii, and ovarian stroma itself. It was originally stressed that Brenner tumors were uniformly benign, but there have been scattered reports in the past several decades of a number of malignant Brenner tumors. Brenner tumors are generally thought to be endocrinologically inert, but several cases in recent years have been associated with postmenopausal endometrial hyperplasia, and a frequent estrogen effect has been attributed to this neoplasm. These lesions are managed by simple excision.

MANAGEMENT OF THE ADNEXAL MASS

Observation versus Surgery

Optimal management for patients with adnexal masses can be achieved by combining all available information from the history, examination, and diagnostic studies to create an accurate differential diagnosis. The presence and severity of symptoms are other important considerations. For example, a patient with a 6-cm unilocular cyst may be initially observed expectantly, whereas a similar patient with severe pain may need urgent surgery. In addition, consultation with additional specialists (gynecologic oncologist, urologist, general surgeon) may be required based on suspicion of malignancy or the differential diagnosis being considered.

Decisions that must be considered are as follows:

1. Does the patient require surgical evaluation (vs observation)?
2. Once a decision for surgery has been made is a specialist referral/consultation required, and what type of surgical procedure is planned (open vs minimally invasive)?
3. If observation has been elected, at what intervals and with what thresholds for changing course would be considered?

Deciding which patient needs surgical exploration can best be done by considering the characteristics of the adnexal mass. In reproductive-age women, 95% of ovarian cysts smaller than 5 cm in diameter are nonneoplastic. In addition, functional cysts are seldom larger than 7 cm in diameter and are usually unilateral and freely mobile. A physician can presume that during the reproductive years, an adnexal mass as described earlier is a functional or hyperplastic change of the ovary rather than a true neoplasm. The transitory existence of functional cysts is of prime importance in distinguishing them from true neoplasms. Tradition and clinical experience have shown that functional cysts usually persist for only a few days to a few weeks, and reexamination during a later phase of the menstrual cycle has been a reliable procedure in confirming this diagnosis. Many gynecologists prescribe oral contraceptives to accelerate the involution of the functional cyst on the presumption that these cysts are gonadotropin dependent. The unconfirmed theory is that the inhibitory effect of the contraceptive steroids on the release of pituitary gonadotropins shortens the life span of these cysts, hastening their

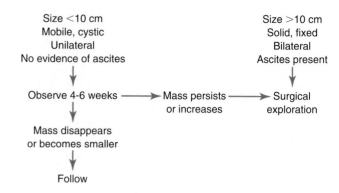

FIGURE 10-9 Management of a premenopausal woman with an adnexal mass.

identification as functional or nonneoplastic lesions. In an era before the use of ultrasound, Spanos conducted a careful study of 286 patients who had adnexal cysts. Combination oral contraceptives were prescribed, and the women were re-examined in 6 weeks. In 72% of the women, the masses disappeared during the observation period. Of the 81 patients whose masses persisted, none were found to have a functional cyst at laparotomy. The fact that five of the removed tumors were malignant underscores the importance of avoiding unnecessary delay in the operative investigation of these patients. In general, masses greater than 10 cm in diameter should be surgically explored regardless of concerns for malignancy because these masses are not likely to be functional and seldom resolve spontaneously. Our practice is to reassess young women with suspected functional cysts with a repeat examination and ultrasound in 6 to 8 weeks. If the cyst resolves, no further therapy is indicated. If the cyst persists, the patient is counseled regarding surgical evaluation (Figure 10-9).

Data also have accumulated showing that some patients with nonfunctional cyst adnexal masses may be conservatively followed with serial observation and not undergo surgery. For example, postmenopausal women with unilocular cysts less than 5 cm and normal CA-125 levels may be considered for observation because the risk for malignancy is very low. In addition, many of the masses will resolve spontaneously. In some older patients with concurrent medical comorbidities, avoiding surgery may be a safer strategy. Patients undergo serial repeat pelvic ultrasound every 3 to 6 months with CA-125 testing. Surgical intervention is recommended if the morphology becomes complex, the size increases, or the CA-125 level increases outside of normal range. Saunders and colleagues at the University of Kentucky recently evaluated a series of 1319 patients (25% premenopausal, 75% postmenopausal) with 2870 septated ovarian cysts without solid or papillary projections. On serial follow-up 39% of cysts resolved (mean duration to resolution of 12 months). Of 1756 cysts that persisted,

TABLE 10-4   Adnexal Mass: Indications for Surgery

Ovarian cystic structure >5 cm that has been observed 6-8 weeks
   without regression
Any solid ovarian lesion
Any ovarian lesion with papillary vegetation on the cyst wall
Any adnexal mass >10 cm in diameter
Ascites
Palpable adnexal mass in a premenarchal or postmenopausal patient
Torsion or rupture suspected

TABLE 10-5   Society of Gynecologic Oncologists and American College of Obstetricians and Gynecologists Referral Guidelines for Women with a Newly Diagnosed Pelvic Mass

PREMENOPAUSAL PATIENTS (<50 YEARS OLD)

CA-125 >200 units/mL
Presence of ascites
Evidence of intraperitoneal or distant metastasis (based on
   examination or imaging studies)
Family history (first-degree relative) of breast or ovarian cancer

POSTMENOPAUSAL PATIENTS (>50 YEARS)

Elevated CA-125 level
Ascites
Evidence of intraperitoneal or distant metastasis (based on
   examination or imaging studies)
Family history (first degree relative) of breast or ovarian cancer

Adapted from ACOG Practice Bulletin, Management of Adnexal mass, Obstet Gynecol 2007;110:207.

128 surgeries were performed and no case of ovarian cancer was identified. The most common histopathologies were serous cystadenoma, mucinous cystadenoma, and endometrioma. The authors suggested that patients with septated cysts without solid components are at low risk for ovarian cancer and may be followed.

Masses that raise a suspicion for malignancy require surgical intervention (Table 10-4). In addition, consultation with a specialist trained in the management of ovarian cancer should be considered. Patients with associated hallmarks of ovarian cancer including peritoneal/omental implants, ovarian caking, and markedly elevated CA-125 levels frequently have advanced ovarian cancer and require care from physicians specialized in surgical debulking techniques. In other tumors with the potential for malignancy, surgical evaluation should be considered and consultation is advised. Conditions raising the concern of possible malignancy include the following:

- Bilateral adnexal masses
- Complex masses, especially including solid components, thick septations, and/or mural nodules
- Premenopausal patients with complex masses that persist or grow following period of observation
- Postmenopausal patients with simple masses greater than 5 cm or complex masses of any size
- Masses associated with elevated tumor markers
- Symptomatic masses

In a joint publication, the American College of Obstetrics and Gynecology (ACOG) and the Society of Gynecologic Oncologists (SGO) suggested referral guidelines to triage patients with adnexal masses to specialists in the care of ovarian cancer. The guidelines are shown in Table 10-5. The SGO performed a multisite, retrospective validation trial assessing the guidelines in 1035 women undergoing surgery for an adnexal mass. The prevalence of ovarian cancer was 31%. When using the referral guidelines, the positive predictive value was 34% for premenopausal and 60% for postmenopausal women. The negative predictive value was approximately 92% for each group. Others have criticized the guidelines for largely detecting cases of advanced cancers and missing many cases of early-stage cancers (where appropriate staging would be desired).

Minimally Invasive Surgery for Adnexal Masses

Minimally invasive surgery (MIS), either laparoscopic or robotic, is the preferred approach for a presumptively benign adnexal mass. With the use of specific ultrasound criteria, benign masses can be predicted with a high degree of certainty, especially in premenopausal women. Careful selection of patients is critical for the appropriate use of MIS for removal of adnexal masses. The patient's age, the clinical examination, tumor markers, and the ultrasound findings provide important information that helps determine the appropriate operative approach. MIS should be used cautiously in the presence of any mass with clinical or ultrasonographic characteristics suggestive of malignancy, especially an adnexal mass in a postmenopausal woman associated with an elevated serum CA-125 value.

All patients scheduled for MIS with an adnexal mass should also consent to possible laparotomy. If the preoperative risk for finding malignancy is high enough, referral to a surgeon prepared to proceed with staging or surgical debulking if malignant disease is uncovered is warranted. Cell washings are obtained from the pelvis and upper abdomen and saved for proper staging if a malignant neoplasm is found. Any lesions or suspicious areas are sampled and sent for frozen section analysis. If an unexpected malignancy is found, appropriate biopsies and photo documentation can be taken and referral can be made to a cancer specialist. The main reasons for conversion from laparoscopy to laparotomy are extensive adhesions or intraoperative complications.

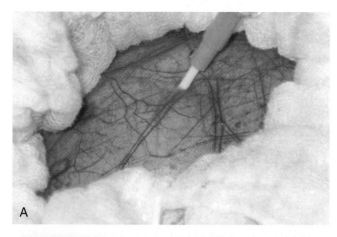

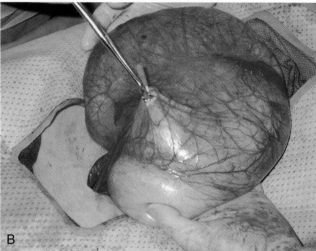

FIGURE 10-10   **A,** Aspiration of a large 40-cm simple cyst at laparotomy. The area around the puncture site is surrounded with dry laparotomy sponges. **B,** Collapsed cyst extracted through an 8-cm incision.

Nezhat and colleagues reported their experience with 1209 patients with adnexal masses who were managed laparoscopically. Of 1011 cases with surgical management, ovarian cancer was discovered intraoperatively in 4. The management of a cystic mass included aspiration of fluid, which was sent for cytologic examination, followed by opening of the cyst and inspection of the wall for any irregular thickening. Frozen section biopsy specimens were obtained if the surgeon thought any surfaces were suspicious. An ovarian cystectomy–oophorectomy was then performed, and tissue was sent for permanent histologic examination. The Nezhat study suggests that experienced surgeons using intraoperative histologic sampling may safely evaluate adnexal masses laparoscopically.

Hasson reported another series of 102 women with ovarian cysts who were managed laparoscopically. In 83 of the women, laparoscopic fenestration and biopsy were done, with or without coagulation or removal of the cyst lining. Only 1 of 56 functional, simple, or

TABLE 10-6   Frequency distribution of Adnexal Masses in Childhood

Mass	Age of Patient at Diagnosis (0-20 yr)	%
Nonneoplastic	335	64
Simple or follicular cyst	117	23
Corpus luteum cyst	143	28
Other*	75	14
Neoplastic	186	36
Benign	144	28
Malignant	42	8
Germ cell	17	3
Stromal	9	2
Epithelial	14	3
Gonadoblastoma	2	1
Total	521	

Modified from Van Winter JT, Simmons PS, Podratz KC: Am J Obstet Gynecol 170:1780, 1994.
*Endometrioma, polycystic ovary syndrome, pelvic inflammatory disease, ectopic pregnancy.

paraovarian cysts recurred during the study. Two of the 18 ovarian endometriomas treated with fenestration and coagulation or removal of the lining recurred, whereas 8 of 9 such lesions recurred with treatment by fenestration alone. There were no surgical complications.

Canis reported his group's experience with 247 adnexal masses suspicious at ultrasound examination and managed laparoscopically. Actually, 17 patients were evaluated by laparotomy and 230 by laparoscopy. The 204 women (82.6%) who were treated by laparoscopy included 7 of 37 malignant tumors and 191 of 210 benign masses. One case of tumor dissemination did occur after a laparoscopic adenectomy and morcellation of a grade 1 immature teratoma. Some surgeons prefer to manage cystic ovarian masses with a mini laparotomy. A small incision (3-5 cm) is made over the mass, and the cyst fluid is aspirated with a long needle, trocar, or suction cannula after draping the field with dry laparotomy pads (Figure 10-10, *A*). The collapsed mass can then be removed through the small incision (Figure 10-10, *B*) and submitted to pathology. Spill is minimal with this approach, but thorough irrigation of the surgical field is recommended prior to closure.

SPECIAL CIRCUMSTANCES

Adnexal Masses in Childhood

The differential diagnosis of an adnexal mass in children and adolescents also includes benign and malignant processes. Table 10-6 outlines the frequencies of adnexal masses in young women and children. Figure 10-11 outlines the process of differentiating between benign and malignant masses in childhood. Whenever possible,

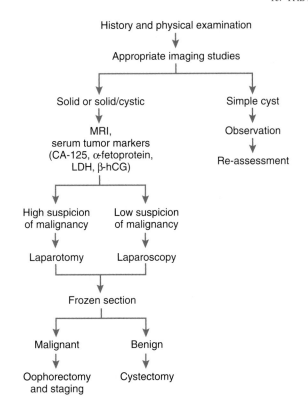

History and physical examination
↓
Appropriate imaging studies
↓
Solid or solid/cystic ← | → Simple cyst
↓
MRI,
serum tumor markers
(CA-125, α-fetoprotein,
LDH, β-hCG)

Simple cyst
↓
Observation
↓
Re-assessment

High suspicion of malignancy ← | → Low suspicion of malignancy
↓
Laparotomy   Laparoscopy
↓
Frozen section
↓
Malignant ← | → Benign
↓
Oophorectomy and staging   Cystectomy

FIGURE 10-11 Management of an ovarian mass during childhood.

TABLE 10-7 Symptoms at Initial Presentation of 521 Adnexal Masses in Children

Symptom	No. of Patients
Pain*	271
Mass†	151
Menstrual irregularity‡	71
Dysmenorrhea	50
Amenorrhea, primary	12
Amenorrhea, secondary	35
Increased abdominal girth	34
Urinary complaints§	16
Hirsutism	13
Premature sexual development	6

From Van Winter JT, Simmons PS, Podratz KC: Am J Obstet Gynecol 170:1780, 1994.
*Mass was secondarily discovered in 150 of these patients.
†Without accompanying pain.
‡Metrorrhagia, menorrhagia, oligomenorrhea.
§Frequency, dysuria, suprapubic pressure.

conservative or minimally invasive surgery is preferred to preserve endocrine and reproductive functions. Dermoid cysts are among the most common ovarian masses in both pediatric and adolescent patients. These tumors are bilateral in 15% to 25% of cases. Two percent of dermoids (teratomas) have malignant components; these are usually found in adolescent patients but can also be found in childhood. A complete workup of a pelvic mass in this age group should include imaging and determination of serum levels of tumor markers such as CA-125, α-fetoprotein, lactate dehydrogenase, and β-hCG. The differential diagnosis should consider acute appendicitis, intussusception, gastroenteritis, chronic constipation, genitourinary problems, and pelvic infection.

In a study by Ehren and colleagues, 63 children and adolescents with benign or malignant ovarian tumors were described. Abdominal pain was the most common complaint; 22% had torsion. The most common sign on initial examination was a palpable abdominal mass (45 of 54 patients). Benign teratoma was the final diagnosis in 41 of the patients (65%), and 29 had calcification apparent on abdominal radiography. All patients younger than 12 years with ovarian neoplasms had germ cell lesions, although an epithelial tumor has been reported in a 4-year-old patient. Two patients experienced precocious puberty, and of note, both had embryonal carcinoma. In this 63-patient study, appendicitis was the most usual misdiagnosis. Twenty-one percent had malignant tumors. Breen and Maxson noted that 35% of ovarian tumors in children were malignant.

Van Winter and associates reported on 521 adnexal masses in infancy, childhood, and adolescence; 92% were benign, including 335 nonneoplastic and 144 of 186 (77%) neoplastic lesions. The frequency of ovarian malignant neoplasms correlated inversely with the patient's age. Germ cell, stromal, and epithelial malignant neoplasms accounted for 40%, 21%, and 33%, respectively, of the 42 cancers. Nonconformance between preoperative and postoperative diagnoses was noted in 94 cases. The most common preoperative diagnosis necessitating reassignment was acute appendicitis. During the last decade of this study, ultrasonography and CT did not miss a single malignant neoplasm. The majority of these patients presented with a pain or a mass (Table 10-7).

Postmenopausal Ovary

During the postmenopausal years, when the ovary becomes smaller and quiescent after cessation of menses, the presence of a palpable ovary must alert the physician to the possibility of an underlying malignant neoplasm. Physiologic enlargement and functional cysts should not be present in late postmenopausal ovaries. The postmenopausal gonad atrophies to a size of 1.5 × 1 × 0.5 cm on average (Figure 10-12), and at that size it should not be palpable on pelvic examination. The possibility of malignant disease must therefore be carefully assessed when an ovary is palpable in a postmenopausal woman. Goswamy and colleagues studied ovaries from 2221

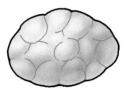

Postmenopausal palpable ovary syndrome
The PMPO syndrome

Normal ovary
Premenopause
3.5 × 2 × 1.5 cm

Early menopause
(1-2 years)
2 × 1.5 × 0.5 cm

Late menopause
(2-5 years)
1.5 × 0.75 × 0.5 cm

FIGURE 10-12 Comparison of the size of the ovary during progressive periods of a woman's life. *(From Barber HRK, Graber EA: Obstet Gynecol Surv 28:357, 1973. Copyright © 1973 The Williams & Wilkins Co, Baltimore.)*

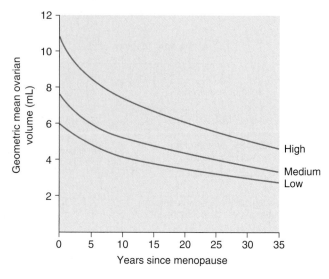

FIGURE 10-13 The 95th centiles for high, medium, and low expected ovarian volumes (geometric means) based on data from 2221 postmenopausal women. *(From Goswamy RK et al: Br J Obstet Gynaecol 95:795, 1988. Reproduced by permission of the Royal College of Obstetrics and Gynaecologists.)*

postmenopausal women with regard to ovarian volumes (Figure 10-13). They noted that there were three ranges of volume and that volume appeared to be increased in obese and multiparous women.

Adnexal masses are usually evaluated by ultrasound, and suspicious masses should be surgically evaluated (Figure 10-14). When surgery is performed, the approach should be made with the assumption that the patient may have an early ovarian carcinoma. Cytologic washings should be obtained and careful exploration of the abdomen should be done, as in any patient being staged for ovarian cancer. If laparotomy is chosen, a vertical abdominal incision is recommended, which allows for careful assessment of the upper abdomen. Small simple cysts are not uncommon in the adnexae of postmenopausal asymptomatic women who undergo pelvic imaging. Wolf and colleagues identified unilocular cysts ranging in size up to 5 cm in 22 of 149 (14.8%) asymptomatic postmenopausal women. Conway and colleagues performed transvaginal sonography on 1769 similar asymptomatic women and found 116 (6.6%) simple cysts up to 5 cm in diameter. Others have had a similar outcome (Table 10-8).

Castillo evaluated 8794 asymptomatic postmenopausal women with ultrasound and identified 215 women with simple adnexal cysts (2.5%). Of 104 women who underwent conservative observation, 44% had spontaneous resolution of the cysts during follow-up, and of women with cysts that did not resolve, 70% of the cysts remained the same size, 17% increased, and 17% decreased. Of 45 women who underwent surgery, 1 was identified with an ovarian cancer. The authors suggested that the risk of malignancy in simple cysts is low and that conservative management is reasonable.

Lerner and colleagues accurately predicted a benign outcome in 247 of 248 patients studied. They used color flow Doppler analysis to improve the accuracy of ultrasonic characterization of ovarian masses. However,

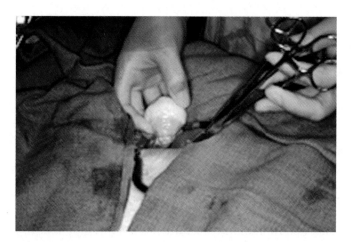

FIGURE 10-14 A 5-cm adenofibroma found in surgery in a postmenopausal woman and detected preoperatively and diagnosed by ultrasonography as a solid mass. *(Courtesy Ibrahim Ramzy, MD, UC, Irvine, California.)*

TABLE 10-8 Frequency of Simple Ovarian Cysts in Asymptomatic Postmenopausal Women

Author	No. of Women	No. of Cysts	% with Cysts
Wolf et al.	149	22	14.8
Conway et al.	1769	116	6.6
Andolf and Jorgensen	534	30	5.6
Aubert et al.	622	36	5.7
Bailey et al.	7705	256	3.3

From Oyelese Y et al: Obstet Gynecol Surv 57:803, 2002. © 2002 by Lippincott Williams & Wilkins, Inc.

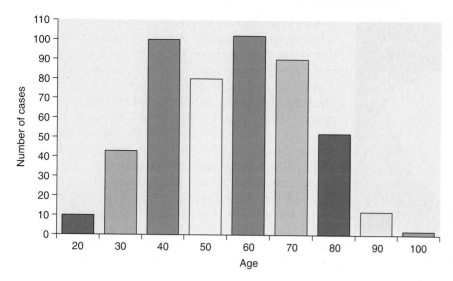

FIGURE 10-15 Epithelial borderline tumors of the ovary. Age distribution. *(From Annual Report Gynecological Cancer. FIGO, Vol 22, 1994.)*

this technique has not been as accurate when used by others. Shalev and coworkers described 55 postmenopausal women who underwent operative laparoscopy for an adnexal cyst that was not complex and when the serum CA-125 level was normal. All of the 55 cysts were benign. During the same period, 75 women underwent exploratory laparotomy for complex cysts or an elevated serum CA-125 level. Of the 75 women, 23 had malignant lesions. Size is an important determinant of malignant potential. Cysts less than 5 cm in diameter are rarely malignant, whereas cysts more than 5 cm in diameter have a high probability of malignancy in the postmenopausal patient.

A diagnosis of ovarian cancer should be considered when a postmenopausal woman presents with a pelvic mass. The presence of ascites, which can be detected clinically or by ultrasound examination, markedly increases the probability of a diagnosis of malignancy. In addition, CA-125, although nonspecific in the population of premenopausal patients, is sensitive in the postmenopausal patient when it is used in combination with a clinical impression and an abnormal ultrasound finding. Early surgical intervention is a key component in the treatment of these patients, and extensive diagnostic testing should be discouraged.

Borderline Malignant Epithelial Ovarian Neoplasms

In the past four decades, clear evidence has been presented that there is a group of epithelial ovarian tumors with histologic and biologic features intermediate between those of clearly benign and those of frankly malignant ovarian neoplasms. These borderline malignant neoplasms account for approximately 15% of all epithelial ovarian cancers. In the younger population, these lesions tend to occur more frequently than the

obviously malignant epithelial ovarian carcinomas, which are seen more frequently in older patients (Figure 10-15). There is a 10-year survival rate of more than 95% for stage I lesions in these borderline neoplasms. However, symptomatic recurrence and death may occur as many as 20 years after therapy in a few patients, and these neoplasms are correctly labeled as being of low malignant potential.

Borderline serous epithelial tumors (Figure 10-16) definitely occupy an intermediate position between the benign serous cystadenomas and the frankly malignant serous cystadenocarcinomas in their histologic features and prognostic aspects. On gross evaluation, the borderline serous tumors are similar to the previously described benign serous cystadenomas, which have papillary projections, but the borderline tumors possibly show an increased incidence of bilaterality. In addition, the papillary component is usually more abundant in the borderline lesions than in the perfectly benign serous cystadenoma. Survival in these lesions differs significantly from that in their obviously malignant counterpart (Figure 10-17).

The histologic criteria characterizing the borderline tumors can be summarized as follows:

- Stratification of the epithelial lining of the papillae
- Formation of microscopic papillary projections or tufts arising from the epithelial lining of the papillae
- Epithelial pleomorphism
- Atypicality
- Mitotic activity
- No stromal invasion present.

In 1973 Hart and Norris reported a series of borderline mucinous tumors confined to either ovary or both

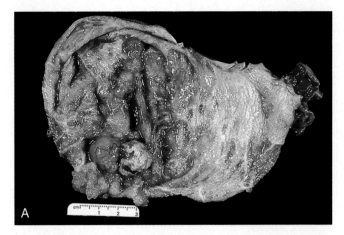

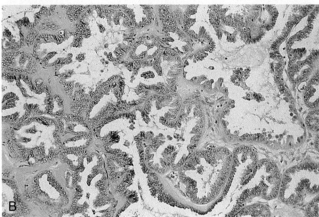

FIGURE 10-16   Borderline serous carcinoma. **A,** Gross appearance.
B, Histologic section showing stratification of the epithelial lining in
papillary projections.

ovaries at the time of diagnosis, with a corrected 10-year
actuarial survival rate of 96%. These neoplasms do not
differ significantly from their benign counterparts in
gross appearance. They are multilocular, cystic, frequently voluminous masses with smooth outer surfaces.
The inner lining, also similar to that of benign mucinous
cystadenomas, is generally smooth, although papillary
structures and solid thickening of the capsule have been
observed in about 25% to 50% of lesions reported (Figure
10-18). On microscopic examination, in contrast to
benign mucinous cystadenoma, the epithelial lining of
the borderline tumor is characterized by stratification of
two or three layers. In the benign tumors, the cells show
no atypia or pleomorphism, but the epithelium of the
borderline lesions does demonstrate atypia, with irregular, hyperchromatic nuclei and enlarged nucleoli. Mitotic
figures are also seen.

Trimble and Trimble reported an excellent review of
epithelial ovarian tumors of low malignant potential in
1994. For serous and mucinous tumors of low malignant
potential, the mean age at diagnosis falls close to 40
years, approximately two decades earlier than the mean
age at diagnosis for invasive epithelial ovarian cancer. In
a meta-analysis of 12 case-control studies conducted in
the United States, Harris and colleagues found a mean
age of 44 years for women with tumors of low malignant
potential compared with a mean age of 52.9 years for
women with invasive ovarian carcinoma. The meta-
analysis conducted by the Collaborative Ovarian Cancer
Group found protective factors against the development
of tumors of low malignant potential to be pregnancy,

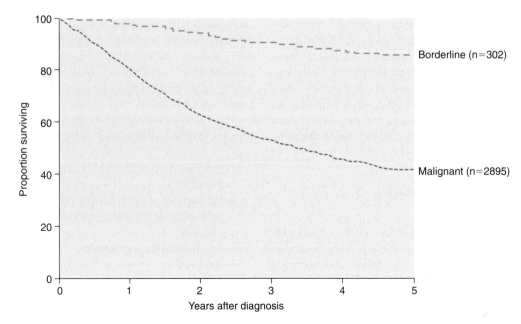

FIGURE 10-17   Carcinoma of the ovary: Patients treated in 1900-1992. Survival by histology (n = 3197). *(From FIGO Report. J Epidemiol Biostat
Vol 3, 1998. Reprinted with permission of the publisher, Taylor & Francis Ltd., http://www.tandf.co.uk/journals.)*

breastfeeding, and use of oral contraceptives. A history of infertility increased the risk of tumors of low malignant potential (odds ratio 1.9), and the use of infertility drugs further increased the risk for development of a tumor of low malignant potential above that of women with no history of infertility (odds ratio 4.0).

Kurman and Trimble reviewed survival in 22 studies of serous tumors of low malignant potential, excluding those patients with invasive peritoneal implants. For 538 patients with stage I disease, survival was 99%, with a mean follow-up of 7 years. Even in the series of 415 patients with stage II and stage III disease, survival was 92% with a mean follow-up of 7 years. In review of the causes of death in this series, 3 patients died of radiation-associated complications, 9 died of chemotherapy-associated complications, 8 died of bowel obstruction, and 8 died of invasive carcinoma; 18 patients were reported as "dying of disease" without additional information. In short, more patients seemed to die with disease than of disease. In addition, more patients died of treatment-related complications than of bowel

obstruction from progressive disease. For treatment of borderline lesions, the physician should strive to completely extirpate all grossly visible tumor. If disease is unilateral, a salpingo-oophorectomy or a carefully performed ovarian cystectomy is appropriate, on condition that a thorough evaluation of the other ovary (biopsy if necessary) is done. Julian and Woodruff evaluated 65 patients who had low-grade papillary serous carcinoma of the ovary and found that 100% of the 50 patients who had unilateral adnexectomy and 90% of the 10 patients who had complete operation (total abdominal hysterectomy and bilateral salpingo-oophorectomy) were alive at 5 years. Lim-Tan and colleagues described 35 patients with ovarian serous borderline tumors treated by unilateral cystectomy or bilateral cystectomy. Tumor persisted or recurred only in the ovary that had been subjected to cystectomy in 2 (6%) of the 33 patients, with stage I tumors in both the ipsilateral and contralateral ovary in 1 patient (3%) and only in the contralateral ovary in the other patient (3%). All the patients were alive without evidence of disease 3 to 18 years after initial operation, with the average follow-up of 7.5 years. Scattered reports of similar smaller series suggest that these lesions may be managed with ovarian cystectomy alone in patients desirous of further childbearing when acceptance of a small risk is appropriate.

If there is bilateral ovarian involvement, especially when papillary projections are found on the external surface of the tumor, or if peritoneal spread is noted, a more radical surgical approach, such as total abdominal hysterectomy with bilateral salpingo-oophorectomy and radical excision of involved pelvic peritoneum, is advocated. Peritoneal cytologic examination, partial omentectomy, and selected pelvic and periaortic lymphadenectomy should also be done in these patients with more advanced disease. Advanced (stage III) borderline lesions can occur with metastases to lymph nodes. The survival rate even with these advanced lesions is appreciable.

Several authors have described patients with ovarian serous borderline tumors with peritoneal implants. Gershenson had a 95% disease-free survival rate at 5 years and a 91% disease-free survival rate at 10 years. However, Bell reported that 13% of patients died of tumor and one patient was alive with widespread progressive tumor. Death resulting from tumor was 4% at 5 years and 23% at 10 years. Drescher and coworkers studied the significance of DNA content and nuclear morphology in these lesions. Their results suggest that measurement of DNA ploidy and nuclear morphology by image analysis can provide important prognostic information in patients with borderline ovarian tumors. Some extraovarian implants are associated with irregular glandular structures in immature, desmoplastic, or inflamed stroma, and these represent a difficult diagnostic problem. Many

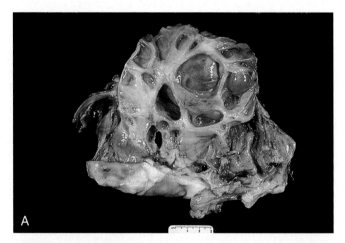

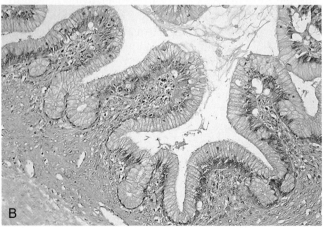

FIGURE 10-18   **A,** Mucinous tumor with low malignant potential. Gross appearance. **B,** Photomicrograph of mucinous tumor seen in Figure 10-18A.

also have a clear pattern of invasion of subjacent tissues and cellular features of malignancy. They thus exhibit a capacity for invasion not seen in the ovarian lesion and may represent an independent or autochthonous origin. Other bland cellular nests of cells in desmoplastic reactive granulation tissue do not invade the underlying tissue and are termed noninvasive compared with the invasive implants. Russell and Merkur reported that invasive implants are associated with a poor clinical outcome compared with the noninvasive group.

Gershenson and colleagues described seven assessable patients with invasive implants who underwent chemotherapy and a second-look surgery. Four of the patients had a response. No clear conclusion could be drawn about which agents were most active. A total of 39 patients with invasive implants were identified at their institution, and 12 (31%) developed progressive disease or a recurrence.

Kurman has identified an aggressive subgroup of proliferative serous lesions, which he calls micropapillary serous carcinoma. Seidman and Kurman found 11 patients with micropapillary projections, and according to Seidman and Kurman, these lesions should be classified as carcinomas, as should serous borderline tumors with invasive implants. The poor prognosis for these patients has prompted some clinicians to prescribe chemotherapy as an adjuvant to surgery.

The role of adjuvant therapy, whether radiotherapy or chemotherapy, in tumors of low malignant potential has not yet been established. Several prospective, randomized studies of adjuvant therapy in patients with invasive ovarian carcinoma have included patients with tumors of low malignant potential. From 1983 to 1992, the Gynecologic Oncology Group (GOG) studied 414 patients with low malignant potential lesions of the ovary. The purpose of the protocol was to evaluate the biologic behavior of these tumors, the effectiveness of melphalan chemotherapy in patients with clinically detectable residual disease after surgical staging and in patients with recurrent disease, and the response rate to cisplatin in patients who failed to respond to melphalan therapy. The preliminary conclusions were that ovarian serous tumors of low malignant potential limited to the ovary rarely recur. Conservative management with unilateral salpingo-oophorectomy or ovarian cystectomy is adequate therapy for women of reproductive age. The effectiveness of melphalan and cisplatin has yet to be analyzed.

It is clear that some patients with advanced disease will ultimately die of their tumor. It is not clear that adjuvant chemotherapy has any impact on survival. A strong clinical need currently exists to develop a mechanism for distinguishing lesions that are biologically aggressive from lesions that persist in a state of equilibrium, posing no threat to the patients' health and welfare.

Fertility Preservation

Operative treatment has traditionally been the mainstay of management in ovarian carcinoma. The technical aspects of the initial laparotomy have a greater bearing on outcome than do many subsequent therapeutic decisions. Hysterectomy with bilateral salpingo-oophorectomy continues to be the most cogent therapy for ovarian carcinoma. The opposite ovary is removed because of the frequency of bilateral synchronous tumors and the possibility of occult metastases, which in the normal-appearing opposite ovary have varied from 6% to 43%, depending on the report and stage of the disease. Because the uterine serosa and endometrium are often sites of occult metastasis and because the prevalence of synchronous endometrial carcinoma is relatively high, hysterectomy is also indicated. Because 3% to 17% of patients with ovarian cancer are less than 40 years of age, some patients may consider options for fertility preservation in the setting of an adnexal mass.

Conservative therapy, designed by preservation of some ovarian tissue, appears to be safe, although no prospective trials have compared conservative surgery with bilateral salpingo-oophorectomy. Trimble and Trimble collected eight series (Table 10-9). In a study of these data, there were only 10 recurrences in 148 patients for an incidence of 6.8%. Zanetta and colleagues published their results with 99 women aged 40 years or younger with stage I ovarian carcinoma. Of the 99 women, 56 underwent fertility-sparing surgery and 43 had more radical surgery with a median follow-up of 7 years; they observed five recurrences (9%) of carcinoma in the women treated conservatively and five recurrences (12%) in those treated more radically. Two recurrences after conservative surgery involved the residual ovary (3.6%). These two women developed a borderline tumor in the contralateral ovary and were treated with surgery. More recent data from Schlaerth and colleagues from Memorial Sloan-Kettering Cancer Center evaluating 123 patients with stage I ovarian cancer, including

TABLE 10-9   Recurrence Rate in Patients with Low Malignant Potential Lesions with Conservative Surgery

Author	Incidence of Recurrence (%)
Casey et al.	0/7 (0)
Chambers et al.	2/20 (20)
Lim-Tan et al.	4/35 (11)
Manchul et al.	0/15 (0)
Rice et al.	0/32 (0)
Sawada et al.	1/5 (20)
Tazelaar et al.	3/20 (15)
Tropé et al.	0/14 (0)
Total	10/148 (7)

Modified from Trimble CL, Trimble EL: Gynecol Oncol 55:S42, 1994.

20 with preservation of the uterus and contralateral ovary, found no difference in 5-year PFS (84% vs 78%) or survival (84% vs 82%) for fertility-preserving versus standard surgical approaches. Wright reviewed a large population database of patients with early-stage ovarian cancer and noted that neither ovarian nor uterine preservation had an effect on survival. Colombo and associates reported data of 99 patients younger than 40 years with stage I ovarian cancer. Conservative surgery was performed in 56 of the patients (36 stage Ia, 1 stage Ib, and 19 stage Ic). Relapses occurred in three patients assigned to stage Ia (grades I, II, and III). One recurrence was in the residual ovary, and the patient was rescued by surgery; the other 2 patients had relapse at distant sites and died as a result of the tumors. Seventeen patients who desired to become pregnant did so, for a total of 25 conceptions.

Some centers are studying the role of ovarian cystectomy alone for low-grade stage I epithelial neoplasms. Others have permitted stage I lesions, grade II and III lesions, and stage Ic neoplasms to undergo ovarian tissue-sparing surgery followed by chemotherapy in an attempt to preserve fertility. These investigations await further observation and confirmation as to long-term safety. Chemotherapy administered after such ovarian tissue-sparing procedures may destroy the remaining ova, especially in patients older than 30 years.

It is estimated that 7% to 8% of stage I ovarian cancer cases occur in women younger than age 35. Considerations for conservative management of stage Ia ovarian cancer are listed in Table 10-10. Unilateral salpingo-oophorectomy may be the definitive treatment of a young woman of low parity found to have a well-differentiated serous, mucinous, endometrioid, or mesonephric carcinoma of the ovary. The tumor must be unilateral, well encapsulated, free of adhesions, and not associated with ascites or evidence of extragonadal spread. Peritoneal washings for cytologic examination should be taken from the pelvis and upper abdomen, and the opposite ovary should be evaluated for disease.

TABLE 10-10 Optimal Requirements for Conservative Management in Epithelial Ovarian Cancer Stage Ia

Well differentiated
Young woman of low parity
Otherwise normal pelvis
Encapsulated and free of adhesions
No invasion of capsule, lymphatics, or mesovarium
Peritoneal washings negative
Adequate evaluation of opposite ovary and omental biopsy result negative
Close follow-up probable
Excision of residual ovary after completion of childbearing

Modified from DiSaia PJ, Townsend DE, Morrow CP: Obstet Gynecol Surv 29:581, 19714. Copyright © 1974 by The Williams & Wilkins Co.

If the opposite ovary is of normal size, shape, and configuration, surgical evaluation is not routinely done. Munnell and others have calculated the incidence of microscopic metastases in the opposite ovary to be approximately 12%. The para-aortic and pelvic wall nodes must be carefully palpated and sampled, and an adequate sample of the omentum must be taken for biopsy. In addition, the preserved pelvic organs should be reasonably normal because there is little to be gained by retaining the opposite ovary in a patient who is not fertile. With the finding of carcinoma in any of these areas, conservative surgery must be abandoned. After the patient has completed childbearing, some consideration should be given to the removal of the other ovary to eliminate the risk of another ovarian malignant neoplasm. Because the incidence of epithelial cancer of the ovary increases when a woman reaches the sixth decade and because a patient with a history of such a lesion harbors the unfortunate milieu that could promote another epithelial lesion, it is reasonable to remove the vestigial ovarian tissue after childbearing.

Cyst Rupture/Spill of Tumor

The subject of tumor spill has been controversial in gynecologic oncology for some time. FIGO staging denotes a change of stage to IC if cyst rupture is noted preoperatively or intraoperatively, and survival data suggest that patients with stage IA disease have survival approaching 94%, whereas it is approximately 84% for Ic disease. In addition to cyst rupture, tumor penetration of the cyst wall and presence of malignant cytology would also change stage to IC (in a tumor otherwise confined to one or both ovaries). Traditionally, upstaging to Ic leads to a recommendation for the use of postoperative chemotherapy also. It is logical to assume that implantation and germination of cancer cells are conceivable and probable when a malignant cyst ruptures at the time of surgery. The data to support the independent prognostic significance of cyst rupture are mixed, however.

Analyses of older studies where complete surgical staging was not performed and contemporary chemotherapy regimens were not used make it difficult to understand the relevance of cyst rupture as a single variable (Table 10-11). Sjöval described 247 patients with stage I disease who were at risk of spill. There was no difference in survival between the patients whose tumors had intact capsules and the patients in whom rupture occurred during surgery (78% and 85%, respectively). However, a significant difference in survival was found between patients in whom rupture occurred before surgery and those with intraoperative rupture (59% and 85%, respectively). The conclusion was that manipulation during surgery that results in puncture or rupture does not have a negative influence on the outcome for

TABLE 10-11   Recurrence Rates as a Function of Cyst Rupture

Series	Ruptured Neoplasm (%)	Unruptured Neoplasm (%)
Purola and Nieminen (1968)	18/30 (60)	83/100 (83)
Williams, Symmonds, and Litwak (1973)	3/7 (43)	57/58 (98)
Parker, Parker, and Wilbanks (1970)	16/27 (59)	12/20 (60)
Dembo et al. (1989)	98/119 (82)	168/199 (84)
Sevelda et al. (1989)	23/30 (76)	23/30 (76)

TABLE 10-12   Frequency of Prior Pelvic Surgery/Hysterectomy (%)

Author (year)	All Ages	>40 yr
Bloom (1962)	10.6	
Grogan (1967)	8.2	
Terz (1967)	8.8	3.8
Gibbs (1971)	11.8	
Kofler (1972)	8.1	8.1
Grundsell (1980)	6.0	4.6
Averette (1994)	18.2	10.1

patients. However, rupture occurring at some interval before surgery may lead to seeding in the peritoneal cavity. Vergote and colleagues assessed 1545 stage I ovarian cancer patients and found that tumor differentiation/grade and cyst rupture were the two most important predictors for disease-free survival. Cyst rupture occurring before definitive surgery heralded a poorer prognosis than that occurring intraoperatively. Bakkum-Gamez and associates reported on 161 patients with stage I ovarian cancer, all of whom underwent thorough surgical staging. In a multivariate analysis, capsular rupture and positive peritoneal cytology were independent predictors of poorer disease-free survival. It is noted that rupture may occur as a result of laparoscopic removal and drainage, may occur by cyst wall weakening (necrosis, tumor penetration), or may be associated with adhesions and adhesion lysis required to remove the cyst. The effect of these confounding variables is difficult to separate, however.

We believe that collection of cytology before the mass is manipulated provides important information. Cysts should be removed intact where possible, recognizing that coexisting conditions (endometriois, adhesions, infection, inflammation) may make this impossible. In some cases, particularly with a large, simple cyst, aspiration by a needle attached to suction (with the area draped off with dry laparotomy pads) has been used to decompress a cyst. Our experience with this type of "controlled spill" is that it appears to be safe and has not adversely affected outcome. In cases of masses with solid components or a high suspicion for malignancy, we favor removing the mass intact. Most authors advocate platinum-based chemotherapy for at least three cycles in patients with stage IC disease secondary to tumor rupture. No prospective study comparing these different approaches has been reported.

Prophylactic versus Risk-Reducing Oophorectomy

The early diagnosis of ovarian carcinoma is as difficult and infrequent now as in the past. Although survival figures for this disease may be recently improving to a slight degree, the prognosis is still grave. The gynecologist frequently counsels women with regard to strategies to reduce the risk of developing ovarian cancer. In one typical clinical scenario, a low-risk patient who is to undergo a hysterectomy for benign indications must be counseled as to the risk and benefits of removing the ovaries at the time of surgery (prophylactic oophorectomy).

At some time during their lives, 1% to 2% of all women develop ovarian carcinoma. The risk increases after 40 years of age, with a peak incidence between 55 and 60 years of age, closely paralleling the peak incidence of menopause in Western countries (Figure 10-19). The function of the ovary lies in its role of ova production for procreation and as the primary site of estrogen production. After the need for ova has passed in a woman's life, only estrogen production remains an essential function. The adverse effects of oophorectomy on several metabolic parameters are well known; understanding of the endocrinology, sexuality, and psychology of the postmenopausal patient (natural or surgical) has increased considerably during the past decade, and good methods of adequate substitution for the loss of ovarian function are now available.

In 1981 Grundsell and associates reported on a series of 352 women with ovarian carcinoma and studied the incidence of previous pelvic surgeries performed on these patients; 21 (6%) had undergone previous pelvic surgery, and 16 (4.6%) of these patients had surgery at some time after the age of 40 years. Others (Table 10-12) have reported similar results (Bloom, Gibbs, Grogan, Kofler, and Terz). McKenzie, Christ, and Paloucek reported that as many as 3.6% of women who have pelvic surgery with preservation of ovarian tissue will need subsequent surgery for benign lesions of the ovary, further influencing the argument for prophylactic oophorectomy.

Averette and Nguyen found that 18.2% of patients reported previous hysterectomy with ovarian conservation in a national survey of 12,316 ovarian cancer cases. Of these, hysterectomies were abdominal in 7.2%, vaginal in 4.2%, and unspecified in another 6.8%. In a subsequent analysis, Boike and associates found that

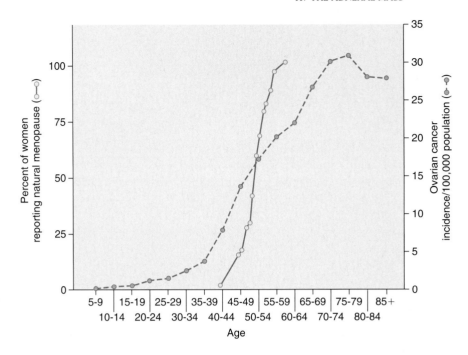

FIGURE 10-19 Incidence of ovarian cancer and the onset of natural menopause vs age.

57.4% of hysterectomies were performed after the age of 40 years. Thus, a potential 1286 ovarian cancer cases could have been prevented if prophylactic oophorectomy had been practiced in women undergoing hysterectomy at the age of 40 years or later. Assuming an annual incidence of 24,000 new ovarian cases and that 5% to 14% of these cases had previous hysterectomies with conserved ovaries, it is estimated that at least 1000 cases could have been prevented if prophylactic oophorectomy were diligently practiced after the age of 40 years.

We are obviously influenced by the frequent task of caring for patients with advanced ovarian carcinoma. The occurrence of this disease in patients who had previous pelvic surgery and in whom the ovaries could have been removed is certainly frustrating. Randall and coworkers have shown that unilateral oophorectomy does not influence the subsequent incidence of ovarian carcinoma.

All patients in whom prophylactic oophorectomy is under consideration should be thoroughly informed about the possible adverse effects and the advantages. The patient must make the decision without undue pressure from her physician. All thoughts of further childbearing must be settled. Open discussion should be encouraged, especially in areas of body image, libido, and other psychosexual concerns. With this as background, we believe that prophylactic oophorectomy should be offered to all perimenopausal patients (40 to 50 years of age) undergoing pelvic surgery.

A second clinical scenario is that in a patient with a strong family history of breast/ovarian cancers or who harbors a known mutation in the BRCA1 or 2 gene.

These high-risk patients frequently seek consultation to undergo surgery to remove the ovaries to reduce the risk of development of ovarian cancer. Risk-reducing salpingo-oophorectomy (RRSO) has been evaluated in several populations of women at high risk for developing ovarian cancer. Women with known BRCA1 mutations are estimated to have a lifetime risk of developing ovarian cancer from 39% to 46% and those with BRCA2 mutations have a risk from 12% to 20%. Removing the ovaries in this high-risk group of patients reduces the risk of ovarian cancer, with 0.8% to 1% of women subsequently developing a primary peritoneal cancer. In addition, premenopausal women undergoing RRSO have a 50% to 80% reduction in the risk of breast cancer. In a consensus statement by the SGO, women at high risk of ovarian cancer based on family history or BRCA1/2 mutation should be offered RRSO when childbearing is complete. It should be noted that in the setting of RRSO, some patients will be identified with an incidental early-stage cancer of the ovary or fallopian tube. RRSO should not be offered routinely for women at average risk for ovarian cancer because there are no data to support improved survival in these patients. Patients undergoing hysterectomy for other reasons (fibroids, endometriosis) should be counseled as to the risk and benefits related to salpingo-oophorectomy. Risk reduction must be balanced against changes in cardiovascular, bone, and sexual health.

For full reference list, log onto www.expertconsult.com ⟨http://www.expertconsult.com⟩.

Epithelial Ovarian Cancer

Eric L. Eisenhauer, MD, Ritu Salani, MD, MBA, and Larry J. Copeland, MD

Malignant neoplasms of the ovary are the cause of more deaths than any other female genital tract cancer. In the United States, there were approximately 21,880 new cases and 13,850 deaths in 2010 as a result of ovarian cancer. Ovarian cancer accounts for 6% of all cancers among women. In the United States, deaths from this cause occur at a rate of 1 every 44 minutes, and this disease will develop in 1 of every 68 women. Doctors and patients alike continue to be frustrated by our lack of understanding of the factors that lead to ovarian cancer and the failure to achieve a significant reduction in mortality.

CLASSIFICATION

The student of ovarian pathology is often confused by the wide variation in histologic structure and biologic behavior. The most popular and practical classification scheme is based on the histogenesis of the normal ovary, shown in Table 11-1. The early development of the ovary may be divided into four major stages. During the first stage, undifferentiated germ cells (primordial germ cells) become segregated and migrate from their sites of origin to settle in the genital ridges, which are bilateral thickenings of coelomic epithelium. The second stage occurs after

TABLE 11-1   Histogenetic Classification of Ovarian Neoplasms

Neoplasms derived from coelomic epithelium
  Serous tumor
  Mucinous tumor
  Endometrioid tumor
  Mesonephroid (clear cell) tumor
  Brenner tumor
  Undifferentiated carcinoma
  Carcinosarcoma and mixed mesodermal tumor
Neoplasms derived from germ cells
  Teratoma
    Mature teratoma
      Solid adult teratoma
      Dermoid cyst
      Struma ovarii
      Malignant neoplasms secondarily arising from mature cystic teratoma
    Immature teratoma (partially differentiated teratoma)
  Dysgerminoma
  Embryonal carcinoma
  Endodermal sinus tumor
  Choriocarcinoma
  Gonadoblastoma
Neoplasms derived from specialized gonadal stroma
  Granulosa–theca cell tumors
    Granulosa tumor
    Thecoma
  Sertoli–Leydig tumors
    Arrhenoblastoma
    Sertoli tumor
  Gynandroblastoma
  Lipid cell tumors
Neoplasms derived from nonspecific mesenchyme
  Fibroma, hemangioma, leiomyoma, lipoma
  Lymphoma
  Sarcoma
Neoplasms metastatic to the ovary
  Gastrointestinal tract (Krukenberg)
  Breast
  Endometrium
  Lymphoma

TABLE 11-2   Probability for Females at Birth Developing Cancer by Age 85 in the United States

All sites	1 in 3
Breast	1 in 9
Cervix	1 in 154
Uterine corpus	1 in 41
Lung	1 in 18
Ovary	1 in 81
Colon–rectum	1 in 26

DevCan 6.6.0, National Cancer Institute 2011. http://surveillance.cancer.gov/devcan.

The specific malignant histologic type has less prognostic significance than clinical stage, extent of residual disease, and histologic grade. Histologic grade is an important independent prognostic factor in patients with epithelial tumors of the ovary (Figure 11-1). Because survival for patients with grade II and III tumors is more closely related, research studies frequently stratify by low-grade (grade I) and high-grade (grade II and III) tumors.

INCIDENCE, EPIDEMIOLOGY, AND ETIOLOGY

Approximately 27% of gynecologic cancers are of ovarian origin (Figure 11-2), but 53% of all gynecologic cancer deaths occur in women who have ovarian cancer. Cancer of the ovaries is the fifth most frequently occurring fatal cancer in women in the United States and also ranks high as a cause of death in Canada, New Zealand, Israel, and countries of northern Europe. Ovarian cancer will develop in approximately 14 of every 1000 women in the United States older than age 40 years (Table 11-2), but only 4 of the 14 will be cured. The remaining patients often develop repeated bouts of intestinal obstruction as the tumor spreads over the surface of the bowel, develop inanition and malnutrition, and quite literally starve. In a review of mortality trends in the United States, age-adjusted (to the 2000 U.S. standard population) ovarian cancer mortality rates from 1975 to 2002 showed the absolute number of deaths increased, consistent with a growing and aging population. Over the past 30 years, mortality rates have decreased for women younger than 65 years, whereas rates increased for women older than 65 years, with some plateauing over the past 10 years. These changes may result from increased use of oral contraceptives in younger patients and a shifting of the survival curve to the right. Even when matched for stage, survival was worse in older women. Some have suggested this may be a result of less aggressive treatment in the older woman and the higher percentage of low-grade disease in younger

arrival of the germ cells in the genital ridges and consists of proliferation of the coelomic epithelium and the underlying mesenchyme. During the third stage, the ovary becomes divided into a peripheral cortex and a central medulla. The fourth stage is characterized by the development of the cortex and the involution of the medulla. The histogenetic classification categorizes ovarian neoplasms with regard to their derivation from coelomic epithelium, germ cells, and mesenchyme (stroma).

The majority (85% to 90%) of malignant ovarian tumors are epithelial. They can be grouped into predominant histologic types as follows:

Serous cystadenocarcinoma	42%
Mucinous cystadenocarcinoma	12%
Endometrioid carcinoma	15%
Undifferentiated carcinoma	17%
Clear cell carcinoma	6%

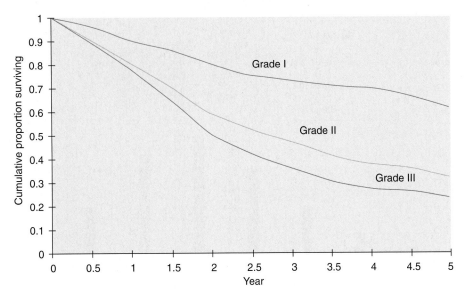

FIGURE 11-1   Serous cystadenocarcinoma of the ovary. Cumulative proportion surviving by degree of differentiation. *(From Annual Report on the Results of Treatment in Gynecological Cancer, Vol 22. Stockholm, International Federation of Gynecology and Obstetrics, 1994.)*

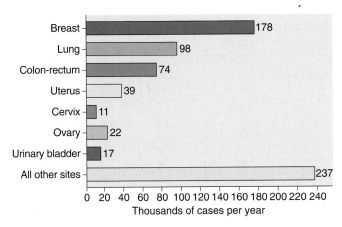

FIGURE 11-2   Leading sites of new cancer cases and deaths: 2010 estimates. *(© 2010 American Cancer Society, Inc., Surveillance and Health Policy Research.)*

TABLE 11-3   Primary Ovarian Neoplasms Related to Age

Type	<20 Yr (%)	20-50 Yr (%)	>50 Yr (%)
Coelomic epithelium	29	71	81
Germ cell	59	14	6
Specialized gonadal stroma	8	5	4
Nonspecific mesenchyme	4	10	9

patients. Age-adjusted death rates were higher in whites than in blacks. Asian/Pacific Islanders, American Indian/Alaskan natives, and Hispanics have lower death rates than blacks.

Malignant neoplasms of the ovaries occur at all ages, including infancy and childhood (Figure 11-3). Throughout childhood and adolescence, the rate of death from ovarian carcinoma in the United States is exceeded by those for leukemia; lymphomas; and neoplasms of the central nervous system, kidney, connective tissue, and bone. The major histologic types occur in distinctive age ranges (Table 11-3). Malignant germ cell tumors are most commonly seen in girls younger than age 20 years, whereas epithelial cancers of the ovary are primarily seen in women older than age 50 years. Beginning with the age group 45 to 49 years, which has a rate of 16.4 cases per 100,000, incidence increases progressively with age. The rate increases after the age of 60 years to about 40 cases per 100,000 and continues to peak to a rate of 61 cases per 100,000 in the age group 80 to 84 years. The largest absolute number of patients with ovarian cancer is found in the age group 60 to 64 years, but more than one third of the cases occur in patients 65 years or older. Elderly women are more likely than younger women to be in advanced stages of ovarian cancer at initial diagnosis, and the 5-year relative survival rate for elderly women is about half the rate (28.4%) observed in women younger than 65 years (56.6%).

Epidemiologic evidence strongly suggests that environmental factors are major etiologic determinants in epithelial cancer of the human ovary. Highly industrial countries have the highest reported incidence, which suggests that physical or chemical products of industry may be causative factors. A notable exception is highly industrialized Japan, where rates for ovarian cancer have been among the lowest recorded in the world. Of interest, the incidence of ovarian cancer increases in Japanese immigrants to the United States and their

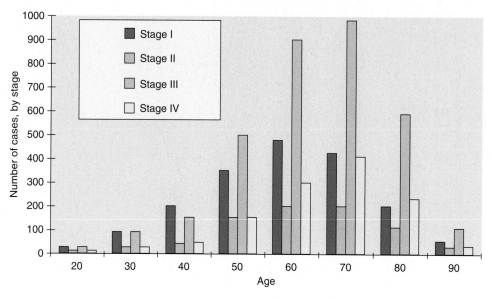

FIGURE 11-3   Obviously malignant ovarian epithelial tumors. Age distribution by stage. *(From Annual Report on the Results of Treatment in Gynecological Cancer, Vol 22. Stockholm, International Federation of Gynecology and Obstetrics, 1994.)*

offspring, eventually approaching that of Anglo-Saxon whites by the second and third generations. This suggests strongly that the causative carcinogens are probably in the immediate environment, such as food, personal customs, and other influences that change gradually during the cultural transition. To date, there are no clues as to which dietary items or other environmental contacts might be specifically carcinogenic for the ovary.

Whittemore and others have shown that the odds for invasive epithelial ovarian cancer vary with the number of term pregnancies each woman experiences. Danforth prospectively examined risk of ovarian cancer in the Nurses' Health Studies and found that women who never breastfed faced a 1.5-fold risk of ovarian cancer compared with women who breastfed for greater than 18 months. These observations coincided with data illustrating a reduction in the disease incidence with the use of oral contraceptives (Table 11-4). The hypothesis that oral contraceptive use reduces the risk of epithelial ovarian cancer was suggested by Casagrande and associates in 1979. In 1982 Rosenberg and colleagues reported a case-control study of women younger than 60 years. Combination oral contraceptives were used by 26% of the cancer patients and 35% of the control subjects. The relative risk estimate for combination oral contraceptive use was 0.6 (Table 11-5). The reduction in risk appears to persist for as long as 10 years after use has ceased and to be greater for longer durations of use, but these results were not statistically significant. Their conclusion was that the use of combination oral contraceptives protects against epithelial ovarian cancer. The theory of

TABLE 11-4   Odds Ratio for Invasive Epithelial Ovarian Cancer According to Parity

No. of Term Pregnancies	Cases	%	Population Studies		Odds Ratio
			Controls	Percentage	
0	322	24	765	14	1.44
1	164	12	605	11	1.6
2	376	28	1515	27	1.53
3	265	19	1259	22	1.48
4	135	10	774	14	1.36
5	56	4	345	6	1.33
6	45	3	346	6	1.29

Modified from Whittemore AS et al: Am J Epidemiol 136:1184, 1992.

TABLE 11-5   How Oral Contraceptive Use Affects the Risk of Ovarian Cancer

Duration of Oral Contraceptive Use	Number of Women Who Developed Ovarian Cancer	Controls	Relative Risk
Never	242	1532	1.4
3-6 months	26	1280	0.6
7-11 months	14	1134	0.7
1-2 years	65	1602	0.7
3-4 years	40	1397	0.6
5-9 years	39	1594	0.4
≥10 years	13	1328	0.2

From the Cancer and Steroid Hormone Study of the Centers for Disease Control and the National Institute of Child Health and Human Development: N Engl J Med 316:650, 1987. Reprinted, by permission, from the New England Journal of Medicine.

"incessant ovulation" suggests that the epithelial lining of the ovary may be sensitive to the events of ovulation, which in turn can act as a promoting factor in the carcinogenic process. Gross and Schlesselman determined the effect of oral contraceptive use on the cumulative incidence of epithelial ovarian cancer from ages 20 to 40 years, 20 to 50 years, and 20 to 55 years. The women were categorized into four groups: positive family history, negative family history, parous, and nulliparous. The Cancer and Steroid Hormone Study data were used in all four groups. The cumulative number of epithelial ovarian cancer cases estimated to occur per 100,000 oral contraceptive users compared with never-users decreased with increasing duration of use. Their results suggest that 5 years of use by nulliparous women can reduce their ovarian cancer risk to the level seen in parous women who never use oral contraceptives, and 10 years of use by women with a positive family history can reduce their risk to a level below that of women whose family history is negative and who never use oral contraceptives. On the basis of these data, the recommendation is strongly made that patients with a family history of ovarian cancer use oral contraceptives when pregnancy is not being sought.

Studies have suggested an association between fertility drug exposure and ovarian cancer. Whittemore and associates noted that infertile women treated with infertility drugs had a 2.8 times increased risk of ovarian cancer compared with women without infertility. The risk was higher among women who did not become pregnant compared with the parous women. Specific drug exposure was not documented. The study by Franceschi and colleagues noted a nonsignificant decreased risk of ovarian cancer in women undergoing ovarian stimulation. Rossing and coworkers examined the risk of ovarian tumors in a cohort of 3837 women evaluated for infertility between 1974 and 1985 in Seattle, Washington. Computer linkage with a population-based tumor registry was used to identify women whose tumors were diagnosed before January 1, 1992. There were 11 invasive or borderline malignant ovarian tumors, compared with an expected number of 4.4 (odds ratio = 2.3, nonsignificant). Nine of the women in whom ovarian tumor developed had taken clomiphene (Clomid), and five had taken the drug during 12 or more monthly cycles. Venn and associates found no influence of ovulation induction on ovarian cancer, and Shishan in a case-control study found no increase in invasive carcinoma, although there was an increase in tumors of low malignant potential in women who used infertility drugs. There was no increase with clomiphene, but treatment with human menopausal gonadotropin was associated with increased risk, which is exactly opposite of Rossing's finding. The largest reported cohort drew 126 women with invasive epithelial ovarian cancer from a cohort of 54,362 women treated at all Danish infertility clinics from 1963 to 1968. The effects of four separate groups of fertility drugs were evaluated individually and in combination (gonadotropins, clomiphene citrate, human chorionic gonadotropin, and gonadotropin-releasing hormone). No convincing associations were found between use of these fertility drugs and ovarian cancer risk. In an earlier study from Denmark, Mosgaard and associates noted an increased risk of ovarian cancer in nulliparous women compared with parous women. Infertile nontreated nulliparous women had an odds ratio of 2.7 compared with noninfertile nulliparous women. The risk of ovarian carcinoma among treated nulliparous and treated parous women was less than that of nontreated nulliparous and parous infertile women. The published data suggest that there is probably little relationship between fertility drug use and ovarian cancer. Further investigations are under way to clarify this association. The concept is appealing when one considers the reduction in incidence noted with the use of oral contraceptives and parity.

Whittemore and associates, in a population-based study, noted protection against ovarian cancer with increasing parity (see Table 11-4). McGowan and colleagues, on the basis of a study of 197 women with ovarian cancer, estimated that nulligravidae were 2.45 times more likely to have malignant ovarian tumors and 2.9 times more likely to have ovarian carcinoma of low potential malignancy than were women who had been pregnant three or more times. The risk of ovarian cancer in their series was reduced to 1.27 among women who had been pregnant at least once. In Gerow's series, women with ovarian cancer demonstrated a marked decrease in the number of live births. One possible interpretation could be that the endocrinologic status of pregnancy protects against ovarian cancer and that the lack of this protection places infertile women at higher risk for ovarian cancer. A second explanation could be that infertility and ovarian cancer result from the same abnormal gonadal status. This theory would explain why infertile women are more at risk than never-married and never-pregnant women.

In the large prospective Cancer Prevention Study II, Rodriguez and coworkers evaluated the use of acetaminophen and a possible relationship to ovarian cancer mortality. Women who reported using acetaminophen daily had a death rate from ovarian cancer 45% lower than that of women reporting no use (relative risk = 0.55; confidence interval [CI] = 0.27-1.09). In a case-control study, Cramer and associates had previously reported that the odds ratio was 0.52 for development of ovarian cancer among women who used the drug at least once a week for at least 6 months; lowest risk was found in women who used the drug daily and for more than 10 years. Cramer also noted that the odds ratio of ovarian cancer was 0.75 (CI = 0.52-1.10) for aspirin and 1.03 for ibuprofen.

Parazzini and colleagues studied the influence of various menstrual factors on the risk of epithelial ovarian cancer. They reported that the risk rose with later age at menopause and with early menarche. Confirmation of this work is not yet at hand. Studies of dietary fat have been inconclusive, and other dietary factors are not well characterized. Although the Women's Health Initiative investigators reported a low-fat diet was associated with up to a 40% reduction in ovarian cancer risk, several large cohort studies have not been able to demonstrate this. Because diet and exercise are potentially modifiable risk factors, continued investigation as to their role is under way by both the Gynecologic Oncology Group (GOG) and others.

Some have suggested that ovarian cancer may be initiated by a chemical carcinogen through the vagina, uterus, and fallopian tubes, and the substance promoting cancer may even be the steroid-rich antral fluid from ruptured follicles. For years, Woodruff and coworkers suggested this hypothesis of migration of chemical carcinogens from the vagina to the pelvic peritoneum. Venter demonstrated with the use of radionuclides that upward migration is possible. Certainly many different chemical substances are regularly used in the vulvovaginal areas, and some of these could be implicated in carcinogenesis. The agent most extensively studied has been talc powder. Many of the studies that noted a slight increased risk of ovarian carcinoma in association with talc did not adjust for other factors (oral contraceptive use, family history) that are related to ovarian cancer. Others included low malignant potential tumors with their invasive cancers or did not correct for integrity of the female genital tract status. The relationship (if any) of talc to ovarian cancer would appear to be minimal at best.

No epidemiologic or experimental evidence exists to incriminate viruses in the development of neoplasms of the human ovary. Attempts to isolate viruses from cultures of human ovarian cancer cells have been unsuccessful to date. Because of its gonadotropic properties, mumps virus is an obvious candidate among known viruses for oncogenic activity in the ovary. Case-control studies have revealed a possible negative association with mumps parotitis, but these historical accounts were not supported by skin tests or serologic evidence of reactivity to mumps virus. Menczer and coworkers have postulated that an immunologic incompetence may enable development of ovarian cancer, possibly through a direct etiologic role of mumps virus. At present, however, the evidence for mumps virus as an etiologic agent in ovarian cancer remains speculative.

Our knowledge of ovarian cancer etiology is limited to fragments of information. The cooperative group clinical trials programs offer an ideal population of women for case-control studies. Each patient should be questioned for a history of pre-existing gynecologic abnormalities, documented by clinical or laboratory data when possible, and for information about exposure to environmental carcinogens. There are many programs of this nature that may lead to better information regarding these mechanisms.

Familial Ovarian Cancer

Familial hereditary ovarian cancer falls into three categories:

- Site-specific familial ovarian cancer;
- Breast-ovarian cancer syndrome, in which there is an increased incidence of breast and ovarian carcinomas alone or in combination; and
- Lynch syndrome type II, in which family members may develop a variety of cancers, including colorectal, endometrial, and ovarian cancer.

Inherited genetic mutations are associated with approximately 10% of women who develop ovarian cancer. The mutation is inherited in an autosomal-dominant fashion (maternal or paternal transmission), and multiple family members are affected over several generations. First-degree relatives (mother or sister) are frequently involved.

True hereditary ovarian cancer and breast cancer mainly result from mutations of BRCA1 and BRCA2 genes. Individuals with these mutations (BRCA1 and BRCA2) generally have a germline mutation (inherited mutated copy of the gene) in contrast to the more common somatic mutation (noninherited, or acquired) in most patients with ovarian cancer. BRCA1 mutations are located on the long arm of chromosome 17q, and BRCA2 mutations are located on chromosome 13q12. Lynch II syndrome arises as a result of inherited mutation in a family of DNA repair genes (MSH2, MLH1, PMS1, PMS2); this group accounts for only a small number of inherited ovarian cancers. Initial evaluation of these germline mutations suggested an estimated risk of ovarian cancer of 32% to 84% for carriers of the BRCA1 mutation if they are from a kindred with multiple cases of breast or ovarian cancer but a much lower rate for carriers of the BRCA2 mutation. With more than 400 mutations identified in BRCA1 and BRCA2 genes along with multiple polymorphisms, estimating risk is difficult. As more data are collected, the risk in patients with this mutation appears lower than was previously thought (65% decreasing to 20%). In most women with a strong family history who do develop ovarian cancer, the disease is sporadic in nature and not inherited. In a population-based study of 432 women with ovarian cancer, 34 (6.9%) gave a family history of the cancer, but only 3 (0.6%) had more than one relative with the disease; after further review, it was likely that only 1 (0.2%) may have had hereditary ovarian cancer. Houlston and colleagues evaluated 391 women who were self-referred to a screening clinic for familial ovarian cancer. Of these, 290 (74%) appeared to have no clear inheritance pattern, and there was no increased risk of cancer in the first-degree relatives. There were 82 (21%) pedigrees compatible with multisite cancer family syndrome with a relative risk of about 6, or development of ovarian cancer in 1 of 16. In the 19 families with site-specific ovarian cancer, the relative risk for first-degree relatives was 39, with a lifetime risk of 1 in 2. Kerlikowske and associates reviewed published studies of familial ovarian cancers and used ovarian cancer incidence data from the Surveillance, Epidemiology, and End Results (SEER) database to estimate lifetime probabilities of ovarian cancer in these families. They noted that the lifetime probability of ovarian cancer for a 35-year-old woman was 1.6% in an individual without a family history of ovarian cancer. It increased to 5% if she had one relative and 7% if she had two relatives with ovarian cancer. Bourne and colleagues identified 1601 high-risk patients on the basis of family history. These patients were then screened for ovarian cancer. In 1156 women who were thought to have sporadic family histories, two cancers (one low malignant potential) were identified (0.17%). Of the 288 with multiple-site designation, three cancers (two low malignant potential) were found (1.04%), and in the women with ovarian cancer, family history was identified in only 1 of 157 (0.63%). Cancers found subsequent to screening consisted of one peritoneal cancer in the sporadic group (0.08%), four (one peritoneal cancer) in the multiple-site group (1.38%), and none in the ovarian-only group. All of these studies were based on family history pedigree and preceded BRCA1 and BRCA2 testing.

Claus and associates, using a previously fit autosomal-dominant genetic model, evaluated the Cancer and Steroid Hormone Study of 4730 breast cancer patients aged 20 to 54 years and 4688 control subjects to estimate the proportions of breast and ovarian cases in the general population that are likely to result from breast and ovarian cancer susceptibility genes. About 10% of patients with ovarian cancer in the general population were estimated to be carriers of a breast or ovarian cancer susceptibility gene; the proportion of ovarian cancer cases predicted to be a result of the susceptibility gene ranged from 14% among patients diagnosed in their 30s to 7% among those diagnosed in their 50s. The risk for ovarian cancer in carriers to the age of 60 years and 80 years was estimated to be about 10% and 27%, respectively. Carriers were predicted to have at least a 15-fold age-specific risk of ovarian cancer compared with noncarriers. Some ethnic groups appear to be at high risk for gene mutation, and the Ashkenazi Jews have been most extensively studied. In a large study by Struewing and associates, 5318 Jewish subjects had BRCA1 and BRCA2 evaluated, identifying only 120 carriers. Carriers had a significantly elevated risk, with an estimated risk of 2% by age 50 years and 16% by age 70 years, compared with the noncarrier risk of 0.4% by 50 years and 1.6% by 70 years. Metcalfe and colleagues performed BRCA testing for three founder mutations in 2080 self-identified Jewish women and found the BRCA mutation rate to be 1% (22 women) in an unselected population.

Frank and associates evaluated 283 women with breast cancer before age 50 or ovarian cancer at any age, and at least one first- or second-degree relative with either diagnosis, for BRCA1 followed by BRCA2 analysis. Mutations were identified in 94 women (39%) including 59 of 117 (50%) from families with ovarian cancer and 35 of 121 (29%) from families without ovarian cancer. In women with breast cancer, mutations in BRCA1 and BRCA2 were associated with a 10-fold increased risk of subsequent ovarian cancer. Mutations were noted in 24 of 38 women (63%) who had ovarian cancer. In women from breast–ovarian cancer families, 30 of the germline mutations occurred in BRCA2. Of note in this study, the authors did not find Ashkenazi ancestry significantly increased in the identification of BRCA1 or BRCA2 mutation, suggesting the importance of a strong family history.

In considering the woman at high risk, two questions should be addressed: (1) Who should be tested? and (2) Are there screening or prophylactic measures that can be applied to decrease the risk? A family history of breast or ovarian cancer, particularly before the age of 50 years in a first-order relative, and Ashkenazi Jewish ancestry, are risk factors for BRCA1 or BRCA2 mutations. Family history, both maternal and paternal, should be obtained (three generations is desired), and age at diagnosis should be noted. Pathology reports or death certificates verify accuracy of history; there can be considerable errors from history alone. Lifetime empirical risks can be determined from this information and may suggest that testing for a gene mutation is indicated. The extensive evaluation of family history and counseling should be done before genetic testing. Interpretation and plan of action that will influence medical management should be discussed in detail before genetic testing is performed. Testing of family members known to have cancer before testing of the cancer-free members is recommended. If a suspect mutation is found in the cancer member, the relatives without cancer can be tested for that specific mutation. If the cancer member does not have a mutation, other relatives probably will not benefit from testing. In one study, women sought DNA testing most commonly because of concern about the potential cancer risk to their children and secondly for their own cancer surveillance and prevention.

In a consensus statement of the Cancer Genetics Studies Consortium, annual or semiannual screening with transvaginal ultrasonography and determination of serum CA-125 levels beginning at age 25 to 35 years are recommended for BRCA1 mutation carriers. Both of these tests carry a relatively high false-positive and false-negative rate with low positive predictive value. Narod and associates found that oral contraceptives protected against ovarian cancer in patients with mutation in either the BRCA1 or BRCA2 gene. It has been suggested that prophylactic oophorectomy after fertility desires have been satisfied would be of benefit in protecting against ovarian cancer. The consensus statement concluded that there is insufficient evidence for or against prophylactic oophorectomy for it to be recommended as a measure to reduce ovarian cancer risk. A National Institutes of Health Consensus Conference recommended that women with two or more first-degree relatives with ovarian carcinoma be offered prophylactic oophorectomy after completion of childbearing or age 35 years. Prophylactic oophorectomy does not prevent subsequent primary peritoneal cancer, where failure rates of 2% to 11% after prophylactic oophorectomy have been reported. Schrag and associates found prophylactic oophorectomy to be associated with a small gain in life expectancy (0.3-1.7 years of life, depending on the cumulative risk of cancer). Rubin and associates identified 53 women with BRCA1 mutations. Compared with matched-control subjects, survival of patients with advanced disease was much better in women with the mutation (77 months vs 29 months; $P < 0.001$).

A recent population-based study of 232 patients with epithelial ovarian carcinomas suggested that previous studies may have underestimated the frequency of BRCA1 and BRCA2 mutations. Of 209 patients with invasive cancer, 32 patients (15%) had mutations of BRCA1 (20) or BRCA2 (12). Based on their data, Pal and colleagues suggested it may be reasonable to offer genetic counseling to any woman with an invasive, nonmucinous epithelial ovarian cancer.

The GOG has conducted a study (GOG#199) of 2605 women at increased risk for developing ovarian cancer, either by known BRCA mutation or family history risk factors. Patients were enrolled after choosing either prophylactic oophorectomy or screening, and both groups followed with CA-125 levels and Risk of Ovarian Cancer Algorithm (ROCA) assessment. The study was designed to evaluate both the prospective incidence of new and occult ovarian cancers and to assess the ROCA and quality of life. Enrollment closed in 2006 and the results are forthcoming.

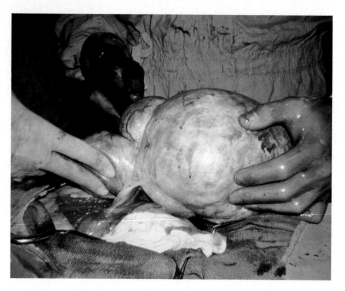

FIGURE 11-4 Large bilateral ovarian neoplasms: low-grade mucinous adenocarcinoma.

TABLE 11-6   Most Frequent Presenting Symptoms of Ovarian Cancer

Symptom	Relative Frequency
Abdominal swelling	XXXX
Abdominal pain	XXX
Dyspepsia	XX
Urinary frequency	XX
Weight change	X

SIGNS, SYMPTOMS, AND ATTEMPTS AT EARLY DETECTION (SCREENING)

Although the wide range of ovarian tumor types generally presents in a similar manner, the diagnosis of early ovarian cancer is often more a matter of chance than a triumph of the scientific method. As enlargement occurs (Figure 11-4), there is progressive compression of the surrounding pelvic structures, producing vague abdominal discomfort, dyspepsia, urinary frequency, and "pelvic pressure" (Table 11-6). The insidious onset of ovarian cancer needs no elaboration. As the neoplasm reaches a diameter of 15 cm, it begins to rise out of the pelvis and may account for abdominal enlargement. The notions that the development of ovarian cancer is "silent" and there are no early symptoms of ovarian cancer are a focus of the patient advocacy "listen for the whisper" educational efforts. Vague symptoms may be present for several months before the diagnosis. Such complaints are usually not recognized as anything more than "middle-age indigestion." A high index of suspicion is warranted in all women between the ages of 40 and 69 years who have persistent gastrointestinal symptoms

TABLE 11-7   Surgical Findings

	Benign	Malignant
Surface papilla	Rare	Very common
Intracystic papilla	Uncommon	Very common
Solid areas	Rare	Very common
Bilaterality	Rare	Common
Adhesions	Uncommon	Common
Ascites (100 mL)	Rare	Common
Necrosis	Rare	Common
Peritoneal implants	Rare	Common
Capsule intact	Common	Infrequent
Totally cystic	Common	Rare

TABLE 11-8   Nonmalignant Conditions That May Elevate CA-125 Concentrations

Gynecologic	Nongynecologic
Acute pelvic inflammatory disease	Active hepatitis
Adenomyosis	Acute pancreatitis
Benign ovarian neoplasm	Chronic liver disease
Endometriosis	Cirrhosis
Functional ovarian cyst	Colitis
Meigs' syndrome	Congestive heart failure
Menstruation	Diabetes (poorly controlled)
Ovarian hyperstimulation	Diverticulitis
Unexplained infertility	Mesothelioma
Uterine myoma	Nonmalignant ascites
	Pericarditis
	Pneumonia
	Polyarteritis nodosa
	Postoperative period
	Renal disease
	Rodent exposure (HAMA response)
	Systemic lupus erythematosus

HAMA, Human antimouse antibody.

that cannot be diagnosed. The majority of such nonspecific complaints are nonmalignant, causing the primary care physician to dismiss the possibility of ovarian cancer in many cases. Too frequently, it is only when the patient has gross abdominal enlargement marking the occurrence of ascites and extension of the neoplastic process to the abdominal cavity that appropriate diagnostic evaluation is undertaken.

Methods for early diagnosis have been investigated in limited studies using cul-de-sac aspiration for peritoneal cytologic assessment and frequent pelvic examinations. All these endeavors have failed to show a significant impact on early diagnosis of this disease. Most ovarian neoplasms grow quickly and painlessly. A persistent ovarian enlargement should be an indication to consider surgery, and the diagnosis rests with the pathologist. The size of the tumor does not indicate the severity of disease, and many of the largest neoplasms are histologically benign, most commonly mucinous cystadenoma. Moreover, many large adnexal masses may be of nonovarian etiology. Nonovarian causes of apparent adnexal masses are diverticulitis, tubo-ovarian abscess, carcinoma of the cecum or sigmoid, pelvic kidney, and uterine or intraligamentous myomas. At the time of surgery, it may be difficult to discern the malignant potential of a particular ovarian neoplasm (Table 11-7). There is sufficient overlap of morphologic criteria to cause confusion. The diagnosis rests with the histologic examination of the specimen, and the error rate of frozen section is about 5%.

Immunologic diagnosis of subclinical ovarian cancer by means of identification of specific tumor-associated antigens in the serum has yet to materialize. Several tumor-associated antigens, including CA-125, have been identified and purified. Recent research identifying patterns of protein fragments (proteomics) in patients with ovarian carcinoma requires validation in larger trials.

It has been suggested that every woman should have a periodic pelvic examination, pelvic ultrasound examination, and CA-125 test to make sure she does not harbor

an occult ovarian cancer. Enthusiasm for early detection of ovarian cancer is laudable. However, it has been calculated that 10,000 routine pelvic examinations would be required to detect one early ovarian cancer in a population of asymptomatic patients. For a low-incidence cancer such as ovarian cancer, cost-effective screening strategies require a positive predictive value (PPV) greater than 10%. This generally requires a technique specificity of greater than 99%, with a high sensitivity of greater than 75%. The majority of early trials of screening techniques did not meet this metric. Jacobs and colleagues studied 22,000 postmenopausal women screened with CA-125 determinations and have reported follow-up observed for a mean of 6.76 years; 767 women (3.5%) had elevated CA-125 values, of whom 49 (6%, or 0.0022% of the total screened) had cancer. One third of these were early stage. Overall specificity was 97%, whereas sensitivity at 1 year and 7 years of follow-up was 75% and 57%, respectively. The PPV of 3% was not high enough to be an effective screening method, and there is no current role for screening with CA-125 levels in unselected women. Many conditions of a benign nature, and most gastrointestinal tract malignant neoplasms, may elevate the CA-125 concentration (Table 11-8). The value of ultrasonography in screening for early ovarian carcinoma has received much attention. Campbell and coworkers reported early detection of five primary ovarian cancers in approximately 5000 women screened by abdominal ultrasonography (Table 11-9). DePriest and associates have reported the largest number of women screened with transvaginal sonography (TVS). All patients were postmenopausal unless a family history of ovarian cancer was present (24% of women). They

TABLE 11-9 Stage and Prevalence of Screen-Detected Primary Ovarian Cancer in 20 Prospective Screening

	Screened	Prevalence of Detected Primary Cancer	Screen-Detected Cancers per 100,000	Stage I
GENERAL POPULATION				
Ultrasound	15,834	8	51	6
Exclude LMP		6	38	4
Multimodal*	27,560	14	51	7
Exclude LMP		13	47	6
HIGH-RISK POPULATION				
Ultrasound[†]	4551	21	461	12
With family history	3146	15	477	9
Exclude LMP		8	254	2

From Bell R et al: Br J Obstet Gynaecol 105:1136, 1998.
*CA-125.
[†]With or without CA-125.
LMP, Low malignant potential.

have screened 6470 women with 14,829 scans; 90 women had persistent abnormalities on transvaginal ultrasonography and underwent surgery. Six primary ovarian cancers were found (five stage I and one stage IIIb), and only four were epithelial. Sensitivity was 86% and specificity was 99%, with a PPV of only 7% but with a negative predictive value (NPV) of 99.9%.

A strategy to improve the effectiveness of ovarian cancer screening would be to target populations at increased risk for the development of the disease, such as individuals with a positive family history of ovarian cancer. Bourne and colleagues reported the results of such a strategy in screening patients with transvaginal ultrasonography in combination with color flow Doppler imaging and morphologic assessment. In the screening of 1601 patients, 57% required repeated transvaginal ultrasonography to confirm the presence of a mass. Six ovarian cancers were diagnosed (two stage I, three low malignant potential tumors, and one stage III). Karlan and associates reported screening of 597 patients with a family history of cancer by CA-125 measurement, transvaginal ultrasonography, and color flow Doppler imaging. Initially, 115 patients had an abnormal finding on transvaginal ultrasonography, and 68 had an abnormal CA-125 level. After repeated transvaginal ultrasonography, because of abnormal findings of color flow Doppler imaging, 19 patients underwent surgery. At the time of the report, one low malignant potential tumor had been diagnosed.

Bell and colleagues reviewed 25 studies on screening for ovarian cancer, 16 studies on women at average risk, and 9 studies on women at higher risk. Many of the studies were small and imprecise on methodology; few gave follow-up details. Some studies used single screening techniques, whereas others used multimodal screening. For women at average risk, 75% of primary cancers were stage I when they were detected with ultrasonography and 50% were stage I when they were detected by multimodal screening (see Table 11-9). In women at higher risk, 60% of tumors detected by screening were stage I; but most important, if low malignant potential tumors were excluded, only 25% were stage I. False-negative rates were higher in the higher risk population than in the group at average risk. The false-negative data, when applied to a population with an annual incidence of 40 per 100,000, imply that 30 to 60 surgical procedures would be carried out for every cancer detected at annual gray-scale ultrasonography (assuming 100% sensitivity), and 2.5 to 15 surgical procedures would be carried out for every cancer detected by multimodal screening. Even if screening detects all ovarian cancers and these are treated with 100% success, the absolute reduction in mortality would be only 1 in about 2500 screened women per year. This is much smaller than the complication rate from unnecessary diagnostic surgery or recall for further tests.

Combining CA-125 levels with TVS has been explored as a means by which to improve predictive value. Skates and colleagues have developed a risk of ovarian cancer (ROC) algorithm based on rising CA-125 that has been validated in a prospective cohort. Although their initial validation PPV was high (19%), it has been incorporated into two large prospective trials to be combined with TVS for better risk prediction in postmenopausal women. These two trials, the United Kingdom Collaborative Trial of Ovarian Cancer Screening (UKCTOCS) and the UT MD Anderson Cancer Center Specialized Program of Research Excellence (SPORE), are ongoing. Prevalence screening from the UKCTOCS trial showed a PPV from the multimodality testing of 35%, with almost half of these cancers detected at stage I or II. Further assessment of the survival impact of these measures is ongoing.

Currently, however, there are no reliable data that screening for ovarian cancer is effective in improving length and quality of life in women with ovarian cancer. Another strategy to improve sensitivity and specificity in screening for ovarian cancer involves the use of multiple serum tumor markers. Because less than 50% of patients with stage I ovarian cancer will have an elevated CA-125 concentration and because CA-125 can be elevated by benign and malignant conditions, the addition of other markers in the screening strategy could potentially improve predictive value. Yurkovetsky and colleagues reported the results of their screening panel of four biomarkers, with 86% sensitivity at 98% specificity for detecting early-stage disease, and additional studies looking at additional biomarkers are ongoing. In addition, recent research in the area of proteomics has injected new hope into a more effective screening tool. These techniques may also offer useful guidelines for predicting therapeutic response and for treatment selection. The National Institutes of Health Consensus Development Conference on ovarian cancer screening in 1994 reached the following conclusions: There is no evidence available yet that the current screening modalities of CA-125 measurement and transvaginal ultrasonography can be used effectively for widespread screening to reduce mortality from ovarian cancer or that their use will result in decreased rather than increased morbidity and mortality. Routine screening has resulted in unnecessary surgery with associated risks. Clearly, it is important to identify and validate effective screening modalities. Currently available technology for screening should be used in the context of clinical trials to determine the efficacy of these modalities and their effect on ovarian cancer mortality. In addition, research must be continued to identify additional markers and imaging techniques that will be useful. Although these same recommendations still hold, we may have better techniques for screening as the data from ongoing trials mature. If a woman has one first-degree relative with ovarian cancer (making her lifetime risk of developing the disease 5%) but no clinical trials are available to her, she may feel that despite the absence of prospective data, this is sufficient risk for her to be screened. This opportunity for screening should be available to the woman and her physician.

If a woman were undergoing pelvic surgery, removal of the ovaries at that time would almost fully eliminate her risk of ovarian cancer (although there remains a small risk of peritoneal cancer). If the woman is premenopausal, discussion of estrogen replacement therapy is important before removal of the ovaries because for some younger women, if estrogen replacement is not used, the risk of premature menopause and the potential for osteoporosis may outweigh the risk of ovarian conservation and the potential for ovarian cancer.

DIAGNOSTIC TECHNIQUES AND STAGING

Routine pelvic examinations detect only 1 ovarian cancer in 10,000 asymptomatic women. However, pelvic examination remains the most practical means of detecting early disease. Pain is usually a late complication; it is seen with early disease only in association with a complication such as torsion; rupture; or, rarely, infection. The physician should have a high index of suspicion for an early ovarian neoplasm in any ovary palpated in a patient 3 years or longer after menopause. These patients should be considered for immediate laparoscopy or laparotomy when ultrasound examination findings suggest malignant change (e.g., complex mass, >5 cm, or intracystic papillations).

To help with evaluating a patient with a complex pelvic mass, the American College of Obstetricians and Gynecologists (ACOG), in conjunction with the Society of Gynecologic Oncologists (SGO), published guidelines in 2002 that could help direct referral to or consultation with a gynecologic oncologist. Physicians should perform a pelvic examination and imaging as appropriate for the patient's symptoms or physical examination findings. For premenopausal women with a suspicious pelvic mass, referral to a gynecologic oncologist should be considered by at least one of the following: CA-125 level higher than 200 U/mL, ascites, abdominal or distant metastases, or one or more first-degree relatives with breast or ovarian cancer. For postmenopausal women with a concerning pelvic mass, consultation should be considered for any CA-125 elevation, ascites, nodularity or limited mobility, evidence of metastasis, or a first-degree relative with breast or ovarian cancer.

Routine laboratory tests are not of great value in the diagnosis of ovarian tumors. The major value of laboratory tests is in ruling out other pelvic disorders. Pelvic ultrasound examination or abdominal radiography may reveal calcifications consistent with myomas or toothlike calcifications consistent with benign teratomas. Intravenous pyelography may be helpful in ruling out disease in adjacent pelvic structures. A barium enema study should be considered in a woman with lower intestinal symptoms. A similar comment can be made for colonoscopy and upper gastrointestinal endoscopy in patients who have lower or upper intestinal symptoms, respectively. Computed tomography (CT) with contrast enhancement may be helpful in identifying the extent of clinical disease; however, a clinical pelvic mass in a postmenopausal woman needs surgical evaluation irrespective of the CT scan findings. Surgical exploration is the ultimate test as to the nature of the disorder. Paracentesis for the purpose of obtaining a cell block and cytologic smear of the peritoneal fluid appears unnecessary and is not indicated. If one is dealing with a self-contained malignant cyst, such a procedure can result in spillage of malignant cells into the peritoneal cavity. Regardless of whether the fluid contains neoplastic cells, laparotomy is still necessary to remove the large benign neoplasm or to define the extent of the malignant process. In addition, up to 50% of ascitic fluid samples from patients with true ovarian malignant neoplasms will be negative for malignant cells on cell block analysis. Diagnostic paracentesis in a patient with ascites and a pelvic abdominal mass is therefore both unnecessary and potentially dangerous (Figure 11-5).

The staging of ovarian cancer is surgical (Table 11-10) and based on the surgical and pathologic findings (Figure 11-6). A longitudinal midline incision is recommended to

TABLE 11-10   Carcinoma of the Ovary: Staging Classification Using the FIGO Nomenclature

FIGO Stage	Description
I	Growth limited to the ovaries
Ia	Growth limited to one ovary; no ascites present containing malignant cells; no tumor on the external surfaces; capsule intact
Ib	Growth limited to both ovaries; no ascites present containing malignant cells; no tumor on the external surfaces; capsules intact
Ic*	Tumor stage Ia or stage Ib but with tumor on the surface of one or both ovaries; or with capsule ruptured; or with ascites present containing malignant cell; or with positive peritoneal washings
II	Growth involving one or both ovaries with pelvic extension
IIa	Extension and/or metastases to the uterus and/or tubes
IIb	Extension to other pelvic tissues
IIc*	Tumor stage IIa or stage IIb but with tumor on the surface of one or both ovaries; or with capsule(s) ruptured; or with ascites present containing malignant cell; or with positive peritoneal washings
III	Tumor involving one or both ovaries with peritoneal implants outside the pelvis and/or positive retroperitoneal or inguinal nodes; superficial liver metastasis equals stage III; tumor is limited to the true pelvis but with histologically verified malignant extension to small bowel or omentum
IIIa	Tumor grossly limited to the true pelvis with negative nodes with histologically confirmed microscopic seeding of abdominal peritoneal surfaces
IIIb	Tumor of one or both ovaries; histologically confirmed implants of abdominal peritoneal surfaces, none exceeding 2 cm in diameter; nodes negative
IIIc	Abdominal implants 2 cm in diameter and/or positive retroperitoneal or inguinal nodes
IV	Growth involving one or both ovaries with distant metastasis; if pleural effusion is present, there must be positive cytologic test results to allot a case to stage IV; parenchymal liver metastasis equals stage IV

From International Federation of Gynecology and Obstetrics: Am J Obstet Gynecol 156:263, 1987.
*To evaluate the impact on prognosis of the different criteria for allotting cases to stage Ic or stage IIc, it would be of value to know if rupture of the capsule was (1) spontaneous or (2) caused by the surgeon and if the source of the malignant cells detected was (1) peritoneal washings or (2) ascites.

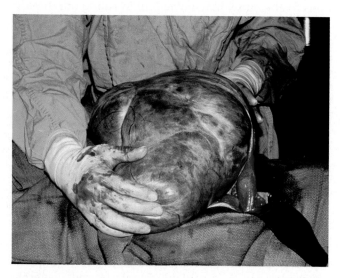

FIGURE 11-5   Large cystic tumors, similar to the illustration, are at risk of perforation and leakage at the time of paracentesis.

facilitate removal of the neoplasm and to permit adequate visualization of the entire abdominal cavity, including the undersurface of the diaphragm. A Pfannenstiel incision is ill-advised in a patient suspected of having an ovarian malignancy. Ovarian cancer is classically a serosal spreading disease (Figure 11-7); thus all peritoneal surfaces must be carefully inspected, especially when disease is thought to be limited to the pelvis. Although lymphatic spread to retroperitoneal nodes is common in ovarian cancer, the disease most often spreads intraperitoneally; free-floating cells shed from the primary tumor are capable of implanting on any peritoneal surface. Any peritoneal fluid (ascites) found when the peritoneal cavity is opened should be aspirated and submitted for cytologic examination. In the absence of peritoneal fluid, four washings should be taken by lavage of the peritoneal surfaces: the undersurface of the diaphragm as the first specimen (Figure 11-8), lateral to the ascending and descending colon as the second and third specimens, and the pelvic peritoneal surfaces as the fourth specimen. These specimens are obtained by lavaging these areas with 50 to 75 mL of saline solution and retrieving the fluid for cell block analysis. Care should be taken to visualize and palpate all peritoneal surfaces, particularly the underside of the diaphragm, the surface of the liver, the lateral abdominal gutters, and the small and large bowel mesentery. Fiberoptic light sources are particularly helpful in properly visualizing the peritoneal surfaces of the upper abdomen through a vertical lower abdominal incision. The omentum should be removed because microscopic disease is often present in the omentum that is not obvious grossly. Recommended surgical therapy is presented in sequence in Table 11-11. If the disease is limited to the pelvis, great care should be taken to avoid rupture of the neoplasm during its

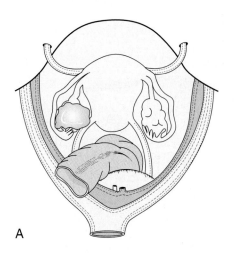

A

One ovary, capsule intact; no tumor on ovarian surface.

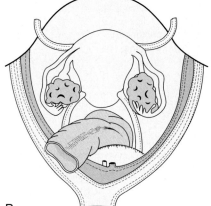

B

Both ovaries, capsule intact; no tumor on ovarian surface.

FIGURE 11-6 Ovarian epithelial carcinoma. **A,** Stage Ia. **B,** Stage Ib. Ovarian epithelial carcinoma. **C,** Stage Ic. **D,** Stage IIa. **E,** Stage IIb. Ovarian epithelial carcinoma.

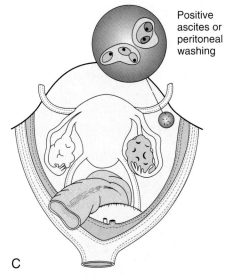

C

One or both ovaries with capsule ruptured or tumor on ovarian surface; malignant cells in ascites or peritoneal washings.

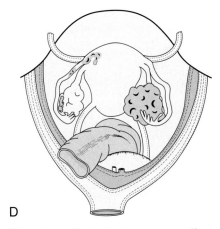

D

Extension and/or implants on uterus and/or tubes; adnexae.

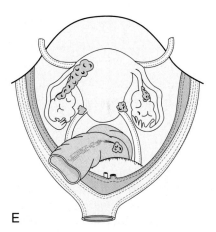

E

Extension and/or implants to other pelvic tissues; pelvic wall, broad ligament, adjacent peritoneum, mesovarium.

Continued

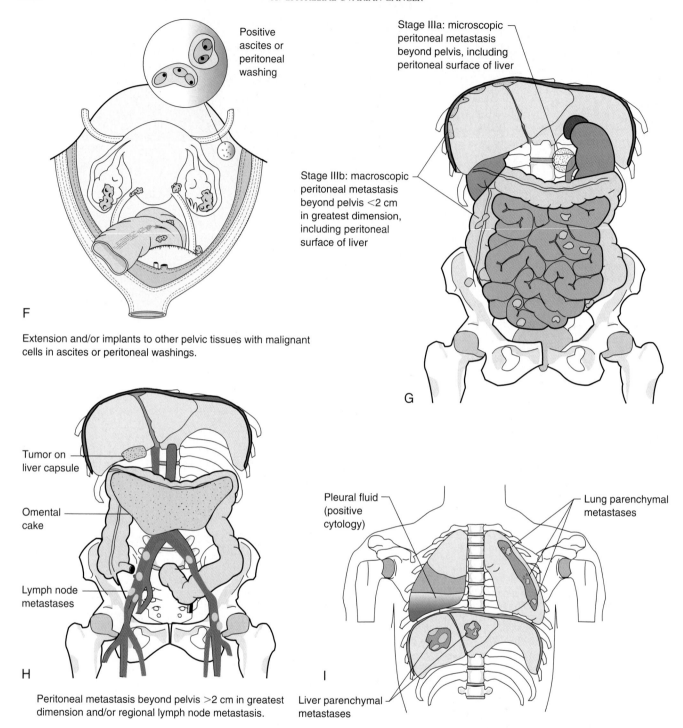

Positive ascites or peritoneal washing

Stage IIIa: microscopic peritoneal metastasis beyond pelvis, including peritoneal surface of liver

Stage IIIb: macroscopic peritoneal metastasis beyond pelvis <2 cm in greatest dimension, including peritoneal surface of liver

F

Extension and/or implants to other pelvic tissues with malignant cells in ascites or peritoneal washings.

G

Tumor on liver capsule

Omental cake

Lymph node metastases

H

Peritoneal metastasis beyond pelvis >2 cm in greatest dimension and/or regional lymph node metastasis.

Pleural fluid (positive cytology)

Lung parenchymal metastases

Liver parenchymal metastases

I

FIGURE 11-6, cont'd   **F,** Stage IIc. **G,** Stages IIIa and IIIb. **H,** Stage IIIc. **I,** Stage IV.

removal. All roughened or suspicious surfaces in the peritoneal cavity should be removed as biopsy specimens. This includes adhesions, which should be excised, not incised, because they often contain microscopic disease. Several studies are under way to investigate the efficacy of "blind" peritoneal biopsies and routine retroperitoneal node dissections in the proper staging of early epithelial cancer of the ovary (Table 11-12). Any abnormal-appearing surface is always regarded as suspicious, and biopsies are readily performed. Proper staging is important for treatment planning and for providing an accurate prognosis (Table 11-13).

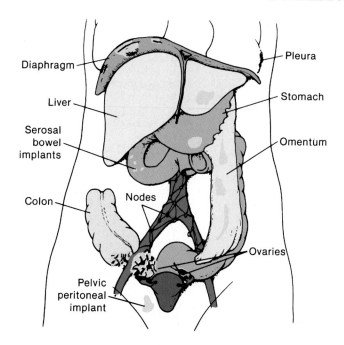

FIGURE 11-7 Spread pattern for epithelial cancer of the ovary. *(From DiSaia PJ: Hosp Pract [Off Ed] 22:235, 1987.)*

THERAPEUTIC OPTIONS FOR PRIMARY TREATMENT

Borderline Malignant Epithelial Neoplasms

Over the past four decades, investigators have described a subset of epithelial ovarian tumors whose histologic and biologic features lie between those of clearly benign and frankly malignant ovarian neoplasms. These borderline malignant neoplasms account for approximately 15% of all epithelial ovarian cancers. They have also been called proliferative cystadenomas and tumors of low malignant potential and are more completely discussed in Chapter 10. Compared with invasive epithelial ovarian cancer, epithelial borderline tumors affect

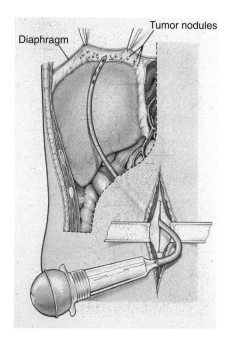

FIGURE 11-8 Technique of obtaining subdiaphragmatic cytologic washings at laparotomy. Saline lavage of the space between the diaphragm and the dome of the liver is easily accomplished; fluid pockets collecting in the lateral recesses are aspirated with a bulb syringe.

TABLE 11-11 Surgical Therapy in Ovarian Cancer

Peritoneal cytologic examination
Determination of extent of disease
    Pelvis
    Peritoneal surfaces
    Diaphragms
    Omentum
    Lymph nodes
Removal of all tumor possible (total abdominal hysterectomy and
    bilateral salpingo-oophorectomy) plus node sampling and
    omentectomy

TABLE 11-12 Aortic Lymph Node Metastases in Epithelial Ovarian Cancer

Series	Stage I		Stage II		Stages III–IV		
	Positive Lymphangiography	Positive Biopsy	Positive Lymphangiography	Positive Biopsy	Positive Lymphangiography	Positive Biopsy	Total
Hanks and Bagshaw (1969)	2/9	—	2/6	—	4/7	—	8/22
Parker et al (1974)	3/13	—	2/29	—	12/27	—	17/69
Knapp and Friedman (1974)	—	5/26	—	—	—	—	—
Delgado et al (1977)	1/5	—	1/5	—	—	3/5	2/10
Buchsbaum et al (1989)*	—	4/95	—	8/41	—	7/46	—
Burghardt (1991)	—	1/20	—	4/7	—	51/78	—
Total	10/141	12/48	61/129				

All patients had optimal carcinoma with metastatic lesions less than 3 cm.

FIGURE 11-9 Algorithm for the management of borderline epithelial ovarian neoplasms. *BSO*, bilateral salpingo-oophorectomy; *TAH*, Total abdominal hysterectomy.

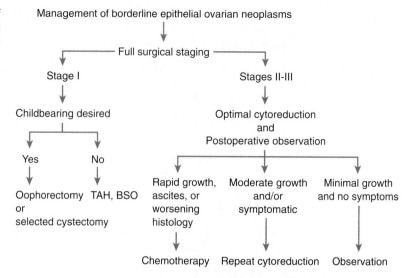

TABLE 11-13 Carcinoma of the Ovary, Obviously Malignant Cases, All Histopathologic Classes: 5-Year Actuarial Survival by Stage

Stage	No.	5-Year Survival (%)
Ia	632	89.6
Ib	69	86.1
Ic	663	83.4
IIa	72	70.7
IIb	93	65.5
IIc	241	71.4
IIIa	128	46.7
IIIb	271	41.5
IIIc	2030	32.5
IV	626	18.6

From Heintz APM, Odicino F, Maisonneuve P, et al: Int J Gynaecol Obstet. 2006 Nov;95 Suppl 1:S161–192.

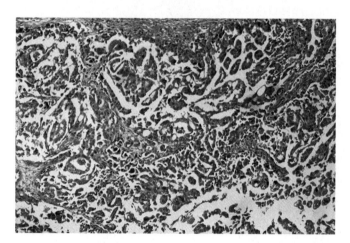

FIGURE 11-10 Papillary serous adenocarcinoma of ovary. Histologic appearance with prominent fibrous stalks and non–mucin-producing epithelial cells.

a younger population and may have a 10-year survival rate approaching 95% (see Chapter 10). Although symptomatic recurrence and death may rarely develop as late as 20 years after therapy, these neoplasms are correctly labeled as being of low malignant potential. Most gynecologic oncologists recommend conservative therapy, especially in patients who are desirous of further childbearing and have stage Ia disease (see Chapter 10). We have found surgical excision of disease the most effective therapy and when necessary have used repeated explorations, reserving chemotherapy for patients who develop ascites or whose tumor changes histologic features or demonstrates rapid growth (Figure 11-9).

Treatment of Malignant Epithelial Neoplasms

The most common epithelial cancers of the ovary are histologically categorized as serous, mucinous, endometrioid, and clear cell (mesonephroid) types (Figures 11-10 to 11-13). Most large studies demonstrate that these different histologic types have similar outcomes with existing therapy, stage for stage and grade for grade. Mucinous and endometrioid subtypes are more commonly found in earlier stages. There are ongoing studies to investigate targeted therapies in certain cell types, most notably mucinous and clear cell cancers. Based on our current data, however, prognosis, survival, and therapy for these various forms of epithelial cancer will be considered collectively.

The unifocal theory of ovarian epithelial cancer growth suggests that the disease initially grows locally, invading the capsule and mesovarium, and then invades adjacent organs by local extension and lymphatic spread. When the malignant neoplasm reaches the external surface of the capsule, cells exfoliate into the peritoneal cavity, where they circulate and implant on free peritoneal surfaces. Local and regional lymphatic metastasis

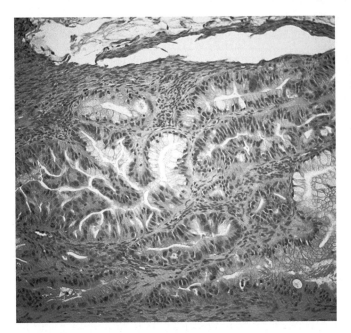

FIGURE 11-11 Mucinous adenocarcinoma of ovary. Microscopic appearance. Note tall, columnar, mucin-producing cells.

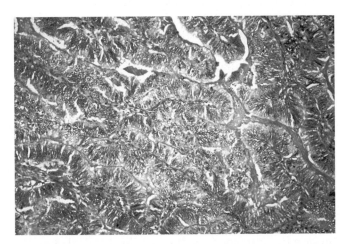

FIGURE 11-12 Endometrioid adenocarcinoma of ovary. Histologic appearance with columnar and pseudostratified epithelial cells showing prominent elongated hyperchromatic nuclei.

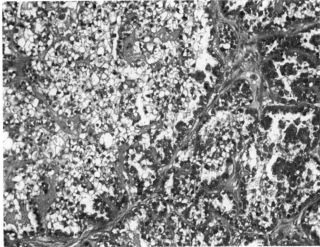

FIGURE 11-13 Clear cell adenocarcinoma of ovary. Microscopic view showing hobnail or peg cells.

TABLE 11-14 Guidelines for Staging in Epithelial Ovarian Cancer

Four peritoneal washings (diaphragm, right and left abdomen, pelvis)
Careful inspection and palpation of all peritoneal surfaces
Biopsy or smear from undersurface of right hemidiaphragm
Biopsy of all suspicious lesions
Infracolic omentectomy
Biopsy or resection of any adhesions
Random biopsy of normal peritoneum of bladder reflection cul-de-sac, right and left paracolic recesses, and both pelvic sidewalls (in the absence of obvious implants)
Selected lymphadenectomy of pelvic and para-aortic nodes
Total abdominal hysterectomy, bilateral salpingo-oophorectomy, and excision of masses when prudent

may involve the uterus, fallopian tubes, and pelvic lymph nodes. Spread to the aortic lymph nodes through lymphatics in the infundibulopelvic ligament is also common.

Woodruff suggested a multifocal mechanism of disease spread, whereby the entire coelomic epithelium can give rise to this lesion after exposure to carcinogenic agents that enter the peritoneal cavity from the vagina through the fallopian tubes. Indeed, the lesion could then originate in a multifocal distribution, "like a measles rash," over large portions of the coelomic epithelium.

Although the early precursors leading to advanced ovarian cancer are incompletely understood, more current molecular evidence favors the unifocal origin theory.

Regardless of origin, the most important prognostic variable for each patient is the extent, or "stage," of disease. A staging system has been devised that allows treatment results in patients with similar prognostic factors to be compared between different institutions. Survival is affected by the cancer stage, the grade of differentiation, the gross findings at surgery (Table 11-14), the amount of residual tumor after surgery, and the additional treatment required.

Stages Ia, Ib, and Ic

Careful surgical staging is critical in the management of stage I invasive ovarian cancer and should include bilateral salpingo-oophorectomy, hysterectomy, omentectomy, and pelvic and aortic lymph node sampling, with

TABLE 11-15   Lymph Node Metastasis in Stage I Ovarian Cancer

Author	Patients
Di Re	16/128
Benedetti–Panici	5/25
Wu	1/7
Burghardt	9/37
Petru	9/40
Knapp and Friedman	5/26
Tsuruchi	1/51
Chen	3/11
Lanza	3/11
Carnino	2/47
Baiocchi	32/242
	86/625 (13.7%)

TABLE 11-16   Frequency of Subclinical Metastasis in Patients with Presumed Early-Stage Ovarian Cancer (Based on 14 Studies)

Localization	Frequency (%)	Range (%)
Peritoneal cytology	22	10-46
Diaphragm	9	0-44
Omentum	5	0.7
Pelvic nodes	8	0-20
Para-aortic nodes	12	0-25
Pelvic peritoneum	9	6-10
Abdominal peritoneum	8	7-9
Bowel mesentery-serosa	6	3-13

peritoneal biopsies and washings. Accurate staging forms the cornerstone of clinical decision-making regarding the type and duration of adjuvant therapy.

Pelvic and aortic lymph nodes may be involved 10% to 20% of the time in apparent stage I disease, and lymphadenectomy is an important diagnostic and therapeutic procedure. Burghardt and colleagues reported on a series of ovarian cancer patients with all sizes of primary tumors who underwent complete pelvic and aortic lymphadenectomies, and the pelvic nodes were frequently positive (15% for stage I, 57% for stage II, and 64% for stage III). Baiocchi and associates reviewed their experience in 242 women who had pelvic and aortic lymphadenectomy in whom cancer was apparently confined to the ovaries (stage I), and nodal metastasis was found in 32 patients (13%). Patients with serous adenocarcinoma had the highest incidence of node metastasis (25%). Those with grade III lesions had 39% metastasis compared with 6% with grade I and grade II cancers. There were 33 women with low malignant potential tumors, and 7 (21%) had nodal metastasis. When only one to three nodes were involved, metastases were usually ipsilateral, but these patients could also have metastases to the common iliac or aortic nodes. Positive aortic nodes were also found in the absence of positive pelvic nodes. Accumulated reports of lymph node metastases in clinical stage I ovarian cancer patients are shown in Table 11-15. Without thorough surgical staging, occult metastasis may be present and missed, leading to inadequate subsequent therapy. Many studies have addressed this item (Table 11-16).

The use of adjuvant therapy and its role in stage I ovarian cancer continues to be investigated. The evolution toward platinum-based chemotherapy in these early-stage patients was demonstrated in three studies by the GOG. The first study by the GOG and the Ovarian Cancer Study Group reported on patients with stage Ia and stage Ib grade I or grade II disease who were randomly assigned to receive oral melphalan for 12 cycles or no further therapy. The 5-year survival in both arms of the study was excellent (>90%) and did not justify the additional toxicity and risks associated with melphalan in this patient population. Another GOG–Ovarian Cancer Study Group trial included high-risk, early-stage patients who had stage Ia and Ib grade III disease and stage Ic and II all grades with no macroscopic residual. These patients were randomly assigned to receive melphalan or intraperitoneal colloidal 32P. Survival and disease-free survival were similar in both arms of the study (approximately 80%), and the frequency of severe side effects was low in both arms. In follow-up, the GOG studied the same high-risk, early-stage population and compared combination chemotherapy (cyclophosphamide plus cisplatin) to intraperitoneal 32P (GOG #95). Survival was slightly better in the combination chemotherapy arm, and although not statistically significant, the lower rate of complications and side effects in the chemotherapy arm led to the conclusion that platinum-based chemotherapy was preferred.

European investigators have also reported their experience with platinum-based therapy in early-stage ovarian cancer. The European gynecologic groups reported a combined analysis of the ICON 1 and the ACTION trials. More than 900 patients with early-stage ovarian cancer received either platinum-based adjuvant chemotherapy or observation until chemotherapy was indicated. After a median follow-up of more than 4 years, the improved overall survival (82% chemotherapy vs 74% observation) and recurrence-free survival (76% vs 65%, respectively) at 5 years favored treatment with platinum-based therapy. Although not all patients had undergone comprehensive staging, a subgroup analysis of these patients was reported. In another European Organization for Research and Treatment of Cancer (EORTC)-ACTION trial of 448 patients, they noted that the benefit of chemotherapy was limited to patients who lacked comprehensive surgical staging, questioning the necessity of adjuvant therapy in the patient with well-staged early ovarian carcinoma.

The next evolution of GOG trials involved the addition of paclitaxel to a platinum-based regimen because the treatment protocols for advanced-stage disease had demonstrated improved survival by replacing cyclophosphamide with paclitaxel. GOG #157 evaluated carboplatin (AUC 7.5) and paclitaxel (175 mg/m^2) in high-risk, early-stage disease, randomly assigning patients to three vs six chemotherapy cycles. Over a 3-year interval, 457 patients were enrolled and evaluated after a median follow-up of 6.8 years. Although the recurrence rate was 24% lower with the six cycles ($P = 0.18$), overall survival was similar for the two arms (hazard ratio [HR] 1.02). The study concluded that the additional three cycles contributed to increased toxicity (11% grade III/IV neurotoxicity versus 2% with only three cycles) without an overall survival advantage. Building on the hypothesis that low-dose paclitaxel may have anti-angiogenesis activity, GOG #175 tested whether the addition of 24 weekly paclitaxel treatments (60 mg/m^2) to the initial three cycles of carboplatin and paclitaxel would improve outcomes. The results of the trial have been reported, and although the recurrence rate was 20% lower in patients receiving extended paclitaxel, the result was not statistically significant and there was no appreciable difference in overall survival.

In the young woman with stage Ia disease who is desirous of further childbearing, unilateral salpingo-oophorectomy may be associated with minimal increased risk of recurrence, provided a careful staging procedure is performed and due consideration is given to grade and apparent self-containment of the neoplasm. After conservative treatment for invasive ovarian cancer, term delivery rates have been reported as high as 30%, and successful pregnancy outcomes have been reported after adjuvant chemotherapy. Conservative surgery is generally not recommended for patients with clear cell or carcinosarcoma or grade III tumors and when disease is present outside the ovaries. A careful discussion regarding the risks and benefits of this approach is essential because Maltaris and colleagues reported that 12% of patients undergoing fertility-sparing ovarian cancer surgery experienced recurrence and 4% of patients died from their disease.

In the management of stage I ovarian cancer the physician must weigh the possible benefits of adjuvant chemotherapy against the risks. It appears reasonable to not recommend adjuvant therapy for patients with stage Ia, Ib, grade I and II lesions who have been comprehensively staged. Patients with stage I, grade III and stage Ic disease present a more difficult problem because the incidence of recurrence in this group approaches 50% in some series. We favor treatment with platinum-based combination chemotherapy despite the fact that no clear data show a survival advantage over single-agent therapy. Because combination therapy is our best

TABLE 11-17   Relationship of Residual Tumor Size and Median Survival (Months)

Author	No. of Patients	Optimal (<2 cm)	Suboptimal (>2 cm)
Griffiths et al	102	28	11
Wharton et al	104	27	15
Hacker et al	47	22	6
Sutton et al	56	39	22

treatment for metastatic disease, it is difficult to withhold the apparent best therapy from a group of patients who may have the best situation for a chemotherapy "cure." In addition, this group is usually younger and better able to tolerate combination chemotherapy.

Stages IIa, IIb, and IIc

In most institutions, the therapy of choice for stage IIa and stage IIb disease is staging surgery followed by platinum-based combination chemotherapy. Although historically the role of pelvic and abdominal irradiation and intraperitoneal 32P has been described, the radioisotope and irradiation treatment approaches have all but faded from frontline therapy for ovarian carcinoma. Careful surgical staging is essential to successful treatment planning. A combined analysis of GOG #95 and #157 revealed that the stage II patients represented a disproportionate percentage of the recurrences. The GOG now includes stage II patients in their clinical trials of patients with advanced-stage disease. Outside of a clinical trial patients with stage II disease should be managed in a similar fashion to optimally debulked stage III disease.

Stage III

In stage III, as in other stages, every effort should be made to remove the uterus with both adnexa. In addition, every reasonable effort should be made to remove all visible ovarian tumors. Retrospective studies have strongly suggested that the survival rate in patients with stage III disease is related to the amount of residual tumor after surgery, such that patients with no macroscopic residual tumor appear to have the best prognosis after primary chemotherapy (Table 11-17 and Figure 11-14). Most centers prefer combination platinum-based chemotherapy, usually carboplatin and paclitaxel, for this group of patients because of the excellent response rates reported in the literature (see later section on combination chemotherapy and intraperitoneal therapy).

The duration of multiple-agent therapy is usually six cycles. If after primary chemotherapy the patient has no clinical evidence of disease (clinical complete response), a second-look procedure was often considered in the past to ascertain the presence of subclinical residual

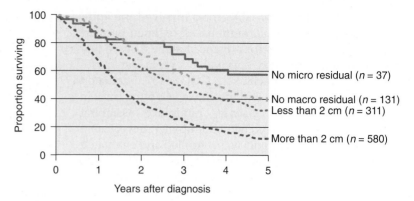

FIGURE 11-14   Survival in patients with stage IIIc disease by completeness of surgery (*n* = 1059). (*Modified from Annual Report on the Results of Treatment in Gynecological Cancer, Vol 23. Stockholm, International Federation of Gynecology and Obstetrics, 1998.*)

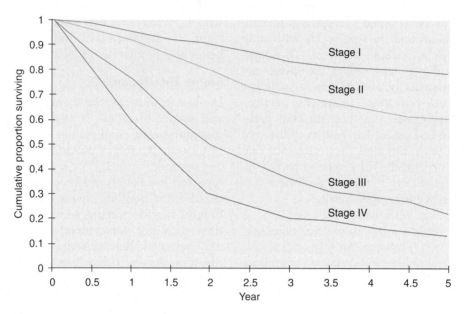

FIGURE 11-15   Obviously malignant cases of ovarian carcinoma. Cumulative proportion surviving by stage. (*From Annual Report on the Results of Treatment in Gynecological Cancer, Vol 22. Stockholm, International Federation of Gynecology and Obstetrics, 1994.*)

disease. However, a secondary exploratory data analysis on a GOG study (#158) suggested no apparent outcome advantage resulted from second-look surgery. For the most part second-look surgery is no longer recommended.

Stage IV

The ideal management of stage IV disease is to remove as much cancer as possible and to administer chemotherapy after surgery. The role and benefit of surgical cytoreduction in these patients is detailed in the next section. The overall survival is worse for this group of patients than for those of other stages, as expected (Figure 11-15).

Maximal Surgical Effort

The goal of primary surgery for advanced ovarian cancer should be to remove all visible tumor and to use all reasonable surgical means to do so (Figure 11-16). In the

1970s Griffiths and coworkers evaluated the importance of postsurgical tumor residual by using a multiple linear regression equation with survival as the dependent variable to control simultaneously for the multiple therapeutic and biologic factors that contribute to the ultimate outcome in the individual patient. The most important factors proved to be histologic grade of the tumor and size of the largest residual mass after primary surgery. The operation itself contributed nothing to survival unless it effected reduction in the size of the largest residual tumor mass below the limit of 1.6 cm.

Cytoreductive or "debulking" procedures have gained considerable attention in the management of ovarian cancer. The concept is to reduce the residual tumor burden to a level that subsequent chemotherapy can be most effective. A careful and persistent surgeon can often remove large tumor masses that on first impression appear to be unresectable. Using the clear retroperitoneal spaces, one can usually identify the infundibulopelvic ligament and ureter and then isolate

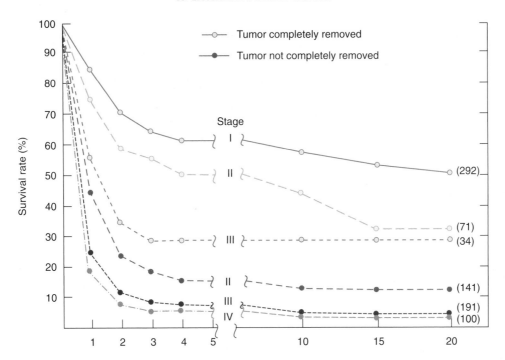

FIGURE 11-16 Survival rates stage for stage in patients in whom all tumor was surgically removed versus patients in whom not all tumor was completely removed. *(From Aure JC, Hoeg K, Kolstad P: Clinical and histologic studies of ovarian carcinoma. Long-term follow-up of 990 cases. Obstet Gynecol 37:1, 1971.)*

the vessels of the infundibulopelvic ligament and the blood supply of the ovary. Once these vessels have been ligated and transected, retrograde removal of large ovarian masses is more easily performed. The ureter is protected throughout the dissection so that the probability of traumatizing this pelvic structure is minimized. A clear space usually exists on the transverse colon whereby large omental "cakes" of ovarian carcinoma can be removed after the right and left gastroepiploic vessels have been ligated (Figure 11-17). Removal of large ovarian masses and omental involvement may reduce the tumor burden by 80% to 99%. The theoretical value of debulking procedures lies in reducing the number of tumor cells and the advantage this affords to adjuvant therapy. This is especially relevant in bulky chemosensitive solid tumors such as ovarian cancer, in which removal of large numbers of cells in the resting phase (G0) may propel the residual cells into the more vulnerable proliferating pool. Several careful retrospective studies have repeatedly demonstrated improved survival rate in patients who can be surgically brought to a status of minimal tumor burden. The GOG has attempted to better define primary cytoreductive surgery with a detailed analysis of the results of surgery in patients with advanced disease. Their initial study compared survival of the patients with stage III disease who were found at surgery to have abdominal disease of 1 cm or less with that of patients found to have disease greater than 1 cm but whose tumors were surgically

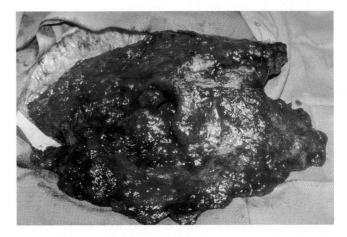

FIGURE 11-17 This photograph demonstrates a large omental cake of ovarian cancer exceeding 25 cm in greatest measurement.

cytoreduced to 1 cm or less. If surgery was the only important factor, survival should have been equivalent in both groups. This was not the case. Patients found to have small-volume disease survived longer than did patients who had cytoreduction to small-volume disease at surgery, suggesting that the tumor biology also carries prognostic significance. In a second study, GOG investigators evaluated the effect of the diameter of the largest residual disease on survival in patients with suboptimal cytoreduction. They demonstrated that cytoreduction so that the largest residual mass was 2 cm or less resulted

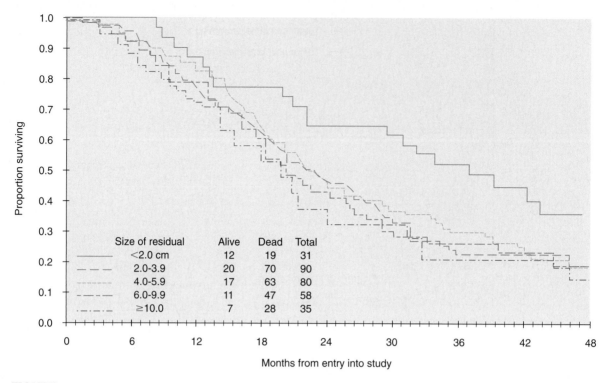

FIGURE 11-18   Survival by maximal diameter of residual disease. *(From Hoskins WJ et al: Am J Obstet Gynecol 170:974, 1994.)*

in a significant survival benefit, but all residual diameters greater than 2 cm had equivalent survival (Figure 11-18). Therefore, unless the mass can be cytoreduced to 2 cm or less, residual diameter did not influence survival. In evaluating optimal and suboptimal cytoreduction, these GOG investigators showed that three distinct groups emerged: microscopic (no visible) residual, residual disease of less than 2 cm, and residual disease of greater than 2 cm (Figure 11-19). It is clear from these studies that patients with microscopic disease had a 4-year survival of about 60%, whereas patients with gross disease 2 cm or less had a 4-year survival of 35%. However, patients whose disease could not be cytoreduced to 2 cm or less had a 4-year survival of less than 20%. Most striking, however, was the failure of cytoreductive surgery to improve survival unless the largest diameter of residual disease was 2 cm or less.

An inverse correlation between the amount of residual disease after surgery and overall survival has been consistently associated. In 2002, Bristow and associates published a meta-analysis of published studies at the time, in which the impact of cytoreduction was clearly demonstrated. By comparing currently available studies of advanced ovarian cancer patients undergoing surgical cytoreduction, they demonstrated that for each 10% increase in the proportion of patients undergoing optimal cytoreduction, median survival increased by 5.5% to 6%. Although the current accepted definition of "optimal

cytoreduction" is no visible residual tumor less than 1 cm in greatest dimension, the best reported outcomes occur in patients who have complete cytoreduction or no visible residual disease.

In an effort to remove visible tumor deposits and achieve optimal cytoreduction, gynecologic oncologists frequently perform radical surgical procedures beyond those required for standard staging. Eisenkop and associates described 163 consecutive patients assigned to stage IIIc and stage IV. Complete cytoreduction could be performed in 86% of patients using an array of radical procedures. Overall median survival was 54 months, but it was 62 months in those whose tumor was optimally debulked. Aletti and colleagues reported that for patients cytoreduced to low-volume residual disease, their favorable survival was directly associated with the need for radical surgery. Two sites that often require radical operations to clear are tumor metastases to the bowel and to the upper abdomen. Multiple investigators have reported the utility and safety of large and/or small bowel resection, which may be necessary in up to 50% of cases to achieve optimal cytoreduction and has been associated with a subsequent improvement in survival. Upper abdominal cytoreduction has also been shown to be safe and effective but may require additional training or assistance. Cliby and colleagues reported procedures such as liver resection, splenectomy, and diaphragm resection to be possible and associated with an

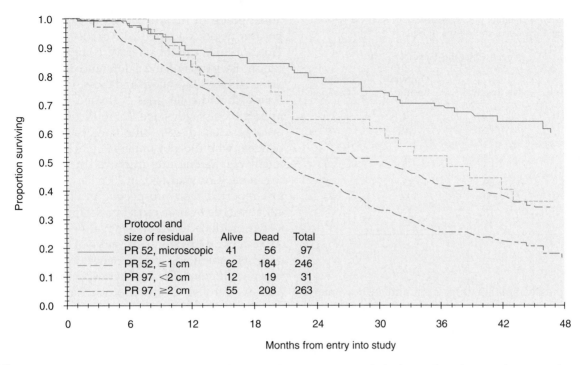

FIGURE 11-19 Survival by residual disease, Gynecologic Oncology Group protocols (PR) 52 and 97. *(From Hoskins WJ et al: Am J Obstet Gynecol 170:974, 1994.)*

acceptable morbidity. Investigators from Memorial Sloan-Kettering Cancer Center demonstrated that the addition of upper abdominal procedures to achieve optimal cytoreduction resulted in a median survival greater than 5 years, which was comparable to that of patients who did not require these extensive procedures for optimal cytoreduction. Improvements in surgical cytoreduction have developed in consort with additional advances in intensive care and postoperative care, allowing additional benefits for our ovarian cancer patients.

The role of cytoreductive surgery in stage IV cancers has been investigated. Several studies have suggested that optimal debulking can be performed in many of these patients with beneficial effect. Liu and associates described 47 patients with stage IV cancers, of which 14 (30%) were optimally debulked to less than 2 cm residual. Median survival was 37 months in the patients in whom the cancer was optimally debulked compared with 17 months in the patients in whom the cancer was suboptimally debulked. A study from Memorial Sloan-Kettering identified 92 patients; optimal debulking was achieved in 45% with a median survival of 40 months compared with 18 months for suboptimal debulking. A recent ancillary study by the GOG demonstrated that the ability to achieve cytoreduction to less than 5 cm residual disease in stage IV patients rendered some survival advantage, although the most favorable subgroup was those patients reduced to no visible residual disease.

Aletti and colleagues also demonstrated that using radical procedures to perform cytoreduction to no visible residual disease resulted in median survival more than 3 years in stage IV patients. For patients known or suspected to have thoracic metastases, the use of video-assisted thoracic surgery (VATS) can be diagnostic and/or potentially therapeutic. Positive findings on VATS may allow for intrathoracic cytoreduction in select cases or may indicate which patients are best served with neoadjuvant chemotherapy as a result of unresectable pleural disease.

The effect of maximal cytoreductive surgery can be seen in the percentage of negative second-look procedures (Table 11-18). Even though cytoreductive surgery seems to have therapeutic value, controversy continues. The primary unresolved issue is whether the poor prognosis with bulky disease is caused by the presence of increased tumor burden (in which case cytoreductive surgery is of potential benefit) or whether it is associated with differences in tumor biology or a decreased sensitivity to chemotherapeutic regimens (if these possibilities are indeed the case, cytoreductive surgery is not likely to have a major impact on survival). The implication is thus that those patients who have disease that can be cytoreduced are a select group with good prognoses on the basis of factors independent of the cytoreductive surgery. It is not clear how many patients with bulky disease can actually successfully undergo cytoreduction

TABLE 11-18 The Effect of Cytoreductive Surgery on Residual Disease as Found By Second-Assessment Surgery

Author (Year)	Negative Second Look (%)		
	No Residual	Optimal Residual	Suboptimal Residual
Barnhill (1984)	67	61	14
Cain (1986)	76	50	28
Smirz (1985)	75	—	25
Webb (1982)	95	36	20
Podratz (1983)	82	44	33
Curry (1981)	79	45	22
Dauplat (1983)	100	100	40
Hoskins (1989)	75	45	25
Mean	81	52	23

of tumor masses smaller than 2 cm and in how many patients such aggressive surgery is medically contraindicated. Furthermore, if chemotherapy is delayed because of complications of surgery, this may have a deleterious effect on long-term survival. Finally, the most appropriate time for cytoreductive surgery has not been determined: before any chemotherapy, after one to three cycles of induction chemotherapy, or after completion of a full 6- to 12-month induction course of chemotherapy. The percentage of patients with advanced ovarian cancer who can effectively undergo cytoreductive surgery seems to range from 43% to 87%, depending on the investigators reporting. This difference may reflect not only the individual skills of the surgeons, but also is influenced by different referral patterns and other selection factors. Neoadjuvant chemotherapy has been investigated as a means by which to address this issue, and these studies are described in the subsequent section.

The role of lymphadenectomy in patients with advanced disease continues to be debated. Lymph node involvement is common in patients with advanced disease (>50%); the question is whether lymphadenectomy improves survival. Burghardt was one of the first to suggest a therapeutic benefit. His data suggested that patients with advanced disease who had involved lymph nodes removed had improved survival compared to similar patients who did not have lymph nodes evaluated. It has been suggested by some that metastases in lymph nodes do not respond to chemotherapy and intraperitoneal metastasis and therefore these potential metastatic sites should be removed. Opponents state that recurrence most frequently occurs in the peritoneal cavity, and therefore lymph node status has little impact on the overall disease course. Several studies have come to somewhat different conclusions. Parazzini and associates evaluated 456 women with stage III-IV disease entered in a prospective randomized chemotherapy trial. There were 161 patients with positive nodes. They noted grade III tumors to have a greater number with positive nodes compared with grade I or grade II tumors. This was also true of stage IV compared with stage III cancer. They did not find a difference in survival between those with positive nodes and those with negative nodes. Scarabelli and colleagues evaluated lymph node status in 98 patients with stage IIIc to IV disease who had no gross residual disease after surgery compared with 44 patients who did not undergo lymphadenectomy. Survival was significantly improved if lymphadenectomy was done (Cox analysis). In 2005 Panici and coinvestigators reported their prospective multicenter analysis of 427 advanced ovarian cancer patients randomly assigned to lymphadenectomy or removal of bulky nodes only. Although progression-free survival was improved in patients undergoing lymphadenectomy, overall survival was not different. The 2005 retrospective analysis of 889 patients enrolled in the Scottish Randomised Trial in Ovarian Cancer (SCOTROC-1) was conducted. The analysis demonstrated that optimal debulking (<2 cm) was more commonly achieved in patients accrued from the United States, Europe, and Australia than in patients recruited from the United Kingdom (71% vs 58%). Comparison of the UK and non-UK patients who had no visible residual disease demonstrated a better survival for the non-UK patients, and the authors attributed this to the fact that non-UK patients more commonly underwent primary lymphadenectomy, suggesting a potential therapeutic benefit. It has been our practice to do pelvic and aortic lymphadenectomy routinely if the patient's tumor can be optimally debulked. Benefits of lymphadenectomy in patients with bulky residual disease remain questionable. It currently seems appropriate that patients with a diagnosis of advanced ovarian cancer should undergo resection of all masses when technically feasible.

Because a suboptimal surgical effort confers no survival benefit and adds only postoperative morbidity, accurate methods to determine which patients could be successfully resected would be useful. Both preoperative imaging and initial laparoscopy have been investigated as methods to determine the likelihood of success. Most imaging series have used preoperative CT scan to assess factors that could predict an optimal cytoreduction. Although sets of radiographic risk factors have been described, these have had poor predictive value because the majority of patients (62%-86%) identified as having "poor prognostic indicators" have been able to undergo optimal cytoreduction. Similarly, laparoscopy in advanced ovarian cancer has limitations in terms of how complete an assessment of the intraperitoneal space is possible, and metastases at port sites have been reported. Cancer recurrence at the site of an open surgical incision is well known but actually is rare even when there is considerable intra-abdominal tumor. Wang and associates reviewed the literature to determine risk factors that may contribute to early recurrence at the port site. Of the gynecologic cancers, ovarian cancer was the most common malignant neoplasm with subsequent port site metastasis. This occurred in patients with and without ascites, in patients with gross tumor within the abdominal cavity, in patients who had undergone diagnostic or palliative procedures, and in early-stage disease. Metastasis to the port site was more common if ascites and intraperitoneal carcinomatosis were present. The earliest time from laparoscopy to port site metastasis was 8 days. Several theories about the mechanism of port site metastasis have been proposed. These include implantation of cancer cells traumatically disseminated at the time of surgical removal of the primary tumor; direct implantation by the instruments; and creation of a pressure gradient by the pneumoperitoneum, with the outflow of gas floating the tumor cells through the port sites. Although laparoscopy has been used successfully in the management of benign adnexal masses, we prefer the open laparotomy approach if ovarian cancer is expected. The European Organization for Research and Treatment of Cancer (EORTC) group reported their experience with interval debulking surgery in patients with advanced ovarian carcinoma. Patients received three courses of cisplatin and cyclophosphamide and were then randomly assigned to receive interval debulking surgery or no further surgery. All patients received six courses of chemotherapy. There were 278 patients evaluated, and median survival was 26% versus 20% (surgery vs no surgery, $P = 0.012$). Debulking surgery was an independent prognostic factor in multivariate analysis. After adjustment for all prognostic factors, surgery reduced the risk of death by 33% ($P = 0.008$).

The GOG conducted a similar study. This study (GOG #152) enrolled 550 patients, all of whom had initial primary surgery by a gynecologic oncologist. Patients who were suboptimally debulked (residual tumor >1 cm) received three cycles of paclitaxel plus cisplatin. Patients were randomized to continued chemotherapy or to a secondary surgical cytoreduction and then continued chemotherapy. Neither the progression-free survival nor the relative risk of death was improved with the additional interval surgery. The authors speculate that the patients in the GOG study may also have undergone more aggressive primary surgery than the patients on the EORTC study, and this may have accounted for the difference in results. Most important, one could summarize these two studies by concluding that patients with advanced ovarian cancer are deserving of at least one maximal effort at cytoreduction, preferably by a gynecologic oncologist.

Although a maximal primary surgical effort appears to be a cornerstone of potential long-term survival, the timing of the surgical effort remains a focus of debate.

In patients with borderline performance status, based upon age, compromising medical disease, and extensive effusions (especially pleural or pericardial), and in patients with extensive abdominal disease, unlikely to be effectively debulked, strong consideration should be given to initiating therapy with neoadjuvant chemotherapy. Following two to four cycles, a good clinical response to chemotherapy may provide an opportunity for an effective surgical debulking with an acceptably low complication rate. Prior to initiating chemotherapy, the diagnosis of ovarian, tubal, or peritoneal cancer should be confirmed by cytology or minimally invasive surgery. Neoadjuvant chemotherapy treatment (followed by surgical debulking) results have been reported in small retrospective reports of between 20 and 90 patients and generally report survival outcomes similar to those of patients who have been suboptimally cytoreduced. A meta-analysis of these studies by Bristow and Chi demonstrated that the use of neoadjuvant chemotherapy was associated with a reduction in survival of approximately 4 months with every preoperative cycle, implying that surgical intervention should be performed as soon as is feasible. However, the preliminary results of a large randomized European trial of patients with advanced ovarian cancer treated with primary surgery followed by chemotherapy versus neoadjuvant chemotherapy for three cycles followed by surgical cytoreduction and three additional cycles of chemotherapy recently demonstrated comparable progression-free and overall survival. Additionally, the results favored the group receiving neoadjuvant chemotherapy because they experienced lower morbidity compared with the primary surgery group. Further analysis of the results of this trial may provide more detailed information regarding candidate selection and outcomes for neoadjuvant chemotherapy. Regardless of approach, patients with advanced ovarian cancer should be assessed by an experienced gynecologic oncologist to determine the best treatment course for each patient. Other areas of investigation include using imaging such as sequential F-18-fluorodeoxyglucose position emission tomography (FDG-PET) to predict response to neoadjuvant chemotherapy. Avril and colleagues found the median overall survival was 38.3 months in metabolic responders (to FDG-PET) compared with 23.1 months in nonresponders, and the 2-year survival was 73% and 46%, respectively.

As discussed previously and later in this chapter, second-look laparotomy is being used less frequently unless a patient is enrolled in a protocol that requires it. Most would agree that it has no or little impact on survival, although status of disease at a certain point in time can be ascertained. Some advocates of second-look laparotomy have suggested that secondary debulking could be beneficial and improve survival. Although there may be a benefit if debulking can be done to microscopic

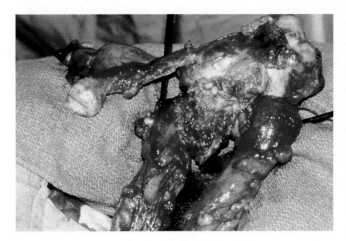

FIGURE 11-20   In situ surgical specimen demonstrating a large left ovarian neoplasm infiltrating a portion of sigmoid colon.

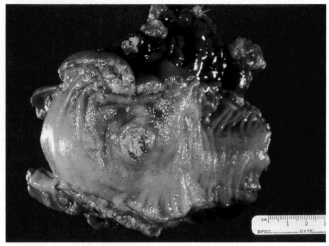

FIGURE 11-21   Portion of colon demonstrating transmural ovarian tumor infiltration.

disease only, it appears from a review of the literature that this can be accomplished in less than 10% of patients clinically free of disease and undergoing second-look laparotomy.

Patients who undergo extensive surgery (Figures 11-20 and 11-21) are at increased risk for wound disruption; therefore, mass closure techniques for abdominal wall closure should be used (Figure 11-22). However, in situations in which edematous bowel is protruding from the abdominal cavity, an interrupted closure with delay of pulling the sutures tight may produce less fascial fracturing and less dehiscence. These patients also require close monitoring for abdominal compartment syndrome in the postoperative period.

Role of Radiation Therapy

With improvements in chemotherapy and surgery for ovarian cancer, radiation therapy no longer plays a central role in primary therapy. The systemic pattern of spread makes effective radiation therapy difficult, and with bulky residual disease, radiation therapy is particularly ineffective. Studies by the GOG and others demonstrated the extent to which the addition of radiation did not improve outcomes, even before the current era of highly active chemotherapy. Some special problems are listed in Table 11-19. The entire abdomen must be considered at risk; therefore the volume that must be irradiated is large, resulting in multiple limitations for the radiotherapist. Dose restrictions are listed in Table 11-20.

Radiation therapy as a second-line treatment in patients with chemotherapy-persistent or recurrent ovarian cancer has its advocates. As noted before, radiation therapy as part of the initial therapy has been abandoned in favor of chemotherapy. The impetus for renewed interest in second-line radiation therapy is that

TABLE 11-19   Special Problems in Ovarian Cancer

Limits of tumor spread often unknown
Variability of radiosensitivity
Total tumor burden usually large
Free mobility of tumor cells within the abdominal cavity
Radiation dosage restricted by neighboring organs
Infrequent detection of early disease

TABLE 11-20   Dose Restrictions

Tolerance of small intestine
Limited tolerance of kidneys
Bone marrow depression
Radiation enteritis caused by large volume of intestine irradiated
Adhesive peritonitis

subsequent chemotherapy for platinum-refractory disease by and large has not been successful. Cmelak and Kapp reported their experience of 41 patients who failed to respond to platinum-based chemotherapy. All were treated with whole-abdomen irradiation, usually with a pelvic boost. The 5-year actuarial disease-specific survival was 40% and 50% in the platinum-refractory patients. If residual tumor was less than 1.5 cm, 5-year disease-free survival was 53%, but it was 0% in patients with greater than 1.5-cm residual disease. Almost one third of patients failed to complete the planned course of whole-abdomen irradiation because of toxicity. Three patients required surgery to correct gastrointestinal tract problems. Sedlacek and colleagues described 27 patients treated with whole-abdomen irradiation after platinum-based chemotherapy. All patients completed the planned course. Although patients with primary microscopic disease had improved survival to the patients with greater than 2-cm residual disease, the survival rate at

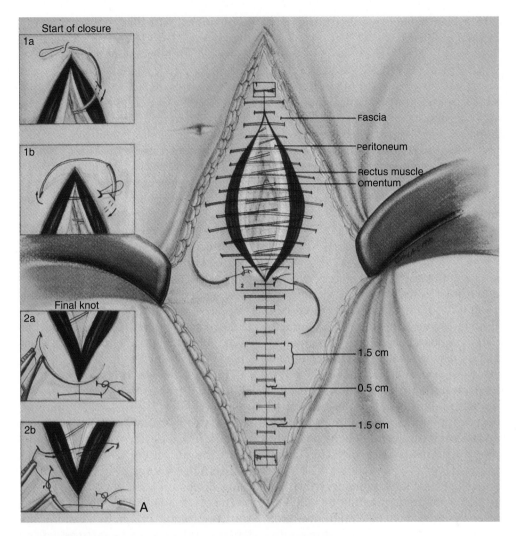

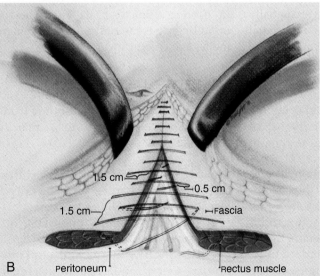

FIGURE 11-22 **A,** Running Smead–Jones closure techniques. After taking initial bite *(1a)*, the needle, with double-stranded suture, is pulled through the open loop end *(1b)*. At completion of the fascial closure, one of the two strands of the looped suture is cut from the needle *(2a)*. A bilateral bite through both anterior fascial layers is taken, and the suture is tied to itself *(2b)*. **B,** A mass closure technique with 0 Maxon loop suture in a running Smead–Jones technique has the value of speed and security in our experience.

5 years was only 15%. Four patients required surgery to correct gastrointestinal problems.

Radioisotopes

Numerous trials have been conducted comparing intraperitoneal 32P with or without pelvic radiation to whole abdominal radiation or single-agent chemotherapy in various clinical settings of ovarian cancer. Because intraperitoneal 32P has failed to demonstrate improved outcomes, can be associated with increased complications, and is "technique-intensive," it has all but evaporated from our contemporary treatment planning.

Chemotherapy

The evolution of chemotherapy for advanced ovarian cancer over the past 30 years has been significant. Ovarian cancer was one of the first solid malignant tumors demonstrating responsiveness to chemotherapy. Effectiveness of the various chemotherapy treatments has been measured by response rates (usually complete plus partial responses), negative second-look rates, progression-free survival (PFS), and overall survival (OS). All of these outcome measures can be subject to error. Even survival outcomes can be compromised by the fact that many patients receive a number of variously active chemotherapy treatments over their treatment history.

The earliest agents used for the treatment of ovarian carcinoma (1970-1980) were predominantly the alkylating agents melphalan (also called phenylalanine mustard, Alkeran, L-PAM, and L-sarcolysin), cyclophosphamide, chlorambucil, and thiotepa. Response rates were usually reported in the 20% to 60% range, but median survival rates for patients with advanced ovarian cancer were often in the range of 10 to 18 months, quite inferior to most outcomes from today's clinical trials. Antimetabolites, such as 5-fluorouracil and methotrexate, were also used in many of the earlier trials, especially in combination with alkylating agents. The contemporary use of these agents in epithelial ovarian cancer is rare to nonexistent.

The late 1970s and 1980s saw the introduction of combination chemotherapy regimens, Hexa CAF (hexamethylmelamine, cyclophosphamide, doxorubicin, and 5-fluorouracil) and CAP (cyclophosphamide, doxorubicin, and cisplatin) being two of the most common. By the early 1980s, combination therapy was the standard treatment for most patients. The 1980s also witnessed the introduction of cisplatin and later carboplatin. The introduction of the platinum compounds increased response rates to the 50% to 80% range and increased median survivals to the 12- to 30-month range in most studies. The wide range was often attributable to select patient populations, with the "suboptimal" debulked patients having the 12- to 18-month survival and the "optimal" debulked patients having the 18- to 30-month survivals. The platinum compounds have remained an integral component of treatment to this day.

The 1990s saw the introduction of paclitaxel, an agent first extracted from the stripped bark of the Pacific yew tree, *Taxus brevifolia*. Paclitaxel, now chemically synthesized, demonstrated a new mechanism of action by promoting microtubular assembly and stabilizing tubulin polymer formation, thus inhibiting rapidly dividing cells from completing the mitotic process. The initial single-agent paclitaxel response rates in patients with refractory ovarian cancer were in the 25% to 35% range. Contemporary drug development is looking at various formulations of the taxane group. One study by Vasey and colleagues demonstrated the substitution of paclitaxel with docetaxel yielded similar survival outcomes, and the toxicity profile favored docetaxel. Other modified taxanes under investigation, such as CT-2103 (Xyotax) and Abraxane, may offer advantages of either greater activity or less toxicity.

The past decade has also seen the introduction of additional cytotoxic agents in ovarian cancer treatment, most noticeably topotecan, a topoisomerase I-inhibitor; a pegylated liposomal encapsulated form of doxorubicin (Doxil); and gemcitabine, a drug first tested in the pancreatic cancer setting. These three drugs were tested in the frontline setting by the GOG 182/ICON-5 clinical trials, discussed later.

The current new therapeutic focus in the clinical trials is in the testing of agents targeting specific molecular targets. One such agent that has considerable attention in current clinical trials is bevacizumab, a VEGF-inhibiting agent initially with demonstrated activity in metastatic colon cancer.

Clinical Trials

The relatively low rates of response to most single agents stimulated investigators to search for combination schedules. In the "modern" era, platinum-based combinations have proved to be the most successful. Pertinent clinical trials relating to early-stage disease are discussed earlier in this chapter, and the following discussion focuses on more advanced disease.

A study by the GOG published in 1986 (GOG #47) comparing doxorubicin (Adriamycin) and cyclophosphamide (AC) with AC and cisplatin (CAP) because primary therapy indicated improvement with the three-drug combination. Response rate, response duration, and progression-free survival were all improved with CAP, although there was no statistically significant increase in overall survival for the whole cohort. When patients with measurable disease were evaluated separately (227 of 440 assessable patients), statistical significance for overall survival was present for the CAP arm, suggesting an advantage for the platinum arm in those patients with suboptimal, measurable residual disease after debulking surgery.

Other studies at that time noted that an alkylating agent was just as effective as combinations (including platinum) containing up to four drugs. In another study by the GOG (GOG #52) of patients with stage III ovarian cancer optimally debulked to 1 cm or less of residual disease, CAP was compared with cyclophosphamide and cisplatin. Progression-free interval and survival were not appreciably different in the two arms. Cyclophosphamide-cisplatin, therefore, became the "standard" arm for many clinical trials in the late 1980s and early 1990s.

Four trials were considered in a meta-analysis that specifically evaluated the benefit of doxorubicin in ovarian cancer. Considering only pathologic complete responses, the study shows a constant small benefit for CAP, higher for the North-West Oncology Group (GONO) and Danish Ovarian Cancer Group (DACOVA) studies. By pulling together these data in a meta-analysis, it was possible to detect a statistically significant benefit of pathologic complete responses (6%) and overall survival (7%) with CAP. However, because in three trials the dose intensity was greater for CAP than for cyclophosphamide-cisplatin, to what extent the benefit of CAP is from greater dose intensity or from doxorubicin itself remains unsolved. A subsequent study by the GOG (GOG #132) evaluated 614 patients with suboptimally debulked cancer who were treated in a three-arm protocol comparing cisplatin alone, paclitaxel alone, and a combination of the two drugs. Neither progression-free survival nor survival was different between the three arms, but crossover to the other drug in the single-drug arms may account for the similarity in the results. Some interpreted the results of this study to indicate that a platinum agent should be a component of primary therapy.

The GOG (GOG #111) then randomized 386 patients with large-volume disease to six cycles of cisplatin 75 mg/m^2 plus cyclophosphamide 750 mg/m^2 every 3 weeks or paclitaxel 135 mg/m^2 during 24 hours followed by cisplatin 75 mg/m^2 every 3 weeks. In the paclitaxel arm, administration of paclitaxel before the cisplatin was important to optimize response and minimize toxicity. In terms of therapeutic efficacy, the cisplatin-paclitaxel arm produced a significantly greater overall response rate (73% vs 60%) and clinical complete response rate, whereas the frequency of pathologic complete response was similar between the two arms. Progression-free survival was significantly greater in the paclitaxel arm (18 vs 13 months). The risk of progression was 32% lower among those treated with the paclitaxel

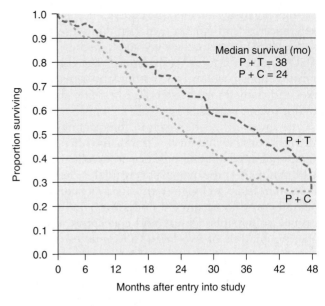

P + T = platin + taxol
P + C = platin + cytoxan

FIGURE 11-23 Survival by treatment group. *(Modified from McGuire WP et al: N Engl J Med 334:1, 1996. Copyright © 1996 Massachusetts Medical society. All rights reserved. Adapted 2006 with permission.)*

regimen compared with the cyclophosphamide regimen. Survival was significantly longer in the paclitaxel arm (38 vs 24 months), and the risk of death was 39% lower among those treated with the paclitaxel regimen (Figure 11-23). A European-Canadian Intergroup trial (OV-10) had a study design similar to GOG #111, testing the replacement of cyclophosphamide with paclitaxel. This study included patients with optimal and suboptimal stage Ib, IIb, III, and IV. Again, the clinical response rate was superior for the paclitaxel arm (59% vs 45%), with a subsequent 25% reduction in the rate of death. The combination of paclitaxel and cisplatin became the standard for combination first-line chemotherapy for the treatment of epithelial ovarian carcinoma.

When combined with cisplatin, paclitaxel requires an extended infusion interval (24 hours) to prevent unacceptable neuropathy. This administration schedule was inconvenient, prompting many community providers to replace cisplatin with carboplatin, with which paclitaxel did not require this extended infusion. Several groups conducted equivalency trials to compare paclitaxel (175-185 mg/m^2) and carboplatin (AUC 5-7.5) with the standard cisplatin-paclitaxel regimen. The GOG conducted GOG #158 on the optimal (<1 cm) patient population as a noninferiority trial. The relative risk (RR) of progression on the paclitaxel plus carboplatin arm was equivalent (RR = 0.88, 95% CI, 0.75-1.03), and toxicity was greater on the paclitaxel plus cisplatin arm. Similar findings regarding therapeutic equivalence and toxicity preference for carboplatin over cisplatin were reported by the Arbeitsgemeinschaft Gynäkologische Onkologie (AGO) Ovarian Cancer Study Group. The combination of intravenous paclitaxel and carboplatin replaced paclitaxel and cisplatin as the standard first-line chemotherapy for ovarian cancer.

Care must always be taken in interpreting response rates as a correlate for survival rates. Too often a chemotherapeutic regimen will produce an excellent response rate but not affect the overall survival rate. Therefore the clinician must await longer-term studies of combination chemotherapy to accurately understand its impact on survival of patients. Omura and colleagues reported a sobering analysis of two large GOG studies of multiagent chemotherapy in epithelial ovarian cancer. In this analysis of 726 women with stage III or stage IV disease, excellent follow-up had been obtained. The authors concluded that the impact of chemotherapy to date had been modest. Less than 10% of their patients were progression free at 5 years, and late failures continued to occur, even beyond 7 years. Sutton and coworkers reported a 7% disease-free survival at 10 years. Unfortunately, the superiority of any particular combination of chemotherapeutic agents as reflected by statistically significant improvement in long-term survival remains unproved. Although carboplatin appears to be the most active agent in epithelial cancer of the ovary, there is still controversy that combining it with other agents improves outcome.

In vitro testing of chemotherapy resistance or sensitivity has been investigated for at least two decades without clarification of its role in either primary or recurrent disease. Multiple technologies are currently in use, and there is a need to identify the relative value of this testing modality.

Maintenance therapy after primary surgery and chemotherapy in patients with a complete clinical response (consolidation chemotherapy) is an area of current controversy. One clinical trial randomized this patient population to 3 versus 12 additional treatments with paclitaxel at 4-week intervals. The study was closed early by the Data Safety Monitoring Board when a planned interim analysis demonstrated a progression-free interval advantage of 7 months for the extra 9 months of treatment. However, a follow-up report failed to demonstrate any survival advantage, which was difficult to interpret because the early closure caused the trial to be underpowered for this endpoint. Additional trials are in progress to clarify the potential role for maintenance therapy.

Two trials evaluating the role of bevacizumab combined with carboplatin and paclitaxel in the first-line setting have recently been reported. Bevacizumab is a potent antitumor therapy that targets vascular endothelial growth factor (VEGF), and for which there are multiple phase II trials demonstrating efficacy in recurrent ovarian cancer. GOG 218 randomly assigned women with advanced ovarian cancer to one of three treatment arms: standard carboplatin and paclitaxel for 6 cycles, carboplatin, paclitaxel plus bevacizumab for 6 cycles, and carboplatin, paclitaxel plus bevacizumab for 6 cycles followed by bevacizumab for up to an additional 16 cycles. Preliminary results demonstrate equivalent progression-free survival in the two nonconsolidation arms, but a significant progression-free survival advantage with the bevacizumab consolidation therapy. A large European trial, ICON 7, reported similar findings of improvement in progression-free survival in patients receiving concurrent plus maintenance bevacizumab. Details of these trials including overall survival results are still pending.

Dose-Intense Chemotherapy

Dose intensity refers to the amount of chemotherapy to which a cancer is exposed per unit of time; this is generally assumed to be reflected by the dose of drug in milligrams per square meter of body surface area per unit of time. The theory is well grounded in preclinical work showing that as the concentration of drug in culture medium increases, the fraction of surviving cancer cells decreases logarithmically. The cell kill for a particular drug frequently follows a sigmoid curve indicating a point at which continued dose escalation will yield little improvement in results. To determine whether dose intensity is important clinically, randomized trials are needed. The GOG did design such a trial in patients with large-volume, advanced disease. A total of 458 patients were entered into the study and were randomly assigned to low-dose cisplatin 50 mg/m^2 plus cyclophosphamide 500 mg/m^2 every 3 weeks for eight cycles or high-dose cisplatin 100 mg/m^2 plus cyclophosphamide 1000 mg/m^2 every 3 weeks for four cycles. Each regimen delivered the same total dose of chemotherapy, but the high-dose schedule was delivered in half the time. The overall response rate of the 130 patients with measurable disease was 65% for the low-dose arm versus 59% for the high-dose arm; clinical complete response rates were 26% and 27%, respectively. These differences were not significant. There was no difference in progression-free or overall survival in the subsets of patients with measurable or nonmeasurable disease. The results of this study did not support the concept that increased dose intensity will produce greater therapeutic effect of cisplatinum or cyclophosphamide. Colombo and associates reported a randomized trial in patients with advanced disease who were given cisplatin 50 mg/m^2 per week for 9 weeks or cisplatin 75 mg/m^2 every 3 weeks for six cycles. The weekly arm delivered the same total dose of cisplatin in half the time, but each arm received the total dose of drug. Within the subsets of patients with small-volume and large-volume disease, no significant differences were observed with regard to either clinical or pathologic complete response rates, progression-free survival, or overall survival. Whereas neither of these randomized trials of pure dose intensity in cisplatin showed an advantage for a higher dose intensity across a clinically relevant range of doses, other lines of evidence have been cited to support the use of higher dose schedules. In trials conducted by the National Cancer Institute (NCI) of the United States, even higher dose intensities of cisplatin in conjunction with hypertonic saline to protect the kidneys had been stated to yield higher response rates than more standard doses. A closer examination of these data reported by Rothenberg and coworkers shows confusing results. In patients with large-volume disease, the NCI regimen complete response rates were no different (11% vs 12%) than the GOG results with cisplatin, doxorubicin, and cyclophosphamide (CAP), as reported by Omura, regimens with a 3.3-fold difference in dose intensity of cisplatin. In patients with small-volume disease, the NCI regimen complete response rates were not statistically different (38% vs 30%) than the GOG results with a two-drug combination of cisplatin plus cyclophosphamide, as reported by Omura in 1989. There appears to be no evidence from these data to support the importance of dose intensity of cisplatin over a 3.3-fold range of doses. At least 11 randomized trials have compared standard doses of carboplatin- or cisplatin-based chemotherapy with double doses of the same platinum analogs. Most of these trials showed no advantage in most outcome parameters. A second meta-analysis of the Levin and Hryniuk meta-analysis (in which it appeared that dose intensity had a positive impact on response rate and survival) suggested that platinum dose intensity is unimportant, although intensity of all administered drugs is important, as is tumor residual volume at initiation of therapy.

Katsumata and colleagues from the Japan GOG reported their results of their phase III trial in advanced ovarian cancer evaluating IV carboplatin and paclitaxel dosed every 3 weeks vs IV carboplatin with weekly dose-dense paclitaxel. For each 3-week cycle of therapy, the weekly dose-dense arm received 240 mg/m^2 of paclitaxel vs 180 mg/m^2 of paclitaxel in the control arm. Progression-free and 3-year overall survival were significantly improved in the weekly paclitaxel arm (28 vs 17 months, 72% vs 65%), with a higher incidence of grade III and IV anemia. The pharmacokinetic and pharmacodynamic issues inherent in a homologous Japanese population make generalization of these results to the Western world problematic. Confirmatory trials in the United States and Europe will soon be under way.

In the last decade, high-dose chemotherapy with autologous bone marrow transplantation (ABMT) or peripheral blood stem cell support has been reported for several solid tumors, and there has been a tendency for improved response rates but a relatively short period of disease-free survival in most of the reports reviewed. Many reports show that even in advanced cases, the most important factor for long-term survival after high-dose chemotherapy is the completeness of the primary cytoreductive surgery. Most of the reports in the literature with high-dose chemotherapy with ABMT have been phase II trials of patients with a mixed response to first-line chemotherapy. The best response and survival have been in those patients who had had a complete response to pretransplantation chemotherapy. The MD Anderson group reported their experience of 96 patients undergoing transplantation, of whom 43% were in clinical remission. Overall 6-year survival was 38% and was 53% in the clinical remission group. Bengala and colleagues reported the results of the European Group for Blood and Marrow Transplantation (EBMT) for 91 patients in first complete remission treated with high-dose chemotherapy and ABMT. Median survival was 44 months, and they were unable to identify a subgroup more likely to benefit. These reported median survivals are not significantly better than that with use of paclitaxel as second-line therapy. However, the toxicity of high-dose chemotherapy is a serious concern, as is the additional expense. Although interesting, it appears that targeting of patients for high-dose therapy with bone marrow support cannot be considered standard therapy and should only be done as part of an established national protocol so that information can be obtained to increase our knowledge of this therapy.

Immunochemotherapy

In the past three decades, there has been considerable interest in combining chemotherapy with immunotherapy for better results in patients with epithelial cancer of the ovary. The GOG and others have investigated immunomodulating agents such as *Corynebacterium parvum* and bacille Calmette-Guérin (BCG). Results have been conflicting as to whether nonspecific immunostimulation combined with chemotherapy improves survival.

The potential role of immune response modifiers in the treatment of ovarian cancer has been investigated. Ovarian cancer is a suitable model for biologic therapies because the peritoneal cavity is capable of mounting an inflammatory response to many stimuli, and this response has been shown to induce an antitumor effect. Early experimental observations confirmed that ovarian cancer is a suitable prototype tumor in which to evaluate novel immunotherapeutic and chemoimmunotherapeutic approaches. Berek and coworkers have reported that

TABLE 11-21   Randomized Trials Comparing Intravenous versus Intraperitoneal First-Line Treatment of Ovarian Cancer Needs Framework

Study Identifier/ Year Published	Control Regimen	Experimental Regimen	Target Population	No. of Patients	Median Duration of Survival for Control Regimen (Months)	Median Duration of Survival for Experimental Regimen (Months)
SWOG/GOG-104 (Alberts et al 1996)	Cisplatin 100 mg/m^2 IV, Ctx 600 mg/m^2 IV q 3 weeks × 6	Cisplatin 100 mg/ m^2 IP, Ctx 600 mg/m^2 IV q 3 weeks × 6	Stage III ≤2 cm residual	546	41	49
Greek (Polyzos et al 1999)	Crbpt 350 mg/m^2 IV, Ctx 600 mg/m^2 IV q 3 weeks × 6	Crbpt 350 mg/m^2 IV, Ctx 600 mg/m^2 IV q 3 weeks × 6	Stage III ≤ or >2 cm residual	90	52	63
GONO (Gadducci et al 2000)	Cisplatin 50 mg/m^2 IV, Ctx 600 mg/m^2 IV, Epidox 60 mg/m^2 IV q 4 weeks × 6	Cisplatin 50 mg/m^2 IP, Ctx 600 mg/m^2 IV, Epidox 60 mg/m^2 IV q 4 weeks × 6	Stage II-IV <2 cm residual	113	25	26
GOG-114/SWOG (Markman et al 2001)	Cisplatin 75 mg/m^2 IV, Tax 135 mg/m^2 (24 hr) IV q 3 weeks × 6	Crbpt AUC 9 IV q 28 days × 2, Cisplatin 100 mg/m^2 IP, Tax 135 mg/m^2 (24 hr) IV q 3 weeks × 6	Stage III ≤1 cm residual	462	51	67
Taiwan (Yen et al 2001)	Cisplatin 50 mg/m^2 IV Ctx 500 mg/m^2 IV Epi/Adr 50 mg/m^2 IV q 3 weeks × 6	Cisplatin 100 mg/m^2 IV Ctx 500 mg/m^2 IV, Epi/Adr 50 mg/m^2 IV q 3 weeks × 6	Stage III ≤1 cm residual	118	48	43
GOG-172 (Armstrong et al 2005)	Cisplatin 75 mg/m^2 IV, Tax 135 mg/m^2 (24 hr) IV q 3 weeks × 6	Tax 135 mg/m^2 (24 hr) IV, Cisplatin 100 mg/m^2 IP, Tax 60 mg/m^2 IV on day 8q 3 weeks × 6	Stage III ≤1 cm	415	49	67

recombinant interferon alfa has clinical activity in patients with small-volume residual disease. Numerous phase II trials, using substances such as tumor necrosis factor, interleukin-2, and the like, along with other studies using combinations of cytokines have failed to demonstrate significantly improved outcomes. Combining biologic immune response modifiers with standard chemotherapy has proved to be more difficult than initially conceived because of overlapping toxicities. In view of this, it seems prudent to await proven efficacy before attempting to launch the phase III trials with biologic immune response modifiers.

Intraperitoneal Chemotherapy

Ovarian cancer is predominantly a disease limited to the peritoneal cavity for most patients. For some chemotherapeutic agents, intraperitoneal (IP) administration offers pharmacokinetic advantages, including high intraperitoneal drug concentration and longer exposure in the peritoneal cavity. Although intraperitoneal chemotherapy proposals date back decades, it has only been over recent years that the accumulated clinical trial data favor this approach.

Results from randomized trials, listed in Table 11-21, summarize the experience of clinical trials conducted since the mid-1980s. These studies, all primary therapy trials, compare IV chemotherapy to combined IV and IP chemotherapy. The initial IP study demonstrating that IP chemotherapy may represent a survival advantage was a combined SWOG/GOG trial (SWOG #8501 and GOG #104). The study compared IV cisplatin and IV cyclophosphamide to IP cisplatin and IV cyclophosphamide in patients with less than 2-cm-diameter residual disease. The IP arm produced a median survival of 49 months compared to 41 months for the IV arm, with an HR of 0.77. However, critics pointed out that the subsequent introduction of paclitaxel to our frontline treatment may have neutralized this apparent advantage for IP therapy. The other concern is that accrual was extended beyond the initial study design for patients with 0 to 0.5-cm residual disease, and still this subgroup failed to demonstrate superior survival (51 months vs 46 months, HR = 0.80). One would have expected the treatment difference to be most pronounced in this patient subgroup. Due in part to these issues, IP therapy was not uniformly supported as producing a survival advantage over the current IV standard, carboplatin-paclitaxel.

Another GOG study, GOG #114, reported in 2003, compared IV cisplatin and paclitaxel (six cycles) to high-dose (AUC = 9) carboplatin IV (two cycles) plus six cycles IV paclitaxel and IP cisplatin in patients with

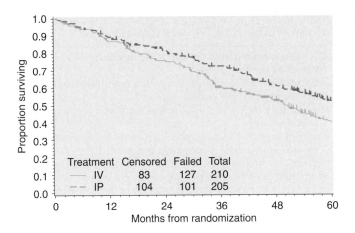

FIGURE 11-24 Overall survival for GOG #172: IP therapy vs IV therapy for optimally debulked advanced ovarian carcinoma.

stage III disease less than or equal to 1-cm diameter residual. The median survival for the IP arm was 67 months versus 51 months for the IV arm and was statistically significant. Because the patients in the IV arm did not receive the extra two cycles of the high-dose carboplatin, critics were hesitant to support IP delivery as the reason for the survival improvement.

The most recently reported GOG study, GOG #172, compared IV paclitaxel (135 mg/m^2/24 hours), followed by either IV cisplatin (75 mg/m^2) on day 2 or by IP cisplatin (100 mg/m^2) on day 2 and IP paclitaxel (60 mg/m^2) on day 8—each arm for six cycles at 21-day intervals. The patient population was similar to GOG #114—stage III, less than 1 cm diameter residual. The median survival for the IP arm was 66.9 months compared to 49.5 months for the IV arm (HR of 0.71), results remarkably similar to the preceding study, GOG #114 (Figure 11-24). This survival advantage prompted an NCI alert that IP therapy should be considered for first-line treatment for women with optimally cytoreduced advanced ovarian cancer. However, this study reported significant toxicity for the IP arm, with double-digit percentage grade III/IV toxicities. Although the greatest experience with an IP platinum agent has been with cisplatin at a dose of 100 mg/m^2, substitution of carboplatin for cisplatin may limit the toxicity. Curiously, in GOG #172, only 42% of patients on the IP treatment received the complete six cycles of IP therapy, and 48% received three or fewer cycles of IP chemotherapy. Patients not able to receive the IP chemotherapy were switched to IV treatment, and 83% of the patients on the IP arm completed six cycles of chemotherapy (IP and/or IV). The authors postulate that the initial cycles of IP chemotherapy may render most of the benefit. Although the IP-treated patients reported a significantly worse quality of life prior to cycle four and 3 to 6 weeks post treatment, there was no difference in quality of life between the IP/IV arms 1 year post treatment, except for moderate neurotoxicity (paresthesias) being more common in the IP arm. Despite the evidence for a survival advantage from IP therapy and the resultant NCI clinical alert, IP therapy has not been accepted universally as a result of issues with catheter placement and therapy-associated toxicities. The GOG is currently evaluating both dosing modifications and substituting carboplatin for cisplatin as the IP platinum agent to improve the tolerance to IP therapy. These trial results are eagerly anticipated because they have the potential again to improve our current standard regimen for this disease.

This study also reported catheter-related complications in 39 of 118 patients (33%). The GOG recommends use of a venous catheter with a subcutaneous access port overlying the lower ribs (Figure 11-25). In patients who have undergone rectosigmoid resection, the catheter tubing should be trimmed at the pelvic brim so as to not contact the anastomosis. The study does not provide information detailing information about IP catheter retention or management in patients converted to IV therapy. Actually, none of the IP studies conducted to date have ruled out the possibility that the presence of an intraperitoneal foreign body is the inciting agent, altering host immune/cytokine response producing the more favorable outcomes. This possibility is being explored as part of the translational research component of an ongoing GOG IP trial (Figure 11-26).

Extraovarian Peritoneal Serous Papillary Carcinoma

Extraovarian peritoneal serous papillary carcinoma is a recognized clinical-pathologic entity in which peritoneal carcinomatosis of ovarian serous type is found in the abdomen or pelvis. Similar tumor deposits may be found on the surface of the ovary, but histologic evidence of primary or in situ ovarian carcinoma is either absent or insignificant. The tumor deposits are rarely noninvasive (borderline). This entity was first reported as "mesothelioma resembling papillary ovarian adenocarcinoma" by Swerdlow in 1959. Parmley and Woodruff, in 1974, demonstrated that pelvic peritoneum had the potential to differentiate into a müllerian type of epithelium. This entity is different from mesothelioma. The malignant neoplasm spreads inside the peritoneal cavity, invading mostly the omentum, with minimal or no involvement of the ovary. Peritoneal studding is commonly present with psammoma bodies. Although usually serous, other cell types have been demonstrated. This entity has been identified in women who have had previous oophorectomies. The GOG has developed criteria for the diagnosis of extraovarian peritoneal carcinoma (Table 11-22).

Experience with extraovarian serous neoplasia of this type has been compared to clinical outcomes of

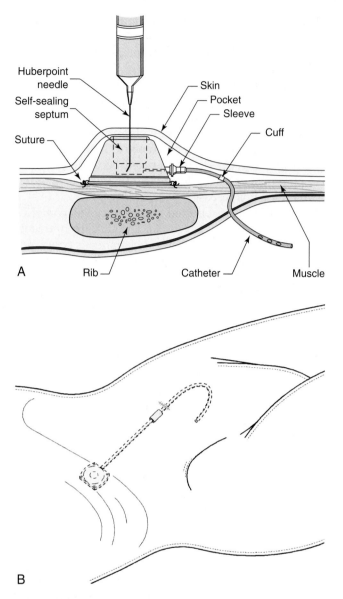

A

B

FIGURE 11-25 **A,** Implanted peritoneal access catheter with subcutaneous self-sealing port providing a path for intraperitoneal therapy. **B,** Intraperitoneal chemotherapy.

TABLE 11-22   Gynecologic Oncology Group Criteria for Diagnosis of Extraovarian Peritoneal Carcinoma

Both ovaries must be either physiologically normal in size or enlarged by benign process.

Involvement in extraovarian sites must be greater than involvement on the surface of either ovary.

Microscopically, the ovarian involvement must be:
    Nonexistent
    Confined to ovarian surface epithelium, or underlying cortical stromal involvement of no more than 5 mm

Histologic characteristics are primarily serous type, similar or identical to ovarian serous papillary adenocarcinoma.

extraovarian peritoneal carcinoma. More than 95% were stage III to IV, ascites was present in 80%, and 95% had elevated CA-125 concentrations. Optimal debulking was performed in about two thirds, and most received platinum-based regimens. Overall, survival was about 2 years; patients with stage III disease had a median survival of 29 months compared with only 15 months for patients with stage IV disease. In those with optimal debulking, survival was 40 months compared with 19 months if suboptimal debulking was done. In a multivariate analysis, only performance status and optimal debulking had a significant effect on overall survival. Of note, 10 of the patients had had previous oophorectomy. A GOG trial of cisplatin and cyclophosphamide in these patients demonstrated a response similar to that in women with papillary serous ovarian cancer.

Our experience has been that these patients generally respond to therapy in a manner similar to patients with serous papillary carcinoma of the ovary. Because many characteristics of this entity and serous ovarian cancer are similar, the GOG accepts patients with extraovarian peritoneal carcinoma into its protocols of epithelial ovarian cancer. CA-125 measurements also appear similar in both groups of patients. There have been reports suggesting a higher incidence of polyclonal cell populations in peritoneal carcinoma than in the generally monoclonal ovarian cancers, which may lead to higher rates of chemoresistance. Although most reports show similar survival between ovarian and peritoneal cancers, this polyclonal nature has been suggested to explain those series showing a decreased survival in peritoneal cancer. There would appear to be an increased incidence of extraovarian peritoneal cancers in patients with a hereditary predisposition for development of ovarian cancer. In Piver's report of women at high risk for hereditary ovarian cancer, extraovarian cancer developed after prophylactic oophorectomy in almost 2%, 10 times greater than the lifetime incidence in the general population. BRCA1 mutations appear to arise in a similar number of women with extraovarian and primary ovarian cancers.

homologous ovarian tumors of similar stage and grade. Fromm and colleagues reported a series of 74 patients identified as having papillary serous carcinoma of the peritoneum. The average age at diagnosis was 57 years, and the majority of the patients were white. Clinical presentation was similar to that of ovarian carcinoma. Clinical response to chemotherapy was seen in 64% of the patients; 41% had partial responses, and 23% had complete responses. Median survival for the total group was 24 months. Dalrymple reported 31 cases of extraovarian peritoneal serous papillary carcinoma with equivalent survival to primary ovarian neoplasms. The Roswell Park Cancer Institute described 73 patients with

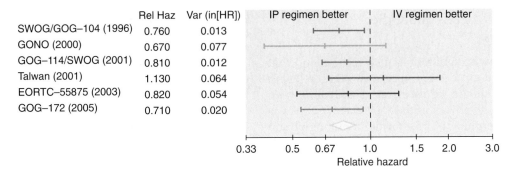

	Rel Haz	Var (in[HR])
SWOG/GOG–104 (1996)	0.760	0.013
GONO (2000)	0.670	0.077
GOG–114/SWOG (2001)	0.810	0.012
Talwan (2001)	1.130	0.064
EORTC–55875 (2003)	0.820	0.054
GOG–172 (2005)	0.710	0.020

$\Mu^2$ heterogeneity (5 d.f.)= 3.1, $P = 0.68$
Hazard ratio is not reported for the GONO study, but it is calculated from the available data reported.
Hazard ratio is not reported for the Greek study.

FIGURE 11-26 Treatment hazard ratios for death intraperitoneal versus intravenous therapy. (*National Cancer Institute Clinical Announcement, December, 2005.*)

Small Cell Carcinoma of the Ovary

Small cell carcinoma of the ovary has been identified as a specific histopathologic entity. This rare and highly aggressive malignant neoplasm primarily affects children and young women between the ages of 10 and 40 years. The first 11 cases were documented by Dickersin and colleagues in 1982. Many, but not all, patients with this lesion have an associated hypercalcemia. Neuron-specific enolase may be both a histologic marker (immunohistochemistry) and a serum marker for this disease. Various chemotherapeutic agents have been suggested with minimal success. Young and associates reported on the poor prognosis of these patients, with only 33% of women with stage Ia tumors alive and no survivors with advanced stage disease. In general, similar chemotherapy regimens used for small cell lung carcinoma will be used to treat this disease. Pautier and colleagues have reported the most promising regimen to date: a combination of cisplatin, doxorubicin, etoposide, and cyclophosphamide, with, if complete remission is achieved, high-dose chemotherapy with carboplatin, etoposide, cyclophosphamide, and stem-cell support. Of 27 patients treated, 21 were stage II to IV and 18 complete responses were seen. Median duration of the 18 complete responses was 30 months, and 10 patients went on to receive high-dose chemotherapy. Overall survival at 3 years was 49%. Further study of this devastating group of tumors is necessary.

FOLLOW-UP TECHNIQUES AND TREATMENT OF RECURRENCES

Ovarian cancer is insidious in that it is late to cause symptoms, and thus follow-up examinations are imperative to detect early recurrence. The optimal follow-up strategy for the asymptomatic patient who has advanced ovarian cancer after initial treatment remains undecided. Important considerations are divided between more passive and active approaches to follow-up. Currently the National Comprehensive Cancer Network (NCCN) practice guidelines in oncology recommend surveillance of patients after the completion of primary therapy, regardless of stage. This follow-up includes a comprehensive physical examination every 2 to 4 months for the first 2 years, every 6 months for the next 3 years, and then annually after 5 years. Laboratory studies, such as blood counts and chemistry profiles, should be done as indicated.

Second-Look Operation (Reassessment Surgery)

Historically, following the completion of primary therapy, a second-look operation was conducted to assess for occult disease. First described in the late 1940s by Owen Wangensteen, the objective of this procedure was to determine response to treatment and the findings would provide insight for both treatment planning and prognostic information. However, presently second-look procedures are not routinely recommended and typically are only utilized in the setting of a clinical trial. The reasons for the change in attitude are several. Regardless of negative second-look laparotomy results half the patients will have recurrence. Second, an exploratory data analysis of a GOG study (protocol 158) did not demonstrate a survival benefit in patients undergoing second-look procedures, even in those with positive findings. Last, these procedures are associated with surgical morbidity and the advent of biochemical markers and improvement in imaging (discussed in greater detail later), which have improved early detection of recurrence, further contributing to the decreased utilization of second-look surgery.

Use of CA-125 Levels and Other Tumor Markers

The oncology practice guidelines also recommend that the measurement of CA-125 level, or other relevant tumor markers, should be assessed at each follow-up evaluation if the level was initially elevated. CA-125 is an antigenic determinant of a murine immunoglobulin Ig1 monoclonal antibody that was raised against an epithelial ovarian carcinoma cell line and is expressed in more than 80% of nonmucinous epithelial ovarian cancers.

Multiple CA-125 determinants are associated with a mucin-like glycoprotein of more than 200,000 daltons. Traces of the antigen are expressed in adult tissues derived from the coelomic epithelium, including mesothelial cells lining the pleura, pericardium, and peritoneum, and from the epithelial component of the female reproductive system. Thus there are other causes of elevated CA-125 levels, which include both gynecologic and nongynecologic conditions. Acute inflammatory processes involving the pelvic area and other regions of the body may increase CA-125. These may include acute hepatitis or pancreatitis, chronic liver disease, colitis, congestive heart failure, diverticulitis, arthritis, and pneumonia, to name a few.

The radioimmune assay was developed to detect CA-125 in serum and body fluids. The day-to-day coefficient of variability for the assay is approximately 15%. Consequently, a doubling or halving of antigen levels has been considered significant. If a cut-off of 35 U/mL is chosen for the upper limit of normal, elevated CA-125 levels should be found in 1% of apparently normal blood bank donors, 6% of patients who have benign disease, 28% of individuals who have nongynecologic malignant neoplasms, and 82% of patients who have surgically demonstrable epithelial ovarian cancer. Niloff and coworkers reported detection of elevated CA-125 in sera from patients who have advanced fallopian tube, endometrial, and endocervical adenocarcinomas. In epithelial ovarian carcinoma, rising or falling levels of CA-125 have correlated with disease progression or regression in more than 90% of patients. In the report by Niloff, when CA-125 levels returned to less than 35 U/mL, findings of second-look surveillance procedures were in fact normal in 14 of 36 cases, but in no instance was a nodule greater than 1 cm found. Persistently elevated CA-125 levels have been associated consistently with persistence of disease. Recurrence of disease has been heralded by elevations of CA-125 in 85% of patients whose tumors shed the antigen. Elevated CA-125 levels preceded disease recurrence by 1 to 14 months with a mean of 5 months in one study reported by Knapp and Friedman. Elevation of CA-125 in hepatocellular disease and in chronic peritonitis is important to note but should not compromise the utility of CA-125 as a marker for monitoring ovarian cancer.

A rapid regression of the serum CA-125 level to normal limits shortly after commencement of chemotherapy has been shown to be associated with a higher frequency of negative results at second-assessment surgery. Levin reported that almost all patients who subsequently come to a negative second-look laparotomy have serum CA-125 levels within normal ranges within 3 months of primary cytoreductive surgery. Buller and colleagues have shown that a favorable outcome is associated with a steep regression curve of serum CA-125 levels after cytoreductive surgery and chemotherapy. These investigators demonstrated that patients in whom the CA-125 level reverts sharply to within the normal range by the third course of chemotherapy after surgery have a survival that is markedly improved over that of the patients who have an elevation of CA-125 levels before their fourth course of chemotherapy. Buller described the regression curve of the serum CA-125 level as "S." Indeed, he has suggested that patients with a delayed "S" curve (regression of the elevated value) possibly should be considered for alternative therapy rather than persisting with the same chemotherapeutic regimens. Hogberg and Kagedal demonstrated that 23 patients with a serum CA-125 half-life shorter than 16 days during induction chemotherapy had an estimated survival of 68% at 59 months after second-look operation. This compared with survival of 18% in 49 patients with a serum CA-125 half-life longer than 16 days. However, one must be aware that normal levels may also accompany disease, with tumors up to 2 cm, in one third or more of cases.

An elevation of CA-125 in the post-treatment surveillance period is usually related to recurrence of tumor, even if clinically otherwise undetectable. It remains controversial if patients should restart chemotherapy based on CA-125 elevation alone. Recently, the EORTC conducted a randomized study of early treatment for ovarian cancer relapse based on CA-125 level alone versus clinical/symptomatic recurrence. They evaluated 527 patients, approximately 265 in each group, and found no difference in overall survival between the two groups, even though patients in the arm evaluating CA-125 levels were treated earlier. Thus they concluded that routine measurement of CA-125 may not be warranted. However, it is important to note that patients in this study were predominantly treated with second-line chemotherapy. Therefore, the role of secondary cytoreductive surgery, discussed in detail later, for asymptomatic recurrences may not have been accounted for and survival benefit of early detection based on CA-125 level may be underestimated for this group. Therefore at this time, construction of the specific plan of follow-up should be individualized to each patient's needs.

In addition to CA-125, other tumor markers are being investigated for the detection of recurrent disease. Currently, the human epididymis protein 4 (HE4) has gained interest as a biomarker of recurrence. In a recent study, HE4 was shown to be elevated several months before CA-125 levels; implying a potential role for early detection of recurrent disease. Other studies have evaluated the markers including glycodelin, MMP7, in addition to HE4 and CA-125. The combination of these biomarkers was found to be useful for the detection of relapse before the onset of clinically detectable disease. However, these tests are in their infancy and larger studies need to be conducted to confirm their efficacy.

Radiographic Imaging

For patients demonstrating a complete response to primary therapy, the NCCN guidelines recommend the use of radiographic imaging as clinically indicated. This may include the use of CT scan; magnetic resonance imaging (MRI) scan; or, more recently, PET/CT scan. The detection of recurrent disease on radiographic imaging varies dependent on modality and the size and location of disease. CT and MRI studies detected recurrent tumor in 66% to 95% of cases. However, most often failed to detect small-volume disease and disease located on visceral surfaces. Recently, PET/CT scan with F-18 fluorodeoxyglucose for the evaluation of recurrent ovarian cancer has been used. This modality has been shown to detect disease recurrence, particularly when patients presented with rising CA-125 levels and negative or equivocal CT scan or MRI. Although one must be aware of the limitations, namely physiologic uptake of the FDG, particularly in the gastrointestinal and urinary systems, and misalignment with CT scan secondary to bowel peristalsis and respiratory movements, FDG-PET/CT has become a more common imaging choice.

FDG-PET/CT scan not only offers the benefit of functional and anatomic imaging, but also allows for the ability to locate small-volume disease in locations not amenable to physical examination and the ability to differentiate metabolically active disease from inactive disease. In an effort to detect small lesions, PET/CT scan was performed for suspected recurrence and confirmed by surgical exploration or clinical follow-up. The investigators reported PET/CT scans had a sensitivity of 93% to 95% and specificity of 97% to 100%, suggesting that PET/CT may be used for post-therapy evaluation of recurrent ovarian cancer. Thus PET/CT scan may provide valuable prognostic information, similar to second-look operations, without the associated morbidity.

However, the role of radiographic imaging for routine surveillance is less clear. In a retrospective case-control study, investigators evaluated survival impact based on the asymptomatic versus symptomatic detection of ovarian cancer. The common practice in this study was CT scanning of the abdomen and pelvis at 6-month intervals for the first 2 years followed by annually for the next 3 years. The authors reported a significant difference in post-recurrence survival favoring those detected asymptomatically on imaging (45 vs 29.4 months). However, these tests are not without costs and should be evaluated in a prospective fashion to determine the true benefit. Until then, the decision to evaluate asymptomatic patients for recurrent disease with imaging should be individualized.

Maintenance Therapy

In addition to surveillance, patients with a complete response following primary therapy may be candidates for maintenance therapy, chemotherapy given with the intention of extending the disease-free interval and improving overall survival. Currently, the role of maintenance therapy, or consolidation therapy, is still under investigation, which includes identifying the ideal agent(s) and dosages, the treatment interval, and the length of treatment.

As one of the most active agents in the primary setting, platinum agents are a natural choice for maintenance therapy. In patients with advanced disease who achieved a complete response after six cycles of chemotherapy, Kim and colleagues evaluated the role of three additional cycles of platinum and paclitaxel compared to observation (control arm). The authors noted that both groups demonstrated similar survival outcomes. Additional studies have evaluated the efficacy of single-agent carboplatin and intraperitoneal cisplatin for maintenance therapy; however, similar to the aforementioned study, no survival advantage was ascertained.

Several randomized studies have also been conducted studying the role of paclitaxel for maintenance therapy. In one randomized study, six additional cycles of paclitaxel were compared to observation. The investigators reported no difference in progression-free or overall survival at 3 years. Weekly paclitaxel (80 mg/m^2) for 12 weeks was evaluated following primary therapy, and the investigators reported a 2-year survival rate of 94% and acceptable tolerability. In contrast, a study by the GOG (protocol 178) compared 3 cycles to 12 cycles of paclitaxel after a complete clinical response. Patients in the 12 additional cycle arm demonstrated a significant progression-free survival benefit of 7 months (28 vs 21 months). However, the survival benefit came with increased treatment-related neuropathy. Currently the GOG (protocol 212) is conducting a study randomly assigning patients to monthly paclitaxel, paclitaxel poliglumex, or observation for 12 months after the completion of primary therapy. Until the results of this trial are available, the role of paclitaxel for maintenance therapy remains to be determined.

In addition to platinum and paclitaxel, studies have been conducted evaluating the impact of numerous other chemotherapy agents, including topotecan, pegylated liposomal doxorubicin, and altretamine, which also failed to demonstrate a survival advantage. Over the past decade, biologic agents have also been investigated, such as oregovomab, a monoclonal antibody targeting CA-125 antigen, and tanomastat, a matrix metalloproteinase inhibitor. However, neither of these agents demonstrated a survival benefit. Recently, the GOG concluded a study (protocol 218) that evaluated the use of bevacizumab (15 mg/kg) as maintenance therapy compared to placebo following primary treatment with carboplatin, paclitaxel, and bevacizumab. This regimen showed a significant progression-free survival benefit favoring the arm administering maintenance bevacizumab. ICON-7 using bevacizumab (7.5 mg/kg) in the maintenance setting likewise showed a significant improvement in progression-free survival. These promising studies suggest that maintenance therapy may become an important area for further study.

Chemotherapy for Recurrent Disease and Targeted Therapies

Advanced epithelial ovarian cancer is a highly chemosensitive solid tumor with responses in the range of 70% to 80% to first-line chemotherapy, including a high proportion of complete responses. Most patients, however, eventually relapse and ultimately die of chemoresistant disease. Even with platinum-based chemotherapy, less than a quarter of the patients with an initial advanced disease diagnosis are alive at 5 years. In all forms of ovarian epithelial cancer, second-line chemotherapy has to date been disappointing. When effective drug combinations are initially used and fail, there is a very limited chance of inducing a sustained remission or cure with a second or third drug or combinations. Response and control of malignant effusions can frequently be achieved, but these are usually of progressively shorter duration. Most gynecologic oncologists attempt to treat these patients with use of a reasonable second-line regimen usually consisting of active chemotherapeutic agents that have not been used in the first treatment plan (Table 11-23). The selection of therapy is based on the following factors: (1) potential for platinum sensitivity; (2) number of previous regimens; (3) potential cumulative toxicities; (4) patient performance status and symptoms; and (5) patient choice.

TABLE 11-23   Agents Used in Epithelial Ovarian Cancer

Active Agents	Inactive Agents
Alkylating agents	BCNU
Bevacizumab	Vincristine
Hexamethylmelamine	6-Mercaptopurine (6-MP)
Doxorubicin	Dactinomycin
Cisplatin	Raltitrexed (Tomudex)
Carboplatin	CI-958
5-Fluorouracil	
Methotrexate	
Etoposide (VP-16)	
Paclitaxel (Taxol)	
Vinorelbine tartrate (Navelbine)	
Gemcitabine	
Topotecan	
Liposomal doxorubicin	
Docetaxel	

TABLE 11-24   Response Rate Versus Interval from Previous Treatment with Platinum-Based Regimen

Interval (Mo)	Total No.	Responding (No.)	Responding (%)
<3	39	4	10
4-6	11	1	9
7-9	11	4	36
10-12	6	1	17
13-15	4	2	50
16-18	4	3	75
19-21	1	1	100
>21	16	15	94

From Blackledge G et al: Br J Cancer 59:650, 1989.

Patients whose disease recurs within 6 months of achieving a complete clinical response to front-line platinum-based therapy are deemed platinum resistant. In comparison, patients who respond and have a progression-free interval of more than 6 months off treatment are defined as platinum sensitive or, more appropriately, chemotherapy sensitive. The response rates to second-line therapy are strikingly different in these two groups of patients. Blackledge and associates, in an analysis of 92 patients receiving five different second-line regimens, found that the interval off platinum-based therapy was a strong predictor of response. This observation held for both platinum-based and non–platinum-based second-line regimens. A response rate of less than 10% was observed for patients with a treatment-free interval of less than 6 months compared with up to 90% for those with an interval more than 21 months (Table 11-24).

Seltzer and coworkers reported a 72% response rate, including a 36% complete response rate, to second-line therapy with cisplatin in 11 patients who had achieved complete response to platinum-based, first-line chemotherapy. Markman and coworkers reported a 77% response rate to cisplatin in patients who had received no treatment for more than 24 months, compared with 27% in women whose treatment-free interval remained 5 to 12 months. Similarly, Eisenhauer and associates reported a 43% response rate to carboplatin in patients whose treatment-free interval was more than 12 months compared with 10% in those whose treatment-free interval was less than 12 months. These findings make it mandatory that we define the populations of patients in clinical trials of second-line therapy. Phase II trials should include multiple adequately sized cohorts, such as patients with platinum-sensitive disease and those with platinum-refractory disease. In addition, patients should probably be stratified by the length of their treatment-free interval. In general, in phase II trials, response rates of more than 25% to 30% are expected for active agents being tested in the platinum-sensitive population, and response rates of greater than 10% to 15% are considered promising in the platinum-resistant population.

A current issue of debate is whether recurrent ovarian cancer is better managed by sequential single-agent therapy or combination chemotherapy. Two European reports suggest combination therapy is superior. One trial (ICON4/AGO-OVAR 2.2) reported on more than 800 patients. The patient population was "very platinum-sensitive," with more than 75% of the patients having more than a 12-month platinum-free interval. After a median follow-up of 42 months, analysis showed the combination had a 2-year survival of 57% vs 50% for the platinum-only treated patients, and the median survival difference was 29 months versus 24 months. This study has been the subject of some criticisms. The study was an analysis of multiple parallel trials conducted by difference groups involving five countries and 119 hospitals. The platinum agent was either cisplatin or carboplatin. The treatments were given monthly. A number of the patients had not previously received a taxane, and there was no difference in outcome if the patient previously received a taxane in their primary therapy. Thus, considering most patients receive a taxane and carboplatin for primary therapy in the United States, the application of this experience to our U.S. population is questioned. Other smaller studies, including a Spanish study (GEICO), also suggested the observation that combination therapy in the refractory setting may offer better outcomes. However, in general, in patients with disease-free intervals of longer than 12 months, the tendency is to retreat with taxane plus platinum combinations.

In addition to the rechallenge with platinum, single-agent paclitaxel is often used in the treatment of recurrent disease. In patients with platinum-sensitive disease, although rechallenge with platinum-based combination is favored, paclitaxel as a single agent has moderate response rates, ranging from 20% to 45%. Even in the platinum-resistant disease setting, standard-dose paclitaxel has been shown to produce response rates of 22% to 23%. Kohn and associates evaluated higher doses of paclitaxel, which required hematologic support, and observed a 48% response rate in platinum-refractory patients. As with other agents, these responses were generally of short duration. Nonetheless, paclitaxel should figure prominently in the consideration of second-line therapy for patients who have platinum-resistant disease. In a phase II GOG study, weekly paclitaxel (80 mg/m^2) in the platinum- and paclitaxel-resistant population demonstrated a response rate of more than 20% and was found to be well tolerated. The importance of dose intensity in this setting is being explored in randomized studies throughout the world. The results will have important implications for paclitaxel dose in combination regimens, which are being evaluated both as first-line and second-line therapy.

Along with platinum and paclitaxel, three chemotherapeutic agents have received the most interest in evaluating their role in the treatment of recurrent ovarian cancer: gemcitabine, pegylated liposomal doxorubicin, and topotecan. In addition to activity in recurrent disease, these agents offer the strategy of extending the platinum-free interval. Discussed in detail later, these agents are now being incorporated into clinical trials, in both primary and recurrent disease settings.

The GOG reported a positive phase II trial with a 5-day topotecan (1.5 mg/m^2) regimen (every 21 days), demonstrating a 33% response rate and median response duration of 11.2 months. Even in patients with platinum-resistant disease response rates range from 13% to 17%. Fatigue, anemia, and thrombocytopenia were the prominent toxicities. A weekly regimen of topotecan, administering 3.5 to 4 mg/m^2 on days 1, 8, and 15 on a 28-day cycle has also been used and data comparing the weekly to 5-day regimen are forthcoming. In a phase II study, the use of 5-day topotecan (1.0 mg/m^2) with carboplatin (AUC of 5) in a platinum-sensitive group not only demonstrated a response rate of 40%, but also was well tolerated. Thus topotecan as part of a combination regimen seems to be a promising therapeutic choice for patients with recurrent ovarian cancer.

Gordon and coinvestigators reported a phase III trial in patients with refractory ovarian cancer comparing pegylated liposomal doxorubicin (Doxil), 50 mg/m^2 every 28 days, to topotecan, 1.5 mg/m^2 per day for 5 days every 21 days. In the platinum-refractory patient group, there was no survival difference. In the platinum-sensitive group, there was a 30% decrease in the risk of death for the pegylated liposomal doxorubicin-treated patients (median survival 108 weeks vs 70 weeks).

Pegylated liposomal doxorubicin has demonstrated response rates up to 26% in the platinum-resistant group, making it an attractive option in this patient population. Recently, pegylated liposomal doxorubicin was studied as combination therapy in recurrent disease. In the CALYPSO trial, carboplatin in combination with either pegylated liposomal doxorubicin or paclitaxel was evaluated in a randomized trial for patients with relapsed, platinum-sensitive disease. Progression-free survival was 11.3 months for the pegylated liposomal doxorubicin arm compared to 9.4 months for the paclitaxel arm, resulting in an 18% reduction in risk of recurrence. Although generally well tolerated, dose-limiting toxicity includes palmar-plantar erythrodysesthesia.

Although gemcitabine has demonstrated modest activity as a single agent in the refractory setting, in combination with a platinum, most commonly cisplatin, the activity appears substantial. Nagourney and colleagues reported results of treatment with cisplatin (30 mg/m^2) plus gemcitabine (600-750 mg/m^2) on days 1 and 8 in a 21-day cycle. They reported 26% complete responses and 44% partial responses (70% overall response rate) with a median time to progression, for responders, of 7.9 months (range 2.1-13.2 months). Neutropenia, anemia, thrombocytopenia, nausea and vomiting, and peripheral neuropathy were problematic toxicities. Additional studies suggest that gemcitabine may reverse cisplatin resistance and may be a useful combination for both platinum-sensitive and platinum-resistant groups.

Bevacizumab for the treatment of ovarian cancer in the recurrent setting has also demonstrated activity. In 62 patients, both platinum-sensitive and platinum-resistant patients, single-agent bevacizumab (15 mg/kg every 21 days) demonstrated a response rate of 21%. In a predominantly platinum-resistant group, bevacizumab (15 mg/kg every 21 days) resulted in a 16% overall response rate. Although gastrointestinal perforation rates ranged from 0% to 11% in these studies, both cohorts were composed of patients who had received multiple chemotherapy regimens prior to the use of bevacizumab. Bevacizumab has also been studied in combination with other agents. The addition of bevacizumab to cytotoxic agents has also been shown to have activity in this setting. Response rates range from 15% to 43% and include combinations with gemcitabine, taxanes, cyclophosphamide, liposomal doxorubicin, 5-fluorouracil, and erlotinib. To further elucidate bevacizumab's role in the recurrent platinum-sensitive population, studies such as the OCEANS trial evaluating bevacizumab with gemcitabine and carboplatin and GOG 213 evaluating bevacizumab with carboplatin and paclitaxel are under way.

Intraperitoneal therapy (discussed elsewhere in this chapter) has been used with several antineoplastic agents as second-line therapy in ovarian cancer. Activity is essentially limited to patients with small-volume residual disease (<0.5 cm in maximal diameter) when the second-line therapy program is initiated. In the absence of a randomized phase III trial, the ultimate impact of these surgically documented responses on survival is difficult to evaluate. Although rare, long-term disease-free survival in patients with small-volume refractory disease has been reported after intraperitoneal therapy.

There is limited evidence of sustained benefit from second-line therapy in patients with ovarian cancer. Overall, only modest response rates with short durations of response have been reported. In addition, there has been a lack of consistency in these studies with regard to key definitions, such as platinum sensitivity compared to platinum resistance. Future second-line trials should clearly define their patients in these two categories. It may also be necessary to discuss paclitaxel-sensitive versus paclitaxel-resistant lesions in the future. Platinum-sensitive patients are appropriate for pilot studies of platinum combinations incorporating different cytotoxic mechanisms of action and dose schedule investigations. Patients with platinum resistance are good candidates for novel investigational approaches and studies of drug resistance. Various other agents, such as hexamethylmelamine, 5-fluorouracil, etoposide, and others will rarely induce modest short-duration responses.

Radiation to the abdomen and pelvis has been used in select second-line situations. Whole-abdomen irradiation with a pelvic boost has been given in patients with minimal disease at second-look surgical reassessment for ovarian carcinoma. With limited follow-up, some studies report as many as 30% of such patients have remained in remission. However, our experience is that with longer follow-up periods, more than 90% of patients will have recurrence, even in this optimal group.

Targeted Therapy

The area with the most rapid development in regard to ovarian cancer treatment is in the area of targeted therapeutics. Secondary to the toxicities and emerging resistance, alternatives or additions to chemotherapy are coming to the forefront. This is best demonstrated with bevacizumab, described earlier, which has been studied in the primary and recurrent setting and in maintenance therapy. Multiple other agents are now under investigation.

Tyrosine kinase inhibitors, which target vascular endothelial growth factor receptors (VEGFR), inhibit an important target in ovarian cancer. The most studied agent in this group, cediranib, has demonstrated response rates of 41% and 29% in platinum-sensitive and platinum-resistant groups, respectively. As a result of this activity, Cediranib is being further evaluated in the phase III randomized trial ICON-6 in conjunction with carboplatin and paclitaxel in the primary setting.

Poly-ADP ribose polymerase (PARP) inhibitors have recently garnered interest in ovarian cancer treatment. PARP is an enzyme responsible for the repair of DNA single-strand breaks. Inhibition of the PARP repair mechanism is particularly effective in tumors where homologous double-stranded repair mechanism is also deficient, such as in patients with BRCA mutations. Olaparib, a PARP-1 inhibitor, was not only well tolerated but demonstrated response rates ranging from 33% to 41% in patients with a known BRCA mutation. Studies have shown that many sporadic epithelial cancers may be BRCA deficient, as a result of inactivation of a BRCA allele despite intact BRCA gene status. Thus the use of PARP inhibitors, alone or in combination, is now being studied in epithelial ovarian cancer irrespective of BRCA status.

Inhibition of the epidermal growth factor receptor (EGFR), which affects cell proliferation, angiogenesis, and apoptosis, has emerged as a possible therapeutic option for patients with ovarian cancer. Agents in this category may inhibit EGFR through tyrosine kinase inhibition (erlotinib, gefitinib, CI-1033) and monoclonal antibodies (trastuzumab, cetuximab). Patients with refractory, recurrent ovarian cancer have demonstrated modest activity to EGFR inhibitors. Currently studies are evaluating the role of EGFR in the recurrent and maintenance setting, both as a single agent and in combination with other cytotoxic or biologic agents. A multitude of other molecular agents have also been evaluated in epithelial ovarian cancer. VEGFs trap, which inhibit VEGF and platelet growth factors, targeted angiogenesis and have shown some activity in the platinum-resistant group and are under further investigation. The mTOR inhibitors (temsirolimus, everolimus, deforolimus) target the PI3K/AKT/mTOR pathway and have recently been studied in phase II evaluations. The use of this agent in combination with other biologic and cytotoxic therapy is currently under way. Other agents being further evaluated include platelet-derived growth factor inhibitors, multikinase inhibitors (sorafenib, dasatinib), and folate receptor inhibitors.

The advent of molecular targets has been promising to date; however, it is still premature in understanding its true role. As information regarding the genetics of cancer and activity at the cellular level increases, this class of agents will have more applicability in cancer care. However, improving our understanding into these agents, providing selective use in specific populations, and maximizing efficiency in conjunction with cytotoxic therapies will be of continued importance.

Surgery for Recurrent Disease

Because recurrence is more the rule than the exception for women with ovarian cancer, in addition to chemotherapy, the role of surgery has been evaluated. The philosophy of secondary cytoreductive surgery is similar to that of primary cytoreductive surgery: Reduce disease burden to enhance the effectiveness of chemotherapy. To date, there are no prospective trials comparing secondary cytoreductive surgery to chemotherapy. Although several retrospective studies have shown benefit in specific groups of patients, the role of secondary cytoreductive surgery may be limited to select patients. Factors associated with a perceived survival benefit including the following: patients with a good performance status; a longer disease-free interval, typically more than 12 months; and patients with disease localized to one or two sites. The most significant contributor to overall survival is the ability to resect all macroscopic disease at the time of recurrent disease. This has been demonstrated in a European multi-institutional review (DESKTOP OVAR) that showed that only patients who were able to undergo complete resection of recurrent disease benefit from surgical intervention. This finding was also reported in a meta-analysis, confirming that the only factor associated with survival benefit was complete resection of disease. Presently, the role of cytoreductive surgery in the recurrent setting is being evaluated in two prospective studies, DESKTOP II and a GOG study (protocol 213). Ideally these studies will help elucidate the ideal patients and the true role of surgery for patients with recurrent ovarian cancer. Until the results are available, therapy should be individualized.

When the focus of care shifts from a curative intent to quality of life, surgery may play a role in the relief of symptoms. Although the risks and morbidity from invasive procedures must be considered, several situations during the terminal stages of the disease may be amenable by surgical intervention. Most commonly, this pertains to patients who develop an intestinal obstruction. Surgery may afford relief of symptoms by resecting the area followed by reanastomosis or performing an intestinal bypass. To decrease morbidity, patients with a distal obstruction may be excellent candidates for a diverting ostomy or intraluminal stent placement. For patients with a more proximal obstruction, endoscopic or percutaneous placement of a gastrostomy tube may provide symptomatic relief. Although occurring less frequently than gastrointestinal blockage, malignant urologic obstructions may also occur with recurrent disease. To minimize morbidity, and depending on the location of the obstruction, treatment options include the placement of ureteral stents, percutaneous nephrostomy tubes, or a suprapubic catheter.

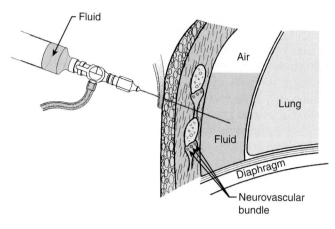

FIGURE 11-27   Thoracentesis.

TABLE 11-25   Relative Survival Percentage* for Women During Three Time Periods

Site	Periods, by Cancer Site		
	1974-1976	1984-1986	2001-2007
All sites	56	58	67
Breast	75	80	90
Colon	50	57	68
Lung and bronchus	16	16	19
Ovary	36	39	44
Pancreas	2	3	6

Source: SEER Program, 1975-2008, National Cancer Institute, 2011.
*5-year relative survival rates based on follow-up of patients through 2008.

Patients with refractory disease may also develop ascites that significantly compromise their quality of life. This may result in a multitude of symptoms, including abdominal pain or discomfort, and respiratory embarrassment. Unfortunately, some patients develop ascites that cannot be controlled by systemic chemotherapy and they may require periodic aspiration. Although a palliative paracentesis may be adequate, patients with refractory, symptomatic ascites may benefit from the use of a long-term catheter. Patients may be found to have pleural effusions during the time of primary or recurrent disease diagnosis, which may present with symptoms of respiratory compromise. This may be a direct result of pleural disease or indirect result secondary to abdominal ascites. Similar techniques for the management of ascites can be used for pleural effusions. Thoracentesis (Figure 11-27), which may be used for immediate relief of symptoms, is often used. When patients develop refractory reaccumulations, they may require insertion of an indwelling pleural catheter or chest tube drainage followed by pleurodesis. Pleurodesis can be performed with the instillation of bleomycin (60-120 mg) or talc into the pleural cavity and offers the highest probability of successful palliation.

REHABILITATION

The nature of ovarian cancer is such that the major vital organs (lungs, heart, liver, and kidneys) remain unaffected. The disease itself and its therapy appear primarily to attack the gastrointestinal tract. Indeed, the terminal event for most patients who succumb to this disease is electrolyte imbalance caused by prolonged gastrointestinal obstruction, malnutrition, and significant protein and electrolyte loss from repeated paracentesis and thoracentesis. It is necessary to support these patients with various forms of alimentation during therapy to sustain them sufficiently to tolerate the somewhat vigorous therapy often prescribed. The placement of semipermanent Silastic intravenous catheters (e.g., Hickman, Broviac, or Groshong) greatly facilitates the ability to support these patients (Figure 11-28). Some clinicians prefer to gain intravenous access by means of a device (Port-A-Cath) implanted in the subcutaneous tissue. Many centers can arrange intravenous alimentation at home for patients who are unable to take sufficient nourishment by mouth. Home pharmacy services are available in many areas, and intravenous medications, including analgesics, can be administered at home by pump infusion devices through these semipermanent intravenous catheters.

In general, the most discouraging aspect in the management of patients with ovarian cancer is the apathy of many physicians. In truth, these diseases are discouraging, but a determined attitude is medically sound and reassuring to the patient. Significant numbers of patients referred to oncologic centers as "unresectable" not only have had their tumor debulked, but also have responded nicely to postoperative therapy. Still other patients have survived complicated combinations of multiple surgical and adjuvant therapies. A positive approach to the disease, which restores hope in the patient with this devastating illness, is justified on that basis alone.

CONCLUSIONS ON MANAGEMENT

Although adenocarcinoma of the ovary remains one of the solid tumors most sensitive to chemotherapeutic regimens, the mortality from this disease remains high. Progress over the past 30 years has been modest and, although there has been some improvement in survival, there is significant opportunity to do better (Table 11-25). There appears, however, to be great promise with newer developments in the management of this disease.

When treating a patient with ovarian cancer, the following general principles should be kept in mind. An

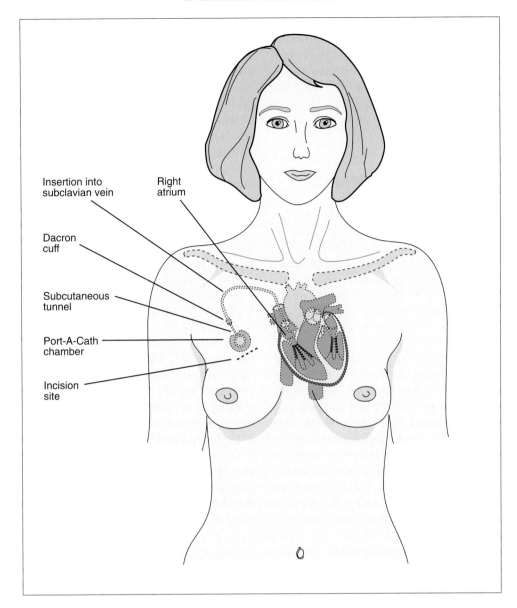

Insertion into
subclavian vein

Right
atrium

Dacron
cuff

Subcutaneous
tunnel

Port-A-Cath
chamber

Incision
site

FIGURE 11-28   Silicone rubber catheter tunneled subcutaneously and positioned in right atrium.

optimal surgical procedure should be carried out when-ever possible. This is defined as the removal of all bulk tumor with the intent to leave no macroscopic residual disease. It is not possible to advocate any one operation for all patients, and the clinician must make a judgment at the time of surgery. Unquestionably, patients with small residual tumor volumes have a better prognosis with any postoperative therapy. Even when optimal debulking is not possible, bilateral salpingo-oophorectomy, total abdominal hysterectomy, and omentectomy may afford significant palliation for the patient. Second, the use of a chemotherapeutic regimen, containing platinum and taxane, plays an integral role in the care of patients with advanced disease. Recent advances in the route of administration

(IP chemotherapy), use of dose-dense paclitaxel, and addition of bevacizumab are encouraging and need to be verified with further clinical trials. Physicians should offer patients treatment on clinical trials whenever available.

Advances in genetics have helped increase our under-standing regarding the natural history of ovarian cancer. Tumor suppressor genes such as BRCA1, BRCA2, and p53 and oncogenes including K-ras and erb-b2 are known to be altered in a fair number ovarian cancer cases. Developing specific targets for known genetic or cellular functions within tumors has become a popular area of interest and shows potential in early studies.

The role of continued surveillance for recurrent disease continues to evolve; thus it is important to counsel patients on symptoms of recurrence, thus providing early intervention. When a recurrence is detected, multimodality treatment options, including surgery and chemotherapy, are available. Although, to date, therapies for recurrent disease have been short-lived with modest efficacy, promising new combinations of chemotherapy and biologic agents are being studied in hopes of improving outcomes.

CURRENT AREAS OF RESEARCH

Over the past several decades, the majority of advances in ovarian cancer treatment have resulted from phase III trial outcomes. These results include the combination of more effective chemotherapeutic agents, more effective route of administration, better understanding of drug resistance, and the addition of biologic response modifiers as a new modality, each strategy improving the outcome for this devastating group of malignant neoplasms.

Chemotherapy has proved curative in some types of advanced cancers and is useful as an adjunct to surgery and radiotherapy in many others. That 90% of the cures with chemotherapy occur in 10% of the tumors that afflict humans is a perplexing biologic problem that appears to be related to the greater propensity of some tissue to develop specific and permanent resistance to chemotherapy of a broad nature. A discussion of tumor cell resistance is beyond the scope of this section; however, understanding and overcoming the mechanisms by which tumor resistance occurs will be necessary to improve treatment outcomes.

Although much has been learned about ovarian cancer and treatment modalities, the surface has just been scratched. With the explosion of new techniques to explore the genetic and molecular biology of this disease, many avenues for research are open and need exploration. The establishment of the GOG tumor and serum bank will continue to allow further investigation into these and many other aspects of molecular biology.

In addition to biologic targets, there are data supporting experimental therapies, such as gene therapy. Although gene therapy in its infancy, if the genetic defect is identified, the gene could be replaced. Many types of gene therapy are possible: immunogene, antioncogene, and tumor suppressor gene; anti-growth factor and cytokine gene drug resistance; and genes that are associated with apoptosis. All of these may be attractive, and preliminary studies have been started. Because of the emergence of chemotherapy resistance, new agents that have non–cross-resistance properties and novel approaches to modulations or targeting are sought. Many new drugs are in the pipeline to be evaluated in phase II studies.

More recently, receiving much deserved attention is a focus on patient's quality of life. Reliable and valid tools for measuring quality of life on multiple facets have been developed and are being incorporated into study protocols by the GOG and other cooperative group studies. These areas of study include symptoms related to cancer and surgical intervention, toxicities associated with therapy, and factors related to psychological stress. Other topics of interest include measurements of pain management, sexual function, and social support. This area is a challenge, and continuing studies will improve our ability to deliver optimal comprehensive care to our patients.

For full reference list, log onto www.expertconsult.com
⟨http://www.expertconsult.com⟩.

Germ Cell, Stromal, and Other Ovarian Tumors

Michael A. Bidus, MD, John C. Elkas, MD, and G. Scott Rose, MD

GERM CELL TUMORS

Classification

The germ cell tumors group of ovarian neoplasms consists of several histologically different tumor types and embraces all the neoplasms considered to be ultimately derived from the primitive germ cells of the embryonic gonad (Figure 12-1). This concept of germ cell tumors as a specific group of gonadal neoplasms has evolved in the last five decades and become generally accepted. This acceptance is based primarily on the common histogenesis of these neoplasms, on the relatively common presence of histologically different tumor elements within the same tumor mass, on the presence of histologically similar neoplasms in extragonadal locations along the line of migration of the primitive germ cells from the wall of the yolk sac to the gonadal ridge and on the remarkable homology between the various tumor types in men and women. In no other group of gonadal neoplasms has this homology been better illustrated. An example of this is the striking similarity between the testicular seminoma and its ovarian counterpart, the dysgerminoma. These were the first neoplasms to become accepted as originating from germ cells. A number of classifications of germ cell neoplasms of the ovary have been proposed over the past few decades. Table 12-1 shows a modification of a classification that was originally described by Teilum and is similar to that proposed by the World Health Organization, which divides the germ cell tumors into several groups and also includes neoplasms composed of germ cells and "sex" stroma derivatives.

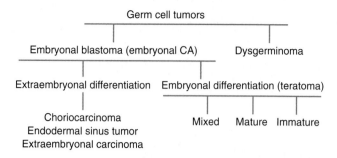

FIGURE 12-1   Classification schema of germ cell tumors of ovary.

TABLE 12-1   Classification of Germ Cell Neoplasms of the Ovary

GERM CELL TUMORS

Dysgerminoma
Endodermal sinus tumor
Embryonal carcinoma
Polyembryoma
Choriocarcinomas
Teratoma
  Immature (solid, cystic, or both)
  Mature
    Solid
    Cystic
      Mature cystic teratoma (dermoid cyst)
      Mature cystic teratoma (dermoid cyst) with malignant
        transformation
  Monodermal or highly specialized
    Struma ovarii
    Carcinoid
    Struma ovarii and carcinoid
    Others
    Mixed forms (tumors composed of types A-F in any possible
      combination)

TUMORS COMPOSED OF GERM CELLS AND SEX CORD–STROMAL DERIVATIVE

Gonadoblastoma
Mixed germ cell–sex cord stromal tumor

Germ cell tumors are classified according to degree of differentiation. Two classes exist:

- Undifferentiated germ cell tumors, which include dysgerminoma and gonadoblastoma; and
- Differentiated tumors, which include all other germ cell tumors.

Differentiated tumors are further classified as to whether the tumor differentiates histologically into embryonic or extraembryonic structures. Extraembryonic tumors include choriocarcinoma, endodermal sinus tumor, and extraembryonal tumors. Embryonal tumors include embryonal carcinoma, polyembryoma, and teratomas that may be mature, immature, monodermal, or

TABLE 12-2   Relative Frequency of Ovarian Neoplasms

Type	%
Coelomic epithelium	50-70
Germ cell	15-20
Specialized gonadal stroma	5-10
Nonspecific mesenchyme	5-10
Metastatic tumor	5-10

highly specialized. Finally, it is important to recognize that germ cell tumors clinically behave in part on whether they are histologically pure, consisting of only one cell type, or mixed. Clinical behavior typically conforms to the most aggressive histologic subtype present in mixed tumors. Treatment therefore should be predicated on this knowledge.

Clinical Profile

Germ cell tumors represent a relatively small proportion (20%) of all ovarian tumors (Table 12-2) but are becoming increasingly important in the clinical practice of obstetrics and gynecology. Of these tumors, 97% are benign and only 3% are malignant. Although rare reports (nine families total) of familial clustering of ovarian and testicular germ cell tumors have been described in the literature, there is no known syndrome or genetic abnormality conferring susceptibility to germ cell malignancies. With respect to race, Asian and black ethnic groups are affected by malignant germ cell tumors three times as frequently as white women. However, a recent review of cases reported to the Surveillance, Epidemiology and End Results (SEER) database from 1988 to 2004 revealed improved survival in white women compared to black women, a finding attributable to a more favorable stage distribution in whites and a more favorable histology. In this study, white patients were twice as likely as black patients to have dysgerminoma and 1.5 times less likely to have immature teratoma. Advanced-stage tumors were more common in black patients. On multivariate analysis, race was not an independent predictor for survival after controlling for staging, histology, and stage of disease.

Most germ cell tumors occur in young women. A SEER database review of malignant germ cell tumors from 1973 to 2002 revealed the highest incidence rates of disease in the 15- to 19-year age group. Survival rates in this study improved over time but were lower for older women and varied by histologic subtype, with dysgerminoma having the most favorable survival rates, and by stage, with worse survival for advanced-stage patients. Another SEER registry analysis of ovarian tumors in patients younger than 19 years old from 1973 to 2005 revealed that germ cell tumors were the most

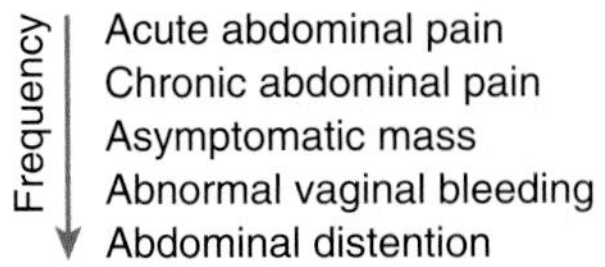

Frequency

Acute abdominal pain
Chronic abdominal pain
Asymptomatic mass
Abnormal vaginal bleeding
Abdominal distention

FIGURE 12-2   Initial symptoms in young patients with malignant germ cell tumors.

common pathologic finding but were associated with excellent 5- and 10-year survival rates in excess of 91%. Similar to prior studies, advanced-stage disease was associated with worse outcomes.

It is not surprising that, because germ cell tumors occur more frequently in young patients, extirpation of the disease involves decisions concerning childbearing and probabilities of recurrence. Recent developments in chemotherapy have dramatically changed the prognosis for many patients who develop more aggressive types of germ cell tumors. Knowledge of the classification of these lesions and how the pathologist arrives at the diagnosis, and the clinical significance of that diagnosis, has great practical value for the practicing obstetrician/gynecologist.

Most of these lesions are found in the second and third decades of life and are frequently diagnosed by finding a palpable abdominal mass, often associated with pain (Figure 12-2). Except for the benign cystic teratoma, ovarian germ cell tumors are usually rapidly enlarging abdominal masses that often cause considerable abdominal pain. At times, the pain is exacerbated by rupture or torsion of the neoplasm. One of the classic initial signs of a dysgerminoma is hemoperitoneum from capsular rupture of the tumor as it rapidly enlarges, although this may occur with any germ cell tumor. Asymptomatic abdominal distention, fever, or vaginal bleeding are occasionally presenting complaints. Isosexual precocious puberty has been described, occurring in young patients whose tumors express human chorionic gonadotropin (hCG).

Because these tumors occur predominantly in the reproductive age group, it is not surprising that they are encountered commonly during pregnancy. Dysgerminomas and teratomas are the most common germ cell tumors diagnosed during pregnancy or after delivery. Surgical evaluation and treatment, including chemotherapy if necessary, can be safely performed in the second and third trimesters. Germ cell tumors are typically rapidly growing, unilateral tumors that present at an early stage (stage I). These tumors spread by direct extension, seeding of abdominal and pelvic peritoneal surfaces, and hematogenous and lymphatic spread. Hematogenous spread to the lungs and liver parenchyma is more common in germ cell malignancies than in epithelial ovarian cancer, as is lymph node spread.

Many germ cell tumors produce serum markers that are specific and sensitive enough to be used clinically in following disease progression. A detailed discussion of individual tumor markers will be presented in the individual sections on specific tumor types.

Staging

Germ cell tumors should be staged surgically in the same manner as epithelial ovarian cancers and in accordance with the International Federation of Gynecologists and Obstetrician (FIGO) guidelines. Because surgical management and adjuvant therapy are predicated in part on stage of disease, accurate staging is essential. Traditionally, all patients with germ cell malignancies except those patients with stage Ia dysgerminoma or stage Ia grade I immature teratoma were treated with adjuvant chemotherapy. Comprehensive staging therefore allows patients to be appropriately risk stratified and selected for surveillance regimens or adjuvant therapy. Proper staging procedures for germ cell tumors consists of a vertical midline incision, a sampling of ascitic fluid if present, cell washings, a careful exploration of the abdomen and pelvic cavity, and random staging biopsies of the omentum, paracolic gutters, pelvic sidewalls, cul-de-sac, vesicouterine reflection, and diaphragm. If extensive disease is present in the abdominal cavity, omentectomy and cytoreduction to optimal residual disease should be performed if possible. Pelvic and para-aortic lymph node sampling should be performed, but a complete lymphadenectomy is not necessary. Bulky lymph nodes, if present, should be removed. Based on an analysis of SEER data, the prevalence of lymph node metastasis in germ cell malignancies is 18% for all patients regardless of histologic subtype. Dysgerminomas have the highest prevalence of disease at 28%, followed by mixed germ cell tumors at 16% and immature teratomas at 8%. After controlling for age, race, stage, and histology, positive lymph nodes remained an independent predictor of poor survival on multivariate analysis.

In spite of the prognostic significance of positive lymph nodes and the obvious benefits of guiding adjuvant therapy, comprehensive surgical staging is frequently not performed. In a paper evaluating compliance with surgical staging guidelines, only 3 patients of 131 with germ cell malignancies had complete staging performed. Failure to perform recommended lymph node sampling was the most common reason for noncompliance (97%), followed by no omentectomy (36%) and no cytologic washing (21%). The decision to proceed with restaging operation for patients who have not been staged at their initial surgical procedure is controversial. Data from the Pediatric Oncology Intergroup suggest that deviations from standard staging requirements do not adversely affect survival.

Treatment Options

Surgery

The initial approach to patients with suspected germ cell tumors is surgical management for both diagnostic and therapeutic intent. The extent of primary surgery is dictated by the findings at surgery and the reproductive desires of the patient. If childbearing has been completed and future fertility is no longer a concern, then a bilateral salpingo-oophorectomy and hysterectomy are performed in addition to a full staging procedure. However, if preservation of fertility is desired, then every attempt should be made to perform a careful staging procedure followed by a unilateral salpingo-oophorectomy. The safety of such an approach has been well established in the literature. In select cases such as stage Ia dysgerminoma and stage Ia grade I immature teratoma, unilateral salpingo-oophorectomy is felt to be curative and is all that is required. All other cases will likely require adjuvant therapy. In all cases of apparent unilateral disease confined to the ovary, the contralateral ovary should be carefully evaluated. Although dysgerminoma is the only germ cell malignancy with a propensity for bilaterality (10% to 20% of cases), other histologic subtypes have occasionally involved both ovaries, so careful inspection is warranted. The contralateral ovary, if abnormal, should be biopsied or a cystectomy should be performed. If frozen section confirms a diagnosis of malignancy, then the ovary should be removed. Frozen section has been shown to be highly accurate for nonteratomatous sex cord stromal and germ cell tumors. If the contralateral ovary appears normal, then it should be left alone. Some clinicians have advocated performing a wedge biopsy of a normal-appearing contralateral ovary in cases of dysgerminoma to detect subclinical or microscopic disease. We recommend avoiding wedge biopsy of a normal-appearing ovary because of the potential for surgical complications such as hemorrhage or adhesion formation that may affect future fertility.

The excellent response of germ cell malignancies to adjuvant chemotherapy has allowed a tailored approach to the surgical management of this disease in women desiring to preserve fertility. Although unilateral salpingo-oophorectomy should be considered the standard procedure in such cases, recently some clinicians have advocated ovarian cystectomy in select cases of immature teratoma. Beiner and colleagues reviewed eight cases of immature teratoma (three grade I, four grade II, and one grade III) treated with ovarian cystectomy. Five of the eight patients received postoperative adjuvant chemotherapy. There were no recurrences in 4.7 years of follow-up, and three patients delivered a total of

seven babies. The authors concluded that ovarian cystectomy with adjuvant chemotherapy appeared to be satisfactory therapy for early-stage immature teratoma if close follow-up was available but that more studies were needed to evaluate cystectomy alone as a surgical management option. This management strategy, although exciting because of the potential for ovarian preservation, should be approached with caution, especially for other histologic germ cell subtypes, which may not share the same prognosis as early-stage immature teratoma.

Patients with bulk disease in the abdomen, pelvis, and retroperitoneum should be surgically cytoreduced to optimal residual disease if at all possible. Although there is scant literature to support such a recommendation, what literature exists suggests a benefit for cytoreduction. In a Gynecologic Oncology Group (GOG) study by Slayton and colleagues, patients with completely resected disease failed subsequent VAC (vincristine, dactinomycin, and cyclophosphamide) chemotherapy in 28% of the cases compared to 68% of cases with incomplete resection of disease. In the same study 82% of cases with bulky residual disease failed chemotherapy compared to 55% with minimal residual disease. Subsequently, the GOG published results showing that patients with clinically nonmeasurable disease after surgery treated with PVB (cisplatin, vinblastine, and bleomycin) remained progression free in 65% of cases compared to 34% of patients with measurable disease. Patients with optimal cytoreduction did better than those with unresectable bulky disease. This study helped establish the efficacy of cisplatin-based chemotherapy for germ cell tumors. Finally, Williams and colleagues showed that patients with completely resected advanced-stage (II and III) disease who were treated with cisplatin, etoposide, and bleomycin had similar tumor-free recurrence rates as those with disease limited to the ovary. These studies provide the bulk of evidence to support the thesis that cytoreduction of advanced-stage disease is advantageous in germ cell cancers.

In patients with bulky metastatic disease, a normal-appearing uterus and contralateral ovary may be preserved, allowing for future fertility options if desired. Tangir and colleagues reviewed 64 patients with germ cell malignancies treated with fertility-preserving surgery. Ten patients were stage III (five IIIc, two IIIb, and three IIIa). Eight of the 10 successfully conceived. Survival data were not included in the analysis. Zanetta and colleagues evaluated 138 women with germ cell malignancies of all stages treated with fertility-sparing surgery, 81 of who received postoperative chemotherapy. Survival was comparable between patients treated with radical surgery and fertility-sparing surgery after a mean follow-up period of 67 months. Low and colleagues retrospectively reviewed 74 patients with germ cell malignancies of all cell types treated with conservative surgery. Forty-seven patients were treated with adjuvant chemotherapy. Fifteen patients had stage III to IV disease. After 52 months of follow-up, patients with advanced disease had a 94% survival, comparable to historical survival rates.

The value of secondary cytoreduction procedures in patients with germ cell malignancies has not been studied. Given the sensitivity of these malignancies to combination chemotherapy regimens, it is highly likely that metastatic lesions will respond to subsequent chemotherapy, making the value of secondary cytoreduction questionable. Limited cytoreduction remains an effective management option for isolated lesions.

In summary, patients with germ cell malignancies should undergo operative evaluation, staging, and cytoreduction. If future fertility is not desired, surgical treatment should be identical to that for epithelial ovarian cancers. If preservation of fertility is desired, conservative management should be used with conservation of the uterus and contralateral ovary and cytoreduction to optimal residual disease should be performed if possible. In spite of the success of surgical management, surgeons should recognize the excellent response of these tumors to chemotherapy when aggressive and potentially morbid resections of metastatic and retroperitoneal disease are considered.

Surveillance for Stage I Tumors

As previously noted, historically in the gynecologic oncology literature only patients with stage Ia dysgerminoma or stage Ia grade I immature teratoma of the ovary have been treated conservatively without adjuvant chemotherapy. This surveillance recommendation has been and continues to be at odds with contemporary management practices in pediatric oncology where patients with grade II and III immature teratomas have been followed with observation only without a compromise in survival. Similarly, male patients with stage I germ cell tumors are followed with observation only as standard practice. Rustin and Patterson published provocative data on their 37-year experience with a liberal surveillance policy for patients with stage I germ cell tumors of the ovary. In their first report, 24 patients with stage Ia germ cell tumor (9 dysgerminoma, 9 pure immature teratoma, and 6 endodermal sinus tumor with or without immature teratoma) were followed without chemotherapy after surgery. Five-year overall survival was 95% and disease-free survival was 68%. Eight patients had a recurrence or developed a second primary germ cell tumor and required chemotherapy. All but one who died of a pulmonary embolus were salvaged with chemotherapy. In their second publication, 37 patients with stage Ia germ cell malignancies were followed with surveillance only after surgery. Twenty-two percent of dysgerminoma and 36% of nondysgerminoma patients had a recurrence. All

but one of these patients were successfully salvaged and cured with cisplatin-based chemotherapy at the time of recurrence. Overall disease-specific survival was 94%. It is unlikely that randomized trials addressing the safety of this approach in ovarian germ cell tumors will be performed. Given the potential serious toxicity associated with bleomycin, etoposide, and cisplatin (BEP) chemotherapy, managing patients with stage 1 germ cell tumors of the ovary with surveillance only is a reasonable option if they have been adequately staged.

Second-Look Laparotomy

The role of the second-look laparotomy (SLL) in germ cell tumors of the ovary is currently being debated. Williams, when reporting the experience of the GOG, noted that in patients with complete tumor resection followed by BEP chemotherapy, 43 of 45 patients had no evidence of tumor or mature teratoma only at the time of the SLL, suggesting that there is no value of SLL in patients with completely resected disease. There were 72 patients with advanced incompletely resected tumors who received chemotherapy followed by SLL. Of 48 patients who did not have teratomatous lesions in their primary surgery, 45 had no tumor. The 3 patients who had persistent tumors died of their disease despite aggressive therapy. These authors think that the role of SLL is rarely, if ever, beneficial if the tumor is almost completely resected initially and followed by adequate chemotherapy. However, patients in this series who had incompletely resected tumors at initial surgery and had teratomatous elements present may have benefited from SLL. There were 24 patients who had teratomatous elements in the primary tumor and 16 who had progressive or bulky mature elements at SLL. Four patients had residual immature teratoma. Fourteen of the 16 with residual teratoma and 6 of the 7 with bulky disease remained tumor free after secondary cytoreduction. Therefore the subgroup of patients that may have significant benefit from SLL are those with incompletely resected disease with teratomatous elements at primary surgery. Other authors in small series have suggested that there is a role for SLL, particularly in patients seen initially with advanced unresected disease. The use of advanced imaging technologies such as positron emission tomography (PET) and computed tomography (CT) imaging may further reduce the impact of SLL. Preliminary studies suggest positive and negative predictive values of 100% and 96%, respectively, for PET imaging in seminomas looking for residual disease after chemotherapy, suggesting the possibility of similar results for germ cell malignancies.

Radiation Therapy

In the past, radiation therapy was traditionally used as adjuvant therapy for patients with germ cell malignancies and dysgerminomas in particular. Historically, dysgerminomas have been extremely sensitive to radiation therapy with overall survival rates of between 70% and 100%. However, with the recent advances and success rates seen with combination chemotherapy, radiation therapy is rarely used today.

Chemotherapy

Tremendous advances have been made in the chemotherapeutic management of germ cell malignancies, such that current management strategies offer even advanced malignancies an excellent chance at long-term control or cure. Historically, VAC was the first combination chemotherapy regimen widely used for treatment of these tumors. However, as a result of the success of cisplatin-based regimens in the treatment of testicular germ cell tumors combined with long-term survival of less than 50% in advanced-stage or incompletely resected ovarian germ cell malignancies, VAC was gradually replaced by PVB (cisplatin, vinblastine, bleomycin). This transition resulted in an improvement in overall survival; however, failures still occurred even in patients with good prognosis at the conclusion of primary surgery.

Based on the success of etoposide therapy in testicular cancer, current combination platinum-based chemotherapy for ovarian germ cell malignancies has evolved to the use of BEP. The GOG prospectively evaluated this regimen in women with stage I to III, completely resected, nondysgerminoma germ cell malignancies given as three cycles of adjuvant chemotherapy. Of 93 patients, 91 were noted to be free of recurrence at follow-up, establishing this regimen as equivalent or superior to PVB. The toxicity profile in this series was acceptable. As a result of these findings, BEP has become the standard chemotherapeutic regimen for the adjuvant treatment of women with germ cell malignancies. Although successful, concern exists over potential long-term pulmonary toxicity of bleomycin and the risk of secondary malignancies associated with etoposide. Traditionally, cisplatin and etoposide are administered over 5 days, whereas bleomycin is administered weekly. Recently Dimopoulos and colleagues demonstrated safety and efficacy of outpatient BEP utilizing a lower dose of bleomycin administered over 3 days in women with early-stage, optimally debulked germ cell malignancies.

Controversy exists regarding the efficacy of high-dose cisplatin used in combination with etoposide and bleomycin (HDBEP). Several adult trials in testicular germ cell malignancies have suggested an improvement in efficacy compared to standard-dose cisplatin, whereas other studies have not seen this association. These studies have not been replicated in adults with ovarian germ cell malignancies. Cushing and colleagues, however, evaluated HDBEP in 74 pediatric patients with ovarian germ cell malignancies and found no difference in overall survival and increased toxicity with the HDBEP regimen. Currently, there is no established role of high-dose therapy in ovarian germ cell tumors.

Current management strategies for germ cell malignancies utilize chemotherapy in an adjuvant setting and to treat recurrent disease. Because approximately 20% of patients with germ cell malignancies treated with surgery alone will be expected to recur, and given the successful long-term outcomes associated with BEP, all patients except those with stage Ia dysgerminoma and stage Ia grade I immature teratoma should be treated with adjuvant chemotherapy to reduce the risk of recurrent disease. Completely resected disease treated in this fashion can be cured nearly 100% of the time. Metastatic or incompletely resected tumors, however, may fare worse but still have excellent long-term survival rates and should be treated aggressively with adjuvant chemotherapy.

Recurrences in Germ Cell Cancer

Even in cases of advanced-stage disease, the majority of patients with germ cell malignancies are cured with a combination of primary surgery and adjuvant combination platinum-based chemotherapy. All patients with germ cell malignancies, especially early-stage disease treated with conservative therapy for curative intent, warrant close follow-up. Recurrences usually occur within 2 years of primary therapy. Patients with early-stage dysgerminoma treated with salpingo-oophorectomy alone can be expected to experience recurrence in 15% to 25% of cases. For all germ cell malignancies, recurrences in many cases can be treated successfully. Recurrences after chemotherapy are defined as platinum resistant or platinum sensitive, a classification with clinical significance because platinum-resistant disease is not thought to be curable. The group at the MD Anderson Hospital noted 42 primary therapy failures in 160 patients with germ cell tumors. Seventeen of these failures were treated with VAC chemotherapy. Using different chemotherapeutic regimens, 12 of 42 (29%) patients are currently disease free. Surgical debulking may have a role in the management of recurrences. In this study, 24 patients had surgery and 12 are alive, all with less than 2 cm of residual disease. None of the 7 patients with more than 2 cm of residual disease survived. More recently, male patients with platinum-resistant or platinum-refractory disease germ cell tumors have been treated with combination chemotherapy consisting of gemcitabine, oxaliplatin, and paclitaxel. This regimen has an acceptable toxicity profile, a 51% overall response rate, and a 39% complete or tumor marker negative response rate. Median response duration was

8 months. For patients with platinum-resistant or platinum-refractory disease, optimal treatment has not been defined and prognosis overall is poor.

Treatment Toxicity

Given the favorable long-term outcomes associated with modern surgical management and combination platinum-based chemotherapy for women with germ cell malignancies, the long-term effects of treatment toxicity cannot be ignored. Because many of these patients desire future fertility and undergo conservative surgery for their disease, meticulous surgical technique is essential to avoid future infertility related to surgically induced pelvic adhesive disease. Equally important is avoiding unnecessary hysterectomies and biopsies of normal-appearing contralateral ovaries. A thorough understanding of the natural history and management options of these tumors is essential. Women with fertility-sparing surgery can be expected to have the same survival outcome as those patients treated with standard surgery. A review of SEER data from 1988 to 2001 involving 760 patients with germ cell malignancies concluded that the overall survival of patients treated with fertility-sparing surgery ($n = 313$) was not statistically different compared to those who were subjected to standard surgery. This study revealed that the use of fertility-sparing surgery also had increased over the study period. Two thirds of the patients had stage I to II disease, and one third had stage III to IV disease. The most common histologic subtype was immature teratoma (55%) followed by dysgerminoma (32%).

The long-term effect of combination chemotherapy in germ cell malignancies is less clear. Of particular concern is the risk of development of acute myelogenous leukemia (AML) associated with etoposide use. This risk appears to be dose and schedule dependent. AML rarely has been noted in patients receiving three cycles or less of etoposide or cumulative doses of less than 2000 mg/m². It is estimated that the risk of developing AML is 0.4% if these cutoff values are used. Leukemia, when it occurs, typically is seen within 2 to 3 years after treatment. Unlike in ovarian epithelial cancer, in which patients may not be expected to survive until the risk of developing AML is real, patients with germ cell malignancies are expected to survive well beyond the time when AML usually occurs. In spite of this risk, an analysis of the risk-to-benefit ratio favors the use of etoposide in advanced germ cell malignancies, in which one case of etoposide-induced AML would be expected to occur for every 20 patients cured.

The long-term effects of chemotherapy on gonadal function appear to be minimal. Most younger patients can expect a return to normal ovarian function and reproductive potential with no additional risk of congenital malformations in their offspring. The most significant risk factor for impaired fertility is age and type of treatment administered. Although ovarian failure is a risk associated with chemotherapy, factors such as older age at treatment, higher drug doses, and long duration of therapy appear to confer higher risk. Childhood cancer patients treated with standard contemporary agents such as BEP have the greatest likelihood of preservation of fertility, resumption of normal menstrual cycles, and normal sexual development by virtue of the higher number of follicles present in young women compared to older women. Although normal menstrual cycles will likely resume in reproductive-age women, data suggest that diminished ovarian reserve resulting in a significant reduction in the probability of pregnancy by 50% is present in these patients as determined by reduced ovarian volume compared to controls, fewer antral follicles on ultrasonography, and lower levels of inhibin B and estradiol on cycle days 2 to 5. Alkylating agents such as cyclophosphamide are far more likely to cause toxicity to the gonads than other chemotherapeutic agents. In one study, alkylating agents had an odds ratio (OR) of 4 for causing premature ovarian failure, compared to platinum agents (OR 1.8) or plant alkaloids (OR 1.2).

There is a convincing body of literature to suggest that gonadotropin-releasing hormone (GnRH) agonists may be cytoprotective for primordial follicles when given during chemotherapy. Most of these data are retrospective; however, recently Badawy and colleagues reported on a prospective randomized trial in 80 breast cancer patients younger than age 40 who were randomly assigned to GnRH agonists with chemotherapy or chemotherapy alone. Ninety percent of study patients resumed menses and 70% resumed spontaneous ovulation within 8 months of completing therapy, compared to 33% and 26% of control patients, respectively. In the setting of germ cell malignancies, in which younger age at diagnosis is the norm, these patients tolerate therapy quite well.

Dysgerminoma

Dysgerminoma is the most common germ cell malignancy, accounting for 1% to 2% of primary ovarian neoplasms and for 3% to 5% of ovarian malignancies. Dysgerminoma may occur at any age from infancy to old age, with reported cases ranging between the ages of 7 months and 70 years, but most cases occurring in adolescence and early adulthood (Figure 12-3). They also present at a relatively early stage:

Stage Ia	65% to 75%
Stage Ib	10% to 15%
Stages II and III	15%
Stage IV	5%

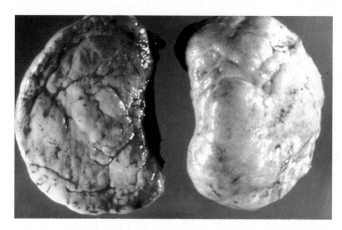

FIGURE 12-3   Large (25 cm) solid mass of the right ovary in a 16-year-old girl with stage Ia dysgerminoma.

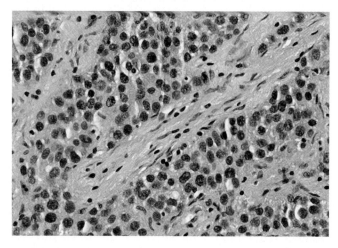

FIGURE 12-4   Dysgerminoma is characterized histologically by the presence of large, round, ovoid, or polygonal cells with stroma infiltrated by lymphocytes.

Dysgerminoma consists of germ cells that have not differentiated to form embryonic or extraembryonic structures (Figure 12-4). The stroma is almost always infiltrated with lymphocytes and often contains granulomas similar to those of sarcoid. Occasionally, dysgerminoma contains isolated gonadotropin-producing syncytiotrophoblastic giant cells. An elevated serum lactate dehydrogenase or human chorionic gonadotropin (hCG) level may be present in these patients. Grossly, the tumor may be firm, fleshy, cream colored, or pale tan; both its external and cut surfaces may be lobulated. A few dysgerminomas arise in sexually abnormal females, particularly those with pure (46, XY) or mixed (45, X, 46, XY) gonadal dysgenesis or testicular feminization (46, XY). In such cases, the dysgerminoma often develops in a previously existing gonadoblastoma. The symptoms of dysgerminoma are not distinctive, and they are similar to those observed in patients with other solid ovarian neoplasms. The duration of symptoms is usually short; however, despite this, the tumor is often large, indicating rapid growth. The most common initial symptoms are abdominal enlargement and the presence of a mass in the lower abdomen. When the tumor is small and moves freely, its capsule is intact. Large lesions, however, may rupture or adhere to surrounding structures. Rupture can lead to peritoneal implantation, resulting in an increase in stage. In several cases, the tumor has been found incidentally at cesarean section or as a cause of dystocia. Dysgerminoma is the most common malignant ovarian neoplasm observed in pregnancy. The relatively common finding of dysgerminoma in pregnant patients is nonspecific and relates to the age of the patient rather than to the pregnant state. Dysgerminoma may also be discovered incidentally in patients investigated for primary amenorrhea; in these cases, it is frequently associated with gonadal dysgenesis and a gonadoblastoma. Occasionally, menstrual and endocrine abnormalities may be the initial symptoms, but these symptoms tend to be more common in patients with dysgerminoma combined with other neoplastic germ cell elements—especially choriocarcinoma. Dysgerminoma is the only germ cell tumor in which the opposite ovary is frequently involved with the tumor process (10% to 20% of cases). Kurman reported a 20% incidence of disease in the serially sectioned normal appearing opposite ovary. Dysgerminomas are notable by their predilection for lymphatic spread and their acute sensitivity to irradiation and chemotherapy. Metastatic spread occurs via the lymphatic system; the lymph nodes in the vicinity of the common iliac arteries and the terminal part of the abdominal aorta are the first to be affected. Occasionally, there may be marked enlargement of these lymph nodes, with a mass evident on abdominal examination. The lesion can spread from these abdominal nodes to the mediastinal and supraclavicular nodes. Hematogenous spread to other organs occurs later. Any organ can be affected, although involvement of the liver, lungs, and bones is most common. Historically, surgery followed by radiation (in both early- and late-stage disease) has resulted in an excellent cure rate. More recently, the use of multiple-agent chemotherapy has produced equivalent results. In the young woman with a unilateral encapsulated dysgerminoma who is desirous of future childbearing, conservative management is indicated. In a review of the literature, more than 400 cases of dysgerminoma were reported. Seventy percent of patients had stage I disease at diagnosis and only 10% involved both ovaries. Because 85% of all patients with dysgerminomas are younger than 30 years, conservative therapy and preservation of fertility are major considerations. Conservative surgery without radiation or adjuvant chemotherapy in stage Ia lesions has resulted in excellent outcomes (Table 12-3). In patients in whom unilateral

TABLE 12-3   Results of Conservative and Nonconservative Surgery in Stage Ia Dysgerminoma of the Ovary

	10-Year Survival	
	Conservative Surgery (%)	Nonconservative Therapy* (%)
Asadourian and Taylor	42/46 (91)[†]	21/25 (84)
Gordon et al.	68/72 (94)[†]	11/14 (79)
Malkasian and Symmonds	23/27 (85)[†]	13/14 (93)
Total	133/145 (92)[†]	45/53 (85)

*Surgery plus radiation.
[†]Includes those salvaged after a recurrence (23/25% to 92%).

salpingo-oophorectomy is performed, careful inspection of the contralateral ovary and exploration to rule out disseminated disease is mandatory. Assessment of the retroperitoneal lymph nodes is an important part of the initial surgical therapy because these neoplasms tend to spread to the lymph nodes, particularly to the high para-aortic nodes. Pelvic nodes on the same side as the primary tumor should also be evaluated through a retroperitoneal incision. Our routine is not to wedge or bivalve the opposite ovary if it has a normal size, shape, and consistency.

Several prognostic factors in dysgerminoma may be important because they might influence conservative therapy in the early stage of disease. Some authors suggest that in patients with large tumors (>10 cm), there is a greater chance of a recurrence; therefore, adjuvant therapy should be given. Today, most agree that tumor size is not prognostically important and these patients do not require additional therapy. The long-term survival is almost 90% in patients who have stage I lesions. There is presently no good evidence that the behavior of an individual tumor can be assessed from its histologic appearance. Some authors consider patients older than 40 years or younger than 20 years to have a worsened prognosis, but this is not consistent in all studies. The presence of other germ cell elements definitely worsens prognosis.

Some recent series are reporting 100% survival with conservative surgery in stage Ia patients. These data strongly support an initial conservative approach with preservation of fertility. More extensive surgery and radiation therapy were not beneficial when patients had disease limited to one ovary. Schwartz and colleagues reported four patients with metastasis to the contralateral ovary and preservation of that ovary with subsequent chemotherapy. All patients were alive and had no disease 14 to 56 months after diagnosis.

De Palo and associates reported on 56 patients who had pure dysgerminomas. In their study 44 patients underwent lymphangiography, and a positive study resulted in the restaging of 32% of patients. Diaphragmatic implants were not found in any patients, and positive cytologic findings were obtained in only 3 patients. The 5-year relapse-free survival rates were 91% in patients with stages Ia, Ib, and Ic; 74% in those with stage III retroperitoneal disease; and 24% in patients who had stage III peritoneal disease. Peritoneal involvement of any kind was associated with a poor prognosis if disease had extended to the abdominal cavity. All patients with stage III disease received postoperative radiation therapy.

These patients should be followed closely and have periodic examinations because approximately 90% of recurrences appear in the first 2 years after initial therapy. Fortunately, most recurrences can be successfully eradicated by salvage therapy including surgery, radiation therapy, and chemotherapy. This knowledge permits the conservative management of patients. Recurrences should be treated aggressively with re-exploration and tumor reduction. The removed tissue should be examined carefully for evidence of germ cell elements other than dysgerminoma. Some presumed recurrent dysgerminomas have been found to be mixed germ cell tumors and should be treated accordingly.

Although radiation therapy has been successful in treating dysgerminomas, more recently chemotherapy appears to have become the treatment of choice because radiotherapy is associated with a high incidence of gonadal failure. The success rate of chemotherapy is as good as that of radiation, and preservation of fertility is possible in many patients, even those with bilateral ovarian disease. Weinblatt and Ortega reported on five children with extensive disease who were treated with chemotherapy as the primary therapeutic modality. Three of the five children were alive and free of disease at the time of the report, suggesting a therapeutic approach to extensive childhood dysgerminoma that spares pelvic and reproductive organs.

Chemotherapy is also being used more frequently with significant success in patients who have advanced disease. Dysgerminomas are typically very sensitive to platinum-based chemotherapy and most patients treated with combination platinum-based chemotherapy will be complete responders. Bianchi and associates reported 18 patients (6 patients with stage Ib or Ic and 12 patients with stage IIb, III, IV, or recurrent disease) who were treated with doxorubicin and cyclophosphamide or cisplatin, vinblastine, and bleomycin. Doxorubicin and cyclophosphamide were highly effective: 7 of 10 patients were disease free; 2 of 3 relapsing patients were saved with VBP therapy. Of the 8 patients treated with VBP, 1 had a recurrence in the brain and was saved with radiation therapy. Four patients who had no residual disease in the remaining ovary or in the uterus are all free of disease, and 1 patient has had a successful pregnancy.

The optimal drug combination has not yet been determined. Because bleomycin can cause pulmonary fibrosis with resultant death, the drug is being used less frequently. Etoposide also appears to be an effective drug in the treatment of dysgerminomas. More recently, patients with advanced disease have received multiple-agent chemotherapy with results equal to or better than results for those treated with radiation. Complete responses in the 80% to 100% range are being reported in patients with stage II to IV disease. This is not surprising—the cure rates for stage III dysgerminomas treated with effective chemotherapy are greater than 90%. Today, chemotherapy appears to be the treatment of choice after surgery in patients with advanced disease. Based on a growing body of literature demonstrating the effectiveness of BEP chemotherapy in patients with ovarian germ cell tumors and seminomas in male patients, our preferred combination chemotherapy regimen for patients with dysgerminoma requiring chemotherapy is BEP.

The common association of dysgerminoma with gonadoblastoma, a tumor that almost always occurs in patients with dysgenetic gonads, indicates that there is a relationship between dysgerminoma and genetic and somatosexual abnormalities. Patients with these genetic abnormalities should be offered gonadectomy after puberty to prevent the development of gonadoblastoma or dysgerminoma. Phenotypically normal females suspected of having a dysgerminoma should be evaluated with a karyotype, especially if ovarian conservation is desired. Patients with pathology reports that reveal streak gonads or gonadoblastomas should also be karyotyped. If a Y chromosome is present, the retained contralateral ovary should be removed to prevent neoplasia. As stated earlier, the treatment of the usual patient with dysgerminoma should be conservative if possible. Historically, the treatment of patients with dysgerminoma associated with gonadoblastoma is radical because of the frequent occurrence of bilateral tumors and the absence of normal gonadal function. Investigation of the genotypes and karyotypes of all patients with this neoplasm is recommended by some, especially if any history of virilization or other developmental abnormalities is elicited. In vitro fertilization (IVF) can be utilized in patients without gonads. Therefore, it may be prudent to preserve the uterus in patients in whom the ovaries must be removed. In most cases, we leave the uterus. This may be particularly important in prepubertal patients, because in these patients other signs of abnormal function (e.g., primary amenorrhea, virilization, and absence of normal sexual development) are lacking.

Often lesions that consist primarily of dysgerminoma elements contain small areas of more malignant histology (e.g., embryonal carcinoma or endodermal sinus tumor). If tumor markers such as alpha-fetoprotein (AFP) or hCG are elevated, a strong suspicion of mixed lesions should be entertained. When the dysgerminoma is not pure and these more malignant components are present, the prognosis and therapy are determined by the more malignant germ cell elements, and the dysgerminoma component is disregarded.

Endodermal Sinus Tumor (Yolk Sac Tumor)

Endodermal sinus tumors are the second most common form of malignant germ cell tumors of the ovary, accounting for 22% of malignant germ cell lesions in one large series. The median age of the patient is 19 years. Three fourths of the patients are initially seen with a combination of abdominal pain and abdominal or pelvic mass. Acute symptoms are typically caused by torsion of the tumor and may lead to the diagnosis of acute appendicitis or a ruptured ectopic pregnancy. These yolk sac tumors are almost always unilateral. The tumor is usually large with most tumors measuring between 10 and 30 cm. On the cut surface, they appear gray–yellow with areas of hemorrhage and cystic, gelatinous changes.

These neoplasms are highly malignant; they metastasize early and invade the surrounding structures. Intra-abdominal spread leads to extensive involvement of abdominal structures with tumor deposits. Metastases also occur via the lymphatic system. AFP levels are often elevated in this group of tumors. Endodermal sinus tumors are characterized by extremely rapid growth and extensive intra-abdominal spread; almost half the patients seen by a physician complain of symptoms of 1 week duration or less.

Endodermal sinus tumors are thought to originate from germ cells that differentiate into the extra embryonal yolk sac because the tumor structure is similar to that found in the endodermal sinuses of the rat yolk sac. The tumors consist of scattered tubules or spaces lined by single layers of flattened cuboidal cells, loose reticular stroma, numerous scattered para-aminosalicylic–positive globules, and, within some spaces or clefts, a characteristic invaginated papillary structure with a central blood vessel (Schiller–Duval body) (Figure 12-5).

Historically, the prognosis for patients with endodermal sinus tumor of the ovary has been unfavorable. Most patients have died of the disease within 12 to 18 months of diagnosis. Until multiple-agent chemotherapy was developed, there were only a few known 5-year survivors. Most of these patients had tumors confined to the ovary. In several cases, the tumor consisted of endodermal sinus tumors admixed with other neoplastic germ cell elements, frequently dysgerminoma. The clinical course in most patients with tumors composed of endodermal sinus tumor associated with dysgerminoma or other neoplastic germ cell elements does not differ greatly from that in patients with pure

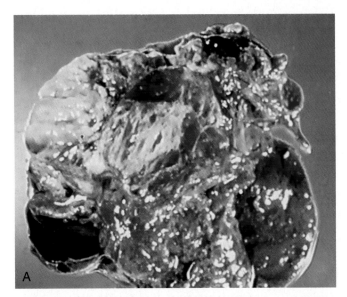

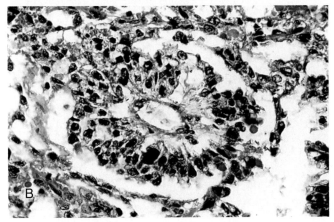

FIGURE 12-5　Endodermal sinus tumor. **A,** Gross appearance with areas of hemorrhage and gelatinous necrosis. **B,** Microscopic appearance with isolated papillary projections containing single blood vessels and having peripheral lining of neoplastic cells (Schiller–Duval body).

endodermal sinus tumors. Frequently, intracellular and extracellular hyaline droplets that represent deposits of AFP can be identified throughout the tumor. Mixed germ cell lesions often contain endodermal sinus tumors as one of the types present.

In the past, the treatment of patients with endodermal sinus tumor of the ovary has been frustrating. Kurman and Norris reported no long-term survivors in 17 patients with stage I tumors who were receiving adjunctive radiation or single alkylating agent, dactinomycin, or methotrexate. Gallion and colleagues reviewed the literature in 1979 and found that only 27% of 96 patients with stage I endodermal sinus tumors were alive at 2 years. The tumor is not sensitive to radiation therapy, although there may be an initial response. Optimal surgical extirpation of the disease has been advocated, but this alone is unsuccessful in producing a significant number of cures.

TABLE 12-4　VAC, VBP, and BEP Regimens

Regimen	Dosage Schedule
VAC	
Vincristine, 1.5 mg/m²	Weekly IV administration for 12 wk (maximum dose 2.5 mg)
Dactinomycin, 0.5 mg	5-day IV course every 4 wk
Cyclophosphamide,	5-day IV course every 4 wk 5-7 mg/kg
VBP	
Vinblastine, 12 mg/m²	IV every 3 wk for 4 courses
Bleomycin, 20 U/m²	IV q wk for 7 courses (maximum dose eighth course given in 30 U/m²) wk 10
Cisplatin, 20 mg/m²	Daily × 5 every 3 wk for 3-4 courses
BEP	
Bleomycin, 20 U/m²	IV q wk × 9 (maximum dose 30 U)
Etoposide, 100 mg/m²	IV days 1-5 q 3 wk × 3
Cisplatin, 20 mg/m²	IV days 1-5 q 3 wk × 3

BEP, Bleomycin, etoposide, cisplatin; VAC, vincristine, actinomycin D (dactinomycin), cyclophosphamide; VBP, vinblastine, bleomycin, cisplatin.

In more recent years, there have been optimistic reports of sustained remissions in some patients treated by surgery and multiple-agent chemotherapy. The GOG used VAC chemotherapy to treat 24 patients who had pure endodermal sinus tumors (ESTs) that were completely resected and 7 whose diseases were partially resected. Of 31 patients, 15 (48%) failed, including 11 of 24 (46%) who had complete resection. Of 15 patients with mixed germ cell tumors containing EST elements treated with VAC, 8 (53%) failed. Subsequently, the GOG treated 48 patients with stages I to III completely resected ESTs with VAC for six to nine courses. Thirty-five (73%) patients were free of disease with a median follow-up time of 4 years. Gershenson and associates reported that 18 of 26 (69%) patients with pure EST were free of tumors after VAC therapy. Gallion and associates reported 17 of 25 (68%) patients with stage I disease who were alive and well 2 years or more after treatment with VAC. Sessa and associates treated 13 patients with pure EST of the ovary, 12 of whom had initial unilateral oophorectomy. All received VBP and are alive at 20 months to 6 years (Table 12-4). Three patients had a relapse but were saved. This experience is important because 9 of these patients had stage IIb or more advanced disease.

Schwartz and colleagues have used VAC for stage I disease but prefer VBP for stage II to IV patients. Of 15 patients, 12 are alive and have no evidence of disease. Their routine is to treat at least one course beyond a normal AFP titer (this has become routine in many centers). One recurrence was treated successfully with BEP. Two early VAC failures were not saved with VBP. The GOG evaluated VBP in stage III and IV and in recurrent malignant germ cell tumors, many with measurable disease after surgery. Sixteen of 29 (55%) ESTs were long-term disease-free survivors. VBP induced a substantial number of durable complete responses, even in patients with prior chemotherapy. Toxicity was significant. Williams noted that in disseminated germ cell tumors (primarily of the testes), BEP was more effective and had less neuromuscular toxicity than had VBP. Williams also reported the GOG experience with 93 patients who were given BEP postoperatively in an adjuvant setting for malignant germ cell cancers of the ovary. Forty-two were immature teratomas, whereas 25 were ESTs and 24 were mixed germ cell tumors. At the time of Williams' report, 91 of 93 had no evidence of disease (NED) after three courses of BEP with a median follow-up of 39 months. One patient developed acute myelomonocytic leukemia 22 months after diagnosis, and a second patient developed lymphoma 69 months after treatment. Dimopoulos and colleagues reported a similar result from the Hellenic Cooperative Oncology Group. Forty patients with nondysgerminomatous tumors were treated with BEP or PVB. With a median follow-up of 39 months, 5 patients developed progressive disease and died. Only one of the 5 who failed received BEP. Most recently, de La Motte Rouge and associates reported on 52 women with endodermal sinus tumor, 35 of which had stage I or II tumors and 17 with stage III or IV disease. All were treated with BEP. After a median follow-up 68 months, the 5-year overall survival and disease free survival rates were 94% and 90%, respectively. In this series, fertility sparing surgery was performed in 41 cases and pregnancy was achieved in 12 of 16 (75%) of women who attempted to conceive, demonstrating that conservative surgery plus chemotherapy resulted in an appreciable number of successful pregnancies after treatment.

From a practical point of view, serum AFP determination is considered to be a useful diagnostic tool in patients who have endodermal sinus tumors and should be considered an ideal tumor marker. It can be useful when monitoring the results of therapy and for detecting metastasis and recurrences after therapy. As noted earlier, many investigators use AFP as a guide to the number of courses needed for an individual patient. In many cases, only three or four courses have placed patients into remission with long-term survival. Levels of hCG and its beta subunit (beta-hCG) have been found to be normal in patients with endodermal sinus tumor.

Embryonal Carcinoma

Embryonal carcinoma is one of the most malignant cancers arising in the ovary (Figure 12-6). The neoplasm closely resembles the embryonal carcinoma of the adult

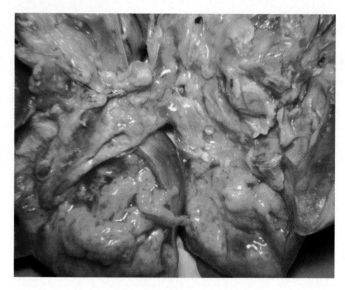

FIGURE 12-6   Gross photograph of embryonal carcinoma of the ovary.

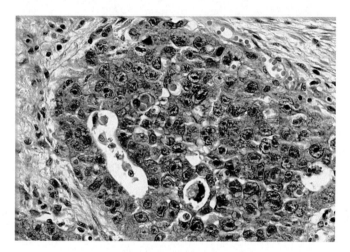

FIGURE 12-7   Microscopic appearance of large primitive cells with occasional papillary or gland-like formations characteristic of embryonal carcinoma.

testes, a relatively common tumor. However, it represents only 4% of malignant ovarian germ cell tumors in the ovary, and its confusion with choriocarcinoma and ESTs in the past accounts for its late identification as a distinct entity. It usually manifests as an abdominal mass or pelvic mass occurring at a mean age of 15 years. More than half of the patients have hormonal abnormalities, including precocious puberty, irregular uterine bleeding, amenorrhea, or hirsutism. The tumors consist of large primitive cells with occasional papillary or gland-like formations (Figure 12-7). The cells have eosinophilic cytoplasm with distinct borders and round nuclei with prominent nucleoli. Numerous mitotic figures, many atypical, are seen; scattered throughout

TABLE 12-5 Comparison of Embryonal Carcinoma with Endodermal Sinus Tumor

	Endodermal Sinus Tumor (71 Cases)	Embryonal Carcinoma (15 Cases)
Median age	19 years	15 years
Prepubertal status	23%	47%
Precocious puberty	0	43%
Positive pregnancy test	None (0/15)	All (9/9)
Vaginal bleeding	1%	33%
Amenorrhea	0	7%
Hirsutism	0	7%
Survival, stage I patients	16%	50%
Human chorionic gonadotropin	Negative (0/15)	Positive (10/10)
α-Fetoprotein	Positive (15/15)	Positive (7/10)

From Kurman RJ, Norris HJ: Cancer 38:2404, 1976.

the tumor are multinucleated giant cells that resemble syncytial cells.

These tumors secrete hCG from syncytiotrophoblast-like cells and AFP from large primitive cells, and these tumor markers can be used to monitor progress during therapy. This tumor probably arises from primordial germ cells, but it develops before there is much further differentiation toward either embryonic or extraembryonic tissue. In a review of 15 patients, Kurman and Norris reported an actuarial survival rate of 30% for the entire group; for those with stage I tumors, the survival rate was 50% (Table 12-5). This result is significantly better than survival with the endodermal sinus tumor for the same period of time and before the advent of vigorous multiple-agent adjuvant chemotherapy. With modern therapy, survival rates should be greatly improved. Optimal therapy, although not yet established, is probably similar to that for endodermal sinus tumor.

The VAC regimen is definitely active in this disease but does not appear to be as reliable for advanced cases as the VBP regimen. It is suggested that patients receiving VAC be watched closely for progression of disease, and the more toxic VBP regimen can be used at that point in the hope of salvage. The total number of courses of VAC therapy needed to achieve optimal numbers of disease-free patients is really not known.

The GOG has evaluated the effectiveness of the VBP regimen in stages III and IV recurrent malignant germ cell tumors of the ovary, including embryonal carcinoma. Ninety-four patients have been treated, and this therapy has produced a substantial number of durable complete responses in patients who previously received chemotherapy. The overall progression-free interval at 24 months is approximately 55%.

Polyembryoma

Polyembryoma is a rare ovarian germ cell neoplasm that consists of numerous embryoid bodies resembling morphologically normal embryos. Similar homologous neoplasms occur more frequently in the human testes. To date, only a few ovarian polyembryomas have been reported. In most cases, the polyembryoma has been associated with other neoplastic germ cell elements, mainly the immature teratoma. Polyembryoma is a highly malignant germ cell neoplasm. It is usually associated with invasion of adjacent structures and organs and extensive metastases that are mainly confined to the abdominal cavity. The tumor is not sensitive to radiotherapy, and its response to chemotherapy is unknown.

Choriocarcinoma

Choriocarcinoma, which is a rare, highly malignant tumor that may be associated with sexual precocity, can arise in one of three ways:

1. As a primary gestational choriocarcinoma associated with ovarian pregnancy
2. As a metastatic choriocarcinoma from a primary gestational choriocarcinoma arising in other parts of the genital tract, mainly the uterus
3. As a germ cell tumor differentiating in the direction of trophoblastic structures and arising admixed with other neoplastic germ cell elements

Choriocarcinomas of the ovary may also be divided into two broad groups:

1. Gestational choriocarcinoma, encompassing the first two groups mentioned above
2. Nongestational choriocarcinoma, a germ cell tumor that differentiates toward trophoblastic structures

The presence of paternal DNA on analysis distinguishes gestational from nongestational choriocarcinoma. Only nongestational choriocarcinoma of the ovary is discussed here. In most cases, the tumor is admixed with other neoplastic germ cell elements, and their presence is diagnostic of nongestational choriocarcinoma. The tumor, in common with other malignant germ cell neoplasms, occurs in children and young adults. Its occurrence in children has been emphasized; in some series, 50% of cases occurred in prepubescent children. This high incidence in children may result from the previous reluctance of investigators to make the diagnosis in adults.

These neoplasms secrete hCG. This is particularly noticeable in prepubescent children, who show evidence of isosexual precocious puberty with mammary development, growth of pubic and axillary hair, and uterine bleeding. Adult patients may have signs of ectopic pregnancies because the nongestational choriocarcinoma, like its gestational counterpart, is associated with an increased production of hCG. Estimation of urinary or plasma hCG levels is a useful diagnostic test in these cases. Historically, the prognosis of patients with choriocarcinoma of the ovary was unfavorable, but modern chemotherapy regimens appear to be effective. Creasman and associates in four cases using the MAC combination chemotherapy achieved prolonged remissions. Some responses have been seen with combination chemotherapy using methotrexate as one of the drugs in the regimen. In most instances, the other drugs used in the combinations have been dactinomycin and an alkylating agent.

Mixed Germ Cell Tumors

Mixed germ cell tumors contain at least two malignant germ cell elements. Dysgerminoma is the most common component (80% in Kurman and Norris' report and 69% in material from the MD Anderson Hospital). Immature teratoma and EST are also frequently identified; embryonal carcinoma and choriocarcinoma are seen only occasionally. It is not unusual to see three or four different germ cell components. In 42 patients treated at the MD Anderson Hospital, 9 patients were treated with surgery alone and another 6 patients received radiation therapy; all developed recurrences. Of 17 patients who received VAC, 9 patients were placed into remission. Five patients received primary treatment of VBP after surgery, and 4 patients are alive and well. Of the original 42 patients, 20 patients (48%) are alive and well. Of 14 patients who had stage I disease and were treated with combination chemotherapy after surgery, 11 (79%) survived. The GOG treated 10 completely resected mixed germ cell tumors with VAC, and 7 are long-term survivors. Of 5 patients who had incompletely resected disease and who were treated with VAC, 4 developed recurrences. Schwartz and colleagues treated 8 patients with mixed tumors with VAC; 7 patients are long-term survivors. Only 1 patient did not respond to PVB therapy. Because the most significant component of mixed tumors usually predicts results, it should determine therapy and follow-up.

Teratoma

Mature Cystic Teratoma

Accounting for more than 95% of all ovarian teratomas, the dermoid cyst, or mature cystic teratoma, is one of the most common ovarian neoplasms. Teratomas account for approximately 15% of all ovarian tumors. They are the most common ovarian tumors in women in the second and third decades of life. Fortunately, most benign cystic lesions contain mature tissue of ectodermal, mesodermal, or endodermal origin. The most common elements are ectodermal derivatives such as skin, hair follicles, and sebaceous or sweat glands, accounting for the characteristic histologic and gross appearance of teratomas (Figure 12-8). These tumors are usually multicystic and contain hair intermixed with foul-smelling, sticky, keratinous and sebaceous debris. Occasionally, well-formed teeth are seen along with cartilage or bone. If the tumor consists of only ectodermal derivatives of skin and skin appendages, it is a true dermoid cyst. A mixture of other, usually mature tissues (gastrointestinal, respiratory) may be present.

The clinical manifestation of this slow-growing lesion is usually related to its size, compression, or torsion, or to a chemical peritonitis secondary to intra-abdominal spill of the cholesterol-laden debris. The latter event tends to occur more commonly when the tumor is large. Torsion is the most frequent complication, observed in as many as 16% of the cases in one large series, and it tends to be more common during pregnancy and the puerperium. Mature cystic teratomas are said to comprise 22% to 40% of ovarian tumors in pregnancy, and 0.8% to 12.8% of reported cases of mature cystic teratomas have occurred in pregnancy. In general, torsion is more common in children and younger patients. Severe acute abdominal pain is usually the initial symptom, and the condition is considered to be an acute abdominal emergency. Rupture of a mature cystic teratoma is an uncommon complication, occurring in approximately 1% of cases, but it is much more common during pregnancy and may manifest during labor. The immediate result of rupture may be shock or hemorrhage, especially during pregnancy or labor, but the prognosis even in these cases is favorable. Rupture of the tumor into the peritoneal cavity may be followed by a chemical peritonitis caused by the spill of the contents of the tumor. This may result in a marked granulomatous reaction and lead to the formation of dense adhesions throughout the peritoneal cavity. Infection is an uncommon complication of mature cystic teratoma and occurs in approximately 1% of cases. The infecting organism is usually a coliform, but Salmonella species infection causing typhoid fever has also been reported. Removal of the neoplasm by ovarian cystectomy or, rarely, oophorectomy appears to be adequate therapy. Malignant degeneration of mature teratomas is a rare occurrence. When it occurs the most common secondary tumor is a squamous cell carcinoma. Prognosis and behavior of this secondary malignancy is similar to that of squamous cell cancers arising in other anatomic sites and appear to be highly dependent on stage. There is no consensus on treatment

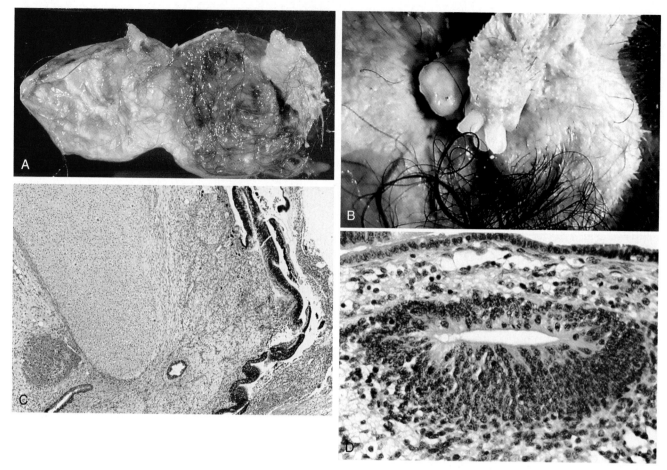

FIGURE 12-8   Benign cystic teratoma. **A** and **B,** Gross appearance. Benign cystic teratoma. **C,** Microscopic view of ectodermal elements (skin and skin appendages). **D,** Immature neural elements evident.

recommendations; however, patients with stage I to II disease treated with platinum-based chemotherapy and whole pelvic radiation have a chance for long-term survival. Although squamous cell carcinoma in this setting is usually an incidental finding at pathology, preoperative risk factors include age greater than 50, tumor size greater than 10 cm, and elevated concentrations of squamous cell carcinoma antigen and CA-125.

Mature Solid Teratoma

Mature solid teratoma is a rare ovarian neoplasm and a very uncommon type of ovarian teratoma. The histologic components in a mixed solid teratoma are similar to those found in an immature solid teratoma, which occurs mainly in children and young adults. The presence of immature elements immediately excludes the tumor from this group; by definition, only tumors composed entirely of mature tissues may be included. The tumor is usually unilateral and is adequately treated by unilateral oophorectomy. Although this neoplasm is considered benign, mature solid teratomas may be associated occasionally with peritoneal implants that consist entirely of mature glial tissue. Despite the extensive involvement that may be present, the prognosis is excellent.

Immature Teratoma

Immature teratomas consist of tissue derived from the three germ layers—ectoderm, mesoderm, and endoderm—and, in contrast to the much more common mature teratoma, they contain immature or embryonal structures. These tumors have had a variety of names: solid teratoma, malignant teratoma, teratoblastoma, teratocarcinoma, and embryonal teratoma. These names have arisen because immature teratomas have been incorrectly considered mixed germ cell tumors or secondary malignant tumors originating in mature benign teratomas. Mature tissues are frequently present and sometimes may predominate. Immature teratoma of the ovary is an uncommon tumor, comprising less than 1% of ovarian teratomas. In contrast to the mature cystic teratoma, which is encountered most frequently during

TABLE 12-6   Immature Teratoma Grading System

Grade	Thurlbeck and Scully	Norris et al
0	All cells well differentiated	All tissue mature; rare mitotic activity
1	Cells well differentiated; rare small foci of embryonal tissue	Some immaturity and neuroepithelium limited to low magnification field in any slide (×40)
2	Moderate quantities of embryonal tissue; atypia and mitosis present	Immaturity and neuroepithelium does not exceed three low-power microscopic fields in any one slide
3	Large quantities of embryonal tissue; atypia and mitosis present	Immaturity and neuroepithelium occupying four or more low magnification fields on a single slide

TABLE 12-7   Immature (Malignant) Teratomas

Grade	No.	Tumor Deaths (%)
1	22	4 (18)
2	24	9 (37)
3	10	7 (70)

From Norris HJ, Zirkin HJ, Benson WL: Cancer 37:2356, 1976.

the reproductive years but occurs at all ages, the immature teratoma has a specific age incidence, occurring most commonly in the first two decades of life and almost unknown after menopause. By definition, an immature teratoma contains immature neural elements. According to Norris and associates, the quantity of immature neural tissue alone determines the grade. Neuroblastoma elements, glial tissue, and immature cerebellar and cortical tissue may also be seen. These tumors are graded histologically on the basis of the amount and degree of cellular immaturity. The range is from grade I (mature teratoma containing only rare immature foci) through grade III (large portions of the tumor consist of embryonal tissue with atypia and mitotic activity). Generally, older patients tend to have lower grade primary tumors compared with younger patients. When the neoplasm is solid and all elements are well differentiated histologically (solid mature teratoma), a grade 0 designation is given (Table 12-6).

Immature teratomas are almost never bilateral, although occasionally a benign teratoma is found in the opposite ovary. These tumors may have multiple peritoneal implants at the time of initial surgery, and the prognosis is closely correlated with the histologic grade of the primary tumor and the implants. Norris and co-workers studied 58 patients with immature teratomas and reported an 82% survival rate for patients who had grade I primary lesions, 63% for grade II, and 30% for grade III (Table 12-7). These results antedate the use of multiple-agent chemotherapy.

Multiple sections of the primary lesion and wide sampling of the peritoneal implants are necessary to properly grade the tumor. In most cases, the implants are better differentiated than the primary tumors. Both the primary lesion and the implants should be graded according to the most immature tissue present. Patients with mature glial implants have an excellent prognosis; immature implants, however, do not.

To date, the histologic grade and fertility desires of the patient have been the determining factors regarding extent of surgical therapy and subsequent adjuvant therapy. Because the lesion is rarely bilateral in its ovarian involvement, the present method of therapy consists of unilateral salpingo-oophorectomy with wide sampling of peritoneal implants. Total abdominal hysterectomy with bilateral salpingo-oophorectomy does not seem to be indicated, because it does not influence the outcome for the patient. Although some authors have advocated cystectomy alone for early-stage, low-grade disease, this management strategy should be approached with caution. Radiotherapy has also been shown to have little value. If the primary tumor is grade I and all peritoneal implants (if they exist) are grade 0, no further therapy is recommended. However, if the primary tumor is grade II or III or if implants or recurrences are grade I, II, or III, triple-agent chemotherapy is frequently recommended. The recommendation to use adjuvant chemotherapy in high-grade stage I disease is based on studies performed before meticulous surgical staging of germ cell malignancies was routine. Cushing and colleagues evaluated surgical therapy alone in 44 pediatric and adolescent patients under the age of 15 who had completely resected immature teratomas of all grades. Thirty-one patients had pure immature teratomas, and 13 patients had immature teratomas with microscopic endodermal sinus tumor foci. The 4-year event-free and overall survival for both groups was 97% and 100%, respectively. The only EST failure was salvaged with subsequent chemotherapy. The authors concluded that surgery alone was curative for most children and adolescents with completely resected ovarian immature teratomas of any grade and advocated avoiding adjuvant chemotherapy in this group. The VAC regimen has proved to be highly effective. DiSaia and associates have reported on several patients with disseminated disease treated with this chemotherapeutic regimen. At second-look laparotomy these patients were free of immature elements but retained peritoneal implants containing exclusively mature elements. This was labeled chemotherapeutic retroconversion of immature teratoma of the ovary, and is a similar if not identical syndrome as the "growing teratoma syndrome" described in testicular nonseminomatous germ cell tumors All these patients have had uneventful follow-ups with the mature implants apparently remaining in static states. Apparently this is a common occurrence.

The GOG treated 20 completely resected immature teratomas with VAC. Only one patient failed, and she was treated primarily at the time of recurrence. Of eight advanced or recurrent lesions that were incompletely resected, only four responded to VAC. The group at the MD Anderson Hospital reported that 15 of 18 patients (83%) with immature teratomas had sustained remission with primary VAC chemotherapy. VBP has been used by the GOG in patients with advanced or recurrent immature teratomas. They treated 26 patients, of whom 14 (54%) were disease-free survivors. Creasman treated 6 patients who had immature teratomas with MAC, and all are long-term survivors. Schwartz and colleagues usually treats stage I patients with six cycles of VAC. Those with more advanced disease were given 12 cycles and a second-look operation. Of 29 patients, 24 were successfully treated. Four of the 5 patients with persistent lesions were successfully saved.

Bonazzi and colleagues from Italy reported their experience with 32 patients with pure immature teratomas. This represents 28% of all germ cell tumors seen by these investigators. Twenty-nine patients had stage I or II and 24 had grade I or II tumors. Twenty-two patients were treated with conservative surgery only (unilateral oophorectomy or cystectomy). Of 32 patients, 30 had fertility-sparing surgery performed. Of 6 patients who wished for subsequent pregnancies, 5 had seven pregnancies with delivery of seven normal infants. Chemotherapy was given to patients after surgery only in the case of stage I and II grade III tumors or in the case of stage III tumors. Ten patients received a cisplatin-based regimen. All 32 patients were alive and disease free at a median of 47 months (11-138 months). Conservative therapy for germ cell tumors is now the norm. Even with advanced disease, unilateral oophorectomy and complete surgical staging with preservation of the uterus and other ovary may be considered.

Today, most investigators treat stage Ia grade I immature teratomas with unilateral oophorectomy alone. Patients with stage Ia grade II or III, and more advanced lesions, are treated postsurgically with VAC. Three courses appear to be as effective as longer chemotherapy regimens, particularly in patients with completely resected disease. Fortunately, most germ cell tumors are early staged; these tumors are most frequently limited to one ovary. Shorter courses of chemotherapy have been shown to produce excellent results. This is important, because menstrual irregularity (even amenorrhea) during chemotherapy may be related to the duration of chemotherapy. Subsequent fertility may be affected. Fortunately, many patients with germ cell tumors have had many successful subsequent pregnancies after therapy. Although this appears to be age related in that the earlier the age at treatment the less vulnerable the patient is to menstrual irregularities and infertility, most patients with germ cell tumors are young and have apparent minimal infertility.

Monodermal or Highly Specialized Teratomas

Struma ovarii. Another tumor thought to represent the unilateral development of benign teratoma is struma ovarii, which consists totally or predominantly of thyroid parenchyma. This is an uncommon lesion and should not be confused with benign teratomas, which contain small foci of thyroid tissue. Between 25% and 35% of patients with strumal tumors will have clinical hyperthyroidism. The gross and microscopic appearance of these lesions is similar to that of typical thyroid tissue, although the histologic pattern may resemble that in adenomatous thyroid. These ovarian tumors may undergo malignant transformation, but they are usually benign and easily treated by simple surgical resection.

Carcinoid tumors. Primary ovarian carcinoid tumors usually arise in association with gastrointestinal or respiratory epithelium, which is present in mature cystic teratoma. They may also be observed within a solid teratoma or a mucinous tumor, or they may occur in an apparently pure form. Primary ovarian carcinoid tumors are uncommon. Approximately 50 cases have been reported. The age distribution of patients with ovarian carcinoid tumors is similar to that of patients with mature cystic teratoma, although the average age may be slightly higher in ovarian carcinoid tumors. Many patient are postmenopausal.

One third of the reported cases have been associated with the typical carcinoid syndrome, despite the absence of metastasis. This is in contrast to intestinal carcinoid tumors, which are associated with the syndrome only when there is metastatic spread to the liver. Excision of the tumor has been associated with the rapid remission of symptoms in all of the described cases and the disappearance of 5-hydroxyindoleacetic acid from the urine. The primary ovarian carcinoids are only occasionally associated with metastasis; metastasis was observed in only 3 of 47 reported cases in one review. The prognosis after excision of the primary tumor is favorable, and in most cases a cure results.

Strumal carcinoid is an even rarer entity and represents a close admixture of the previously discussed struma ovarii and carcinoid tumors. Strumal carcinoids may actually represent medullary carcinoma, resulting in thyroid tissue. Most cases follow a benign course.

TUMORS OF GERM CELL AND SEX CORD DERIVATION

Tumors of germ cell and sex cord derivation are unique, rare tumors that are composed of two distinct populations of cells closely admixed but with different origins. The two histologic types of tumors that fall into this category are gonadoblastomas and mixed germ cell–sex cord stromal tumors. Gonadoblastomas are benign tumors of the ovary that occur in dysgenetic gonads and are frequently associated with the development of a malignant germ cell component. The risk of developing a malignant germ cell component increases with age, such that prepubertal girls at the time of gonadectomy are very unlikely to have an associated malignant germ cell tumor, whereas the risk of malignancy approaches 100% for women in their 20s. Mixed germ cell–sex cord stromal tumors occur in chromosomally normal gonads. Malignant germ cell tumors occur less frequently than in gonadoblastomas.

Gonadoblastoma

Gonadoblastoma is a rare ovarian lesion that consists of germ cells that resemble those of dysgerminoma, and gonadal stroma cells that resemble those of a granulosa or Sertoli tumor. Sex chromatin studies usually show a negative nuclear pattern (45, X) or a sex chromosome mosaicism (45, X/46, XY). Gonadoblastomas usually arise in dysgenetic gonads, but the presence of dysgenetic gonads, a Y chromosome, or a Y fragment is not required; very rare cases of gonadoblastomas have been reported in normal women with normal ovaries and a normal karyotype. Because patients with XY gonadal dysgenesis have a very high risk of gonadoblastoma and a nearly 100% risk of associated malignant germ cell tumor with advancing age, these patients are recommended to undergo prophylactic bilateral oophorectomy after puberty. Patients who have a gonadoblastoma usually have primary amenorrhea, virilization, or developmental abnormalities of the genitalia. It is poorly understood as to why some patients with these lesions become virilized and others do not. Although there is a correlation between the virilization of patients with gonadoblastoma and the presence of Leydig or lutein-like cells, this relationship is not constant and some virilized patients are free of these cells. The discovery of gonadoblastoma is made in the course of investigation of these conditions. Another common initial sign is the presence of a pelvic tumor. Most patients with gonadoblastoma (80%) are phenotypic women, and the remainder are phenotypic men with cryptorchidism, hypospadias, and internal female secondary sex organs. Among the phenotypic women, 60% are virilized, and the remainder appear normal. The prognosis of patients with gonadoblastoma is excellent if the tumor and the contralateral gonad, which may be harboring a macroscopically undetectable gonadoblastoma, are excised. Bilateral involvement is identified in approximately 50% of cases. The association with dysgerminoma is seen in 50% of cases and with other more malignant germ cell neoplasms in an additional 10%. In view of this, the concept that these lesions represent an in situ germ cell malignancy appears valid. When gonadoblastoma is associated with or overgrown by dysgerminoma, the prognosis is still excellent. Metastases tend to occur later and more infrequently than in dysgerminoma arising de novo. Complete or partial regression of virilization usually occurs after excision of the gonads. Exogenous estrogen therapy is given for periodic bleeding. We leave the uterus even after removing both gonads. Cyclic hormone therapy is indicated in these young women. Ovum transfer has been successful in patients who have had both ovaries removed. Although gonadoblastomas themselves are benign, treatment should follow the usual tenets for surgical management of ovarian malignancy if a malignant component is identified.

Mixed Germ Cell–Sex Cord Stromal Tumors

Mixed germ cell–sex cord stromal tumors are less common than gonadoblastomas and occur in phenotypically normal women with normal karyotypes and normal gonads. These tumors are usually identified in girls younger than age 10; however, they rarely may be seen in reproductive-age women. Although clinically benign, these mixed tumors are associated with a malignant germ cell component in 10% of cases. When this tumor is identified in postpubertal girls, the risk of a malignant germ cell tumor rises to 80%. Isosexual precocity may be seen. Similar to gonadoblastoma, the most common germ cell tumor identified is dysgerminoma. However, unlike gonadoblastoma, in which the sex cord element is usually mature, in mixed tumors the sex cord element is usually less mature. Histologic features may resemble characteristics of multiple sex cord stromal tumors (SCST) such as retiform patterns or annular tubules and may not be characteristic of a single sex cord stromal tumor type. They are usually large and unilateral tumors and metastasize or recur infrequently. Because of the unilateral nature, unilateral oophorectomy and staging if a malignant germ cell component is identified is all that is required. Because these patients are usually young and are phenotypically, anatomically, and karyotypically normal, surgical management should be guided by fertility preservation and appropriate staging if malignancy is identified.

TUMORS DERIVED FROM SPECIAL GONADAL STROMA

Classification, Clinical Profile, and Staging

This category of ovarian tumors includes all those that contain granulosa cells, theca cells and luteinized derivatives, Sertoli cells, Leydig cells, and fibroblasts of gonadal stromal origin. These tumors originate from the ovarian matrix and consist of cells from the embryonic sex cord and mesenchyme. As a group, SCSTs are found in all age groups, with the age-related incidence increasing throughout the fifth, sixth, and seventh decades. These tumors account for approximately 5% of all ovarian tumors; however, functioning neoplastic groups of this variety comprise only 2%. Approximately 90% of hormonally active ovarian tumors belong to this category and are associated with physiologic and pathologic signs of estrogen and/or androgen excess, including isosexual precocity, hirsutism, abnormal bleeding, endometrial hyperplasia or carcinoma, and breast cancer risk. Of ovarian cancers, 5% to 10% belong in the sex cord stromal group; most of these (70%) are granulosa cell tumors, which are low-grade malignancies with a relapse rate of 10% to 33%. Because SCSTs have a propensity for indolent growth, they tend to recur late. The average time to recurrence is between 5 and 10 years; some recur as late as 20 years after the initial diagnosis. Most authors report a 10-year survival of 90% for stage I and 0% to 22% for stage III. Prognostic factors shown to be responsible for survival in multivariate analysis by Chan and colleagues include age younger than 50, tumor size less than 10 cm, and absence of residual disease. An analysis of SEER data from 1988 to 2001 including 376 women with SCST confirmed age younger than 50 and early-stage disease (I and II) as significant prognostic factors for improved survival. Observational studies have shown an improvement in relative and overall survival for SCST over time, likely attributable to the increased recognition of the importance of cytoreduction and residual disease on overall survival and accurate staging resulting in more favorable stage at diagnosis. SCSTs are staged surgically in accordance with FIGO guidelines and staging recommendations for ovarian epithelial tumors.

Treatment

The definitive treatment of SCST is based on findings encountered during complete surgical staging, the reproductive desires of the patient, and the histologic type of tumor. The majority of SCSTs are benign or low malignant potential tumors. As a result, surgical therapy is adequate in most cases and remains the cornerstone of treatment. In patients who desire to retain fertility, unilateral salpingo-oophorectomy with preservation of the uterus and contralateral ovary and full surgical staging is appropriate therapy for patients with stage Ia disease. Advanced-stage disease and disease in older women should be managed with complete staging and hysterectomy with bilateral salpingo-oophorectomy. Although scientific evidence suggesting benefit is lacking, most authors recommend aggressive attempts at complete cytoreduction if possible when faced with advanced-stage, metastatic, or bulky disease. Secondary cytoreduction is controversial, although there may be a survival or palliative benefit for patients with focal recurrent disease.

Although contemporary surgical practice mandates routine staging lymphadenectomy, the therapeutic value of routine lymphadenectomy is uncertain. There is no doubt that staging lymphadenectomy is prognostic and is clinically useful in guiding adjuvant therapy decisions. Brown and colleagues recently reported on 262 patients with SCST of the ovary. Fifty-eight patients underwent lymphadenectomy as part of staging, and none were found to have positive lymph nodes. Of the 117 patients who eventually had a recurrence, 6 patients (5.1%) had nodal metastasis at the time of recurrence. Three of these patients had negative nodes at the time of initial staging. These authors concluded that lymphadenectomy could be omitted as part of surgical staging of ovarian SCST because lymph node metastasis at time of diagnosis is rare. Similar findings have been reported by Chi and colleagues, who noted no lymph node metastasis in 16 of 68 patients with granulosa cell tumors who underwent pelvic lymph node dissection as part of surgical staging or 13 of 68 patients who underwent para-aortic lymph node sampling. Thirty-four patients ultimately experienced recurrence, 33 of which were incompletely staged at their initial operation. Only 15% of recurrences involved the retroperitoneum. In spite of these provocative reports, we continue to recommend full surgical staging including lymphadenectomy for the four SCST that may behave in a malignant fashion:

1. Granulosa cell tumor
2. Sertoli–Leydig cell tumor, grade II or III
3. Sex cord tumor with annular tubules (not associated with Peutz–Jegher's syndrome)
4. Steroid cell tumor (not otherwise specified)

Two special clinical situations require additional surgical evaluation. Because estrogen-secreting ovarian tumors are associated with endometrial hyperplasia or cancer in 25% to 50% and 5 to 10% of cases, respectively, surgical evaluation should include dilation and curettage of the uterine cavity, regardless of the benign or malignant nature of the ovarian primary. If malignancy in the uterus is encountered, it should be managed accordingly. Additionally, because sex cord tumors with annular tubules (SCTAT) associated with Peutz–Jegher's syndrome (discussed later) can be associated with adenoma malignum of the cervix, it is imperative that the endocervix be evaluated with an endocervical curettage. Although these ovarian tumors are benign, postoperative follow-up and surveillance of the cervix is required.

Patients with early-stage disease (Ia or Ib) may be treated with surgical therapy alone and expect an excellent prognosis. However, those with stage Ic or greater disease should have strong consideration given for adjuvant therapy despite the lack of any objective evidence suggesting benefit. Adjuvant therapy may consist of radiation or chemotherapy. The effectiveness of radiation therapy for SCST is controversial and unclear. There are small case series in the literature that would suggest that isolated incompletely resectable primary disease or pelvic recurrent disease may respond to radiation therapy. Because of the size and retrospective nature of these reports, no definitive conclusion can be drawn regarding the utility of radiation in this setting. Although experience with chemotherapy is likewise limited, active regimens are BEP or VAC. Recently, Brown and colleagues published results demonstrating taxane activity in patients with SCST. In this study, a 42% response rate was noted in the setting of recurrent, measurable disease. Specific adjuvant therapy for individual tumor subtypes will be discussed later. In a subsequent study, Brown and colleagues directly compared BEP to taxanes in women with SCST. In this study, there was no difference in progression free survival, overall survival, or response rates in patients with newly diagnosed tumors treated with BEP compared to taxanes. In patients with recurrent measurable disease, BEP had a higher response rate compared to the taxane regimens (71% vs 37%), a finding not statistically significant. In this study, the presence of a platinum compound in the taxane regimen correlated with response, suggesting that a platinum and taxane combination is active in SCST tumors and may have equivalent efficacy but with lower toxicity when compared to the standard BEP.

Granulosa–Stromal Cell Tumors

Granulosa–stromal cell tumors include granulosa cell, theca cell tumors, and fibromas and account for the majority of SCST. They occur about as frequently in women in the reproductive age group as they do in women who are postmenopausal, with a peak incidence in perimenopausal women. Only about 5% of granulosa cell tumors occur before puberty (Table 12-8). Most granulosa and theca cells produce estrogen, but a few are

TABLE 12-8   Granulosa Cell Tumor: Age Distribution of 118 Cases

Age	No.
Child	3
12-40	27
41-50	28
51-60	32
60-79	28
Total	118

Based on data from Evans AJ III et al: Obstet Gynecol 55:213, 1980.

androgenic. The exact proportion of these neoplasms that have function is not known, because the endometrium is often not examined microscopically and appropriate preoperative laboratory tests are not done. About 80% to 85% of granulosa cell and theca cell neoplasms are palpable on abdominal or pelvic examination, but occasionally an unsuspected tumor is found when a hysterectomy is done on a patient who has abnormal bleeding as a result of endometrial hyperplasia or endometrial carcinoma. Most patients present either with nonspecific symptoms such as awareness of an abdominal mass, abdominal pain, abdominal distention, or bloating. Some patients present with an acute abdomen as a result of internal tumor rupture and hemorrhage with resultant hemoperitoneum. About 15% of patients with cystic granulosa cell tumors are first examined for an acute abdomen associated with hemoperitoneum. Granulosa cell tumors vary greatly in gross appearance (Figure 12-9). Sometimes they are solid tumors that are soft or firm, depending on the relative amounts of neoplastic cells and fibrothecomatous stroma that they contain. They may be yellow or gray, depending on the amount of intracellular lipid in the lesion. More commonly, the granulosa cell tumor is predominantly cystic and, on external examination, may resemble mucinous cystadenoma or cystadenocarcinoma. However, when sectioned, this cyst is generally found to be filled with serous fluid or clotted blood. Granulosa cell tumors occur in two subtypes: adult and juvenile. Adult granulosa cell tumors account for approximately 95% of all granulosa cell tumors. They occur more commonly in the postmenopausal patient and are the most common tumor that produces estrogen. Abnormal endometria in these patients are not uncommon, such as hyperplasia or even carcinoma of the endometrium. A study by Evans and associates from the Mayo Clinic of 76 patients who had granulosa cell tumors and in whom endometrial tissue was available shows a high incidence of endometrial stimulation (Table 12-9). In another study, one third of patients had atypical endometrial cells. In postmenopausal women, vaginal bleeding is common as a result of stimulation of the endometrium. Approximately 10%

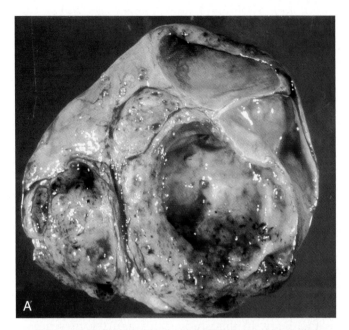

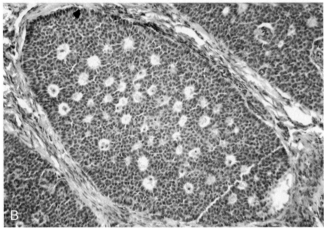

FIGURE 12-9 Granulosa cell tumor of the ovary. **A,** Gross appearance. **B,** Microscopic appearance with Call–Exner bodies.

TABLE 12-9 Granulosa Cell Tumor (76 Patients)

Endometrial Histology	No.	%
Proliferative endometrium	19	25
Atrophic endometrium	5	7
Hyperplastic endometrium	42	55
Adenocarcinoma	10	13

Based on data from Evans AJ III et al: Clinicopathological review of 118 granulosa and 82 theca cell tumors. Obstet Gynecol 55:213, 1980.

of patients with this lesion will harbor an endometrial carcinoma, usually of the well-differentiated type. Other estrogenic effects may also be noted (e.g., tenderness or swelling of the breast), and vaginal cytology may show an increase in maturation of the squamous cells. Rarely, androgenic effects may be present in which hirsute

changes may be present, or progestational effects may be noted on histologic evaluation of the endometrium. Histologically, fibrothecomatous components are common, and the cytoplasm is usually scanty. The typical coffee-bean grooved cells are present. Cells may be arranged in clusters or rosettes surrounding a central cavity and, when present, resemble primordial follicles called Call–Exner bodies and are common. Adult granulosa cell tumors are typically low-grade malignancies that demonstrate indolent growth and present as stage I disease in more than 90% of cases. Unilateral disease is most common, but bilateral disease may be found in up to 10% of cases. The most important prognostic factor is surgical stage.

In juvenile granulosa cell tumors, the great majority are found in young adults, and most occur during the first three decades of life. Most juvenile granulosa cell tumors are hormonally active, producing estradiol, progesterone, or androgens. Most of the juvenile granulosa cell tumors that occur in children result in sexual precocity with the development of breasts and pubic and axillary hair. Irregular uterine bleeding may also be present. Thyromegaly may also occur. Juvenile tumors that are hormonally active may have a more favorable prognosis than inactive tumors, presumably resulting from earlier presentation as a result of the signs and symptoms associated with hormonal activity. Like the adult subtype, most of these tumors are limited to one ovary. Ninety-eight percent present with stage I disease. Histologically, thecomatous components are common; cytoplasm is abundant. Mitosis may be numerous; the nuclei are dark and do not usually have the grooved coffee-bean appearance. Pleomorphism may also be present. Juvenile tumors rarely demonstrate Call–Exner bodies. Even though these tumors appear to be less well differentiated than the adult type, the cure rate is quite high. In contrast to adult cell types that are typically indolent and recur late, juvenile types are aggressive in advanced-stage disease with recurrence and death occurring within 3 years after diagnosis.

On the basis of their differentiation, granulosa cell tumors should be divided into two general categories: well differentiated and moderately differentiated. The former pattern may have various presentations, including microfollicular, macrofollicular, trabecular, solid-tubular, and watered silk. Tumors in the moderately differentiated category have a diffuse pattern that has also been designated "sarcomatoid." Although many authors have made attempts, no distinct correlation between histologic structure and prognosis has yet been substantiated. It is important that undifferentiated carcinomas, adenocarcinomas, and carcinoids should not be misdiagnosed as granulosa cell tumors, which they may superficially resemble. Each of these tumors has a strikingly different prognosis. One characteristic feature is

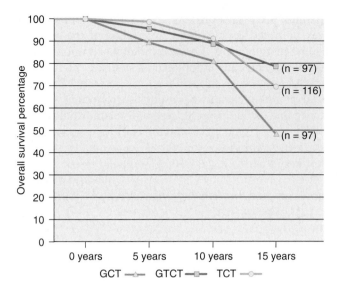

FIGURE 12-10   Granulosa–theca cell tumors from Emil Novak Ovarian Tumor Registry (1999). *(Modified from Cronje HS, Niemand I, Bam RH, Woodruff JD: Am J Obstet Gynecol 180:323, 1999.)*

the appearance of the nuclei. Oval or angular, grooved nuclei are typical of granulosa cell tumors (coffee-bean appearance). Call–Exner bodies also have diagnostic importance, but unfortunately they are not often sharply defined.

True granulosa tumors are low-grade malignancies, the majority of which are confined to one ovary at the time of diagnosis. Only 5% to 10% of the stage I cases will subsequently recur, and they often appear more than 5 years after initial therapy. The prognosis for these patients is excellent: long-term survival rates from 75% to 90% have been reported for all stages (Figure 12-10). These lesions are adequately managed during the reproductive years by removing the involved ovary and ipsilateral tube with full surgical staging. The uterus and uninvolved adnexa should be removed in the perimenopausal and postmenopausal age groups, which is the treatment for other benign or low malignant potential tumors. In a series from the Mayo Clinic, 92% of the patients had survived 5 to 10 years (76 patients, 82% of whom had stage I lesions). The recurrence pattern in this same series (18.6% overall recurrence rate) revealed that 23% of the recurrences were more than 13 years after initial therapy. Most of the recurrences occurred in preserved genital tract structures. These kinds of data have prompted some authors to recommend that the preserved internal genitalia be removed in the perimenopausal patient in whom preservation may have been appropriate during the childbearing period. In spite of recommendations for full staging, an analysis of current practice patterns by Abu-Rustum and colleagues revealed that 55 of 68 patients (81%) with

granulosa cell tumors were incompletely staged at primary surgery.

Several studies address prognostic factors in granulosa cell tumor of the ovary. The most important prognostic factor is stage. Other than stage, mitotic activity, DNA ploidy and S-phase fractions have been evaluated. In a study of 54 patients from Sweden, patients with mitotic rates of 4/10 high-power fields (hpf) had no deaths, whereas all patients with 10/10 hpf died, with the longest survival being 4 years. Patients with mitotic rate of 4–10/10 hpf had a median survival of 9 years. Fortunately, most patients had mitotic counts of 4/10 hpf. In a small study, about two thirds of the patients studied were found to have euploid tumors. Only 1 patient died of disease, whereas 4 of 5 patients with aneuploid tumors died of disease. S-phase fraction did not correlate with any clinical or histologic parameters. Recently the Hellenic Cooperative Oncology Group reported on 34 patients with adult granulosa cell tumors of the ovary. In this study, stage and the presence of residual disease were noted to have prognostic significance for overall survival on univariate analysis. Tumor rupture during surgery was prognostic for disease free survival. Thirteen patients with unresectable disease were evaluated for response to chemotherapy. Six of seven patients who responded to first-line platinum-based chemotherapy had complete responses to therapy, demonstrating the importance of platinum agents in treating this tumor type.

Inhibin is a nonsteroidal polypeptide hormone that is secreted by granulosa cells of the ovary. This hormone secretes throughout the menstrual cycle and during pregnancy but not in the postmenopausal woman. As a result, inhibin has been suggested as a tumor marker for granulosa cell tumors. In collective series, the relationship of tumor to the level of inhibin appears to be very good. However, there have been many reports denying the specificity of this substance, which may also be secreted by many other ovarian neoplasms, including mucinous ovarian epithelial neoplasms. Nevertheless, serum inhibin levels have an important role as a marker for monitoring patients under therapy and for detection of tumor recurrence. Although both inhibin A and inhibin B have utility as tumor markers, inhibin B has increased sensitivity (89% vs 67%) with equivalent specificity (100%) for the diagnosis of recurrent granulose cell tumor and should be used preferentially when available. Other tumor markers include müllerian inhibiting substance (MIS) and estradiol. Estradiol is not used clinically because of poor sensitivity, and MIS, although demonstrating excellent specificity, is only used for research purposes. Tumor markers, when elevated in the surveillance setting, are typically followed by imaging to localize disease recurrence. In this setting, PET/CT has been shown to have variable F-18 fluorodeoxyglucose avidity, ranging from none to mild avidity, resulting in a potential false-negative study result.

Often, recurrent tumors have been treated effectively by means of reoperation, radiation therapy, chemotherapy, or a combination thereof. Although radiation therapy has been advocated for these tumors by many authors, careful search of the literature shows little evidence relating enhanced curability to the use of radiation therapy. A prospective study has never been done to compare one form of therapy with another for patients who have advanced or recurrent disease. The question of adjuvant radiotherapy in the postmenopausal woman found to have granulosa cell tumor is often an issue.

We recommend no further therapy for patients who have stage I lesions. Adverse prognostic factors that have been reported include large tumor size, bilateral involvement, intra-abdominal rupture of the neoplasm, nuclear atypia, and a high mitotic rate. There appears to be agreement that the histologic pattern of the neoplasm has no predictive value. Stage II or III or recurrent granulosa cell tumors are probably best treated with systemic chemotherapy. Metastatic and suboptimally reduced disease should also be aggressively treated with combination chemotherapy because response rates as high as 83% have been reported. Although the optimal chemotherapeutic regimen has not yet been determined, the following drugs have been used singly or in combination and appear to be effective: doxorubicin, bleomycin, cisplatin, and vinblastine. Colombo and associates reported 11 previously untreated women with recurrent or metastatic granulosa cell tumor of the ovary who were treated with VBP. Nine patients responded; 6 patients had a complete pathologic response. Patients received between two and six courses of chemotherapy. The GOG has evaluated BEP in a nonrandomized study of advanced or recurrent granulosa cell tumors of the ovary. Fifty-seven evaluable patients received four cycles of BEP followed by a reassessment laparotomy. Only 38 patients agreed to a second-look laparotomy, and 14 (37%) had negative results. Obviously, BEP is an active combination in these patients with advanced disease.

The natural history of patients with recurrences is prolonged, thus making analysis of any therapy very difficult in terms of overall survival. This is especially true of therapy utilized in an adjuvant setting. Although responses have been reported with paclitaxel alone, paclitaxel and carboplatin in combination, BEP, gonadotropin-releasing hormone agonists, medroxyprogesterone acetate, megestrol, and alternating megestrol and tamoxifen, there are no good data to guide therapy in this setting. The role of biologic agents in the treatment of recurrence is unclear. Although some studies have shown significant expression of PDGFR alpha and beta in granulosa cell tumors, raising the possibility of response to drugs such as imatinib mesylate, other investigators have documented low levels of c-kit, c-Abl, and PDGFR, suggesting limited efficacy of this class of agent.

Thecomas

Thecomas do not occur as frequently as do granulosa cell tumors, but they have similar appearances. They are solid fibromatous lesions that show varying degrees of yellow or orange coloration. Whereas granulosa cell tumors are found to be bilateral in 2% to 5% of patients, thecomas are almost always confined to one ovary. On microscopic examination, most tumors in the granulosa–theca cell category are found to contain both cell types. If more than a very small component of granulosa cells is present, the term granulosa cell tumor, rather than granulosa–theca cell tumor, is generally applied. The designation theca cell tumor or thecoma should be reserved for neoplasms that consist entirely of benign theca cells.

Thecomas consist of neoplastic cells of ovarian stromal origin that have accumulated moderate to large amounts of lipid. Sometimes such tumors contain clusters of lutein cells, in which case the term luteinized thecoma is often used. Occasionally, tumors fall into a gray zone between thecomas and fibromas. Although the latter also arise from ovarian stromal cells, they differentiate predominantly in the direction of collagen-producing fibroblasts. Tumors in the gray zone may be designated as thecoma-fibromas. They are almost always unilateral and virtually never malignant. Several tumors have been reported in the literature as malignant thecomas, but at least some of these are better interpreted as fibrosarcomas or diffuse forms of granulosa cell tumors. In cases in which preservation of fertility is important, a thecoma may be treated adequately by unilateral oophorectomy. However, total hysterectomy with bilateral salpingo-oophorectomy is recommended in most postmenopausal and perimenopausal women. As thecomas are typically one of the most hormonally active SCSTs, 15% to 37% and 25% of cases are associated with endometrial hyperplasia and carcinoma respectively, and endometrial sampling should be performed. Patients typically present with abnormal bleeding and an abdominal or pelvic mass.

Fibromas and Sclerosing Stromal Cell Tumors

Fibromas are the most common SCST and occur primarily in postmenopausal women, although they can occur in any age group. They are not hormonally active tumors. Fibromas are benign tumors; however, recently cellular fibromas have been described and are considered to be of low malignant potential. Fibrosarcomas by contrast are rare but considered highly aggressive tumors. Behavior of these tumors is correlated with mitotic activity and degree of anaplasia.

Fibromas may be associated with ascites or hydrothorax as a result of increased capillary permeability thought to be a result of vascular endothelial growth factor (VEGF) production. Meigs' syndrome (ovarian fibromas, ascites, and hydrothorax) is uncommon and usually resolves after surgical excision of the fibroma. Gorlin's syndrome represents an inherited predisposition to ovarian fibromas and basal cell carcinomas, and occurs rarely. Because of the benign nature of fibromas, surgical excision is all that is required.

In contrast to most SCSTs, sclerosing stromal cell tumors typically present in the second and third decades of life, although they can occur in adolescents and premenarchal girls. They may be clinically undetectable or grow to very large size. They are considered benign, occur unilaterally, and are hormonally inactive except in very rare cases. Clinical symptoms include premature menarche, menstrual irregularities, pain, and uncommonly, ascites. Imaging characteristics reveal predominately solid masses with hypervascularity although complex cystic masses may be seen. Tumor markers are not elevated.

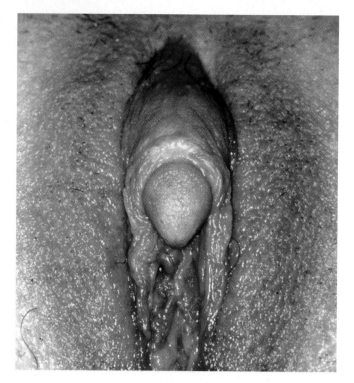

FIGURE 12-11   Enlarged clitoris in a patient with a Sertoli–Leydig cell tumor (arrhenoblastoma).

Sertoli–Leydig Cell Tumors

Sertoli–Leydig cell tumors contain Sertoli cells or Leydig cells in varying proportions and degrees of differentiation. These tumors are thought to originate from the specialized gonadal stroma. The cells were able to differentiate into any of the structures derived from the embryonic gonadal mesenchyme. Because less well-differentiated neoplasms within this category may recapitulate the development of the testes, the terms androblastoma and arrhenoblastoma have been used as synonyms for Sertoli–Leydig cell tumors. However, their connotation of associated masculinization is misleading because some of these tumors have no endocrine manifestation and others may even be accompanied by an estrogenic syndrome. Nevertheless, the World Health Organization has selected androblastoma as an alternate term for Sertoli–Leydig cell tumor. These neoplasms account for less than 0.5% of all ovarian tumors but are among the most fascinating from pathologic and clinical viewpoints. They are typically unilateral tumors and confined to the ovary in 97% of cases. They occur in all age groups but are most often encountered in young women (between the ages of 20 and 30), who usually become virilized (Figure 12-11). In immunocytochemical studies, testosterone appears to be localized predominantly within the Leydig cells. Estrogen and androstenedione appear in many of the same cells. Thus one can see the multifaceted clinical presentation of this

fascinating neoplasm. Classically, there is progressive masculinization that is heralded by hirsutism, temporal balding, deepening of the voice, and enlargement of the clitoris. Other patients may manifest secondary amenorrhea, breast atrophy, and marked increase in libido.

Sertoli–Leydig cell tumors can be described in terms of differentiation and the presence or absence of heterologous elements, distinctions that have clinical relevance. Sertoli–Leydig cell tumors with heterologous elements may contain various unusual cell types, but the degree of differentiation of the tumors is probably of greater importance in determining its prognosis than is its content of unexpected tissue. In the report by Young and Scully, only 29 of 220 tumors of this type have been clinically malignant. None of the 27 well-differentiated tumors and only 4 of 100 tumors of intermediate differentiation were known to be clinically malignant. Fifty-nine percent of poorly differentiated tumors and 19 percent of heterologous tumors displayed malignant behavior. Zaloudek and Norris reported on 64 intermediately and poorly differentiated neoplasms. Only 3 of 50 patients with stage I disease developed a recurrence (Table 12-10). The 5-year survival rate in all of their patients was 92%.

The overall 5-year survival rate of patients with Sertoli–Leydig cell tumors has been reported to range from 70% to more than 90%. Because these tumors occur predominantly in young women and are bilateral in less

TABLE 12-10   Management of Germ Cell and Sex Cord Stromal Tumors

Neoplasms	Suggested Surgery	Postoperative Chemotherapy	Reassessment Laparotomy
Dysgerminoma	Unilateral S&O when confined to one ovary—preserve normal-appearing ovarian tissue	BEP 3 cycles if the patient is not adequately staged or if stage II-IV	Not necessary unless a recurrence is suspected
Endodermal sinus	Debulk—attempt to preserve fertility	BEP 3-4 cycles; follow with AFP titers	Same as above
Embryonal carcinoma	Same as above	BEP 3-4 cycles; follow with β-hCG titers	Same as above
Malignant teratoma	Same as above	BEP or VAC 3-4 cycles	Same as above
Granulosa cell	Unilateral S&O for young patients with stage Ia disease; otherwise TAH, BSO	BEP 3-4 cycles; GnRH agonists for advanced disease	Same as above
Sertoli–Leydig cell	Same as above	BEP or VAC 3-4 cycles for advanced disease	Same as above

BEP, Bleomycin, etoposide, and cisplatin; GnRH, gonadotropin-releasing hormone; S&O, salpingo-oophorectomy; VAC, vincristine, dactinomycin, and cyclophosphamide.

than 5% of cases, conservative removal of the tumor and adjacent fallopian tube is justifiable if preservation of fertility is an important consideration and if there is no evidence of extension beyond the involved ovary. Removal of the tumor will halt, but not fully reverse, the masculinizing process. Like granulosa cell tumors, they are considered to have low malignant potential. There are no solid data to suggest that adjuvant therapy has any value in preventing a recurrence in patients with stage I lesions. Tumors with poor differentiation, heterologous elements, advanced stage, or recurrent lesions should be treated with adjuvant chemotherapy. Once again the VAC regimen of chemotherapy is often recommended. In the unusual patient who has an advanced or recurrent Sertoli–Leydig cell tumor, chemotherapy appears to be effective, although the experience is very limited. The combination of cisplatin and vinblastine and bleomycin therapy appears to be active in this disease. At least one case report has noted an elevated serum AFP as an early indication of a recurrence. Gershenson reported on nine patients with a poor prognosis after sex cord stromal tumors were treated with BEP chemotherapy. The overall response rate was 83%, but the regimen lacked durability. The median survival time was 28 months, and only two of the nine patients had no evidence of disease at the time of the report.

Sex Cord Tumor with Annular Tubules

Sex cord tumor with annular tubules (SCTAT) represents a unique ovarian tumor that appears as a histologic intermediate between granulosa and Sertoli–Leydig cell tumors. This tumor typically presents in the third to fourth decade of life and is usually unilateral. Presenting complaints are usually abnormal vaginal bleeding or postmenopausal bleeding, a testament to the endocrine activity of these tumors. Both estrogen and progesterone production have been reported. SCTAT tumors are distinguished on the basis of association with Peutz–Jegher's syndrome (PJS). Tumors associated with PJS are benign but are associated with adenoma malignum of the cervix in 15% of cases. Because adenoma malignum has a relatively high mortality rate, these patients deserve careful evaluation and follow-up. In contrast, SCTAT, which is not associated with PJS, has a 20% malignancy rate. There is limited experience in the literature with these tumors. Clinically, they should be managed in a similar manner to other SCSTs. Combination chemotherapy (BEP) may be helpful in patients with advanced disease. As SCTAT represents an intermediate cell type between granulosa cell and Sertoli–Leydig cell tumors, SCTAT may express inhibin or MIS. The utility of these tumor markers in this disease is uncertain.

Gynandroblastoma

Rarely, a gonadostromal tumor contains unequivocal granulosa cell elements combined with tubules and Leydig cells that are characteristic of arrhenoblastomas. Designated as gynandroblastomas, these mixed tumors may be associated with either androgen or estrogen production, and they can be expected to behave as low-grade malignancies similar to the individual components.

Steroid Cell Neoplasms

Steroid cell neoplasms (also known as lipid cell neoplasms) are a heterologous group of tumors that have in common a parenchyma composed of polygonal cells that contain lipid. They include neoplasms that have been designated as hilus cell tumors, Leydig tumors, adrenal rest tumors, stromal luteomas, or masculinovoblastomas. Stromal luteomas are benign tumors which account for 25% of steroid cell neoplasms and occur 80% of the time in postmenopausal women. They commonly present with postmenopausal bleeding, thought to result from a hyperestrogenic state from either direct secretion of estrogens by the tumor or secretion of androgens with subsequent conversion to estrogen. Estrogen secretion predominates, however. Leydig cell tumors are unilateral and are found commonly in the medulla or hilus regions of the ovaries. These tumors are androgen secreting tumors and are not thought to be malignant. Reinke crystals, which normally occur in mature Leydig cells of the testes, are often found in these neoplasms, and their presence may be interpreted as signifying a benign lesion. Steroid cell tumors (not otherwise specified [NOS]) are tumors that cannot be characterized as stromal luteomas or Leydig cell tumors. They are androgenic tumors that may be associated with paraneoplastic manifestations such as hypercalcemia, erythrocytosis, or ascites. In 20% of cases they will have spread to contiguous organs at the time of surgery. Tumors that have microscopic cellular pleomorphism with high mitotic activity or the presence of necrosis should be considered malignant.

TUMORS DERIVED FROM NONSPECIFIC MESENCHYME

Benign and malignant tumors, including fibromas, hemangiomas, leiomyomas, soft tissue sarcomas, lymphomas, and rare neoplasms, may arise in the ovaries from nonspecific supporting tissues that are common to most organs. The most common and most important tumors in this category are the fibroma and the lymphoma.

The mixed mesodermal sarcoma of the ovary (analogous to its uterine counterpart) has been more widely recognized in the last decade. This neoplasm is rare and is usually fatal. A review by Hernandez and colleagues suggested that 50% of the patients have stage III tumors when first seen, and the patients are most commonly diagnosed in the sixth decade of life. Various forms of combination chemotherapy, including a vigorous regimen with VAC, have been advocated with varied results. Many of these lesions are carcinosarcomas, and the metastatic sites are made up predominantly of adenomatous components so that treatment with platinum and Taxol similar to high-grade epithelial ovarian carcinoma has been utilized with reasonable success. This is particularly true when the sarcomatous elements are limited to the primary lesion in the ovary.

MALIGNANT LYMPHOMA

Lymphoma is a rare tumor of the ovary and most commonly represents ovarian involvement in overt systemic disease, almost always of the non-Hodgkin's type. There has been debate as to whether lymphoma can arise de novo in the ovary; lymphoid aggregates do exist in normal ovarian tissue, which could give rise to such a lesion.

Patients with disease localized to one ovary usually do well with unilateral surgical resection followed by systemic chemotherapy. The use of chemotherapy is based on the principle that ovarian lymphoma must be considered a localized manifestation of systemic disease. The prognosis for such patients is much better than that of patients with obvious systemic disease.

METASTATIC TUMORS TO THE OVARY

The ovary is frequently the site of metastasis from certain primary carcinomas. Approximately 10% of ovarian tumors are not primary in origin. The most common metastasis is in the form of a carcinoma that arises in the endometrium. There is no doubt that cancer of the endometrium metastasizes to the ovaries, but it may be difficult to distinguish metastasis of an endometrial cancer from a separate ovarian tumor. This is particularly true in the case of ovarian endometrioid carcinoma, which, according to Scully, is associated with a similar tumor in the endometrium in one third of cases.

There are four possible pathways of spread to tumors to the ovary:

1. Direct continuity
2. Surface papillation
3. Lymphatic metastasis
4. Hematogenous spread

Lymphatic metastasis is undoubtedly the most common pathway for spread to the ovary. The rich network of lymph nodes and lymphatic channels in the pelvis readily explains the metastatic pathway of tumors in the uterus and contralateral ovary. The rare finding of clusters of tumor cells limited to lymphatics in the medulla of the ovary in cases of breast carcinoma confirms that this is the pathway of spread to the ovary. As yet, no one has convincingly described the pathway of metastasis to the ovaries from cancer of the stomach. It is known that the lymphatic channels that drain the upper gastrointestinal tract ultimately link up with the lumbar chain of lymph nodes. Ovarian lymphatics drain into the lumbar nodes. This could be the route of spread to the ovaries in these cases.

The latest reports confirm adenocarcinoma of the colon as the most frequent nongynecologic primary site of metastatic disease to the ovary, with breast cancer in second place. These lesions are characterized microscopically by the presence of large acini similar to those of primary intestinal carcinomas. Grossly, they may form

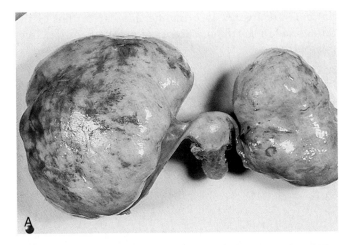

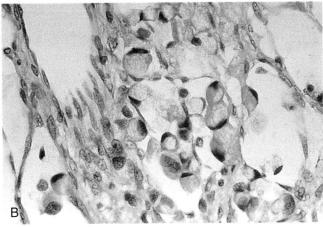

FIGURE 12-12 Metastatic tumor to the ovary from adenocarcinoma of the colon. **A,** Gross appearance. **B,** Histologic appearance. Note the large acini similar to those of the intestinal carcinoma.

solid metastases but more often appear as large, partly cystic tumors with areas of hemorrhage and necrosis (Figure 12-12). In such cases, they are easily confused with cystic forms of primary ovarian cancers. Metastatic adenocarcinomas of large intestinal origin have become more common than Krukenberg tumors in the past two decades with the gradual decline in the incidence of carcinoma of the stomach. The term Krukenberg tumor should be reserved for metastases that contain significant numbers of signet-ring cells in a cellular stroma derived from the ovarian stroma. This restriction is important, because tumors with these microscopic characteristics also have distinctive gross pathologic and clinical features. Almost all metastasize from the stomach, but some arise in the breast, intestine, or other mucous gland–containing organs. Krukenberg tumors form a solid, often uniform mass, the sectioned surface of which typically exhibits gelatinous necrosis and hemorrhage. Metastases from carcinomas of the breast are among the more common surgical specimens of the ovary, especially if one includes those found

incidentally. They are almost always incidental findings in therapeutic oophorectomy and rarely form symptomatic masses that require surgical removal.

Cases of metastatic ovarian carcinoma have occurred in which a clinical presentation was consistent with hormonal activity. Both androgen and estrogen excretion have been described. Endometrial hyperplasia has been described in postmenopausal patients with metastatic ovarian carcinomas, presumably indicating estrogen activity within the metastatic lesion or its normal tissue capsule.

MALIGNANT OVARIAN TUMORS IN CHILDREN

Ovarian tumors, cysts, and torsion are more frequent indications for surgical intervention in infancy and childhood than is commonly realized. They may produce symptoms similar to appendicitis, and it is not always appreciated how often they mimic this condition. Pain is the most frequently reported symptom. The proportion of all tumors of the abdomen in this age group that are ovarian in origin has not been reported. A palpable abdominal mass is found in half of the patients with neoplasms. Approximately 10% of the patients have isosexual precocity, which includes patients who demonstrate precocious puberty and those with an early onset of sexual development. The initial signs are areolar pigmentation and breast development. Some patients have vaginal discharge or bleeding, and others have pubic hair. These changes usually completely regress after surgical extirpation of the responsible endocrine-secreting tumor. Granulosa–theca cell tumors are by far the most common ovarian neoplasms found in these patients with isosexual precocity and adnexal enlargement. Most ovarian cancers in children are of germ cell origin. Cangir and associates reported on 21 girls younger than 16 years, with a median age of 13.5. Of the 21 patients, 8 had malignant teratomas, 6 had mixed germinal tumors, 6 had ESTs, and 1 had a stromal cell tumor (Sertoli–Leydig type). Eight patients were at stage I; 1 patient was at stage II; 7 patients were at stage III; and 5 patients were at stage IV. Ablin reported on a study of 17 children with ovarian germ cell tumors treated with multiple-agent chemotherapy. Of the 17 patients, 13 showed complete responses to therapy, suggesting that survival rates in this group of patients have improved significantly with modern chemotherapy. Lack and co-workers reported that granulosa–theca cell tumors in the premenarche patient accounted for 4% of childhood ovarian tumors at their institution from 1928 to 1979. The average age of diagnosis of their 10 patients was 5 years, and precocious "pseudopuberty" was the most common presentation. These 10 lesions were solitary; 5 were on the right side and 5 were on the left side, with an average diameter of 12 cm. All 10 patients survived at least 10 years, and salpingo-oophorectomy was curative despite tumor spillage in two patients.

Fortunately, the most common germ cell neoplasm is the benign teratoma. A significant number of other patients have benign functional cysts of the ovary. All patients are treated in a manner similar to that of the adolescent or the older patient in the early reproductive-age period.

For full reference list, log onto www.expertconsult.com ⟨http://www.expertconsult.com⟩.

Fallopian Tube Cancer

Michael A. Bidus, MD, G. Larry Maxwell, MD, and G. Scott Rose, MD

INCIDENCE AND EPIDEMIOLOGY

Adenocarcinoma of the fallopian tube is one of the rarest malignancies of the female genital tract. Its frequency in relationship to all gynecologic cancers has traditionally been considered to be 1% or less, with an average annual incidence in the United States of 3.3 per 1 million women. The incidence of fallopian tube cancer (FTCA) in Finland is reported to have increased more than fourfold, from 1.2 to 5.4 per 100,000 from the 1950s to the 1990s, but a similar trend has not been reported elsewhere. Factors thought to be associated with the increase were a decrease in parity, higher socioeconomic status, possibly pelvic inflammatory disease, and improved diagnosis and increased longevity. FTCA has been associated with BRCA mutations in several recent case series, and the incidence in this subset of women is reported to be as high as 3%, an estimated 120-fold increase in risk compared with the general population.

FTCA is initially seen in many cases as an unexpected operative finding at the time of laparotomy for a pelvic mass because of its low incidence and difficulty in distinguishing preoperatively fallopian tube masses from ovarian or uterine pathology. Cases have been reported in patients undergoing prophylactic salpingo-oophorectomy for hereditary ovarian cancer syndrome or tubal sterilization. Chronic tubal inflammation has been reported to be associated with fallopian tube carcinoma. The initial connection was with tuberculosis, and sporadic case reports of fallopian tube carcinoma with coexisting tubercular salpingitis continue to be published. Although histologic features of old pelvic inflammatory disease are frequently noted on examination of the tube and changes consistent with chronic healed salpingitis have been found in the contralateral tube of patients with unilateral FTCA, it has not been determined whether such inflammatory changes are precursors to the development of carcinoma. There is currently no suspected infectious agent thought to be a co-carcinogen in FTCA, as with human papillomavirus and cervical cancer.

Nulliparity has been reported in up to one third of FTCA cases, and infertility has been associated in some series. Age-related incidence resembles the pattern seen among women who develop ovarian or endometrial malignancies, with cases occurring rarely at a young age and incidence increasing to a peak in the 60s to early 70s. Two thirds of the patients are postmenopausal (Figure 13-1). The similarities of age group incidence, low parity, and infertility status suggest that the etiology may be similar to that of ovarian and endometrial carcinoma. Some studies have demonstrated similar genetic abnormalities, such as c-crb, B-2, p53, and K-ras mutations. These abnormalities are also common in ovarian and endometrial carcinomas.

FIGURE 13-1 Carcinoma of the fallopian tube: patients treated in 1996-1998. Distribution by age groups. *(FIGO report. Int J Gynecol Obstet, Nov 2006, vol. 95, Suppl #1. © International Federation of Gynecology and Obstetrics. Reprinted with permission.)*

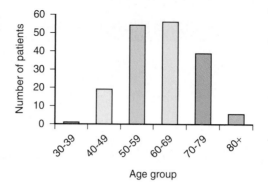

Age group	Patients (n)	Percentage (%)
30-39	1	0.6
40-49	19	10.9
50-59	54	30.9
60-69	56	32.0
70-79	39	22.3
80+	6	3.4
Total	175	100.0

MOLECULAR BIOLOGY AND GENETICS

Some studies have demonstrated a number of genetic abnormalities in FTCA that are similar to those noted in ovarian cancer, such as gene mutations, alterations in gene copy number, and loss of heterozygosity. Gene mutations include ERBB-2 (HER-2/neu), TP53 (p53), and K-RAS (K-ras) mutations. All FTCAs show a high frequency of copy number aberrations, with similar alterations noted by several authors. The most frequent changes detected in FTCA are gains at 3q (70%) and 8q (75%), with high-level amplifications in several cases. Other common gains occur at 1q, 5p, 7q, 12p, and 20q. The most frequent losses are found at 18q, 16q, 17p, 8p, and 5q. Similar alterations are reported in ovarian cancer, with amplifications of 8q, 1q, 20q, and 3q and under representation of 18q. Loss of heterozygosity at 13q has been reported in BRCA-related fallopian tube and ovarian cancers, but the significance of this genetic alteration is unclear.

Alterations in protein levels documented by immunohistochemical staining occur similarly in fallopian tube and ovarian cancer, with an increase in the proliferation-related protein MKI67 (Ki-67) and decreases in the cell cycle inhibitory proteins CDKN1A (p21) and CDKN1B (p27). Other proteins elevated in both cancer types include TP53, MYC (c-myc), ERBB-2, AKT2, WT1 (Wilms tumor 1), and PCNA. Mutation of the tumor suppressor gene TP53 is the most frequent genetic abnormality associated with FTCA. Elevated levels of p53 are associated with decreased survival and are also increased in tubal dysplasia associated with FTCA.

Although the exact molecular events responsible for the development of FTCA have yet to be fully described, an increasing body of evidence suggests that the development of high-grade serous carcinomas such as that seen commonly in FTCA may follow a stepwise progression on a cellular level from normal to serous intraepithelial carcinoma and finally invasive carcinoma. Such histologic changes are accompanied by defined molecular changes. As previously noted,

mutations in TP53 occur commonly in invasive serous carcinoma of the fallopian tube and result in overexpression of mutated p53 protein in cancer cases compared to controls. These findings are present in early-stage disease, suggesting that abnormal p53 accumulation is an early event in fallopian tube carcinogenesis. Conversely, HER-2/neu overexpression has been shown to be absent in normal controls and early-stage FTCA but overexpressed in greater than 50% of advanced-stage disease, suggesting a role in progression of disease.

In recognition of the important role of p53 in the development of serous FTCA, multiple investigators have focused attention on the p53 status of fallopian tubes removed from patients undergoing risk-reducing salpingo-oophorectomy (RRSO). In such cases high nuclear staining for p53 has facilitated the diagnosis of difficult to diagnose occult early serous carcinomas. However, these investigations also found regions of benign, normal-appearing tubal mucosa with high nuclear staining for p53. Crum and colleagues termed these foci of benign cells "p53 signatures." These regions, although histologically bland, share many features with invasive high-grade serous carcinomas of the tube such as DNA damage, secretory cell type, and reproducible p53 mutations and have been hypothesized to be the cells of origin or precursor cells for invasive cancer. The p53 signature is a relatively common finding (20%) in the fallopian tubes of high-risk women undergoing RRSO; however, cells displaying these signatures do not invariably progress to malignancy. Additionally, available data suggest that p53 signatures occur with similar frequency in the distal fallopian tubes of both high- and low-risk women. It appears that additional downstream events such as BRCA mutation or decreased expression of p27 are required to facilitate transit from precursor cells to cancer. It is interesting to note that the distal fallopian tube in patients with Li-Fraumeni syndrome (a rare familial disorder characterized by an inherited germline mutation in TP53) is known to contain abundant regions with p53 signatures. The fact that ovarian and fallopian tube carcinomas are not associated with

TABLE 13-1   Cancers Detected Using Standard Pathologic Evaluation in Patients Undergoing Prophylactic Bilateral Salpingo-Oophorectomy for Hereditary Cancer

	Reference					
	Fishman et al (2005)	Meeuwissen et al (2005)	Barakat et al. for the Society of Gynecologic Oncologists (2003)	Kauff et al (2002)	Rebbeck et al (2002)	Total
Patients screened	580	133	180	98	259	1250
Cancers detected	10	2	3	3	6	24
Cancers detected (%)	1.7	1.5	1.7	3.1	—	1.9
Fallopian tube cancer	3	1	1	1	0	6
Fallopian tube cancer/all	30	50	33	33	—	25 cancers (%)
Ovarian cancer	4	0	2	2	6	14
Peritoneal papillary serous	3	0	0	0	0	3 carcinoma
Metastatic	0	1	3	0	0	4

Li-Fraumeni syndrome is consistent with the hypothesis that additional genetic events are required in addition to TP53 overexpression to produce a malignant phenotype. Determination of the genetic and molecular alterations of fallopian tube carcinoma compared with normal mucosa and alterations associated with other intraperitoneal cancers may lead to a better understanding of disease development and the relationship among these cancer types.

HEREDITARY CANCER

FTCA has been found with increased incidence (1.7% to 3%) at centers that have established screening programs for women at high risk for gynecologic malignancy, both in patients observed using a screening protocol and in patients electing prophylactic surgery (Table 13-1). The lifetime risk of FTCA in BRCA mutation carriers has been reported to be 0.6% to 3%. Fishman and colleagues, in the largest series to date, reported 10 cancers in 581 BRCA mutation carriers (1.8%) undergoing RRSO, of which 3 were FTCAs (30%). Barakat and colleagues reported 3 cancers in 180 cases (1.7%), with 1 of 3 from the fallopian tube. Meeuwissen and colleagues found 2 cancers in 133 patients in their series, with 1 of 2 (50%) being a fallopian tube malignancy. Rebbeck and colleagues, however, found 6 ovarian cancers in 259 patients and no FTCA.

Several authors have recently noted a marked increase in the detection of occult gynecologic cancers, including FTCAs and carcinoma in situ (CIS), at the time of RRSO if extensive sectioning of the pathologic specimen is performed. FTCA and peritoneal papillary serous carcinoma, rather than ovarian cancer, comprise the majority of gynecologic malignancies in these high-risk women. Colgan and colleagues found 5 in 60 (8%) FTCAs in their series in 2001, with 2 in 5 (40%) cases

with disease confined to the fallopian tube; 1 case with disease of the fallopian tube and ovary; and 1 case with disease of the fallopian tube, ovary, and uterine serosa. These findings have been confirmed by others. Olivier and colleagues reported 5 cancers in 58 patients, with 2 (40%) cancers of the fallopian tube and 1 of the fallopian tube and ovary. Leeper and colleagues reported 5 in 30 (17%) patients with occult malignancy at the time of RRSO, with 3 in 5 (60%) being FTCA. Powell and colleagues found 7 cancers in 67 (10%) patients, with 4 in 7 (57%) from the fallopian tube. Consolidating the data reported in the literature, 22 (10.2%) cancers have been detected in 215 hereditary cancer patients undergoing RRSO, with 11 (50%) arising in the fallopian tube (Table 13-2).

Precancerous changes of the fallopian tube without the presence of cancer have also been noted with increased frequency in high-risk women. Carcangiu and colleagues evaluated normal-appearing fallopian tubes in RRSO specimens (after excluding cancers discovered at surgery) to look for epithelial changes and found that 4 in 22 (18%) BRCA1 patients had CIS or atypical hyperplasia, whereas 0 in 4 BRCA2 patients had cellular changes. Similar findings have been reported by Shaw and colleagues, who showed CIS in 8% of BRCA cases and 3% of controls. In this series 79% of patients with CIS also demonstrated p53 signature overexpression, a rate that approximates the p53 overexpression seen in high-grade serous carcinoma.

FTCA may be associated with BRCA mutations more frequently than ovarian cancer, with 16% to 43% of patients found to carry a mutation in recent series. BRCA1 appears to be associated with FTCA at a higher rate than BRCA2, although most papers linking BRCA2 with FTCA to date are case reports. The presence of a BRCA mutation also affects the histologic type of cancer that develops. In a series of 50 BRCA-associated FTCAs, Piek and colleagues noted no nonepithelial

TABLE 13-2   Cancers Detected Using Serial Sectioning of the Pathologic Specimens in Patients Undergoing Prophylactic Bilateral Salpingo-Oophorectomy for Hereditary Cancer

	Reference				
	Olivier et al (2004)	Leeper et al (2002)	Powell et al (2005)	Colgan et al (2001)	Total
Patients screened	58	30	67	60	215
Cancers or carcinoma in situ detected	5	5	7	5	22
Cancers detected (%)	8.6	16.7	10.4	8.3	10.2
Fallopian tube/invasive (carcinoma in situ)	2	3 (2)	4 (3)	2 (1)	11
Fallopian tube cancer/all cancers (%)	40.0	60.0	57.1	40.0	50.0
Ovarian cancer	2	1 (LMP)	3	1	7
Peritoneal papillary serous carcinoma	—	1	—	—	1
More than one site	1	—	1	2	4

malignancies, and 94% of the cases were papillary serous cancers compared with 62% of sporadic intraperitoneal malignancies. Improved survival of BRCA mutation carriers with FTCA, with a median survival of 148 months compared with 41 months in sporadic cases, has been reported.

Peritoneal washings and serial sectioning of pathologic specimens should be considered essential in high-risk patients because they have improved detection of both FTCA and occult ovarian cancer. Prior to the recent association of BRCA1/2 mutations and FTCA, oophorectomy was considered by some to be adequate prophylactic surgery in high-risk patients. There has been one case report of FTCA after oophorectomy only, and the tubal epithelium is clearly at risk in these patients. Salpingectomy, along with oophorectomy, must be a part of prophylactic surgery. Hysterectomy has also been advocated to avoid the possible risk of cancer in the interstitial portion of the tube, although this remains controversial. It has recently been shown by Cass and colleagues that FTCA is a distal and mid-tube process in their series of 50 patients, and there have been no documented cases of cancer arising in the interstitial portion of the tube. Restaging, which can be done laparoscopically, is necessary if occult tumor is found at the time of RRSO, with more than half the cases (5 in 8) of apparent early-stage FTCA upstaged in the report by Leblanc and colleagues. Patients with FTCA or CIS appear to be at significant risk for carrying a BRCA mutation, so BRCA testing should be offered to allow appropriate counseling regarding the potential increased risk of other BRCA-associated cancers in the patient and her family.

Patients with Peutz–Jeghers syndrome may also have a genetic predisposition to tumors of the female genital tract, including the fallopian tube. They have an increased incidence of the rare tumors adenoma malignum and ovarian sex cord tumor with annular tubules. There have also been reports of mucinous metaplasia and carcinosarcoma in the fallopian tubes of these patients.

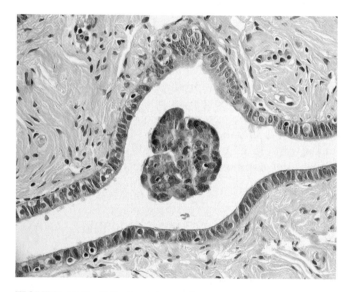

FIGURE 13-2   Fallopian tube carcinoma in situ seen adjacent to carcinoma in the lumen of the tube. (*Courtesy Keith Kaplan.*)

CARCINOMA IN SITU

CIS of the fallopian tube is a diagnosis that histologically requires the epithelial cells of the endosalpingeal lining to form papillae with cytologically malignant mitotically active nuclei. CIS was present in 18% of fallopian tubes removed at RRSO in BRCA mutation carriers in one report and can also be seen side by side with invasive adenocarcinoma (Figure 13-2). The epithelial cells lose their polarity and grow in papillae without stromal. Nuclei are hyperchromatic, large, and irregular, and mitoses are numerous, but the basement membrane is intact. Atypical hyperplasia or dysplasia of the fallopian tube epithelium in high-risk women undergoing RRSO has been reported to occur in 2 in 22 (10%) specimens by Carcangiu and colleagues and in 6 in 12 (50%) of the tubes by Piek and colleagues. Piek and colleagues also reported atypical hyperplasia, considered to be less severe than dysplasia, in another 5 of the 12 patients. Of note, morphologically normal, hyperplastic, and dysplastic epithelium in the RRSO patients had molecular alterations consistent with cellular proliferation, a higher proportion of Ki-67–expressing cells, and lower fractions of cells expressing p21 and p27 compared with control patients. Tamoxifen therapy has also been associated with diffuse bilateral atypical hyperplasia and adenocarcinoma in situ of the fallopian tube in case reports. The role of the patients' genetic predisposition versus an effect of tamoxifen therapy on the tubal epithelium remains unclear. Controversy also remains regarding the terminology of hyperplastic and dysplastic changes of the epithelium and the premalignant potential of hyperplastic changes of the tubes in RRSO patients.

Mucinous metaplasia and neoplasia have been described. There are case reports of these changes noted at the time of tubal ligation and in patients with Peutz–Jegher's syndrome.

Treatment of tubal CIS, if it exists alone, involves removal of the tube or tubes, with a staging procedure including careful inspection of the ovaries to rule out metastatic disease. The incidence of bilaterality of CIS is unknown and is an important consideration of this disease, which may be found incidentally in a portion of a tube removed for an ectopic pregnancy. The decision regarding therapy in this setting must consider the patient's desire for future fertility, in addition to a possible genetic predisposition for breast and gynecologic cancer. Careful surveillance for gynecologic and breast cancers, with the offer of bilateral salpingo-oophorectomy at the completion of childbearing, is probably warranted, as for women with hereditary breast and ovary cancer syndromes. When CIS is found in the portion of the tube removed at tubal ligation, the authors have routinely recommended, at a minimum, bilateral salpingo-oophorectomy because preservation of fertility is not an issue.

INVASIVE CARCINOMA

Signs and Symptoms

Most patients who have these malignancies will have symptoms such as vaginal bleeding or discharge and/or lower abdominal pain. Less frequent symptoms include abdominal distension and urinary urgency. In many cases, these symptoms are vague and nonspecific. Vaginal bleeding is the most common symptom of tubal carcinoma and is present in approximately 50% of the patients. Because this lesion occurs most frequently in the postmenopausal patient, postmenopausal bleeding is common; as a result, carcinoma of the endometrium is the first consideration in the differential diagnosis. One must seriously consider the diagnosis of fallopian tube carcinoma when the result of the dilation and curettage is negative and symptoms persist. Vaginal bleeding is caused by blood that accumulates from the lesion in the fallopian tube, which subsequently passes into the uterine cavity and finally exits into the vagina. Pain is frequently a symptom in tubal carcinoma, is usually colicky, and often accompanies the vaginal bleeding. The pain is caused by distension of the tubal wall and stimulation of peristaltic activity. This pain, in many cases, is relieved with the passage of blood or watery discharge. Vaginal discharge, which is usually clear, occurs in approximately 25% of patients with tubal carcinoma.

The triad of pain, metrorrhagia, and leukorrhea is considered pathognomonic for tubal carcinoma, but it occurs infrequently. Pain with bloody vaginal discharge is a more common finding. Pain combined with a profuse, watery vaginal discharge referred to as hydrops tubae profluens, is reported to be present in less than 5% of cases. If a patient is examined during the time that hydrops tubae profluens is present, a palpable pelvic mass is frequently found. The mass can decrease during the examination while the watery discharge continues. With the cessation of watery discharge and decrease in pelvic mass, the pain also decreases. Hydrops tubae profluens is caused by the effusion produced by the tumor that accumulates within the tube and causes the distension, which in turn produces the colicky pain. A pelvic mass, which is often interpreted as a pedunculated fibroid or ovarian neoplasm, is the most common physical sign. It is found in more than half of patients, with an abdominal mass noted in another 25% of patients, usually adnexal in location (Figure 13-3). Ascites were

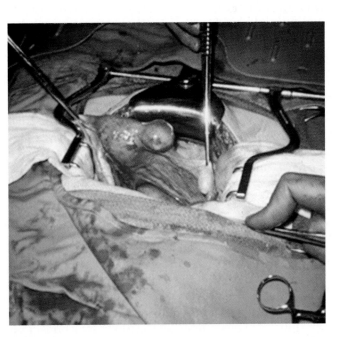

FIGURE 13-3   Primary tubal carcinoma. The right ovary is normal.

reported to be present in 5% of patients in a meta-analysis by Nordin in 1994. Presentation with symptoms consistent with pelvic inflammatory disease should raise suspicion for FTCA in a postmenopausal patient. Presentation with metastasis to an inguinal node has been reported, as have several cases of paraneoplastic cerebellar degeneration.

Delay of diagnosis appears to be common. In a study by Eddy and associates, symptoms had been present for as long as 48 months. Half of the patients had symptoms for 2 months or longer. Semrad and colleagues noted a delay from the onset of symptoms to the diagnosis of an average of 4 months in about half of their patients. Peters and colleagues reported that 14% of patients were asymptomatic in their series of 115 patients.

Malignant cells are found in 11% to 23% of cervical cytologic preparations in patients with tubal cancer. In patients with hydrops tubae profluens, the chance of obtaining malignant cells should be relatively high. The identification of psammoma bodies in cervical cytology of postmenopausal women is often a sign of uterine or clear cell carcinoma, with serous fallopian tube or ovarian cancer occasionally being identified as the source.

Diagnosis

More than 80% of patients have either a pelvic or an abdominal mass noted before surgery. Between 10% and 25% will have abnormal cervical cytology suggestive of adenocarcinoma. Because uterine and ovarian pathologies are much more common than tubal disease, it is not surprising that patients with pelvic masses are thought to have abnormalities other than tubal ones. Patients with abnormal cytology are likewise believed to have the more common diagnosis of a cervical or uterine malignancy instead of a primary tubal malignancy.

Ultrasound, both abdominal and vaginal, is reported to be accurate in noting changes in adnexal size and its morphology. Patlas and colleagues reported that transvaginal sonography in five of seven patients with FTCA showed normal ovaries in association with a discrete solid adnexal mass in four. In the three patients without a discrete adnexal mass, there were more extensive changes, including large, solid adnexal masses of unknown origin or gross peritoneal carcinomatosis. Presence of small cystic or solid masses shaped like a sausage, a snail, or a gourd, regardless of clinical stage, are other reported findings. Kurjak and colleagues reported improved identification of FTCA using three-dimensional ultrasound compared with two-dimensional ultrasound. The three-dimensional ultrasound allowed precise depiction of tubal wall irregularities such as papillary protrusions and pseudosepta. Multiple sections of the tube demonstrating sausage-like structures also enabled determination of local tumor spread and capsule

infiltration. Study of the vascular architecture was further enhanced using three-dimensional power Doppler imaging. Other authors have not confirmed these findings, and the role of advanced ultrasound techniques in the evaluation has not been determined.

Reports that have appeared in the literature evaluating use of ultrasound in conjunction with CA-125 testing as a method of screening for gynecologic malignancy have noted higher than expected incidence of FTCA. In the large cancer screening project of the Royal London Hospital, 22,000 patients were screened with CA-125, and if the serum CA-125 was elevated, patients underwent pelvic ultrasound. Of 15 patients with pelvic malignancies identified through the elevated CA-125 screening, 3 (20%) had primary FTCA. The ratio of epithelial ovarian cancers to FTCAs in volunteers for ovarian cancer screening was 6:1, which is 25-fold greater than the expected ratio. Two of the patients had stage I disease, and 1 patient had stage II. A large screening program for high-risk women that uses both CA-125 and ultrasound every 6 months, the National Ovarian Cancer Early Detection Program, has been ongoing in the United States since 1990. Fishman and colleagues recently reported that 12 gynecologic malignancies were discovered by screening 4426 high-risk women who elected not to have a prophylactic RRSO. Four cancers (33%) arose in the fallopian tube, 4 (33%) were primary peritoneal serous carcinoma, 2 (16%) were ovarian, and 2 (16%) were uterine. Unfortunately, all the cancers detected were stage III at the time of diagnosis except for the uterine cancers, casting doubt on the value of CA-125 and transvaginal ultrasound for detecting early-stage disease.

Both of these large screening trials found a much higher ratio of FTCA to ovarian cancer than expected based on the reported incidence of FTCA in the general population. This is in contrast to the findings of Nagall and colleagues, who did not report an increased proportion of FTCAs in a screening program of women in the general population in Kentucky. The reason for the different ratios of FTCA to ovarian cancer in these screening trials is unclear. Whether the English study was subject to selection bias, leading to high-risk women being screened, is unknown. It may be that the diagnostic criteria for gynecologic cancers favor assessment of advanced-stage intraperitoneal cancers as ovarian in origin, and the ratio of FTCA to ovarian cancer in the general population may be higher than previously reported.

Successful use of other radiologic imaging modalities to identify FTCAs has been described in case reports. There have not been trials evaluating diagnostic imaging of FTCA prospectively, but the data on ovarian cancer are applicable to all intraperitoneal cancers because the radiologic findings are similar. The Radiology Diagnostic Oncology Group found that magnetic resonance imaging (MRI) is superior to Doppler ultrasound and computed tomography (CT) in diagnosis of malignant ovarian masses and that CT and MRI are preferred over ultrasound for staging. Positron emission tomography–CT with 2-fluoro-2-deoxy-d-glucose may prove to be a sensitive and accurate method for detection of metastatic disease, which may influence the clinical management of recurrent fallopian tube carcinoma.

Immunohistochemical staining for CA-125 is positive in 87% of tumors. The use of serum CA-125 levels becomes a valuable tool in monitoring these patients during and after therapy for evidence of a recurrence. It has also been evaluated in screening programs for ovarian cancer, as noted, and has been reported to be a harbinger of FTCA in this setting. Its usefulness as a screening tool remains to be determined.

Histologic diagnosis may be difficult because of the similarities of FTCA to metaplastic processes associated with inflammation of the tubal epithelium found in pelvic inflammatory disease or tuberculous salpingitis and other gynecologic cancers. Another complicating factor can be multifocal neoplasia, which can occur both within the fallopian tube and in the other genital organs and the peritoneal cavity. Synchronous cancers in the fallopian tube have been reported in up to 10% of ovarian cancers. Hu and colleagues suggested diagnostic criteria for the diagnosis of tubal cancer:

- The main tumor grossly should be in the tube
- Histologically, the tubal mucosa should be involved with a papillary pattern
- If the tubal wall is involved to a large extent, transition from benign to malignant tubal epithelium should be identified

When the ovaries are involved, differentiation between a primary tubal malignancy and a primary ovarian malignancy should be attempted. When ovarian cancer extends to the tube, serosal involvement is usually evident and the mucosa of the endosalpinx may not be involved. In such situations, the correct diagnosis is apparent. In some cases of tubal cancer, the benign to malignant transition may not be readily apparent. It may be that these strict diagnostic criteria favor assessment of advanced-stage intraperitoneal cancers as ovarian in origin. Of interest, in tubal carcinoma there is usually intraperitoneal involvement before the ovaries are affected. Because of the possibility of early intraperitoneal cytologic spread even with only mucosal involvement, the role of peritoneal cytology is important in this disease entity. In patients with disease limited to the tube, the exact extent should be ascertained. If an in situ lesion is present or invasion is limited to the lamina propria, the prognosis is good. When the muscularis is invaded or the cancer is located in the fimbria, the prognosis worsens, even with disease limited to the tube.

The late stage of the disease mimics late-stage ovarian cancer with intraperitoneal spread. It appears that FTCA, like ovarian cancer, also has a propensity for lymph node metastasis. This has been described even with apparent stage I/II disease and with well-differentiated tumors. Klein and associates noted that the frequency of lymph node metastasis increased with intra-abdominal disease. Six of eight patients with stage III disease had lymph node metastasis. Patients frequently have para-aortic lymph node involvement only, whereas the majority of patients who had pelvic node metastasis had both pelvic and para-aortic involvement. Deffieux and colleagues found that the left para-aortic chain above the level of the inferior mesenteric artery is the most frequently involved in patients with primary tubal carcinoma who have para-aortic lymph node metastasis.

Most carcinomas of the tube are cystic adenocarcinomas (Figure 13-4), comprising 71% of cancers in one report with endometrioid, transitional cell, and mixed cell–type carcinomas each accounting for approximately 5% to 10% of tumors. The more indolent female adnexal tumors of probable wolffian origin made up half of the endometrioid tumors at one referral center. Other rare epithelial cell types include clear cell carcinomas and adenosquamous carcinomas. Low malignant potential tumors have been reported. Sarcomas have been removed, and several case reports of other rare tumor types have been published.

Cass and colleagues found that FTCA appears to arise primarily in the distal portion of the tube, with 8 of 10 cases in the distal and mid-portion of the tube and 2 cases involving the entire tube. Occult cancers were found only in the distal portion of the tube. There were no cases of only proximal involvement. Multifocal skip lesions; diffuse precursor lesions; and benign findings such as transitional cell metaplasia and p53 signature

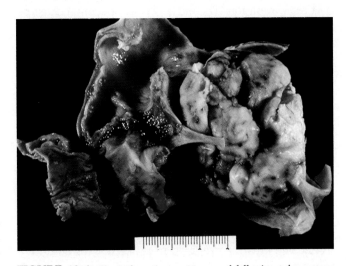

FIGURE 13-4 Typical cystic appearance of fallopian tube cancer. *(Courtesy Keith Kaplan.)*

regions, which may mimic early tubal carcinoma, were noted in the fallopian tubes of BRCA mutation carriers. Transitional cell metaplasia is present in up to 26% of RRSO specimens and is multifocal in up to 67% of cases. Metaplastic foci stain negative for p53 and MIB-1, a marker of proliferation. p53 signature foci stain positive for p53 but negative for MIB-1. When cancer is present, both tubes are equally affected. Bilaterality has been noted in 10% to 25% of patients. Tumors are usually large and noted on the pelvic examination; however, a number of cases of clinically occult cancers have been reported in patients undergoing RRSO. Overexpression of p53 was found in 70% of cancers and associated dysplastic epithelium but in only 10% of surrounding normal epithelium in one report. The changes were present in both BRCA1 carriers and noncarriers. Meticulous histologic evaluation of the fallopian tube in apparent benign cases, including serial sectioning in high-risk patients, is obligatory.

Because occult carcinoma may be found in as many as 17% of specimens in patients undergoing RRSO, it is essential that these specimens undergo extensive histologic evaluation aided by immunohistochemical evaluation in cases in which occult malignancy is suspected. Multiple protocols exist. Pathologic detection of disease is dependent on the thoroughness of evaluation. Two guiding principles should be adhered to in such cases. First, the surgeon must ensure that at least 2 cm of infundibulopelvic ligament be resected and submitted for evaluation with the ovaries and fallopian tubes because microscopic ovarian tissue may extend proximally into the ligament beyond that which is grossly visible. In cases in which the uterus is left in situ, up to 6 mm of tube may remain in the transmural portion of the myometrium. If complete resection is desired, hysterectomy should be performed. Second, the entire tube, ovary, and mesosalpinx should be thinly sliced and totally embedded for evaluation. The entire RRSO specimen must be sliced thinly at intervals of no greater than 3 mm and evaluated. Deeper sectioning is only performed in areas suspicious for neoplasm or when additional sections are needed for immunohistochemical evaluation. This protocol has been evaluated by Rabban and colleagues in 102 women with BRCA germline mutations and found to be highly accurate. The authors advise against performing multistep sectioning at deeper levels as long as there is an optimal dissection protocol and the tissue is sliced at intervals of 2 to 3 mm.

Therapy

Because the diagnosis is rarely established preoperatively, one must be prepared to proceed with definitive therapy at the time of exploratory laparotomy for any adnexal mass or when this lesion is found coincidentally with other disease. In 1991 the International Federation of Gynecology and Obstetrics (FIGO) established a staging classification for tubal carcinoma for the first time. It follows the general outline of ovarian carcinoma. Alvarado-Cabrera and colleagues proposed that depth of invasion into the lamina propria and muscularis layers of the fallopian tube and fimbrial involvement in stage I disease be incorporated into the staging classification because these features have prognostic significance (Table 13-3).

Therapy guidelines should be essentially the same as those for ovarian carcinoma, and a total abdominal hysterectomy with bilateral salpingo-oophorectomy and surgical staging, including lymph node sampling, is optimal therapy. The safety of unilateral salpingectomy or salpingo-oophorectomy in appropriately staged young patients who desire fertility and whose disease apparently is confined to one tube has not been established. Removal of the remaining tube and ovary (or ovaries) should be performed at the completion of childbearing.

Even with apparent early disease, this malignancy can be bilateral. Peritoneal cytologic specimens should be obtained on opening the peritoneal cavity, not only from the pelvis, but also from the lateral paracolic gutters and supradiaphragmatic areas. Prognostic correlation with peritoneal cytologic findings has been noted in a report from the Mayo Clinic. Patients with negative cytologic findings had a 5-year survival of 67% compared with 20% in patients with positive cytologic findings. A partial omentectomy should be performed also. Any disease outside the areas already extirpated should be removed if technically feasible. Debulking, as described in ovarian carcinoma, would also be applicable to this malignancy. Carcinomatous reduction to 1 cm or smaller was feasible in two thirds of patients reported by Podratz and colleagues. Optimal debulking appears to enhance survival, as in ovarian cancer. Patients with an earlier stage and complete surgical removal have a better survival than do patients with advanced disease and suboptimal removal.

The role of lymphadenectomy in staging FTCA is well established. Pelvic and para-aortic lymph node sampling (above the inferior mesenteric artery) are required for staging, even for patients with apparent early-stage disease, because of the risk of early lymphatic spread. Of patients subjected to routine lymphadenectomy, 42% to 59% will show metastatic disease, a rate higher than that seen with ovarian cancer. Even in apparent early-stage disease, the propensity for retroperitoneal nodal spread is high. The therapeutic value of systematic complete lymphadenectomy remains controversial with a paucity of clinical data to support its use. In recurrent disease, FTCA tends to recur more often in retroperitoneal nodes and extraperitoneal sites than ovarian carcinoma.

TABLE 13-3   International Federation of Gynecology and Obstetrics Fallopian Tube Staging*

Stage	Definition
0	Carcinoma in situ (limited to tubal mucosa).
I[†]	Growth limited to the fallopian tubes.
Ia	Growth is limited to one tube, with extension into the submucosa or muscularis but not penetrating the serosal surface; no ascites.
Ib	Growth is limited to both tubes, with extension into the submucosa or muscularis but not penetrating the serosal surface; no ascites.
Ic	Tumor stage Ia or Ib but with tumor extension through or on to the tubal serosa; or with ascites present containing malignant cells, or with positive peritoneal washings.
II	Growth involving one or both fallopian tubes, with pelvic extension.
IIa	Extension or metastasis to the uterus or ovaries.
IIb	Extension to other pelvic tissues.
IIc	Tumor stage IIa or IIb, with ascites present containing malignant cells or with positive peritoneal washings.
III	Tumor involves one or both fallopian tubes, with peritoneal implants outside the pelvis or positive retroperitoneal or inguinal nodes. Superficial liver metastasis equals stage III. Tumor appears limited to the true pelvis but with histologically proven malignant extension to the small bowel or omentum.
IIIa	Tumor is grossly limited to the true pelvis, with negative nodes but with histologically confirmed microscopic seeding of abdominal peritoneal surfaces.
IIIb	Tumor involving one or both tubes, with histologically confirmed implants of abdominal peritoneal surfaces, none exceeding 2 cm in diameter. Lymph nodes are negative.
IIIc	Abdominal implants >2 cm in diameter or positive retroperitoneal or inguinal nodes.
IV	Growth involving one or both fallopian tubes, with distant metastases. If pleural effusion is present, there must be positive cytology to be stage IV. Parenchymal liver metastases equals stage IV.

*Staging for fallopian tube is by the surgical pathologic system. Operative findings designating stage are determined before tumor debulking.
†Alvarado-Cabrera et al have proposed that stage I disease be further subdivided based on no extension (0), extension into the lamina propria (1), and extension into the muscularis (2), with disease of the fimbria designated as a separate substage, 1(f).
(With permission of the International Federation of Gynecology and Obstetrics.)

Postoperative therapy is most often needed, as in ovarian carcinoma. Patients with stage Ia tumor without spread to the muscularis layer had 100% 5-year survival in the report by Alvarado-Cabrera and colleagues and need not be treated. In contrast, patients with invasion of the muscularis layer or tumor in the fimbria, who had a 5-year survival of 71% to 72%, should receive additional therapy.

Fallopian tube cancers are often incorporated with ovarian cancer in chemotherapy trials because of the small number of FTCAs and the apparent similarity of FTCA to ovarian cancer, and data regarding adjuvant, maintenance, and intraperitoneal chemotherapy for ovarian cancer are considered applicable to FTCA. Additionally, the usual tenets of ovarian cancer treatment for recurrent disease with respect to platinum sensitivity or resistance also apply to FTCA. Adjuvant therapy with a combination platinum/paclitaxel-based chemotherapy regimen, as in ovarian cancer, is typically used; case reports and one series reporting the outcomes of platinum/paclitaxel therapy in FTCA have also been published. Historically, the use of alkylating agent chemotherapy did not improve survival in this group of patients. Wagenaar and colleagues have reported the results of a phase II European Organization for Research and Treatment of Cancer trial of cyclophosphamide (C), doxorubicin (Adriamycin, A), and cisplatin (P) treating 24 patients with stage III to IV FTCA. Median overall survival at 3 and 5 years was only 25% and 19%, respectively. The group at the MD Anderson Hospital treated 18 patients with cisplatin, Adriamycin, and cyclophosphamide (Cytoxan) (CAP), with a mean survival rate of 44 months. No patient responded to second-line therapy.

Gemignani and colleagues reported initial results of combination platinum and paclitaxel chemotherapy in 24 patients (one received paclitaxel only because of hearing impairment) with this regimen in FTCA. Seven patients with stage I and II disease had been treated, with one (14%) recurrence at a median follow-up of 42 months. In four earlier studies, adjuvant therapy in early-stage disease (I and II) had not been shown to benefit survival, although survival rates in the 50% to 60% range indicate that there was probably undetected disease outside the pelvis.

Combination platinum/paclitaxel therapy has been reported to produce complete responses and long-term survivals in advanced-stage FTCA patients. Seventeen patients with stage III and IV disease were treated using platinum/paclitaxel therapy, with a 90% 3-year survival. Five of eight patients with suboptimal cytoreduction at the time of laparotomy developed recurrence, and four were re-treated with the same combination. Only two patients had died of disease at a median survival time of 51 months, so the authors were optimistic that the combination regimen would improve survival for FTCA, as it has for ovarian cancer. In an earlier report by Barakat and colleagues, 38 patients were treated with cisplatin-based combination chemotherapy, with an overall survival of 51% at 5 years. Patients with stages II to IV disease who had completed resected tumors had a 5-year survival of 83%, compared with 28% if gross disease remained after surgery. It appears that cisplatin-based chemotherapy improves long-term survival in patients with advanced disease, but it may not be as effective as platinum combined with paclitaxel. This conclusion has been supported recently by Leath and colleagues, who reported in their series of 38 patients that those treated with paclitaxel and platinum had superior overall survival compared to those patients treated with cisplatin alone or melphalan. Recently, Pectasides and colleagues reported a retrospective analysis of 64 patients treated in contemporary practice with carboplatin and paclitaxel. Among patients with measurable disease, they reported a 68% complete response and 25% partial response rates. Five-year survival for the entire reported cohort was 70%; however, when stratified by stage, the median survival for stage I/II patients was not reached and was 62 months for stage III/IV patients. In this study, stage and residual disease were prognostic for both overall survival and for time to progression.

The role of second-look laparotomy (SLL) has not been defined in tubal carcinoma, but it would be expected to be similar to that in ovarian cancer, in which there appears to be limited benefit. The clinical utility of SLL is related to the effectiveness of second-line treatment options. In the absence of effective second-line therapy, the utility of SLL must be questioned. Barakat and associates noted in their patients undergoing SLL that the absence of gross residual disease following primary surgery was the best predictor of disease-free status at SLL. These patients also had a significantly better 5-year survival rate (83%) than did those with gross residual disease (28%). The group at the Memorial Sloan-Kettering Cancer Center evaluated 35 patients with SLL following cytoreductive surgery and platinum-based chemotherapy. Twenty-one patients were tumor-free at the time of SLL. None of five patients with stage I or grade 1 tumors had disease at SLL. The absence of gross disease at the completion of primary surgery was the best predictor of disease-free status at SLL. Of the patients who were negative at SLL, only 4 (19%) had a recurrence of their tumor (mean follow-up of 50 months). Eddy and co-workers noted their experience with 8 patients. Their results mimic those of ovarian cancer. The procedure may be prognostic, although 2 of 5 patients with negative SLL had a recurrence. Combined series in the literature note that of all patients with complete clinical responses who underwent SLL, 63% were pathologically negative for disease. Of those pathologically negative patients, 22% ultimately had a recurrence. This, of course, is much better than in ovarian cancer. Approximately 30% of those found to have persistent disease at SLL were alive after 5 years. Whether an SLL has any appreciable

effect on long-term survival is unknown. Although a negative SLL is associated with longer survival in fallopian tube cancer compared to those found to harbor residual disease, this alone is inadequate justification for recommending SLL. As such, SLL should be reserved for clinical trials.

Radiation therapy after surgery had been used frequently to treat FTCA before the advent of platinum- and taxane-based therapy, but it is not used frequently today. Much of the data regarding radiation therapy precede the era of surgical staging of apparent early-stage disease, making it difficult to draw conclusions regarding efficacy in properly staged patients. Given these constraints, Rosen and colleagues retrospectively compared patients with stage I and II disease who received adjuvant therapy with radiation or chemotherapy treated at multiple centers over a 25-year period ending in 1999 and found no significant difference in median survival time. They found significantly improved survival in patients undergoing surgery that included lymphadenectomy, presumably as a result of exclusion of advanced-stage disease in this group. They also reported that practice patterns had changed dramatically over the course of their study, with no radiation therapy for patients with stage II disease after 1988 and for patients with stage I disease after 1995. Baekelandt and colleagues, in their review of 151 patients treated over many years, concluded that radiation therapy in FTCA should be abandoned because of frequent recurrences in patients receiving pelvic radiotherapy and an unacceptable complication rate in patients treated with whole abdominal radiation. Schray and colleagues, however, reported in 1987 that 8 of 10 (80%) patients with stage I and II disease who received whole abdominal radiation (2 with intraperitoneal P-32) survived disease free, whereas only 4 of 11 (36%) patients treated with pelvic radiation remained disease free.

Radiation therapy appears to have fallen out of favor and was used in only 4% of patients reported in the Surveillance, Epidemiology, and End Results (SEER) database in 2002 and in 4 of 105 patients in the FIGO report for 1995 to 1998. Radiation is unlikely to be compared with combination chemotherapy in a prospective randomized trial, but preliminary data evaluating whole abdominal radiation following combination chemotherapy that indicate it may be more efficacious in preventing recurrence in ovarian cancer may be applicable in FTCA.

Finally, given the explosion of clinical knowledge and experience in using biologic and small molecule therapy in the treatment of ovarian cancer, it should be mentioned that there are minimal specific trial data on these new treatment modalities in FTCA. Current clinical trials utilizing these agents for ovarian cancer include patients with FTCA and conclusions, when published, will likely be extrapolated to FTCA patients. One of the most promising agents for adjuvant and maintenance therapy in trials at this time is bevacizumab, a monoclonal antibody against VEGF. In a retrospective analysis of 26 patients with FTCA, VEGF was found to be reactive on immunohistochemical staining in 85% of cases, although this did not display prognostic significance. A single case report has been published describing a complete clinical response to single-agent bevacizumab in a patient with chemotherapy-refractive FTCA who remained disease free on maintenance therapy for greater than 26 months after achieving a clinical remission.

Prognosis

Survival with fallopian tube carcinoma has traditionally been reported as poorer than for ovarian cancer, but this has changed in two recent reports (Table 13-4). Five-year relative survival from the SEER database was reported by Kosary and Trimble as follows: stage I, 95%; stage II, 75%; stage III, 69%; and stage IV, 45%. Only 39% of patients had stage I or II disease, in contrast to earlier series in which more than half the patients had stage I or II disease, even though almost half of those diagnosed with stage I or II disease did not undergo surgical evaluation of lymph nodes. Most women with stage I or II disease were treated with surgery alone, whereas most women with stage III or IV disease were treated with surgery and chemotherapy.

Survival may improve further as a larger proportion of patients is staged and treated appropriately. Heintz and colleagues reported the FIGO 5-year survival data on patients treated from 1996 to 1998, with results as follows: stage I, 79%; stage II, 82%; stage III, 61%; stage IV, 29%; and an overall survival of 69%, a 24% increase from the previous 3-year reporting period. The report by Heintz and colleagues had 57% of patients staged as stage I or II, with poorer survival when compared with the SEER data, suggesting that a greater number of patients were understaged in their report.

Survival was better stage for stage with FTCA compared with ovarian cancer in both of these reports. Factors that contribute to the improved survival rates are improved therapeutic regimens that include chemotherapy with platinum and paclitaxel as primary therapy, upstaging of patients with apparent stage I and II disease, improved debulking, and the difficulty of distinguishing the primary site of advanced-stage intraperitoneal cancer with possible misclassification of more aggressive FTCAs. Recently, Wethington and colleagues reported a retrospective review of SEER data for patients with fallopian tube or ovarian cancer from 1988 to 2004. Compared to ovarian cancer patients, those with fallopian tube carcinoma were more likely to present with earlier stage tumors. When stratified by stage, those with stage I/II tumors had similar survival. Those patients with stage III/IV FTCA had a better overall survival (54% vs 30%) compared to stage III/IV ovarian cancer patients. Other recent large retrospective reviews report worse survival for patients with early-stage disease, but these studies cover many years, with a large percentage of patients not receiving adequate staging or platinum and paclitaxel therapy. The wide disparity in reported results from these and other studies are explained in part by inherent biases present in retrospective reviews, lack of uniformed and consistent staging likely resulting in stage migration, inconsistent adjuvant chemotherapy and/or radiation use, nonstandardized chemotherapy regimens used, and lack of central pathology review. As such, the issue of relative survival between FTCA and ovarian cancer remains unresolved.

Stage and the amount of residual disease at the time of debulking have consistently been found to be important prognostic factors, and some reports also have found age, grade, lymphovascular space involvement, and a closed fimbriated end of the fallopian tube to be significant. Depth of invasion and involvement of the fimbria have also been reported as prognostic factors in stage I tumors, and it has been suggested that these factors be incorporated into FIGO staging by subdivision of stage I into substages based on no invasion, invasion into the lamina propria, or invasion into the muscularis layer of the tube. In patients with invasion into the tubal muscularis layer, there was a statistically significant increase in the risk of death from tumor. In these patients, the 5-year survival was only 60%, compared with 100% survival among patients who had no muscularis involvement.

Similar to ovarian cancer, serum concentrations of CA-125 in patients with FTCA have been shown to be prognostically important. In the largest study published to date, evaluating 53 patients and 406 serum samples of CA-125 in only FTCA patients, pretreatment serum CA-125 levels were shown to be a prognostic factor for disease-free and overall survival, independent

TABLE 13-4 Diagnosed and Treated After Adoption of International Federation of Gynecology and Obstetrics Staging

Stage	Kosary and Trimble (2002)			Heintz et al (2003)		
	No. of Patients	% of All Cases	5-Year Survival (%)	No. of Patients	% of All Cases	5-Year Survival (%)
I	102	30.5	95	42	40.8	79
II	29	8.7	75	17	16.5	82
III	52	15.6	69	35	34.0	60
IV	151	45.2	45	7	6.8	29
Overall	334	—	—	103	—	69

of surgical stage. Presurgery CA-125 was noted to be elevated in 80% of patients with FTCA, and serum levels during therapy correlated well with response to treatment. All patients with a complete or partial response to treatment had declining CA-125 levels, and 2 of 2 patients with progressive disease had rising CA-125 levels. During follow-up, rising CA-125 levels were shown to have a sensitivity and specificity of 92% and 90%, respectively, for recurrent disease. A rising CA-125 preceded clinically evident disease by a median of 3 months.

SARCOMAS AND OTHER TUMORS

Sarcomas of the fallopian tube are rare. Although carcinosarcoma (mixed mesodermal or müllerian tumor) represents the largest number of sarcomas, fewer than 60 have been reported in the literature. Although 25 of the reported cases were found to contain heterologous elements, with non-müllerian tissue present this has not been shown to affect survival. Sarcomas have been reported in adolescents and in the elderly. Most patients present with symptoms similar to those of adenocarcinoma, are mainly in the sixth decade of life, and have low parity.

Treatment should be surgery initially, as in adenocarcinoma of the fallopian tube. Adjunctive chemotherapy with a platinum-based regimen is recommended. Sit and colleagues reported a median survival of 19 months with paclitaxel/platinum versus 23 months with platinum/ifosfamide in carcinosarcoma of the fallopian tube. Duska and colleagues reported combination paclitaxel/platinum therapy in 28 patients with carcinosarcoma of the ovary, with a complete response rate in 16 of 28 (55%), and a partial response rate in 6 patients, for a total response rate of 72%. Overall median survival was 27 months.

Prognosis in carcinosarcoma is guarded. Weber, in a review of the earlier literature, noted a survival rate of 63% at 1 year and only 47% at 2 years. Imachi noted a mean survival of all patients of only 16 months. Early-stage carcinosarcomas of the ovary have been reported to have the same prognosis as early-stage epithelial ovarian cancer when 382 cases were compared with epithelial ovarian cancer cases in the SEER database. Advanced-stage carcinosarcoma of the ovary was reported to have a 60% increased risk of death when compared with advanced-stage epithelial ovarian cancer. Presumably, carcinosarcoma of the fallopian tube has a similar prognosis, stage for stage, although there are not enough cases to make a similar evaluation of carcinosarcomas of the fallopian tube. Leiomyosarcoma of the tube has been reported but is rarer than is the carcinosarcoma. Optimal surgery combined with adjuvant therapy seems appropriate. Adjuvant therapy has yet to be defined. Pure embryonal rhabdomyosarcoma and chondrosarcoma of the tube have been reported. Trophoblastic lesions of the tube are very uncommon. Gestational trophoblastic neoplasia has been reported, including placental site nodule, placental site trophoblastic tumor, epithelioid trophoblastic tumor, and choriocarcinoma.

Metastatic tumors involving the tube are usually from the ovary or the endometrium. Low-grade stroma sarcoma may extend to involve the tube. Blood-borne metastases from breast or colon carcinoma or other extrapelvic tumors may also occur.

Other rare tumors that have been reported in the fallopian tube include neuroendocrine carcinoma, parafallopian tube transitional cell carcinoma, malignant carcinoid tumor, mixed malignant germ cell tumor, T-cell lymphoma, and marginal zone B-cell lymphoma. Benign lesions such as leiomyoma, serous cystadenofibroma, schwannoma, extraskeletal chondroma, and müllerianosis of the mesosalpinx have all been reported.

For full reference list, log onto www.expertconsult.com ⟨http://www.expertconsult.com⟩.

Breast Diseases

Mary L. Gemignani, MD

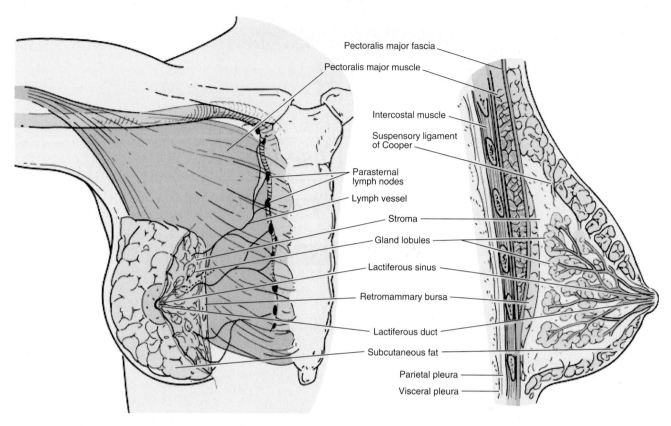

Pectoralis major fascia

Pectoralis major muscle

Intercostal muscle

Suspensory ligament
of Cooper

Parasternal
lymph nodes

Lymph vessel

Stroma

Gland lobules

Lactiferous sinus

Retromammary bursa

Lactiferous duct

Subcutaneous fat

Parietal pleura

Visceral pleura

FIGURE 14-1 Anatomy of the female breast.

Breast cancer remains the most common cancer in women and is second only to lung cancer as the leading cause of cancer-related death in the United States. It is estimated that in 2010 there will be 207,090 new cases of breast cancer diagnosed in women and 39,840 cancer-related deaths. The lifetime risk among women of developing breast cancer is 12.5% (1 in 8); the lifetime risk of dying from breast cancer is 3.6% (1 in 28). Although breast cancer remains a serious health concern around the world, breast cancer mortality is declining in the United States and other industrialized countries. This decline is thought to be secondary to the increased use of mammographic screening and early detection of breast cancer, and the use of effective adjuvant therapies.

Obstetricians and gynecologists serve as primary care physicians for many women during the reproductive and perimenopausal years. According to the American College of Obstetricians and Gynecologists (ACOG), the diagnosis of breast disease, the education of women on breast self-examination, and their referral for mammographic screening are central to the obstetrician/gynecologist's role in women's health care. In this role, they have the unique opportunity to intervene in educating women and aiding in the screening and detection of breast diseases.

This chapter presents an overview of breast cancer screening, benign and malignant conditions of the breast, and the role of the obstetrician/gynecologist in the diagnosis of and education of women about breast disease.

ANATOMY OF THE BREAST

The adult breast lies between the second and sixth ribs in the vertical plane, and between the sternal edge (medially) and mid-axillary line (laterally). The average breast measures 10 to 12 cm in diameter and 5 to 7 cm in thickness. It is concentric, with a lateral projection into the axilla named the axillary tail of Spence (Figures 14-1 and 14-2).

The breast consists of three major structures: skin, subcutaneous fatty tissue, and breast tissue (parenchyma and stroma). The skin contains hair follicles, sebaceous glands, and eccrine sweat glands. The glandular breast is divided into 15 to 20 segments (lobes) that are separated by connective tissue and converge at the nipple in a radial arrangement. These lobes are made up of 20 to 40 lobules, which in turn consist of 10 to 100 alveoli (tubulosaccular secretory units). Five to 10 major milk-collecting ducts drain each segment and open at the nipple into subareolar lactiferous sinuses.

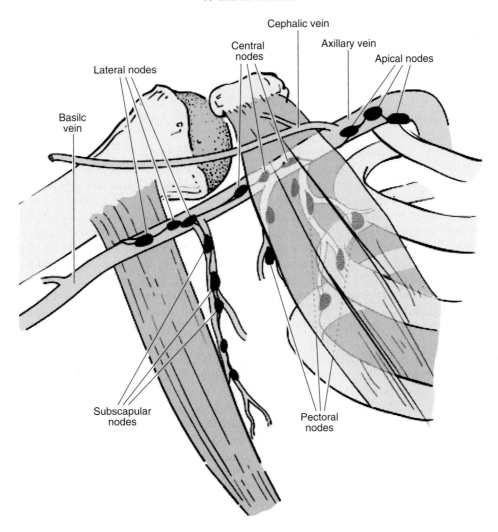

FIGURE 14-2   Axillary nodes.

A superficial pectoral fascia envelops the breast; the undersurface of the breast lies on the deep pectoral fascia. The superficial pectoral fascia is continuous with the superficial abdominal fascia of Camper. Between these two fascial layers are fibrous bands called Cooper suspensory ligaments that provide support for the breast. The space between the deep layers of the superficial fascia of the breast and the deep investing fascia of the pectoralis is the retromammary bursa.

The epidermis of the nipple (mammary papilla) and areola is pigmented and wrinkled, and consists of keratinized, stratified squamous epithelium that contains smooth muscle fibers in dense connective tissue. These fibers are responsible for the erection of the nipple. Two receptor-type nerve endings (Ruffini-like bodies and end bulb of Krause) are present on the nipple and associated with the tactile reception of stretch and pressure.

The areola has no hair follicles; it has sebaceous glands (at its margin), apocrine sweat glands, and accessory areolar glands (Montgomery glands) that open on the surface of the areola as small elevations called Morgagni tubercles. Montgomery glands are large sebaceous glands capable of secreting milk; they represent an intermediate stage between the sweat and the mammary glands.

The blood supply of the breast is mostly from superficial vessels. The principal blood supply is derived from the internal thoracic (mammary) and lateral thoracic artery and their tributaries. The posterior intercostal arteries of the second to fourth intercostal spaces also give off tributaries called the mammary branches. Approximately 60% of the breast, mainly the medial and central parts, is supplied by the anterior perforating branches of the internal mammary artery. About 30% of the breast, mainly the upper outer quadrant, is supplied by the lateral thoracic artery.

The superficial veins follow the arteries and drain through perforating branches of the internal thoracic vein, tributaries of the axillary vein, and perforating branches of posterior intercostal veins. The veins anastomose circumferentially around the nipple, which is called the circulus venosus.

Subepithelial or a papillary plexus of lymphatics of the breast are confluent with the subepithelial lymphatics over the surface of the body. These valveless lymphatic vessels communicate with subdermal lymphatic vessels and merge with Sappey's subareolar plexus. The subareolar plexus receives lymphatic vessels from the nipple and the areola and communicates by way of the vertical lymphatic vessels that are equivalent to those connecting the subepithelial and subdermal plexus elsewhere in the body. Lymph flows unidirectionally from the superficial to the deep plexus and from the subareolar plexus through the lymphatic vessels of the lactiferous duct to the perilobular and deep subcutaneous plexus. Lymph flow from the deep subcutaneous and intramammary lymphatic vessels moves centrifugally toward the axillary and internal mammary lymph nodes. It is estimated that about 97% of the lymph flows to the axillary nodes and 3% to the internal mammary chain.

Axillary lymph nodes may be divided into three anatomic levels defined in reference to the pectoralis minor muscle. Level I nodes are the axillary vein lymph nodes that lie along the axillary vein from the lateral extent of the pectoralis minor muscle to the latissimus dorsi muscle. In this area, deep to the floor of the axilla, subscapular nodes that lie on the subscapularis muscle are identified.

Level II nodes are designated by their location underneath the pectoralis minor muscle. Medial to the pectoralis minor are level III nodes, which include apical or subclavicular nodes and are adjacent to Halstead's ligament.

Interpectoral nodes are called Rotter's nodes. They lie between the pectoralis major and minor muscle.

EMBRYOLOGY AND DEVELOPMENT OF THE BREAST

The mammary glands are highly specialized skin derivatives of ectodermal origin. The epithelial ridge that develops into breast tissue undergoes a series of proliferations to form the lactiferous ducts. Primitive breast tissue is under the gonadal control of fetal androgen production, which causes a suppression of breast growth during the period of gestation when the tissue is under the simultaneous influence of increasing levels of growth-promoting estrogen and progesterone. After birth, breast tissue remains dormant until adolescence, when estrogen produces a proliferation of ductal epithelium and progesterone produces rapid growth of the acini. However, breast growth and development are not totally dependent on estrogen and progesterone

levels. Insulin, cortisol, thyroxine, growth hormone, and prolactin are also required for complete functional development. Minor deficiencies in any one of these hormones can be compensated for by an excess of prolactin.

PREGNANCY AND BREAST FEEDING

Increasing amounts of estrogen, progesterone, and human placental lactogen produce active growth of functional breast tissue during the course of pregnancy. Estrogen production is under the control of the fetus. Estrogen influences progesterone production, uteroplacental blood flow, mammary gland development, and fetal adrenal gland function. By the 20th week of pregnancy, most of the estrogen excreted in maternal urine comes from fetal androgens. About 90% of maternal estriol is derived from fetal precursors. Serum prolactin rises from nonpregnant levels of 10 ng/mL to term levels of 200 ng/mL. Amniotic fluid prolactin levels are more than 100 times greater than the levels in maternal or fetal blood early in pregnancy. It is not known whether the fetal pituitary gland or the trophoblast secretes the hormone into the amniotic fluid. Elevated levels of estradiol parallel those of prolactin and indicate that estriol may be responsible for increases in prolactin. Although estrogen may initiate prolactin secretion, high levels block its physiologic effects. Prolactin secretion is also controlled by the prolactin-inhibiting factor. A decrease in estrogen level after delivery and suppression of the prolactin-inhibiting factor by suckling increase prolactin levels. If breast feeding does not occur, serum prolactin levels decrease to nonpregnant levels in about 1 week.

The release of oxytocin from the posterior pituitary gland affects contraction of the duct system, stimulating the delivery of milk to the nipples. However, after 3 to 4 months of breast feeding, suckling appears to be the only stimulus required for lactation.

BENIGN BREAST CONDITIONS

Fibrocystic Changes

Fibrocystic change is the most common benign breast condition in women. It consists of no single entity and encompasses a histologic spectrum of changes in the breast, some of which are normal and some of which are abnormal. It is a result of fluctuating hormone levels and is most common in premenopausal women between the ages of 20 and 50. It is often associated with pain and tenderness (mastodynia) and tends to be bilateral. Most women will report symptoms during the premenstrual phase of the cycle, which suggests that progesterone may play a role in the development and symptoms of cystic alterations in breast tissue. However, the proportional effect of both estrogen and progesterone on the cause of benign breast conditions is unclear.

Pain results from breast stromal edema, ductal dilation, and associated inflammatory response. An increase in breast size is also frequently reported. The differential diagnosis for breast pain includes other conditions affecting the anterior chest wall, such as intercostal neuralgia, myalgia, and chronic costochondritis. Women with large, pendulous breasts will have associated stretching of Cooper ligaments and associated breast pain.

Etiologic factors are still inconclusive. The ingestion of foods and medications containing methylxanthines has been implicated through an inhibition of 3858-cyclic adenosine monophosphate (cAMP) phosphodiesterase and 3858-cyclic guanosine monophosphate (cGMP) phosphodiesterase. This inhibition will lead to accumulation of increased amounts of cAMP and cGMP. High levels of cAMP and cGMP have been detected in patients with fibrocystic change. In some studies, reduction of dietary methylxanthines has been associated with symptomatic subjective reduction in pain, tenderness, and palpable nodularity. Other studies have failed to show an effect from decreased consumption of dietary methylxanthines, however.

Fibrocystic change is not a risk factor for cancer in the majority of women. In 1985 the Cancer Committee of the College of American Pathologists published a consensus statement and discouraged the use of the term *fibrocystic disease*; they prefer the terms *fibrocystic changes* or *fibrocystic condition*. Histologically, two changes are noted with fibrocystic change: nonproliferative changes and proliferative changes. The nonproliferative changes include cystic changes with formation of microcysts (2 mm or less in size), macrocysts, and fibrosis.

Proliferative Changes

Proliferative changes include hyperplasia and adenosis. Hyperplasia is proliferation of ductal epithelium, which results in layering of the cells. Atypia may be associated with this proliferation. If atypia is noted, this confers a five-fold increase in breast cancer risk for the patient. Hyperplasia with atypia is the only fibrocystic change associated with an increased risk factor for breast cancer. If atypia is noted on a core biopsy, a surgical excision of the area is recommended because it is thought that there is a 25% chance of finding a coexistent carcinoma.

Adenosis is also a proliferative lesion caused by changes in the acini in the distal mammary lobule. Sclerosing adenosis refers to the dense, fibrotic tissue surrounding these small ducts. These lesions may present as a palpable mass in women in their 30s and 40s.

A papilloma can result from this ductal proliferation. Papillomas are papillary lesions with a branching fibrovascular core surrounded by epithelium. These lesions are associated with serosanguineous nipple discharge in 25% to 50% of presentations. Ninety percent of the time there is a small palpable mass adjacent to the areola. Intraductal papillomas are rarely associated with carcinoma but require surgical excision to rule out the possibility of misdiagnosis of a malignancy.

Management of fibrocystic changes includes regular physical examinations, appropriate imaging, and supportive measures to help control symptoms. Recommendations for use of a good support bra may be helpful, especially in physically active women. Dietary restrictions of methylxanthines may produce subjective improvement in 65% of patients. The use of vitamins A and E has been reported in some studies to be helpful. For vitamin E, the mechanism of action is unknown, although an alteration in serum gonadotropins and adrenal tropines has been shown to occur in patients taking high doses of vitamin E. Diuretic therapy during the premenstrual period has been reported to provide temporary relief and requires cyclical use. Fluid retention is a result of cyclical hormonal stimulation.

Oral contraceptives suppress symptoms of fibrocystic changes in the majority of patients (70% to 90%). Symptoms often recur after discontinuation. Other medications such as danazol (17α-norethisterone) in doses of 100 to 400 mg per day should be reserved for patients in whom other agents have been ineffective. Their side-effect profile can lead to poor compliance. A 3- to 6-month course can provide significant reduction in symptoms, and its effect can last several months after its discontinuation. As with other progestogens, the mechanism of its effect on fibrocystic disease is unclear. Brookshaw described 514 patients who had benign breast disease treated with varying doses of danazol for as long as 6 months. For the best results, treatment was necessary for 4 to 6 months at a dose of 200 to 400 mg/day, with a complete response rate of 68%. Tamoxifen, a selective estrogen receptor modulator (SERM) that is used as a preventive agent and a hormonal therapy agent in premenopausal women with breast cancer, has been considered in women with severe mastopathy and mastodynia. The effectiveness of tamoxifen was studied by Ricciardi and Ianniruberto with use of 10 mg/day from day 5 to day 25 of the menstrual cycle for 4 months. The response rate was 72%.

Sclerosing Lesions

Sclerosing lesions have been described by a variety of names, including sclerosing papillary proliferation, non-encapsulated sclerosing lesion, indurative mastopathy, and radial scar. They are important because they may simulate carcinoma on mammographic, gross, and microscopic examinations. These lesions are typically less than 1 cm in diameter. On gross examination, they are irregular, gray or white, indurated with central retraction and have an appearance identical to scirrhous carcinoma. On microscopic examination, the lesion has a stellate configuration and consists of a central, fibrotic core containing entrapped glandular elements. The surrounding breast tissue typically shows varying degrees of intraductal hyperplasia and adenosis. The significance of this lesion relative to subsequent development of carcinoma is controversial. Available evidence suggests that these lesions are part of the fibrocystic complex. It is likely that their premalignant potential is the same as that of the constituent parts. Local excision of these lesions is the treatment of choice.

Fibroadenoma

Fibroadenomas are benign fibroepithelial tumors and are the second most common benign lesion of the breast. They are the most common lesion found in women younger than age 25. They will persist during the menstrual years of a woman's life, but regression after menopause has been reported. Patients typically present with a mobile, smooth, painless, palpable mass. Ultrasound examination along with physical examination can help in making the diagnosis. Mammographically, fibroadenomas may appear as round, oval, or lobulated masses with circumscribed margins. In older women, they can have a rim of coarse calcifications. Fine-needle aspiration (FNA) will reveal benign ductal epithelial cells and elongated dense stromal cells. Microscopically fibrous tissue comprises most of the fibroadenoma. Carcinoma arising in fibroadenomas is rare.

Fibroadenomas can be followed without the need for complete surgical excision. This can be achieved with physical examination or ultrasound examination if they are not palpable. However, surgical excision should be performed in the following situations:

- The mass continues to enlarge
- The results of FNA or core biopsy are inconclusive or yield atypia
- The patient desires surgical excision

Table 14-1 lists proliferative breast disease and breast cancer risk. Table 14-2 shows breast diagnoses grouped by cancer risk.

Phyllodes Tumor

Phyllodes tumors are uncommon, slow-growing fibroepithelial tumors. Previously referred to as cystosarcoma phyllodes, this name contributed to confusion in

TABLE 14.1 Proliferative Breast Disease and Breast Cancer Risk

Characteristic	Relative Risk (Confidence Interval)
Proliferative disease, no atypia	1.3 (0.6911.9)
Complex fibroadenoma*	1.46 (0.5314.0)
Atypical hyperplasia	2.53 (1.016.3)
Neither proliferative disease nor complex fibroadenoma	1.27 (0.8911.8)

Modified from Dupont WD, Page DL, Parl FF et al: Cancer 85:1277, 1999.
Contains cysts, sclerosing adenosis, epithelial calcification, or papillary apocrine changes.

TABLE 14-2 Breast Diagnosis Grouped by Cancer Risk

Cancer Risk	Diagnosis
No increased risk	Adenosis, sclerosing or florid
	Apocrine metaplasia
	Cysts, macro or micro
	Duct ectasia
	Fibroadenoma
	Fibrosis
	Hyperplasia (mild)
	Mastitis
	Periductal mastitis
	Squamous metaplasia
Slightly increased	Hyperplasia, moderate or florid
	Papilloma, solid or papillary, with fibrovascular core
Moderately increased	Atypical hyperplasia
	Ductal
	Lobular

understanding this entity. Although very similar to a fibroadenoma, the stromal component is hypercellular with increased pleomorphism and mitotic activity. Phyllodes tumors can occur in women of any age but more commonly occur in premenopausal women.

Malignant behavior in phyllodes tumors is rare in premenopausal women. Malignant phyllodes tumors are noted when there is a combination of increased mitotic activity, invasive borders, or marked pleomorphism. Incomplete excision is a major determinant for local recurrence. Treatment is total surgical excision with a wide margin of healthy tissue.

Adenoma

Adenoma of the breast is a well-circumscribed tumor composed of benign epithelial elements with sparse, inconspicuous stroma, a feature that differentiates this lesion from fibroadenoma, in which the stroma is an integral part of the tumor. For practical purposes, adenomas may be divided into two major groups: tubular adenomas and lactating adenomas. Tubular adenomas in young women are well-defined, freely movable nodules that clinically resemble fibroadenomas. Lactating adenomas manifest as one or more freely movable masses during pregnancy or the postpartum period. They are grossly well circumscribed and lobulated; on cut section they appear tan and softer than tubular adenomas. On microscopic examination these lesions have lobulated borders and are composed of glands lined by cuboid cells with secretory activity identical to the lactational changes normally observed in the breast tissue during pregnancy and the puerperium.

It should be noted that breast biopsy in a pregnant or lactating woman calls for meticulous hemostasis because of the increased vascularity and risk of postoperative hematoma formation. The lactating breast is predisposed to postoperative infection because milk is a good culture medium. Anesthesia by local injection may be difficult in the enlarged breast but is the method of choice. Incisional biopsy under local anesthesia is an option when excisional biopsy is a problem. Because of the significant risk of infection and milk fistula, the patient who is lactating should cease lactating before biopsy is performed.

Superficial Thrombophlebitis

Superficial thrombophlebitis is also known as Mondor disease of the breast. It is an uncommon benign inflammatory process. It can occur spontaneously but usually is associated with breast trauma, breast surgery, or pregnancy. It is a thrombophlebitis of the thoracoepigastric vein, which drains the upper-outer quadrant of the breast. Patients present with acute pain and a linear, tender fibrotic band with skin retraction over the distribution of the thoracoepigastric vein.

Treatment is conservative, with analgesics and application of heat. The condition resolves in 1 to 3 weeks. Skin retraction superficial to the area of inflammation can remain if the inflammation is extensive. Biopsy is not necessary.

Mastitis

Mastitis usually occurs in relation to lactation. It can occur in nonpuerperal periods in association with galactorrhea. Skin organisms, *Staphylococcus aureus,* and *Streptococcus* species may cause infection of the nipple and breast ducts. Presence of milk in the ducts can provide an excellent medium for infection.

Women with mastitis may continue to breast feed. Antibiotic therapy with dicloxacillin sodium (250 mg qid) or penicillin G is indicated. If there is no response, an abscess that may require surgical drainage must be excluded. Inflammatory carcinomas can mimic mastitis,

and if no resolution of infection is noted despite continued antibiotics, a skin biopsy may be indicated.

Galactoceles are milk-filled cysts. They are usually tender and present after the abrupt termination of breast feeding. Aspiration of the cyst is often necessary for symptomatic relief. If reaccumulation occurs, however, surgical excision may be required to avoid infection.

Duct Ectasia

Duct ectasia is a condition that usually occurs in perimenopausal or postmenopausal women. Patients present with a tender, hard, erythematous mass adjacent to the areola in association with burning, itching, or a pulling sensation in the nipple area. A thick, greenish-black discharge may be present. The pathogenesis of this condition has not been fully established. Available evidence suggests, however, that the primary event is periductal inflammation and that ductal ectasia is the ultimate outcome of this disorder. The postulated sequence of events in the evolution of this disease is periductal inflammation leading to periductal fibrosis that subsequently results in ductal dilation. However, the etiology of the initial inflammatory response remains obscure. Histologic evaluation of the area shows dilated, distended terminal-collecting ducts obstructed with inspissated lipid-containing epithelial cells and phagocytic histiocytes. This process tends to occur in a segmental fashion extending from the involved nipple area to adjacent ducts. Occasionally, a small abscess forms at the base of the nipple. Treatment is excisional biopsy.

Younger women can present with inflammation of the ducts in the region of the nipple, which may produce fissures and fistulae with connection from the nipple ducts to the skin at the edges of the areola. Prior periductal mastitis leads to the squamous epithelium of the terminal dilated portion of the collecting ducts to undergo squamous metaplasia. Keratin is formed in the duct, accumulates, and can cause an abscess at the base of the nipple. Excision of the area usually is necessary.

Fat Necrosis

Fat necrosis is a relatively uncommon benign condition occurring as a response to breast trauma. Patients present with a hard mass that can mimic a carcinoma. The irregular mass is palpable and may involve skin retraction. Multiple calcifications can be seen on mammography.

The histology is active chronic inflammatory cells, with lymphocytes and histiocytes predominating. In the later stages, a collagenous scar is noted, with "oil cysts" or free lipid material released by lipocyte necrosis. Fat necrosis does not increase the risk of carcinoma, and its clinical importance is in the differential diagnosis of a carcinoma.

Nipple Discharge

Nipple discharge has been reported in 10.0% to 15.0% of women with benign breast disease and in 2.5% to 3.0% of those with carcinoma. Galactorrhea presents as bilateral milky nipple discharge consisting of lipid droplets; the condition is usually idiopathic but can be found after discontinuation of oral contraceptives or as a persistent discharge after pregnancy. Plasma prolactin levels should be determined because of the possibility of a prolactin-producing pituitary adenoma.

The discharge is classified according to its appearance as milky, green, bloody, serous, cloudy, or purulent. The drainage should be classified according to whether it is unilateral, bilateral, spontaneous, or recurrent. This information is obtained at the time of a thorough history and physical examination. For example, if the drainage first appeared in the patient's bra or nightgown on awakening, this finding is significant. The presence of a mass should also be investigated. The risk of cancer is increased when the discharge is unilateral from a single duct, when it occurs in a postmenopausal patient, or when a mass is present.

Unilateral, Spontaneous Nipple Discharge

In cases of unilateral, spontaneous nipple discharge, several causes are included in the differential. The most common cause of nipple discharge is mammary-duct ectasia, which produces a multicolored (green, yellow, white, brown, gray, or reddish-brown) nipple discharge. The reddish-brown discharge is often mistaken for a blood discharge. It is thought to result from an increase in glandular secretions, with the production of an irritating lipid fluid that can produce a nipple discharge. Guaiac testing of the discharge can help to diagnose whether it is bloody.

The next most common cause of a multicolored, sticky nipple discharge is nonpuerperal mastitis. The persistent type involves inflammation in deeper portions of the breast; the transient types are associated with periareolar inflammation. If the inflammation develops into an inflammatory mass, surgical excision and drainage are necessary. Medical management with local care, avoidance of all nipple manipulation, and administration of nonsteroidal anti-inflammatory agents and an antistaphylococcal antibiotic are often successful when infection is suspected.

Bloody nipple discharge warrants surgical evaluation. Intraductal papillomas are the most common cause of bloody nipple discharge. During the breast examination, physicians should look for an associated periareolar mass. The examination consists of gently and carefully palpating the subareolar region to identify the pressure point that produces the discharge. It is important to

TABLE 14-3   Characteristics of Nipple Discharge

Color	Likely Cause	Percentage Caused by Cancer
Milky (galactorrhea)	Pituitary adenoma, pregnancy, oral contraceptives	Rare
Green, yellow, sticky	Ductal ectasia	Rare
Clear, watery	Ductal carcinoma	30-50
Bloody, sanguineous	Fibrocystic changes, ductal papillomas	25
Pink, serosanguineous	Fibrocystic changes, ductal papillomas	10
Yellow, serous	Fibrocystic changes, ductal papillomas	5
Purulent	Bacterial infection	Rare

reproduce the discharge and demonstrate the breast quadrant from which it emanates. All significant nipple discharges warrant referral for tissue biopsy. Although a mass is usually present when the discharge is a result of cancer, there is no palpable mass in 13% of cancers with nipple secretions. Bloody discharge occurring in the third trimester of pregnancy may be regarded as physiologic, however, and does not require intervention unless persistent for several months after delivery. There are no contraindications to breast feeding in these patients. In addition, physicians should not rely solely on the cytology of the discharge because there is an 18.0% false-negative rate and a 2.6% false-positive rate with standard cytology alone.

Galactography (injecting radiopaque contrast into the discharging duct and then performing mammography) offers better visualization of small intraductal papillomas but cannot differentiate between benign and malignant lesions. A surgical procedure is still necessary. Mammography has a 9.5% false-negative rate and a 1.6% false-positive rate for detecting cancer in patients with a nipple discharge. Table 14-3 reveals characteristics of nipple discharge.

HISTORY AND PHYSICAL EXAMINATION

Obtaining a thorough history, including a family history and information on menstrual status, pregnancies and lactation, hormone use, and prior breast surgeries and trauma, is essential. In addition, ascertaining whether the patient performs breast self-examinations and determining the presence and characterization of nipple discharge or a breast mass are important.

Bilateral breast examination is best performed following menstruation and before ovulation. At this time, breast engorgement and tenderness are less likely to be present.

A multipositional breast examination should be performed, including examination in the upright and supine positions. Breast retraction and subtle changes in the skin and nipple may be missed if the patient is examined in only one position.

The patient should be in the sitting position during the inception of the physical breast examination. In this position, asymmetry, skin or nipple retraction, and nipple ulceration should be most apparent (Figure 14-3, A). When the patient's arms are raised (Figure 14-3, B), skin changes in the lower half of the breast or in the inframammary fold become accentuated. Contraction of the pectoralis major muscle, affected by the patient pushing her hands against her hips (Figure 14-3, C), may demonstrate an otherwise undetected skin retraction. Next, palpation of the breast with the patient still upright may allow detection of subtle lesions that would be more difficult to palpate if she were supine (Figure 14-3, D). Examination of the supraclavicular areas and both sides of the neck for the purpose of detecting suspicious lymphadenopathy is also best done when the patient is in the upright position.

The axilla should be examined with the patient in the upright position. The patient's right arm should be fixed at the elbow and held there by the physician's right hand. This allows relaxation of the chest wall musculature (Figure 14-3, E). Palpation with the left hand permits assessment of the lower axilla, and with extension higher toward the clavicle, the middle and upper portions of the axilla can be assessed. The left axilla is examined with the right hand after relaxation of the patient's left arm in the physician's left hand. If lymph nodes are palpable, the clinician must assess their level and size and whether they are suspicious, single or multiple, and mobile or fixed to underlying structures.

The second phase of the breast examination is conducted with the patient in the supine position and with the patient's arm raised above the head (Figure 14-3, F). Digital palpation is carried out using the index and middle fingers, and by applying varying amounts of pressure with the flats or pads of the fingers. A thorough examination systemically covers the entire breast and chest wall. The examination can be done in a clockwise direction or by rows (stripwise). It is important to carefully examine beneath the nipple–areolar complex and within the axilla.

An inflammatory appearance of the breast should raise suspicion of an inflammatory carcinoma. The classic appearance of inflammatory breast cancer includes a red, swollen breast with skin edema ("peau d'orange"). The breast is generally not tender. If the inflammation persists following a short course of antibiotics to rule out cellulitis, biopsy of the breast and skin

is warranted. Inflammatory breast cancer is often a clinical diagnosis, and a benign skin biopsy should not dissuade the clinician from undertaking further evaluation and treatment. Any asymmetric skin changes or changes of the nipple–areolar complex should arouse suspicion. Paget's disease of the nipple suggests the presence of intraductal or invasive cancer involving the nipple, and cancer should be excluded by a nipple biopsy of the abnormal area following a mammogram.

It is important to instruct patients in the technique of breast self-examination. Physician-directed discussion on breast self-examination is the most effective approach. Physicians have the opportunity to reinforce what is normal versus abnormal to patients during the examination. If no abnormal findings are noted on examination, it is critical to document negative findings. The date of the last mammogram, discussion of cancer screening, and plans for follow-up should also be recorded.

Hormones (hormone replacement therapy [HRT] or oral contraceptive pills [OCP]) should not be renewed without a documented annual breast examination or mammography if indicated. A great deal of litigation results from failure to diagnose breast cancer. The Physician Insurers Association of America's breast cancer claims study, conducted in 1988, determined that 75% of successful malpractice lawsuits involved primary care physicians with practices in family medicine, internal medicine, or obstetrics and gynecology. It is important that the medical chart include careful documentation because approximately one-third of the cases reported in the Physician Insurers Association of America's study resulted from inadequate documentation.

Clinical breast examination and breast self-examination as methods for screening for breast cancer mainly aim at detection of palpable breast lesions. However, there are no published reports demonstrating these methods as being effective in breast cancer mortality risk reduction.

A Cochrane systematic review published in 2003 included two large population-based studies from Russia and Shanghai, China that compared breast self-examination with no intervention. In both trials, almost twice as many biopsies with benign results were performed in the screening group compared to the control group (RR 1.89; 95% CI, 1.79-2.00). No randomized trials on clinical breast examination are available. The United States Preventive Services Task Force (USPSTF) in their most recent update recommended against breast self-examination based on a systematic review of published reports.

For breast cancer screening, the American Cancer Society (ACS) recommends clinical breast examination every 3 years for women aged 20 to 39 years and annually beginning at age 40 years.

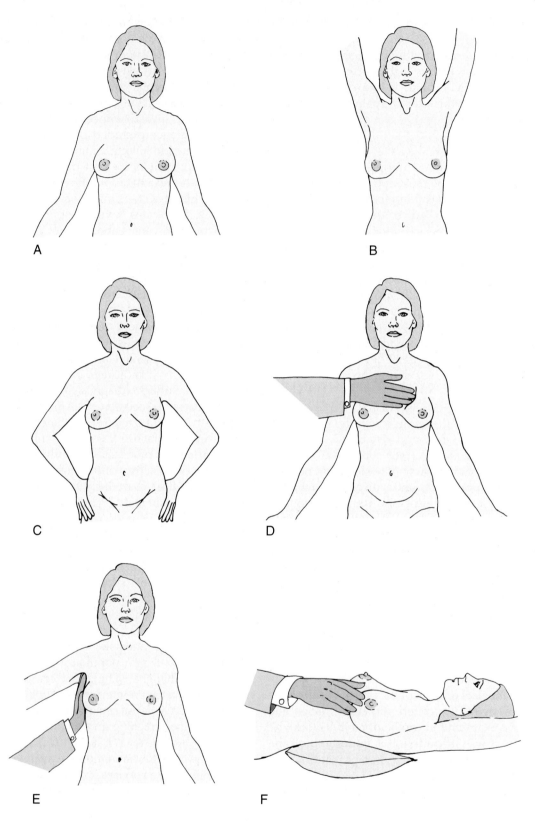

FIGURE 14-3   Physical examination of the breast. **A,** Upright position. **B,** Arms raised. **C,** Pushing hands against hips. **D,** Palpation in upright position. **E,** Palpation of the axilla. **F,** Palpation in supine position.

MAMMOGRAPHY

The primary goal of mammography is to screen asymptomatic women to help detect breast cancer at an early stage. The goal of screening mammography is to find cancers before they are clinically palpable, more likely to be small, and less likely to have nodal involvement. Most studies of mammography use mortality as the end point, and the value of screening is often limited to mortality rates. Few studies factor the effects of early detection on quality of life or the fact that treatment at earlier stages carries less morbidity and has more treatment options.

In general, a routine screening mammogram consists of a mediolateral oblique (MLO) view and a craniocaudal (CC) view of each breast. With modern low-dose screening, the dose is less than 0.1 rad per study (for comparison, a chest radiograph delivers 0.025 rad per study). The effectiveness of screening also varies depending on the density of the breast.

Breast composition may be one of four patterns of increasing density:

1. Almost entirely fat
2. Scattered fibroglandular densities
3. Heterogeneously dense
4. Extremely dense

The greater the breast density, the lower the sensitivity of the mammogram. Because some palpable cancers are invisible on mammography, a negative study cannot always exclude cancer. It is important to note that the false-negative rate for mammograms is 10% to 15% and that a normal mammogram does not eliminate the need for further evaluation of a dominant mass in the breast. If the clinical examination is suspicious, a negative mammogram result should not delay further investigation.

Mammographic screening in women 40 years or older has reduced mortality by 20% to 30%. The efficacy of screening mammography in decreasing breast cancer mortality has been demonstrated in numerous studies. In the 1960s the Health Insurance Plan of Greater New York performed a study of physical examination and mammography in a study group of 30,756 women and a control group of 30,239 women between the ages of 40 and 64 years. At 10 years follow-up, the study group had a 30% decrease in breast cancer mortality compared with the control group.

A total of eight large randomized trials on mammographic screening have been conducted. Six of the eight trials revealed a statistically significant reduction in mortality with mammographic screening. The reduction in mortality was not as evident among women between the ages of 40 and 49 compared with women older than 50 years of age. The relative mortality reduction appears

TABLE 14-4 Randomized Population-Based Mammography Trials

Trial	Relative Risk (95% CI)
Malmö	0.96 (0.68-1.35)
Canada	1.08 (0.84-1.40)
Göteborg	0.55 (0.31-0.95)
Stockholm	0.73 (0.50-1.06)
Kopperberg	0.58 (0.45-0.76)
Östergötland	0.76 (0.61-0.95)
New York	0.79 (0.64-0.98)
Edinburgh	0.87 (0.70-1.08)

CI, *Confidence interval.*

later in women between the ages of 40 and 49 at randomization compared with women 50 years or older. It is also likely that the small numbers of women between 40 and 49 years of age in the existing randomized trials may have contributed to this difference.

In a meta-analysis of eight randomized, controlled trials of mammographic screening, a statistically significant 18% reduction in mortality in women aged 40 to 49 years was noted. Combined data from five Swedish trials yielded a statistically significant mortality decrease of 29% (Table 14-4).

A more recent Cochrane systematic review was published in 2006. Because of the inclusion criteria they chose for the review, they reported on six randomized trials, and reported an overall 20% risk reduction in mortality from breast cancer (RR, 0.80; 95% CI, 0.73-0.88).

Screening Interval

For several years, there has been a significant debate about the appropriate age at which to commence mammographic screening. In 1997 the ACS and the National Cancer Institute (NCI) modified the guidelines for mammographic screening for women between the ages of 40 and 49, recommending regular mammograms for women in this age group. The recommended intervals differ: The ACS recommends a yearly mammogram starting at age 40, whereas the NCI recommends a mammogram every 1 or 2 years. ACOG recommendations on mammography are similar to the NCI guidelines. Table 14-5 lists recommendations by society.

Most recently, the USPSTF published its recommendations (in 2009). After reviewing the evidence regarding the efficacy of breast self-examination, clinical breast examination, and mammography in reducing breast cancer mortality, it recommended starting mammography at age 50 and performing biennial screening. It recommended against breast self-examination and routine mammography in women younger than age 50.

The risk reduction afforded by mammography in the 39 to 49 age group (RR, 0.85; 95% CI, 0.75-0.96) was the

TABLE 14-5   Recommendations for Mammographic Screening for Breast Cancer

Age (Years)	American College of Obstetricians and Gynecologists	American Cancer Society	National Cancer Institute	U.S. Preventive Services Task Force
40-49	1-2 years	Annually	1-2 years	Discuss w/MD
50-74	Annually	Annually	1-2 years	2 years

TABLE 14-6   Screening Guidelines for Women Younger Than Age 40

Condition	Timing of Annual Mammography
Lobular cancer in situ or breast cancer diagnosis	At time of diagnosis
First-degree relative with premenopausal breast cancer	10 years earlier than relative's age at diagnosis, but not younger than 25 years
Mantle irradiation for Hodgkin's disease	8 years after completion of radiation therapy
BRCA1 or BRCA2 mutation	Age 25-35 years; specific age chosen based on adequacy of mammography imaging in the first study and patient choice

Data from American College of Obstetricians and Gynecologists. Primary and preventive care: periodic assessments. ACOG Committee Opinion 246. Washington, DC: ACOG; 2000.

same as the risk reduction obtained in the 50 to 59 age group (RR, 0.86; 95% CI, 0.75-0.99). The USPSTF emphasized that because the absolute risk of developing breast cancer in women in their 40s is low compared with the other age groups, it felt that the net benefit of mammography was small and that the decision to start mammography earlier than age 50 should be based on a discussion with the patient about risks and benefits. The task force estimated that it would take 1904 invites for screening to prevent 1 breast cancer death in the 39 to 49 age group. The task force cites the risk of false-positive mammography results (up to 56%) as a potential harm and considers pain, anxiety, distress, and other psychologic responses as potential harms. However, the task force states that these harms are transient and thus do not represent a substantial deterrent to the continued use of mammography for screening. These new recommendations have caused much controversy and debate in the medical community and lay press since they were announced. The majority of clinical societies did not change their recommendations after these guidelines were issued. Other groups, including the ACS, still recommend annual screening mammography beginning at age 40 years.

Annual screening mammography may commence earlier than age 40 in a few special circumstances (Table 14-6).

Breast Imaging Reporting and Data System

In the past, a lack of uniformity in mammography terminology and reporting often led to confusion as to the malignant nature of a lesion. In 1994 the Mammography Quality Standards Act was passed by Congress and is administered by the U.S. Food and Drug Administration (FDA). It requires that mammography facilities monitor the results of their breast cancer detection programs, including the number of recommended biopsies and the size, number, and stage of cancers detected. The American College of Radiology (ACR) uses a terminology and lexicon system called BI-RADS for reporting abnormalities seen on mammography (Table 14-7). This standardized reporting system—the Breast Imaging Reporting and Data System—was developed in 1995. Each category leads to a fixed assessment and specific management recommendations. In addition, associated findings, such as skin or nipple retraction, skin thickening, skin lesions, axillary adenopathy, and the presence of architectural distortion should also be reported.

The predictors of malignancy for the BI-RADS categories are 0% to 2% for category 3 and approximately 98% or greater for category 5. Category 4 is less predictable. Liberman and colleagues and Orel and colleagues have placed the risk of malignancy for this category at around 30%.

The ACR Task Force has published a new edition of the BI-RADS classification system that, in particular, will attempt to provide data on category 4 in terms of risk of malignancy. In the new edition of BI-RADS, category 4 is divided into three parts based on the pre-biopsy risk for malignancy of the lesion—4a (small), 4b (low, medium, and high), and 4c (substantial)—in an effort to better guide clinicians and to collect meaningful data about this category. By subdividing the category, the ACR hopes to provide better communication to the referring physician about the prebiopsy risk of malignancy. Additionally, the fourth edition of the lexicon also addresses the assignment of categories to ultrasound and magnetic resonance imaging (MRI) findings. One recent retrospective study evaluated interobserver variability and positive predictive value of BI-RADS categories 4A, 4B, and 4C. The risk of malignancy was found to be 6%, 15%, and 53%, respectively. Table 14-7 shows BI-RADS reporting.

TABLE 14-7 American College of Radiology BI-RADS Assessment Categories

BI-RADS Category	Assessment
ASSESSMENT IS INCOMPLETE	
0	Need additional imaging evaluation and/or prior mammograms for comparison
ASSESSMENT IS COMPLETE: FINAL CATEGORIES	
1	Negative
2	Benign finding(s)
3	Probably benign finding; initial short-interval follow-up suggested
4*	Suspicious abnormality; biopsy should be considered Optional subdivisions: 4A: Finding needing intervention with a low suspicion for malignancy 4B: Lesions with an intermediate suspicion of malignancy 4C: Findings of moderate concern, but not classic for malignancy
5	Highly suggestive of malignancy; appropriate action should be taken
6	Known biopsy; proven malignancy; appropriate action should be taken

D'Orsi CJ, Bassett LW, Berg WA, et al: Breast Imaging Reporting and Data System: ACR BI-RADS-Mammography (ed 4), Reston, VA, American College of Radiology, 2003. Reprinted with permission of the American College of Radiology. No other representation of this material is authorized without expressed, written permission from the American College of Radiology.
*By subdividing Category 4 into 4A, 4B, and 4C, it is encouraged that relevant probabilities for malignancy be indicated within this category so the patient and her physician can make an informed decision on the ultimate course of action.
BI-RADS, Breast Imaging Reporting and Data System.

Diagnostic Mammography

Abnormalities found on mammographic screening may need further evaluation with additional mammography views or other imaging modalities, such as ultrasound or MRI. In some screening programs, the mammograms are reviewed by the radiologist as they are performed, and if additional views are needed, they are performed on the same day. In other programs, if additional studies are required, the patient is called back for them at a later date. In several studies, the frequency of "call-backs" has ranged from 5% to 11%.

Mammographic Lesions

A "mass" is defined as a space-occupying lesion seen in two different projections. If a possible mass is seen on only one view, it is called a "density" until its three-dimensionality is confirmed. A description of the shape and the margins of the lesion are also necessary. The highest frequency of carcinoma is noted in masses that have an irregular shape or spiculated borders. These

TABLE 14-8 Morphology of Microcalcifications and Associated Lesions

Morphology	Description/Associated lesion
Typically benign	Includes skin (lucent-centered) Vascular (parallel tracks) Coarse "popcorn-like" (fibroadenomas) Large rod-like (secretory disease) Eggshell or rim (fat necrosis) Milk of calcium (within tiny cysts) Dystrophic (after trauma or irradiation)
Intermediate	Amorphous/indistinct (round or "flake-shaped," small or hazy in appearance)
Higher probability of malignancy	Pleomorphic or heterogeneous (granular) varying in size and shape, <0.5 mm) Fine/linear/branching (casting) Linear and discontinuous

lesions are associated with pleomorphic calcifications that appear discontinuous and linear in distribution. This discontinuous linear pattern suggests irregular filling of a duct with abnormal cells.

Microcalcifications

The BI-RADS lexicon describes calcification morphology (shape) and distribution. Calcifications may be scattered or clustered, coarse or fine, and old or new. Comparison with prior mammograms is often necessary (Table 14-8).

Breast Ultrasound and Magnetic Resonance Imaging

Breast ultrasonography can be used to distinguish between solid and cystic masses in the breast. It can be used to evaluate a focal mass identified on a mammogram or a palpable mass. It is also used as an adjuvant for biopsy. Because of its low specificity, it is not thought to be a good modality for screening. It cannot replace mammography because it has no ability to detect microcalcifications. Ultrasound can complement mammography in young women with dense breasts because dense breasts limit the accuracy of the mammogram.

MRI has a high sensitivity in the diagnosis of breast cancer, ranging from 86% to 100%, but a low specificity, ranging from 37% to 97%. Because of this low specificity, it is of limited value in screening. It is an expensive test that requires intravenous contrast, and the technology for performing biopsy under MRI guidance is not widely available. Current uses include evaluation of breast implants for rupture, evaluation of pectoralis involvement with extensive breast cancer, and evaluation of post-lumpectomy bed fibrosis. Other uses include evaluation of occult breast cancers and evaluation of multifocal disease in those patients who are considering breast conservation. Studies on the use of MRI for surveillance of women at high risk for hereditary breast cancer have been published recently. Warner and colleagues compared breast MRI with mammography, screening ultrasonography, and physical examination in 196 women at high risk for developing breast cancer. These women had proven mutations in the BRCA genes or strong family histories of breast and or ovarian cancer. Six invasive cancers were found, including two cancers not identified through other modalities (i.e., mammography, ultrasound, and physical examination). A study of 236 women with BRCA mutations and MRI in conjunction with mammographic screening and clinical breast examination detected 22 cancers; 77% were detected by MRI, and 32% were detected by MRI alone.

A multi-institutional Dutch national study trial for MRI screening in women with a familial or genetic predisposition that was published in 2004 included 1909 women; of them, 358 were BRCA mutation carriers. Forty-five cancers were diagnosed, and 22 of these (49%) were detected by MRI alone. This demonstrates the greater sensitivity of MRI over the use of mammography alone in screening for breast cancer in these high-risk women.

Overall, MRI has proved to be an extremely valuable tool in screening women at the highest risk for developing breast cancer. Determining the optimal point in time to perform the MRI in relation to the mammogram has not been determined.

The ACS has issued guidelines about the use of MRI for screening in high-risk women. A guideline panel was assembled to review evidence and develop new recommendations for women at different levels of risk. Based on this panel screening, MRI is recommended for women with an approximately 20% to 25% or greater lifetime risk of developing breast cancer. This includes women with strong family history of breast and/or ovarian cancer, and women with a history of treatment for Hodgkin's disease. The panel considered that there was insufficient evidence to recommend for or against screening with MRI for women with a personal history of breast cancer, CIS, atypical hyperplasia, and extremely dense breasts on mammography.

DIGITAL MAMMOGRAPHY

In 1991 the NCI convened a panel of experts on breast imaging. The panel placed high priority on the development of digital mammography. Four full-field systems were developed and underwent FDA testing. The benefits of digital mammography over traditional film mammography concern image acquisition and facilitation of storage. In addition, digital-image processing allows manipulation of image contrast and may enhance subtle contrast differences. In January 2000 the General Electric Senographe 2000D was approved by the FDA.

Pilot studies and U.S. Department of Defense full-field digital mammography screening trials of digital mammography versus conventional film mammography found that the two modalities are similar in terms of the number of cancers diagnosed. However, the researchers noted a lower recall rate with digital mammography. Since its introduction, population-based screening trials comparing screen-film and full-field digital mammography have been conducted. In the Oslo I Study conducted in Norway, full-field digital and screen-film mammography were performed in 3683 women aged 50 to 69 years. The investigators found no statistically significant difference in cancer detection rates between the two modalities. The Oslo II Study yielded similar results in cancer detection rates. Full-field digital mammography did yield higher cancer detection rates, but this difference between film and digital mammography was not statistically significant. In Canada and the United States, 49,528 women were enrolled in the Digital Mammographic Imaging Screening Trial (DMIST). All participants underwent both digital and film mammography in random order. The investigators noted that, although the diagnostic accuracy of digital and film mammography was similar, the accuracy of digital mammography was better in women younger than age 50 years, women with radiographically dense breasts, and premenopausal or perimenopausal women. Thus, in women who met those criteria, the investigators recommended digital mammography. How feasible this is remains a question, however. It is thought that fewer than 10% of facilities in the United States currently have digital mammographic systems. The cost of installing a digital mammographic system can significantly increase the cost of performing mammograms. However, when both technologies are available, the use of digital mammography can be tailored to the individual.

With ongoing research into this new technology, new adjunct technologies may be developed. For example, telemammography will make telemedicine consultations possible. Computer-aided diagnosis may facilitate second opinions for digital mammographic studies.

DIAGNOSTIC EVALUATION

Palpable Mass

The workup of a patient with a dominant mass should include a bilateral mammogram. In addition to gaining valuable information about the characteristics of the mass, a secondary purpose in this setting is to screen the normal surrounding breast and the contralateral breast for nonpalpable mammographic abnormalities (densities or calcifications). Evaluation of a palpable mass is important to determine whether the mass is cancerous even if the mammogram is negative.

Fine-Needle Aspiration or Biopsy

FNA can be extremely useful in providing a cytologic analysis of a palpable breast mass. Many palpable thickenings and all dominant masses should be considered for FNA because it can differentiate between solid and cystic masses. In addition, FNA can diagnose and treat simple cysts and provide cellular material for cytologic analysis. The FNA should be performed after radiologic examination because the resultant hematoma could mask an underlying abnormality.

The breast is prepped with alcohol; with the physician facing the patient, the lesion is stabilized with the physician's opposite hand. Usually, a 21-gauge or 25-gauge needle on a 10-cc syringe is used. Approximately 3 cc of air is aspirated into the syringe to facilitate expulsion of the contents onto the slide following the procedure. The needle is introduced into the lesion, and suction is applied on the syringe. If the mass is cystic, the fluid is completely evacuated and the lesion should completely disappear. The syringe is withdrawn, and the fluid is discarded if it is serous and nonbloody. The patient should return in 4 to 6 weeks for re-examination.

If the lesion encountered is not cystic or suspected to be solid, an FNA biopsy can be performed in the same manner. After insertion into the lesion, multiple passes (10-15) through the lesion with changes in direction allow extensive sampling and create a "feel" for the mass (carcinomas are usually hard and gritty). The goal of sampling is to obtain material in the hub of the needle, not to fill the syringe. Care should be taken to release the suction before withdrawing the needle to prevent aspiration into the syringe. The sample is then ejected onto a glass slide, gently smeared with another slide, and placed in sterile jars containing 95% ethanol for transport to the cytology laboratory. Alternatively, it can be placed in a specimen jar containing cytofixative. The needle should be removed from the syringe, the medium aspirated into the syringe, the needle replaced; and the medium then ejected into the jar.

An FNA requires a cytopathologist experienced in breast pathology. The false-negative rate can range from 3% to 35% depending on the expertise of the aspirator and cytopathologist, the size of the lesion, the location within the breast, and the cellular composition of the lesion. Negative findings of an FNA sample in the presence of a suspicious mass should not preclude further diagnostic evaluation. A diagnosis of atypical cells following an FNA warrants a surgical biopsy. Any mass

remaining after aspiration of a cyst should be excised. Similarly, a cyst that recurs in the same location after one or two aspirations should be excised.

The false-positive rate of an FNA sample is less than 1%, but in the United States most surgeons will not perform definitive surgery such as a mastectomy without a prior surgical biopsy, core-needle biopsy, or frozen-section diagnosis at the time of surgery. An FNA sample that is positive for adenocarcinoma could, however, provide a preliminary diagnosis and guide subsequent management.

Patients with palpable solid masses can have a biopsy of the mass in the office with use of a Tru-cut 14-gauge biopsy device. The breast is prepped sterilely, and a local anesthetic is used to infiltrate the skin. A small nick is made in the skin with a scalpel to accommodate the biopsy instrument. A core biopsy of the solid mass is obtained. The instrument has a "firing range" and therefore should be kept parallel to the chest wall to avoid penetrating trauma. The specimen is placed in formalin and sent for pathologic examination. It is believed that if the specimen "floats" in the solution, it is likely non-diagnostic fat. Tumor specimens will have a grayish appearance and will typically "sink" in the solution.

Needle Localization and Excision

Needle localization is a technique that allows surgical excision of a lesion that is nonpalpable. The technique uses a hook-wire system to target the lesion, and image guidance can be provided by mammogram, ultrasound, and in some cases MRI. In mammography-guided needle localization, coordinates of the lesion are obtained by placing the breast in an alphanumeric grid. The needle is inserted and, when adequate placement is noted, the hook wire is deployed and the needle removed. Two mammographic views are then obtained.

The mammography films are available intraoperatively and show the relationship between the lesion and localizing hook. Excision with needle localization allows the surgeon to minimize the amount of breast tissue removed by following the needle to the targeted lesion. After removal, a specimen radiograph is obtained to ensure that successful removal of the lesion has been performed. Radiologists and surgeons experienced in needle localization and excisions report only 0.2% to 0.3% of lesions missed with this approach. The specimen radiograph helps to ascertain the lesion was not missed.

Image-Guided Percutaneous Breast Biopsy

With the current advancements available in breast imaging, percutaneous image-guided breast biopsy is increasingly being used as an alternative to surgical biopsy. Percutaneous biopsy methods differ with respect to the method of imaging guidance, and the tissue-acquisition device used. The use of image-guided percutaneous biopsy has advantages over surgical excision for the diagnosis of breast lesions. It is less invasive, and because less tissue is removed, it will result in less scarring on subsequent mammograms. Regardless of whether the diagnosis is benign or malignant, the patients who have percutaneous biopsies will undergo fewer operations. In addition, in cases of malignancy, the discussion and surgical treatment plan can be streamlined. The choice of which image-guided modality to use depends on the lesion. Stereotactic biopsy is best for calcifications. If a lesion is seen on ultrasound, it is best to use that modality because it is easier to use and has been reported to be less costly.

Stereotactic Biopsy

Stereotactic-guided core needle biopsy uses specialized mammography equipment to calculate the location of a lesion in three dimensions. Stereotactic biopsy can be performed with the patient prone on a dedicated table or with the patient sitting in an upright unit. Some patients may not be candidates for this approach. A patient may be too large to be accommodated by the system. The thickness of the breast must be adequate to accommodate to the automated biopsy device. Abnormalities just under the skin may also pose technical problems. A vague asymmetric density or diffuse group of widely separated calcifications may present difficulties. Patients who cannot remain prone or are unable to cooperate for the 20- to 40-minute duration of the procedure may not be candidates.

An automated core needle or directional vacuum-assisted biopsy probe is used to obtain the tissue specimens. Multiple tissue specimens are obtained for pathologic analysis. Many reports in the medical literature state the procedure has a sensitivity of 70% to 100% and a specificity of 85% to 100%. Studies have shown 99% accuracy with a 14-gauge needle obtaining five specimens. Radiography should be performed routinely on women with specimens of breast microcalcifications to determine whether calcifications were obtained.

Ultrasound-Guided Biopsy

The use of ultrasound imaging for percutaneous biopsy of lesions seen on ultrasound has certain advantages. For example, it requires no specialized equipment, requires no radiation exposure, and has the ability to sample areas that may be inaccessible with stereotactic biopsy (such as the axilla). A 14-gauge automated needle is used, and real-time imaging allows accurate positioning. Multiple tissue core samples are sent for pathologic analysis.

Tissue-Acquisition Devices

Available tissue-acquisition devices include fine needles, automated core needles, directional vacuum-assisted probes, and biopsy cannulas. Excellent results have been obtained using the 14-gauge automated needle for biopsy of masses under ultrasound or stereotactic guidance. Most centers use larger tissue-acquisition devices instead of fine needles because of accuracy of tissue diagnosis when a larger volume of tissue is obtained. Compared with the automated needle, the vacuum device acquires larger samples of tissue, has a higher frequency of retrieval of calcifications, and may provide more accurate lesion characterization. Accurate placement of a localizing clip through the biopsy probe is necessary to facilitate subsequent localization if needed.

Surgical Excision/Breast Biopsy

ACOG has stopped short of recommending that open biopsy be performed by every obstetrician and gynecologist.

A biopsy can be performed on an outpatient basis under local anesthesia in the majority of patients. It is important to choose the appropriate incision and location. Unless the lesion is close to the nipple or suspected to be a fibroadenoma, the incision should be made in close proximity to the mass and not circumareolar. The surgeon should keep in mind the possibility of subsequent mastectomy when placing the incision. Many times, the biopsy is part of the treatment. The specimen should be adequately oriented for margin analysis by the pathologist and also sent for the appropriate markers such as estrogen-receptor (ER) and progesterone-receptor (PR) status and HER2/neu. Orientation of the specimen is important because a re-excision of a close or involved margin may need to be performed.

The incision should be closed with fine suture material with a subcuticular closure. Hemostasis needs to be ascertained before closing and is usually achieved with electrocautery. Weck clips can be placed in the cavity bed if a diagnosis of breast cancer is known and breast conservation is planned. No particular immobilization is required, but a good support bra is recommended to minimize hematoma, induration, and discomfort.

Certain benign lesions on core needle biopsy have a relatively high incidence of coexisting carcinoma found on subsequent surgical excision. The small volume of tissue obtained on core needle biopsy in these cases may not be adequate to rule out cancer. Atypical ductal hyperplasia is the most commonly encountered of these lesions. About 25% of atypical ductal hyperplasia on core biopsy specimen will have carcinoma on excisional biopsy. Radial scars are reported to have a coexistent carcinoma in 20% and therefore also require surgical excision. The

TABLE 14-9 Major Risk Factors for Breast Cancer

Age
Family history of breast cancer
Benign breast disease
   Proliferative changes
   Atypical hyperplasia
Endogenous endocrine factors
   Early menarche
   Late menopause
   Long menses duration
   Nulliparity
   Late maternal age at first pregnancy
Exogenous hormones?
   Oral contraceptives
   Estrogen replacement therapy

tissue obtained from a core needle biopsy may not be concordant with the imaging findings. In a study by Dershaw and colleagues, repeated biopsy for nonconcordance found carcinoma in 47% of cases. A diagnosis of lobular carcinoma in situ (LCIS) should not be accepted as consistent with imaging findings because these lesions do not have a classic characteristic mammographic appearance. These lesions on core biopsy are often followed by a recommendation for surgical excision.

EPIDEMIOLOGY OF BREAST CANCER

Table 14-9 lists major risk factors for breast cancer.

Risk Factors and Assessment

Age

The incidence of breast cancer increases with age. Age is the most significant risk factor for breast cancer.

Family History

Hereditary breast cancers account for 5% to 10% of all breast cancers and are thought to be attributable to highly penetrant mutations in breast cancer–susceptibility genes. Two such tumor-suppressor genes, BRCA1 and BRCA2, have been well characterized. Breast cancer has also been noted to occur in association with other cancers, such as in Li-Fraumeni syndrome and Cowden syndrome.

Prospective data from the Nurses' Health Study noted that the risk of breast cancer doubled among women whose mother had breast cancer diagnosed before the age of 40 years or who had a sister with breast cancer. The risk decreased with advanced maternal age; however, it remained elevated even with maternal diagnosis at age 70 years (RR 1.5; 95% CI, 1.1-2.2). The data did show that the risk associated with a mother or sister with history of breast cancer is smaller than previously suggested. In the population of middle-aged women, the authors found that only 2.5% of breast cancer cases were attributed to a positive family history. In the large Cancer Prevention Study II by the ACS, the authors evaluated the association of fatal breast cancer and family history. They found that family history of breast cancer in a mother or sister was significantly related to fatal breast cancer risk after multivariate analysis. Association was significantly modified by age with a risk ratio of almost 5 in women younger than 40 years at enrollment compared with 1.28 in women aged 70 years or older.

Personal History

A patient's history of prior breast biopsy is important. Although the number of breast biopsies undergone does not increase a woman's risk of breast cancer, certain pathologic entities do play a role. Atypical ductal or lobular hyperplasia and LCIS are considered markers of increased risk of developing invasive breast cancer. A personal history of breast cancer increases the risk for development of another breast cancer. Women treated for breast cancer are at risk for the development of a contralateral breast cancer. Various studies have shown this risk to be between 0.5% and 1.0% per year. In addition, patients treated with breast conservation (lumpectomy and radiation therapy) are at risk for an ipsilateral recurrence. In these women, this risk could be 10% at 10 to 15 years post-treatment.

Reproductive History

Early menarche, late menopause, and nulliparity are thought to be risk factors for breast cancer. Age at first pregnancy is also thought to be a relative risk (RR) factor for breast cancer.

Early age at first pregnancy is often associated with a lower risk for breast cancer. For a woman younger than 19 years of age at first full-term birth, a 50% reduction in the risk of breast cancer compared with that of a nulliparous woman is predicted. If the first full-term pregnancy occurs at age 30 to 34 years, the risk of breast cancer is approximately the same as that noted in nulliparous women. Pregnancy in women after age 35 years is associated with an increased risk compared with that of a nulliparous woman. Pregnancies that are not full term do not show this protection.

Some have suggested that the time interval between the onset of menarche and the first full-term pregnancy is the important factor with regard to the endocrine milieu. This importance has a possible explanation in the "estrogen open window hypothesis." There is, however, some inconsistency in reported data in regard to relationship of age at first full-term pregnancy. The association depends somewhat on control subjects used, and later studies have suggested a less-strong association.

Breast feeding has been reported to reduce risk of breast cancer. Studies in the United States have suggested only a weak protective effect and do not demonstrate an association between reduction in risk and duration of breast feeding.

The effect of menopause as it relates to breast cancer risk has been examined. Late menopause poses an increase in risk of breast cancer. Early exposure to the hormone milieu is thought by some to be an important etiologic factor. In one large international case-control study, it was noted that for each 2-year delay in the onset of menstruation, breast cancer risk was reduced by about 10%. The later a woman's menopause occurs, the higher her risk for breast cancer. For every 5-year difference in age at menopause, the risk for breast cancer changes about 17%. The effect of this later age at menopause in regard to increasing breast cancer is not seen for 10 to 20 years after menopause. It has been suggested that the total duration of menstruation may also be important because the risk increases in the woman who has menstruated more 30 years compared with those who have had less than 30 years of menstruation. Among women who have undergone a natural menopause, the risk among those whose menopause occurred at age 55 years is about twice that of women whose menopause occurred before age 44 years.

Data from observational studies demonstrate that bilateral oophorectomy before natural menopause has been reported to reduce risk of breast cancer compared with those who had a later natural or artificial menopause.

Exogenous Hormone Use

The role of exogenous estrogens in the promotion of breast cancer is still controversial. Studies of OCPs and HRT have yielded conflicting results. Studies of HRT and breast cancer risk indicate that women who are currently using HRT are at increased risk for breast cancer development. A meta-analysis of the largest studies, however, suggests that the increased risk is only about 10%. Women who have taken HRT in the past but are not currently using HRT are not at increased risk. Long-term use of HRT (>10 years) has been associated with a relative increase in breast cancer risk, and the highest risk was noted in those patients using HRT with progestins (RR, 1.41). Of note, multiple studies have shown that patients who develop breast cancer while taking HRT have smaller, less aggressive cancers and a lower risk of death from breast cancer.

Results from the Women's Health Initiative (WHI) randomized controlled trial were reported. Between 1993 and 1998, 16,609 women with an intact uterus were randomly assigned to receive combination HRT (0.625 mg/day conjugated equine estrogens and 2.5 mg/day medroxyprogesterone acetate) or placebo.

The planned duration of the trial was 8.5 years; however, the data and safety monitoring board of the committee recommended halting the trial because the incidence of invasive breast cancer had exceeded the stopping boundary that had been set at the initiation of the trial. This occurred after a mean of 5.2 years of follow-up. The increased risk of breast cancer reported hazard ratio was 1.25 (95% CI, 1.00-1.59). There was also a reported increased risk of coronary heart disease (HR, 1.29; 95% CI, 1.02-1.63) and stroke (HR, 1.41; 95% CI, 1.39-3.25). Beneficial effects included decreased risk in colorectal cancer (HR, 0.63; 95% CI, 0.43-0.92) and hip fracture (HR 0.66; 95% CI, 0.45-0.98). Based on the data, the safety monitoring board initially did not recommend stopping the estrogen-alone arm in women who had had a hysterectomy. Results of the estrogen-only arm and the WHI study have been reported. The study included 10,739 postmenopausal women (aged 50-79 years) with prior hysterectomy. These women were randomly assigned to receive 0.625 mg/day of conjugated equine estrogen or placebo. In February 2004 the National Institutes of Health decided to terminate the intervention phase of the estrogen-only study, which had been scheduled for a close-out interval of October 2004 to March 2005. With an average follow-up of 6.8 years, there was an increased risk of stroke (HR, 1.39; 95% CI, 1.10-1.77), a decreased risk of hip fracture (HR, 0.61; 95% CI, 0.41-0.91), and no effect on coronary heart disease incidence (HR, 0.91; 95% CI, 0.75-1.12). The investigators noted a possible reduction in breast cancer risk (HR, 0.77; 95% CI, 0.59-1.01) that warrants further investigation.

The annual increased risk for an individual woman is still relatively small. The increased risk for breast cancer is apparent after 4 years of HRT use. ACOG stresses the importance of addressing the reasons for initiating or continuing on HRT. It is no longer recommended to prevent heart disease in healthy women (primary prevention) or to protect women with pre-existing heart disease (secondary prevention). In addition, it is no longer recommended solely for prevention of osteoporosis.

HRT is highly effective in treating vasomotor symptoms with limited effective alternative therapies. In this setting, short-term use (<5 years) can be considered because data on short-term use does not show an increased association with breast cancer. A recent study surveyed attitudes of obstetricians and gynecologists toward hormone therapy after the WHI results were published. Respondents to the survey remained skeptical of the results; 49.1% did not find them convincing. There was strong support for the use of HRT for vasomotor symptoms, vaginal dryness, and osteoporosis, but most of the physicians surveyed did not find it useful for prevention of cardiovascular disease or dementia.

In the past, most studies addressing OCP use and breast cancer risk concluded that there was a significant increase in risk associated with OCP use. However, the majority of studies regarding OCP use and breast cancer risk have demonstrated little association with breast cancer incidence rates. In women who have used OCP for extended periods (>10 years), a minimal, nonsignificant increase in breast cancer cases has been reported, seen most commonly in the group of women who began using OCP at a young age (<20 years). Past or present use of OCP at the time of diagnosis of breast cancer does not affect mortality from breast cancer. The presence of a family history of breast cancer does not appear to further increase the risk of breast cancer associated with either OCP or HRT use.

Prior Exposure to Radiation Therapy

Exposure to ionizing radiation such as occurs in treatment with mantle radiation for Hodgkin's disease poses a risk for breast cancer. This is noted 7 to 10 years after completion of radiation therapy. The cumulative probability of breast cancer at age 40 approaches 35% in these women. The risk of breast cancer associated with radiation exposure decreases with increasing age at exposure.

Other Factors

Breast cancer is more frequent in Jewish women than in non-Jewish women and more frequent in black women than in Caucasian women. Women of Ashkenazi Jewish descent have a 1 in 40 (2.5%) risk of carrying a mutation in *BRCA1* and *BRCA2* genes, thus accounting for the increased risk in these women. Asian women have a low incidence of breast cancer. Japanese women show lower rates of breast cancer than Caucasian women. Although postmenopausal breast cancer is less common in Japanese women who have migrated to Western countries than among the general populations of these countries, after two or three generations the incidences of breast cancer in these women approach that of white women. The Western diet, with its increased intake of animal fat, has been implicated in these studies.

Alcohol consumption has been reported to increase breast cancer risk in a dose-related manner. Women who drink approximately one drink per day have a slightly elevated risk of breast cancer over nondrinkers. This risk is significantly higher with moderate-to-high alcohol consumption (two to five drinks per day).

Relative Risk

RR is a ratio that depicts the likelihood over time of an event's occurrence in a study population relative to that in a reference population. It is often used to quantify risk factors for breast cancer. Absolute risk is a percentage that depicts the likelihood over time of the occurrence of an event. For rare events, these two are the same, but for common events they are not. It is best to discuss risk with patients in terms of absolute rather than relative risk.

Several models exist to estimate a woman's risk of breast cancer. The Gail model, developed for use in the National Surgical Adjuvant Breast and Bowel Project (NSABP P-1) Breast Cancer Prevention Trial, is available from the NCI and provides a measurement of absolute risk over time for breast cancer. However, in familial-type hereditary cases, it underestimates the risk of breast cancer by overlooking age at onset, bilaterality of disease among affected family members, and breast cancer in non–first-degree relatives (Table 14-10).

BRCA1 and BRCA2

BRCA1 and *BRCA2* are breast cancer–susceptibility genes that have expanded our knowledge of familial breast cancer. Linkage studies done in 1990 in early-onset breast cancer families led to cloning of the *BRCA1* gene at the University of Utah in Salt Lake City in 1994. The *BRCA1* gene consists of 22 coding exons distributed over approximately 100 kb of genomic DNA on chromosome 17q21. It is thought to be responsible for approximately 45% of early-onset hereditary breast cancers and nearly 90% of hereditary ovarian cancers in families with a high incidence of breast and ovarian cancers. Two specific mutations, 185delAG and 5382insC, are present in approximately 1.00% and 0.25% of the Ashkenazi Jewish population, respectively. They are thought to be founder mutations (i.e., an altered gene or genes seen with a high frequency in a population originating from a small ancestral group, one or more of whose founders were carriers of the mutant gene).

BRCA2 was isolated on chromosome 13q12-13 in 1995. The *BRCA2* gene is composed of 26 coding exons distributed over approximately 70 kb of genomic DNA. This gene appears to account for 35% of families with early-onset breast cancer. It confers a lower risk of ovarian cancer compared with breast cancer. A single mutation, 6174delT, is found in approximately 1.4% of the Ashkenazi Jewish population. Together, both *BRCA1* and *BRCA2* mutations are found in approximately 1 in 40 Ashkenazi Jewish individuals. For both genes, the estimated penetrance is 70% to 90% for breast cancer by age 70, but the risk of breast cancer by age 50 may be lower for *BRCA2* mutations.

The likelihood of a patient having a *BRCA1* or *BRCA2* mutation is dependent on certain factors, such as age at the time of diagnosis of breast or ovarian cancer and the number and age of first- and second-degree relatives in the same parental lineage and ethnicity with breast

TABLE 14-10   Breast Cancer Risk Factors

PERSONAL AND FAMILY HISTORY FACTORS WITH RELATIVE RISK OF >4.0

- Certain inherited genetic mutations for breast cancer
- Two or more first-degree relatives with breast cancer diagnosed at an early age
- Personal history of breast cancer
- Age (≥65 years vs <65 years, although risk increases across all ages until age 80 years)

PERSONAL AND FAMILY HISTORY FACTORS WITH RELATIVE RISK OF 2.1-4.0

- One first-degree relative with breast cancer
- Nodular densities seen on mammogram (>75% of breast volume)
- Atypical hyperplasia
- High-dose ionizing radiation administered to the chest
- Ovaries not surgically removed before age 40 years

PERSONAL AND FAMILY HISTORY FACTORS WITH RELATIVE RISK OF 1.1-2.0

- High socioeconomic status
- Urban residence
- Northern U.S. residence

REPRODUCTIVE FACTORS THAT INCREASE RELATIVE RISK

- Early menarche (<12 years)
- Late menopause (≥55 years)
- No full-term pregnancies (for breast cancer diagnosed at age 40+ years)
- Late age at first full-term pregnancy (≥30 years)
- Never breast fed a child

OTHER FACTORS THAT AFFECT CIRCULATING HORMONES OR GENETIC SUSCEPTIBILITY

- Postmenopausal obesity
- Alcohol consumption
- Recent hormone replacement therapy
- Recent oral contraceptive use
- Being tall
- Personal history of cancer of endometrium, ovary, or colon
- Jewish heritage

Data from Hulka BS, Stark AT: Lancet 346:883, 1995. Kelsey JL: Epidemiol Rev 15:256, 1993.
American Cancer Society. Breast cancer facts & figures 2001-2002. Atlanta (GA): ACS; 2001.

TABLE 14-11   American Society of Clinical Oncology (ASCO) Guidelines for Recommending Genetic Testing for Families with High Probability (>10%) of Having *BRCA1* Mutation

Three or more kindred with breast cancer before age 50

Two or more breast cancers and one or more ovarian cancer diagnosed at any age

Sister pairs with two breast cancers, two ovarian cancers, or a breast and an ovarian cancer, all diagnosed before age 50

---

or ovarian cancer. The parental lineage can be either maternal or paternal. The American Society of Clinical Oncology issued guidelines for recommending genetic testing for families with high probability (>10%) of having a mutation for *BRCA1* (Table 14-11).

Patients with a high-risk family history should be referred for genetic counseling and testing. The decision to undergo genetic testing is a complex one because it can affect an individual's personal, psychological, social, financial, and ethical well-being.

Women who have a negative genetic test result should still be considered at risk on the basis of age and environment and because of the possibility of other genetic factors or unknown mutations.

Natural History

The most common site of origin of breast cancer is the upper-outer quadrant (38.5%), followed by the central area (29%), upper-inner quadrant (14.2%), lower-outer quadrant (8.8%), and the lower-inner quadrant (5%). These percentages correlate with the amount of tissue that is present in these quadrants. Metachronous bilateral carcinoma of the breast has been observed in 5% to 8% of patients.

Metastasis to the ipsilateral axilla is the most common route of spread. Metastasis to the internal mammary nodes is more frequent with inner-quadrant lesions and is more likely to occur when involvement of the axillary nodes is also present.

Pathology

Ductal Carcinoma in Situ

Ductal carcinoma in situ (DCIS) is an abnormal proliferation of malignant epithelial cells within the mammary ductal–lobular system without invasion into the surrounding stroma. It is classified as a heterogenous group of lesions with different growth patterns and cytologic features. Classification of DCIS has traditionally been based on architectural pattern. The most common types are comedo, cribriform, micropapillary, papillary, and solid. The increased use of screening mammography during the past two decades has led to a marked increase in the number of patients with a diagnosis of DCIS, and in many centers today one DCIS is diagnosed for every two or three mammographically detected invasive breast cancers. Today, about 85% of all DCIS are detected solely based on mammography. Age-specific time trends illustrate that the greatest increase has been in women older than 40 years who are more likely to have mammography. In 1980 only 2% of 10,000 cancer cases were DCIS. Between 1973 and 1992, age-adjusted DCIS incidence increased almost sixfold, whereas the incidence of invasive cancer has increased only by one third. This increase is almost entirely a result of mammography screening.

Indeed, autopsy series suggest that latent DCIS is relatively common, ranging from 6% to 18% of women who died of causes other than breast cancer. The natural history of DCIS is only partially understood, particularly for small, mammographically detected lesions. The microcalcifications in DCIS are most often secondary to calcification of necrotic cellular debris within the involved ducts, and their extent and characteristics are better defined with magnification views of the microcalcification.

The potential of DCIS to progress to invasive breast cancer is an unresolved issue. Because DCIS has historically been treated with mastectomy, little information on the risk of progression to invasive disease is available. The retrospective study by Page and colleagues of benign breast biopsy specimens revealed 25 patients who were subsequently identified with DCIS; 7 (28%) had progressed to invasive disease during the period of observation.

Paget's Disease

Paget's disease is involvement of the nipple with intraductal carcinoma. In the absence of a palpable mass, invasive carcinoma occurs in less than 40% of cases. The malignant cells are large and pale-staining, and are seen in the basal layer and upper portions of the epidermis. Diagnosis is made through a nipple biopsy.

Lobular Carcinoma in Situ

Foote and Stewart initially described LCIS in 1941 as a noninvasive lesion arising from the lobules and terminal ducts of the breast. LCIS is characterized by a solid proliferation of small cells with round to oval nuclei that distort the involved spaces in the terminal duct–lobular units. Three important features of LCIS are as follows:

1. It is usually an incidental microscopic finding that is not detected clinically or by gross pathologic examination.
2. It is multicentric, and the associated cancer may be ductal or lobular.
3. The risk for subsequent cancer is the same for both breasts.

It is unfortunate that Foote and Stewart chose the name they did because it has led to a great deal of confusion over the past several decades. LCIS is a marker for breast cancer risk and is not a malignant finding.

Invasive Duct Carcinoma

Invasive duct carcinoma is the most common group of malignant mammary tumors and comprises 65% to 80% of all mammary carcinomas. Included in this group are special subtypes: tubular, medullary, metaplastic, mucinous (colloid) papillary, and adenoid cystic carcinoma. Each subtype constitutes only 1% to 2% of all invasive breast cancers, except medullary carcinoma, which constitutes 7%, and the rare adenoid cystic carcinomas, which constitute less than 0.1%.

Many of these subtypes, such as tubular and medullary carcinomas, carry an excellent prognosis. Metaplastic carcinomas, however, often have aggressive behavior. These tumors are characterized by the presence of homologous (epithelial) or heterologous (mesenchymal) elements. Two types have been described: squamous and pseudosarcomatous metaplasia.

Invasive duct carcinoma not otherwise specified (NOS) is a generic term that includes tumors that may express more than one element of the specific forms of duct carcinoma.

Infiltrating Lobular Carcinoma

Infiltrating lobular carcinoma has been reported to constitute 10% to 14% of invasive carcinomas. These carcinomas are characterized by uniform cells with small, round nuclei and limited cytoplasm. The presence of intracytoplasmic mucin vacuoles often gives the cells the appearance of signet-ring cells. The cells tend to grow circumferentially around ducts and lobules with a linear arrangement. This pattern is referred to as "single-file" or targetoid growth. There is often an associated desmoplastic stromal reaction.

Inflammatory Carcinoma

Inflammatory carcinoma is characterized by cutaneous findings present with an underlying invasive carcinoma. Usually the invasive tumor is a poorly differentiated infiltrating duct carcinoma. Upon microscopic evaluation, skin involvement often reveals tumor emboli in dermal lymphatics with an associated lymphocytic reaction in the dermis.

Metastases from Extramammary Tumors

The most common primary site of an occult extramammary tumor is the lung. Other primary sites include the ovaries, uterus, kidneys, and stomach. In those previously diagnosed, melanoma, prostate, cervix, uterus, and urinary bladder are the most common sites. Metastatic ovarian cancer may simulate papillary or mucinous carcinoma of the breast. A workup and history are often helpful in difficult cases. Often, identification of an in situ component helps to provide definitive evidence of a mammary origin.

Biologic Markers and Prognostic Factors

Axillary Lymph Node Status

The most important prognostic factor is nodal status. The presence of metastasis, and the number of lymph nodes involved, is significant and correlates with local failure and distant metastases. It is predictive of overall survival.

Tumor Size

Tumor size correlates with the incidence of lymph node metastases. The size of the tumor is also important, even in the absence of lymph node involvement. Patients with tumors less than 1 cm in size, or with good histologic types measuring less than 3 cm, do very well.

Histologic Grade

Histologic grade also correlates with breast cancer outcome. Poorly differentiated tumors have been associated with more aggressive behavior.

Molecular Profiling

Molecular classification of breast cancer into different subtypes can be used to stratify breast cancers into different groups. The luminal subtype makes up the hormone-receptor–expressing breast cancers. Generally, these have overall better prognosis than the other groups currently identified. The HER2/neu subtypes make up the tumors with HER2/neu overexpression. These subtypes confirm the clinical impression that tumors with HER2/neu overexpression are more aggressive tumors, are more likely to be grade III, and have a higher degree of concomitant *TP53* mutations. The basal-like subtype of breast cancer was named because of the similarity in expression pattern of this subtype to that of basal epithelia cells. Basal subtypes lack estrogen-receptor expression, have low HER2/neu expression, and are more likely to be aggressive tumors. Some authors have reported that these tumors are often seen in patients with BRCA mutations. Multiple studies have demonstrated that this subtype often carries a poor prognosis because this subtype is more likely than other subtypes to have tumors that are grade III and that have TP53 mutations. Ongoing validation studies are being conducted on the presence of these subtypes as independent prognostic indicators and on the impact of molecular classification on clinical decision making.

ERs/PRs

The hormone receptors can be measured by immunohistochemical (IHC) studies using monoclonal antibodies directed against the receptors. Positivity correlates with response to antihormonal agents and better prognosis.

HER2/neu

HER2/neu is an oncogene whose protein product may function as a growth factor receptor. It can be detected by IHC demonstration of the protein product or by gene amplifications. Overexpression or amplification has been shown to correlate with a poor prognosis; however, the studies differ with regard to the method of detection used and the interpretation of results. HER2/neu overexpression has been used as a predictor of response to certain chemotherapeutic agents. Particularly, increased response to doxorubicin-based therapy has been reported in the treatment of patients with positive nodes and overexpression of HER2/neu.

p53

A tumor-suppressor gene, p53 has a protein product that is a nuclear transcription factor with many functions, including regulation of the cell cycle and apoptosis. Most clinical studies have used IHC to study protein expression. Accumulation of p53 protein has been reported to correlate with reduced survival in some studies.

Staging of Breast Cancer Using the Tumor–Node–Metastasis System

The American Joint Committee on Cancer (AJCC) determines staging of breast cancer. The AJCC staging system is a clinical and pathologic staging system based on the tumor–node–metastasis (TNM) system. The new updated AJCC staging system incorporates sentinel node staging. It distinguishes micrometastasis from isolated tumor cells on the basis of size and histologic evidence of malignant activity. In the current AJCC staging system, supraclavicular lymph node metastasis is now classified as N3 disease rather than M1 disease, as in the old system (Tables 14-12 and 14-13).

TREATMENT OF BREAST CANCER

Most patients with intraductal carcinoma and stage I and stage II breast cancer have the options of breast-conservation therapy and mastectomy. For patients with invasive breast cancer, the axillary nodes can be addressed with a sentinel lymph node (SLN) biopsy and, possibly, an axillary dissection. For patients with more extensive disease, a mastectomy may be necessary. The use of postmastectomy chest-wall irradiation in these patients may also be considered.

Surgery

Mastectomy

William Halsted performed a radical mastectomy in 1894. The guiding principle at this time was centered on the belief that cancer originates in the breast and spreads in a stepwise fashion to the regional lymph nodes first, and then to distant sites. Removal of all the breast tissue, pectoral muscles, and axillary contents

TABLE 14-12   American Joint Committee on Cancer Staging for Breast Cancer

DEFINITION OF TNM

Primary Tumor (T)

Definitions for classifying the primary tumor (T) are the same for clinical and for pathologic classification. If the measurement is made by physical examination, the examiner will use the major headings (T1, T2, or T3). If other measurements, such as mammographic or pathologic measurements, are used, the subsets of T1 can be used. Tumors should be measured to the nearest 0.1 cm increment.

TX	Primary tumor cannot be assessed
T0	No evidence of primary tumor
Tis	Carcinoma in situ
Tis (DCIS)	Ductal carcinoma in situ
Tis (LCIS)	Lobular carcinoma in situ
Tis (Paget's)	Paget's disease of the nipple NOT associated with invasive carcinoma and/or carcinoma in situ (DCIS and/or LCIS) in the underlying breast parenchyma. Carcinomas in the breast parenchyma associated with Paget's disease are categorized based on the size and characteristics of the parenchymal disease, although the presence of Paget's disease should still be noted.
T1	Tumor ≤20 mm or less in greatest dimension
T1mi	Tumor ≤1 mm in greatest dimension
T1a	Tumor >1 mm but ≤5 mm in greatest dimension
T1b	Tumor >5 mm but ≤10 mm in greatest dimension
T1c	Tumor >10 mm but ≤20 mm in greatest dimension
T2	Tumor >20 mm but ≤50 mm in greatest dimension
T3	Tumor >50 mm in greatest dimension
T4	Tumor of any size with direct extension to the chest wall and/or to skin (ulceration or skin nodules)
T4a	Extension to chest wall, not including only pectoralis muscle adherence/invasion
T4b	Ulceration and/or ipsilateral satellite nodules and/or edema (including peau d'orange) of the skin, which do not meet the criteria for inflammatory carcinoma
T4c	Both T4a and T4b
T4d	Inflammatory carcinoma

Regional Lymph Nodes/Clinical

NX	Regional lymph nodes cannot be assessed (e.g., previously removed)
N0	No regional lymph node metastasis
N1	Metastasis to movable ipsilateral level I, II axillary lymph nodes(s)
N2	Metastases in ipsilateral level I, II axillary lymph nodes that are clinically fixed or matted; or in clinically detected* ipsilateral internal mammary nodes in the absence of clinically evident lymph node metastases
N2a	Metastasis in ipsilateral level I, II axillary lymph nodes fixed to one another (matted) or to other structures
N2b	Metastasis only in clinically detected* ipsilateral internal mammary nodes and in the absence of clinically evident level I, II axillary lymph node metastasis
N3	Metastases in ipsilateral infraclavicular (level III axillary) lymph node(s) with or without level I, II axillary lymph node involvement; or in clinically detected* ipsilateral internal mammary lymph node(s) with clinically evident level I, II axillary lymph node metastases; or metastases in ipsilateral supraclavicular lymph node(s) with or without axillary or internal mammary lymph node involvement
N3a	Metastasis in ipsilateral infraclavicular lymph node(s).
N3b	Metastasis in ipsilateral internal mammary lymph node(s) and axillary lymph node(s)
N3c	Metastasis in ipsilateral supraclavicular lymph node(s)

Pathologic (PN)[†]

pNX	Regional lymph nodes cannot be assessed (e.g., previously removed, or not removed for pathologic study)
pN0	No regional lymph node metastasis identified histologically.
	Note: Isolated tumor cells clusters (ITCs) are defined as small clusters of cells not greater than 0.2 mm, or single tumor cells, or a cluster of fewer than 200 cells in a single histologic cross section. ITCs may be detected by routine histology or by immunohistochemical (IHC) methods. Nodes containing only ITCs are excluded from the total positive node count for purposes of N classification but should be included in the total number of nodes evaluated.
pN0(i-)	No regional lymph node metastasis histologically, negative IHC
pN0(i+)	Malignant cells in regional lymph node(s) no greater than 0.2 mm (detected by H&E or IHC including ITC
pN0(mol-)	No regional lymph node metastasis histologically, negative molecular findings (RT-PCR)
pN0(mol+)	Positive molecular findings (RT-PCR), but no regional lymph node metastases detected by histology or IHC
pN1	Micrometastases; or metastases in 1-3 axillary lymph nodes; and/or in internal mammary nodes with metastases detected by SLNB but not clinically detected[‡]
pN1mi	Micrometastases (greater than 0.2 mm and/or more than 200 cells, but none greater than 2.0 mm)
pN1a	Metastases in 1-3 axillary lymph nodes, at least one metastasis greater than 2.0 mm
pN1b	Metastases in internal mammary nodes with micrometastases or macrometastases detected by SLNB but not clinically detected[‡]
pN1c	Metastases in 1-3 axillary lymph nodes and in internal mammary lymph nodes with micrometastases or macrometastases detected by SLNB but not clinically detected

Continued

TABLE 14-12   American Joint Committee on Cancer Staging For Breast Cancer—cont'd

pN2	Metastases in 4-9 axillary lymph nodes; or in clinically detected§ internal mammary lymph nodes in the absence of axillary lymph node metastases
pN2a	Metastases in 4-9 axillary lymph nodes (at least one tumor deposit greater than 2.0 mm)
pN2b	Metastases in clinically detected§ internal mammary lymph nodes in the absence of axillary lymph node metastases
pN3	Metastases in 10 or more axillary lymph nodes; or in infraclavicular (level III axillary) lymph nodes; or in clinically detected§ ipsilateral internal mammary lymph nodes in the presence of one or more positive level I, II axillary lymph node(s); or in more than three axillary lymph nodes and in internal mammary lymph nodes with micrometastases or macrometastases detected by SLNB but not clinically detected‡; or in ipsilateral supraclavicular lymph nodes
pN3a	Metastases in 10 or more axillary lymph nodes (at least one tumor deposit larger than 2.0 mm); or metastases to the infraclavicular (level III axillary) lymph nodes
pN3b	Metastases in clinically detected§ ipsilateral internal mammary lymph nodes in the presence of one or more positive axillary lymph nodes; or in more than three axillary lymph nodes and in internal mammary lymph nodes with micrometastases or macrometastases detected by sentinel lymph node biopsy but not clinically detected§
pN3c	Metastasis in ipsilateral supraclavicular lymph nodes
Distant Metastasis (M)	
M0	No clinical or radiographic evidence of distant metastases
cM0(i+)	No clinical or radiographic evidence of distant metastases, but deposits of molecularly or microscopically detected tumor cells in circulating blood, bone marrow, or other nonregional nodal tissue that are no larger than 0.2 mm in a patient without symptoms or signs of metastases
M1	Distant detectable metastases as determined by classic clinical and radiographic means and/or histologically proven larger than 0.2 mm

(From: Edge SB, Byrd DR, Compton CC, Fritz A, et al: AJCC Cancer Staging Manual, seventh edition. New York: Springer, 2009.)

*Clinically detected is defined as detected by imaging studies (excluding lymphoscintigraphy) or by clinical examination and having characteristics highly suspicious for malignancy or a presumed pathologic macrometastasis based on fine needle aspiration biopsy with cytologic examination. Confirmation of clinically detected metastatic disease by fine needle aspiration without excision biopsy is designated with an (f) suffix, for example, cN3a(f). Excisional biopsy of a lymph node or biopsy of a sentinel node, in the absence of assignment of a pT, is classified as a clinical N, for example, cN1. Information regarding the confirmation of the nodal status will be designated in site-specific factors as clinical, fine-needle aspiration, core biopsy, or sentinel lymph node biopsy. Pathologic classification (pN) is used for excision or sentinel lymph node biopsy only in connection with a pathologic T assignment.

†Classification is based on axillary lymph node dissection with or without sentinel lymph node biopsy. Classification based solely on sentinel lymph node biopsy without subsequent axillary lymph node dissection is designated (sn) for "sentinel node," for example, pN0(sn).

‡"Not clinically detected" is defined as not detected by imaging studies (excluding lymphoscintigraphy) or by clinical examination.

§"Clinically detected" is defined as detected by imaging studies (excluding lymphoscintigraphy) or by clinical examination and having characteristics highly suspicious for malignancy or a presumed pathologic macrometastasis based on fine needle aspiration biopsy with cytologic examination.

RT-PCR, Reverse transcriptase-polymerase chain reaction.

TABLE 14-13   Stage by Tumor, Node, Metastasis (TNM)

Stage 0	Tis, N0, M0
Stage I	T1f, N0, M0
Stage IIA	T0, N1, M0
	T1*, N1, M0
	T2, N0, M0
Stage IIB	T2, N1, M0
	T3, N0, M0
Stage IIIA	T0, N2, M0
	T1*, N2, M0
	T2, N2, M0
	T3, N1, M0
	T3, N2, M0
Stage IIIB	T4, N0, M0
	T4, N1, M0
	T4, N2, M0
Stage IIIC†	Any T, N3, M0
Stage IV	Any T, Any N, M1

(From: Edge SB, Byrd DR, Compton CC, Fritz A, et al: AJCC Cancer Staging Manual, seventh edition. New York: Springer, 2009.)

*T1 includes T1mic.

†Stage IIIC breast cancer includes patients with any T stage who have pN3 disease. Patients with pN3a and pN3b disease are considered operable and are managed as described in the section on stage I, II, IIIA, and operable IIIC breast cancer. Patients with pN3c disease are considered inoperable and are managed as described in the section on inoperable stage IIIB or IIIC or inflammatory breast cancer.

was the standard surgical treatment. Over the next several decades, two simultaneous trends existed. One involved less radical surgery, which included removal of the breast and axillary contents, but preserved the pectoral muscles and more skin. This was described by Patey and Dyson in 1948 and is the modern-day modified radical mastectomy. The other trend involved more extensive surgery, the extended radical mastectomy, which included en-bloc removal of the internal mammary chain at the time of radical mastectomy. Retrospective studies found that survival rates were similar regardless of the extent of the operative procedure when the Halsted radical mastectomy was compared with any of the modified approaches; as a result, a modified approach was accepted in 1979 by the NCI Consensus Conference.

Breast-Conservation Therapy

The shift toward less radical surgery at the time of mastectomy occurred for several reasons. As earlier diagnosis of breast cancer with smaller tumors and less

TABLE 14-14 Prospective Randomized Trials Comparing Conservative Surgery

	N	Years	Overall Survival (%)	
			Conservative Surgery and Radiation	Mastectomy
Milan Cancer Institute	701	18	65	65
Institut Gustave-Roussy	179	15	73	65
National Surgical Adjuvant Breast Project B-06	1219	12	63	59
Project B-06 National Cancer Institute	237	10	77	75
European Organization for Research and Treatment of Cancer	874	8	54	61
Danish Breast Cancer	904	6	79	82

Modified from Winchester DP, Cox JD: CA Cancer J Clin 48:83, 1998.

involvement of pectoral muscles occurred, the need for radical procedures decreased. In addition, even with radical mastectomy, not all patients were cured, and although regional recurrences were low, patients died of distant disease. The morbidity of the radical mastectomy was well documented, including lymphedema, immobility of the shoulder, and disfigurement. A shift to breast conservation followed the same trends. The initial trials with radiation therapy using radium implants at the Princess Margaret Hospital in Toronto had promising results.

This led to randomization studies comparing breast-conservation therapy with mastectomy. Table 14-14 lists randomized trials that compared radical and modified radical mastectomy in stage I and stage II carcinoma of the breast.

In breast-conserving surgery, a wide-local excision is performed with excision of the tumor and a 1- to 2-cm rim of normal tissue. This excision is referred to as "lumpectomy" or a "tumorectomy." This differs from a quadrantectomy, in which a resection of the tumor with the overlying skin and the involved quadrant of the breast is performed. The six randomized trials differed with respect to the type of wide-local excision performed and with respect to tumor size in the patients who were randomized. In the Milan trial, a quadrantectomy was performed. In the Insitut Gustave Roussy trial, the "tumorectomy" performed was removal of the tumor and a 2-cm margin of normal tissue. In the United States, the NSABP B-06 trial did not specify the margins on the lumpectomy specimen, providing they were grossly free of tumor. In the NCI study there was a significantly higher local recurrence rate in the breast-conservation group, but only gross tumor removal was required for study entry. Whole-breast irradiation (45-50 Gy) was used in all trials, with a boost to the primary site given in five of the six trials.

In all trials, the authors noted comparable disease-free survival in both arms. The only difference noted was in local recurrence. In addition to the randomized trials, there are many nonrandomized reports published with similar results in survival between breast conservation and mastectomy.

In a meta-analysis of nine prospective randomized trials comparing conservative surgery and irradiation with mastectomy, no survival differences were found in seven of the trials. Local recurrence was reported in 6.2% of patients treated with mastectomy and in 5.9% of those treated with breast-conservation surgery. No difference was seen in the incidence of contralateral breast cancer or a second malignant neoplasm that was not breast cancer. The incidence of recurrence in the treated breast ranged from 3% to 19%. Most failures in the treated breast can be salvaged with mastectomy, which can result in a 70% survival at 5 years. Mastectomy did not prevent local recurrences, which developed in 4% to 14% after this treatment.

In 1992 the American Colleges of Surgeons, Radiologists, and Pathologists, along with the ACS and the Society of Surgical Oncology, began the process of describing standard practice for breast-conservation treatment. Many retrospective and prospective randomized trials suggested equally effective results in appropriately selected patients with early-stage breast cancer, regardless of whether they were treated with mastectomy or breast-conservation surgery. The results of these deliberations were published in 1998.

Radiation therapy is an important component of breast conservation. Adequate surgical margins are required to be negative on pathologic inspection. After healing, the radiation therapy is planned. Treatment to the entire breast should be at a dose of 1.8 to 2.0 Gy per day for a total of 45 to 50 Gy. A 10- to 15-Gy electron-therapy boost is often given to the lumpectomy bed. More recently, data on hypofractionation, which increases the daily dose and shortens the radiation therapy time, have been reported and demonstrate equivalence to standard radiation techniques.

Breast conservation depends on the use of radiation. The question of whether lumpectomy alone would yield similar results has been addressed through randomized trials. Local recurrence rates of 18% to 40% with lumpectomy alone have been reported compared with 2% to 14% with lumpectomy and radiation. In these studies, a significant reduction in relapse was noted in the lumpectomy-and-radiation arm.

The NSABP B-17 trial is the only prospective randomized trial of lumpectomy alone versus lumpectomy and radiation (50 Gy) in patients with DCIS. There were 818 women randomly assigned, and surgical margins were histologically tumor free. Mean follow-up was 90 months (67-180 months). Incidence of noninvasive ipsilateral breast tumor was reduced from 13.4% to 8.2% ($P = 0.007$), and incidence of invasive ipsilateral breast tumor was reduced from 13.4% to 3.9% ($P < 0.001$). All women benefited from radiation therapy regardless of clinical or mammographic tumor characteristics. No difference in mortality was noted. In a subsequent report, only marked-to-moderate comedo necrosis was found to be a high-risk predictor. Mortality from breast carcinoma after DCIS for the entire cohort was found to be only 1.6% at 8 years. In cases of invasive recurrence, patients in the lumpectomy-plus-radiation arm can be salvaged with mastectomy.

Interest in partial-breast radiation for early-stage breast cancers has prompted single-institution studies to use brachytherapy catheters, the MammoSite balloon (Proxima Company, Alpharetta, GA), and three-dimensional external-beam partial-breast treatment. The FDA-approved MammoSite Radiation Therapy System is a means of administering brachytherapy internally in prescribed doses over a 5-day period. During the lumpectomy, a deflated balloon is placed inside the surgical cavity. A tube connects the balloon to the outside of the breast and may be inflated with saline to fill the cavity. Radiation is delivered within the inflated balloon over 1 to 5 days, after which the balloon is deflated and then removed.

These approaches are being studied as an alternative to the standard 5- to 6-week whole-breast radiation treatment. To shorten the radiation course, the proportion of breast tissue to be radiated is significantly less. Data on local recurrences after radiation show that the majority of recurrences after lumpectomy and whole-breast radiation occur in the same quadrant, hence the reason to consider partial-breast radiation. In this manner, a greater dose will be delivered to the lumpectomy site and the surrounding tissue in a shorter course of therapy. Currently, the National Surgical Adjuvant Breast and Bowel Project and Radiation Therapy Oncology Group (NSABP-RTOG) cooperative groups are opening a phase III trial comparing whole-breast radiation therapy to some form of partial-breast radiation. The partial-breast treatment will be delivered using brachytherapy catheters, MammoSite balloon, or external three-dimensional conformal treatment. Randomization to either whole- or partial-breast radiation will occur at entry into the trial. Patients are currently being enrolled in this study.

Overall, it appears that the clinician can now be confident in recommending lumpectomy plus irradiation to patients because it seems to be equivalent to mastectomy in terms of survival and optimal local-regional control.

Patient Selection

Possible contraindications can interfere with offering a patient breast-conservation therapy. Cosmetic result should be considered when deciding whether to offer breast-conserving surgery; tumor size in relation to breast size is an important consideration. In addition, other factors that may affect the ability to receive irradiation must be considered (i.e., history of prior breast or chest irradiation, concurrent pregnancy, and autoimmune connective-tissue disease). Particularly, with a history of systemic lupus erythematosis, radiation may not be a possibility. Women with multiple cancers in the breast are not candidates for this approach and require a mastectomy. In addition, patients with extensive calcifications on a mammogram suggesting a diffuse process may be better treated with mastectomy.

An area of controversy remains over the status of negative margins at the time of lumpectomy. Patients with positive resected margins should undergo re-excision. If resected margins remain positive on re-excision, mastectomy is the preferred treatment. Gage and colleagues noted the 5-year actuarial breast cancer recurrence rate to be 3% for negative margins, 9% for focally positive margins, and 28% for diffusely positive margins. Recent data suggest that systemic therapy may decrease the 5-year breast cancer recurrence rate in patients with positive margins. Status of surgical margins is probably the most important aspect of pathologic evaluation of breast tumor excision specimens in patients being considered for conservative surgery.

Extensive intraductal component (EIC) is a condition that exists when greater than 25% of the tumor is associated with DCIS. In these cases, the invasive component may be outside the area of the intraductal carcinoma. This has been reported to have a higher relapse rate with breast conservation; however, it is thought to be secondary to margin status because margin involvement may be an indication of residual intraductal carcinoma. In DCIS, Silverstein and associates developed the Van Nuys prognostic index (VNPI). The system combines the scores for histologic grade, tumor size, and margin status of a lesion in order to obtain an overall score. It considers margins of 1 cm to indicate a decreased rate of local relapse, even with no radiation.

Management of the Axilla

The axilla is a pyramidal space between the arm and thoracic wall. It contains the axillary vessels and their branches, the brachial plexus and its branches, and lymph nodes embedded in fatty tissue. The primary route of lymphatic drainage of the breast is through the axillary lymph nodes. The lymph nodes are also divided into levels based on location relative to the pectoralis minor. Level 1 lymph nodes lie lateral to the lateral border of the pectoralis minor muscle. Level 2 nodes lie behind the pectoralis minor muscle, and level 3 nodes are medial to the medial border of this muscle.

In an axillary dissection, nerve branches of the brachial plexus are encountered. The lateral and medial pectoral nerves supply the pectoralis muscles. The thoracodorsal nerve runs downward and innervates the latissimus dorsi. The long thoracic nerve is located on the medial wall of the axilla on the serratus anterior. It arises from the C5 to C7 roots, and injury to these nerves results in paralysis to part or all of the serratus anterior. The functional deficit is inability to raise the arm above the level of the shoulder.

At the time of Halsted's radical mastectomy procedure, a complete axillary dissection was performed. The status of the axilla is the most important prognostic factor for breast cancer. In the past, the use of axillary dissection has been demonstrated to significantly decrease local recurrence, which may ultimately translate to a survival advantage.

Clinical examination of the axilla is inaccurate, because even in patients with a T1 lesion there is a 10% risk of lymph node metastasis. Before the use of sentinel lymph node biopsy, there was no accurate method to adequately stage the axilla without an axillary dissection. Axillary lymph node sampling (i.e., removal of only a few lymph nodes) was inadequate.

Metastatic involvement of lymph nodes usually occurs in a stepwise manner. Rosen and co-workers demonstrated the incidence of skip metastasis to be less than 2%. A complete level 1 and level 2 lymph node dissection provides excellent local control, and local recurrence after this procedure has been shown to be less than 1%.

The NSABP B-04 trial was begun in 1971, and the NSABP designed this trial to determine the value of prophylactic regional node dissection. Patients with clinically uninvolved axillary nodes (clinical stage I) were randomly assigned for treatment among radical mastectomy, total mastectomy plus irradiation of the chest wall and regional lymphatics, and total mastectomy alone. Women who had clinically involved axillary nodes (clinical stage II) were randomly assigned to treatment with either radical mastectomy or total mastectomy and irradiation to the chest wall and all lymph node drainage areas for the breast. If ignoring occult axillary metastases permitted continuing dissemination, the patients treated with total mastectomy alone should fare poorly; if having still-functioning nodes improves host defenses, the patients treated with total mastectomy alone should fare better than the others.

A total of 1665 patients were entered and observed for 72 months with no difference found among the three treatment arms in stage I. Overall, patients assigned stage II survived less well, but again there was no difference between the two treatment alternatives. Only 60

(16%) of the 365 patients who did not undergo prophylactic axillary dissection developed progression in the axilla as a first sign of failure and underwent axillary dissections, predominantly in the first 30 months of follow-up, but also as long as 112 months after surgery. In the group in which prophylactic axillary dissection was done, the incidence of positive nodes was 39%. More than half of the patients who should have had positive axillary nodes did not develop clinical evidence of such.

In 1985 Fisher and co-workers reported on this same group of 1665 women observed for a mean of 126 months. There were no significant differences between the two groups of patients who had clinically positive nodes treated by radical mastectomy or by total mastectomy without axillary dissection but with regional irradiation. Survival at 10 years was about 38% in both groups.

The morbidity associated with axillary lymphadenectomy is not inconsequential. About 10% to 15% of patients will develop lymphedema. In addition, numbness, pain, or weakness contribute to a significant decrease in the quality of life in these patients.

Sentinel Lymph Node Biopsy

Sentinel lymph node biopsy in breast cancer evolved out of efforts to minimize the morbidity associated with axillary lymph node dissection while still providing important staging information. Initial studies in melanoma carried out by Morton and colleagues in 1992 demonstrated the feasibility of the concept. Methods used include blue dye or radioisotope.

Several studies have confirmed the accuracy of SLN biopsy. In the majority of the studies, successful identification of the SLN occurs between 92% and 98% of the time. The combination of blue dye and isotope has been reported to be better for identification of the SLN; when used in combination, the positive predictive value of the technique approaches 100%, with a negative predictive value close to 95%. The false-negative rate is about 5% to 10% in most studies.

The validity of the SLN concept lies in the ability of the SLN to predict the status of the regional lymphatic basin. Turner and colleagues performed IHC staining of all lymph nodes, sentinel and nonsentinel, in a series of patients undergoing standard axillary dissection with negative nodes. Of 157 SLNs, 10 (6%) demonstrated IHC positivity compared with 1 of 1087 (0.09%) of the non-SLNs. This provided validity to the SLN concept.

Overall, greater scrutiny is paid to SLNs through serial sectioning and IHC stains. This is possible because only a few SLNs are obtained at the time of the procedure and would not be cost-effective in a standard axillary dissection that yields an average of 20 nodes.

The SLN biopsy procedure is widely used in invasive breast cancer and selectively in DCIS. In certain situations, however, a standard axillary dissection should still be considered, such as when bulky positive axillary nodes are present.

In intraductal carcinoma, an SLN biopsy or axillary dissection is generally not indicated. There are special circumstances of intraductal carcinoma, such as high-grade DCIS or extensive DCIS, in which a microinvasive component may be associated with the intraductal carcinoma. In these circumstances, and particularly if a mastectomy is being performed, an SLN biopsy may be considered.

Adjuvant Therapy

The National Comprehensive Cancer Network (NCCN) first published its comprehensive statement about the adjuvant therapy of early breast cancer in November 2000. Since that time, refinements have occurred. The most significant change in the 2005 guidelines relating to the adjuvant therapy of breast cancer was the inclusion of HER2 as a parameter for treatment selection and recommendations about trastuzumab as adjuvant therapy (Table 14-15). The use of trastuzumab was suggested for patients with HER2 3+ expression, or fluorescent in situ hybridization amplification of 2.1-fold or greater, who had tumors greater than 1 cm in size. The NCCN guidelines for chemotherapy are described in detail on the 2006 NCCN website (http://www.NCCN.org).

Multiple randomized studies have demonstrated that the addition of chemotherapy improves overall survival in patients with breast cancer. The decision to use adjuvant chemotherapy or hormonal therapy depends on certain factors, such as the size of the primary tumor, the expression or lack of expression of ER or PR, lymph node status, HER2/neu status, and the presence or absence of metastatic disease.

Adjuvant treatment in breast cancer was first used more than 100 years ago. In 1894 Beatson reported on the results of oophorectomy and response rate in the metastatic breast cancer setting. Initially, the use of systemic therapy involved the use of single-agent chemotherapy; later, multiagent chemotherapy was used. As in most breast cancer trials, the initial reports were of patients with metastatic disease.

Multiple randomized studies have demonstrated that the addition of chemotherapy improves overall survival in patients with breast cancer. The decision to use adjuvant chemotherapy or hormonal therapy depends on certain factors, such as the size of the primary tumor, lymph node status, and the presence or absence of metastatic disease. In addition, the expression or lack of expression of ER or PR (ER/PR status) is also an important factor.

Adjuvant chemotherapy is standard treatment for patients with positive nodes or large tumors. The combination of CMF (cyclophosphamide, methotrexate, and 5-fluorouracil [5-FU]) has been used for many years in the treatment of patients with breast cancer. An anthracycline-based regimen, such as FAC (5-FU, adriamycin, and cyclophosphamide) has been used in patients with high-risk factors for recurrence. The use of paclitaxel is also considered in this setting. For patients with intermediate-risk factors, such as ER-negative tumors (>1 cm in size) and negative nodes, chemotherapy is considered.

The Early Breast Cancer Trialists' Collaborative Group was formed in 1985 to analyze all available, properly conducted randomized trials. A second overview was done in 1990 and a third in 1995. In women younger than age 50, administration of multiagent chemotherapy decreased the annual risk of relapse by 35% and mortality by 27%. With 10 years of follow-up, this translates

TABLE 14-15   2005 National Comprehensive Cancer Network Guidelines Relating to Adjuvant Therapy

		ER- or PR-Positive, HER-2–Positive	ER- or PR-Positive, HER-2–Negative	ER- or PR-Positive, HER-2–Positive	ER- or PR-Positive, HER-2–Negative
NN or N1ni	T1*	No adjuvant therapy (if NN) ± E (if N1mi)			
	T1b*	No adjuvant therapy (if NN) ± E (if N1mi)		± C	± C
	T1b†	E ± C	E ± C	± C	± C
	T1c	E + C + Tr	E ± C	C + Tr	C
	T2	E + C + Tr	E ± C	C + Tr	C
NP	T	E + C + Tr	E ± C	C + Tr	C
NN OR N1MI	T1AB	ER- or PR-positive, no adjuvant therapy	ER- or PR-negative		
	T1 OR T2 11-30 MM	± E ± C	± C		
	T2 > 30 MM	E + C	C		
NP	T	E + C	C		

From 2005 National Comprehensive Cancer Network guidelines relating to adjuvant therapy of breast cancer available at http://www.adjuvantonline.com/BreastHelpV8Dec05/NCCN2005.html.

Favorable: well differentiated.

†*Unfavorable: moderately or poorly differentiated, angiolymphatic invasion, HER-2–overexpressing.*

±*, Use of this therapy optional ("consider"); C, polychemotherapy; E, endocrine therapy; ER, estrogen receptor; PR, progesterone receptor; Tr, trastuzumab.*

into absolute gains of 7% in patients with node-negative tumors and 11% in those with node-positive tumors. For women older than the age of 50 years, the benefits of chemotherapy were smaller but still significant. Annual risk reduction was 20% for recurrence and 11% for mortality. At 10 years of follow-up, this risk reduction translated into absolute gains of 2% in patients with node-negative tumors and 3% in patients with node-positive tumors. It is important to note that in the overview, different regimens of CMF were used, but the greatest benefit was seen in those using CMF for 6 months or longer.

The question of whether to use CMF or FAC in high-risk patients (tumors = 2 cm in size or ER/PR-negative with negative nodes) has been addressed. Although the anthracycline regimen is more toxic than CMF, trials have shown superiority with this regimen. Presently, other factors are used to determine which regimen to recommend in this subgroup. The most promising candidate factor is HER2/neu overexpression because increased response rates with an anthracycline-based therapy have been reported in cases where there is overexpression of HER2/neu.

Postmenopausal women with negative nodes and ER-negative tumors greater than 1 cm in size are also considered for chemotherapy.

The question of whether to use CMF or FAC in high-risk patients (tumors at least 2 cm or ER- or PR-negative with negative nodes) has been addressed. Although the anthracycline regimen is more toxic than CMF, recent trials have demonstrated its superiority. Determining whether to use FAC also is based on other factors. Tumors with HER-2/neu overexpression have an associated increased response rate with an anthracycline-based therapy.

The use of taxanes, such as docetaxel and paclitaxel as adjuvant treatment, in combination with anthracycline-based chemotherapy, is currently being investigated. Several randomized trials have been conducted to test the feasibility and effectiveness of anthracycline and/or taxanes administered in a dose-dense fashion. Dose density refers to the frequency of administration of a drug or regimen compared with standard regimens. These trials have resulted in an overall modest, beneficial impact on disease recurrence in patients with early breast cancer. The most benefit was seen in patients with node-positive disease and/or hormone receptor–negative tumors and HER2/neu overexpression. The Cancer and Leukemia Group B (CALGB) trial 9741 compared concurrent versus sequential regimens in patients with node-positive breast cancer. In the trial's 2 × 2 factorial design, the regimens consisted of concurrent four cycles of doxorubicin and cyclophosphamide, followed by four cycles of paclitaxel in Q2-week and Q3-week regimens. This was compared with sequential treatment consisting

of four cycles of doxorubicin, followed by four cycles of paclitaxel and four cycles of cyclophosphamide in Q2-week and Q3-week regimens. The dose-dense treatment (Q2 week) significantly improved disease-free survival and overall survival compared to the Q3-week regimen. There was no difference between sequential and concurrent schedules.

The use of trastuzumab (Herceptin) in addition to combination chemotherapy has also associated with a decrease in relapse in HER-2/neu-positive breast cancers. Trastuzumab is a humanized anti-HER2 antibody against the extracellular domain of the 2-neu oncoprotein. Its use in the metastatic setting has been reported to demonstrate an increase in response rate and prolongation of disease-free and overall survival.

Four major adjuvant trials, Herceptin Adjuvant (HERA), National Surgical Adjuvant Breast and Bowel Project (NSABP) B-31, North Central Cancer Treatment Group (NCCTG) N9831, and Breast Cancer International Research Group (BCIRG) 006, have investigated the use of trastuzumab in the adjuvant setting. These trials have shown that trastuzumab reduces the 3-year risk of recurrence by about 50% in this population. More than 13,000 women with HER-2/neu-positive breast cancers were enrolled and received 1 year of adjuvant treatment with trastuzumab. These trials used different chemotherapy regimens but had similar improvements in recurrence-free survival. Cardiac events were at an acceptable level; however, they did note a slightly higher incidence (0.6% to 3.3%) of congestive heart failure that was responsive to treatment. There was an overall survival benefit in the NSABP B-31 and NCCTG N9831 trials and a trend toward an overall survival benefit in the HERA and BCIRG trials.

Recently, lapatinib (Tykerb) in combination with capecitabine was approved by the FDA for treatment of patients with advanced or metastatic breast cancer whose tumors overexpress HER2 and who have received previous therapy, including an anthracycline, a taxane, and trastuzumab.

Node-Positive Breast Cancer

The Canadian consensus states that chemotherapy should be offered to all premenopausal women with stage II breast cancer. Polychemotherapy is preferred to prolonged single-agent therapy. A 6-month course of CMF or a 3-month course of AC was suggested. CMF of 6 months' duration was just as effective as four courses of AC (NSABP Protocol B-15). Other studies have shown 6 months of CMF to be as effective as 12 to 24 months of CMF. Full standard doses should be used if possible. In the Milan study of 20 years of follow-up, only those who received 85% of the planned CMF dose benefited from adjuvant chemotherapy.

The 10th St Gallen (Switzerland) expert consensus meeting in March 2007 refined and extended a target-oriented approach to adjuvant systemic therapy of early breast cancer. Target definition is inextricably intertwined with the availability of target-specific therapeutic agents. Since 2005 the presence of HER2 on the cell surface has been used as an effective target for trastuzumab much as steroid hormone receptors are targets for endocrine therapies. An expert panel reaffirmed the primary importance of determining endocrine responsiveness of the cancer as a first approach to selecting systemic therapy. Three categories were acknowledged: highly endocrine responsive, incompletely endocrine responsive, and endocrine nonresponsive. The panel accepted HER2-positivity to assign trastuzumab and noted that adjuvant trastuzumab has only been assessed together with chemotherapy. They largely endorsed previous definitions of risk categories. While recognizing the existence of several molecularly based tools for risk stratification, the panel preferred to recommend the use of high-quality, standard histopathologic assessment for both risk allocation and target identification. Chemotherapy, although largely lacking specific target information, is the only option in cases that are both endocrine receptor–negative and HER2-negative. Chemotherapy is conventionally given with or preceding trastuzumab for patients with HER2-positive disease and may be used for patients with endocrine-responsive disease in cases where the sufficiency of endocrine therapy alone is uncertain. Recommendations are provided not as specific therapy guidelines but rather as general guidance emphasizing main principles for tailoring therapeutic choice.

Estrogen Receptor-Positive Breast Cancer

ERs are proteins found in hormonally dependent tissue, both malignant and nonmalignant. The amount of receptor present in the breast cancer specimen is predictive of the success or failure of endocrine therapy. The identification of the ER protein in certain human mammary cancers, and the subsequent explanation of the role of estrogen in tumor growth, clarified a clinical relationship that had been observed for a century. In 1896 Beatson produced regression of mammary cancer by oophorectomy. Huggins and Bergenstal demonstrated in 1952 that some mammary and prostatic cancers were not autonomous but under the partial control of the endocrine system. Regressions of mammary cancers were continually obtained by removing the source of endogenous circulating hormones by oophorectomy, adrenalectomy, and hypophysectomy. Alternatively, breast cancer regressions were also achieved by administering large doses of estrogen, androgen, progesterone, and glucocorticoids.

The choice of a particular endocrine therapy has been in large part empiric, guided by certain clinical features such as menopausal status, disease-free interval, site of the dominant lesion, and response to previous therapy. As a result of basic investigations by Jensen, Smith, and DeSombre of steroid hormone metabolism, there has been development of a series of assays that can identify with considerable accuracy breast cancers that are not autonomous and that will respond to endocrine manipulation. Such a method of predicting a priori those cancers that will be responsive to changes in the endocrine milieu greatly enhances the usefulness of hormone therapy and allows recommendation of such treatments on a plausible biochemical basis.

Knowledge of the ER content of either the primary or the recurrent mammary cancer must be viewed within the proper clinical perspective. This one determination is but a single piece in the mosaic of the subcellular biochemistry of breast cancer. To deprecate the clinical importance of this determination because some patients with significant ER content will not respond to hormone treatment (because of eventual escape from hormone regulation or because of lack of understanding of the role of other steroid or protein hormone receptors) begs the question. Knowledge of the ER content of either a primary or a metastatic tumor does not allow the physician to predict the hormone dependency of a tumor with enough accuracy for it to be rationally used in the selection of appropriate palliative treatment. It does, however, allow a good assessment of the likelihood that the patient with breast cancer would benefit from endocrine therapy.

Ovarian Ablation

Ovarian suppression is one of the oldest methods for treating premenopausal metastatic breast cancer. This can be accomplished surgically, by use of luteinizing hormone–releasing hormone analogs or radiation. In 1996 the Collaborative Group published an overview of randomized trials concerning ovarian ablation in early breast cancer. There were 12 of 17 studies available for evaluation, all of which were begun before 1980. There were 2102 randomized women younger than 50 years and 1354 women aged 50 years and older. In women younger than 50 years, there were six fewer recurrences or deaths per 100 women allocated to ovarian ablation (45% vs 39% alive without recurrence) 15 years after randomization. Historically, ovarian ablation was used to treat premenopausal patients with metastatic or recurrent breast cancer. In this review, the benefit of ablation was most noticeable in patients with positive nodes. In patients with negative nodes, the overall survival at 10 years was not statistically significant between the two groups. There were only 473 women in the node-negative group. This group speaks to the possible role of prophylactic ovarian ablation.

The overview meta-analyses of 1995 showed a 25% reduction in relapse and 24% reduction in mortality over the control group. A prospective randomized European study by Soreide and colleagues showed equal efficacy when ovarian ablation was compared to tamoxifen in the 320 premenopausal node-positive patients.

Tamoxifen

Many prospective, double-blind, randomized studies have been performed to evaluate the role of adjuvant tamoxifen among women with early breast cancer. In 1998 the Collaborative Group published an update on 55 such trials of 37,000 women. In the 18,000 women with ER-positive tumors, the reduction in the recurrence rate at 1, 2, and 5 years of tamoxifen use was 21%, 28%, and 50%, respectively. These figures are all highly significant. Those women with ER-positive tumors with at least 100-fmol receptor per milligram of cytosol protein had a greater reduction in recurrence than those with positive receptors but less than 100 fmol (60% vs 43% after 5 years of tamoxifen). The reduction in mortality was also greater in those with a higher receptor level (36% vs 23%). Those patients with ER-positive, PR-negative tumors had results (reduction of recurrences and mortality) similar to those of patients with ER-positive tumors (progesterone-receptor status unknown). Among the 800 women with ER-poor tumors, the reduction in recurrence was only 10%, irrespective of length of time of tamoxifen treatment. Although this reduction is statistically significant, the apparent benefit is small and the lower confidence limit is close to zero. Irrespective of the duration of tamoxifen use, the mortality reduction was only 6%. In the 2000 women with ER-poor, PR-poor tumors, tamoxifen had no apparent effect on recurrence or mortality rates (about 1%), but in the 602 women with ER-poor, PR-positive tumors, recurrence reduction was 23% and mortality reduction was 9%. There were 12,000 women with unknown ER status. It can be estimated that about two thirds of these women would have ER-positive tumors if measured. The data suggest highly significant benefits among women with unknown ER status.

In trials of 5 years of tamoxifen use, the absolute improvement in the 10-year recurrence risk was greatest for women with node-positive disease compared with those with node-negative status. The absolute improvement was 5.6% in node-negative disease compared with 10.5% in node-positive disease. In trials of 5 years, adjuvant tamoxifen reduced recurrence, and mortality appeared equally large in the absence or presence of chemotherapy.

Although the benefit of tamoxifen appears greater in the postmenopausal women, there was a 45% reduction in those younger than 50 years. This was true for those younger than 40 years (54% reduction) and in those aged 40 to 49 years (41%). Tamoxifen also reduced the incidence of contralateral breast cancer (47%) in those who took tamoxifen for 5 years. Risk reduction was independent of age.

The studies also evaluated possible adverse effects. There was only a slight nonsignificant excess of colorectal cancers in those allocated to tamoxifen. There was a significant increase in endometrial cancer (relative risk, 21.58), and the relative risk was 4.2 with 5 years of use. This was based on only 32 endometrial cases among the control group. The normal incidence of endometrial cancer in the United States is 1 per 1000. The absolute excess of deaths from endometrial cancer during the decade after randomization was about 1 to 2 per 1000 (annual excess of about 0.2 per 1000). There was no difference in the tamoxifen group versus the control group for the aggregate of all cardiac or vascular deaths or non-breast cancer and nonendometrial cancer deaths. There was about 1 extra death per 5000 women years of tamoxifen attributed to pulmonary embolus.

It appears that up to 5 years of tamoxifen use reduces recurrence and mortality in women with ER-positive tumors, irrespective of age and menopausal status and whether the lymph nodes are positive or negative, even if cytotoxic chemotherapy has been given. There is no clear evidence of benefit in women with ER-poor tumors.

Aromatase Inhibitors

Aromatase inhibitors suppress estrogen levels by inactivating aromatase, the enzyme responsible for synthesizing estrogens from androgens. In contrast to tamoxifen, these compounds lack partial agonist activity. The Anastrozole, Tamoxifen Alone or in Combination (ATAC) trial compared 5 years of tamoxifen versus anastrozole versus the combination. Anastrozole was found to have a significantly better survival, prolonged time to recurrence, reduced distant metastases, and lower incidence of contralateral breast cancer compared with tamoxifen. Letrozole, another aromatase inhibitor, was compared to tamoxifen in the multicenter Breast International Group trial of 8028 postmenopausal women with metastatic breast cancer. Letrozole reduced significantly the risk of recurrent disease when compared with tamoxifen, especially at distant sites in these postmenopausal women. Another international study of 5187 women administered letrozole after completing 5 years of tamoxifen. The results from the data indicated a nearly 50% lower recurrence rate. As a result, letrozole is now an accepted treatment choice for those postmenopausal women with hormone receptor–positive breast cancers who have utilized tamoxifen for a 5-year period. The American Society of Clinical Oncology now recommends aromatase inhibitors be used to lower the risk of recurrence in receptor-positive postmenopausal breast cancers as initial therapy or after treatment with tamoxifen. The duration of therapy has not yet been established.

Three double-blind, randomized, prospective studies—ATAC, the Intergroup Exesmestane Study (EIS), and the MA-17 trial—have confirmed the superiority of aromatase inhibitors over tamoxifen in early-stage cancers in postmenopausal women. All three studies have demonstrated an increase in disease-free survival. Short-term side effects were acceptable, but all had a negative impact on bone health. Based on the results of these trials, patients who are postmenopausal have the option of starting on anastrozole as first-line therapy after initial diagnosis. Patients who have been on tamoxifen for 2 to 3 years can be switched to an aromatase inhibitor to complete a total of 5 years of therapy. Patients who have completed 5 years of tamoxifen have the option of no further therapy versus letrozole. The optimal duration of letrozole in this setting has not been defined.

There have been several studies of chemohormone therapy in patients with breast cancer. Many of these studies have included both node-negative and node-positive patients. In a recent Cochrane Database Systems review published in 2008, for patients who are premenopausal and ER-positive, investigation of suppression of estrogen synthesis by luteinizing hormone–releasing hormone (LHRH) agonists or ovarian ablation with either surgery or radiotherapy shows that the use of an LHRH agonist with or without tamoxifen is likely to lead to a reduction in risk of recurrence and a delay in death.

However, based on the current available evidence from multiple randomized trials, the evidence is insufficient to support LHRH agonists over chemotherapy in regard to recurrence-free survival or overall survival.

Gene Expression Assays

Two gene-expression assays, used to determine the risk of breast cancer recurrence in patients with stage I or II node-negative breast cancer, are currently available. Oncotype DX (Genomic Health Institute, Redwood City, CA) is an assay performed on RNA extracted from paraffin-embedded tumor tissue. It analyzes the expression of 21 genes: 16 cancer-related genes and 5 reference genes. The results are used to calculate a recurrence score to identify the likelihood of cancer recurrence in patients treated with tamoxifen. The results of two studies evaluating the ability of Oncotype DX to predict the risk of breast cancer recurrence suggest that patients with ER-positive, node-negative breast cancer and a low recurrence score may need only adjuvant treatment with tamoxifen, whereas intermediate- and high-risk patients may require additional treatment with adjuvant

chemotherapy. MammaPrint, an oligonucleotide microassay performed on fresh-frozen tumor samples, analyzes the expression of 70 genes. Studies have found that MammaPrint allows young patients (<61 years) with early-stage breast cancer to be categorized as having a high or low risk of distant metastasis. High-risk patients may then be managed with more aggressive therapy.

Metastatic Disease

The goal of therapy in metastatic disease is palliation of symptoms because cure is unlikely. The majority of patients with metastatic disease receive antihormonal therapy. First-line agents include tamoxifen or aromatase inhibitors such as letrozole or anastrozole. These agents offer a 20% response with ER/PR-positive tumors. Disease stabilization is the goal of therapy, and because these therapies are less toxic than chemotherapy, most patients will remain on them for prolonged periods. Upon failure of these agents, however, chemotherapy is the next step.

High-Dose Chemotherapy

Five large randomized trials have been conducted addressing the use of high-dose chemotherapy with bone-marrow or stem-cell rescue in metastatic breast cancer. Only one trial, conducted in South Africa, showed a lower rate of relapse. The other four trials showed no increase in overall survival. The investigators of the trial conducted in South Africa subsequently admitted to fraud. Thus it is felt that high-dose chemotherapy offers no survival advantage over conventional treatment approaches.

Neoadjuvant Chemotherapy

Preoperative or neoadjuvant chemotherapy is attractive because it may reduce the amount of disease present and thereby facilitate obtaining clean surgical margins when the disease is still confined to the breast. This is often the case in inflammatory breast cancer or in N2 disease in which neoadjuvant chemotherapy may improve surgical resectability. A significant response of 50% to 90% has been seen with this approach.

Downstaging of the tumor, and the axillary lymph nodes, has been reported.

Radiation Therapy

As discussed, radiation therapy is used in conjunction with lumpectomy for patients opting for breast conservation. The dose used is 1.8 to 2.0 Gy per day for a total of 45 to 50 Gy to the entire breast. A 10- to 15-Gy electron-therapy boost is often given to the lumpectomy bed.

Postmastectomy chest-wall irradiation is used with increasing frequency. Patients with large tumors (T3 lesions) and more than three positive nodes or presence of extranodal extension are offered chest-wall radiation because they are at risk for local–regional failure. Chest-wall radiation is 50 Gy over 5 weeks, with a 10-Gy boost to the mastectomy scar. Women with a high risk of local recurrence will benefit from radiation therapy postmastectomy. This finding applies to women with four or more positive nodes or advanced primary cancer. In women with one to three positive nodes, the benefits of the use of postmastectomy irradiation are uncertain and should be tested in randomized controlled trials. For patients with a chest-wall recurrence, the option of surgical debulking followed by chest-wall irradiation is used.

Radiation therapy can also be used in the palliative setting. It can be used for metastatic lesions to the bone or brain and can help to alleviate the patient's symptoms.

Breast Reconstruction

Breast reconstruction represents a major advance in cancer rehabilitation for patients undergoing a mastectomy. Previously, a 2-year surveillance period was recommended before reconstruction for detection of local disease recurrence. Immediate reconstruction has not interfered with disease detection, however, and it has the advantage of combining the two procedures into one. In addition, a greater amount of skin can be saved with planned immediate reconstruction, and the scar tissue that would be encountered with delayed procedure can be avoided.

A delayed reconstruction can be performed if the patient is ambiguous about the reconstruction or if operative risk is increased with prolonged anesthesia. It is also considered in those patients with locally advanced disease if a delay in adjuvant irradiation or chemotherapy is anticipated because of the reconstruction.

Reconstruction options include expandable breast prosthesis (implant) and autologous tissue transfer. Tissue-transfer operations may yield the greatest symmetry between breasts, especially with larger breasts; however, they take longer, require greater surgical expertise, involve a longer recovery, and result in another scar at the donor site. The donor site may be the latissimus dorsi, transverse rectus abdominus, or gluteal muscle.

SPECIAL ISSUES

Hereditary Breast Cancer

One of the most characteristic features of hereditary breast cancer is its tendency to manifest at a young age. In the Breast Cancer Consortium's study of

BRCA1-linked families that transmit BRCA1 mutations, more than 80% of breast cancers occurred in women younger than 50 years of age.

Pathologic Features

Most BRCA1-associated breast cancers have been reported to be of an infiltrating ductal type with an over-representation of poorly differentiated high-grade types. The tumors tend to be ER/PR-negative. Less than 20% of these cancers are ER/PR-positive, even when age matched with non–BRCA1-associated controls. In BRCA2 there is less of this over-representation of aggressive histology. Overall, BRCA2-associated breast cancers tend to be ER/PR-positive.

Stage

Most studies demonstrate that BRCA-associated breast cancers are seen at a stage comparable to non–BRCA-associated breast cancers. The incidence of axillary metastasis does not appear to be significantly different in patients with BRCA-associated breast cancers. In the literature, conflicting study data exist regarding the prognosis of patients with BRCA-associated breast cancer. Some studies have conferred a worse prognosis in patients with certain mutations in BRCA1. Some of these reports have been of highly selected groups of women, and thus further study is necessary in larger series of women with BRCA1 and BRCA2 mutations.

Treatment

Although some researchers have questioned the role of breast-conservation therapy in women with hereditary predisposition, there is no reason to suspect a unique survival advantage for mastectomy in these women.

Studies that have examined the outcomes of breast-conservation therapy in women with BRCA mutations are small with variable follow-up. Local ipsilateral recurrence appears to be about 15% at 5 years. Although this is higher than would be expected for patients treated with breast-conservation therapy, it is within the range observed for treatment of young women with breast cancer. It is likely to be an influence of the age at diagnosis and not because of radiation resistance.

After breast-conservation therapy, however, the breast tissue remains at risk for developing a second primary. Women with BRCA mutations may be at risk for a late ipsilateral recurrence because of the development of a second primary breast cancer.

The degree of contralateral risk needs to also be addressed with patients. Some studies have reported an estimated average risk of 2.5% to 5.0% per year in BRCA1 mutation carriers, and this risk may be higher with younger age at diagnosis. In patients with *BRCA2*, the risk appears lower, estimated at 1.8% per year. Unlike the *BRCA1*-associated risk, in *BRCA2* the age dependence is unknown.

Chemoprevention

Chemoprevention is the principle that cancer prevention can be achieved through pharmacologic intervention. It refers to the use of a medication in a healthy patient to reduce the risk of a particular cancer. It is an option for all women with significant risk for future breast cancer development. Currently, the only FDA-approved medication for prevention of breast cancer is tamoxifen. Tamoxifen is a SERM that acts as an antiestrogen in breast tissue. It has been used in the adjuvant setting in breast cancer since 1972 for both metastatic and early breast cancers. A reduction of 40% to 50% in contralateral breast cancer was seen in the adjuvant setting; thus it was thought to be an ideal agent to use in a chemopreventive setting.

The trial to determine the role of tamoxifen in chemoprevention was performed by the NSABP. In this randomized, double-blinded trial, women with a projected risk of breast cancer of greater than 1.66% over a 5-year period received either tamoxifen or a placebo for a period of 5 years. The Gail model was used to assess the risk. This multivariate logistic regression model combines risk factors to estimate the probability of recurrence of breast cancer over time. Variables included in the model are age, number of first-degree relatives with breast cancer, nulliparity or age at first live birth, number of breast biopsies, pathologic diagnosis of atypia or hyperplasia, and age at menarche; the model then predicts the risk for breast cancer in 5 years or life expectancy. Participants eligible for this study were 60 years of age or older, between the ages of 35 and 59 years with a 5-year predicted risk of breast cancer of at least 1.66%, or had a history of LCIS. A total of 368 invasive and noninvasive breast cancers occurred, of which 244 were in the placebo group and 124 in the tamoxifen group. With invasive cancer, there was a 49% reduction in the overall risk (P <0.0001), with a cumulative incidence through 69 months of 43.4 per 1000 women and 22.0 per 1000 women in each of the two groups, respectively. For the noninvasive breast cancer, reduction was 50% (P <0.002). Reduction in noninvasive cancers was related to a decrease in the incidence of both DCIS and LCIS. Tamoxifen reduced the recurrence of ER-positive tumors by 69%, but there was no difference in recurrence of ER-negative tumors. There was, however, no survival difference between the two groups, with only nine deaths attributed to breast cancer, six in the placebo group and three in the tamoxifen group.

Additionally, there was a 2.5-fold greater risk for development of endometrial cancer in the tamoxifen group compared with patients receiving placebo. There appeared to be no difference in ischemic heart disease or fatal myocardial infarction in the tamoxifen group versus the control group. Vascular events, including stroke, venous thrombosis, and pulmonary embolism, were greater in the tamoxifen-treated patients compared with those receiving placebo (91 vs 52). There was a reduction in the risk of fracture of the hip, radius, and spine in the tamoxifen group compared with the placebo group, although the reduction was not statistically significant.

When an independent reviewing agency verified a 50% reduction in both invasive and noninvasive breast cancer cases in the population taking tamoxifen, the trial results were unblinded earlier than expected. Shortly thereafter, the use of tamoxifen was approved for chemoprevention. In patients who are desirous of tamoxifen for risk reduction, a discussion of the risks and benefits is important.

Two other chemoprevention trials using tamoxifen have been reported: the Italian tamoxifen-prevention study and the Royal Marsden Hospital tamoxifen trial in the United Kingdom. These two trials did not reveal a statistically significant reduction in breast cancer risk in women randomly assigned to tamoxifen. However, the studies differed in respect to subject numbers, median age, eligibility criteria, risk, and use of HRT.

Another SERM, raloxifene, is approved by the FDA for use in osteoporosis. In studies in which raloxifene was used for the treatment of osteoporosis, a secondary finding was a noted reduction in breast cancer risk of 50% to 70% in the population taking the medication. The women in the trials were at fairly low risk of breast cancer development. Results from the randomized double-blind trial to compare raloxifene with tamoxifen in a population of postmenopausal women at increased risk for breast cancer development, the study of tamoxifen and raloxifene (STAR) trial/P-2 study, were recently reported.

The STAR trial randomized 19,747 postmenopausal women with an increased 5-year Gail risk to receive either tamoxifen or raloxifene. There were 163 and 168 invasive breast cancers in each group, respectively. The conclusion was that they were equivalent in reducing risks of breast cancer in postmenopausal women at high risk. Raloxifene had a better side-effect profile, with fewer uterine cancers and thromboembolic events compared with tamoxifen. The risk reduction is thought to be about 50%, which is extrapolated from the P-1 study of tamoxifen and placebo. There was no placebo arm in this study; the conclusions were based on raloxifene having the same risk reduction as tamoxifen in the STAR trial.

In the NASBP P-1 study there was an increased risk of developing endometrial cancer with tamoxifen use (annual risk, 2.3/1000 women vs 0.9/1000 women in the placebo group). All cases of endometrial cancer in the patients taking tamoxifen were early stage. Another important side effect noted was a higher incidence of thromboembolic phenomena. Raloxifene does not increase the risk of endometrial cancer and thus may prove to be an adequate alternative to tamoxifen in a chemopreventive role. An ideal SERM would have anti-estrogenic effects on breast and uterine tissues but estrogenic effects on bone and the cardiovascular system among others. Current investigations into other SERMs are being conducted.

Surveillance versus Prophylactic Surgery in High-Risk Patients

Patients with a genetic predisposition to breast cancer often ask about risk reduction. Many of these patients are young women. The diverse issues related to prophylactic mastectomy include both physical and psychologic factors. Appropriate counseling is very important because these women often experience regret after the procedure. Prophylactic mastectomy has been reported to have a risk reduction of approximately 90% in larger studies. However, this reduction often relates to the type of mastectomy performed (e.g., subcutaneous mastectomy may not remove all breast tissue).

Women with a genetic predisposition to breast cancer are also candidates for chemoprevention with tamoxifen or, if they are postmenopausal, for consideration for the STAR trial. In the NSABP P-1 trial, women who had *BRCA* mutations were not protected by tamoxifen. However, because the number of such patients was small and confidence intervals were wide, more data are needed. In addition, it is likely that chemoprevention may have no significant impact in *BRCA1,* where the tumors are predominantly ER negative. The data are still inconclusive regarding *BRCA*-predisposition genes and the use of tamoxifen for chemoprevention.

Participation in a screening program is another option. Many women considering prophylactic mastectomy are young and have dense breasts on mammography. The use of bilateral breast MRI is recommended for these women.

These women are also at risk for developing ovarian cancer, and prophylactic oophorectomy at approximately age 40 years is an option. In addition, prophylactic oophorectomy before the age of 40 has been reported to decrease the risk of breast cancer significantly. But even prophylactic risk-reducing salpingo-oophorectomy does not exclude the risk of primary peritoneal cancer, which is estimated at 2%. Ovarian cancer screening programs currently use serum CA-125 and pelvic ultrasonography. Ovarian screening is not recommended for the general population, however, because of the low specificity of the tools currently available.

CONCLUSIONS

Screening for breast cancer is clearly indicated for all women at the appropriate age. Determining a woman's unique risk factors will help to determine both the age at which that screening should begin and the intensity of that screening. It will also help to identify those women who need to be counseled regarding options for prevention of breast cancer. The hope is that by correctly identifying high-risk populations and then applying appropriate screening schedules and chemopreventive agents, many cases of breast cancers will be averted completely and that those that still occur will be found at the earliest stages. The role of the obstetrician and gynecologist in providing information on breast cancer diagnosis and screening is very important. In addition, the understanding of breast disease, both benign and malignant, is crucial not only in the diagnosis of disease, but also in helping to guide women in their treatment and follow-up.

For full reference list, log onto www.expertconsult.com ⟨http://www.expertconsult.com⟩.

Cancer in Pregnancy

Krishnansu S. Tewari, MD

BACKGROUND AND EPIDEMIOLOGY OF CANCER IN PREGNANCY

Cancer in pregnancy poses significant challenges to both the clinician and the mother. This is undoubtedly the result of the trend to defer childbearing into the fourth decade of life, when the incidence of some of the more common malignant neoplasms begins to rise (Figure 15-1). The tragedy of the presence of a malignant neoplasm discovered during pregnancy raises many issues (Table 15-1). Fortunately, the peak incidence years for most malignant diseases do not overlap the peak reproductive years (Table 15-2). Thus, as in any unusual situation that physicians rarely encounter, clear therapeutic decisions are not readily at hand. However, a significant number of well-studied reviews can provide some guidance in this dilemma. The largest series ever reported was that of Barber and Brunschwig in 1968, which consisted of 700 cases of cancer in pregnancy. The most common malignant neoplasms in that series were breast tumors and leukemias–lymphomas as a category, melanomas, gynecologic cancer, and bone tumors, in that order. Other authors suggest that gynecologic malignant neoplasms are second only to breast carcinoma and remind us that cancer of the colon and thyroid are also seen in pregnancy (Table 15-3).

The incidence of cancer in pregnancy is unclear but is estimated to be one in 1000. From historical case series collected at a variety of referral institutions, many commentators have concluded that cervical cancer is the most frequent malignancy to complicate pregnancy. This finding is likely to be inaccurate because the incidence of cervical cancer in the United States and in most developed nations is steadily declining. In a 1984 population-based study, Haas reviewed the National Cancer Registry of the German Democratic Republic for the years between 1970 and 1979, and from a total of 31,353 cancer cases and 2,103,112 live births among women between the ages of 15 and 44 years, 355 pregnant women were diagnosed with a malignancy. Dinh and Warshal emphasized that in the Haas study, the incidence of cancer in pregnancy per 1000 live births rose from 0.02 for women aged 15 to 19 years to 2.3 for women aged 40 to 44 years. In order of decreasing frequency, cancer of the cervix, breast, ovary, lymphoma, melanoma, brain, and leukemia were found to complicate pregnancy.

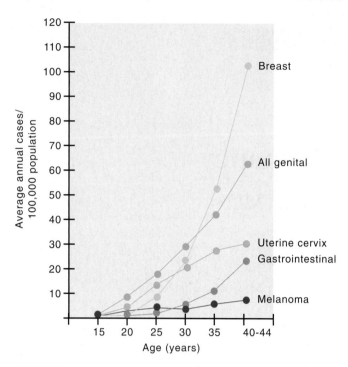

FIGURE 15-1 Incidence by age of more common malignancies seen in pregnancy. *(Data from the American Cancer Society Facts and Figures, 1995.)*

TABLE 15-1 Cancer in Pregnancy: Issues to Consider

Oncologic Issues	Obstetric Issues	Ethical, Religious, Medicolegal, and Socioeconomic Issues
Timing of surgery	Fetal effects of therapy	Pregnancy termination
Type of therapy	Antepartum fetal surveillance	Independent advocate for the fetus
Maternal effects of therapy	Corticosteroid administration	Fetal viability
Maternal surveillance	Amniocentesis	Maternal risk
Fertility-sparing therapy	Timing of delivery	Healthcare costs
	Route of delivery	Principle of beneficence
	Neonatal effects of therapy	Right to autonomy
	Long-term effects of therapy	Mother's overall prognosis*

Important to take into account the estimated length of time the mother will realistically live to spend with the baby.

TABLE 15-2 Probability of Developing Invasive Cancers (%) Over Selected Age Intervals in Females, United States, 2003-2005

	Birth-39 Years	40-59 Years
All sites	2.07 (1 in 48)	8.97 (1 in 11)
Breast	0.48 (1 in 208)	3.79 (1 in 26)
Melanoma	0.27 (1 in 370)	0.58 (1 in 189)
Uterine cervix	0.15 (1 in 651)	0.27 (1 in 368)
Leukemia	0.12 (1 in 835)	0.14 (1 in 693)
Non-Hodgkin lymphoma	0.08 (1 in 1191)	0.32 (1 in 316)
Colon and rectum	0.07 (1 in 1343)	0.72 (1 in 138)
Uterine corpus	0.07 (1 in 1499)	0.72 (1 in 140)
Lung and bronchus	0.03 (1 in 2997)	0.81 (1 in 124)
Urinary bladder	0.01 (1 in 10,185)	0.12 (1 in 810)

Modified from The American Cancer Society, Surveillance and Health Policy Research, 2009.

TABLE 15-3 Distribution of Tumor Types Among 215 Women Diagnosed with Cancer in Pregnancy from 1998 to 2008 in Belgium, the Netherlands, and the Czech Republic

	No.	Percent
Breast cancer	99	46
Hematologic malignancies	40	18
Dermatologic malignancies	21	10
Cervical cancer	17	8
Brain tumor	8	4
Ovarian cancer	8	4
Colorectal cancer	5	2
Other (sarcoma, lung, liver, kidney, GI, etc.)	17	8

Modified from van Calsteren et al: J Clin Oncol 2010;28:683.

Data from the Surveillance, Epidemiology, and End Results (SEER) program in the United States from 1992 to 1996 estimate that among women aged 15 to 44 years, in order of decreasing frequency, cancer of the breast, melanoma, thyroid, cervix, lymphoma, and ovary are coincident with pregnancy. The Centers for Disease Control and Prevention have highlighted pregnancy trends in the United States over the preceding 25 years. Although the birth rate for women younger than 30 years of age rose slowly until the early 1990s, it has steadily declined since then. In contrast, the birth rate for women older than 30 years of age has risen steadily over the past two decades by an average of 67%. Because of the changing attitudes regarding the role of women as part of the workforce, the delay in childbearing observed in this country will be associated with at least three considerations that are germane to the subject of this chapter.

1. As many malignancies manifest with advancing age, it is reasonable to expect an increase in the occurrence of some specific types of cancers during pregnancy.
2. Theoretic concerns regarding possible effects of pregnancy-derived hormones among cancer survivors contemplating pregnancy will need to be addressed.
3. With the popularization of investigational fertility-sparing medical and surgical therapy for nulliparous patients with seemingly early lesions who strongly desire to retain childbearing capacity, there exists an increased potential for

the oncologist to encounter recurrent disease irrespective of whether pregnancy occurs.

The enormous physiologic changes of pregnancy suggest many possible influences on the malignant state. First, it has been assumed by many that malignant neoplasms arising in tissues and organs influenced by the endocrine system are possibly subject to exacerbation with pregnancy, and this has often been erroneously extrapolated to a recommendation for "therapeutic" abortion. Second, the anatomic and physiologic changes of pregnancy may obscure the subtle changes of an early neoplasm. Third, the increased vascularity and lymphatic drainage may contribute to early dissemination of the malignant process. Although all these hypotheses are interesting, the validity of each is variable, even within the same organ.

Several additional points must be emphasized when caring for the pregnant patient with symptoms suggestive of cancer or in whom the diagnosis has been established. Although pregnancy is usually characterized by extensive medical observation, a delay in diagnosis can occur if attention is not paid to the subtle presentation of malignancies. Thus, although pregnancy has not been shown to increase the virulence of any tumor type, many pregnancy-associated cancers portend a poor prognosis for the mother. Even though many essayists have claimed that the conduct of the pregnancy is not affected by the cohabitation of malignancy, the oncologist must recognize that some tumor types have been shown to metastasize to the placenta and even to the fetus. In all cases of pregnancy complicated by malignancy, it is advisable to have a multidisciplinary team of specialists involved in the care of the patient.

When considering therapy in pregnancy, surgery is rarely contraindicated, with the optimal time being in the second trimester. Chemotherapy for the most part should have restricted use during the first trimester but can generally be safely administered thereafter. Certain diagnostic imaging procedures can be safely performed during pregnancy, but in most cases radiation therapy should be postponed until after delivery. Aggressive nutritional support is a mandatory requirement for the pregnant mother afflicted with cancer. In the majority of cases, with a proper coordination of effort, the pregnancy need not be terminated in order to begin treatment.

THE MORE COMMON SOLID TUMORS IN PREGNANCY

Cervical Cancer

Cervical cancer complicates approximately 1 in 1200 pregnancies. As a consequence of widespread cytologic screening, the dramatic decrease in invasive cervical cancer observed in recent years has been paralleled by a rise in cervical intraepithelial neoplasia (CIN), especially in younger women. Because the peak incidence for both CIN and childbearing occurs during the third decade in life, abnormal Papanicolaou smears are common among gravid women, occurring at a rate of 0.5% to 5%. The diagnosis of cervical dysplasia in pregnancy may occur in up to 5% of some populations. For these reasons, screening for cervical neoplasia is an essential component of prenatal care. All pregnant women should have a cervical smear submitted for cytology. The ectocervix and endocervical canal should be sampled adequately. Patients noted to have a visible lesion should undergo cervical biopsy straight away because cervical smears taken directly from tumors often contain only inflammatory cells. A recent review from the Magee Gynecologic Cancer Program in Pittsburgh noted that in some populations up to 20% of pregnant women have an abnormal Pap result during pregnancy. Nearly 3% of newly diagnosed cervical cancer cases occur in pregnant women, probably because it is the one cancer that is screened for as part of routine prenatal care.

In concordance with the known risk factors for invasive cervical cancer, pregnant women who develop CIN tend to marry at an earlier age, have a higher parity, and are diagnosed at an earlier age than nonpregnant women with CIN. Hacker and colleagues compiled data from nine reports and noted that the average age of patients with carcinoma in situ (CIS) during pregnancy was 29.9 years, and the average parity was 4.0. Among nonpregnant women, the average age of CIS is 35 years. The investigators noted that the median age of patients diagnosed with invasive carcinoma of the cervix during pregnancy is 33.8 years (range 17-47 years) and the average parity is 4.5. The average parity among pregnant women with cervical cancer was 5.4 in a study reported by Creasman and colleagues; in this group, increasing parity was not associated with a more advanced lesion, nor did it have an impact on prognosis.

Human Papillomavirus in Pregnancy

Although the human papillomavirus (HPV) is strongly associated with cervical dysplasia and carcinoma in both nonpregnant and pregnant women, a significant relationship between pregnancy and HPV prevalence has not been established. Eversion of the endocervical epithelium results in exposure to the acidity of the vaginal environment, producing a high degree of squamous metaplasia. This metaplasia is important because HPV requires active cellular machinery to reproduce and transform cells. Schneider and colleagues examined the negative cervical smears of 92 pregnant and 96 nonpregnant, age-matched control subjects for the presence of HPV DNA by Southern blot hybridization. The investigators demonstrated both an increased prevalence of HPV (preferentially the oncolytic HPV subtype 16) and a higher replication rate of viral DNA during pregnancy. Using the ViraPap/ViraType dot blot DNA hybridization procedure, Smith and co-workers detected an increase in HPV prevalence with advancing gestational age, suggesting that as estrogen levels rise, pregnant women may be more vulnerable to HPV infection. Using similar hybridization methods, however, Kemp and colleagues and Chang-Claude and colleagues were unable to demonstrate a higher prevalence of HPV infection during pregnancy.

Castellsague and colleagues performed a prospective study in Barcelona to quantitate the mother-to-child transmission of HPV subtypes. This study included 66 HPV-positive and 77 HPV-negative pregnant women and their offspring. To estimate HPV prevalence and genotypic distribution in pregnancy the investigators also carried out a related screening survey of cervical HPV-DNA detection among 828 pregnant women. Exfoliated cells from the mouth and external genitalia of the infants were collected at birth and at several intervals up to 2 years of age. At 418 infant visits and a mean follow-up time of 14 months, 19.7% of infants born to HPV-positive mothers and 16.9% of those born to HPV-negative mothers tested HPV positive at some point during the infants' follow-up. The most frequently detected genotype both in infants and in mothers was HPV-16. Of note, there was a strong and statistically significant association between mother's and child's HPV status at the 6-week postpartum visit in that children of mothers who were HPV positive at the postpartum visit were five times more likely to test HPV positive than children of corresponding HPV-negative mothers ($P = 0.02$). The authors concluded that the risk of vertical transmission of HPV genotypes is relatively low and that vertical transmission may not be the sole source of HPV infections in infants. There exists the potential for horizontal mother-to-child transmission.

Evaluation of the Papanicolaou Smear in Pregnancy

The cytopathologist frequently encounters atypical cells when reviewing the cervical smear from a pregnant patient. Cells within the endocervical canal that undergo the Arias–Stella reaction may contain a vacuolated clear or oxyphilic cytoplasm, intraglandular tufts, hobnail patterns, delicate filiform papillae, intranuclear pseudoinclusions, cribriform intraglandular growth, and even occasional mitotic figures. Distinguishing features of dysplastic and frankly malignant cells would include an infiltrative pattern, spectrum of cytologic atypia, a high nuclear-to-cytoplasmic ratio, and increased mitotic activity. Other atypical cells exfoliated by the endocervix in pregnant women include small decidualized cells

with sharp cytoplasmic borders and hypochromatic nuclei, but unlike dysplastic cells, decidualized cells contain regular chromatin and distinct nuclei. Finally, large, multinucleated trophoblastic cells may be discharged from the uterus. At this time, it is not clear if liquid-based cytology can decrease the false-positive rate. Nevertheless, careful inspection of the cervical smear maintains its reliability as a screening test for dysplasia among pregnant patients.

The Performance of Colposcopy in Pregnancy

Colposcopy is facilitated by the pregnancy-induced eversion of the normal cervical ectropion. However, pregnancy results in dramatic alterations in the colposcopic appearance of the cervix, the most significant changes resulting from the elevated levels of circulating estrogen, which produces a significant increase in cervical volume through hypertrophy of the fibromuscular stroma. The increased vascularity produces a bluish hue, which is then exaggerated with application of acetic acid to the metaplastic epithelium in pregnancy. Toward the end of the first trimester, eversion and metaplasia produce areas of fusion of columnar villa and distinct islands or fingers of immature metaplastic epithelium. Fine punctation and even mosaicism may accompany metaplasia, which in and of itself produces an acetowhite effect. Tenacious endocervical mucus develops, which further hinders colposcopic examination. Finally, stromal edema, enlargement of glandular structures, acute inflammatory responses, and stromal decidualization may occur in the second and third trimesters, which, although physiologic, may appear suspicious to the inexperienced colposcopist. For these reasons, colposcopy in pregnancy is difficult and should be reserved for an experienced gynecologist.

The aim of colposcopy in pregnancy is to exclude cancer, and only one directed biopsy of the site compatible with the most advanced area of dysplastic change should be performed to establish the histologic level of disease. Because of false-negative results ranging from 8% to 40%, random or nondirected biopsies should be avoided. Great care must be exercised because the increased vascularity may lead to precipitous, heavy bleeding. A Tischler or baby Tischler biopsy forceps should be used, followed by immediate placement of a cotton-tipped applicator above the cervical epithelium. If bleeding occurs, it may be controlled with three silver nitrate sticks or with dehydrated Monsel's solution. An endocervical curettage, however, is best avoided during pregnancy.

Yoonessi and colleagues conducted a retrospective analysis of suspected CIN associated with pregnancy and concluded that colposcopic examination with or without directed biopsy eliminated the need for cervical conization in 104 of 107 patients. In their classic paper,

Hacker and colleagues noted that serious morbidity, such as hemorrhage, preterm labor, miscarriage, or infection, only infrequently occurs when directed biopsies are performed. For 1064 reported colposcopic examinations during pregnancy, the diagnostic accuracy was 99.5% and the complication rate was 0.6%. No case of frankly invasive carcinoma was missed, and the two cases of microinvasion missed on colposcopic biopsy both had a colposcopic pattern suggestive of microinvasion, which was confirmed by subsequent conization. Thus, in experienced hands, colposcopy reduces the need for cone biopsy in pregnancy, with a false-negative rate of less than 0.5%.

Recently, Wetta and colleagues presented the University of Alabama experience on 625 pregnant women with CIN. The most common referral cytology was low-grade squamous intraepithelial lesions (LSIL; 41%) followed by atypical squamous cells of undetermined significance (ASC-US; 34.1%) and high-grade squamous intraepithelial lesions (HSIL; 13.6%). Of the 269 patients with ASC-US and LSIL cytology, 20 of 78 patients who underwent cervical biopsy were diagnosed with CIN II-III. Of the 128 patients with HSIL, 31 of 60 patients who underwent cervical biopsy were diagnosed with CIN II-III. Repeat colposcopy in the third trimester was performed on 47 patients and only 3 of 13 patients who had a repeat biopsy had CIN II-III. The authors concluded that pregnant patients with ASC-US or LSIL cytology rarely have colposcopically suspected CIN II-III at their initial colposcopy that warrants a cervical biopsy. The investigators consider it reasonable to defer the initial colposcopy in these cases until at least 6 weeks postpartum.

Onuma and colleagues have evaluated the diagnosis of ASC-H (atypical squamous cells, with possible HSIL) in 60 patients. Among 30 who had histologic follow-up, 3 women (10%) had HSIL and 13 (43%) had LSIL. Among 32 women who had cytologic follow-up, 2 (6%) had HSIL, 3 (9%) had LSIL, 1 (3%) had ASC-H, and 3 (9%) had ASC-US. High-risk HPV DNA was detected in 24 of 43 patients (56%). The authors suggest that ASC-H in pregnant women has a lower predictive value for an underlying HSIL compared with the general population. Although a positive high-risk HPV DNA test result was not a good indicator for underlying SIL, a negative result appeared useful for ruling out an underlying HSIL. The authors advocated for a more conservative follow-up for pregnant women with ASC-H and support using high-risk HPV DNA testing as an adjunctive test.

The Natural History of Cervical Intraepithelial Neoplasia in Pregnancy

It appears that in the immunocompetent host evaluated colposcopically and pathologically by experienced eyes, CIN rarely, if ever, progresses to microinvasive disease during pregnancy. In fact, there appears to be a subset of patients who will experience disease regression following delivery of the neonate. Postpartum regression rates for abnormal cervical cytology consistent with dysplasia (combining both low- and high-grade squamous intraepithelial lesions) have ranged from 25% to 77%. This wide range is hard to explain, with some authors postulating that regression occurs in at least one third of patients as a consequence of resolution of pregnancy-induced changes in the maternal immunologic system. An Italian study published in 2008 detailed the natural history of CIN in 78 pregnant women. Among those with CIN II-III ($n = 36$, 46.2%), no invasion was suspected during pregnancy, and at the postpartum evaluation, no invasive or microinvasive cancer was diagnosed. Of note, there were 19 (52.7%) cases of persistent CIN II-III and 42 (53.8%) regressions. The authors noted that CIN I has a significantly higher tendency to spontaneous regression in comparison to nonpregnant women with CIN I. High-risk HPV testing may improve the follow-up of patients with SIL in pregnancy and postpartum to assist in the diagnosis of persistent infections.

Some authors have advanced the theory that vaginal birth trauma may result in the complete debridement of dysplastic tissues. This phenomenon was observed by Ahdoot and colleagues in a prospective collection of abnormal cytology during pregnancy and in the postpartum period. The investigators observed a 60% regression rate among women with HSILs who delivered vaginally versus 0% in those with HSILs who delivered by cesarean section ($P < 0.0002$). A study by Siristatidis and colleagues demonstrated a 66.6% regression rate among women with HSILs who delivered vaginally versus 12.5% of those with HSILs who delivered by cesarean section ($P < 0.002$). In direct contradistinction, the cytologic study by Murta and colleagues (LSILs in pregnancy) and the pregnancy-related histologic investigations by Murta and colleagues (CIN II/III), Yost and colleagues (CIN II/III), and Coppola and colleagues (CIS) failed to show any statistically significant difference in postpartum regression rates for those patients who delivered vaginally versus those who labored and went on to deliver by cesarean section versus those who underwent elective cesarean delivery.

A recent report by Ueda and colleagues describes the experience with CIN in pregnancy at Osaka University Hospital. The investigators observed regression of CIN in 34 (76%) of 45 cases of vaginal delivery and in 6 (50%) of 12 cases of cesarean delivery, indicating that the outcome of an initially diagnosed CIN and the delivery routes appear not to be significantly related. However, a different result was obtained when only those patients whose CIN lesions persisted until the delivery were analyzed. Among the 35 such cases in the vaginal delivery group, 24 cases (69%) regressed following the delivery; in 8 such cases from the cesarean delivery group, only

2 cases (25%) regressed following delivery. There was also significantly more frequent postpartum regression of biopsy-proven CIN lesions following vaginal delivery compared to cesarean section ($P = 0.042$; OR 6.55; 95% CI, 1.13-37.8).

Conization and Related Procedures in Pregnancy

The performance of a cone biopsy during pregnancy is a formidable undertaking, and one must weigh the risks of the procedure against the anticipated yield of micro-invasive carcinoma, which would remain otherwise undetected. Maternal risk appears to be restricted to either immediate or delayed hemorrhage, occurring in up to 14% of cases and exceeding 400 mL when the procedure is performed during the third trimester. Averette and colleagues reported the largest series of cold knife cervical conization biopsies in pregnancy and noted that 9.4% of the study group ($n = 180$) required a blood transfusion. Maternal death has not been reported. Injury to the pregnancy resulting in spontaneous abortion, intrauterine infection, and preterm birth, however, places the fetus at considerable risk. Rogers and Williams presented a series of 72 pregnancy conizations and reported a perinatal complication rate of 19.4%. Across the literature, the risk of pregnancy loss when the procedure is performed during the first trimester ranges from 15.2% to 33%. Overall, cone biopsy in pregnancy is associated with a 3% to 6% risk of perinatal death as a consequence of profuse hemorrhage or from delivery of a previable or extremely premature fetus through an incompetent cervix. A further point that needs emphasizing is that 30% to 57% of pregnant cones will have dysplasia and/or microinvasive tumor at the endocervical or ectocervical margins. For this reason, the procedure should not be considered therapeutic in the pregnant patient.

The large-loop electrosurgical excision of the transformation zone (LLETZ) may be used in the operating room to excise a shallow cone of sufficient breadth and depth to permit treatment decisions during pregnancy. Robinson and colleagues reported on 20 women who underwent LLETZ from 8 to 34 weeks of gestational age and noted significant morbidity in patients treated between 27 and 34 weeks of gestational age, including two blood transfusions, three preterm births, and one unexplained intrauterine fetal demise 4 weeks postprocedure. Mitsuhashi and Sekiya performed a LLETZ on 9 women during the first 14 weeks of pregnancy, none of whom experienced spontaneous abortion, premature delivery, or excessive bleeding. These preliminary results would suggest that LLETZ can be performed safely during the first trimester of pregnancy, but there are insufficient data to determine whether this procedure can replace the traditional cold knife cone biopsy. LLETZ is also associated with a significant proportion of patients left with residual disease.

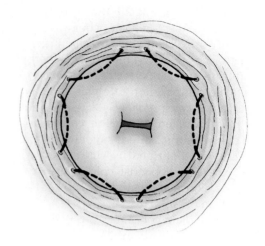

FIGURE 15-2   The location of six hemostatic sutures is shown. *(From Creasy RK, Resnick R: Maternal–Fetal Medicine: Principles and Practice. Philadelphia, Saunders, 1987.)*

Hacker and colleagues commented that most authors reserve conization for patients in whom the transformation zone was not fully visualized, microinvasion was shown on biopsy or suspected colposcopically, or possible adenocarcinoma was found on biopsy. If colposcopy is unsatisfactory, one alternative to a full cone is a wedge resection of the cervix, removing only areas incompletely visualized colposcopically. Another option is to place six hemostatic sutures, evenly distributed around the perimeter of the cervix close to the vaginal reflection (Figure 15-2). These sutures reduce blood flow to the cone bed, evert the squamocolumnar junction, and facilitate performance of a shallow "coin" biopsy with little interruption of the endocervical canal (Figure 15-3).

To offset the risk of cervical incompetence, Goldberg and colleagues performed 17 cone cerclages between 12 and 27 weeks of gestation. All procedures were performed with the patient under general anesthesia. Following injection of the entire ectocervix with vasopressin (20 units in 60 mL of normal saline), lateral hemostatic 2-0 polyglycolic acid sutures were placed at the 10 o'clock and 2 o'clock positions on the cervix, and a standard McDonald cerclage using no. 1 nylon suture material was inserted as high and as close to the internal cervical os as technically possible without reflection of the bladder. Once the cervical cone was excised, the McDonald suture was tied with the knot placed anteriorly and an iodoform vaginal pack inserted for 24 hours. All 17 patients had uneventful pregnancies, delivering viable infants at or beyond 34 weeks of gestation.

Tsuritani and colleagues have reported on the safety and efficacy of CO_2 laser conization in pregnant women with CIN III/CIS ($n = 30$) and microinvasive carcinoma

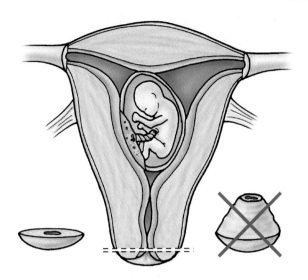

FIGURE 15-3 Demonstration of shallow "coin" biopsy appropriate in pregnancy. *(From Creasy RK, Resnick R: Maternal–Fetal Medicine: Principles and Practice. Philadelphia, Saunders, 1987.)*

(MIC, $n = 19$). The median gestational age was 17 weeks and the median length of cervix resected was 14 mm. Median duration of surgery was 20 minutes and median blood loss was 78 mL. Laser conization identified one case of International Federation of Gynecology and Obstetrics (FIGO) Ia2 carcinoma and three cases of FIGO IB1 disease. Of the 35 women who were able to be followed through until delivery, 27 (77.1%) delivered vaginally. Although 8 (22.9%) had a cesarean section and 6 (17.1%) delivered preterm, no CO_2 conization–related obstetric complications were observed.

Fambrini and colleagues have performed CO_2 laser conization in 26 pregnant patients with biopsy-proven CIS/CIN III whose colposcopic evaluation was suspicious for invasion. The procedures were performed during the 18th week of gestation and no major intraoperative or postoperative complications occurred. Two cases of occult FIGO stage IA1 carcinoma with free surgical margins were diagnosed. Twenty patients (76.9%) delivered vaginally, whereas six patients underwent cesarean section for indications not related to the prior conization. After a mean postpartum follow-up of 18 months, 92.3% of patients were cytologically and colposcopically negative for persistent or recurrent disease. Two cases of persistent CIN were managed successfully by reconization.

Management of Cervical Intraepithelial Neoplasia in Pregnancy

An algorithm that illustrates several key points concerning the management of CIN in pregnancy is proposed in Figure 15-4. The critical issue is to exclude the coexistence of microinvasive disease with pregnancy. This is because everything else, the gamut between cellular atypia and CIS, can be followed expectantly during pregnancy, with treatment deferred following its conclusion. We emphasize the following steps:

- Step 1. All abnormal cervical smears in pregnancy (excluding HPV-negative atypia) should prompt an evaluation by colposcopy.
- Step 2. An experienced colposcopist must accurately assess the disease in order to determine whether a directed biopsy is indicated.
- Step 3. In cases involving a CIS on directed biopsy, a coordinated effort between the gynecologist and the pathologist should be undertaken to determine whether an excisional biopsy is required to exclude invasion.

Management of Squamous Cell Abnormalities

In 2006 the American Society for Colposcopy and Cervical Pathology (ASCCP) updated their recommendations for cervical cancer screening in pregnancy and management of CIN and AIS in pregnancy. Highlights of these recommendations (which were published in 2007) include the following:

For squamous cell abnormalities:

- Expectant management during pregnancy is acceptable for CIN I-III and CIS.
- In patients for whom there is no concern for microinvasion, serial colposcopy during pregnancy (e.g., every trimester) is not necessary.
- Definitive management of CIN/CIS should be deferred to the postpartum period in most cases.

Pregnant women with normal prenatal cytologic screening traditionally undergo repeat screening during the postpartum period. Patients with a prenatal Papanicolaou test consistent with ASC-US may undergo reflex testing for oncolytic HPV subtypes if the Hybrid Capture II test (Digene Corporation) is available. Patients who test HPV negative may be re-evaluated with cervical cytology 6 to 8 weeks after delivery. Pregnant women who are found to have cytology consistent with ASC-US and are high-risk HPV positive should be referred for colposcopic evaluation. Patients with cytology consistent with atypical squamous cells favoring a high-grade lesion, LSILs, HSILs, and squamous cell carcinoma (and all Papanicolaou tests suggesting glandular cell abnormalities) should be referred for colposcopic evaluation. Because of the high prevalence of HPV in cytologic smears consistent with intraepithelial lesions and carcinoma, HPV testing is not indicated.

If the colposcopic impression is normal or consistent with CIN I, the Papanicolaou test with or without

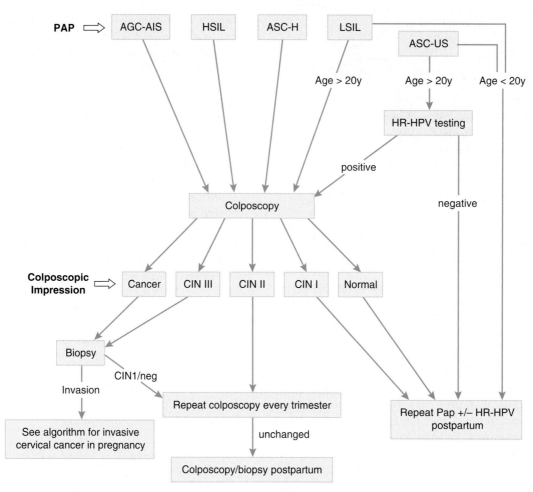

FIGURE 15-4   Management of abnormal cytologic findings in pregnancy. *CIN*, Cervical intraepithelial neoplasia; *ECC*, endocervical curettage; *Pap*, Papanicolaou smear.

colposcopy can be repeated in the postpartum period provided that the original Papanicolaou test was not consistent with a high-grade lesion; if colposcopy was performed because of HSILs or squamous cell carcinoma, the colposcopic evaluation should be repeated each trimester of the pregnancy, with a directed punch biopsy taken if the impression is consistent with progressive disease (above CIN II).

Patients for whom colposcopy is consistent with CIN II or greater should undergo a single directed biopsy. If this reveals CIN III or worse, the patient should undergo repeat colposcopic evaluation each trimester, with definitive treatment reserved for after delivery, provided there is no evidence for disease progression.

Patients whose biopsies are suspicious for microinvasion should undergo one of the excisional procedures described previously (i.e., conization or LLETZ with or without cerclage, coin biopsy, or wedge biopsy). If microinvasion is excluded, the patient should be observed during the pregnancy with colposcopy. If microinvasion is established either by directed punch

biopsy or by excisional biopsy, recommendations specific for malignant disease must be sought (see later).

In some circumstances, the colposcopic evaluation will be unsatisfactory, in that the entire transformation zone cannot be completely evaluated. If there is no evidence of a severe lesion in the evaluable areas, and the original Papanicolaou test was not consistent with squamous cell carcinoma or adenocarcinoma in situ (AIS), close observation with repeat colposcopy during each trimester of the pregnancy may be considered. Under more dire scenarios, a coin biopsy of the cervix or a wedge biopsy of the hidden part of the transformation zone may be necessary.

Management of Glandular Cell Abnormalities

Cervical smears containing glandular cell abnormalities may be reported as atypical cells not otherwise specified (AGC-NOS), atypical cells favor neoplasia, AIS, or even adenocarcinoma. Of note, 40% of cervices associated with an atypical glandular cells of undetermined significance (AGUS) smear will have a significant tissue abnormality, with greater than 50% harboring an SIL. The significance of an AGUS Papanicolaou result in the pregnant and in the postpartum woman is not yet clear. In a recent manuscript by Chhieng and colleagues, 30 pregnant women and 5 within the immediate postpartum window were evaluated for a cytologic diagnosis of AGUS. Of 27 women for whom there was follow-up, 17 underwent colposcopic examination and biopsy. Five women (29.4%) had CIN, including three high-grade and two low-grade lesions on biopsy. It is interesting that the remaining patients (70.6%) had benign pathology, which included chronic cervicitis ($n = 5$), endocervical and/or endometrial polyps ($n = 4$), Arias–Stella reaction ($n = 2$), and microglandular hyperplasia ($n = 1$); of the 10 patients who had repeat Papanicolaou tests, only 2 had persistent AGUS/ASC-US. Nevertheless, the finding that up to 30% of pregnancy-associated AGUS patients had a significant preneoplastic lesion warrants careful evaluation.

The clinician's diagnostic armamentarium is limited during pregnancy. In the absence of a visible lesion or a significantly expanded cervix (i.e., the barrel-shaped cervix), all patients with AGUS smears should undergo colposcopic evaluation with directed biopsy. Patients diagnosed with a squamous lesion or AIS should be evaluated by colposcopy during subsequent trimesters. It is not known whether a patient with AIS on directed biopsy should undergo wedge resection of that area to rule out invasion in a nearby "skip" lesion. A diagnostic LLETZ and/or cold knife cervical conization during pregnancy is best reserved only for those few cases in which an AIS or squamous lesion suspicious for microinvasion is encountered on directed biopsy.

If colposcopy is unrevealing, however, the concern is raised that an endocervical lesion high in the canal or even within the endometrial compartment is being missed. Nevertheless, an endocervical curettage, cervical dilatation with fractional uterine curettage, and/or endometrial aspiration biopsy is best deferred until the postpartum period, when even a full cervical conization can be performed if needed. Therefore, in these clinical scenarios, consultation with the cytopathologist should be arranged to determine if the original Papanicolaou slide contains troublesome features such as inflammatory cells, polyps, glandular hyperplasia, or the Arias–Stella reaction, any of which could confuse the picture, especially when dealing with an AGC-NOS Papanicolaou smear. Gravid women with a negative colposcopic survey for an atypical glandular cell (AGC) favoring neoplasia cervical smear can be evaluated safely in pregnancy with either endovaginal ultrasonography or magnetic resonance imaging (MRI) of the pelvis to search for a lesion within the endometrium or endocervical canal. In these latter circumstances, referral to a gynecologic oncologist should be contemplated.

The 2006 ASCCP management schema for AIS includes the following:

- Expectant management during pregnancy is acceptable for AIS.
- In patients for whom there is no concern for microinvasion, serial colposcopy during pregnancy (e.g., every trimester) is not necessary.
- Definitive management of AIS should be deferred to the postpartum period.

Intrapartum Hysterectomy

Some authors have described a program in which an intrapartum hysterectomy (following either vaginal or cesarean birth) is performed for patients with CIS or AIS who have completed childbearing and/or have proved to be noncompliant. Because there is not sufficient evidence to suggest that an immunocompetent patient is at risk for rapid progression of disease during pregnancy, the need to remove the diseased segment of the cervix is not urgent. Intrapartum hysterectomies, both elective and nonelective, can be associated with significant blood loss. Furthermore, among inexperienced obstetricians, the bladder is particularly at risk for injury. One must balance the noncompliance of a given patient with the possibility that microinvasion may not have been sufficiently excluded during pregnancy, especially in cases of CIS or AIS with positive margins. The observation that postpartum regression may also occur with even CIS argues against the routine performance of an intrapartum hysterectomy for the management of CIN in pregnancy.

Invasive Cervical Cancer

Presenting symptoms in order of frequency among pregnant women with cervical carcinoma include abnormal vaginal bleeding (63%), vaginal discharge (13%), postcoital bleeding (4%), and pelvic pain (2%). Of importance, in the review by Hacker and colleagues, 18% of patients were asymptomatic, as were 30% of the patients in the study by Creasman and colleagues. When bleeding occurs, this symptom must be investigated and not automatically attributed to the pregnancy. Examination during the first trimester will not lead to abortion. Third-trimester bleeding can be adequately assessed in the operating room as a double setup procedure. Many times, visual inspection is all that is needed for diagnosis of this malignant neoplasm. The International Federation of Gynecology and Obstetrics (FIGO) staging system applies also in pregnancy. To avoid the risks of radiation exposure to a developing fetus, we recommend an ultrasound of the kidneys to evaluate for the presence of hydronephrosis and an MRI of the pelvis when there is concern for parametrial extension of the tumor. Chest radiography may be performed with appropriate

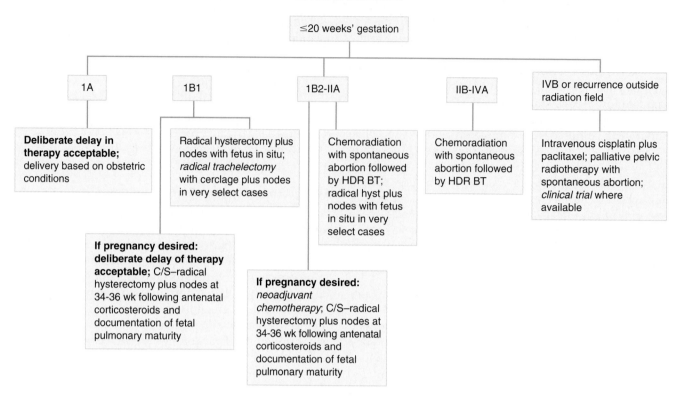

FIGURE 15-5 Suggested therapy for cervical cancer in pregnancy. *B,* Brachytherapy (mg/hr) vaginal radium in two applications; *WP,* whole-pelvis irradiation (cGy).

abdominal shielding to exclude pulmonary metastases. An algorithm for the suggested management of invasive cervical cancer in pregnancy appears in Figure 15-5.

A working group was set up in 2007 in France to propose national recommendations for the management of pregnant patients with invasive cervical cancer. The management of cervical cancer during pregnancy is affected by five factors:

- FIGO stage (and tumor size)
- Nodal status
- Histologic subtype of the tumor
- Gestational age at diagnosis
- Patient's wishes regarding continuation of pregnancy

In patients with early-stage disease diagnosed during the first two trimesters of pregnancy, there is an increasing tendency to preserve the pregnancy while awaiting fetal maturity in patients with absence of nodal involvement.

Microinvasive Disease

The diagnosis of microinvasive carcinoma in pregnancy is typically established with colposcopic directed biopsy, and in a minority of cases in which the colposcopic biopsy cannot exclude microinvasion, a shallow coin biopsy or the cervix or wedge excision of the area under suspicion as outlined earlier is suggested. This is the only absolute indication for conization during pregnancy. Conization distinguishes patients who have "early stromal invasion" and who can proceed to term without appreciable risk to their survival from those with frank invasion in whom consideration must be given to early interruption of the pregnancy. We advise patients with early stromal invasion (i.e., FIGO stage Ia1) that the pregnancy may continue safely to term, provided the surgical margins are free. Cesarean section is not thought to be necessary for this group of patients, and the route of delivery should be determined by obstetric indications. Patients with FIGO stage Ia2 or occult Ib1 lesions should undergo cesarean delivery when fetal pulmonary maturation is demonstrable, followed by an immediate modified radical abdominal hysterectomy with bilateral pelvic lymphadenectomies. We advocate the deployment of a vertical uterine incision so as to leave the lower uterine segment undisturbed for subsequent detailed pathologic examination. It is interesting that the physiologic changes of pregnancy actually enhance the performance of radical surgery by providing the surgeon with multiple levels of distinct tissue planes.

Recently, reports of laser conization for microinvasive disease have originated from Japan. As described earlier,

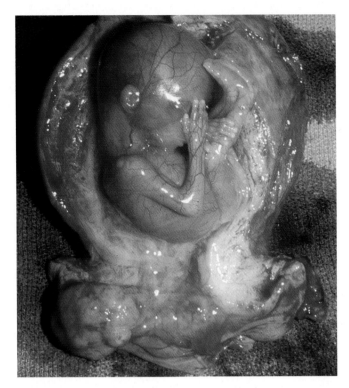

FIGURE 15-6   An 18-week-old fetus. Cervical cancer with a vaginal cuff and an extruding placenta are seen in a radical hysterectomy specimen from a 32-year-old patient.

Tsuritani and colleagues have included 19 women with microinvasive carcinoma in their series of 49 women and considered CO_2 laser conization within 20 mm of length to be safe in pregnant patients. Yahata and colleagues have reported their experience with four patients diagnosed with stage IA1 cervical adenocarcinoma who underwent KTP laser conization and vaporization from 16 to 23 weeks of gestation. All patients delivered at term, at which point they underwent radical hysterectomy with lymphadenectomy ($n = 3$) or cold knife conization ($n = 1$). None have developed recurrent disease during a 2- to 13-year follow-up period.

Cesarean–Radical Hysterectomy with Pelvic Lymphadenectomies

In deciding on therapy for frankly invasive cervical cancer in pregnancy, the physician must consider both the stage of disease and the duration of pregnancy. The decision can often be influenced by the religious convictions of the patient and family and the desire of the mother for the child. For FIGO stage I and FIGO stage IIa lesions, radical hysterectomy with bilateral lymphadenectomy is acceptable during any trimester (Figure 15-6). We prefer the surgical approach because of the overall result, which includes ovarian preservation, improved sexual function, and elimination of unnecessary delays for the patient. The complication rate of

radical surgery for cervical carcinoma in pregnant patients does not exceed that in nonpregnant patients when normal surgical principles are scrupulously followed.

Monk and Montz examined their institutional experience in treating invasive cervical cancer complicating intrauterine pregnancy with radical hysterectomy. They identified 13 patients treated with radical hysterectomy and bilateral pelvic lymphadenectomy with the fetus in situ and 8 others treated with cesarean delivery followed by radical hysterectomy and bilateral pelvic lymph node dissection. The mean operative time was 281 minutes, and the mean blood loss was 777 mL for radical hysterectomy with the fetus in situ plus lymphadenectomy and 1750 mL when cesarean section preceded the cancer operation. The surgical morbidity was minimal for the whole group, and after documentation of fetal maturation, seven healthy infants were delivered. Twenty patients (95%) are alive and free of disease with a mean follow-up of 40 months. The authors concluded that radical surgery offers immediate treatment for early-stage cervical cancer during intrauterine pregnancy, with low associated morbidity, acceptable survival, and preservation of ovarian function.

Radical Trachelectomy with Lymphadenectomy

In recent years, several reports have appeared describing the successful performance of radical trachelectomy during pregnancy. Abu-Rustum and colleagues treated a 37-year-old pregnant woman at 15 weeks of gestational age for a FIGO stage IB1 poorly differentiated lymphoepithelioma-like cervical carcinoma found on conization. The procedure was performed abdominally and included bilateral pelvic lymphadenectomies and permanent cerclage placement. The final pathology revealed 7-mm (out of 19 mm) invasion with no lymphovascular involvement, negative margins, and negative nodes. The pregnancy was delivered by elective planned cesarean hysterectomy at 39 weeks of gestational age. This procedure has also been safely performed during the 19th week of gestation by Mandic and colleagues. Once again the abdominal approach was used, and the patient underwent successful cesarean section at 36 weeks of of gestation. At the time of manuscript acceptance, the patient was in the 15th week of a new pregnancy and had normal cytologic screening and no evidence of metastatic/recurrent carcinoma. Finally, Gurney and Blank have described a patient diagnosed with FIGO IB1 disease at 21 weeks of gestational age who underwent postpartum radical abdominal trachelectomy. Ungar and colleagues reported five cases of radical abdominal trachelectomy during pregnancy and the birth of two healthy term infants.

The first case of vaginal radical trachelectomy was reported by van de Nieuwenhof and colleagues to have occurred at 16 weeks of gestation for a FIGO stage IB1 lesion. This patient underwent an uneventful cesarean section followed by radical hysterectomy at 36 weeks of gestational age, and at 9 months of follow-up both mother and infant were doing well.

Alouini and colleagues reported laparoscopic pelvic (with and without aortic) lymphadenectomy during pregnancy in eight patients from 12 to 32 weeks of gestation. There were no surgical or general anesthetic maternal or fetal complications. The mean number of lymph nodes removed was 18 (range, 11-28), and in five patients (stage IB1, $n = 4$; stage IB1, $n = 1$) there was pathologic evidence of nodal metastases. One patient experienced a spontaneous abortion following radical trachelectomy, whereas the remaining seven reached fetal maturity and had healthy babies by cesarean section. Laparoscopic staging with retrieval of 19 negative nodes for a FIGO stage IB1 carcinoma complicating a twin pregnancy was safely performed at 17 weeks of of gestation by Favero and colleagues.

Finally, Silva and colleagues explored the possibility of sentinel node mapping in pregnant patients with cervical cancer. They reported the first case of sentinel node detection using technetium-labeled radiocolloid. Histologic analysis of the operative specimen demonstrated a poorly differentiated squamous carcinoma with metastasis in the sentinel and a neoplastic embolus in a blood vessel of the placental bed.

Whole-Pelvis Radiotherapy with Intracavitary Brachytherapy

Radiation therapy is equally efficacious in treating patients with early-stage (i.e., FIGO stage Ib1) cervical cancer in pregnancy and, together with radiosensitizing chemotherapy, is the treatment of choice in more advanced stages (FIGO stage Ib2-IVa). In the first and second trimesters when the pregnancy is to be disregarded, treatment should begin with whole-pelvis irradiation. Spontaneous abortion usually occurs during therapy, and the treatment is then completed with intracavitary radium or cesium applications. Spontaneous abortion usually occurs at about 35 days in the first trimester and at 45 days in the second trimester after onset of radiotherapy. Some second-trimester patients will go 60 to 70 days before abortion occurs. An alternative approach in the patient who has not aborted is to evacuate the uterus by means of a hysterotomy followed by conventional intracavitary irradiation delivered within 1 to 2 weeks.

If spontaneous abortion does not occur by completion of the external beam therapy, as occurs commonly after the 16th week of gestation, a modified radical hysterectomy without pelvic lymphadenectomy should be done to excise the remaining central neoplasm. This strategy delivers potentially curative doses of radiation to pelvic lymph nodes with microscopic foci of metastatic tumor followed by surgical resection of the remaining central tumor because the gravid uterus is not suitable for intracavitary radium or cesium. Although some clinicians prefer an extrafascial hysterectomy after 5000 cGy of whole-pelvis irradiation in patients who have early lesions, we prefer the more extensive modified radical hysterectomy. This approach accomplishes adequate excision of the cervix and accompanying medial parametria and upper vagina, which includes all the tissues that would have been effectively irradiated by the pear-shaped isodose distribution of a tandem and ovoid application of radium or cesium. Those who advocate an extrafascial hysterectomy centrally often advise further vaginal vault irradiation after the surgical procedure to treat the upper vagina and medial parametria more completely.

Sood and colleagues assessed the effects of pregnancy on tumor control, survival, and morbidity associated with radiation therapy administered to pregnant patients. They identified 26 women treated primarily with radiation therapy before the era of concurrent chemoirradiation and matched these patients with 26 control subjects based on age, histology, stage, treatment, and year of treatment. Patients were treated with external beam radiation (mean dose 46.7 Gy) and intracavitary radiation (mean dose 56.5 Gy to point A). Three patients diagnosed during the first trimester were treated with radiation with the fetus in situ, and all had spontaneous abortions 20 to 24 days after the start of radiation (mean dose 34 Gy). In all these cases, radiation was interrupted for only 3 days or less. There were no statistically significant differences in recurrence rates or survival between the pregnant group and the control subjects.

Benhaim and colleagues have reported two patients with locally advanced disease who were treated with chemoradiation during the first trimester with the fetus in utero. The first patient (FIGO stage IVA) was treated at 12 weeks of gestation and experienced recurrence at 20 months. The second patient (FIGO stage IIB) was also treated at 12 weeks of gestation and underwent completion surgery (radical hysterectomy with lymphadenectomy) and has survived disease free for 2 years.

Episiotomy Site Recurrence

Patients in whom the diagnosis of invasive cervical cancer is made in the postpartum period may have undergone vaginal delivery. This group of patients warrants immediate therapy and specialized surveillance. Recurrence of cervical cancer at the episiotomy scar is a rare event and is thought to occur through implantation at the time of vaginal delivery from an occult tumor, with subsequent early, isolated recurrence as opposed to regional spread. At least 15 cases have appeared in the literature since 1986, including one patient who experienced relapse along a perineal laceration scar (Table 15-4). In the majority of these patients, the primary diagnosis of cervical cancer was made during the postpartum period, with recurrence at the episiotomy site typically occurring within 6 months of primary treatment.

In a matched case-control study of women with cervical cancer diagnosed during pregnancy ($n = 56$) or within 6 months of delivery ($n = 27$), Sood and colleagues noted that among the patients diagnosed postpartum, 1 of 7 who was delivered by cesarean section developed a local and distant recurrence, whereas 10 of 17 (59%) of those who delivered vaginally developed recurrences ($P = 0.04$). In multivariate analysis, vaginal delivery was the most significant predictor of recurrence. We recommend delivery by cesarean section when the diagnosis is known antenatally, and in those patients diagnosed in the postpartum period, vigilant examination of the episiotomy and vaginal laceration sites is warranted. Although the mode of delivery in the setting of known microinvasive disease may be based on obstetric indications, it should be pointed out that among the 14 cases of episiotomy site recurrences, there was 1 patient who had been diagnosed with a stage Ia endocervical adenocarcinoma.

Neither the time of diagnosis nor time to recurrence appears to affect survival after episiotomy site recurrence. Goldman and Goldberg noted that no patient who received chemotherapy or radiotherapy for recurrent disease without excision survived 1 year. The treatment policy should include wide local excision of the entire nodule with adjuvant external radiotherapy plus brachytherapy. Of seven patients treated by this method, 71% were without evidence of disease at longer than 1 year.

There have been at least two cases of cervical cancer with concomitant episiotomy metastasis in the literature. Baloglu and colleagues reported one of these patients for whom the diagnosis was unknown antenatally. This patient was diagnosed with locally advanced disease and an episiotomy site metastasis and received primary chemoradiation. She was without evidence of recurrence at 1 year of follow-up when their report was published. Women diagnosed with cervical cancer in the postpartum period should have the episiotomy and/or vaginal laceration site carefully examined if they experience vaginal delivery.

Planned Delay of Therapy

Historically, when invasive carcinoma was diagnosed before 20 weeks of gestation, recommendations included immediate treatment of the tumor, either by radical hysterectomy or radiation therapy, leaving the fetus in utero in both instances. This dogma has been challenged during the preceding decade, with multiple reports of a safe outcome for mother and child with a deliberate

delay in therapy to permit gestational advancement (Table 15-5). For example, Duggan and colleagues reported a mean diagnosis-to-treatment interval of 144 days (range, 53-212 days) in eight patients with FIGO stage Ia or FIGO stage Ib cervical cancer who postponed therapy to optimize fetal outcome. All these women were rendered disease-free after a median follow-up of 23 months. Sorosky and colleagues identified eight pregnant women with FIGO stage I squamous cell cervical carcinoma who declined immediate therapy in order to improve fetal outcome. They were observed prospectively until the late third trimester, with a mean diagnosis-to-treatment interval of 109 days (range, 21-210 days). No clinical progression of disease was detected, and following therapy all were alive and disease free after a mean follow-up of 37 months (range, 13-68 months). Takushi and colleagues reported a delay in treatment of 6 to 16 weeks for four women with FIGO stage Ia2, Ib1, or 1b2 lesions. No disease progression was documented and following cesarean–radical hysterectomy all patients have been disease-free at a follow-up period of 70 to 156 months.

Although most patients with FIGO stage Ib disease have fared well with deliberate delays in therapy, four patients are noted in whom progression of disease was observed ($n = 2$) or in whom recurrence and death from disease occurred ($n = 2$). Five patients with FIGO stage II disease who opted to delay therapy were reported by Lee and colleagues, and although they did not progress during the pregnancy, it should be noted that their cancers were diagnosed in the third trimester and the treatment delays were relatively limited. Long-term follow-up data were not presented for this subset of patients. Thus, for patients with FIGO stage Ia1-Ib1 squamous cell lesions diagnosed before and after 20 weeks of gestation, a limited treatment delay to await fetal maturity may be acceptable. The counseling in such situations should be analogous to obtaining an informed consent from the mother.

Neoadjuvant Chemotherapy in Pregnancy

Patients with advanced disease (i.e., FIGO stage Ib2 and greater) should be offered immediate therapy. A novel approach to patients with locally advanced disease who refuse interruption of pregnancy was first reported by our group in 1998. Two women with FIGO stage Ib2 and FIGO stage IIa lesions refused interruption of their pregnancies and received neoadjuvant chemotherapy consisting of vincristine (1 mg/m^2) and cisplatin (50 mg/m^2) during the early second and third trimesters. Both patients experienced significant tumor regression, rendering radical hysterectomy feasible at the time of cesarean delivery following documentation of fetal pulmonary maturation at 32 weeks of and 34 weeks of gestation. At the time of publication, one patient had remained

TABLE 15-4   Treatment Modalities and Survival of Patients with Episiotomy Site Recurrence

Authors	Year	Stage	Prenatal Cytology	Pathology	Time of Initial Diagnosis	Primary Treatment	Disease-Free Interval	Treatment of Recurrence	Status
Burgess and Waymont	1987	Ib	SCCA	SCCA	7 months pp	XRT, BT	17 months	Exenteration	n/r
Copeland et al	1987	Ib	Normal	Adenocarcinoma	3 months pp	RH	3 months	WE, XRT, BT	NED > 5 years
Gordon et al	1989	Ib	Normal	Adenocarcinoma	Biopsy at delivery	RH	5 months	WE, XRT	NED 10 months
van Dam et al	1992	IIIa	n/r	SCCA	Biopsy at delivery	RH	1 month	WE, XRT, BT	NED 3.5 years
		Ib	Normal	SCCA	6 weeks pp	Chemotherapy, XRT, BT	0 months	BT	n/r
Khalil et al	1993	IIIb	Not done	Adenocarcinoma	9 weeks pp	XRT, BT	3 months	WE, XRT, BT	NED >10 years
Cliby et al	1994	Ib	HSIL	SCCA	8 weeks pp	XRT, BT	3 months	Chemotherapy, XRT	DOD 4 months
		Ib	Not done	SCCA	Biopsy at delivery	RH	9 weeks	Chemotherapy	DOD 6 months
		Ib	Not done	SCCA	Biopsy at 36 weeks	RH	24 months	Chemotherapy, WE, XRT	NED 1 year
		Ib	Not done	SCCA	Biopsy at delivery	RH	3 months	XRT	DOD 3.5 years
		Ib	Not done	SCCA	5 weeks pp	RH	1 month	WE, XRT	DOD 6 months
van den Broek et al	1995	Ia1	Normal	Adenocarcinoma	3 months pp	Total abdominal hysterectomy	6 weeks	WE, interstitial implants	DOD 1 year
Goldman and Goldberg	2003	Ib	Normal	SCCA	1 week pp	RH	5.5 years	WE, XRT, BT	DOD 4.5 years
Heron et al	2005	Ib	AGUS	Villoglandular	Biopsy at 31 weeks	RH, BPLND	44 months	XRT, WE	NED 10 months
Baloglu et al	2007	IIIA	Unknown	SCCA	8 months pp	ChemoRT	NED 1 year f/u		

(Modified from Goldman NA, Goldberg GL: Obstet Gynecol 101:1127, 2003.)

AGUS, Atypical glandular cells of undetermined significance; BPLND, bilateral pelvic lymphadenectomy; BT, brachytherapy; DOD, died of disease; f/u, follow-up; HSIL, high-grade squamous intraepithelial lesion; n/r, not reported; NED, no evidence of disease; pp, postpartum; RH, radical hysterectomy; SCCA, squamous cell carcinoma; WE, wide excision; XRT, whole pelvic radiotherapy.

TABLE 15-5 Deliberate Delay of Definitive Therapy for Frankly Invasive Cervical Carcinoma in Pregnancy

Authors	Year	Stage	No.	Delay	Maternal Outcome
Prem et al	1966	I	4	6 wk	NED 5 yr
		I	5	11-17 wk	NED 3-5 yr
Dudan et al	1973	Ib	2	2 and 6 mo	Progression
Lee et al	1981	Ib	1	12 wk	NED 10 yr
		Ib	2	11 wk	No progression
		II	5	1-11 wk	No progression
Nisker and Shubat	1983	Ib	1	24 wk	DOD
Greer et al	1989	Ib	5	6-17 wk	NED 1-3 yr ($n = 4$), DOD ($n = 1$)
Monk and Montz	1992	Ib	4	10-16 wk	NED 3.5 yr
Hopkins and Morley	1992	Ib	5	12 wk	NED 5 yr ($n = 40$)
Mack et al	1981	Ib	3	10-16 wk	NED
Duggan et al	1993	Ib1	5	7-24 wk	NED 3 yr
Sivanesaratnam et al	1993	Ib	2	2 and 4 wk	NED 5 yr
Allen et al	1995	Ib	2	18-19 wk	NED 5 yr
Sorosky et al	1995	Ib1	7	7-29 wk	NED 1.5-5.5 yr
Sood et al	1996	Ib	3	3-32 wk	NED 1-30 yr
Tewari et al	1997	Ib2	1*	11 wk	NED 2 yr
		IIa	1*	18 wk	DOD 9 mo
van Vliet et al	1998	Ib	5	2-10 wk	DOD ($n = 1$), NED 1.5-9 yr
		IIa	1	2 wk	NED 12 yr
Marana et al	2001	IIb	1*	21 wk	DOD 18 mo*
Takushi et al	2002	Ib1	2	13 and 15 wk	NED 8 and 9 yr
		Ib2	1	6 wk	NED 7 yr
Germann et al	2005	Ib1	9	4 mo	NED 5 yr
Traen et al	2006	IB1	1	19 wk	NED

Modified from Tewari et al: Cancer 82:1529, 1998.
DOD, Died of disease; NED, no evidence of disease.
*Treated with neoadjuvant chemotherapy during pregnancy.

without evidence of recurrence for more than 2 years; unfortunately, the second patient experienced a lethal relapse 5 months after primary therapy. Both children have experienced normal development. Another early report was by that of Marana and colleagues, who treated a pregnant woman with a FIGO stage IIb tumor with bleomycin (30 mg on day 1) and cisplatin (50 mg/m^2 on day 2 and day 3) from 17 weeks to 38 weeks of gestation and achieved both tumor regression and a healthy infant, who continued to thrive long after the mother succumbed to recurrent disease 13 months after delivery. Although such a treatment approach remains investigational, the use of neoadjuvant chemotherapy while awaiting gestational advancement may be entertained when the pregnant woman with cervical cancer, for whom a treatment delay is ill-advised, refuses interruption of therapy.

Since these initial publications there have been at least eight additional cases of patients who received neoadjuvant chemotherapy during pregnancy for cervical cancer. Most patients were treated for locally advanced disease (FIGO IB2-IIIB), but two patients received neoadjuvant chemotherapy for FIGO stage IB1 lesions. Neoadjuvant therapy was usually administered during the mid-second trimester to the early third trimester (range, 17-33 weeks of gestation) and single-agent cisplatin

(e.g., 75 mg/m^2 q 10 days) has been used most often. The combination of cisplatin (50 mg/m^2) plus vincristine (1 mg/m^2) q21 days has also been of continued interest in some cases. Obstetric outcomes have been universally favorable, as have maternal outcomes, although there was one case of rapid tumor progression. It should be emphasized, however, that despite the good results, follow-up in several cases has been of short duration. Neoadjuvant chemotherapy should be considered for those patients with locally advanced disease diagnosed in the early- to mid-second trimester who are adamant about continuing the pregnancy. Once again these patients need to be counseled regarding the investigational nature of this treatment modality under the clinical circumstances in question.

Prognosis for Patients with Cervical Cancer in Pregnancy

The overall prognosis for all stages of cervical cancer in pregnancy is similar to that in nonpregnant women (Table 15-6). The favorable overall prognosis for pregnant patients is related to a greater proportion of pregnant patients with stage I disease. In a report by Allen and colleagues of 96 cases of cervical cancer occurring in pregnancy, the disease-free survival rate for 87 patients who were available for analysis was noted to be 92.3%

TABLE 15-6   Long-Term, Cause-Specific Actuarial Survival for Cervical Cancer in Pregnancy Treated from 1960 to 2004 Compared with 2 Controls Matched for Age, Disease Stage, Histopathology, and Treatment Year

Year	Cases ($n = 41$)	Controls ($n = 82$)
0	1.0	1.0
2	0.89	0.87
4	0.86	0.79
6	0.82	0.75
8	0.81	0.73
10	0.79	0.73
12	0.77	0.73

From Pettersson BF et al: Cancer 116:2343, 2010.
Log-rank test (p = 0.85)

for FIGO stage Ia1, 68.2% for FIGO stage Ib, 54.5% for FIGO stage II, and 37.5% for FIGO stage III. The overall survival rate was 65.5%, which is slightly better than that reported by Hacker and colleagues. They also observed an association of advanced clinical staging with diagnosis in the third trimester and postpartum. Of 49 cases of FIGO stage Ib cervical carcinoma, 64.5% were diagnosed in the third trimester and postpartum; of 22 cases of FIGO stage II cervical carcinoma, 77.3% were diagnosed in the third trimester and postpartum; and all 9 cases of stage III cervical carcinoma were diagnosed in the third trimester and postpartum. Of the 32 patients who underwent pelvic lymphadenectomy, 10 were noted to have positive nodes. This increase in frequency has not been our experience.

Zemlickis and colleagues compared 40 women who had carcinoma of the cervix in pregnancy with 89 nonpregnant women matched for age, stage, and tumor type. Long-term survival was similar between the two groups. When pregnant women were compared with a series of 1963 cervical cancers in women younger than 45 years treated during the same time, the pregnant women were three times more likely to have stage I disease and had a lower chance of having FIGO stage III to IV cancers.

In 1993 Sivanesaratnam and colleagues reported surgical management of early invasive cancer of the cervix in a series of 18 patients who underwent radical hysterectomy and pelvic lymphadenectomy, with a 5-year survival of 77.7%. A comparable group of nonpregnant patients who also underwent radical surgery had a survival of 92.3%. Nisker and Shubat also reported that there was a slightly better survival in the nonpregnant group than in the pregnant group. These reports are in contrast to the previous reports by Creasman and colleagues, Sablinska and colleagues, and Lee and colleagues, who found no appreciable difference in the 5-year survival rates of pregnant versus nonpregnant patients with cervical cancer.

A multicenter, retrospective study conducted by the Korean Gynecologic Oncology Group (KGOG-1006) contained 40 pregnant subjects treated from 1995 to 2003. Each case was matched to three controls on the basis of age, stage, histology, and date of treatment. Among 12 patients who delayed treatment for fetal maturity, two died of disease. There was no difference in overall survival between pregnant and nonpregnant patients with stage IB lesions.

Pettersson and colleagues recently published a 90-year experience from the Radiumhemmet. The 10-year actuarial survival rate improved significantly during the study period from 27% (1914-2004) to 79% (1960-2004). The 10-year cause-specific cumulative actuarial survival rate for 41 pregnant women treated during 1960 to 2004 did not differ statistically from the rate for an age-matched, stage-matched, and histopathology-matched control series of nonpregnant women treated at the Radiumhemmet during the same period. The authors concluded that during the study period, the incidence of cervical cancer during pregnancy declined, the cases were discovered at earlier stages, and survival improved.

For more advanced disease, pregnancy may have an unfavorable effect on prognosis as a result of problems with radiation dosimetry in pregnancy and the need to interrupt radiation therapy more frequently because of genital tract sepsis. Clinical stage remains the most important determinant of prognosis.

Obstetric Outcomes

Dalrymple and colleagues analyzed the obstetric outcomes among women in California with pregnancy-associated cervical cancer. Using computer-linked infant birth/death certificates, discharge records, and cancer registry files, cases were identified and then assigned to a prenatal or postpartum cancer diagnosis group. Among 434 cases, those diagnosed prenatally ($n = 136$) had higher rates of cesarean section, hospitalization longer than 5 days, low birth weight, very low birth weight, prematurity, and fetal deaths compared to pregnant controls without cancer. No neonatal deaths were attributable to elective premature delivery. Very low birth weight, prematurity, and fetal death rates remained elevated among those diagnosed postpartum.

Ovarian Cancer

Ovarian cancer is reported to occur in 1 per 10,000 to 1 per 25,000 pregnancies. Pregnancy does not alter the prognosis of most ovarian malignant neoplasms, but complications such as torsion and rupture may increase the incidence of spontaneous abortion or preterm delivery. In a survey by Kohler of the largest studies in the literature, about 1 in 600 pregnancies will be complicated by an adnexal mass. More contemporary accounts suggest that adnexal masses may complicate as many as 1 in 190 pregnancies. At least one third of pregnant women are asymptomatic, with the adnexal mass often discovered during obstetric ultrasonography.

Most cysts in pregnant patients are follicular or corpus luteum cysts and are usually no more than 3 to 5 cm in diameter. Functional cysts as large as 11 cm in diameter have been reported but are rare. More than 90% of these functional cysts will disappear as pregnancy progresses and are undetectable by the 14th week of gestation. It appears that the size of the adnexal mass at the time of diagnosis is inversely related to the likelihood of spontaneous regression. Only 6% of masses smaller than 6 cm persisted during serial examinations, but 39% of masses greater than 6 cm persisted. The complication rate increases with increasing size of the mass. In addition, a solid or complex ultrasonographic appearance and the presence of bilateral adnexal/ovarian abnormalities may also be indications to proceed with laparotomy. Adnexal masses with blood flow characterized by a high resistive index by Doppler ultrasonography are less likely to be malignant, independent of size. MRI may be useful when ultrasonographic findings are equivocal.

The most pressing problems associated with ovarian tumors in pregnancy are the initial diagnosis and the differential diagnosis. When the tumor is palpable within the pelvis, it must be differentiated from a retroverted pregnant uterus, a pedunculated uterine fibroid, a carcinoma of the rectosigmoid, a pelvic kidney, and a congenital uterine abnormality (e.g., rudimentary uterine horn). Analysis of serum tumor markers is a complex undertaking and can be misleading because the titers for each of the markers, especially α-fetoprotein and β-human chorionic gonadotropin (hCG), and even CA-125, are routinely elevated in pregnancy for reasons unrelated to malignancy.

A proposed management algorithm for the adnexal mass in pregnancy appears in Figure 15-7. Our experience has been that patients operated on around the 18th week of gestation have negligible fetal wastage associated with the exploration. Therefore 18 weeks of gestation appears to be a judicious period for laparotomy in terms of its safety both for the fetus and for the elimination of functional ovarian cysts. If the cyst is complex and suspicious for malignancy and increases in size, the patient should undergo exploration earlier than 18 weeks. Whenever exploration is conducted, our recommendation is that the uterus not be manipulated during surgery (i.e., the so-called hands-off-the-uterus approach) in an effort to minimize its irritability.

Torsion is common in pregnancy, with 10% to 15% of ovarian tumors reportedly undergoing this complication. Most torsions (i.e., 60%) occur when the uterus is rising at a rapid rate (8-16 weeks) or when the uterus is involuting (in the puerperium). The usual sequence of events is sudden lower abdominal pain, nausea, vomiting, and in some cases shocklike symptoms. The abdomen is tense and tender, and there is rebound tenderness with guarding. If exploration must be undertaken during the first trimester and extraction of the ovary (or ovaries) is required, supplemental progesterone can be administered to decrease the likelihood of pregnancy loss.

In many instances, the presence of an ovarian tumor may not be suspected until delivery (Figure 15-8). The large uterus obscures the growth of the ovarian neoplasm. The tumor may be growing in the abdomen behind the large uterus and may not fall back into the cul-de-sac until it is large. If there is a mechanical obstruction of the birth canal, exploratory laparotomy is indicated for both delivery of the baby and management of the ovarian neoplasm. Allowing labor to proceed when an ovarian neoplasm is causing obstruction of the birth canal may result in rupture of the ovarian cyst. Even if the cyst is not ruptured, the trauma of labor may cause hemorrhage into the tumor followed by necrosis and suppuration.

Asymptomatic Adnexal Masses

Before detailing the clinical approach to managing the different ovarian malignancies that may occur during pregnancy, some consideration should be given to asymptomatic adnexal masses. Admittedly, asymptomatic masses can be malignant; however, the vast majority are likely to be benign, particularly in the pregnant population. There has been a movement during the past decade that has challenged the dogma of operating on every asymptomatic mass greater than 5 cm that persists into the second trimester. Most of these masses can be followed conservatively in the absence of symptoms and in the absence of concerning sonographic ovarian and extraovarian findings (e.g., ascites).

Endovaginal pelvic ultrasonography is essential in the evaluation of adnexal masses. Approximately 10% of masses are complex, and the examination should determine the origin of the mass and its location, size, and internal structure (e.g., vegetations, septations). The mass should be classified unilocular, unilocular-solid, multilocular, multilocular-solid, or solid. Color Doppler imaging may be used to obtain a vascular road map of an ovarian mass. Pelvic MRI with gadolinium injection can be performed after the first trimester and should only be used during pregnancy to remove further doubt regarding possible malignancy or to provide additional information if ultrasonography is inconclusive.

Laparoscopic Management of the Ovarian Mass

Laparoscopy was previously thought to be contraindicated in pregnancy because of the unknown effect of the pneumoperitoneum on the gravid uterus, the possible

FIGURE 15-7   Management of an ovarian mass in pregnancy.

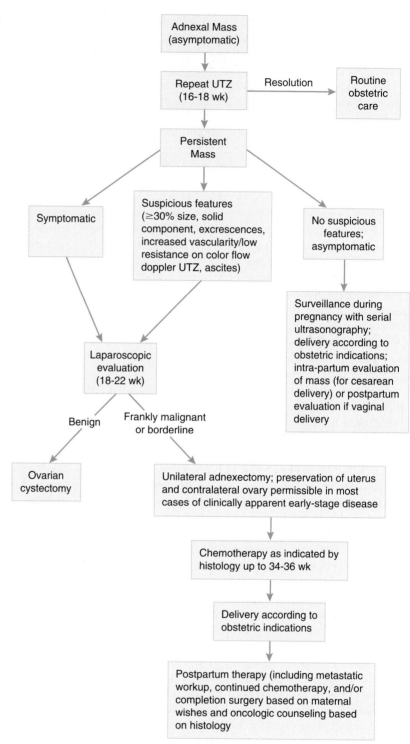

injection of carbon dioxide into the amniotic cavity, and the potential for acidosis in the fetal environment as a result of maternal conversion of carbon dioxide into carbonic acid. Growing evidence, however, suggests that laparoscopy can be performed safely during pregnancy.

The recommended time for laparoscopic intervention mirrors that for open procedures and is between 16 and 20 weeks of gestation. There have been reports of laparoscopy up to the 28th week of gestation, but this would appear to be the upper limit. Larger uteri increase surgical difficulty, and surgery after 23 weeks can be linked

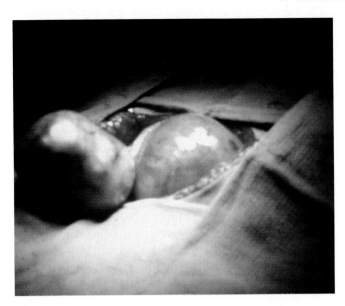

FIGURE 15-8 Benign cystic teratoma: Gross appearance at 18 weeks of gestation.

to adverse fetal outcomes and preterm labor. Intervention before the second trimester is not advisable because this does not give time for the ovarian mass to resolve on its own and could compromise ovarian hormone production before the placenta is fully functional.

The table should be tilted to the left or the right with the patient supine to move the uterus away from the site of trocal insertion. The left upper quadrant or subxyphoid insertion of the trocar should be used with at least 6 cm between the point of entry and the top of the fundus. The open Hasson technique is preferred over the Veress technique, although both have been used successfully in pregnancy. Ultrasound guidance may be used with the Veress technique together with elevation of the abdominal wall to reduce the risk of uterine injury.

Intra-abdominal pressure should be kept below 15 mm Hg with the patient in Trendelenburg position to ensure adequate venous return and uteroplacental blood flow during the operation. Positioning in this manner may require positive pressure ventilation to maintain adequate lung volumes. Depending on the circumstances and gestational age, fetal monitoring may be advisable.

Ovarian Masses Specific to Pregnancy

Two adnexal conditions may specifically be associated with pregnancy. The operating surgeon must be cognizant of their possibility so that unnecessary oophorectomies will not be performed. The luteoma of pregnancy can vary in size from microscopic to 20 cm in diameter and usually consists of multiple, well-circumscribed nodules that can be bilateral in one third of cases. The luteoma may be associated with significant elevations in plasma testosterone and other androgens in about 25% of the cases. Maternal hirsutism or virilism may occur during the latter half of pregnancy, which may cause virilization in up to 70% of female infants born to masculinizing mothers. If the lesion is not recognized grossly, a biopsy may be taken for definitive diagnosis. Because these regress spontaneously postpartum, nothing further needs to be done. Theca-lutein cysts may occur when hCG concentrations are abnormally elevated, such as in a molar pregnancy, fetal hydrops, or multiple gestations. These are usually multiple and thin-walled. Sometimes, massive bilateral theca-lutein cysts manifest that are considerably different from the solid nodules of the luteoma of pregnancy. These also regress postpartum and should not be resected unless acute complications develop.

Histologic Types of Ovarian Tumors

Struyk and Treffers reported on 90 pregnancies complicated by ovarian tumors. No functional cysts were noted in patients operated on after the 18th week. In eight patients, ovarian tumor enlargement was noted during a period of observation; two were malignant, one serous cystadenoma occurred, and five were teratomas. Fifty-four percent of the tumors were diagnosed in the first trimester. Severe pain occurred in 26%, torsion in 12%, obstruction of labor in 17%, and rupture in 9%. Only 37% of the patients had no complications. Fetal wastage was high, with death in utero occurring in three cases and neonatal death in seven cases.

Thornton and Wells reviewed 131 ovarian enlargements in pregnancy, 81 of which were removed (including 1 carcinoma and 6 borderline lesions). Thirty-nine were greater than 5 cm in diameter and had simple internal echo patterns and smooth walls; 3 of these were borderline malignant neoplasms. Hoffman reviewed 13 reports of ovarian neoplasms removed in pregnancy and found benign cystadenomas or cystic teratomas most frequently diagnosed. The Hoffman review also included a summary of 127 malignant ovarian lesions found during pregnancy. A recent literature review by Kwon and colleagues describing the various histologies of ovarian tumors found in pregnancy appears in Table 15-7. Borderline and frankly malignant epithelial lesions were the most commonly encountered during pregnancy.

Borderline Ovarian Tumors

Adnexal masses greater than 6 cm that persist into the second trimester warrant removal at approximately 18 weeks of gestational age. Between 2% and 5% of these lesions will be malignant, with dysgerminoma being most common. Among epithelial tumors, serous carcinoma and serous tumors of low malignant potential are readily encountered. Thirty-five cases of serous ovarian

TABLE 15-7 Distribution of Ovarian Cancers in Pregnancy by Histology

Histology	Dgani et al, 1989 (%)	Copeland and Landon, 1996 (%)	Zanotti et al, 2000 (%)	PUMCH, 2003 (%)	Behtash et al, 2008 (%)	Kwon et al 2010 (%)
Epithelial—borderline	65	37.5	33-40	50	39.1	81.5
Epithelial—invasive	35	—	66	27.3	21.7	55.5
Germ cell	17	45	30-33	40.9	47.8	18.5
Sex cord–stromal	13	10	17-20	9.1	13	0
Other	5	7.5	12-13	0	0	0

Modified from Kwon YS et al: J Korean Med Sci 25:230, 2010.

tumors of low malignant potential in conjunction with pregnancy have been reported since 1988. In the 33 cases in which a FIGO stage was assigned, 30 were stage I (14 stage Ia, 1 stage Ib, 4 Stage Ic, and 11 nonsubstaged I). All 33 patients for whom follow-up data were available were found to be alive without disease (range 1 year to 20 years and 5 months). Recent evidence suggests that the hormonal influence of pregnancy can effect histologic changes in serous low malignant potential tumors that, if not sorted out and characterized appropriately, could be mistaken for frankly invasive carcinoma. The group at the MD Anderson Hospital and Tumor Institute collected 10 cases from 1944 to 1993 and conducted a slide review, noting some very peculiar histologic features distinct from those seen in nonpregnant patients, including epithelial atypia and proliferation, eosinophilic cells, mucin production, decidual changes, and frequent microinvasion. Although these lesions remained within the spectrum of low malignant potential tumors, the histologic features were worrisome for a more aggressive clinical course, yet all 10 patients remained disease free following a variety of treatment modalities. We advise prompt recognition of these histologic findings following cystectomy and/or oophorectomy during pregnancy so as to classify them accordingly as being borderline rather than to confuse them with low-grade serous papillary carcinomas. Of additional interest is that in two cases the tumor was resected both during pregnancy and after parturition (2 months and 3 years), and there was significant regression of the epithelial proliferation, the number of eosinophilic cells, and the amount of mucin production the second time around; this regression following parturition supports a hormonal etiology of these unusual histologic features. In contrast to frankly malignant ovarian carcinomas, unilateral adnexectomy is all that is required during pregnancy for the serous low malignant potential tumor.

Frankly Malignant Ovarian Tumors

Malignant ovarian tumors account for only 2% to 5% of all ovarian neoplasms found in pregnancy. The incidence for all pregnancies is 1 in 8000 to 1 in 20,000 deliveries. The diagnosis is usually fortuitous in that the patient undergoes laparotomy for an adnexal mass that is subsequently found to be malignant. In many instances, the close observation of the pregnant patient has led to the discovery of a lesion in the earlier stages. These include not only malignant germ cell tumors and sex cord–stromal cell cancers, but also some epithelial malignancies. If an ovarian malignant neoplasm is found at the time of abdominal exploration, the surgeon's first obligation is to properly stage the disease, as outlined in Chapter 10. Although the gravid uterus hinders the surgeon's ability to access the retroperitoneum, every effort should be made to remove the tumor intact. The contralateral ovary should be carefully inspected and biopsied if anything suspicious is detected. In the scenario of a clinical stage I ovarian carcinoma, unilateral adnexectomy, omentectomy, unilateral pelvic and aortocaval lymph node sampling, peritoneal biopsies, and four-quadrant washings can be safely carried out during pregnancy, with chemotherapy reserved for those patients who are upstaged on histopathologic analysis. The chemotherapy regimen is similar to what is used for advanced disease (e.g., a platinum compound and a taxane for the epithelial cancers); however, for patients with FIGO stage Ia-Ib, grade I non–clear cell tumors, no chemotherapy will be recommended.

Malignant Germ Cell Tumors in Pregnancy

Fortunately, ovarian germ cell neoplasms in pregnancy are usually benign. Dermoid cysts are by far the most common neoplastic cysts found in pregnancy; however, malignant ovarian germ cell tumors such as the dysgerminoma, embryonal carcinoma, immature teratoma, and yolk sac tumor (formerly called "endodermal sinus tumor") have also been reported. Although a considerable number of these cancers present with early-stage disease (in both pregnant and nonpregnant patients), there are several reports of advanced cancers associated with pregnancy. Combination chemotherapy during pregnancy has been given without deleterious effects on the fetus.

The management of malignant ovarian germ cell tumors is predicated on the histologic identity of the tumor (see Figure 15-7). Patients with clinical stage Ia

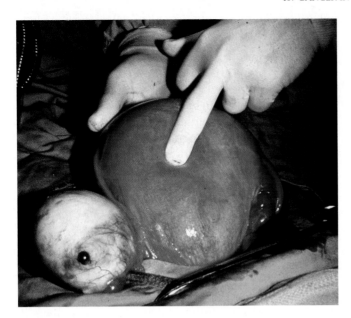

FIGURE 15-9 Immature teratoma in pregnancy.

dysgerminoma and those with clinical stage Ia-Ib grade I immature teratoma require surgical staging to determine the need for adjuvant chemotherapy (Figure 15-9). All other histologic types require adjuvant chemotherapy, and therefore unilateral adnexectomy is all that is typically accomplished at the time of laparotomy, along with removal of all gross metastatic disease. Because most malignant germ cell tumors will be unilateral (the dysgerminoma is the exception in 10% of cases), it is inappropriate to remove both ovaries. Even when the opposite side may harbor an occult dysgerminoma, it is often not necessary to remove the entire contralateral ovary. If, however, both ovaries are grossly involved by malignancy and the pregnancy is in the second trimester and thus free from hormonal support by the corpus luteum, both ovaries should be extracted. The prognosis for this stage is not improved with more extensive surgery. Chemotherapy regimens currently used for this disease comprise bleomycin, etoposide, and cisplatin. This regimen has been used safely during pregnancy.

Combined chemotherapy has improved survival markedly for malignant germ cell ovarian tumors and can permit preservation of childbearing capacity and maintenance of the existing pregnancy if the disease is stage I. If the diagnosis is made during the first or second trimester, the patient must decide whether to permit the pregnancy to continue to viability before adjuvant chemotherapy is instituted. Because these tumors characteristically grow rapidly and often recur within months when therapy is withheld, delays in initiating systemic therapy can be harmful. Indeed, the high success rate obtained with adjuvant chemotherapy has been recorded with use of this modality in the immediate postoperative period. The effect of a treatment-free interval of several months before the commencement of adjuvant chemotherapy has not been tested adequately. Thus the patient with a malignant ovarian germ cell tumor discovered early in pregnancy and in need of chemotherapy is faced with a dilemma for which no data are available. Malone and colleagues described a patient with stage Ic endodermal sinus tumor diagnosed in the 25th week of gestation who received two cycles of combination chemotherapy consisting of vinblastine, bleomycin, and cisplatin and delivered a healthy boy by cesarean section at 32 weeks of gestation. She subsequently completed three more cycles of chemotherapy and remained well at the time of Malone and colleagues' report 18 months after initial diagnosis. To our knowledge, this was the first report of a case of a patient who had endodermal sinus tumor treated with combination chemotherapy during pregnancy that apparently had a successful outcome for both mother and infant. Subsequently, we and others have had similar experiences. Therapeutic decisions for patients who have more advanced stages of these tumors are also difficult and controversial. Many such patients can be cured with early adjuvant chemotherapy after surgery. As in earlier stages, the uterus and opposite ovary can be preserved if metastatic tumor is not found in these locations. Some clinicians preserve the uterus and opposite ovary under all conditions in the hope that postoperative chemotherapy will sterilize those organs also. No long-term follow-up of this approach is available. Delays in withholding chemotherapy are not warranted, and uterine evacuation is often requested because of fear of potential teratogenic effects when chemotherapy is required during the first trimester. The subject of adjuvant chemotherapy in pregnancy is discussed later, but we emphasize that all chemotherapeutic agents are theoretically teratogenic. Although retrospective studies have not shown frequent congenital abnormalities in patients treated in the second and third trimesters, many newer agents have not been used frequently in pregnancy.

Dysgerminoma in Pregnancy

Ovarian dysgerminomas are unique among the malignant germ cell tumors because of their overall good prognosis in FIGO stage Ia treated by surgery alone. Dysgerminoma is particularly common and accounts for 30% of ovarian malignant neoplasms in pregnancy. We believe that these tumors can be managed with a unilateral adnexectomy and continuation of the pregnancy without additional therapy in FIGO stage Ia. Optimal staging should include a pelvic and periaortic lymphadenectomy on the side of the tumor mass because dysgerminomas metastasize primarily through the lymphatic system to the ipsilateral pelvic and periaortic lymph nodes. Because lymphangiography and computed tomography (CT) are contraindicated when the pregnancy is to be continued, patients who have not had adequate exploration at initial surgery should be considered for re-exploration before further therapy and continuation of the pregnancy are recommended. Appropriate diagnostic studies, including lymphangiography and CT scan of the abdomen and pelvis, may be performed in the postpartum period. A mass on scan or a suspicious lymph node on lymphangiography should be evaluated at re-exploration.

Emergency surgical intervention and obstetric complications are common in patients with dysgerminomas. Karlen and associates reviewed 27 cases of dysgerminoma associated with pregnancy. Torsion and incarceration were found commonly in this group of patients who had rapidly enlarging neoplasms averaging 25 cm in diameter. Obstetric complications occurred in nearly half the patients, and fetal demise occurred in one quarter of the reviewed cases. There were recurrences in 30% of 23 stage Ia tumors treated by unilateral oophorectomy, which calls into question the philosophy of treating these patients conservatively. The extent of exploration was not known in most cases, however, and therefore accuracy of staging cannot be assessed. This information is essential for appropriate interpretation of the findings. In our experience, lesions that are confined to one ovary have a 10% recurrence rate. Although most of these lesions recur in the first 2 years after surgery, we believe that this group of patients can continue their pregnancy safely with completion of their proper evaluation in the puerperium. Because radiation therapy and chemotherapy are successful in curing greater than 75% of patients, even those with metastatic or recurrent dysgerminoma, and because there is a low incidence of recurrence in patients with FIGO stage Ia disease, we maintain a philosophy of conservatism for the treatment of these tumors.

Sex Cord–Stromal Tumors in Pregnancy

Granulosa and Sertoli–Leydig cell tumors together account for only 2% to 3% of all ovarian neoplasms. Although granulosa cell tumors are most commonly discovered in perimenopausal or postmenopausal women, 10% to 20% are encountered during the reproductive years. Sertoli–Leydig cell tumors occur in women in the reproductive age group in 74% of cases. Of note, sex cord–stromal tumors are rarely found in pregnancy. It is critical that these entities are distinguished from ovarian decidualization, luteoma of pregnancy, or even benign granulosa cell proliferations observed with pregnancy. Typically, the sex cord–stromal ovarian tumors behave as they do in nonpregnant women, presenting with early-stage disease and having a slow, low-grade, and indolent course. Thus, because their biologic behavior is akin to that of neoplasms of low malignant potential, it

is recommended that they be managed conservatively (i.e., unilateral adnexectomy without comprehensive surgical staging) as in the young nonpregnant patient (see Figure 15-7). It is important, however, to resect all visible tumor whenever possible.

Young and colleagues reported a series of 17 granulosa cell, 13 Sertoli–Leydig cell, and 6 unclassified sex cord–stromal tumors diagnosed during pregnancy or the puerperium. Eleven patients had abdominal pain or swelling when they were first seen by a physician, 5 were in shock, 2 had virilization, and 1 had vaginal bleeding. Three asymptomatic patients underwent exploration because of palpable masses, and one underwent exploration because of an adnexal mass found on ultrasound examination. In 13 patients, the tumors were discovered during cesarean sections; 5 patients had dystocia, and the tumors were incidental findings in 8 patients. All the tumors were FIGO stage I, but 13 of the tumors had ruptured. All but 1 were unilateral. Hemoperitoneum was present in 7 cases.

Young and colleagues uncovered four major sources of difficulty in the interpretation of their series of 36 cases:

1. The young age of the patients
2. An alteration in the histologic appearance of the tumors during pregnancy
3. A decreased frequency of associated endocrine manifestations
4. Pregnancy-induced changes in other neoplastic and non-neoplastic lesions of the ovary that cause them to simulate sex cord–stromal tumors both morphologically and in terms of endocrine function

Indeed, the pregnancy-associated tumors commonly exhibited alterations related to the pregnant state that tended to obscure characteristics and familiar features that are apparent in tumors removed from nonpregnant patients. The most striking changes included intercellular edema and increased extent of luteinization in the granulosa cell tumors and of Leydig cell maturation in the Sertoli–Leydig cell tumors. It is important to note that the edema often blurred the architectural patterns of the tumors and distorted the cytologic features of the neoplastic cells. The marked luteinization and Leydig cell maturation interfered with the recognition of these cells. The end result was that these pregnancy-associated changes made identification of the tumor type more difficult.

Granulosa cell tumors are clinically estrogenic in approximately two thirds of cases, and Sertoli–Leydig cell tumors are virilizing in nearly 50% of cases. These hormonal manifestations often suggest the correct diagnosis to the gynecologist. However, during pregnancy the hyperestrogenic clinical manifestations do not appear, with none of the 17 tumors in the series by Young and colleagues associated with estrogenic manifestations. It is quite probable, however, that many of these tumors were secreting estrogens in large quantities. Furthermore, only 16% (n = 5) of the 36 sex cord–stromal tumors were associated with clinical evidence of excess androgens (virilization in 4 cases, and hirsutism in only 1 case). This low frequency may have been the result of the placenta's ability to aromatize androgens produced by the tumor. In fact, one of the masculinizing tumors was the largest in their series (32 cm in maximal diameter) and may have been secreting androgens in such great abundance that the aromatizing capacity of the placenta was exceeded.

Several other types of ovarian neoplasms and non-neoplastic disorders are more frequently associated with virilization during pregnancy than Sertoli–Leydig cell tumors. Tumors with functioning, proliferative ovarian stroma such as the Krukenberg and the mucinous cystic tumors may be confused morphologically with sex cord–stromal tumors. Other primary ovarian tumors that can cause virilization include luteinized thecomas and Leydig and lipid cell tumors. Finally, as described earlier, two non-neoplastic lesions of the ovary that develop during pregnancy and can be associated with virilization include the luteoma of pregnancy and the hyperreactio luteinalis (multiple luteinized follicle cysts). All these virilizing tumors and lesions must be considered in the differential diagnosis when confronted with virilization of the pregnant mother, so as to not make an erroneous clinical diagnosis of a sex cord–stromal tumor.

With one exception, the patients in the study by Young and colleagues were initially treated by conservative surgical procedures. Two of them received chemotherapy and two received radiation therapy postoperatively. Hysterectomies and salpingo-oophorectomies were performed as second operations in 8 cases; no residual tumor was found in any of these specimens. Only 1 patient had a recurrence, which was treated surgically. Follow-up for the average of 4.7 years was available for 30 of the 36 patients; all of them were free of disease at their last examination. Adjuvant therapy has not been demonstrated to improve the outcome in this group of patients and is not recommended during pregnancy.

Chemotherapy for Nonepithelial Ovarian Cancer During Pregnancy

A recent literature review by Azim and colleagues identified 18 cases of nonepithelial ovarian malignancies treated with systemic chemotherapy during pregnancy. Most patients had a yolk sac tumor (n = 10) and were treated after the first trimester with the bleomycin, etoposide, and cisplatin (BEP) regimen or the cisplatin, vinblastine, and bleomycin (PVB) regimen. Other histologies

reported included 3 cases of dysgerminoma, 3 cases of immature teratoma, 1 mixed germ cell tumor, and 1 Sertoli–Leydig tumor. Fifteen of the 18 women completed their pregnancy without complications; there was 1 case of premature delivery following maternal dehydration at 28 weeks after BEP, 1 case of pregnancy-induced hypertension after three cycles of BEP, and a third patient developed oligohydramnios after three cycles of etoposide-platinum. Postnatal chemotherapy-induced adverse events were restricted to one baby who developed minor anemia and transient respiratory distress at delivery at the 35th week of gestation. This baby had been exposed to three cycles of carboplatin plus paclitaxel for a maternal dysgerminoma and the condition resolved quickly and the authors reported normal development at 20 months of follow-up.

Epithelial Ovarian Cancer in Pregnancy

Very few series of malignant ovarian carcinomas in pregnancy have been published. Reported in 2002, the most recent series contains nine ovarian cancers concurrent with pregnancy from Libya and Saudi Arabia. Among these cases were included seven epithelial cancers (four serous, two mucinous, one undifferentiated), one dysgerminoma, and one granulosa cell tumor. As expected, the latter two lesions occurred in younger women, aged 18 and 21 years, respectively. All seven women with epithelial cancers were multiparous (range 3-10), which is of some interest given the epidemiologic data suggesting increasing parity to be inversely related to the risk of developing ovarian carcinoma. Four patients with FIGO stage Ia tumors, including two with epithelial lesions, underwent unilateral adnexectomy prior to 25 weeks of gestation. None of the patients with more advanced disease who went on to receive chemotherapy did so during pregnancy. The obstetric outcome was favorable for all patients except for one with a FIGO stage Ia serous cystadenocarcinoma whose infant died from complications of meconium aspiration. It is of sufficient interest that five of the epithelial tumors were early stage (three FIGO stage Ia and two FIGO stage Ic) and one was assigned FIGO stage IIa. The only death occurred in a patient with a FIGO stage III undifferentiated carcinoma. Thus fully six of seven women with epithelial ovarian cancers were diagnosed with early or locally advanced disease only, which does not reflect what is typically observed in the general population. It is quite certain that antenatal care including serial physical examinations and ultrasonography contributed to these early pick-ups.

Once the diagnosis of ovarian carcinoma is made during pregnancy, appropriate therapy should not be withheld (see Figure 15-7). In those patients who present with metastatic disease manifest as malignant ascites and carcinomatosis, surgical exploration is warranted, with an attempt to remove as much of the tumor burden as is feasible. Depending on the degree of tumor involvement of the uterus and the mother's desire for the pregnancy, uterine preservation may be considered, and if so the "hands-off" approach to the uterus, and removal of mobile intraperitoneal deposits, can be attempted. Certainly, the typical aggressive cytoreductive approach (e.g., bowel resection, splenectomy) taken in nonpregnant women with advanced-stage ovarian carcinoma can result in significant morbidity, and if the pregnancy is to be continued, we advise against this approach unless the patient has presented with a bowel obstruction.

An untested option in this group of patients is measurement of the serum CA-125 and aspiration of ascites fluid under ultrasound guidance for cytologic analysis. Once malignancy is confirmed and considered likely to be of ovarian origin, systemic chemotherapy during the second and third trimesters in a "neoadjuvant" fashion can be considered, with plans for interval cytoreductive surgery following delivery. The standard regimen for metastatic epithelial ovarian cancer in nonpregnant patients includes platinum-based chemotherapy. Regimens containing cisplatin alone and cisplatin plus paclitaxel, and even administration of a full six cycles of carboplatin and paclitaxel (the current standard among nonpregnant women), have been used during the second and third trimesters of pregnancy. Because there does not appear to be any significant risk to the fetus when these drugs are used in the second and third trimesters, pregnant patients diagnosed during these periods should be offered the opportunity to receive platinum-based therapy without terminating their pregnancy. Postpartum, the patient may return to the operating room to undergo definitive surgical staging or comprehensive tumor debulking.

Patients remote from term (e.g., during the first trimester) with metastatic disease should be advised to undergo hysterectomy with the fetus in situ in conjunction with tumor debulking. Because the prognosis for women with advanced carcinoma is poor, patients must be counseled regarding the realities of how much time they would have with their child when making decisions regarding pregnancy termination.

It should be noted that there are at least two reports of an advanced-stage epithelial carcinoma of the ovary in which the uterus and pregnancy were preserved at 15 and 20 weeks of gestation. Patients were treated with six cycles of single-agent cisplatin or four courses of carboplatin plus paclitaxel followed by cesarean section and completion hysterectomy. One patient was disease free at a short follow-up of 6 months, whereas the other recurred in the pelvis at 24 months following delivery. This second patient underwent secondary cytoreduction and was re-treated with platinum-based therapy and has remained disease free at 42 months. Although some have advocated sparing the uterus if it appears to be uninvolved and the pregnancy is remote from term, this approach should be used with extreme caution when dealing with advanced-stage epithelial ovarian cancer for which the outcome remains exceedingly poor irrespective of pregnancy status.

Chemotherapy for Epithelial Ovarian Cancer During Pregnancy

Azim and colleagues have collected 20 patients from the literature who were treated with chemotherapy during pregnancy for epithelial ovarian cancer. The histologic subtypes included serous ($n = 13$), mucinous ($n = 3$), endometrioid ($n = 2$), clear cell ($n = 1$), and undifferentiated ($n = 1$). The chemotherapy regimens used included cyclophosphamide plus cisplatin ($n = 5$); single-agent cisplatin ($n = 4$); single-agent carboplatin ($n = 3$); paclitaxel plus carboplatin ($n = 2$); and cyclophosphamide, doxorubicin, and cisplatin ($n = 2$). There also was one case each of the use of the following regimens: cisplatin plus paclitaxel, cisplatin plus docetaxel, carboplatin plus cyclophosphamide, and single-agent paclitaxel. Seventeen of the patients received their first cycle during the second trimester and three in the third trimester. Sixteen patients delivered at week 34 or after, and 16 had experienced no pregnancy-related complications. There was 1 case each of intrauterine growth restriction, premature rupture of the membranes, and pre-eclampsia. Nineteen fetuses had a normal outcome, with 9 of these children reported to be normal at 1 year or greater follow-up. There was one neonatal death from multiorgan failure in a baby with congenital anomalies identified before starting cisplatin plus docetaxel at week 20.

Intravenous carboplatin plus paclitaxel is the most commonly used regimen for epithelial ovarian cancer. Although use of platinum derivatives appears to be feasible during the second and third trimesters, their administration does raise concern regarding the transplacental transfer of these drugs in late pregnancy, and the short- and long-term effects have not been well-studied. Intraperitoneal chemotherapy in combination with intravenous chemotherapy has been associated with higher survival rates for patients with epithelial ovarian cancer. In patients opting for this type of therapy, delivery should be induced as soon as fetal pulmonary maturation can be documented before starting intraperitoneal therapy. Catheters can be placed at the time of cesarean section or laparoscopically in the postpartum period if the pregnancy was delivered vaginally.

A recent trial by the Gynecologic Oncology Group demonstrated an improvement in progression-free survival among patients treated with intravenous carboplatin plus paclitaxel and the anti-angiogenesis agent bevacizumab. To date there are no reports of use of bevacizumab in pregnancy and we cannot comment on its potential for maternal, fetal, and neonatal effects.

Other Types of Malignant Ovarian Tumors

Some ovarian cancers are particularly aggressive and chemotherapy should be started immediately upon diagnosis. These include small cell ovarian cancer and metastatic Krukenberg tumors. The only long-term survivor of an advanced-stage small cell ovarian cancer was reported by Tewari and colleagues, who described a patient diagnosed with the disease during pregnancy. Once the histology was confirmed the patient returned to the operating room in the second trimester and underwent cytoreductive surgery with the fetus in situ and postoperatively was treated with a six-drug regimen that contained both epithelial-cell and germ-cell activity. Another patient diagnosed with small cell ovarian cancer with hypercalcemia underwent conservative surgery during pregnancy followed by chemotherapy and died of disease 10 months after diagnosis. Taylor and colleagues reported the surgical removal of a Krukenberg tumor at 15 weeks of gestation followed by treatment with 10 cycles of 5-fluorouracil, folinic acid, and irinotecan every 2 weeks until the 36th week of pregnancy. The neonate was born without complications and at age 4 months showed normal development.

Summary of the Adnexal Mass and Ovarian Cancer in Pregnancy

The problem of an adnexal mass in pregnancy is simple. One must have a high index of suspicion for malignancy, make the diagnosis early, and treat promptly. The difficulty arises when both patient and physician resist abdominal exploration during pregnancy because of fear of precipitating fetal wastage. However, the potential danger to the mother far exceeds the imagined danger to the child. Most of the difficulties seen with ovarian tumors are those of omission rather than of commission. The probability of ovarian cancer must be kept foremost in the minds of physicians caring for these patients. At laparotomy, most malignant ovarian tumors apparently confined to one ovary will require complete surgical staging. A technique of "hands off the uterus," whenever possible, appears to reduce postoperative uterine contractions.

Breast Cancer

Pregnancy-associated breast cancer (PABC) is defined as breast cancer diagnosed during pregnancy or lactation up to 12 months postpartum. The disease is a disaster for all involved. Both patient and physician find it difficult to accept this dreaded disease in a healthy young pregnant woman. Because breast cancer is rare in women younger than 35 years, this problem, fortunately, is a rare complication of pregnancy, with an incidence of approximately 1 case for every 3000 deliveries. Conversely, of all patients with breast cancer, 1% to 2% are pregnant at the time of diagnosis. PABC provides a challenging scenario for the mother and oncologist. It is the second most common malignancy to complicate pregnancy, but, unlike cervical cancer, it is not screened for during pregnancy, and because delays in diagnosis are common and the diagnosis itself is elusive, often patients are diagnosed with advanced tumors for which prognosis is poor. Furthermore, the management of breast cancer often involves a coordination of surgery, radiotherapy, chemotherapy, and even hormonal therapy, all of which may affect the pregnancy. Finally, there are several distinct hormonal issues related to pregnancy that may have an influence on the course of breast cancer.

In a population-based cohort study using data from Swedish registries from 1963 to 2002 encompassing women aged 15 to 44 years at the date of breast cancer diagnosis, Andersson and colleagues noted that the incidence of PABC increased from 16.0 to 37.4 per 100,000 deliveries comparing the first and last calendar periods under study. The authors attributed the increasing incidence in Sweden partly to the trend of postponement of childbearing to an older age.

Historically, PABC has been associated with a poor prognosis, with accounts from the 19th century describing exceedingly rapid growth and a malignant course. In 1943 Haagensen and Stout reinforced this feeling of doom when they decided that the outcome for this group of patients was so poor that they recommended surgical treatment not be offered. Contemporary opinion for the most part maintains the dismal prognosis associated with PABC. It must be acknowledged that the literature comprises mainly single-institution retrospective experiences and case reports. The only series containing greater than 100 patients are four in number (White, Bunker and Peters, Ribeiro and Palmer, Clark and Reid), none of which were published after 1978.

Although the overall survival rate for breast cancer is greater than 60%, the overall survival rate in pregnancy is reported by some to have dropped to 15% or 20%. Pregnant patients tend to have a higher incidence of positive axillary lymph nodes. Locoregional spread of the tumor portends a poor prognosis and in all likelihood suggests that the neoplasm has metastasized at the time of the initiation of therapy. The advanced stage of the presentation of disease in the pregnant patient has been attributed to multiple factors. First, the engorged breast can successfully obscure a lesion for a much longer period. Survivals are lower for cases diagnosed late in pregnancy than for those recognized in the first trimester. Others emphasize the 30 to 50 multiples of increase in serum levels of estrogens and progesterone. In addition, there may be increased vascularity and lymphatic drainage from the pregnant breast, assisting the metastatic process to regional lymph nodes. If a lesion is detected early (present <3 months, smaller than 2 cm, and no positive nodes), the chance of survival (70% to 80%) is the same for the pregnant and the nonpregnant patient. If, however, there is involvement of the subareolar region; diffuse inflammatory carcinoma; edema or ulceration of the skin; fixation of the tumor to the breast wall; or involvement of the high axillary, supraclavicular, or internal mammary nodes, the prognosis is poor for the pregnant and the nonpregnant patient both.

Presentation

At least 10% of patients with breast cancer who are younger than 40 years will be pregnant at diagnosis. PABC typically presents as a painless mass or thickening. In some cases, there may be an associated nipple discharge, and in the lactating breast the infant may exhibit the "milk rejection sign," effectively refusing the breast that contains the cancer. The mean breast weight normally doubles in pregnancy from 200 to 400 grams, resulting in breast firmness and increased breast density. Mammographic evaluation of the pregnant breast is difficult to interpret, and the clinical examination may be deceptive. This has profound implications in terms of delays in diagnosis and treatment, which, as discussed earlier, are not uncommon in PABC. Many patients with PABC will have a delay in diagnosis ranging from 1 to 2.5 months during pregnancy and up to 6 months during lactation. In a 1991 series from the Memorial Sloan-Kettering Cancer Center in New York, 44 of 56 patients did not have the diagnosis of cancer made until the postpartum period. Overall, in a review of the literature by Puckridge and colleagues, a delay of 2 to 15 months longer from manifestation of the first symptoms to the diagnosis of cancer occurs in PABC. Given the tumor-doubling time of 130 days, a 1-month delay in primary tumor treatment increases the risk of axillary metastases by 0.9%, and a 6-month delay increases the risk by 5.1%. For this reason particularly, PABC has been considered an ominous diagnosis, but when age and stage are taken into account, there is no difference in the survival of PABC cases compared with non-PABC cases. Pregnancy is not thought to be an independent risk factor.

Evaluation

A proposed management algorithm for PABC appears in Figure 15-10. Early diagnosis has been associated with improved survivals and relies on the liberal use of imaging strategies and the core and fine-needle biopsy techniques for this group of patients. Mammography in conjunction with abdominal lead shielding can be safely used during pregnancy but, as discussed earlier, the engorged and lactating breast increases tissue density and may mask abnormalities. Ultrasonography yields equivalent information with no known adverse effects to the fetus. Fine-needle aspiration may be difficult to interpret cytologically secondary to cellular changes that take place during pregnancy and lactation and is often associated with an increase in the false-negative rate. Core biopsy remains the gold standard in making the diagnosis. When necessary, an open biopsy under local anesthesia is also appropriate. Stopping lactation with ice packs and breast binding or bromocriptine (2.5 mg three times daily for 1 week) beforehand will reduce the risk of a milk fistula. The breasts should be emptied of milk before the biopsy, and a pressure dressing will decrease the risk of hematoma that may develop from the hypervascularity of the pregnant breast.

Approximately 75% to 90% of PABCs are ductal carcinomas, mirroring what is observed in the nonpregnant population. Historically, there was a perceived increase in inflammatory carcinoma of the breast during pregnancy; however, this has since been refuted in contemporary series, in which the incidence ranges from 1.5% to 4.2% among pregnant and nonpregnant patients. Several studies have demonstrated adverse pathologic features in PABC. Most patients with PABC have estrogen receptor (ER)–negative and progesterone receptor (PR)–negative tumors. This may be a result of the production of false-negative results by the ligand-binding assay used for ER and PR when high circulating levels of estrogen and progesterone downregulate receptors. Immunohistochemistry has not been able to detect a difference in the number of hormone receptor–positive tumors when PABC cases are compared with cases of breast cancer in nonpregnant patients of similar ages. Additionally, higher levels of c-ERBB-2 overexpression and p53 mutations have been reported in lactational carcinomas but not in tumors diagnosed during pregnancy. Furthermore, there have been reports of increased HER-2/neu–positive tumors compared with nonpregnant control subjects. It is interesting that the HER-2/neu oncogene product p105 is overexpressed not only in ductal carcinomas but also in fetal epithelial cells and the placenta and that toward the end of the third trimester of pregnancy, serum levels of p105 normally rise.

It is known from epidemiologic studies that there is an increased incidence of breast cancers in certain families; the risk increases 5 to 10 times if a patient's mother or sister has had the disease. It is interesting that women with a genetic predisposition to breast cancer may be overrepresented among cases of PABC, with a significant family history of breast cancer being three times more common in women with PABC than among nonpregnant patients with breast cancer. Along these lines, PABC has been associated with a higher rate of BRCA2 allelic mutation compared with sporadic breast cancer.

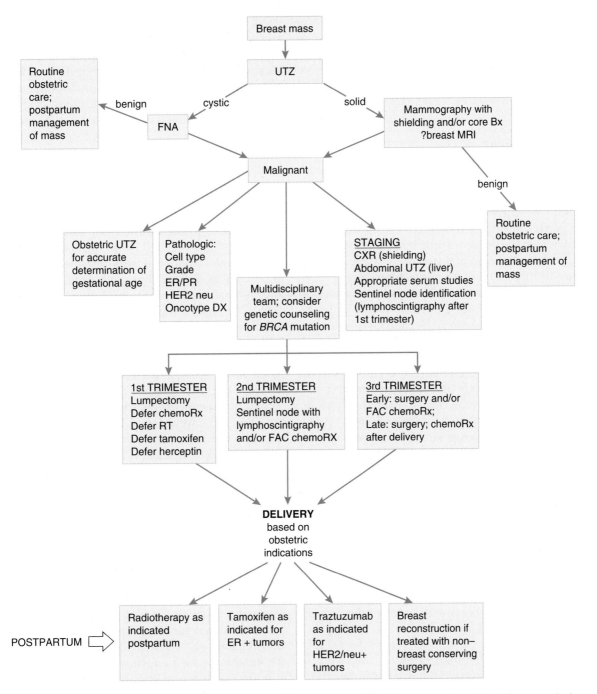

FIGURE 15-10 Management algorithm for pregnancy-associated breast cancer. *ER,* Estrogen receptor; *FAC,* 5-fluorouracil, doxorubicin (Adriamycin), and cyclophosphamide; *FNA,* fine-needle aspiration; *UTZ,* ultrasound.

Indeed, a Swedish report of 292 women with breast cancer before the age of 40 demonstrated a greater likelihood of known *BRCA1* and *BRCA2* carriers to develop cancer during pregnancy.

Staging of breast cancer currently uses a complicated system jointly recommended by the International Union Against Cancer and the American Joint Committee on Cancer (AJCC) (see Table 14-12). The Haagensen clinical staging for breast cancer is more useful in pointing out the unfavorable prognostic indicators in this disease process. Lateral and posteroanterior chest radiographs in conjunction with lead shielding are considered safe during pregnancy, with an estimated fetal dose of only 0.6 mGy. Provided a catheter is placed to allow rapid drainage of radioactive material from the bladder, a low-dose labeled technetium-99 bone scan is also safe. The low-dose bone scan exposes the fetus to 0.0008 Gy instead of the standard 0.0019 Gy. The higher radiation exposure to the fetus excludes the use of CT in planning a metastatic workup, but MRI may be used to study the thorax and abdomen and to image the skeleton. MRI is preferred to ultrasonography for hepatic imaging and is also the safest and most sensitive way to study the brain.

Surgical Management

Surgery is the definitive treatment for PABC (see Figure 15-10). The extent of surgery in the treatment of breast cancer is being debated throughout the world, and that issue cannot be adequately addressed here. Lumpectomy or partial mastectomy is more commonly used, especially when the lesion is not large, although the preferred surgical treatment for stage I, stage II, and some stage III tumors involves mastectomy, thus avoiding the need for adjuvant radiotherapy in most cases (i.e., early-stage breast cancer). Because nodal metastases are commonly identified in PABC, and because nodal status dictates the choice of adjuvant chemotherapy, axillary dissection has been routinely recommended, especially in light of the potential risk to the fetus from radioisotope if sentinel node biopsy was attempted.

The timing of surgery for cancer diagnosed late in pregnancy is another source of debate. Some reports suggest that patients treated postpartum survive longer than those treated in the second and third trimesters. This suggests that postponement of therapy for patients near term may be of benefit. These reports fail to consider the possibility that patients selected for postponed treatment might have been those with small, more favorable cancers discovered late in pregnancy, whereas larger, aggressive, anaplastic cancers with rapid progression received immediate treatment. If such treatment bias exists, prompt treatment would not be expected to correlate with good results, and treatment after delivery would appear favorable because of a preponderance of favorable patients in that group.

Sentinel Lymph Node Identification

Keleher and colleagues assessed the risk to the embryo/fetus associated with sentinel lymph node (SLN) biopsy and lymphoscintigraphy of the breast in pregnant patients. Following peritumoral injection of 92.5 MBq (2.5 mCi) of filtered ^{99m}Tc sulfur colloid the day before surgery in two nonpregnant women with breast cancer, they calculated the absorbed dose to the embryo/fetus for three theoretic extreme scenarios of biodistribution and pharmacokinetics and described the maximum absorbed dose to the fetus being 4.3 mGy calculated for the worst-case scenario. The authors concluded that breast lymphoscintigraphy during pregnancy presents a very low risk to the embryo/fetus. In 2008 Khera and colleagues searched a prospectively accrued breast database for cases of SLN biopsy in patients with PABC and identified 10 patients. The mean gestational age at the time of biopsy was 15.8 weeks. All patients were successfully mapped, and a positive SLN was identified in 5 patients (50%). Nine patients (90%) delivered healthy babies without reported complications, and 1 patient elected to terminate the pregnancy in the first trimester to start chemotherapy. The authors concluded that SLN biopsy can be safely performed in pregnancy with minimal risk to the fetus.

Spanheimer and colleagues measured abdominal, perineal, and urinary radiation in 14 women with breast cancer and total uterine doses were calculated. The average dose to the uterus from bladder radioactivity determined from voided urine was 0.44 ± 0.44 microGy. The average radiation dose to the uterus of 1.14 ± 0.76 microGy was derived through an average of abdominal and perineal doses plus contribution from the bladder dose. One patient was 16 weeks pregnant at the time of SLN biopsy and the total calculated uterine dose was 1.67 microGy, suggesting that pregnancy does not significantly alter measured uterine radiation. When compared with average background radiation (i.e., 3,000 microGy per year or 8.2 microGy per day), it was concluded that the measured uterine dose of radiation from lymphoscintigraphy for SLN biopsy was significantly less than the average daily background radiation.

In a recent report by Gentilni and colleagues, 12 patients with PABC received low-dose (10 MBq on average) lymphoscintigraphy using ^{99m}Tc human serum albumin nanocolloids. The SLN was identified in all patients. In 10 patients, the SLN was pathologically negative. One patient had a micrometastasis in an SLN, and another who had a metastasis in the SLN underwent axillary clearance. Eleven healthy babies were born with no malformations and appropriate birth weight. One baby who underwent lymphatic mapping during the 26th week of gestation was operated on at the age of 3 months for a ventricular septal defect and at 43 months was in good health. The malformation was suspected at the anatomy scan performed during the 21st week of gestation, well before lymphoscintigraphy. At a median follow-up of 32 months, no overt axillary recurrence appeared in the patients with negative SLNs. This experience, together with those described earlier, supports the safety and efficacy of SLN identification in women with PABC when performed with a low-dose lymphoscintigraphic technique.

Breast Reconstruction

Although the performance of a transverse myocutaneous flap of the rectus abdominis muscle (TRAM flap) is a satisfying, one-step, immediate reconstruction of good aesthetic quality without need for prosthetic materials, this is not recommended in patients with PABC who undergo mastectomy. The procedure should be deferred to the postpartum period. The problem of residual functional capacities of the abdominal wall deprived of a part or of all its rectus muscle also has important implications for future pregnancies. In fact, for some authors in the past, the desire for future childbearing was a contraindication to TRAM flap breast reconstruction because it was thought that the abdominal wall, weakened by rotation of one or both of its rectus muscles, would not be capable of withstanding the stress induced by pregnancy. To avoid the development of a hernia in the abdominal wall at the donor site, an interval of at least 12 months between breast reconstruction with a TRAM flap and pregnancy is recommended.

Adjuvant Therapy

Women with early lesions may opt for a tissue-sparing procedure. In these cases, local irradiation is often required. Radiotherapy to the breast, chest wall, or axillary lymph nodes, even with shielding, results in a significant fetal dose because of scatter in excess of that which is considered safe. The doses of internal scatter of radiation have been calculated. At 12 weeks of gestation, the fetus would receive 10 to 15 cGy. In the third trimester, this dose can be as high as 200 cGy. This is because, although during the first trimester the fetus is in a safer position and can be better shielded, it is more sensitive to the effects of radiation. In contrast, as the fetus enlarges and is less sensitive to radiation, it moves upward out of the pelvis, where it is less readily shielded and exposed to higher levels of ionizing radiation. Local irradiation should be deferred until after delivery of the fetus (see Figure 15-10). Women treated with adjuvant radiation during the postpartum period will not be able to lactate from the irradiated breast.

Locally advanced disease is difficult to manage with the pregnancy in place. Chemotherapy or local radiotherapy, followed in 6 weeks by mastectomy, is the usual treatment plan for these lesions. For advanced disease, chemotherapy has been used after the first trimester when the mother is reluctant to terminate the pregnancy and the disease appears to be progressing at an alarming rate. The issue of whether chemotherapy should be administered to patients with node-positive breast cancer in pregnancy is complicated by reports suggesting that both single-agent and combination chemotherapy may significantly improve survival in premenopausal patients in an adjuvant setting. Follow-ups of 10 and 15 years are always necessary in breast cancer, but it would appear that the premenopausal patient is the best candidate for aggressive adjuvant chemotherapy and a resulting improved survival rate. This is especially pertinent to patients in whom positive nodes are discovered at the time of the initial procedure.

Table 15-8 contains reports of chemotherapy use during pregnancy, with favorable neonatal outcomes noted when treatment was administered only after the first trimester.

In a recent review by Azim and colleagues, the authors identified 56 different reports that have described the systemic treatment of PABC and separated them into four groups, as described in the following discussion.

TABLE 15-8 Congenital Anomalies After in Utero Exposure to Breast Cancer Chemotherapy

Authors	Year	n	Treatment	Trimester	Outcome
Tobias and Bloom	1980	1	AV, prednisone	2	No anomaly
Murray et al	1984	1	AC, radiation	1	Imperforate anus, rectovaginal fistula
Mulvihill et al	1987	1	CMF, melphalan	n/s	Spontaneous abortion
Zemlickis et al	1992	2	CMF, melphalan (both cases)	1	Spontaneous abortion
		1	CAFV, tamoxifen	1	No anomaly
		1	CAF, tamoxifen	3	No anomaly
		1	CMF	3	No anomaly
Cullins et al.	1980	1	Tamoxifen	1, 2, 3	Goldenhar syndrome
Tewari et al	1997	1	Tamoxifen	1, 2	Ambiguous genitalia
Turchi and Villasis	1988	1	CAMF	1	No anomaly
Berry et al	1999	24	CAF	2, 3	No anomaly
Isaacs et al	2001	1	Tamoxifen, 0.0017 Gy RT	1, 2, 3	Preauricular skin tags
Andreadis et al	2004	1	FEC,* 28 Gy RT,† tamoxifen,‡ zoledronic acid‡	1, 2, 3	No anomalies
Gonzalez-Angulo et al	2004	1	Neoadjuvant paclitaxel	2, 3	No anomalies
Warraich and Smith	2009	1	T, tamoxifen	1 ,2, 3	Pulm hypoplasia
Baele et al	2009	1	T, tamoxifen	1, 2	Resp failure
Azim Jr et al	2009	1	T	Preconcep	No anomaly

Modified from Woo et al: Arch Surg 138:91, 2003.

A, *Doxorubicin (Adriamycin); C, cyclophosphamide; E, epirubicin; F, 5-fluorouracil; M, methotrexate; T, trastuzumab; n/s, not specified; RT, radiotherapy; V, vincristine.*
First trimester only.
†*Second trimester.*
‡*Second and third trimesters.*

Neoadjuvant/Adjuvant Chemotherapy for PABC

The FAC regimen (5-fluorouracil, doxorubicin, and cyclophosphamide) is the most commonly administered regimen in the neoadjuvant/adjuvant setting. The safety of this regimen was prospectively examined by Hahn and colleagues at the MD Anderson Hospital and Tumor Institute in Houston. Fifty-seven patients were treated, and the regimen was well tolerated and did not adversely affect the pregnancy. All women had live births, with three congenital defects reported, including Down syndrome, clubfoot, and congenital bilateral ureteral reflux. The investigators did not consider these anomalies to have resulted directly from chemotherapy exposure when the incidences were compared to those in the general population. Eighteen of the children have been followed until school age, and only two required special attention schools (including the child with Down syndrome).

Peccatori and colleagues from the European institute of oncology in Milan prospectively evaluated the safety of weekly epirubicin (35 mg/m^2) starting in the second trimester in 20 women with PABC. The schedule was selected to potentially allow lower-peak plasma concentration of the drug, thus lowering the risk of maternal myelotoxicity and possible placental transfer of the drug. There were no grade III/IV toxicities and only one congenital anomaly (polycystic kidney). All children have had normal development at 2 years median follow-up.

Based on these two studies and other retrospective series and case reports from the literature, Azim and colleagues suggested that anthracycline-based regimens are probably safe starting in the second trimester. FAC is the most commonly studied regimen, but offering epirubicin instead of doxorubicin is an option.

In recent years, taxanes have been incorporated into the adjuvant and neoadjuvant settings to improve outcomes. There have been seven reports of docetaxel treatment and two reports of paclitaxel therapy for PABC. In six of these cases, the taxane was given as a single agent. None of the nine cases were associated with a poor obstetric or fetal outcome. Although the experience using taxanes in PABC is clearly limited, this early evidence is reassuring.

The CMF regimen (cyclophosphamide, methotrexate, 5-fluorouracil) has been used for many years as standard adjuvant therapy in breast cancer. As a result of the potential for teratogenicity by methotrexate (after first-trimester exposure), this regimen is not recommended for PABC.

Chemotherapy for Metastatic Breast Cancer

In contrast to early PABC for which neoadjuvant/adjuvant therapy is administered in a good prognosis setting, patients with metastatic disease have fewer options because treatment of the mother must take priority, especially in pregnancies remote from term. Anthracyclines remain the most studied agents for management of metastatic breast cancer, but data are extremely limited in PABC. Patients with bone metastases are frequently treated with bisphosphonates to decrease the risk of skeletal events. There has been some concern for the development of genital and skeletal defects with bisphosphonate use in pregnancy. In addition, the potential for hypocalcemia exists with bisphosphonate therapy, which may lead to stimulation of uterine contractions. There has been very limited experience in PABC, but no adverse events associated with bisphosphonate use have been reported. Among 21 pregnant women exposed to bisphosphonates for osteoporosis during the first trimester, there were no adverse events for the fetus or to the conduct of the pregnancy.

HER2/Neu Targeted Agents in Pregnancy

Trastuzumab and lapatinib are two HER2/neu targeted agents that have been used increasingly in recent years for the management of breast cancer. Azim and colleagues identified 13 cases of trastuzumab use for PABC and 1 report of lapatinib therapy for a patient with metastatic breast cancer who inadvertently became pregnant during therapy. For this patient, lapatinib was discontinued at 11 weeks of gestation and the pregnancy continued with normal outcome.

For the 13 patients exposed to trastuzumab, only 1 patient elected to undergo therapeutic abortion. Eight patients received the drug as a single agent, while others were treated in combination with taxanes, vinorelbine, or tamoxifen. Metastatic disease was the setting for 3 patients, and 7 patients received the drug during the preconception period and the first trimester. There were 5 cases of anhydramnios, 1 case of oligohydramnios, 1 case of intrauterine growth restriction, and 1 case of preterm premature rupture of the membranes. Four neonatal deaths were reported secondary to respiratory and renal failure. Three additional babies developed transient respiratory and/or renal failure but recovered. None of the reports described any fetal or maternal serious cardiac events despite the pivotal role of HER2/neu in cardiogenesis and cardiac repair pathways.

The increased risk of oligo/anhydramnios is thought to result from the effect of trastuzumab on the fetal renal epithelium in which HER2/neu is strongly expressed. Some have correlated the effect of trastuzumab to an inhibition of the vascular endothelial growth factor (VEGF), which regulates the production and reabsorption of amniotic fluid. Prolonged exposure to trastuzumab was consistently associated with serious adverse events both on the pregnancy and on the fetus in these cases. Azim and colleagues have advised that in the case of accidental pregnancy, the drug should be discontinued and the patient should be counseled that brief exposure to the drug is unlikely to be detrimental to the fetus and pregnancy. Elective administration of trastuzumab during pregnancy is not advisable.

Hormonal Treatments for PABC

Preclinical models have shown that in utero exposure to tamoxifen increases the incidence of genital abnormalities. Tewari and colleagues reported the first case of fetal teratogenicity developing from maternal exposure to tamoxifen. The drug was discontinued at 20 weeks of gestation, but the fetus developed ambiguous genitalia with labial fusion and clitoralmegaly. A second case has been reported in which tamoxifen was stopped at 26 weeks of gestation and the fetus developed Goldenhar syndrome. A third patient had the drug discontinued during the first trimester and the pregnancy outcome was normal, and at 27 months follow-up the baby's development was without sequela. The literature contains only one patient who elected to receive tamoxifen as a therapeutic intervention for metastatic PABC, and the pregnancy resulted in a normal baby. There are also two cases in which tamoxifen was administered in conjunction with trastuzumab, and pregnancy was accidentally discovered at 20 weeks of gestational age. In both cases, fetal mortality was reported, but this was likely secondary to trastuzumab exposure. Finally, normal outcomes have been reported in two cases in which tamoxifen was given together with FAC and with CMF plus vincristine.

As with trastuzumab, we recommend active contraception use during tamoxifen therapy, and in those cases in which pregnancy inadvertently occurs, the drug should be discontinued. Although 85 pregnancies with normal fetal outcomes are contained in a tamoxifen chemoprevention study, women should be counseled regarding the possibility of genital or more complex malformations associated with in utero exposure to this drug.

Prognosis of PABC

Thirty-two women with PABC referred to two European Union oncology centers between 1995 and 2007 were analyzed by Halaska and colleagues. Sixteen cases were diagnosed during pregnancy, and 16 were diagnosed within 1 year after delivery. The investigators matched each patient for age at diagnosis, tumor size, and stage to a control group of 32 nonpregnant patients. Overall survival was similar in the PABC and non-PABC patients ($P = 0.449$). The subgroup of patients with PABC diagnosed within 1 year after delivery showed a shorter time to relapse than controls or patients in whom PABC was diagnosed during pregnancy ($P = 0.0178$). Such findings concerning poorer prognosis among postpartum

diagnoses had not been identified in previous series and warrant continued attention.

Cardonic and Iacobucci analyzed the maternal and fetal outcomes of 130 women with PABC that were reported to the voluntary Cancer and Pregnancy Registry and followed prospectively. Among the 130 patients, 120 were diagnosed with a primary tumor, 8 with recurrent disease, and 2 with a new primary malignancy. The mean maternal age at diagnosis was 34.8 years and the mean gestational age at diagnosis was 13.2 weeks. For 113 women who were followed for a mean of 3.14 years, recurrence was reported in 30 women at a mean of 16.2 months from delivery. Twenty-one patients are deceased at a mean interval of 24.71 months from delivery to death. Only 42% were diagnosed with an ER-positive tumor, and 35% of cases had PR-positive disease. Human epidermal growth factor receptor 2 was positive in 25% of patients. Survival by stage for a primary diagnosis in pregnancy included: stage I, 100%; stage II, 86%; stage III, 86%; and stage IV, 0%. These survival rates are similar to what is observed in the nonpregnant breast cancer population.

A very large study was conducted by Rodriguez and colleagues evaluating 797 PBAC cases identified by linking the California Cancer Registry (1991-1997) with the California Patient Discharge Data Set; 4177 age-matched, non-PBAC breast cancer controls were also identified. PABC cases were significantly more likely to have more advanced-stage, larger primary tumor, hormone receptor–negative tumor, and mastectomy as a component of their treatment. In survival analysis, PABC had a higher death rate than non-PABC (39.2% vs 33.4%, $P = 0.002$). In multivariable analysis, advancing stage, African-American ethnicity (68% increased risk over non-Hispanic whites), hormone receptor–negative tumors (20% increased risk), and pregnancy (14% increased risk) were all significant predictors of death.

Lactation

Whether breast feeding is safe or possible has also been debated. Many have postulated that breast cancer is at least in part of viral origin, and the possibility exists that the contralateral breast will be contaminated with the causative agent, which will be passed to the fetus. This theory has never been borne out in fact, but most surgeons recommend artificial feeding of the infant, ostensibly to avoid vascular enrichment in the opposite breast, which may also contain a neoplasm.

Reports by Higgins and Haffty and by Tralins suggest that successful lactation in the breast treated by lumpectomy and irradiation is possible. Apparently, the location of the breast incision is important. It is not surprising that circumareolar incisions were associated with diminished ability to lactate because such incisions interrupt a large number of major milk ducts. Radial incisions in the breast interrupt fewer ducts but may be, however, cosmetically inferior. In addition, the size, shape, and orientation of the nipple are important to allow its normal mechanical function. Patients whose nipples did not extend sufficiently, were not oriented properly, or were not supple found that the infant would not nurse from the treated breast. Finally, concerns have been expressed by some clinicians that attempts to breast feed after conservative surgery may lead to a greater incidence of mastitis secondary to disruptions of the ductal system.

Hormonal Considerations: Pregnancy Preceding Breast Cancer

PROTECTIVE EFFECT OF HUMAN CHORIONIC GONADOTROPIN

The hormonal issues specific to breast cancer appear in Figure 15-11. Epidemiologic data have demonstrated a 50% reduction in the risk of breast cancer in women who complete full-term pregnancies before 20 years of age. The benefit is seen among all ethnic groups worldwide and increases with increasing parity. There is a declination in risk reduction beyond the age of 30 years. Both human and animal breast tissues and human breast cell lines contain low levels of receptors that bind hCG and its structural and functional homolog luteinizing hormone. These gonadotropins exert numerous anticancer effects in breast cancer models and cells, prompting some investigators to speculate that the elevated levels of hCG associated with full-term pregnancies may exert a protective effect against the later development of breast cancer.

RECENT ANTECEDENT PREGNANCY

The previous discussion notwithstanding, concerns have been raised that the protective benefit of pregnancy on the risk of later breast cancer may be biphasic, with a transient increase in the risk of breast cancer shortly after pregnancy, followed by a greater long-term reduction in risk. Russo and colleagues have postulated that this may occur via the short-term stimulation of any existing malignant clones under the influence of the hormonal milieu of pregnancy, but longer term inhibition of breast carcinogenesis is a consequence of induction of differentiation of normal mammary stem cells in the later stages of pregnancy that otherwise have the potential for neoplastic change.

Further extrapolation leads to the possibility that a recent childbirth before the diagnosis of breast cancer may increase a woman's risk of dying from the disease. Whiteman and colleagues observed 4299 U.S. women ages 20 to 54 years enrolled between 1980 and 1982 as incident breast cancer patients in the population-based, case-control study known as the Cancer and Steroid Hormone Study. The 15-year survival rates were 38%, 51%, and 60% among women aged 20 to 45 years whose last birth was 12 months or less, 13 to 48 months, and more than 48 months before diagnosis, respectively, compared with 65% among nulliparous women. Phillips and colleagues prospectively studied 750 women diagnosed with breast cancer before age 45 years who were part of the population-based Australian Breast Cancer Family Study and demonstrated that the proximity of last childbirth to subsequent breast cancer diagnosis was a predictor of mortality independent of histopathologic tumor characteristics. Specifically, compared with nulliparous women, the investigators found that women who gave birth within 2 years before diagnosis were more likely to have axillary node–positive (58% vs 41%, $P = 0.01$) and ER-negative (58% vs 39%, $P = 0.005$) tumors. The unadjusted hazard ratios for death were 2.3, 1.7, and 0.9 for patients who gave birth less than 2 years, 2 to 5 years, and 5 or more years before diagnosis, respectively.

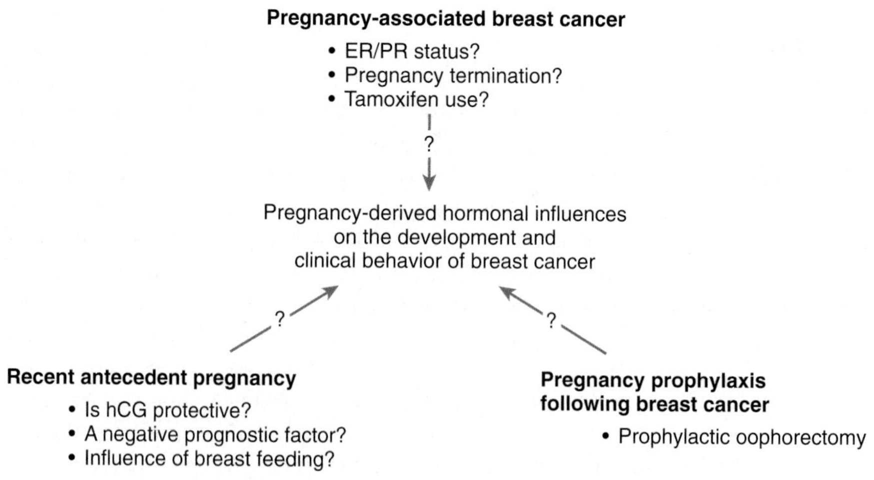

FIGURE 15-11 Hormonal considerations in breast cancer. *ER,* Estrogen receptor; *hCG,* human chorionic gonadotropin; *PR,* progesterone receptor.

Pregnancy-associated breast cancer
- ER/PR status?
- Pregnancy termination?
- Tamoxifen use?

Pregnancy-derived hormonal influences on the development and clinical behavior of breast cancer

Recent antecedent pregnancy
- Is hCG protective?
- A negative prognostic factor?
- Influence of breast feeding?

Pregnancy prophylaxis following breast cancer
- Prophylactic oophorectomy

BREAST FEEDING

In an effort to determine what contribution (if any) breast feeding has on the subsequent development of breast cancer, the Collaborative Group on Hormonal Factors in Breast Cancer examined the individual data from 47 epidemiologic studies in 30 countries that included information on breast feeding patterns. In total, 50,302 women with invasive breast cancer were compared with 96,973 control subjects. The investigators noted that women with breast cancer had fewer births than did control subjects (2.2 vs 2.6) and that fewer parous women with cancer than parous control subjects had ever breast fed (71% vs 79%), with their average lifetime duration of breast feeding being shorter (9.8 vs 15.6 months). The relative risk for breast cancer decreased by 4.3% for every 12 months of breast feeding, and a relative risk reduction of 7.0% was seen for each birth. Thus the longer women breast fed, the more they were protected against breast cancer. The lack of or short lifetime duration of breast feeding typical of women in developed countries may contribute greatly to the high incidence of breast cancer in industrialized nations.

Hormonal Considerations: Pregnancy Coincident with Breast Cancer

Although there is no clear evidence that pregnancy adversely affects the course of this disease, the suspicion persists. It has been established that once the diagnosis is made, stage for stage, the pregnant patient does as well as the nonpregnant patient. However, the low incidence of stage I lesions in pregnancy strongly suggests an acceleration of the disease process in the preclinical period. Many cell kinetic studies of breast cancer suggest that lesions are harbored within the breast for 5 to 8 years before becoming clinical entities. Because the period of gestation is no longer than 9 months, it is difficult to believe that the sole explanation for the high incidence of advanced disease in pregnancy is related to late diagnosis caused by the engorged breast.

The massive endogenous hormone production in pregnancy may adversely affect the course of breast cancer. Urinary excretion of all three major fractions, estrone, estradiol, and estriol, rises progressively after the eighth week of gestation, although there is a disproportionate rise in estriol production by the placenta. Serum concentrations of total estrogens rise nearly 2000-fold, from 4 µg/dL early in pregnancy to mean values of 8 to 22 mg/dL at term. The ability of estrogens to promote growth of breast cancer in animals and humans has been amply illustrated. Whether the stimulatory effect of increased estrogen production has an adverse effect on prognosis or whether the disproportionate rise of estriol, a relatively weak estrogen and a possible antagonist of estrone and estradiol, confers some measure of protection is unknown.

Additional hormone substances secreted in increased quantities in pregnancy that might influence neoplastic growths in the breast include the glucocorticoids and prolactin. Elevated corticosteroid levels are a regular accompaniment of pregnancy and might influence the outcome of breast cancer. Mean production of 17-hydroxycorticosteroids increases from 12 mg/24 hours to approximately 18 mg/24 hours in late pregnancy. Because glucocorticoids can reduce cellular immunity and perhaps promote the implantation and growth of malignant neoplasms, this increased production has grave clinical implications.

Similarly, elevated levels of prolactin produced by the hypophysis and of human placental lactogen by the placenta late in pregnancy and during milk production might affect breast cancer adversely. Prolactin promotes the growth of dimethyleneanthracene-induced mammary tumors in mice. Its role is not established in humans, but it is a subject of current investigation. The levels of prolactin in patients with breast cancer are not appreciably different from those in control subjects, and prolactin suppression with ergot compounds or with L-dopa has not proved to be of therapeutic value. However, the observation that women with bone pain from metastatic breast cancer sometimes obtain relief from prolactin suppression implicates prolactin as a possible promoter of breast cancer in humans.

Estrogen-Receptor and Progesterone-Receptor Status

A recent paper by Middleton and colleagues detected ER positivity in 7 and PR positivity in 6 of 25 patients with PABC whose tumors were studied by immunohistochemistry. Although most tumors associated with PABC are ER/PR negative, a proportion will be ER positive, thus bringing to the discussion the possibility of tamoxifen use during pregnancy (see later). There has been one report of acquired resistance to tamoxifen during the treatment of a patient with PABC, in which the investigators suggest that the changing expression of ER isoforms in pregnancy may have contributed to drug resistance.

Pregnancy Termination

Historically, pregnancy was of concern to surgeons primarily because the risk of excess hemorrhage and shock with mastectomy was increased greatly in the gravid state. Billroth advocated premature induction of labor for this reason but did not find that abortion contributed to cure. More contemporary commentators have argued that the striking rise in estrogen production during pregnancy is of sufficient concern to warrant pregnancy termination and that future pregnancy avoidance should be an important principle of continuing care. Indeed, although many clinicians think that localized breast cancer in the first trimester is a valid reason to recommend termination, reports by Peters and Rose-mond illustrate that therapeutic abortion has no effect on survival, and the presence of a fetus does not compromise proper therapy in early stages. Similarly, therapy for localized disease in later pregnancy can be carried out when the diagnosis is made without pregnancy termination. Of interest, in an updated presentation of 413 patients with PABC referred to the Princess Margaret Hospital in Canada between 1931 and 1985, Clark and Chua observed that therapeutic abortion in breast cancer with coincident, lactational, and subsequent pregnancies is associated with decreased survival. The reasons for this remain unclear. Therapeutic abortion is not currently believed to be an essential component of effective treatment of early disease, despite the theoretic advantage of removing the source of massive estrogen production.

It is critically important to emphasize that treatment of breast cancer should not be delayed provided there are no major obstetric issues. In advanced breast cancer, therapeutic abortion is usually a necessity to achieve effective palliation. In the first trimester of pregnancy, the termination can be accomplished by suction curettage of the uterus; later in pregnancy, termination is accomplished by dinoprostone (Prostin) suppositories, oxytocin (Pitocin) administration, hysterotomy, or hysterectomy. When pregnancy enters the third trimester, the decision for preterm delivery depends heavily on the patient's wishes and the urgency for palliation. A short wait until a viable fetus can be obtained might not be accompanied by significant progress of the neoplasm. Continued gestation represents no threat to the fetus, and the risk of transplacental metastases to the fetus is negligible.

Tamoxifen

Tamoxifen citrate is a nonsteroidal weak estrogen that has found successful applications for each stage of breast cancer in the treatment of selected patients. Tamoxifen was originally introduced for the treatment of advanced disease in postmenopausal women; however, the drug is now also available for the palliative treatment of premenopausal women with ER-positive disease. The proven efficacy of tamoxifen and the low incidence of side effects made the drug an ideal agent to test as an adjuvant therapy for ER-positive women with axillary lymph node–positive breast cancer. Tamoxifen is a selective ER modulator that is often prescribed for up to 5 years following completion of primary therapy.

The long-term effects of tamoxifen use and whether it may increase gynecologic cancers in daughters are unknown. In pregnant rats, tamoxifen administration has been associated with breast cancer in the female offspring. Cunha and colleagues examined 54 genital tracts isolated from 4- to 19-week-old human female fetuses and grown for 1 to 2 months in untreated athymic

nude mice or host mice treated by subcutaneous pellet with the antiestrogen clomiphene, tamoxifen, or the synthetic estrogen diethylstilbestrol. The investigators noted that condensation and segregation of the uterine mesenchyme was greatly impaired and that the fallopian tube epithelium was hyperplastic and disorganized with distortion of the complex mucosal plications in drug-treated specimens as compared with untreated age-matched control subjects.

Table 15-8 also summarizes six reports of tamoxifen use during pregnancy. In 1997 Tewari and colleagues described the first patient to have given birth to a child with congenital anomalies following systemic tamoxifen therapy through 20 weeks of gestation. This 46, XX child had ambiguous genitalia, including labial fusion and clitoramegaly; her internal genitalia were normal according to ultrasonography. Another fetus exposed to tamoxifen during all the first, second, and early part of the third trimesters was born at 26 weeks with oculoauriculovertebral dysplasia (i.e., Goldenhar syndrome). A third case appeared in 2001 and involved a fetus delivered at 31 weeks of gestation whose mother was given tamoxifen as sole systemic therapy and locoregional irradiation before pregnancy was determined. In addition to moderate hyaline membrane disease and necrotizing enterocolitis that was attributable to prematurity, the child had preauricular skin tags, but an appropriate birth weight and no major malformations. At 2 years of follow-up, this last child was meeting all developmental milestones. The presentation of these three cases has prompted the creation of a tamoxifen registry. It is not clear whether women with ER-positive tumors receiving tamoxifen should temporarily discontinue the medication if and when they become pregnant.

Hormonal Considerations: Pregnancy Following Breast Cancer

It has been estimated that only 7% of fertile women go on to conceive following the diagnosis and treatment of breast cancer. Nevertheless, a patient with breast cancer may have several concerns regarding future fertility, not least of which is whether she will remain fertile following treatment. In addition, the risk of recurrence conferred by subsequent pregnancy needs to be addressed because several authors have postulated that the immunosuppressant and hormonal effects of pregnancy so close to diagnosis may have a significant deleterious effect. Finally, a patient may express fear that a child may inherit a genetic predisposition toward the later development of breast cancer. The recommendations given to such patients should be influenced by two major considerations:

1. Whether pregnancy promotes recurrence of cancer
2. The probability of having been cured

Thirty percent of women younger than age 40 years will become amenorrheic following chemotherapy for breast cancer, and 90% of women older than age 40 years will cease menstruating. For those who continue to ovulate and who are desirous of future childbearing, it has been common practice to recommend a waiting period of 2 years following the diagnosis of breast cancer before attempting to conceive because most recurrences occur within the first 2 years of diagnosis. In 1985 Nugent and O'Connell described a poor prognosis for women with early subsequent pregnancy, but many investigators have since refuted this. Of note, women who have a subsequent pregnancy have equivalent or possibly better survival when matched for stage. Gelber and colleagues evaluated 94 patients from the International Breast Cancer Study Group who became pregnant after the diagnosis of early-stage breast cancer and compared them to 188 control subjects (i.e., no subsequent pregnancy) matched for nodal status, tumor size, age, and year of diagnosis. The overall 5- and 10-year survival rates from the diagnosis of early-stage breast cancer among the study group was 92% and 86%, respectively, whereas that of the comparison group was 85% and 74%, respectively. Some have speculated an antitumor effect of the pregnancy, but of course this could reflect the "healthy mother" bias, in that only those select women who feel healthy will go on to conceive. Although it may be presumptuous to conclude on the basis of retrospective studies that pregnancy protects against recurrence after mastectomy, it is reasonably safe to conclude that it does not promote it. In summary, therefore, it would appear that future pregnancies are safe for the mother unless she has an ER-positive tumor and has not been placed into remission. Consequently, if a pregnancy occurs, there appears to be no justification for recommending its termination in patients without evidence of recurrence. The converse, that pregnancy with recurrence should be terminated in most instances and that an uneventful pregnancy in no way guarantees against a subsequent recurrence, is also true. Indeed, there are cases on record in which multiple pregnancies have eventually been followed by recurrence.

Prophylactic Oophorectomy

Surgical castration for patients with early-stage breast cancer has been advocated to prevent further pregnancy, which might cause recrudescence of the disease through hormone stimulation. Oophorectomy also serves to eliminate the ovarian source of estrogen production, ideally preventing or delaying subsequent recurrence. Neither argument is substantiated by data to support a role for "prophylactic castration." In many patients, chemotherapy will cause a cessation of ovarian hormone production. As discussed earlier, pregnancy after treatment for breast cancer has no influence on the disease, and a few reports even suggest that future pregnancies

might be protective. The rationale for eliminating the ovarian source of estrogens in the primary treatment of early disease is based on an observation that castration in the presence of observable recurrent disease results in partial or complete temporary tumor regression in approximately one third of cases. This argument has been refuted by two large clinical trials conducted in the United States that failed to demonstrate a significant benefit from castration and adjuvant therapy. For example, the National Surgical Adjuvant Breast and Bowel Project (NSABP) conducted a randomized trial of prophylactic castration in premenopausal women involving 129 women who were castrated and 70 control women. After an observation period of 10 years, there was no evidence that those who were castrated derived any benefit from the procedure.

Survival Among Patients with Pregnancy-Associated Breast Cancer

Most of the datasets from the preceding few decades show that women with PABC have the same survival stage for stage as nonpregnant women with breast cancer. Women with PABC may do poorly in the aggregate because these patients tend to present with advanced disease. Table 15-9 is adapted from Keleher and colleagues and shows selected 5-year survival data by axillary nodal status for women with PABC. Holleb and Farrow reported a series of 283 patients with carcinomas of the breast in pregnancy, including 73 who had inoperable disease and 210 who underwent surgery with or without postoperative radiation. Of those patients with inoperable disease, 93% died within 2 years of the diagnosis, including all 7 of those who had interruption of pregnancy. The majority of the remaining 210 patients underwent radical mastectomy and were given postoperative radiation therapy. Of 28 patients with a diagnosis in the first trimester, 7 survived for 5 years. Peters and Meakin described 70 patients with breast cancer in pregnancy, all of whom were treated with preoperative, postoperative, or palliative radiotherapy in conjunction with radical mastectomy. The overall survival rate in this series was 32.9% at 5 years and 19.5% at 10 years. Of 12 patients treated during the first and second trimesters, 3 survived 5 years; only 1 of the 9 patients treated during the third trimester survived 5 years, and she had active disease at the time of the report. The remaining 49 patients who were treated postpartum had a 39% 5-year survival rate, prompting the author to suggest that a delay in the treatment of breast carcinoma until after delivery should be considered.

It is now recognized that the independent variable of youth results in an unfavorable prognosis in patients with breast cancer, presumably because of the likelihood of more aggressive tumors in these young women. Previously, only young patients had an opportunity of

TABLE 15-9   Literature Review of Case-Control Series of Patients with PABC

Author	Years	PABC	Matched Patients	Outcome
Petrek, et al 1991	1960-1980	56	166	No survival difference
Zemlickis, et al 1992	1958-1987	118	269	No survival difference
Ishida, et al 1992	1970-1988	192	192	Worse prognosis in PABC group
Chang, 1994	1979-1988	21	199	No survival difference
Nugent, 1995	1970-1979	19	157	No survival difference
Lethaby, 1996	1976-1985	20	362	Worse survival when diagnosed during lactation; no difference when diagnosed during pregnancy
Bonnier, et al 1997	1960-1993	154	308	Worse prognosis in PABC group
Ibrahim, et al 2000	1992-1996	72	216	No survival difference
Zhang, et al 2003	1957-1990	88	176	No survival difference
Halaska, 2008	1995-2007	32	32	No survival difference

Modified from Halaska MJ et al: Breast J 15:416, 2009.

having breast cancer coincident with pregnancy, but as women postpone childbearing, pregnancy coincident with breast cancer will become more common. Physicians must treat patients with breast cancer in pregnancy aggressively and with curative intent.

EVALUATION AND THERAPEUTIC MODALITIES

Anesthesia and Surgery in the Pregnant Patient

Anesthesia

Anesthetic considerations in the pregnant patient must take into account both the potential teratogenicity of the anesthetic agents and the maternal physiologic changes that result from both the pregnancy and the use of anesthetic agents. The vast majority of analgesics and anesthetics are category C drugs (Table 15-10). When a drug has demonstrated teratogenicity in animals, it is likely to have the same effect in humans. Therefore, although category C drugs lack human studies, the existing animal studies may be useful in predicting risk to the fetus. A consensus statement published in 1998 in the pages of *The New England Journal of Medicine* did not list any anesthetic agents as definitive causes of fetal anomalies. Inhalational and local anesthetics, muscle relaxants, narcotic analgesics, and benzodiazepines are known to be safe in pregnancy.

The hyperdynamic cardiovascular system of pregnancy is characterized by an increased cardiac output and increased resting heart rate. The total blood volume is increased by 40% and that of the red blood cells by 25%, resulting in the physiologic anemia of pregnancy that decreases the hematocrit by approximately 30%. As the pregnancy progresses, a decrease in blood return to the heart from the inferior vena cava occurs via increasing intra-abdominal pressures caused by the enlarging uterus.

TABLE 15-10   Drug Safety Categories in Pregnancy

Category	Description
A	Safety established using human studies
B	Presumed safety based on animal studies
C	Uncertain safety; no human studies; animal studies show adverse effect
D	Unsafe; evidence of risk that may in certain clinical circumstances be justifiable
X	Highly unsafe

A 30% to 40% increase in the tidal volume occurs during normal pregnancy as oxygen consumption increases and the abdominal organs undergo mechanical displacement by the gravid uterus. Anesthesiologists may expect a compensatory respiratory alkalosis in pregnancy with a P_aco_2 of 30 to 35 mm Hg. Cricoid pressure should be applied during intubation to prevent aspiration, the risk of which is increased as a result of the pregnancy-associated decrease in lower esophageal sphincter pressure and delayed gastric emptying. Small-diameter endotracheal tubes are recommended to facilitate intubation later in pregnancy when airway edema is increased. Intraoperatively, the end tidal CO_2 is monitored.

Surgery

With the improvements in neonatal care, fetal survival rates continue to increase, and although actual figures vary between different neonatal intensive care units, survival rates greater than 90% can be expected beyond 28 weeks of gestation. Table 15-11 contains neonatal intensive care unit survival statistics based on gestational age and birth weight. Patients in need of surgery during the second trimester can be permitted a short delay to attain fetal viability in many cases. When the clinical suspicion for malignancy is high or the diagnosis is established by biopsy, it is recommended that surgery

TABLE 15-11 Survival with Selected Neonatal Morbidity for Very Low Birth Weight Infants Born in the Nichd Neonatal Research Network Between January 1, 1997 and December 31, 2002

	501-750 g (n = 4046)	751-1000 g (n = 4266)	1001-1250 g (n = 4557)	1251-1500 g (n = 5284)
Survived	55	88	94	96
Overall survival with morbidity	65	43	22	4
BPD alone	42	25	11	4
Severe IVH	5	6	5	4
NEC alone	3	3	3	2

Modified from Fanaroff AA et al. Am J Obstet Gynecol 196:147.e1-147.e8, 2007.
BPD, Bronchopulmonary dysplasia; IVH, intraventricular hemorrhage; NEC, necrotizing enterocolitis; NICHD, National Institute of Child Health and Human Development.

TABLE 15-12 Recommendations for Laparoscopy in Pregnancy

16-20 weeks of gestational age
Tilting table to left or right
Left upper quadrant or subxyphoid insertion (6 cm between point of entry and top of fundus)
Open Hasson technique preferable
Ultrasound guidance with elevation of abdominal wall if Veress technique used
Intra-abdominal pressure 15 mm Hg
Trendelenberg position
Fetal monitoring as indicated

not be delayed in the first or third trimesters. If an asymptomatic and clinically isolated adnexal mass is discovered during the first trimester, as discussed earlier, it is reasonable to repeat an imaging study around 17 to 18 weeks of gestation to determine the need for surgery.

Pregnant patients undergoing surgery during the second trimester before fetal viability (approximately 23-24 weeks of gestation) should have the fetal heart tones documented by Doppler preoperatively and postoperatively. Later in pregnancy, continuous fetal heart rate monitoring can be used perioperatively. Following documentation of an adequate amniotic fluid volume of approximately 10 to 18 mL via ultrasonography, preoperative and postoperative prophylactic indomethacin at a rectal dose of 25 to 50 mg can be used to minimize uterine contractions in patients undergoing surgery before 30 weeks of gestation. The use of indomethacin is not advisable beyond this period because of concerns of premature closure of the patent ductus arteriosus. It must be recognized that although prophylactic tocolytic agents can decrease uterine irritability, they have not been shown to decrease the incidence of preterm birth in patients undergoing surgery. The liberal use of lower-extremity sequential compression devices intraoperatively and during periods of bed rest is advisable. Finally, an external tocodynamometer can be used in the postoperative period to monitor uterine irritability and preterm uterine contractions.

Laparotomy

Historically, laparotomy during pregnancy was a frequent cause of fetal wastage. A 17% loss rate was reported by Brant in 1967 following appendectomy during pregnancy. In 1973 Saunders and Milton observed a 23% rate of fetal wastage after laparotomy. In modern hospitals, however, loss of the fetus as a consequence of laparotomy is uncommon. For example, Kort and colleagues reported in 1993 that for 78 women who underwent

nonobstetric operations, the perinatal mortality rate was not increased provided that fetal viability was established preoperatively. The most common indications for surgical treatment in their series were appendicitis, adnexal mass, and cholecystitis. Nonobstetric surgery was associated with an increased risk of preterm labor, and the authors identified no measurable benefit from the use of perioperative prophylactic tocolytic agents. The premature delivery rate was 21.8% after major surgery, which was twice the rate in pregnant control subjects.

With rare exceptions, when laparotomy is required to evaluate the pregnant woman for suspected or known malignancy, we use the midline, vertical approach. This permits excellent visualization and inspection of the entire pelvis and upper abdomen and, perhaps as important, facilitates the "hands-off-the-uterus" approach we have toward surgery in the gravid patient.

Laparoscopy

Laparoscopy can be used to evaluate adnexal masses during pregnancy and has been shown to be well tolerated by both the mother and the fetus. By the end of the second trimester, the enlarging uterus interferes with the laparoscopic view, and a celiotomy is generally required. Two million deliveries in Sweden from 1973 to 1993 were the subject of a review by Reedy and colleagues, who evaluated 2233 laparoscopic and 2491 open laparotomy cases. The outcome measures included gestational age at delivery, birth weight, intrauterine growth restriction, congenital malformations, stillbirths, and neonatal deaths. Although both groups were at increased risk for preterm delivery and neonatal birth weights less than 2500 g, there were no statistically significant differences between the two. Highlights from the Society of American Gastrointestinal Endoscopic Surgeons recommendations for the conduct of laparoscopy in pregnancy appear in Table 15-12.

For seemingly isolated 6- to 10-cm adnexal masses that persist into the second trimester, we defer laparoscopic evaluation until 18 weeks of gestation and typically use pelviscopy to determine which direction (i.e., transverse or midline-vertical) to make the laparotomy incision. For persistent masses greater than 10 cm, we recommend proceeding directly to laparotomy via a vertical incision in an effort to maximize exposure and allow surgical removal of the mass without any manipulation of the uterus.

Diagnostic and Therapeutic Radiation in Pregnancy

The primary concern of both the oncologist and the obstetrician regarding radiation therapy during pregnancy is its possible effect on the baby. The embryo undoubtedly represents the most radiosensitive stage of human life because many of the cells are differentiating and thus relatively more sensitive to radiation injury. In addition, the high rate of mitotic activity in the cells of the embryo contributes to its radiosensitivity because the mitotic phase of the cell is the most radiosensitive period in the life cycle of the cell. Of note, if the embryonic cell is genetically altered or killed during development, the fetus will be deformed or will not survive. Finally, there is the concern that irradiation of the fetal and maternal gonads may contribute to reproductive difficulties in the future, of both the mother and her offspring.

Radiobiology

For the fetus, the most sensitive period is day 18 through day 38. After day 40, primary organ systems have developed, and much larger doses of x-rays or gamma rays are necessary to produce serious abnormalities. Three periods of fetal development are highly significant from a radiologic point of view.

1. Preimplantation. In this phase, radiation produces an all-or-none effect, in that it either destroys the fertilized egg or does not affect it significantly.
2. Organ system formation. This is the period from day 18 through day 38, when doses of 10 to 40 cGy may cause visceral organ or somatic damage. Microcephaly, anencephaly, eye damage, growth restriction, spina bifida, and foot damage are reported with doses of 4 cGy or less. Cause and effect have not been proved with these lower doses.
3. Period of fetal development after day 40, when larger doses are likely to produce external malformations but organ systems, especially the nervous system, may still be undamaged.

The dose to the fetus is related to internal scatter of radiation after it enters the supradiaphragmatic tissues. Some scatter may also come from the treatment head of the machine and the collimator. Zucali and colleagues used a tissue-equivalent phantom to measure scatter dose to the uterus. In this study, doses of 1.5% of the total dose were measured at the estimated top of the uterus, with less than 1% being measurable in the true pelvis. This occurs even with abdominal shielding.

It is estimated that 1 cGy of radiation produces five mutations in every 1 million genes exposed. Fortunately, most mutants are recessive. Mutant effects are not seen in the first generation and may not be expressed for many generations until two people with the same mutation mate. Most estimates of genetic damage are empiric, but it is estimated that to double the rate of gene mutation, 25 to 150 cGy must be given from birth to the end of reproductive age.

Constant changes are being made in what is considered the permissible body dose of radiation. Some authorities cite 14 cGy in the first 30 years of life; others cite 10 cGy or less as the maximum. This includes medical and background sources. Radiation doses in excess of 200 cGy during the first 20 weeks of gestation will result in congenital malformations in the majority of fetuses exposed (frequently microcephaly and mental retardation). With doses above 300 cGy, there is increasing risk of abortion. If therapeutic irradiation is necessary for a pregnant patient and therapeutic abortion is refused, delay in the initiation of treatment until at least the mid-second trimester is recommended. Irradiation of even supradiaphragmatic structures during pregnancy will deliver fetal doses ranging from 1.2% to 7.1% of the total treatment dose.

Radiation-Induced Anomalies

There are varying sensitivities within the tissues in the human embryo. Various abnormalities have been attributed to irradiation of the embryo; microcephaly and associated conditions are most common. Other abnormalities of the central nervous system, the eye, and the skeleton have also been ascribed to irradiation. However, an accurate prediction of incidence with regard to dose has not been possible. It is widely accepted that irradiation of human beings, especially of their gonads, has certain undesirable effects. Any irradiation of gonadal tissue involves possible genetic damage because the photons can cause gene mutation or chromosome breakage with subsequent translocation, loss, deletion, and abnormal fusion of chromosome material. The effect is basically additive and cumulative; the changes are generally in direct proportion to the total dose. Unfortunately, there is no threshold for genetic damage, and even relatively small doses of irradiation can cause gene mutations, most of which can be harmful.

Doses greater than 50 cGy may produce significant mental retardation and microcephaly, even in the second trimester (Figure 15-12). An analysis of children exposed

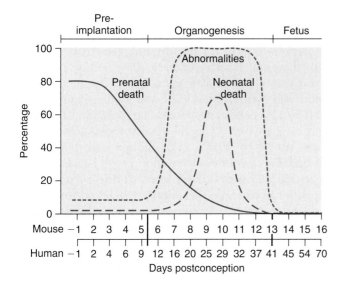

FIGURE 15-12 Incidence of abnormalities and of neonatal and prenatal death in mice given a dose of 200 cGy at various times post fertilization. The lower scale consists of Rugh's estimates of the equivalent stages for the human embryo. *(From Hall EJ: Radiobiology for the Radiologist. New York, Harper & Row, 1973; after Russell LB et al: J Cell Comp Physiol 43[Suppl 1]:103, 1954, and Rugh R: AJR Am J Roentgenol 87:559, 1962.)*

TABLE 15-13 Effects and Risks After Exposure to Ionizing Radiation in Utero and Spontaneous Frequency (Without Exposure)

Time after Conception (Weeks)	Effect(s)	Risk Per 0.01 Gy	Spontaneous Frequency
0-2	Prenatal death*	0.01-0.001	0.3-0.6
3-8	Malformation	0.005†	0.06
8-15	Mental retardation, IQ decrease‡	0.004	0.005
16-25	Mental retardation, IQ decrease§	0.001	0.005
0-38	Leukemia, solid tumors in childhood	0.003-0.004	0.002-0.003

From Kal HB, Struikmans H: Lancet Oncol 6:328, 2005.
*Based on experimental data.
†Above threshold dose of 0.1-0.2 Gy.
‡Reduction of 21 IQ points per 1 Gy above threshold of about 0.05 Gy; threshold dose for mental retardation about 0.06 Gy.
§Reduction of 13 IQ points per 0.1 Gy above threshold dose of about 0.05 Gy; threshold dose for mental retardation about 0.25 Gy.

in utero to the atomic bomb in Hiroshima and Nagasaki shows a 30 in 1600 incidence of severe mental retardation. Most of the mentally retarded children were exposed at 8 to 15 weeks of life; no cases were reported before the eighth week of gestation. A rough linear relationship is suggested, with a probability of mental retardation occurring at 0.4% per cGy (rad).

As noted previously, the exposure dose that is associated with developmental abnormalities remains controversial. Hammer-Jacobsen suggests that 10 cGy received in the first 6 weeks of gestation should be considered a threshold for therapeutic abortion. Others disagree and suggest that the minimal level increases as the pregnancy progresses. Low-dose exposure (<100 cGy) seems acceptable only in the third trimester. Evidence suggests that an exposure of even 3 to 5 cGy can result in an increase in benign or malignant tumors in the child after birth.

Most of the data to date on the effects of irradiation on the fetus are from single-dose exposure; few data are available concerning the effects of fractionated irradiation. Reported cases of fractionated irradiation during pregnancy show a low incidence of fetal anomalies.

Diagnostic Radiology

The metastatic evaluation using diagnostic imaging and the treatment of malignancy by radiotherapy in the pregnant woman underscores an inherent maternal–fetal conflict, in that the mother would be the major beneficiary, whereas the fetus could be at substantial risk. Several recommendations have been widely applied in this scenario, including delaying radiation therapy for breast cancer until after delivery, avoidance of sentinel node identification procedures during pregnancy, and termination of pregnancy when doses greater than 0.05 to 0.1 Gy are received by the fetus. It must be recognized that these recommendations are not based on sufficient knowledge of the radiation risks to the unborn child. Although individual doses are highest in association with radiation therapy, the greatest risk to both the general population and the cancer patient comes from diagnostic procedures. Most radiologic diagnostic procedures should be avoided during the first and second trimesters of pregnancy. The exposure to the fetus and gonads will vary with the procedure performed and the precautions taken. A chest radiograph will result in an exposure of 300 mcGy per plate, whereas a barium enema study will result in a total dose to the gonads and pelvis of 6 cGy. In a pregnant patient, the barium enema study is obviously a greater threat because of the greater dose and the area irradiated.

The International Commission on Radiological Protection prepared two reports on medical irradiation in pregnant women. The biologic effects of prenatal irradiation of the embryo and fetus were derived from animal studies, data from survivors of nuclear explosions, data from children exposed in utero to diagnostic radiographs, and data on children who were exposed to radiation from the Chernobyl accident in utero. As outlined in Table 15-13, lethality, malformations, mental retardation, and cancer induction comprise the expected effects of radiation exposure of the fetus.

Ionizing Radiation

In diagnostic radiograph or CT, ionizing radiation passes through the body to create an image, whereas ionizing radiation from radiopharmaceuticals used in nuclear medicine procedures are retained in the tissues for a period of time and are subsequently removed by elimination from the body and by radioactive decay.

Nonionizing Radiation

Both ultrasonography imaging and MRI form images using nonionizing radiation; however, theoretic risks to the fetus exist. Thermal effects occur in tissues with the absorption of ultrasonic energy, whereas cavitation (i.e., mechanical) effects may occur through motion initiated by the ultrasonic. Both thermal and cavitation effects occur only with very high-intensity ultrasonography, and no confirmed biologic effects associated with the use of diagnostic ultrasonography with standard power levels have been reported. Potential injury at the cellular level in MRI may result from exposure to high static magnetic fields. In addition, heating can result from energy deposited by radiofrequencies used to generate the pulse sequences. The diagnostic magnets create static magnetic fields from 0.1 to 1.5T, and no adverse behavioral or physiologic effects are anticipated with fields up to 2T. Of note, there have been no immediately observable adverse effects or delayed sequelae encountered among fetuses from an MRI examination. Table 15-14 lists the imaging modalities used to diagnose metastatic disease.

Ionic or nonionic iodinated intravenous contrast media used in CT appear to be safe for the fetus; however, only animal studies have been performed using iodinated contrast agents. These agents are pregnancy category B drugs. Gadolinium-based contrast medium is not advisable during pregnancy because the gadolinium crosses the placenta, is filtered through the fetal kidneys, and is then reingested through the amniotic fluid. Gadolinium is a category C drug. The accuracy of bone scans is improved through the addition of single-photon emission computed tomography imaging. MRI is the most sensitive for studying the bone marrow, whereas CT is highly sensitive for cortical destruction. Positron emission tomography scanning with 2-[fluorine-18]fluoro-2-deoxy-D-glucose is being used with increasing frequency in the metastatic workup, although the potential dose to the fetus precludes its use when the pregnancy is to be preserved.

Radionuclides

Most diagnostic nuclear medicine procedures use short-lived radionuclides (e.g., ^{99m}Tc), resulting in a dose to the fetus generally less than 0.01Gy. Special mention should be made regarding whole-body radionuclide scanning using iodine-131 for the metastatic workup of thyroid carcinoma. It is well established that oral administration of radioactive iodine to a mother will have deleterious effects on the thyroid gland of the fetus, with placental transfer of radioactive iodine occurring as early as 8 weeks after conception. The fetal thyroid gland will concentrate iodine and synthesize thyroxine by 11 to 12 weeks of gestation. The radiation dose delivered by 2 μCi of ^{131}I to the fetal thyroid gland ranges from 10,000 to 40,000 cGy. Stoffer and Hamburger studied 237 cases in which radioactive ^{131}I at doses from 10 to 150 μCi was administered during pregnancy. In 55 patients, therapeutic abortion was performed on medical recommendation, and among the remaining 182 pregnancies, there were 2 spontaneous abortions, 2

TABLE 15-14   Imaging Modalities Used for Treatment Planning in Oncology

Site of Anatomic Interest	Imaging Modality	Type of Radiation
Brain	CT scan	Ionizing
	MRI	Nonionizing
	FDG-PET	Ionizing
Chest	Chest radiograph	Ionizing
	CT scan	Ionizing
	MRI	Nonionizing
	FDG-PET scan	Ionizing
	Gallium scan	Ionizing
	Mammography	Ionizing
Abdomen	Ultrasound	Nonionizing
	CT scan	Ionizing
	MRI	Nonionizing
	FDG-PET	Ionizing
	Intravenous pyelography	Ionizing
	Upper gastrointestinal with small bowel follow through	Ionizing
Pelvis (not bony pelvis)	Ultrasound	Nonionizing
	CT scan	Ionizing
	MRI	Nonionizing
	FDG-PET	Ionizing
	Barium enema	Ionizing
	Cystography	Ionizing
Skeletal	Radiograph	Ionizing
	Bone scan/SPECT	Ionizing
	CT scan	Ionizing
	MRI	Nonionizing
	FDG-PET	Ionizing
Lymph nodes	Lymphangiography	Ionizing
	CT scan	Ionizing
	MRI	Nonionizing
	Lymphoscintigraphy	Ionizing
	Sentinel node examination	Nonionizing and ionizing

Modified from Nicklas AH, Baker ME: Semin Oncol 27:623, 2000.
CT, Computed tomography; FDG-PET, 2-[fluorine-18]fluoro-2-deoxy-d-glucose positron emission tomography; MRI, magnetic resonance imaging; SPECT, single-photon emission computed tomography.

stillborn infants, and 2 infants born with abdominal or chest anomalies. Of note, there were 6 infants with hypothyroidism (3%), 4 of whom exhibited mental deficiencies. Pregnancy is a contraindication to the administration of ^{131}I.

Radiation Therapy

When the patient wishes to continue her pregnancy, delay of initiation of therapeutic radiation as long as possible without compromising cure is recommended. Fortunately, most cancers in pregnant women that require radiation therapy are remote from the pelvis. Any radiation therapy to the abdomen should be postponed until after delivery, if at all possible. Therefore, with the exception of a locally advanced cervical tumor, radiation therapy can be used during pregnancy provided that the fetal dose is precisely estimated during the radiation planning sessions. The dose to the fetus can be calculated from the internal scatter, which largely depends on the source of irradiation and on the size of the treatment fields and their proximity to the fetus. Leakage radiation from the tube head of the linear accelerator, scatter from the collimator, and blocks also contribute to the fetal dose. Leakage and scatter can be reduced by proper shielding with four to five half-value layers of lead stacked over the patient's uterus.

Kal and Struikmans tabulated the dosimetry data and pregnancy outcomes of women who received radiation therapy during pregnancy for breast cancer (Figure 15-13), Hodgkin disease, and brain or head and neck tumors (Table 15-15). Successful radiotherapy of breast cancers during pregnancy with fetal doses below the deterministic threshold (0.039-0.18 Gy) have resulted in the birth of healthy children. Similarly, several healthy children, some who have been observed for up to 11 years, have been delivered following radiation therapy for Hodgkin disease during pregnancy with fetal doses ranging from 0.014 to 0.136 Gy. Radiation treatment portals are now more restricted in size, and patients with stage I and II Hodgkin disease currently receive polychemotherapy followed by involved field radiotherapy, thus resulting in potentially less harm to the unborn child. Finally, the successful radiotherapeutic

management of neck and cranial tumors in pregnancy suggests that high doses can be achieved with fetal exposures of less than 0.1 Gy, a dose below the deterministic threshold.

Radiation-Induced Carcinogenesis

The subject of the carcinogenic effects of x-ray radiation was first raised nearly half a century ago by Stewart and Webb from Oxford University in the United Kingdom. Monsoon and Macmahon summarized the bulk of the data accumulated before the 1980s in their monograph that focused on prenatal x-ray exposure and cancer in children. Most of the available information on radiation-induced embryonic damage during the preceding two decades is derived from animal studies, extended follow-up of individuals exposed to atomic bomb explosions in Japan, and statistical analyses.

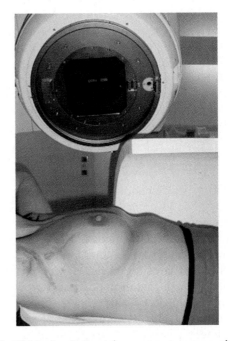

FIGURE 15-13 Irradiation of a pregnant woman after breast-conserving treatment. Shielding of leakage radiation is done with a mobile lead screen usually used for shielding of personnel in the brachytherapy room. *(From Kal HB, Struikmans H: Lancet Oncol 6:328, 2005.)*

TABLE 15-15   Radiotherapy During Pregnancy

Malignancy	n	Median Dose (Gy)	Shielding Used (N)	Median Estimated Fetal Dose (Gy)	Mean Gestational Age (Weeks)	No. Reported Cases with Adverse Outcomes in Offspring
Breast	23	41	2	0.15	17.5	2
Hodgkin lymphoma	58	36	31	0.085	20	3
Brain	7	42	2	0.03	21	1
Melanoma	2	43.5	2	0.05	23	2

Modified from Luis SA et al: J Med Imaging Radiation Oncol 53:559, 2009.

Of interest is a paper by Chen and colleagues, who studied the records of 37 women radiated for Hodgkin disease around the time of pregnancy and of 345 women who were not pregnant. They detected a higher risk of breast cancer after irradiation around the time of pregnancy, suggesting that pregnancy represents a time of increased sensitivity of breast tissue to the carcinogenic effects of radiation.

Genetic Damage and Infertility

In addition, the possibility that human exposure to ionizing radiation might have a detrimental genetic consequence remains a matter of concern and uncertainty. There is concern because recessive mutations may not become apparent for several generations, and there is uncertainty because although there are no human data available, experimental animal studies have demonstrated significant radiation-induced genetic effects. There appears to be no apparent threshold dose for genetic damage, but the effect of any particular radiation dose is considerably reduced if that dose is administered during a prolonged period. Of importance also for patients planning childbearing after significant exposure of gonadal tissue to irradiation is that the genetic effect of radiation on the gonad may be minimized by delaying conception after exposure. In humans, pregnancy should be delayed 12 to 14 months after significant exposure.

Chemotherapy

Because nearly all antineoplastic drugs have been shown to be teratogenic in animal studies, the available data suggest endangerment to human fetuses even for drugs for which no human data are available. Their use often evokes moral, philosophic, and emotional decisions. Both mother and fetus are at risk, with abortion, intrauterine fetal demise, malformations, and growth restriction being foremost considerations. These potential dangers to the fetus must be weighed against the possible detrimental effect to the mother of withholding these agents. The long-term effect on the fetus is unknown. The problem of long-term observation has been dramatically emphasized by the occurrence of adenosis of the vagina in young women exposed to diethylstilbestrol in utero during the first trimester of pregnancy. A similar long-term effect is possible when chemotherapeutic agents are used in pregnancy.

All chemotherapeutic agents profoundly affect rapidly growing tissues, and a high rate of cell division is characteristic of the fetus. Following this reasoning, one would expect a much greater effect than is actually observed. Unquestionably, the first trimester of pregnancy is when the fetus is most vulnerable to cancer chemotherapeutic agents. The two aspects to the problem of fetal damage are as follows:

1. Death of the fetus
2. Induction of fetal abnormalities inadequate to cause fetal death

Most of the available data suggesting the teratogenicity and mutagenicity of chemotherapeutic agents have been derived from experiments in laboratory animals. The rat, the mouse, and the rabbit have placentas very similar to the human placenta, and because the teratogenic effects of a drug are species specific, these animals provide models in which to study chemotherapy exposure in utero. These experiments indicate potential danger to the human fetus only. Teratogenic properties of chemotherapeutic agents also are predicated on the type, dose, and threshold dose of the drug. When considering an extrapolation of animal data to humans, it is important to note that the therapeutic doses used in humans are often lower than the minimum teratogenic dose studied in animal models. Thus teratogenic data are useful only if the dose resulting in injury to the model does not also cause maternal toxic effects. Another important caveat is that many antineoplastic exposures in pregnancy that have resulted in malformations or even fetal deaths have typically been associated with multiagent therapy, sometimes also with concomitant radiation therapy, so that it is difficult to single out one specific agent as the cause of an adverse outcome. It is important to note that, in the majority of exposures, even during the first trimester, the outcome of the fetus is unremarkable. Still, unless the mother's life is in grave danger, we do not recommend chemotherapy use during the first trimester.

Teratology and Embryology

Teratology is the study of the causes, mechanisms, and manifestations of abnormal fetal development. Environmental factors, such as infectious diseases, drugs, chemicals, and radiation, have been shown to cause abnormal development by inducing chromosome abnormalities, specific gene changes, vascular changes, or mechanical disruption. In many instances, the exact cause of a fetal abnormality is unknown. Although different classes of teratogens have been established, certain general principles apply to all. There are three stages of embryonic development. In the first 2 weeks of life, the blastocyst is resistant to teratogens. It is during this period that a large insult is necessary to kill the blastocyst. A surviving blastocyst will not manifest any organ's specific abnormalities as a result of that teratogen. Early embryonic cells have not differentiated sufficiently, so if one cell dies, another can take over. The second stage is organogenesis, or the process of organ differentiation. The most critical period extends from the third to eighth weeks of development (fifth through tenth weeks of gestational age), when susceptibility to teratogenic agents is maximal. In the human fetus, the period of organogenesis usually ends by the 13th week of gestation. The third and final period of growth, organ development, is characterized by increase in fetal and organ size. However, brain and gonadal tissue are exceptions because they continue to differentiate beyond the second period. Exposure to the teratogenic agent beyond the third period can affect general fetal growth but will not produce organ-specific morphologic malformations.

Figure 15-14 depicts prenatal development from implantation, through embryonic progression, and into the fetal period. Drug responses vary among individuals because of differences in absorption, protein binding, and excretion rate and differences in placental transfer and fetal metabolism of the teratogen. Both polygenic and mendelian factors can be responsible for different responses to identical doses of a teratogen in two fetuses of the same species. Administration of small intermittent doses of a teratogen may enable a system to safely metabolize the teratogen and prevent malformation. The effect would be different if the total dose were administered at one time. However, small constant doses of a teratogen may interfere with cellular metabolism and cause more serious malformations than might be expected.

Transplacental Studies

Antineoplastic agents and their metabolites can be detected in placental tissue, amniotic fluid, umbilical cord blood, and breast milk. By enzyme-linked immunosorbent assay and spectrometry, Henderson and colleagues measured cisplatin–DNA adducts in placental tissues but were unable to do so in the umbilical cord tissues or in amniotic cells. Karp and colleagues reported high levels of doxorubicin in placental tissue; the drug was absent in umbilical cord tissue or in the blood of a healthy child born 48 hours after maternal treatment. Separately, Roboz and colleagues and Barni and colleagues were unable to identify doxorubicin in the amniotic fluid after maternal administration. Transplacental conduct of antineoplastic drugs may occur. Although

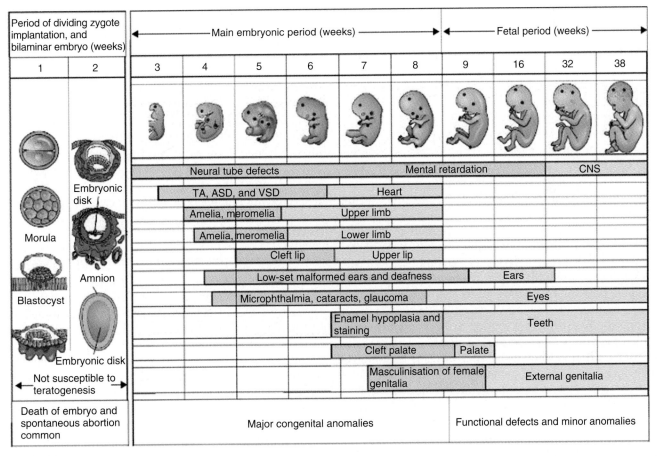

FIGURE 15-14   Crucial periods in prenatal development. Dots on the developing fetus show common sites of action of teratogens. Horizontal bars indicate fetal development during a highly sensitive period *(purple)* and a less sensitive period *(green)*. *ASD,* Atrial septal defect; *CNS,* central nervous system; *TA,* truncus arteriosus; *VSD,* ventricular septal defect. *(From Moore P (ed): The Developing Human, 6th ed. Philadelphia, Saunders, 1998.)*

doxorubicin was not detected by liquid chromatography in the amniotic fluid, fetal brain, or fetal gastrointestinal tract 15 hours following its administration to the mother, d'Incalci and colleagues found the drug in the fetal liver, kidney, and lungs after elective termination. It would have been interesting to have had data from the fetal myocardial tissue. A metabolite of doxorubicin was present in the umbilical cord, placental tissue, and neonatal spleen of a stillborn baby delivered 36 hours after maternal treatment. Egan and colleagues reported a case in which milk and plasma concentrations of doxorubicin and cisplatin were measured after intravenous administration of these agents to a lactating patient who had ovarian cancer. Although the concentrations of doxorubicin in milk at times exceeded those detected in concomitant plasma samples, the total amount of drug delivered in the milk was negligible. However, the authors concluded that it is prudent to advise lactating women who are receiving these antineoplastic drugs to refrain from breast feeding.

Classes of Antineoplastic Agents

ANTIMETABOLITES

Antimetabolites are small, weakly acidic molecules that are cell cycle nonspecific, inhibiting cellular metabolism by acting as false substrates during RNA and DNA synthesis. Examples of these agents include methotrexate, 5-fluorouracil, aminopterin, cytarabine, thioguanine, and mercaptopurine. The aminopterin syndrome has been reported after in utero exposure during the first trimester and is characterized by cranial dysostosis with delayed ossification, hypertelorism, wide nasal bridge, micrognathia, and ear anomalies. Similar malformations have been associated with methotrexate administration when doses greater than 10 mg per week are used during the first trimester. There have been 53 reported cases of exposure to 5-fluorouracil during human pregnancy; when used after the first trimester (usually in combination with other agents), the development of intrauterine growth restriction without anomalies manifested in 11% of cases ($n = 6$). There have been four reports of limb malformations following cytarabine administration during the first trimester; among 89 additional cases in which the drug was given during all trimesters (usually in combination with other agents), adverse fetal events included transient cytopenia (5%), intrauterine fetal demise (6%), intrauterine growth restriction (13%), and two neonatal deaths from sepsis and gastroenteritis. Finally, 49 women have been treated with mercaptopurine during pregnancy, including 29 who were exposed to the drug during the first trimester, none of whom gave birth to an anomalous neonate.

There is no doubt that the antifolics aminopterin and methotrexate almost invariably result in spontaneous abortion or an abnormal fetus when they are given in the first trimester of pregnancy. These drugs should not be given to the pregnant woman in the first trimester unless there is life-threatening disease that can be counteracted by the drug. If an antifolic is used and the mother does not have a spontaneous abortion, therapeutic abortion should be seriously considered. A small amount of data seems to indicate that aminopterin and methotrexate do not cause harm when they are given after the first trimester of pregnancy.

ALKYLATORS

Alkylating agents are an integral component of many combination chemotherapy regimens and include cyclophosphamide, busulfan, ifosfamide, chlorambucil, carmustine, and dacarbazine. First-trimester use of cyclophosphamide has resulted in absent toes, eye abnormalities, low-set ears, and cleft palate. When used during the second and third trimesters, cyclophosphamide appears to be safe, although from a combined experience involving 92 cases, there have been 2 fetal demises, 7 cases of growth restriction, and 1 neonatal death. A very interesting case involves the twins reported by Reynoso and colleagues who were exposed to cyclophosphamide throughout the pregnancy. The girl had no abnormalities, but the twin boy was born with esophageal atresia, right-arm deformity, abnormal inferior vena cava, and growth restriction and went on to develop thyroid cancer at 11 years of age. There have been 19 reported cases of combined regimens containing dacarbazine in pregnancy, resulting in 1 case of growth restriction and possibly 1 minor malformation. Of interest, although there have been eight reports of busulfan use during the first trimester without anomalies, two patients who received the drug during the second trimester delivered anomalous neonates (one case each of pyloric stenosis and unilateral renal agenesis with liver calcifications).

Anthracycline and Antitumor Antibiotics

These high-molecular weight antibiotics interpose between DNA strands and include doxorubicin (Adriamycin), idarubicin, epirubicin, dactinomycin, bleomycin, and mitoxantrone. Turchi and Villasis collected 28 cases of doxorubicin and daunorubicin treatment after the first trimester. Following one elective termination, two spontaneous abortions, and two maternal deaths from malignancy with the fetus in utero, 21 pregnancies were delivered without complications. Two of three limb abnormalities seen following doxorubicin exposure during the first trimester ($n = 25$) may be confounded by concomitant radiation or cytarabine treatment.

It has been recognized for a number of years that children and adults receiving anthracyclines are at risk of developing dose-related cardiotoxicity as a result of free radical damage that results in myocardial apoptosis and hypertrophy. It is not known whether in utero exposure to these agents places the fetus at risk for this complication. Meyer-Wittkopf and colleagues performed serial fetal echocardiograms on a pregnant patient receiving doxorubicin and on unexposed fetuses and were unable to detect any significant differences in systolic function. Postnatal echocardiograms revealed no evidence of myocardial damage up to 2 years after birth. There have been at least two cases of transient right-sided cardiomyopathy after second-trimester exposure to anthracyclines, including one case involving idarubicin, which is more lipophilic and favors increased placental transfer. Until more information becomes available, we suggest that pregnant women requiring an anthracycline be given doxorubicin. Although the cardiac profile of fetuses exposed to anthracyclines appears to be safe in the majority of cases, because cancer treatment advances at a faster pace than the accumulation of safety data in human pregnancy, caution is always warranted before new agents are given to pregnant women.

Plant Alkaloids

The vinca alkaloids are highly protein-bound and include vincristine, vinblastine, and vinorelbine. They have been regarded as less potent teratogens than the antimetabolites. One of 29 patients treated with a four-drug regimen containing vincristine during organogenesis was delivered with malformations including an atrial septal defect and no radii or fifth digits. There have been a total of 11 exposures to either vincristine or vinblastine during pregnancy, and excluding those malformations found only in first-trimester use, there have been 9 cases of growth restriction, 2 fetal demises, and 2 neonatal deaths.

Taxanes

Paclitaxel and docetaxel inhibit microtubule disassembly, a process that is important for cell division and intracellular and intercellular functions. Because of their unique mechanism of action, many commentators have been concerned that taxanes may be detrimental to the fetus in many aspects. Animal studies have demonstrated lethality of paclitaxel to chick, rat, and rabbit embryos. Of note, when administered during the period of organogenesis, few malformations have been recorded. There have been only a handful of scattered reports of paclitaxel use during pregnancy in which the drug, when administered after the first trimester, has been shown to be safe for the fetus. As experience with these relatively newer chemotherapeutic agents increases, we anticipate an increase in the reporting of taxane use during pregnancy.

Platinum Analogs

The precise mechanism by which the platinum agents exert their antineoplastic effect has not been fully elucidated but may be similar to that of the classic alkylators. Drugs in this group include cisplatin, carboplatin, and oxaliplatin. There have been reports of exposure to single-agent cisplatin or cisplatin-based regimens, which have resulted in sensorineural hearing loss and cerebral atrophy resulting from impaired anterior cerebral circulation, respectively. In both of these cases, the babies were born before 30 weeks, so the complications associated with extreme prematurity may be confounding the clinical picture. Nevertheless, close assessment of the fetal central nervous system may be advisable when cisplatin is used during pregnancy. Among 24 cases of cisplatin exposure, 5 have been complicated by growth restriction, fetal demise, hearing loss, and ventriculomegaly. The two reports that have appeared in the literature describing carboplatin use during pregnancy have been associated with unremarkable neonatal outcomes at up to 30 months of age.

Pharmacokinetics, Sublethal Fetal Effects, and Maternal Risks

The increased blood volume and increased renal clearance of pregnancy should be considered when treating the mother for life-threatening disease. Together, these physiologic changes, along with the more rapid turnover of the hepatic mixed function oxidase system, may lead to a decrease in active maternal drug concentration. For example, because pregnant women receive similar weight-based dosages (adjusted with the continuing weight gain of pregnancy) as nonpregnant women, the increased drug clearance from the body may lead to a reduced area under the concentration versus time curve. In addition, changes in the gastrointestinal function may have an impact on drug absorption of some agents. Fortunately, with the pregnancy-associated decrease in plasma albumin, the unbound active drug concentration should rise, and thus the efficacy of the drug should not be compromised when administered during pregnancy. As long as the increase in drug balances potential decrease in serum levels, toxicity should not be increased. This may indeed be the case, as Zemlickis and colleagues have noted higher concentrations of free cisplatin in pregnant women compared with those who were not pregnant, but all were asymptomatic. Countering this is the argument that estrogens are known to increase other plasma proteins, and thereby decrease active drug fractions. Accordingly, Cardonic and Iacobucci have reported more frequent nausea, vomiting, fatigue, alopecia, and neutropenia during postpartum chemotherapy compared with identical antenatal treatment. The volume of distribution, peak drug concentrations, and half-life of administration are likely to be changed during pregnancy, although to date we do not have pharmacokinetic data on pregnant patients receiving chemotherapy.

Concerns regarding sublethal fetal effects of maternally administered chemotherapy have been raised. When a multidrug regimen was used in a pregnant woman with leukemia, Morishita and colleagues reported consistently normal fetal hematopoiesis via percutaneous umbilical cord blood sampling 2 and 5 weeks following treatment. Chemotherapy-induced neonatal alopecia is also a reasonable concern parents may have, but this condition has been reported only in three newborns and involved administration of bleomycin, etoposide, and cisplatin or doxorubicin, cyclophosphamide, and 5-fluorouracil. Microscopic scanning of the hair of neonates exposed to chemotherapy for maternal acute monocytic leukemia by Gokal and colleagues did not reveal any cytotoxic damage.

Attention must also be directed to specific maternal risks associated with chemotherapy administration during pregnancy. The safe use of recombinant erythropoietin in pregnancy has been reported to offset the triple insult of pregnancy-associated dilutional anemia, iron-deficiency anemia, and chemotherapy-induced marrow suppression. Along similar lines, granulocyte-colony stimulating factor has been used without adverse sequelae during human pregnancy to counter the maternal and fetal susceptibilities to infection brought about by the generalized immunosuppression of pregnancy and chemotherapy-induced neutropenia. Finally, because the pulmonary damage associated with bleomycin use is exacerbated by oxygen therapy, we do not advise the administration of oxygen during labor in women who have received bleomycin during pregnancy.

Estimating the Stillbirth Rate

The background stillbirth rate associated with chemotherapy administration throughout pregnancy can be estimated. In 1992 Zemlickis and colleagues reported their experience with 21 pregnancies after in utero exposure to chemotherapy. Of the 13 women exposed during the first trimester, 2 of 5 whose pregnancies continued to term had major malformations in their infants, 4 had spontaneous abortions, and 4 had therapeutic abortions. Of four women with second-trimester exposure to chemotherapy, two had normal live births, one had a stillbirth, and one had a therapeutic abortion. All four pregnancies exposed to chemotherapy during the third trimester resulted in healthy live births. However, infants exposed to chemotherapy had statistically significantly lower birth weights than did matched-control infants, owing to significantly lower gestational age and substantial intrauterine growth restriction. The rate of stillbirth was 1 per 11; this was too small a series for comparison with matched control subjects. However, the authors analyzed 223 births in their community occurring to women who had any form of cancer in the same 30-year period, and found 10 stillbirths among the 223 deliveries, significantly more than in the general population (P <0.0005); this stillbirth rate was calculated at a relative risk of 4.23 (95% CI 2.0-7.8).

Occupational Exposure

In a 1985 case-control study, Selevan and colleagues examined the relationship between fetal loss and occupational exposure to antineoplastic drugs in nurses in 17 Finnish hospitals. The pregnancies studied occurred in 1973 through 1980 and were identified using national sources. Each nurse with fetal loss was matched with three nurses who gave birth. A statistically significant association was observed between fetal loss and occupational exposure to antineoplastic drugs during the first trimester of pregnancy, with an odds ratio equaling 2.30 (95% CI 1.20-4.39). Analyses suggested associations between fetal loss and cyclophosphamide, doxorubicin, and vincristine, although the independent effect of each individual drug could not be specifically identified because many nurses reported handling more than one of these agents.

Recommendations on the Use of Chemotherapy During Pregnancy

In summary, the administration of chemotherapy during the first trimester can be associated with morphologic abnormalities and fetal loss. Although first-trimester use of chemotherapy is inadvisable, if a pregnant patient has an aggressive hematologic malignancy, chemotherapy at full doses can often be safely administered, even during the first trimester, if cure of the hematologic malignancy is considered reasonable.

Chemotherapy administered in the second and third trimesters appears not to be associated with a significant risk of structural anomalies, but some reports suggest an association with preterm delivery, fetal death in utero, and intrauterine growth restriction. The background incidence of growth restriction varies according to the population, geographic location, and standard growth curves used as a reference. We must also keep in mind that the mother's underlying illness may affect perinatal complications. When more than one regimen is available and effective for a particular cancer, clearly the agents for which the most extensive investigation during pregnancy has been conducted should be selected. Some form of antepartum fetal surveillance is advisable, and close coordination with a perinatologist can determine the need and schedule for serial ultrasonography and fetal heart rate monitoring (Table 15-16). Placental pathology is mandatory in all cases following delivery or termination.

TABLE 15-16 Examples of Tests Used in The Antepartum Fetal Surveillance of Pregnant Patients with Cancer

Test	Parameters
Biochemical parameters	Progesterone; E3; hCG; Triple screen (E3, hCG, α-fetoprotein); Human placental lactogen
Fetal movements	Kick counting after 25 weeks of gestation
Electronic fetal heart rate monitoring	Nonstress test; Contraction stress test; Sinusoidal rhythms (correlate with fetal anemia)
Ultrasonography	Accurate pregnancy dating; Confirm fetal well-being (viability); Uterine and adnexal abnormalities; Cervical length; Serial growth assessment; Assessment of the placenta; Assessment of fetal anomalies; Four-dimensional imaging
Fetal echocardiography	Evaluation for fetal cardiac defects
Color Doppler	Systolic:diastolic ratio in the umbilical cord artery; Systolic:diastolic ratio in the fetal middle cerebral artery ultrasound
Fetal biophysical profile	Fetal breathing movements; Gross body movement; Fetal tone; Qualitative amniotic fluid volume; Reactive fetal heart rate
Chorionic villus sampling	9 weeks
Amniocentesis	Genetic: 16-20 weeks; Pulmonary maturation: third trimester
Percutaneous umbilical blood sampling	Fetal hematocrit; Fetal infection
Fetal fibronectin	22-34 weeks
Fetal pulse oximetry	Acidemia with $P_{a}O_2$ <30%

E3, Estriol; hCG, human chorionic gonadotropin.

Timing of Delivery

We recommend withholding chemotherapy after 35 weeks of gestation so as to avoid the maternal nadir period because spontaneous labor may occur before the bone marrow has recovered. Chemotherapy administered to the mother within 3 weeks of delivery may not be adequately excreted by the fetus and therefore persist in the newborn.

The preterm pregnancy is also problematic. Iatrogenic preterm delivery is not advisable, and impending preterm delivery should be treated aggressively. In pregnant patients for whom preterm delivery seems inevitable, it is important to withhold chemotherapy 3 weeks before delivery where possible. Preterm babies have limited ability to metabolize drugs because of immaturity of the hepatic and renal systems. Neonates exposed to chemotherapy 3 weeks before delivery should be assessed for transient bone marrow suppression, and long-term neurologic and developmental follow-up is recommended.

Breast Feeding

Durodola reported one case of neonatal neutropenia occurring in a breast fed infant whose mother was treated with cyclophosphamide during late pregnancy and early lactation. As described earlier, some drugs have been detected in the placental tissues and the breast milk. The ability of a drug to cross the placenta, however, has not correlated with its ability to pass into breast milk. Drug concentrations in breast milk are related to the dose and timing of therapy. Because there are no breast feeding data available for most agents, we consider breast feeding to be contraindicated during therapy.

Long-Term Neonatal Follow-up

Although children and adults treated for lymphoma are at risk for secondary leukemia within 10 years, the risk of secondary malignant disease after in utero exposure to chemotherapy is unknown. No cases of secondary leukemia in exposed fetuses have been reported. As described elsewhere, only one case of malignant disease (i.e., thyroid cancer at age 11 years and neuroblastoma at age 14 years) in an anomalous child exposed to chemotherapy in utero has been published. It must be acknowledged, however, that there is a paucity of satisfactory long-term results among children exposed to chemotherapy in utero.

In one of the few studies to address this important subject, Aviles and Neri reported the outcomes of 84 children born to mothers with hematologic malignancies who received chemotherapy during pregnancy, including 38 during the first trimester (acute leukemia, $n = 29$; Hodgkin disease, $n = 26$; malignant lymphoma, $n = 29$). These children were examined for physical health, growth, and development and for hematologic, cytogenetic, neurologic, psychologic, and learning disorders. The occurrence of cancer or acute leukemia in these children was also considered by the investigators. In addition, some of their subjects had become parents, and their children were also considered in the analysis. In all the children studied, including the 12 second-generation children, the birth weight was normal, as was the learning and educational performance. Specifically, school performance and standardized intelligence testing did not differ significantly from unrelated matched children and unexposed siblings. No congenital, neurologic, laboratory, or psychologic abnormalities were observed. Tolerance of infections was also normal, as was secondary sexual development among the older children. With a median follow-up of 18.7 years (range, 6-29 years), no cancer or acute leukemia was detected.

The lack of adequate observation of the long-term status of the fetus or infant prevents any definite conclusions as to the relative safety or danger of anticancer chemotherapy during pregnancy, even in the second and third trimesters. It is surprising how often the detailed status of the fetus is not mentioned in available reports. The infant is often described as "normal," with few if any details on the physical or laboratory profile of the baby. Long-term observation is necessary to establish normalcy because many of the defects may not be obvious on inspection and may emerge as derangements of growth, development, function, reproduction, and heredity.

Supportive Therapy

Granulocyte-colony stimulating factors (G-CSF), recombinant erythropoietin, and antibiotics are associated with very limited data sets in the medical literature. Among seven reports of G-CSF use during pregnancy (all following the first trimester), there were no adverse pregnancy- or neonatal-related events. Use of G-CSF appears to be reasonable for those patients in desperate need of this drug. Although recombinant human erythropoietin (rhEPO) does not cross the placenta, evidence for its safety remains scarce and blood transfusion should remain the first line of therapy for pregnant patients with severe anemia, particularly during the first trimester. Among the multitude of antibiotics available, penicillins are able to cross the placenta freely, but harmful fetal effects have not been reported. The combination of amoxicillin plus clavulonate is a regimen used frequently in patients receiving chemotherapy, but it is associated with an increased incidence of necrotizing enterocolitis in the newborn and therefore should be avoided during pregnancy. Cephalosporins and metronidazole can be safely used during pregnancy; however, aminoglycosides, quinolones, timethoprim, and tetracycline should not be administered. Aminoglycosides can cause 8th cranial nerve damage, whereas quinolones have been linked to congenital arthropathy in animal models. Like methotrexate, trimithoprim is a folate antagonist and is therefore contraindicated during pregnancy. Finally, tetracyclines are hepatotoxic to the mother and inhibit fetal bone growth. Although no adverse events have been reported with imipenum and meropenem, available data in human pregnancy are even more limited.

Serum Tumor Markers in Pregnancy

Table 15-17 contains serum tumor marker ranges for pregnant and nonpregnant women. Although the serum CA-125 has been found to fluctuate during pregnancy, comprehension of the established trends may assist in following pregnant women with a history of epithelial ovarian cancer and those being evaluated during pregnancy for a pelvic mass. Specifically, the CA-125 values are highest during the first trimester, with levels as high as 1250 U reported. The values decrease during the late first trimester and should remain below 35 U/mL of serum until delivery, at which point the CA-125 transiently increases 1 hour postpartum. It should be mentioned that Jacobs and Bast have reviewed the literature and found cases in which the maternal serum CA-125 remained within normal limits throughout uncomplicated pregnancies.

Bon and colleagues evaluated the concentrations of maternal CA-125 and CA-15-3 (a breast cancer tumor marker) in normal and 120 pathologic pregnancies (e.g., spontaneous abortion, fetal death, growth restriction, chromosomal and structural abnormalities, and pre-eclampsia). The maternal CA-125 serum values were higher during the first and third trimesters during pregnancy, and the CA-15-3 serum levels were higher only during the third trimester. Neither antigen showed any relation with a pathologic outcome of pregnancy.

Of interest, Kiran and colleagues performed simultaneous measurements of CA-125, CA-15-3, CA-19-9, and carcinoembryonic antigen (CEA) in the maternal serum and umbilical cord blood in 53 pregnancies that were terminated by cesarean section. CA-19-9 is a pancreatic cancer tumor marker, and CEA is a marker of mucinous adenocarcinomas with levels that are normal or marginally elevated in normal pregnancy. With the exception of CEA, which was more elevated in the multigravida, all marker levels in maternal serum were significantly different to those of the umbilical cord, irrespective of fetal sex, fetal weight, and maternal parity.

Mammalian α-fetoprotein is classified as a member of the albuminoid gene superfamily. Molecular variants and genetic variants of α-fetoprotein differing in messenger ribonucleic acid (mRNA) kilobase length have been extensively described in the biomedical literature. Following the discovery of the molten globule form in 1981, the existence of transitory, intermediate forms of α-fetoprotein was acknowledged and their physiologic significance was realized. The maternal serum

TABLE 15-17   Serum Tumor Markers in Nonpregnant and Pregnant Patients

Marker	Malignancy	Normal Levels	Effect of Pregnancy
CA-125	Serous papillary ovarian carcinoma and tumors of low malignant potential	<35 U/mL	Elevated during the first trimester
Human chorionic gonadotropin	Gestational trophoblastic neoplasia, malignant germ cell tumors of the ovary	<5 IU/L	Peak at 14-16 wk: 12,000-270,000 IU/L
α-Fetoprotein	Malignant germ cell tumors of the ovary, hepatocellular carcinoma	<15 ng/mL	Peaks at 200-300 mg/dL at 13 wk
Lactate dehydrogenase	Dysgerminoma, tumors of the liver	45-90 U/L	Fluctuates minimally
Inhibin	Granulosa cell tumors of the ovary	33-45 pg/mL	Increased with pre-eclampsia
Testosterone	Sertoli cell tumors of the ovary	30-95 ng/dL	May rise four- to ninefold over nonpregnant levels during normal pregnancy
DHEA-S	Tumors of the adrenal gland	35-430 mcg/dL	Can be increased (usually not >700 mcg/dL)
Carcinoembryonic antigen	Colorectal carcinoma, mucinous cystadenocarcinoma of the ovary, pseudomyxoma peritoneii	<5 ng/mL	Normal or marginally elevated levels
CA-27.29	Breast cancer	≤38 U/mL	Not well studied
CA-15-3	Breast cancer	<40 U/mL	Elevated during third trimester in one study
CA-19-9	Pancreatic cancer	<40 U/mL	Not well studied
Prolactin	Pituitary tumor (prolactinoma)	<20 ng/mL	20-400 ng/mL
Total thyroxine	Thyroid carcinoma	5-12 mcg/dL	Increased due to increases in serum thyroxine-binding globulin

CA, *Cancer antigen*; DHEA-S, *dehydroepiandrosterone sulfate.*

α-fetoprotein is a useful marker for women harboring a malignant germ cell tumor containing an endodermal sinus tumor or embryonal component. Initially produced by the yolk sac, and later by the fetal liver and gastrointestinal tract, α-fetoprotein is also the predominant protein synthesized during fetal development. Maternal serum α-fetoprotein levels are routinely measured between 16 and 20 weeks of gestation to screen for neural tube defects. Pregnant women with marked elevations of serum α-fetoprotein should have a germ cell cancer or liver tumor included in the differential diagnosis.

As Boulay and Podczaski point out in their excellent review on ovarian cancer complicating pregnancy, the use of α-fetoprotein levels to monitor women with a history of endodermal sinus tumor who subsequently become pregnant poses a distinct clinical dilemma. One way to distinguish between ovarian (i.e., yolk sac) α-fetoprotein and fetal (i.e., liver) α-fetoprotein is to divide the heterogeneous human α-fetoprotein into various subfractions stratified by differential reactivity with lectins, such as concanavalin A. Assay chromatography with concanavalin sepharose A will separate the α-fetoprotein into either the yolk sac or liver variant because the yolk sac form of α-fetoprotein contains the carbonal sugar and is the type produced by the endodermal sinus tumor.

The use of the hCG level to monitor pregnant women in remission following treatment for gestational trophoblastic disease is also problematic. The hCG steadily increases during the first trimester of pregnancy and may reach levels beyond 100,000 U at 10 weeks of gestation. Accordingly, women with a history of trophoblastic neoplasia must undergo transvaginal ultrasonography to document intrauterine pregnancy, and a metastatic workup should be conducted if the hCG remains markedly elevated during pregnancy or if focal symptoms manifest.

The glycolytic enzyme lactate dehydrogenase (LDH) is involved in the conversion of pyruvate to lactate. LDH is also a marker for gonadal and extragonadal dysgerminomas. Because the enzyme is ubiquitous, the heterogeneity afforded its multiple molecular forms permits electrophoretic separation into five isoenzymes. Isoenzyme fractions 1 and 2 are specifically elevated in women with dysgerminomas. During pregnancy and the puerperium, LDH values fluctuate very little, unless the patient has pre-eclampsia. In 1992 our group used the LDH level to observe two women with dysgerminoma diagnosed during pregnancy; in both cases, the LDH value was correlated to disease activity.

Inhibin is a glycoprotein hormone produced by normal ovarian granulosa cells and testicular Sertoli cells. In the ovary, it inhibits the secretion of follicle-stimulating hormone. Patients with granulosa cell tumors have elevated serum levels of inhibin, and this finding has been used to detect recurrent tumor. In pregnancy, serum levels of inhibin do not rise significantly unless the patient has pre-eclampsia or gestational hypertension. The use of an inhibin monoclonal antibody can preferentially mark inhibin secreted from granulosa cell tumors and Sertoli–Leydig cell tumors.

HEMATOLOGIC MALIGNANCIES IN PREGNANCY

Leukemia

Arising from bone marrow progenitor cells that have arrested along a line of differentiation, the leukemias manifest clinically when the arrested cells proliferate, overtake the bone marrow, and spill out into the peripheral blood. Without immediate therapy, patients with acute leukemia, particularly acute myelogenous leukemia (AML), survive a median of 3 months. In the United States, there are 30,000 new cases of leukemia and 20,000 deaths are attributable to the disease each year. Table 15-18 summarizes a classification scheme for the leukemias, with the major subtypes being AML (comprising 46% of all leukemias), chronic lymphatic leukemia (29%), chronic myelocytic leukemia (CML, 14%), and acute lymphatic leukemia (11%). Leukemia is estimated to occur in 1 in 75,000 pregnancies, with AML accounting for more than 60% of reported cases, of which there are approximately 500.

The attainment of a morphologic normal bone marrow containing less than 5% blasts, the absence of any signs of extramedullary leukemia, and the return of normal neutrophil counts (>1500/μL) and platelet counts (>150,000/μL) is the treatment goal of acute leukemia. Auer rods must not appear in the peripheral blood, and anemia, if present, does not preclude complete remission

TABLE 15-18   Classification of the Leukemias

Acute	Chronic
Acute myelogenous leukemia	Chronic myelogenous leukemia
Acute promyelocytic leukemia	Chronic myelomonocytic
Acute myelomonocytic leukemia	leukemia
Acute monoblastic leukemia	Chronic lymphatic leukemia
Acute erythroleukemia	T cell
Acute megakaryoblastic leukemia	B cell
Acute lymphatic leukemia	Prolymphocytic leukemia
Common	Sézary syndrome
T cell	Hairy cell leukemia
B cell	
Pre-B cell	
Acute mast cell leukemia	

From Jandl JH: Blood: Textbook of Hematology, 2nd ed. Boston, Little, Brown, 1996.

because this is often slow to recover. Bone marrow aspiration is performed weekly during the induction phase.

Because of severe myelosuppression caused by intensive chemotherapy, the achievement of complete remission is predicated on supportive care and the necessary maintenance of more than 500/μL circulating neutrophils and more than 20,000 circulating platelets to prevent infectious and hemorrhagic deaths. Cytosine arabinoside and daunorubicin are used to induce remission in AML, with postremission therapy requiring maintenances doses of cytosine arabinoside. When the analysis of the cerebrospinal fluid establishes central nervous system involvement, intrathecal chemotherapy with or without cranial radiation is administered. Finally, the treatment and maintenance of acute lymphatic leukemia uses multiagent regimens involving vincristine and central nervous system prophylaxis.

The ability to enter into complete remission is age dependent, with the overall rate for acute leukemia being 65%. Median survival is approximately 2 years, with 25% of patients becoming long-term, disease-free survivors. The prognosis for patients undergoing treatment of leukemia following therapy for another disease, or in the recurrent setting, is very poor. Indeed, the majority of adult patients who achieve remission subsequently experience recurrence. The long-term survival rate seen in children is not obtained in adults.

Leukemia in Pregnancy

In the pregnant patient, persistent fever, weight loss, lymphadenopathy, and/or an abnormal differential on the complete blood count should prompt an investigation and raise the clinician's suspicion for leukemia. As in the case of non-Hodgkin lymphoma (NHL) in pregnancy, patients with acute leukemia are often very ill, and the primary concern is to save the mother's life through induction chemotherapy or radiotherapy. Therefore, if the patient is remote from delivery, appropriate treatment will place the fetus at risk of exposure to chemotherapeutic agents and/or radiation therapy. Chronic myelogenous leukemia in pregnancy, however, can be managed similar to Hodgkin disease, with a justifiable delay in definitive treatment of several weeks if indicated. The outcome of pregnancy-associated acute leukemia is only worse when compared with nonpregnant cases when therapy is delayed. Regardless of gestational age, the induction of remission with combination chemotherapy is the primary objective. Seventy-five percent of pregnant women enter into complete remission following therapy for acute leukemia, owing to their favorable age. During the first and early second trimesters, termination of pregnancy should be seriously considered, especially in the acutely ill mother. When the diagnosis is made later in pregnancy, it should be recognized that there are obvious advantages of delivery before the onset of chemotherapy, and this should be encouraged, if possible.

The average age of the patient with acute leukemia in pregnancy is 28 years. Premature labor is common in these women, and the average period of gestation is approximately 8 months. Postpartum hemorrhage occurs in 10% to 15% of cases. The fibrinogen level in patients with acute leukemia in pregnancy may be reduced from the level anticipated at that stage of gestation. Frenkel and Meyers stated that pregnancy exerts no specific effect on the course of acute leukemia except that early gestation poses an obstacle to vigorous treatment of leukemia. Other authors have observed that infants born of mothers with leukemia are as well as normal control subjects. Lilleyman and colleagues and Bitran and Roth have written comprehensive reports on this subject.

The following factors are associated with the delivery of a normal baby:

- Antimetabolite drugs not administered
- Radiotherapy to the uterus not given
- The fetus reaches the age of viability

The decision to interrupt a pregnancy in patients discovered to have leukemia is primarily based on the desires of the patient. Prompt therapy is always advisable for the possibility of obtaining remission. However, the physician's advice to the patient should be influenced by the aggressiveness of the disease process. For instance, patients with CML are less likely to be harmed by deferring termination of pregnancy than are patients with acute myelocytic leukemia demonstrating symptoms and having a somewhat fulminating course.

Chemotherapy for Acute Leukemia in Pregnancy

There are many reports of successful chemotherapy for patients who have acute leukemia in pregnancy, and there has been little if any significant increase in fetal wastage or congenital anomalies. In 1984 Catanzarite and Ferguson published a review of management and outcome of acute leukemia in pregnancy for the years 1972 to 1982. The investigators collected 14 pregnancies reported in patients cured of acute lymphocytic leukemia, of which there was 1 early spontaneous abortion and 13 term infants. All mothers survived. They also collected 47 reports of pregnancy in association with acute leukemia. In 40 pregnancies in which acute leukemia was treated, there were 5 abortions, 3 perinatal demises, 1 infant "live-born in grave condition," and 31 surviving infants. Median maternal survival was at least 6 months and possibly longer than 12 months from delivery. In the remaining 7 cases, the leukemia was untreated. Despite this, there were 2 perinatal deaths, 1 abortion, and 4 living infants.

During the years of Catanzarite and Ferguson's study, effective combination chemotherapy was in widespread use. Previous reviews covered cases reported before the introduction of effective combination chemotherapy. There were fewer than 300 reported pregnancies, with a 36% to 69% perinatal mortality and a median maternal survival from diagnosis of shorter than 6 months. Advances in the fields of hematology and oncology, maternal and fetal medicine, and neonatology have resulted in marked improvements in both perinatal survival statistics and median maternal survival.

In women who refuse pregnancy termination or in whom delivery is not expected imminently, induction of remission should be attempted. When combination therapy is used during the first trimester (and for acute leukemia in pregnancy, this is not a contraindication), the stillbirth rate is 25%—this decreases to 13% in the second and third trimesters. A combination of cytarabine, doxorubicin, and etoposide has been used with good results for both mother and fetus, and when possible we recommend this regimen. Delivery should be timed to precede the next course of chemotherapy; however, the majority of patients should be counseled to expect preterm delivery, either spontaneous or induced. It is mandatory to perform a hematologic evaluation of the newborn because the drugs used cross the placenta and can result in pancytopenia. Although no growth or developmental abnormalities have been demonstrated, the follow-up of children exposed to in utero chemotherapy for the management of acute leukemia has been limited.

Acute Myeloid Leukemia

AML is the most common leukemia diagnosed during pregnancy. Azim and colleagues identified 87 patients (88 pregnancies) treated with systemic therapy during pregnancy in their literature review. Among those treated during the first trimester, nearly 50% had poor fetal outcomes. Among those treated after the first trimester, the combination of cytarabine and daunorubicin was most commonly used during the induction phase. Out of 32 patients exposed to these two agents starting from the second trimester, only 15 had normal pregnancy outcomes. It is unclear whether this is secondary to cytarabine or daunorubicin. Previous reports of single-agent cytarabine have been associated with normal pregnancy outcomes, whereas single-agent daunorubicin has been associated with one case of maternal–fetal death. Idarubicin is also used for AML induction therapy and is more lipophilic compared to other anthracyclines; therefore placental transfer of this drug is more likely to occur. There have been seven pregnant women exposed to idarubicin and cytarabine following the first trimester from which reports of stillbirth, limb deformities, and cardiomyopathy have appeared. It is of significant concern that the combination of cytarabine with daunorubicin or idarubicin is associated with significant fetal morbidity and mortality, even if administered after the first trimester. However, doxorubicin is an active agent in AML and has been associated with normal pregnancy outcomes both in AML and in PABC. Given the poor safety data of daunorubicin and idarubicin and probably noninferiority of doxorubicin when compared to other anthracyclines, Azim and colleagues consider it the treatment of choice for gestational AML for patients wishing to preserve the pregnancy.

Acute Lymphoblastic Leukemia

Approximately one third of gestational leukemia is of acute lymphoblastic leukemia (ALL). Many of the patients in the literature treated with chemotherapy during the first trimester were unintentionally exposed. The not unexpected findings of limb and ear and Madelung deformities along with a case of esophageal atresia and even stillbirth emphasize the importance of active contraception in patients with ALL during the maintenance phase. Azim and colleagues have identified 21 patients treated after the first trimester. As was observed with daunorubicin and idarubicin exposure during the second trimester in patients with AML, these agents have also been associated with adverse fetal outcomes when given for ALL. Acute cardiac failure, premature delivery, and intrauterine fetal demise have been reported. Fortunately, data on doxorubicin in ALL is reassuring and again Azim and colleagues consider this agent as the anthracycline of choice during pregnancy after the first trimester.

Acute Promyelocytic Leukemia

Acute promyelocytic leukemia (APL) accounts for 13% of AML cases and commonly occurs in young adults. The specific chromosomal translocation, t(15/17), is found in the neoplastic promyeloctic proliferation that characterizes this disease. Disseminated intravascular coagulation (DIC) is a lethal complication of AML. All-trans retinoic acid (ATRA) targets t(15/17) and reduces the incidence of DIC and consequently increases the likelihood of achieving long-term remission. Azim and colleagues collected 22 cases of ATRA treatment during pregnancy, in which 14 patients received single-agent therapy and 8 were treated with a combination of ATRA plus idarubicin or daunorubicin. No congenital anomalies or spontaneous abortions have been reported to have occurred among newborns exposed to single-agent ATRA in utero. One baby who had been diagnosed earlier with Potter syndrome during the first trimester before exposure to ATRA died after the mother went into spontaneous labor; this newborn had been exposed to ATRA for 1 day during week 29 of gestation. Although two patients exposed to ATRA during the first trimester have been reported to have had normal outcomes, there are data that link first-trimester retinoic acid ingestion to craniofacial, cardiac, and brain malformations (i.e., retinoic acid embryopathy).

Among those patients treated with combined therapy, atrial septal defects were reported in two newborns exposed to ATRA plus idarubicin. Postnatal fetal death secondary to pulmonary hemorrhage was reported in a newborn exposed to ATRA plus daunorubicin and cytarabine. In those patients with APL who received chemotherapy alone, once again, daunorubicin has been associated with a high incidence of complications, including intrauterine fetal demise, spontaneous abortion, bone marrow aplasia, cerebral bleeding, and child maceration.

Management of Chronic Leukemia

Chronic myelocytic leukemia represents approximately 90% of all chronic leukemias in pregnancy. An additional 5% of the chronic leukemias in pregnancy are chronic lymphocytic leukemias. Several reports show that pregnant patients with chronic granulocytic leukemia treated during the first trimester with chemotherapy and radiation therapy to the spleen will usually deliver apparently healthy, viable babies if the uterus is protected with lead shields. Lee and co-workers reported 12 cases of leukemia associated with pregnancy. Using lead shields to protect the uterus from radiation therapy to the spleen, six of seven women with chronic leukemia who also received chemotherapy went on to deliver six apparently healthy infants. Another study that showed similar results was reported by Levin and Collea. The prognosis for these patients is poor; median survival is 45 months.

There has been some experience in treating CML during pregnancy with interferon-α. Mubarak and colleagues reported the outcomes of three women, ages 23 to 32 years, with Philadelphia chromosome–positive CML who received interferon-α during the first trimester of pregnancy. No maternal complications occurred, and three normal-appearing babies were delivered, one of whom had a transient mild thrombocytopenia. Subsequently, these children were followed for 4, 12, and 30 months, and all had normal growth and development.

Chronic Myeloid Leukemia

CML is rare among pregnant women. The disease accounts for only 15% of adult leukemias, with only 10% occurring during the childbearing years. The main driving force for development and maintenance of the leukemic clone is the BCR/ABL fusion gene, which is a target of imatinib mesylate. Complete responses with this agent are dependent on the continuous administration of this drug. Pye and colleagues have identified 55 pregnant women exposed to imatinib, 40 of whom

(72%) delivered live births without any congenital anomalies. Seventy-five percent of the congenital anomalies encountered in this series ($n = 9$) were in fetuses exposed to imatinib during the first trimester. Exomphalos occurred in 3 neonates; renal agenesis/malformation in 2; hypospadias in 2; cleft palate, hydrocephalus, meningocele, pyloric stenosis and premature closure of skull bones in 1; and warfarin syndrome in 1. Among the 38 patients (21%) exposed to imatinib throughout the course of pregnancy, 7 had a spontaneous abortion and 1 developed the previously mentioned warfarin syndrome secondary to warfarin exposure. Azim and colleagues identified 26 additional cases of gestational imatinib exposure. Sixty percent were exposed during the first trimester and discontinued the drug when pregnancy was diagnosed. In these patients, 1 preterm delivery, 2 cases of newborn hypospadias, and 1 child with a fatal meningocele were reported. Nine patients became pregnant while taking imatinib and continued the pregnancy to term with no adverse events. Four patients who started imatinib therapy during the second and third trimesters were able to control their disease without affecting the pregnancy outcome. A total of 11 newborns have been followed for more than 1 year with no delayed adverse effects reported. It would appear that early exposure to imatinib is associated with a high risk of spontaneous abortion and congenital anomalies. Imatinib therapy during the second and third trimester does not appear to add significantly to the risk associated with first-trimester exposure.

In the pre-imatinib era, both interferon-(IFN) alpha and hydroxyurea (HU) were used to treat patients with CML. IFN was considered the standard of care for those patients not eligible for bone marrow transplantation. Because of its high molecular weight, IFN is unlikely to cross the placenta. Approximately 15 patients have been exposed during the first trimester with no congenital anomalies reported. Preclinical data also support the safe use of IFN throughout the course of pregnancy.

Preclinical models have been less favorable for HU with significant evidence for teratogenicity in all animal species. Congenital anomalies of the heart, central nervous system, skeleton, and neural tube defects have been described. Among the 49 pregnant patients with CML exposed to HU in the literature review by Azim and colleagues, there was one neonatal death on day 10 of life secondary to intracranial bleeding not associated with congenital anomalies. Three intrauterine fetal deaths were reported, two cases of hip dysplasia, and one case each of pilonidal sinus and unilateral renal dilatation. Although chromosomal anomalies have not been reported in humans following HU exposure in utero, this drug should not be the treatment of choice for CML during pregnancy, particularly in light of its nonsuperiority to other agents used to treat this disease.

Hairy Cell Leukemia, Multiple Myeloma, and Chronic Lymphocytic Leukemia

Hairy cell leukemia (HCL), multiple myeloma (MM), and chronic lymphocytic leukemia (CLL) are among the rarest hematologic malignancies encountered during pregnancy. A few cases of IFN therapy for HCL and MM have been reported with normal outcomes. The standard of care for HCL is cladribine, but its use during pregnancy has not yet been reported. For the rare patient of childbearing age who develops CLL during pregnancy, a watch-and-wait approach is advisable in the absence of symptoms. Chlorambucil has been associated with normal pregnancy outcomes for patients with symptomatic CLL.

Hodgkin Disease

The importance of staging in Hodgkin disease was recognized by Peters as early as 1950, when she devised the first clinical staging classification. Lymphangiography then made possible the earlier detection of retroperitoneal lymph node involvement, and it became important to distinguish two subgroups: those with widespread disease confined to lymphatic organs, and those with spread of disease beyond the lymph nodes, thymus, spleen, and Waldeyer's ring to one or more extralymphatic organs or tissues, which is now recognized as stage IV disease. The subtype classification scheme for Hodgkin lymphoma appears in Table 15-19. The staging system as proposed by the Cotswolds meeting appears in Table 15-20. Surgical staging has gained popularity in Hodgkin disease, and when evaluating young women in whom preservation of ovarian function is desired and pelvic irradiation is planned, surgical oophoropexy can be performed at the time of staging laparotomy.

The feature of the disease most helpful in selecting therapy and estimating the prognosis at the time of onset is its clinical extent. In general, the more widespread the disease, the poorer the prognosis, even if all apparent disease is confined to the lymphoid regions. The poorer prognosis of patients who have involvement of sites beyond the usual lymphoid tissues is well known.

Five-year survival rates of 50% are often reported for patients who have widespread lymph node disease, and rates of 8% are reported for those who have involvement of extranodal sites such as the lung, liver, bone, and bone marrow. Survival depends more on the patient's age and stage than on the subtype. Overall, 36% survive for 20 years, and about 70% do not have a relapse after primary treatment. Those 17 to 34 years old have an 80% long-term survival, compared with 35% for those 60 years or older.

The treatment of Hodgkin disease has undergone radical changes in the past 40 years. Present recommendations are based on the assumptions that radiotherapy is the mainstay of treatment of early-stage disease, combination chemotherapy is the primary treatment of advanced-stage disease with parenchymal organ involvement, and a combination of the two is required for patients with bulky disease (e.g., a large mediastinal mass) or generalized abdominal lymph node involvement. Aggressive therapy has resulted in considerable improvement in overall survival rates for patients with Hodgkin disease. The most successful and widely tested combination of drugs has been developed at the National Cancer Institute (DeVita and colleagues), and consists of six 2-week cycles of therapy with nitrogen mustard, vincristine, procarbazine, and prednisone, the so-called MOPP program, although other combinations have been used successfully.

The major technical factors that determine the efficacy of radiation therapy in Hodgkin disease are the total

TABLE 15-19   Classification of Hodgkin Disease

Subtype	Frequency (%)	Characteristics
Nodular sclerosis	40	Mediastinal and pulmonary involvement
Mixed cellularity	30	Often advanced at presentation
Lymphocyte predominance	15	Rare classic Reed–Sternberg cells
Lymphocyte depletion	15	Oldest median age, worst prognosis

TABLE 15-20   Staging of Hodgkin Disease as Proposed in the Cotswolds, England, 1990

Stage*	Characteristics
I	Involvement of a single lymph node or lymphoid region (e.g., spleen, thymus, Waldeyer's ring) or a single extralymphatic site (Ie)
II	Involvement of two or more lymph node regions on the same side of the diaphragm; localized contiguous involvement of only one extranodal organ or site and lymph node region(s) on the same side of the diaphragm (IIe)
III	Involvement of lymph node regions on both sides of the diaphragm, which may also include spleen (IIIs) or one extranodal localized contiguous site (IIIe), or both (IIIes)
III1	With or without involvement of splenic, hilar, celiac, or portal nodes
III2	With involvement of para-aortic, iliac, and mesenteric nodes
IV	Diffuse or disseminated involvement of one or more extranodal organs or tissues

From Peleg D, Ben-Ami M: Obstet Gynecol Clin North Am 25:365, 1998.
*Applicable designations: a, no symptoms; b, night sweats, fever, weight loss; cs, clinical staging; e, involvement of a single extranodal site contiguous or proximal to a known nodal site; ps, pathologic staging (by laparotomy); x, bulky disease (diameter > one third of mediastinum).

radiation dose per field; the size, shape, and number of treatment fields; and the beam energy. Permanent eradication of any given site of involvement can be achieved consistently with doses of 3500 to 4500 cGy delivered at a rate of 1000 cGy/week. The desirability of irradiating apparently uninvolved lymph node regions has long been advocated by experienced radiotherapists. This approach is based on the knowledge of the clinical behavior of Hodgkin disease, the inadequacies of our diagnostic techniques to discover minute or microscopic foci of the disease, the advantage and efficacy of avoiding patchwork and overlapping fields, and the possible reseeding of previously irradiated regions from unrecognized and untreated sites. Extended field irradiation, so-called total lymphoid or total radial therapy, is technically demanding and potentially hazardous.

Hodgkin Disease in Pregnancy

With a peak incidence between the ages of 18 and 30 years, Hodgkin disease commonly affects young people. It is now being cured and controlled for long periods with irradiation and chemotherapy. Hodgkin disease in pregnancy occurs in approximately 1 in 6000 deliveries. Young women diagnosed with Hodgkin disease are usually asymptomatic. The nodular sclerosis subtype of Hodgkin disease is the most common subtype encountered in pregnancy and carries a favorable prognosis.

Most reports suggest that the onset of Hodgkin disease during pregnancy does not adversely affect survival. Chemotherapy and radiation therapy to the abdomen can usually be postponed until the pregnancy is terminated. The drugs commonly used for Hodgkin disease are contraindicated in the first trimester of pregnancy and are preferably withheld until the postpartum period. The amazing successes achieved with early stages of this disease allow much more flexibility and improved regard for the fetus. Pregnancy itself does not appear to adversely affect the course of the disease, and interruption of pregnancy during the course of the disease is not definitely indicated. The management of the pregnant patient with Hodgkin disease should be individualized and should involve a multidisciplinary team of physicians and other professionals. Three of four patients diagnosed with Hodgkin disease will be cured.

Management of Hodgkin Disease in Pregnancy

Hodgkin lymphoma is the second most commonly diagnosed cancer in people aged 15 to 29 years and is the most common lymphoma diagnosed during pregnancy. The literature contains 68 pregnancies in 67 women with Hodgkin lymphoma who received systemic chemotherapy and/or immunotherapy. Twenty-six of these cases were published by Aviles and colleagues, and an additional 42 were identified in the review by Azim and colleagues. In the former study, most patients had advanced disease and nodular sclerosis histology. More than one third of patients were treated during the first trimester without sequelae (i.e., no low birth weight or anomalies). These results are challenged by the finding of six congenital anomalies and three spontaneous abortions occurring in the 17 patients exposed to chemotherapy during the first trimester in the report by Azim and colleagues. The standard Hodgkin lymphoma regimen ABVD (doxorubicin, bleomycin, vinblastine, and dacarbazine) was given to 16 of the 42 patients. Those treated after the first trimester had normal pregnancy outcome with no adverse fetal events with the exception on one case of intrauterine fetal demise in the third trimester, one case of atrial septal defect, and one case of hemolytic anemia with jaundice at birth. It seems reasonable to start treating patients with the standard ABVD regimen in the second trimester.

For patients with localized disease in the cervical, occipital, or axillary regions, radiotherapy has been reported to be safe because the average embryo dose does not exceed 0.1 to 0.2 Gy in such sites. This represents the threshold dose at which stochastic effects (e.g., mental retardation, organ malformation) could manifest.

The complexity of the management of Hodgkin disease during pregnancy cannot be overstressed. Thorough staging of the pregnant patient is significantly compromised without termination of the pregnancy by one means or another. Surgical staging of the pregnant patient after the 18th week of pregnancy is feasible and often avoids the necessity of many of the diagnostic techniques that might be harmful to the fetus, such as lower-extremity lymphangiography, intravenous pyelography, and bone and liver scans. Splenectomy is often performed at these staging procedures, and no contraindication in pregnancy is known. The purpose of staging with this disease is to achieve the best differentiation between those curable with local therapy (radiation) and those who require systemic therapy (chemotherapy or radiation) for cure. Once a criterion for systemic therapy has been uncovered, no additional diagnostic procedures are required.

Treatment is obviously easier if the pregnancy is terminated, but that may not be an option. Current data suggest that the course of Hodgkin disease does not seem to be affected by an ongoing pregnancy. Other studies have also noted a survival rate of pregnant women with Hodgkin disease comparable with that of nonpregnant patients with Hodgkin disease. Hodgkin lymphoma is not associated with an increase in miscarriage, stillbirths, or congenital anomalies unless treatment is started in the first trimester. Metastasis to the placenta has been reported, although it is rare.

Hodgkin lymphoma is a potentially curable disease, and stage I and II disease typically are treated with

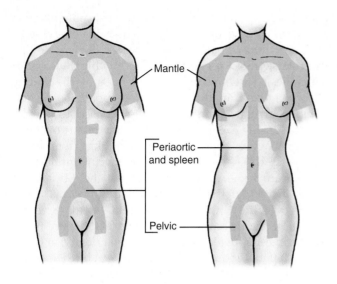

FIGURE 15-15 Schematic representation of "mantle" and "inverted Y" fields for total lymphoid irradiation. **A,** Two-field technique, with a small extension to include the splenic pedicle, used in splenectomized patients. **B,** Three-field technique usually used when the spleen is still present. *(From Rosenberg SA, Kaplan HS: Calif Med 113:23, 1970.)*

megavolt radiotherapy unless bulky disease is present. Given in fractions over 3.5 to 4.5 weeks, a dose of 3500 to 4500 cGy is prescribed. In early-stage disease, the lymphoid areas that need to be irradiated include the mediastinum, Waldeyer's ring and axilla (i.e., mantle field), and the para-aortic area and splenic pedicle (spade field). When necessary, total nodal irradiation includes the pelvis (inverted Y field), as illustrated in Figure 15-15.

Pregnant women with Hodgkin lymphoma present with typical manifestations, with painless enlargement of lymph nodes above the diaphragm, usually the cervical, submaxillary, or axillary nodes. In patients without obvious lymphadenopathy, a delay in diagnosis is not uncommon because symptoms of fatigue, weight loss, chest discomfort, and anemia may be overlooked and considered "normal" during pregnancy. The role of staging laparotomy in Hodgkin disease is diminishing, and if necessary, it should be delayed until after delivery, at which time bilateral oophoropexy can be performed. It has been our practice to bring the ovaries as close to the midline as possible behind the uterus, where they can be shielded underneath a protective block placed between the two arms of the Y.

Pohlman and Macklis carefully reviewed previously published guidelines for Hodgkin disease associated with pregnancy and have proposed the following management scheme, which we have endorsed (Figure 15-16). The earlier the pregnancy, the stronger the recommendation for pregnancy termination so that proper staging and treatment can begin. Patients diagnosed during the first trimester of pregnancy may be observed until the second trimester, when therapy can commence. Those first-trimester patients with B symptoms, bulky or advanced-stage disease, or rapid progression have an indication to initiate treatment immediately and should undergo therapeutic abortion. If the mother does not wish to sacrifice the pregnancy, single-agent vinblastine, which has a 7% anomaly rate when used in the first trimester, should be administered until the second trimester or until significant disease progression. If combination chemotherapy is required, the doxorubicin (Adriamycin), bleomycin, vinblastine, and dacarbazine (ABVD) regimen without dacarbazine during the first trimester should be given and then standard ABVD subsequently.

Patients presenting in the second or third trimester can be closely observed, and the fetus should be delivered as soon as viability and pulmonary maturation are demonstrable. Delivery should be delayed as long as possible after the last dose of chemotherapy (before the next dose) to decrease the risk of marrow suppression in the neonate. It may be worthwhile to consider a cesarean section so that surgical staging can be performed at the same time. Umbilical cord blood should be collected and stored as a possible source of human leukocyte antigen–compatible stem cells. Because the drugs used in Hodgkin disease can reach significant levels in breast milk, mothers receiving chemotherapy must avoid breast feeding.

If treatment is necessary during the second and third trimesters of pregnancy, the standard ABVD regimen should be used. Postchemotherapy-involved field radiation therapy can be postponed until after delivery but should be initiated within 9 weeks following the last cycle of chemotherapy. Mantle and spade field radiotherapy with extensive abdominal shielding is also an acceptable alternative until the third trimester, when the uterus starts to impinge on the field. The inverted Y field is not an option at any time during pregnancy.

Among those women with refractory or relapsed Hodgkin disease for whom the ABVD regimen and/or radiotherapy are not treatment options, MOPP and MOPP-like regimens have demonstrable efficacy with limited adverse effect on the fetus if administered after the first trimester.

Several older series that predate modern therapy suggest that Hodgkin disease has no biologic effect on pregnancy and vice versa. More contemporary reports have substantiated these claims. Investigators from the Hospital for Sick Children and Princess Margaret Hospital in Toronto identified 48 women with 50 pregnancies from 1958 to 1984 and matched them with three nonpregnant control subjects of similar age, stage, and year of diagnosis. Twelve women were diagnosed with

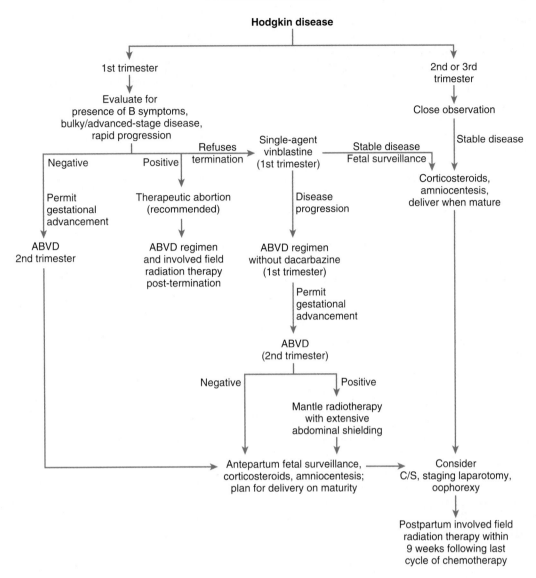

Hodgkin disease

1st trimester

2nd or 3rd trimester

Evaluate for presence of B symptoms, bulky/advanced-stage disease, rapid progression

Close observation

Negative | Positive

Refuses termination

Single-agent vinblastine (1st trimester)

Stable disease Fetal surveillance

Stable disease

Permit gestational advancement

Therapeutic abortion (recommended)

Disease progression

Corticosteroids, amniocentesis, deliver when mature

ABVD 2nd trimester

ABVD regimen and involved field radiation therapy post-termination

ABVD regimen without dacarbazine (1st trimester)

Permit gestational advancement

ABVD (2nd trimester)

Negative | Positive

Mantle radiotherapy with extensive abdominal shielding

Antepartum fetal surveillance, corticosteroids, amniocentesis; plan for delivery on maturity

Consider C/S, staging laparotomy, oophorexy

Postpartum involved field radiation therapy within 9 weeks following last cycle of chemotherapy

FIGURE 15-16 Management algorithm for Hodgkin disease in pregnancy. *ABVD*, Doxorubicin (Adriamycin), bleomycin, vinblastine, and dacarbazine.

Hodgkin disease before conception, 10 during pregnancy, and 27 following delivery or pregnancy termination. No statistically significant difference in stage at diagnosis, maternal outcome, or pregnancy outcome was identified between any of these subgroups and the similar control group. It should be noted that 16 patients received radiotherapy while pregnant and 5 received combination chemotherapy and radiotherapy while pregnant.

In an investigation focusing on fetal effects of therapy, Ebert and colleagues identified 24 cases in the literature between 1983 and 1995. Among 15 women who received cyclophosphamide, vincristine, procarbazine, and prednisone (COPP, $n = 1$), mechlorethamine, vincristine, procarbazine, and prednisone (MOPP, $n = 4$), doxorubicin (Adriamycin), bleomycin, vinblastine, and dacarbazine (ABVD, $n = 7$), or MOPP/ABVD ($n = 3$) beginning in the first ($n = 5$), second ($n = 8$), and third ($n = 2$) trimesters, all had healthy infants who went on to develop normally during a median follow-up of 9 years (range, 0-17 years) after delivery. Of the remaining 9 women, most received one of the aforementioned regimens during the first trimester and either had therapeutic abortions or experienced spontaneous abortions, delivering fetuses with multiple anomalies.

In a study from Stanford University, the outcome of 17 pregnancies associated with Hodgkin disease between 1987 and 1993 was reported. Patients received radiation therapy ($n = 6$), chemotherapy ($n = 4$), or combined modality therapy ($n = 5$), although the specific timings of therapy in relation to pregnancy were not stated. Excluding 4 women who had a therapeutic/spontaneous abortion, no congenital anomalies were noted at delivery, and all children were reported to be healthy at the time of last follow-up. With a median follow-up of 35 months (range, 6-79 months), 15 of the 17 mothers remain in complete remission.

A final report of interest was provided by Sutcliffe, who describes three women with stage II nodular sclerosing Hodgkin disease who received ABVD chemotherapy during the second and third trimesters of pregnancy. Two of these patients also received mantle field radiation therapy following delivery. All three delivered healthy infants between 32 and 35 weeks of gestation. The chromosomal analyses of all three children were normal, and at more than 1 year, 5 years, and 7 years of follow-up, all three mothers and children remain healthy.

Non-Hodgkin Lymphoma

Forty-five thousand new cases of NHL are diagnosed in the United States each year. The mean age at diagnosis is 42 years. NHLs comprise a mixed family of diseases characterized by clonal neoplasms arising from one of the cellular constituents of the lymph node. Approximately 85% of NHLs are B-cell tumors; 15% are T-cell tumors; and a small percentage arise from other cells, primarily macrophages. A multitude of infectious agents (e.g., the Epstein–Barr virus, the human T-cell leukemia/lymphoma virus), noninfectious agents (e.g., radiation, radiation therapy, chemotherapy), and diseases (e.g., ataxia telangiectasia, Sjögren syndrome, systemic lupus erythematosus) are associated with NHLs. Most patients present with painless lymphadenopathy, but NHLs may arise outside the lymphoid system in any tissue accessible to lymphocytes, most commonly in the gastrointestinal tract, pharynx, central nervous system, skin, and bone. Because the disease is usually widespread when peripheral lymph nodes have become involved, staging laparotomy is not used. The prognosis of NHL has been divided into favorable, intermediate, and poor. The Working Formulation is a classification scheme for NHL that is used in determining prognosis and treatment (Table 15-21). Unfortunately, NHLs are cured in less than 25% of the general population, although women of reproductive age have a 50% cure rate.

Early-stage (I/II), low-grade NHL is treated with extended field or total lymphoid irradiation, with 5-year survival rates of 84%. Intermediate-grade tumors are managed with combination chemotherapy (prednisone, methotrexate, doxorubicin, cyclophosphamide, etoposide, cytosine arabinoside, bleomycin, vincristine, and leucovorin—ProMACE-CytaBOM) with or without radiotherapy, resulting in sustained remissions at 4 years in approximately 45% of patients.

TABLE 15-21   Working Formulation for Classification of Non-Hodgkin Lymphoma

	Histologic Type	Description	Prognosis
I	Low grade	Small lymphocytic cell Follicular (nodular) small cleaved cell Follicular mixed small cleaved cell	Favorable
II	Intermediate grade	Follicular large cell Diffuse small cleaved cell Diffuse mixed small and large cell Diffuse large cell cleaved/noncleaved	Intermediate
III	High grade	Diffuse large cell, immunoblastic Small noncleaved cell (Burkitt/non-Burkitt) Lymphoblastic (convoluted/nonconvoluted)	Unfavorable
IV	Miscellaneous	Composite Mycosis fungoides Extramedullary plasmacytoma Histiocytic Unclassified	—

(From Peleg D, Ben-Ami M: Obstet Gynecol Clin North Am 25:365, 1998.)

Non-Hodgkin Lymphoma in Pregnancy

Most women with NHL in association with pregnancy have an aggressive histologic subtype and advanced-stage disease, possibly as a result of a delay in diagnosis in many cases. An unexpectedly high incidence of breast, uterine, cervical, and ovarian involvement among pregnant women has been noted when NHL is associated with pregnancy, with the predilection for these organs attributed to hormonal influences and increased blood flow to these organs. In a review of 96 women with pregnancy-associated NHL, Pohlman and colleagues reported fully 50% of women presenting with stage IV disease. Seven percent of pregnancies ended in therapeutic abortion, and 4% of women experienced a spontaneous abortion. Eleven percent of infants were born prematurely, and 7% died. Only 31 mothers were known to have achieved a complete remission, and for 90 subjects in whom their long-term outcome was known, only 39 were alive and disease free a median of 21 months (range, 2-132 months) after delivery, 4 were alive with disease, and 47 had died with median of 6 months (range, <1 to 36 months) after delivery. Women who were diagnosed during the third trimester of pregnancy appeared to have a better outcome than those diagnosed earlier. Seventy-one of 96 children were reported alive, although the follow-up period for the majority was either less than 1 month or unknown.

Aviles and colleagues reviewed the outcome of both mother and fetus in 19 pregnancies between 1975 and 1986. All patients received doxorubicin-based combination chemotherapy during pregnancy, including 8 who received chemotherapy during the first trimester. Three mothers and their fetuses died during induction, and the 16 remaining women delivered healthy infants between 35 and 39 weeks of gestation. Eight of 12 mothers remained in complete remission 4 to 9 years after delivery, whereas 7 mothers died of lymphoma and 1 was lost to follow-up.

Overall, the prognosis for all patients with NHL is worse than the prognosis for patients with Hodgkin disease. This is explained, in part, by the dissemination of disease at presentation. For this reason, although many dispute the claims that NHL arising in pregnancy is more virulent, the management of NHL in pregnancy needs to be aggressive. A delay in treatment cannot be justified, and a woman who has not completed the first half of pregnancy should be advised to undergo therapeutic abortion unless she is willing to expose herself and her fetus to the risks of combination chemotherapy. After 24 weeks of gestation, premature delivery may be necessary, depending on the mother's medical condition.

Patients with localized disease should receive three to eight cycles of cyclophosphamide, doxorubicin, vincristine, and prednisolone (CHOP) chemotherapy and then, following delivery but within 9 weeks of the last dose of chemotherapy, involved field radiation therapy should be prescribed. Patients with advanced-stage disease should be treated with six to eight cycles of CHOP chemotherapy. Because high-dose methotrexate is an integral component of most effective regimens for Burkitt lymphoma, therapeutic abortion for women diagnosed in the first trimester is essential. Finally, for women with relapsing NHL associated with pregnancy, treatment should not be compromised because the disease is highly aggressive, and therapeutic abortion is generally advisable during the first half of pregnancy because the fetal effects of standard salvage chemotherapy regimens are unknown.

A special consideration can be made for pregnant patients with indolent or low-grade NHLs. These patients may be safely observed until delivery or significant disease progression, provided they are asymptomatic, have a relatively normal complete blood count, and show no impending organ compromise. Such a profile has not yet been reported for NHL associated with pregnancy.

Ward and Weiss reviewed the cases of 42 patients with NHL during pregnancy. Twenty-four of the cases were reported from 1976 to 1985. Three first-trimester cases resulted in two surviving infants. Twenty-one second- and third-trimester cases resulted in 15 surviving infants. Infants who were born to mothers who were untreated or treated with surgery had a 38% prenatal mortality rate, whereas 87.5% of infants of mothers treated with chemotherapy survived. Eight of the 21 second- and third-trimester patients received single-agent or combination chemotherapy. Four of these patients survived. Spitzer and co-workers reported that radiotherapy treatments given to 6 women in the second or third trimester of pregnancy resulted in no harm to the fetus, yet 4 of the mothers died of their disease. Of the 4 cases with a successful delivery and maternal survival, 2 were treated with combination chemotherapy, 1 with chemotherapy and radiotherapy, and 1 with radiotherapy alone. High-grade lymphomas have a particularly poor outcome. In the review by Ward and Weiss, none of the patients diagnosed with Burkitt lymphoma during pregnancy ($n = 18$) survived; however, only 5 of the patients were treated with chemotherapy. Only 5 cases ended with fetal survival. The most important factor influencing the well-being of the fetus is the health of the mother.

Seventy-five cases of pregnant women receiving systemic therapy for NHL have appeared in the literature. The majority of patients have had diffuse large B-cell lymphomas, and the CHOP regimen is the most widely used. Most patients have been treated after the first trimester, although at least four were exposed to CHOP unintentionally during the first trimester. All patients have had a normal course and outcome of pregnancy with no fetal mortality or congenital anomalies encountered. It appears that CHOP is a safe regimen in pregnancy. The combination of CHOP plus bleomycin has also been used safely during pregnancy.

For patients with indolent and aggressive NHL, rituximab (an anti-CD20 monoclonal antibody) has been shown to improve outcomes. There have been seven patients exposed to rituximab during pregnancy, six in combination with chemotherapy. One patient was exposed to rituximab during the first trimester, and the remaining six had the drug initiated during the second trimester. Five patients had normal pregnancy outcomes, including the patient who had first-trimester exposure. There was one case of postnatal B-cell depletion and one case of transient pulmonary insufficiency secondary to prematurity, which resolved after 46 days.

In summary, if the hematologic malignant disease is early stage or low grade, treatment can be deferred or nontoxic therapy can be used. However, many NHLs present with dissemination or aggressive histologic features, for which the most effective therapy is chemotherapy. The mother deserves the most effective chemotherapeutic regimen, despite its teratogenic potential.

OTHER TUMORS IN PREGNANCY

Melanoma

Melanoma accounts for 1 of every 50 cancer-related deaths in the United States. The incidence is rising, with approximately 10,000 cases occurring annually among women aged 20 to 40 years. Congenital nevi may be found within the first 6 months of life and have the highest chance of all nevi for malignant degeneration. Congenital melanocytic nevi may be found in up to 2% of newborns, and giant congenital nevi may cover large areas of the body. Nevi arising later in life are known as the common mole or acquired melanocytic nevi.

The common mole represents more than 95% of nevi and may be subdivided into junctional nevi, compound nevi, and dermal nevi. The blue nevus is another type that usually appears on the dorsal aspects of the extremities and has a very low tendency to become malignant. Nevertheless, any nevi, whether congenital, acquired, or blue, that undergoes suspicious changes should be biopsied. The "ABCD" warning signs that herald changes in nevi that are associated with melanoma are asymmetry, irregular borders, color changes, and moles that increase in diameter. All melanomas masquerade as nevi before diagnosis. The average individual has 15 to 20 nevi, and removal of all these lesions prophylactically is hardly practical. Lesions on the feet, palms, genitals, and areas of persistent irritation from clothing are potentially dangerous nevi and should be removed during childhood.

There are five main types of melanoma, the most common of which is the superficial spreading melanoma, which accounts for 70% to 75% and tends toward horizontal growth prior to becoming invasive. Approximately 15% of melanomas are nodular and become invasive early. In sun-damaged areas, a lentigo maligna may develop, and in darker-skinned persons the acral-lentiginous melanoma can be found on palms and soles. Finally, the least common are the amelanotic melanomas, which are difficult to diagnose.

Staging of Melanoma

Reference may be made to the final version of the AJCC staging system for cutaneous melanoma that was published in 2001. Both depth of penetration of the lesion and the extent to which the lesion has involved local and regional tissues are brought into the staging system. This new system is a blend of the Clark and Breslow microstaging classifications (Table 15-22). The Clark microstaging classification provides a histologic staging scheme for classifying melanomas on the basis of level of penetration of the melanoma under the epidermis and dermis. Prognosis for the patient relates well to this

TABLE 15-22   Microstaging Systems for Melanoma

Level	Clark et al	Breslow et al
I	All tumor cells above basement membrane (in situ)	<0.75-mm depth of invasion
II	Tumor extends to papillary dermis	0.76- to 1.5-mm depth of invasion
III	Tumor extends to interface between papillary and reticular dermis	1.51- to 2.25-mm depth of invasion
IV	Tumor extends between bundles of collagen of reticular dermis	2.26- to 3.0-mm depth of invasion
V	Tumor invasion of subcutaneous tissue	>3-mm depth of invasion

(From Tewari KS: Cancer of the vulva. In Manetta A (ed): Cancer Prevention and Early Diagnosis in Women. Philadelphia, Mosby, 2004.)

microstaging system. Data indicate that a Clark level I melanoma should be viewed as an in situ lesion requiring no lymph node dissection. Clark's level II indicates superficial dermal penetration, with lymph node metastases in 1% to 5% of patients not justifying an elective lymph node dissection. At the other end of this pathologic spectrum are melanomas of Clark's level IV and level V, which metastasize to regional lymph nodes in approximately 40% and 70% of patients, respectively, necessitating lymphadenectomy as part of initial therapy.

An alternative classification suggested by Breslow (see Figure 8-27) and used by some clinicians is a simple micrometer measurement of lesion thickness. Lesions greater than 4 mm have a high incidence of distant metastasis. Lesions 1.5 to 4 mm have a 57% incidence of regional node involvement and 15% incidence of distant metastasis. Lesions between 0.76 and 1.5 mm have a 25% incidence of regional node involvement and an 8% incidence of distant metastasis. Lesions 0.75 mm or less are usually not associated with any spread.

Melanoma in Pregnancy

It is rare that pregnancy adversely affects a malignant process, but for many years melanoma was placed in this category. The average age of the patient with melanoma is 45 years, and 35% of women will be diagnosed during childbearing years. This is suggested by many case reports in which pregnancy has been incriminated in the induction or exacerbation of a melanoma. Partial or complete regressions of melanoma after delivery have been reported. In contrast, Stewart describes a case in which a tumor recurred three times; each recurrence was a few weeks after the patient delivered a child. Female patients have improved survival compared with male control subjects matched for age and tumor thickness.

This suggests that some hormonally based mechanisms are operational in the biologic behavior of melanoma. Contemporary studies fail to substantiate any effect previously attributed to pregnancy.

After the second month of pregnancy, the pituitary gland increases production of melanocyte-stimulating hormone. Melanocyte-stimulating hormone activity is also increased by the pregnancy-associated increase in adrenocorticotropic hormone. This results in the increased pigmentation that is characteristic of pregnancy and often found in the nipples, vulva, linea nigra, and pre-existing nevi. In animal studies, the high circulating levels of estrogens in pregnancy have been shown to control melanocyte activity. These observations have led some to believe that pregnancy can have an inciting influence or a deleterious impact on the course of melanoma and have given rise to several myths about this disease in relationship to pregnancy, including the following:

- Pregnancy increases the risk of developing malignant melanoma.
- Pregnancy worsens the prognosis.
- Future pregnancies have an adverse effect both on prognosis and on recurrence.
- Oral contraceptives and hormone replacement therapy are contraindicated in women with a history of melanoma because of theoretic stimulatory effects of hormones on melanocytes.

None of these claims are substantiated by the medical literature.

Historical Series of Melanoma in Pregnancy

The original report published by Pack and Scharnagel in 1951 contained 1050 patients with melanoma. Ten of these patients were pregnant, 5 of whom died within 3 years of diagnosis. Later authors would cite these observations, which suggested that melanomas in pregnancy grow with unusual rapidity and metastasize widely. Subsequently, many series have challenged the findings of Pack and Scharnagel.

In 1960 George and co-workers gave a comprehensive report of 115 patients with melanoma in pregnancy compared with 330 control subjects from the same institution. In disagreement with an earlier report from their institution, they found that spread to regional nodes appeared to be more rapid in the pregnant patient but that there was no significant difference stage for stage in the outcome for the patient. This was directly contradictory to the earlier philosophy popularized by Pack and Scharnagel that melanoma is indeed aggravated by the pregnant state.

In 1961 White and co-workers reported a study of 71 young women (aged 15-39 years), 30 of whom had

melanoma during pregnancy. The 5-year survival rate in the pregnant group was 73%, and for the 41 nonpregnant patients the survival rate was 54%. They concluded that on the basis of the 5-year survival rates in pregnant and nonpregnant women with age and stage of disease taken into account, survival was equal in the two groups. No deleterious effect of pregnancy on survival of women with melanoma was demonstrated in this series.

Reintgen and colleagues described 58 women who were pregnant when the disease was diagnosed and another 43 patients who became pregnant within 5 years of diagnosis. Control groups were extracted from a total of 1424 women who were registered at the Duke University Melanoma Clinic. The mean age of patients in the series was 28 years. Both actuarial disease-free intervals and survivals were calculated for the study populations and their respective control groups. There was no statistical difference in survival between patients who had mole changes and diagnosis of melanomas during pregnancy and the control population. The results of the study also indicated no difference in survival for women who became pregnant within 5 years of diagnosis.

Despite these equivalency studies, many authorities continue to recommend survivors of melanoma to avoid pregnancy for approximately 3 years after complete surgical excision because this is the period of highest risk of relapse. Obviously, each case must be individualized, and the recommendation should be heavily influenced by the size, depth of invasion, and any detected dissemination. The role of previous pregnancy as a protective factor in melanomas has been suggested by some but also remains controversial. Patients surviving disease free for 5 years have a 95% chance of long-term cure. Conversely, after a woman has had a diagnosis of having a cutaneous melanoma, subsequent pregnancy has no effect on recurrence rates or survival.

Contemporary Studies of Melanoma in Pregnancy

Contemporary studies also note no survival difference in patients with melanoma who are pregnant compared with nonpregnant patients. MacKie and associates evaluated 388 women with stage I melanoma divided into four groups: 85 treated before pregnancy, 92 treated while pregnant, 143 treated after completion of all pregnancies, and 68 treated between pregnancies. Of interest, poor prognostic factors (e.g., tumor thickness and tumor occurring at a poor prognostic site, such as the head, neck, and trunk) occurred more frequently in the pregnant patient than in the nonpregnant patient. However, in multivariate analysis, pregnancy status was not significantly related to prognosis.

In 1998 Grin and colleagues critically reviewed controlled clinical trials to assess the effect of pregnancy on

TABLE 15-23 Multivariable Cox Regression Analysis for the 2101 Women with Melanoma with Known Breslow Thickness, Clark's Level, and Tumor Site

Variable	Hazard Ratio	95% Confidence Interval	P
Pregnancy at the time of diagnosis of primary melanoma*	1.08	0.60-1.93	0.804
Breslow thickness (per additional category)	2.16	1.80-2.58	<0.0001
Axial site vs limb site of primary melanoma	2.51	1.78-3.56	<0.0001
Clark's level (>3 vs <3)	1.39	0.92-2.14	0.12
Age (per year increase)	1.02	0.99-1.05	0.06

From Lens MB, Rosdahl I, Ahlbom A et al: J Clin Oncol 22:4369, 2004.
Pregnant women at the time of diagnosis of melanoma (n = 185) vs nonpregnant women at the time of diagnosis of melanoma (n = 5348).

the prognosis of melanoma and examined the available epidemiologic data to evaluate the risk of melanoma after exposure to oral contraceptives and hormone replacement therapy. The investigators concluded that pregnancy before, during, or after the diagnosis of melanoma did not influence 5-year survival rates, and exposure to oral contraceptives and hormone replacement therapy did not appear to increase the risk of melanoma.

In a recent paper retrospectively evaluating a cohort of 185 women diagnosed with melanoma during pregnancy and 5348 women of the same childbearing age with melanoma not associated with pregnancy, Lens and colleagues noted no statistically significant difference in overall survival between pregnant and nonpregnant groups (Table 15-23). Women with higher Breslow tumor thickness category had a significantly higher risk of death than those with lower Breslow category. Also, women with axial tumors (head and neck, and trunk melanomas) had a poorer prognosis than those with tumors localized on the extremities. Neither pregnancy status at the time of diagnosis of melanoma nor pregnancy status after the diagnosis of melanoma was a significant predictor of survival.

The cumulative retrospective case-controlled studies have involved more than 450 pregnant women with melanoma. The anatomic location of the primary tumor does not differ between pregnant and nonpregnant women, and no analysis identified any differences in survival from nonpregnant women. Multivariate analyses have been performed and have revealed that the stage of disease at diagnosis, and not the pregnancy, is the only consistent finding that influences prognosis. Thus we conclude that pregnancy does not confer a worse prognosis for this diagnosis when matched for stage of disease.

Management of Melanoma in Pregnancy

It is essential that all physicians and midwives conduct a full examination of the skin of their patients. A changing skin lesion should be subjected to an excisional biopsy. Early diagnosis of stage I disease will often lead to curative therapy. Irrespective of pregnancy, treatment of melanoma is related to depth and stage. Lesions less than 1 mm in thickness usually require a wide, deep local excision with a 1-cm margin, and those between 1 and 4 mm need a 2-cm margin of excision. Whereas a wide excision is curative for stage I lesions, the role of IFN-α for stage II and stage III disease is currently under investigation. Although the use of IFN-α in pregnancy has been reported for the management of chronic leukemia, there has been no published experience using this drug for melanoma in pregnancy.

A changing skin lesion should be subjected to excisional biopsy. Early diagnosis of stage I disease will often lead to curative therapy. Irrespective of pregnancy, treatment of melanoma is related to depth of invasion and stage. Lesions less than 1 mm in thickness usually require a wide, deep excision with a 1-cm margin, and those between 1 and 4 mm need a 2-cm margin. Wide, deep local excision can be performed safely before 30 weeks of gestation, and for those beyond 30 weeks of gestation sentinel node identification can be offered after delivery.

Melanomas constitute nearly 50% of all tumors that metastasize to the placenta and account for nearly 90% of those that metastasize to the fetus. Although there have been no reported adverse fetal effects associated with IFN therapy for melanoma during the second trimester, experience with this drug in pregnancy is limited (de Carolis S et al. 2006). Pregnant women with advanced or recurrent disease should undergo ultrasound examination during pregnancy for assessment of any obvious fetal tumor masses. Attention should be directed to placental thickness, the fetal liver, and size of the fetal spleen.

Contemporary studies note no survival difference in patients with melanoma who are pregnant compared with nonpregnant patients. Multivariate analyses demonstrated that the stage of diseased at diagnosis, and not the pregnancy, is the only consistent finding that influences prognosis. In a recent series by Pages and colleagues, 22 patients were included: 10 with AJCC stage III and 12 with AJCC stage IV melanoma. Three patients elected to withhold therapy during pregnancy, 14 underwent surgery, 4 received chemotherapy, and 1 was treated with brain radiotherapy. The median gestational age was 36 weeks. Neither neonatal metastases nor deformities were observed, although placental metastases were found in 1 case. Among 18 newborns, 17 are currently alive at a median follow-up at 17 months; 1 experienced sudden infant death. The 2-year maternal survival rates were 56% for stage III and 17% for stage IV.

Pregnancy does not confer a worse prognosis for melanoma when matched for stage of disease. At delivery, cord blood should be examined for malignant cells and the placental tissue should be sent for detailed pathologic evaluation.

The value of regional lymphadenectomy in clinically negative nodes has been controversial. The debate has been defused to some degree with the development of lymphatic mapping to identify the sentinel lymph node. Pathologic evaluation of the sentinel node is predictive of regional lymph node metastasis in 96% to 98% of cases. Thus SLN identification and evaluation are indicated for lesions penetrating beyond 1 mm. Lloyd and colleagues emphasize that data regarding the effect of radioactive colloid on the fetus are insufficient to permit its use in pregnant women. The dose to the patient from lymphoscintigraphy is 0.4 mSv, with a dose to the uterus of 0.5 mGy. Most of the injected radioactivity stays at the injection site or moves to the sentinel node(s), which are resected the following day during surgery. Despite the small amounts of injected activity, the local dose rate at the injection site is high, and injection sites close to the fetus (over the lower abdomen or back) combined with next-day rather than same-day resection may result in greater doses to the fetus at any stage of the pregnancy.

It is our practice to perform a wide, deep local excision only in women at less than 30 weeks of gestation, and for those beyond 30 weeks of gestation we offer sentinel node identification after delivery. Because small quantities of radioactivity can be excreted into the breast milk, breast feeding is contraindicated if sentinel node identification is performed postpartum.

Melanoma Metastatic to the Products of Conception

The reported low incidence of metastasis of malignant neoplasms to products of conception is probably caused by several factors. One factor is the unexplained resistance of the placenta to invasion by maternal cancer, as demonstrated in many animal studies. Metastasis of maternal cancer to products of conception is rare despite the sizable number of pregnancies at risk. However, although melanoma accounts for only a small number of all cancers associated with pregnancy, almost half of all tumors metastasizing to the placenta and nearly 90% metastasizing to the fetus are melanomas.

A few cases of transplacental transmission of melanomas with subsequent death of the fetus or newborn child from disseminated melanoma have been described, but this situation is extremely rare and occurs only when the mother has widespread blood-borne metastatic disease during pregnancy. Schneiderman and colleagues reported a case of a primary fetal melanoma fatal to a newborn. Microscopic metastases were present in the lungs and liver, and the placenta showed widespread metastases to the chorionic villi but no evidence of invasion of the intervillous spaces. The mother had no evidence of disease 1 year after delivery. To date, no instances of metastasis from fetus to mother have been documented. Moller and associates reported a case of maternal melanoma with metastasis to the placental intervillous sinuses. Tumor cells were also present in the fetal cord blood. The mother died postpartum and the infant survived. Cord blood should be examined for malignant cells, and placental tissue should be carefully inspected. A further discussion on the predilection of melanoma to metastasize to the placenta and the fetus is presented in a separate section in this chapter.

Thyroid Cancer

Papillary, follicular, and anaplastic carcinomas are the most common primary thyroid malignant neoplasms, with medullary carcinoma accounting for only 5%. The disease usually manifests as a relatively asymptomatic nodular mass in the thyroid gland. The lesion is multifocal, as seen on careful sectioning in approximately 30% to 40% of patients, but in only 5% do these become clinically evident if thyroid tissue remains after surgery. Laboratory indices of thyroid function are contributory only if they indicate a hyperthyroid state, thus supporting the diagnosis of a toxic adenoma. Although studies show that these tumors involve regional lymphatics microscopically in 50% to 70% of patients, this subclinical involvement does not affect the prognosis. The growth of papillary carcinoma may depend on thyroid-stimulating hormone (TSH), and therefore thyroid hormone administration to suppress TSH is used routinely as an adjuvant in all patients. The prognosis for patients who have this cancer is favorable, especially in the younger age group. Specifically, in women younger than 49 years, a 90% to 95% survival rate at 15 years is consistently reported.

Papillary and follicular thyroid carcinomas are two to three times more common in women than in men (5.5 vs 2.4 per 100,000, respectively). This female predominance is especially notable during the reproductive years, such that the diagnosis of thyroid carcinoma in pregnancy does occur. In fact, approximately 10% of differentiated thyroid carcinomas in women of reproductive age are diagnosed during pregnancy or within the first year after delivery. The actual incidence of thyroid cancer in pregnancy has not been established.

During pregnancy, nonpathologic enlargement of the thyroid gland to twice its normal size is not uncommon.

Histologic examination shows this enlargement to be caused by an apparent hyperplasia of the follicular cells and abundant colloid formation. A mild suppression of TSH and slight elevation of free thyroxine is common in early pregnancy as a result of the stimulation of the TSH receptor by hCG. A rise in thyroxine-binding globulin during pregnancy results in elevated levels of total thyroid hormone.

Thyroid Cancer in Pregnancy

Because papillary carcinomas are the most common lesions to occur in the reproductive age group, a solitary nodule in an otherwise normal gland is the most common presentation of thyroid carcinoma in pregnancy. Sam and Molitch noted that the incidence of thyroid nodules during pregnancy may be increased, with some data suggesting a higher incidence of malignancy in these nodules. In a 1994 series of 30 pregnant women with thyroid nodules, Rosen and Walfish observed a 43% incidence of malignancy. In 1997 Doherty and colleagues reported the incidence of malignancy to be 39% among 23 women with pregnancy-associated thyroid nodules. In contrast, the incidence of malignancy of thyroid nodules in the nonpregnant population ranges from 8% to 17%. hCG may stimulate the growth of thyroid nodules by cross-reacting with the thyrotropin-stimulating hormone receptor.

Thyroid function tests and a fine-needle aspiration should be performed in the pregnant patient with a newly discovered thyroid nodule. The latter procedure is especially important when the nodule is greater than 2 cm in size. If the results of cytologic examination are benign, a course of thyroid suppression using 0.2 mg of L-thyroxine daily is indicated for the duration of the pregnancy. Repeated cytologic evaluation may be necessary if the nodule does not diminish on suppression or if it enlarges during pregnancy, because 6% of needle aspirations give a false-negative result. The theoretic risk of two false-negative diagnoses is about 0.05%, thus providing excellent confirmation of a conservative approach if the aspirate is repeatedly negative.

If the fine-needle aspiration reveals a papillary or follicular carcinoma, we advise patients to undergo surgery in the second trimester (Figure 15-17). If the carcinoma has been discovered in the third trimester, the workup and treatment can be delayed until after delivery. Rapidly growing tumors and medullary carcinomas should be removed on discovery, regardless of gestational age. Short treatment delays to permit gestational advancement may be acceptable for some patients with medullary carcinomas, but as soon as fetal maturity can be demonstrated labor should be induced or a cesarean section should be performed. Surgery is the only known effective therapy for medullary carcinomas and results

in a 50% survival rate at 5 years. A prophylactic lymph node dissection on the site of the lesion is indicated. Fetal loss associated with surgery has been reported only with extensive neck exploration. Following tumor resection, suppressive doses of thyroid hormone should be administered, keeping in mind that thyroid hormone requirements may be higher in pregnancy.

Radioactive iodine is contraindicated during pregnancy and lactation. Even though trace doses are used in these uptake studies, there is still a theoretic risk of a destructive effect on the fetal thyroid and a concern for teratogenesis within the fetus. A whole-body ^{131}I can be performed 3 months after discontinuation of lactation, and if necessary, iodine-131 ablation is recommended.

The Undifferentiated Lesion

In the uncommon situation of an anaplastic carcinoma of the thyroid, the main concern is to keep the mother alive until the pregnancy has come to term because these tumors are almost uniformly lethal lesions. Between 90% and 95% of patients are dead within 1 year of diagnosis. The standard treatment in these patients is radical thyroidectomy followed by radiation therapy. This obviously presents a difficult situation for the patient in the first or second trimester, and one must carefully discuss the situation with the patient and the family. Treatment of pregnant patients who have progressive, local, unresectable, or metastatic thyroid carcinoma has to be individualized and tailored to the wishes of the patient. Surgical removal of these poorly differentiated lesions will achieve the best local control. The role of radiation therapy and chemotherapy remains investigational.

Prognosis Among Pregnant Women with Thyroid Cancer

Pregnancy does not negatively influence the prognosis of patients with well-differentiated thyroid carcinoma. For example, Moosa and Mazzaferri found no difference in the outcome between 61 pregnant women with thyroid cancer and a group of age-matched, nonpregnant control subjects. In addition, pregnancy has not been shown to increase the recurrence rate of women previously treated for thyroid cancer. Hill and coworkers described 70 women who conceived after the diagnosis of thyroid cancer and compared them with 109 women who remained childless. There was no difference in the overall recurrence rate. The authors concluded that subsequent pregnancy did not alter the course of the disease. Rosvoll and Winship reviewed the cases of 60 women treated for thyroid carcinoma who subsequently became pregnant and concluded that

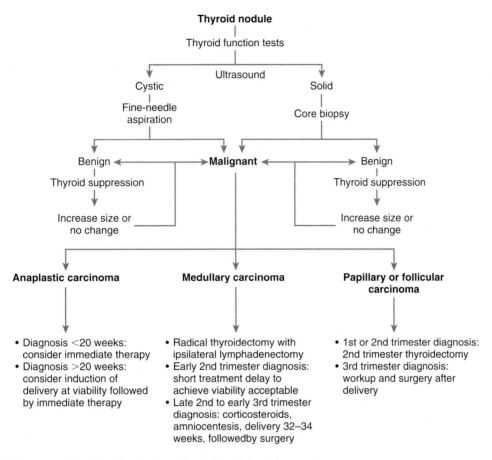

FIGURE 15-17   Management algorithm for the thyroid nodule and thyroid cancer in pregnancy.

a history of thyroid cancer is not an indication for avoidance of pregnancy or for therapeutic abortion. Friedman suggested that pregnancy was not contraindicated if the disease-free interval was at least 3 to 5 years. However, even in patients who had residual or recurrent disease, the prognosis did not appear to be altered by the pregnancy.

Thyroid cancer is among the fastest-rising types of cancer among women in North America. In 2010 Holt summarized the Endocrine Society Guidelines for the management of thyroid dysfunction during pregnancy and postpartum. With respect to thyroid nodules or thyroid cancer, the guidelines stipulate the following:

1. Thyroid nodules measuring 1 cm or larger should be evaluated by fine-needle aspiration biopsy.
2. Individuals with nodules that are malignant or show rapid growth should be offered surgery in the second trimester of pregnancy.
3. It may be appropriate for patients with follicular neoplasia or early-stage papillary thyroid cancers to wait until postpartum for thyroidectomy because these lesions are not expected to progress

rapidly and the risk of surgery may outweigh the benefits of immediate intervention.
4. Patients with known thyroid cancer should maintain a low but measureable TSH and normal thyroxine (T4) values on levothyroxine while pregnant.
5. RAI therapy should not be provided to women who are breast feeding.

After RAI therapy, women should wait 6 to 12 months before becoming pregnant.

Recently the risk of complications of thyroid and parathyroid surgery during pregnancy was evaluated in a retrospective, U.S. cross-sectional analysis of hospital discharge data from the Healthcare Utilization Project National Inpatient Sample (HCUP-NIS). A total of 201 pregnant and 31,155 age-matched nonpregnant women controls who had undergone thyroid or parathyroid surgery were identified. Of the 201 pregnant women, 45.8% underwent surgery for thyroid cancer. Thyroidectomy during pregnancy was associated with a higher risk of complications from surgery for malignant (21% vs 8%) or benign (27% vs 14%) disease. After controlling for other risk factors associated with adverse outcomes, pregnant patients remained twice as likely to have surgical complications as their nonpregnant counterparts. Among the pregnant patients who had thyroid or parathyroid surgery, 5.5% had fetal complications (e.g., fetal distress, abortion), and 4.5% had maternal complications (cesarean section, hysterectomy).

RARE GYNECOLOGIC MALIGNANCIES IN PREGNANCY

Vulvar Cancer

Fewer than 50 cases of invasive cancer of the vulva associated with pregnancy have been reported in the literature. Lutz and colleagues estimated an incidence of 1 case per 8000 deliveries at his institution; our experience has been less frequent, at about 1 per 20,000 deliveries. The most common of these are invasive epidermoid carcinomas, followed by melanomas, sarcomas, and adenoid cystic adenocarcinomas. In recent years, reports of pregnancies complicated by recurrent vulvar carcinoma, metastatic vulvar melanoma, a rapidly enlarging myxoid leiomyosarcoma of the vulva, and primary choriocarcinoma of the vulva have also appeared. The majority of patients have been between 25 and 35 years of age; the youngest patient was 17 years. With the increasing frequency of the diagnosis of CIS of the vulva, the occurrence of preinvasive disease with pregnancy is common today. As is the practice with CIN, therapy for the vulvar counterpart is delayed until the postpartum period. Adequate biopsies of the most suspicious areas are essential to rule out invasive disease. The presence of intraepithelial neoplasia should not prohibit vaginal delivery but should prompt a careful colposcopic evaluation of the lower genital tract to exclude other preinvasive or invasive foci.

HISTORICAL SERIES OF VULVAR CANCER IN PREGNANCY

Gitsch and colleagues presented a concise review of therapy and outcome for this group of patients, correctly noting that the reports have been inhomogeneous. In a review of the literature, Barclay found 31 women with vulvar cancers associated with pregnancy. The vulvar cancers were actually diagnosed and treated during pregnancy in only 12 of these women; another 2 were treated after termination of pregnancy. In 1974 Barclay furnished further details on 9 patients, 1 of whom was treated with radiation therapy during pregnancy. Five patients were treated surgically before delivery, and 3 women underwent vulvectomy in the postpartum period. With extended follow-up, none of the patients experienced recurrent disease, although 1 woman developed a cervical carcinoma that was irradiated. Lutz and colleagues reported 3 cases diagnosed during pregnancy but treated postpartum. Although no one survived, details concerning the stage, treatment, and survival time were not provided.

MANAGEMENT OF VULVAR CANCER IN PREGNANCY

Invasive vulvar malignant disease diagnosed during the first, second, and early third trimesters is usually treated as indicated in the nonpregnant patient some time after the 18th week of pregnancy. T1 lesions should be managed by radical wide excision with ipsilateral groin dissection if the depth of invasion is greater than 1 mm. Larger and/or more deeply invasive tumors require a radical vulvectomy and bilateral inguinofemoral lymphadenectomy. Patients with palpable inguinofemoral nodes undergoing surgery early in pregnancy present a unique challenge because skin bridge metastases are more likely to occur in patients with bulky positive nodes. Such patients are advised to have the groin dissected using an en bloc approach because of the need to delay radiation therapy for many months. When the diagnosis is made after 36 weeks of gestation, we recommend a wide local excision with definitive surgery postponed until the postpartum period. This avoids the greatly enhanced vascularity in vulvar tissues during the later months of gestation and into the immediate postpartum period. A short delay does not appear to seriously prejudice the course of the disease.

Women treated during pregnancy may be allowed to attempt vaginal delivery provided the vulvar wounds are well healed, and there are no indications for additional therapy. Patients with high-risk surgicopathologic features warranting adjuvant radiation should undergo cesarean delivery as soon as fetal pulmonary maturation can be documented. Following delivery of the baby, the ovaries should be transposed to the paracolic gutters, and pelvic and/or groin irradiation can be administered postpartum.

Because this disease occurs more frequently in lower socioeconomic groups, who often do not seek prenatal care, many of these cases are diagnosed at the time of delivery or later. In this group of patients, definitive therapy should be started within 1 week after delivery during the same hospitalization. The pregnant state does not appear to significantly alter the course of the malignant process; survival of these patients stage for stage is similar to that of nonpregnant patients.

Bakour and colleagues have carefully considered the subject of future pregnancies in this group of patients and have found no contraindications after surveying the literature. In fact, they feel that these young patients who have undergone such extensive surgery obtain a great boost psychologically when they realize this possibility. There have been several reports of patients treated for carcinoma of the vulva with radical vulvectomy and bilateral inguinal lymphadenectomy who subsequently became pregnant and had normal deliveries. Whether the patient should deliver vaginally or by cesarean section is a decision that rests with the obstetrician, but it is heavily influenced by the state of the postsurgical vulva. In most instances, the vulva is soft and does not impede a vaginal delivery. In other instances, there may be a high degree of vaginal stenosis or other fibrosis, which makes cesarean section the more appropriate means of delivery.

Primary Invasive Vaginal Tumors

Cancer of the vagina has been found mainly in women older than 50 years. The diagnosis of vaginal cancer during pregnancy is exceptionally uncommon, even with the clear cell adenocarcinoma of the vagina alleged to be associated with the diethylstilbestrol-exposed offspring. Although all these clear cell adenocarcinomas have occurred in women younger than 34 years, the incidence in association with pregnancy has fortunately been rare.

Senekjian and colleagues described 24 women who were pregnant when clear cell adenocarcinoma of the vagina or cervix was diagnosed; 14 were in the first trimester, 6 in the second, and 4 in the third. Among the stage I and stage II tumors, 16 (73%) were vaginal and 6 (27%) were cervical. Thirteen long-term survivors were reported among the 16 early vaginal lesions. No significant differences were observed when the group of 24 patients with pregnancy-associated tumors and 408 never-pregnant (age-corrected) patients were compared with regard to maternal hormone history, symptoms, stage, location, predominant histologic or cell type, greatest tumor diameter, surface area, depth of invasion, grade, and number of mitoses. The overall 5- and 10-year actuarial survival rates (86% and 68%, respectively) for the group pregnant at diagnosis did not differ significantly from the rates for the never-pregnant group analyzed concomitantly ($n = 408$). Pregnancy did not seem to adversely affect the outcome of clear cell adenocarcinoma of the vagina and cervix. Jones and colleagues reported a diethylstilbestrol-related clear cell carcinoma of the vagina in a patient whose tumor, observed directly over an extended period, did not appear to be influenced by elevated plasma estrogen levels during the period when the pregnancy was carried to term.

Primary squamous cell carcinoma of the vagina discovered during pregnancy is exceedingly rare. In 1976 Collins and Barclay identified 10 patients from the literature, and although 3 responded well to radiation therapy, a rapidly progressive downhill course was described for 4 patients available for detailed analysis. In 1977 Lutz and colleagues reported a 24-year-old patient diagnosed at 24 weeks of gestation with a stage II squamous cell carcinoma of the vagina, who despite immediate radiotherapy following preterm delivery, suffered a fatal recurrence 7 months later. Three additional cases have been reported by Palumbo and colleagues, Beck and Clayton, and Baruah and Sangupta, manifesting between 8 and 24 weeks of gestation and all resulting in maternal death within 18 months of diagnosis; in 2 of the cases, pregnancy termination had been performed so as to not delay radiotherapy.

Finally, Steed and colleagues reported a 28 year old with antepartum bleeding at 20 weeks of gestation who was found to have a 6-cm diameter anterior vaginal wall squamous cell carcinoma extending to the right lateral fornix. This patient opted to continue the pregnancy and received corticosteroids, followed by cesarean delivery at 32 weeks of gestation. Before delivery, gold seeds were placed transvaginally to demarcate the tumor edges. Amazingly, although the patient was debulked of multiple, enlarged, positive pelvic lymph nodes, following treatment with chemoirradiation and brachytherapy she had remained disease-free for 3 years at the time of publication. This report brings the total to 15 cases of primary invasive squamous cell carcinoma of the vulva complicating pregnancy, with an overall survivorship of 38%, similar to what is observed in nonpregnant patients.

Both cervical cancer and vaginal cancer are staged clinically, and the management principles to be discussed in detail when cervical carcinoma complicates pregnancy also may be applied to vaginal tumors. Treatment of clear cell adenocarcinoma of the cervix and upper vagina is surgically similar to that of squamous cell cancers. Specifically, very early lesions involving the upper vagina may be treated by radical abdominal hysterectomy with pelvic lymphadenectomy, whereas all others are best managed radiotherapeutically. The pregnancy should be disregarded if the diagnosis is made in the first or early second trimester. Should the pregnancy be further along, the decision for appropriate time of intervention depends on the preferences of the patient and the oncologist. Patients early in pregnancy who resist termination should be given corticosteroids and delivered as soon as fetal pulmonary maturation is demonstrable. The impact of a delay in therapy on the prognosis is impossible to predict. In instances in which there is extensive involvement of the vagina by any lesion, one should seriously consider evacuation of the uterus by a hysterotomy or cesarean section and institution of appropriate radiation therapy.

A few scattered reports of sarcoma botryoides of the cervix and vagina in pregnancy were recorded during the 1960s by Roddick and Honig and Schwartz and colleagues. When these sarcomatous lesions occur in the upper half of the vagina with or without cervical involvement, the most appropriate therapy has been a radical abdominal hysterectomy, upper vaginectomy, and bilateral pelvic lymphadenectomy followed by postoperative adjuvant chemotherapy. In 2003 the first primary vaginal leiomyosarcoma diagnosed during pregnancy was reported by Behzatoglu and colleagues in a 21-year-old woman who presented during the third trimester with a 1.5-cm firm, fleshy, pedunculated mass arising from a short stalk on the right vaginal wall. Previously, female genital tract leiomyosarcomas that have been associated with pregnancy had originated from the uterus or vulva ($n = 10$). Finally, some malignancies have been reported in pregnancy to involve the vagina secondarily by direct extension (e.g., tumors of the cervix), via lymphatic spread (e.g. endometrial carcinoma), or through hematogenous dissemination (e.g., gestational choriocarcinoma and placental site trophoblastic tumor). In fact, secondary involvement from an extravaginal site is more common than the development of a primary vaginal neoplasm, irrespective of pregnancy. Although pregnancy-associated vaginal cancer is rare, the entity must remain part of the differential diagnosis of bleeding in pregnancy. Steed and colleagues emphasize that visualization of the entire vagina and cervix is necessary during speculum examination, and the procedure should be performed in every pelvic examination and for all investigations carried out for antepartum bleeding.

Endometrial Cancer

Endometrial carcinoma in conjunction with pregnancy is extremely rare. Most of the reported cases have been diagnosed at examination of uterine contents obtained by curettage for elective pregnancy termination or spontaneous abortion. Leiomyosarcoma (including a myxoid leiomyosarcoma), endometrial stromal sarcoma, and carcinosarcoma have also been reported during pregnancy. They are usually incidental findings noted in surgical specimens. The recommended therapy for endometrioid adenocarcinomas associated with pregnancy is total hysterectomy with bilateral salpingo-oophorectomy and adjuvant radiotherapy when indicated.

In 1972 Karlen and associates reviewed the literature since 1900, summarized five acceptable cases, and added a sixth. In 2004 Itoh and colleagues collected a total of 29 patients (including one of their own), 11 of whom were older than 35 years. Twenty-one of the 29 cases had no or minimal myometrial invasion, 18 of which were histologically FIGO grade I, and 3 were FIGO grade II. This group includes a 28 year old who received conservative treatment with high-dose medroxyprogesterone acetate following a uterine curettage that had revealed diffuse complex hyperplasia with atypia and a focus of well-differentiated adenocarcinoma showing stromal invasion. This patient subsequently conceived, and following delivery at term she underwent a total abdominal hysterectomy. Pathologic examination of the uterus revealed a persistent well-differentiated endometrioid adenocarcinoma limited to the endometrium. This case serves to illustrate a very important point. As more women opt for conservative management of invasive cancers in an effort to preserve fertility, we may anticipate a larger number of referrals than what was seen previously for patients with persistent or even recurrent malignancy during pregnancy.

All 21 patients with favorable histopathologic features were alive at the time of their report, ranging from 3 months to 10 years after treatment. Therefore, most cases of endometrial carcinoma associated with pregnancy are characterized by well-differentiated tumors, an endometrioid histology with no or minimal myometrial invasion, and favorable outcome, consistent with the typical clinicopathologic features of type I endometrial carcinoma that develops in obese women. It has been hypothesized that the elevated serum progesterone level during pregnancy inhibits the growth of endometrial carcinoma cells, and this may contribute to the good outcomes observed among these 21 patients. This has prompted several authorities to argue that adenocarcinoma in pregnancy does not occur and that the reported cases were misdiagnosed Arias–Stella reactions.

However, the remaining 8 of the 29 reported patients have had well-documented deep myometrial invasion or extrauterine extension. The FIGO grade distribution included grade I ($n = 3$), grade II ($n = 2$), and grade III ($n = 3$, including one serous papillary carcinoma), and the FIGO stage ranged from Ic to IV. Two of these eight patients died of disease, and it is notable that the patient submitted by Itoh and colleagues had deep myometrial invasion and negative expression of ER and PR. Of note, higher grade tumors or nonendometrioid adenocarcinomas are often negative for ER or PR expression, and this group of endometrial carcinomas associated with pregnancy is characterized by high-grade histology, including nonendometrioid type, deep myometrial invasion, advanced stage, and poor outcome consistent with the type II carcinoma manifesting in nonobese patients. Thus not all endometrial carcinomas associated with pregnancy have a favorable prognosis.

Fallopian Tube Cancer

The fallopian tube can become secondarily involved by malignancy through direct extension of an ovarian tumor or from an endometrial carcinoma. Primary fallopian tube carcinoma was described by Starr and colleagues as a disease of recent vintage, having been first reported in 1847 by Raymond and later, in 1861, by Rokitansky. The disease is the least common gynecologic tumor. The mean age ranges from 50 to 55 years. Thus the possibility of its presence in pregnancy is extremely remote. Cases have been reported to be associated with pregnancy; in these instances, the neoplasm is usually unilateral and most often adenocarcinoma.

The clinical presentation of carcinoma of the tube is variable and nonspecific even without an associated pregnancy. The usual watery, blood-tinged vaginal discharge would be obviated in pregnancy because at 12 weeks of gestation the communication between the uterine cavity and the fallopian tube is blocked. In most instances, the diagnosis is established at laparotomy, and the treatment is total abdominal hysterectomy with bilateral salpingo-oophorectomy and postoperative radiotherapy or chemotherapy, depending on the operative findings and the residual disease after surgery. Several instances are reported in the literature of incidental findings of CIS of the tube noted in specimens submitted after postpartum tubal ligation. In these instances, a total abdominal hysterectomy with bilateral salpingo-oophorectomy has been recommended; however, simple removal of the fallopian tubes may be a reasonable alternative.

Adolph and colleagues reported the first case of a recurrent fallopian tube carcinoma associated with pregnancy in 2001. The patient originally underwent a limited surgical procedure to preserve fertility, followed by chemotherapy, and subsequently experienced an intraperitoneal recurrence 1 year later during her 16th week of pregnancy. Following a cesarean section at term, she underwent optimal cytoreductive surgery and was alive with stable disease 6 months following salvage chemotherapy when the paper was published. This case is included with some detail to emphasize a point made earlier, in that as fertility-preserving oncologic procedures become more widely accepted for certain early-stage malignancies, the probabilities increase for having to manage recurrent disease in pregnancy. The criteria through which surgeons determine candidacy for fertility preservation must be carefully devised and rigorously adhered to.

Trophoblastic Tumors of the Fallopian Tube: "Ectopic" Pregnancy

Although choriocarcinoma most frequently arises in the uterus, a primary choriocarcinoma of the fallopian tube may be associated with ectopic pregnancy. In these scenarios, the biologic behavior is very aggressive, with distant metastases manifesting in 75% of cases. A review of the world literature of 93 reported cases by Ober and Maier in 1981 yielded 58 acceptable cases, to which the authors added 18 from the files of the Armed Forces Institute of Pathology. Since that time, there have been approximately 15 additional reports, bringing the total to 91 cases of primary choriocarcinoma of the fallopian tube. The mean age is 33 years, with 66% of patients presenting with acute symptoms consistent with a ruptured ectopic pregnancy. The remainder typically have presented with a gradually expanding adnexal mass clinically indistinguishable from an ovarian tumor. Endovaginal ultrasonography may offer an image compatible with an extrauterine pregnancy in the left appendages, and the quantitative serum β-hCG is elevated. Grossly, the tumor appears as a hemorrhagic friable mass, occasionally containing spongy tissue resembling the placenta. Smaller tubal choriocarcinomas are difficult to distinguish on gross inspection from the common ectopic pregnancy. Histopathologic features and the distribution of metastases are similar to gestational choriocarcinoma arising in the uterus.

The surgical approach has not been uniform, with some women undergoing unilateral salpingectomy only or unilateral adnexectomy or total abdominal hysterectomy with bilateral salpingo-oophorectomy. Most patients have gone on to receive polychemotherapy. In the review by Ober and Maier, it was noted that of 47 acceptable cases treated before modern chemotherapy, the mortality rate was 87% ($n = 41$). Of 16 cases treated with modern chemotherapy, the salvage rate was 94% ($n = 15$). Fewer than 10 patients have been cured by unilateral salpingectomy or unilateral salpingo-oophorectomy alone. Whenever possible, a histologic examination of the tubes should be performed in all cases of ectopic pregnancies. Serial measurements of the β-hCG is an essential component of the surveillance of all patients treated for ectopic pregnancy and especially for those treated with methotrexate or by salpingotomy alone.

Primary choriocarcinoma of the fallopian tube coexistent with a viable intrauterine pregnancy was first reported by Lee and colleagues in 2005, and a heterotopic pregnancy of a primary placental site trophoblastic tumor of the fallopian tube and an intrauterine pregnancy was first reported by Su and colleagues in 1999.

Placental and Fetal Tumors

The placenta may be the site of origin of gestational trophoblastic neoplasia (GTN) or can be secondarily involved by other malignancies. The disease spectrum of GTN encompasses molar pregnancies (e.g., complete, partial, invasive), nonmetastatic GTN, gestational choriocarcinoma (i.e., metastatic GTN), and placental site trophoblastic tumors. These entities are discussed in a separate chapter. The occurrence of gestational choriocarcinoma and placental site trophoblastic tumors in the fallopian tube has been addressed earlier in this chapter under the section concerning tumors of the fallopian tube in pregnancy. The following sections will have as their focus the occurrence of a twin pregnancy complicated by a complete mole and a normal fetus, placental and fetal metastases, and primary fetal cancers that may manifest in utero.

Complete Hydatidiform Mole with Coexistent Fetus

Ultrasonography depicting the combination of a live fetus and a molar-appearing placenta suggests three distinct possibilities:

1. A singleton pregnancy consisting of a partial mole with a live fetus
2. A twin pregnancy comprising one placenta exhibiting a complete mole (no fetus) and the other placenta sustaining a normal twin
3. A twin pregnancy with a partial mole and fetus in one sac and a normal twin in the other sac

The first possibility involves a triploid fetus that usually dies during the first trimester. The third possibility is easily eliminated by the presence of two fetuses.

The incidence of complete hydatidiform mole with coexistent fetus (CMCF) ranges from 1 in 10,000 to 1 in 100,000 pregnancies. The true incidence is difficult to establish, and the observed increased incidence of iatrogenic multiple gestations in recent years is expected to result in a higher incidence of CMCF. Vaisbuch and colleagues have conducted a comprehensive review of the literature, and after exclusion of duplicate publications they have identified 130 cases, some of which include higher-order gestations (e.g., triplets and quadruplets). Fifty-three elected to terminate. Thirty-three live births (25%) occurred. The calculated incidences of specific complications included 30% pre-eclampsia, 33% persistent GTN, and 22% metastatic GTN.

Steller and colleagues discovered eight well-documented cases of twin pregnancy with CMCF. They compared the clinical features of these eight patients with 71 women with singleton complete hydatidiform mole. Although the presenting symptoms were similar in both groups, a twin pregnancy with CMCF was diagnosed at a later gestational age (20.1 weeks vs 13 weeks), had higher pre-evacuation β-hCG levels, and had a greater propensity to develop persistent GTN (55% vs 14%).

Bristow and colleagues reported 25 cases from the literature and 1 of their own, of whom 19 were evacuated before fetal viability and only 7 resulted in a liveborn infant. Although the previable and viable group were unremarkable with respect to mean age, gravidity, parity, uterine size, and presence of theca-lutein cysts, significant differences in gestational age at diagnosis (17.4 weeks vs 29.4 weeks) and pre-evacuation serum hCG levels (>1,000,000 mIU/mL vs 170,000 mIU/mL) were observed. In addition, previable cases were also associated with higher frequencies of pre-eclampsia (31.6% vs 14.3%) and persistent GTN (68.4% vs 28.6%). Clinical factors that required termination of the pregnancy might have been surrogates for aggressive

TABLE 15-24 Evolution to Gestational Trophoblastic Neoplasia after Twin Pregnancy with Complete Hydatidiform Mole and Coexistant Fetus

Author	Number of Pregnancy	GTN(%)
Steller et al.	22	12 (55)
Fishman et al.	7	4 (57)
Matsui et al.	18	9 (50)
Sebire et al.	77	15 (19)
Hancock et al.	9	3 (33)
Niemann et al.	8	2 (25)
Massardier et al.	14	7 (50)

From Massardier J et al: Eur J Obstet Gynecol Reprod Biol 143:84, 2009.

trophoblastic growth and therefore persistent disease and the subsequent need for adjuvant systemic therapy. Bruchim and colleagues reported a 53.3% incidence of persistent GTN (including four patients with pulmonary metastasis) when they analyzed 15 cases of CMCF that had resulted in a live neonate delivered at a mean age of 34.3 weeks of gestation. Although CMCF is associated with a higher risk of persistent GTN when compared with the risk attributable to a singleton complete hydatidiform mole, the issues regarding pregnancy termination are unclear. It does not appear that advanced gestational age is an independent risk factor for developing persistent GTN in the setting of a CMCF. Once fetal anomalies and an abnormal karyotype are excluded, with some degree of caution the literature supports continuing the pregnancy provided there is no evidence of pre-eclampsia and the mother strongly wishes to do so. A declination in serum levels of hCG may also be included in the criteria through which expectant management can be offered. Patients should be informed that only 25% of such pregnancies will result in a live birth and that there may be some serious consequences of premature delivery and prematurity.

The overall risk of developing persistent GTN ranges from 19% to 57% (Table 15-24), irrespective of whether the pregnancy is terminated or carried to viability and/or term. Therefore, the major obstacles to continuing the pregnancy are the development of a paraneoplastic medical complication, catastrophic vaginal hemorrhage, and formation of metastatic foci antenatally. In the exceedingly rare situation in which metastatic GTN coexists with a normal gestation, intravenous systemic chemotherapy is necessary during pregnancy, unless the disease is discovered when the baby is of advanced gestational age, in which case delivery followed by immediate systemic therapy might be an option.

Presenting symptoms of a complete hydatidiform mole with coexisting fetus are similar to those seen with complete hydatidiform moles alone (i.e., size greater than dates, abnormal vaginal bleeding). A twin pregnancy with a complete hydatiform mole and coexisting

TABLE 15-25 Recommendations for Continuation of Pregnancy in the Setting of a Twin Pregnancy with Complete Hydatidiform Mole and Coexisting Fetus

Normal fetal karyotype
No anomalies
No early pre-eclampsia
No observance of decrease in levels of hCG

fetus may be diagnosed later in gestational age (e.g., 20 weeks vs 13 weeks), have a higher pre-evacuation β-hCG level, and have a greater propensity to develop persistent gestational trophoblastic neoplasia necessitating chemotherapy.

Once fetal anomalies and an abnormal karyotype are excluded, the literature supports continuing the pregnancy provided there is no evidence of pre-eclampsia and the mother strongly wishes to do so. In cases of twin pregnancy with a complete hydatidiform mole and coexisting live fetus, continuation of pregnancy is acceptable with a normal fetal karyotype, no anomalies, no early pre-eclampsia, and declination of hCG levels (Table 15-25); the risk of persistent trophoblastic disease may rise to 57%. The overall risk of developing persistent GTN is 33% irrespective of whether the pregnancy is terminated or carried to viability and/or term. The major obstacles to continuing the pregnancy are the development of a paraneoplastic medical complication, catastrophic vaginal hemorrhage, and formation of metastatic foci antenatally.

A series of 14 cases were recently reported by Massardier and colleagues. In 10 cases (71%) the diagnosis was made by ultrasonography, with the differential diagnoses including partial hydatidiform mole and mesenchymal dysplasia. Eight patients elected to terminate the pregnancy and 6 chose to continue. Of the latter, there were 3 intrauterine deaths/spontaneous abortions and 3 (21%) normal live births. Only 1 patient delivered after 37 weeks of gestational age. Seven patients (50%) were diagnosed with gestational trophoblastic neoplasia, and none of the 14 had a fatal evolution. Of note, vaginal bleeding, pre-eclampsia, and hyperthyroidism did not have an impact on the risk of persistent GTN, nor did continuation of the pregnancy increase that risk.

Placental and Fetal Metastases

The patient afflicted with cancer in pregnancy commonly asks whether the disease can spread to her child. Although cancer during pregnancy is not uncommon, metastases to the placental tissue or the fetus rarely occur. Most malignancies, when matched stage for stage, portend the same prognosis for the woman whether she is pregnant or not. Exceptions include hepatocellular cancer, lymphoma, thyroid, colon, and nasopharyngeal cancers. In addition to the primary cancer sites, metastatic disease to the products of conception predicts an ominous course for the mother. Metastatic lesions to the fetus or placenta remain a poorly understood subject.

The first report of metastases to the placenta and/or fetus appeared in 1866. In this case, Friedreich observed a mother with disseminated "hepatic" carcinoma that spread to and killed the fetus. There have been no other reports of "hepatic" metastases to the products of conception, and we suspect that Friedreich's patient had a melanoma, which is most likely to behave in this clinical manner. Indeed, melanoma is the most common cancer to metastasize to the placenta and fetus. Rothman and associates reported 35 cases of disseminated maternal malignant disease with either placental or fetal involvement. In only two instances was tumor demonstrated on both the maternal and fetal sides of the placenta and in the fetus. It is rare for the fetus to be involved if there is invasion only of the maternal side of the placenta. Of 6 cases in the literature when the villus itself was invaded, there was only 1 case of demonstrable fetal disease. In another report by Potter and Schoeneman, 24 cases of maternal cancer metastasizing to the fetus or placenta were reviewed. Melanoma, by far the most common tumor to spread to the fetus or placenta, was found in 11 cases. Breast cancer was found in 4 cases. Eight infants were found to have cancer at birth, and 6 of these subsequently died of their malignant neoplasms. Two infants with metastatic melanoma were noted to have complete tumor regression and ultimately survived. Seven of 8 occurrences of metastasis to the fetus were found in cases of maternal melanoma, and there was 1 case of lymphosarcoma. Finally, Holland reported a case in which maternal, placental, and fetal disease was documented.

Since Friedreich's initial report, there have been fewer than 90 cases of maternal malignancy metastatic to the gestation (Table 15-26). Because of its generous blood flow, large surface area, and favorable biologic environment for growth, one would consider the placenta to be an ideal site for metastases, and therefore the relative paucity of such events remains unclear. Why have the products of conception been privileged in this way? Perhaps immunologic rejection of tumor cells, uteroplacental circulatory mechanisms, or even a protective role of the trophoblast limit the establishment of metastatic foci. Cancers that have been reported to metastasize to the intervillous space or to the placenta proper include sarcomas, carcinomas, lymphomas, leukemias, and melanomas. Of note, 30% of the cases are melanomas, followed by breast cancer (18%) and then the hematopoietic malignancies (13%).

Nearly half of the reports contain cases of known malignancy diagnosed before the onset of pregnancy. Unfortunately, 93% of such women died of their disease, sometimes within hours of delivery. Gestational

TABLE 15-26   Most Common Cancers in Pregnancy to Affect the Placenta and/or Fetus

Cancer Type	Cases Reporting Placental Involvement	Cases Reporting Only Fetal Metastasis	Cases Reporting Both Placental and Fetal Metastasis	Total Cases Affecting Placenta and/or Fetus	Percentage of Total Cases
All cancers	72	10	6	88	100
Melanoma	21	3	3	27	31
Breast	15	0	0	15	17
Lung	8	1	1	10	11
Leukemia	6	0	0	9	10
Lymphoma	3	2	2	7	8

From Alexander A et al: J Clin Oncol 21:2179, 2003.

reactivation of malignancy has been reported in women who had been disease free for 5 years before becoming pregnant. Contrasting with the unfavorable prognosis for mothers with placental metastases, the prognosis for the infant has been excellent, with 53 of the reported cases revealing no evidence of disease in the baby. In addition, since 1966 no infant has succumbed to metastatic disease, although several reports contained fetal demises as a consequence of complications of prematurity. More recently, the first case of maternal pulmonary adenocarcinoma metastatic to the fetus has been reported; the involved scalp was widely excised and skin graft coverage was applied at 3 months of life, and at the time of publication the child was 5 years old and disease free.

Another unusual scenario is that of GTN metastatic to the fetus, with 15 to 20 cases reported to date. It is interesting that widely metastatic disease in the delivered neonate can occur in the absence of metastatic GTN in the mother. There are also reports of acute leukemia developing postnatally in the child of a mother with acute leukemia. In one report by Cramblett and associates, the child developed acute leukemia 9 months after delivery; in another report by Bernard, disease manifestation occurred 5 months after delivery. Transplacental transmission of maternal B-cell lymphoma was reported by Maruko and colleagues when a 29-year-old mother developed the disease at 29 weeks and her infant developed malignant lymphoma at 8 months of life. Hypotheses relating to familial, hereditary, environmental, and viral factors can be advanced in these circumstances, but the weight of evidence suggests that acquisition of maternal malignant disease by the fetus is extremely unlikely.

Guidelines for the evaluation of children born to women with cancer are sparse in the literature. Tolar and Neglia recommend that any child born to a mother with active or suspected malignancy should initially have a thorough physical examination with a complete blood count, comprehensive metabolic panel, liver function tests, coagulation battery, serum LDH, uric acid levels, and a urinalysis. In addition, the placenta should be macroscopically and microscopically examined for tumor involvement. It has been our practice to also obtain imaging studies, including an MRI of the brain and CT scans of the chest, abdomen, and pelvis, when maternal breast cancer, hematopoietic malignancy, or melanoma is at issue or in the setting of confirmed placental metastases. Continued surveillance should be ongoing during the first year of a child's life because some cases of maternal to fetal metastases have not presented until several months after birth. Because not all cases with documented placental involvement have corresponding fetal metastases, infants with an initially negative workup should not be prophylactically treated but should be closely observed with frequent physical examinations, laboratory tests, and imaging studies as clinically indicated.

Primary Fetal Tumors

Benign tumors such as teratomas or lymphangiomas may progress rapidly in utero, distorting the fetal anatomy and resulting in intrauterine fetal and obstetric complications and morbidity. In addition, several developmental tumors, including hamartomas and vaginal adenosis, are not malignant in utero but may undergo malignant degeneration following delivery. Benign and malignant tumors present diagnostic problems and therapeutic challenges. Both typically appear as heterogeneous masses with solid and cystic components when viewed by ultrasonography. The extent and tissue characteristics of these lesions may be further evaluated by MRI, and the diagnosis can occasionally be guided by a cytologic analysis of fluid aspirated from a cystic lesion. Jauniaux and Ogle maintain that expectant management should be the rule in the initial phase, with serial ultrasound evaluations to detect rapid enlargement, metastasis, or secondary fetal complications such as nonimmune hydrops.

The sacrococcygeal teratoma is a tumor arising from totipotential embryonic cells of the coccyx and has an incidence of 1 in 35,000 to 40,000 deliveries. There is a 4:1 female to male predominance, although the sex ratio in the incidence of malignant tumors is equal. With routine prenatal ultrasound, these lesions are being diagnosed increasingly when views of the spine to rule out neural tube defects are obtained. The advent of antenatal ultrasound has shifted the management focus from birth to the antenatal period, in which the fetal mortality rate ranges from 30% to 50%. The most common cause of perinatal loss is premature labor secondary to polyhydramnios, with one series reporting the combination of hydrops and placentomegaly as a very ominous sign with 100% mortality. On this basis, fetal surgery with tumor resection has been advocated in selected cases if the hydrops appears before 28 weeks and the tumor is deemed resectable. Because of the risk of dystocia and traumatic hemorrhage, cesarean section has been the rule for tumors greater than 5 cm. Following birth, complete excision of the tumor should not be delayed, and those who survive surgery should have a favorable prognosis. Residual tumor, however, may lead to malignant change, and although the recurrence risk is extremely low, isolated cases have been reported.

Congenital neuroblastoma is a cancer of neuronal lineage that may occur along the sites of the sympathetic ganglia from the neck to the presacral region, including the adrenal medulla. They typically contain Schwann cells and are the most common malignant tumor of the newborn, representing 30% to 40% of all congenital tumors. The genetic defect is characterized by the loss of locus p36 on chromosome 1. The clinical features are a function of the size, location, and humoral activity of the neuroblastoma, with catecholamine or vasoactive intestinal polypeptide characterizing their biologic behavior. Fetal neuroblastomas are well encapsulated and may displace the kidney inferiorly and laterally, with a predilection for the right side. The presence of calcification by ultrasonography has been associated with improved survival. Of note, neuroblastoma cells may infiltrate the placenta beyond the fetal capillaries and villous trophoblast, with metastasis to maternal tissue. Postpartum symptoms attributable to catecholamine production may be observed in the mother and include sweating, flushing, palpitations, and hypertension.

Concordance for neuroblastoma in monozygotic twins has been rarely reported, with the cause for the shared pathology unestablished. In 2001 Anderson and colleagues described a case of infant monozygotic twins developing neuroblastomas that were morphologically, clinically, and molecularly indistinguishable but with a delay of 6 months between times of presentation. Both tumors had metastasized and had amplification of MYCN and deletion at 1p36. The twin who developed neuroblastoma first had constitutional karyotype abnormalities in at least 5% of peripheral blood mononuclear cells. The second twin had a normal constitutional karyotype and lacked rearrangements or deletions. The authors proposed an acquired neuroblastoma predisposition specific for the first twin and in utero metastatic spread of tumor cells to the second twin (i.e., twin-to-twin metastasis) via the shared placental circulation.

Acute congenital leukemia is the second most common fetal cancer, occurring at an incidence of 1 in 4.7 million live births per year. The diagnosis requires the proliferation of blast cells together with anemia, thrombocytopenia, and leukocytosis. Important congenital infections including cytomegalovirus, rubella, and toxoplasmosis must be excluded. In utero, hepatosplenomegaly and nonimmune hydrops are common at presentation.

Sporadic heritable retinoblastoma is a malignant tumor of the retina that is inherited in an autosomal-dominant manner. The mutant retinoblastoma gene is mainly derived from the father and may be related to exposure of paternal germ cells to carcinogens. Primary hepatic malignant tumors of the fetus may present with an abdominal mass, and in cases of hepatoblastoma the serum levels of α-fetoprotein are markedly elevated and reflect the tumor burden. Finally, rhabdomyosarcoma is the most common soft tissue sarcoma in children and is commonly located at the level of the head and neck. It is associated with a loss of heterozygosity of the short arm of chromosome 11. Only a few cases have been described during pregnancy, during which time the tumors manifested as rapidly growing masses of irregular contour.

For full reference list, log onto www.expertconsult.com
〈http://www.expertconsult.com〉.

Complications of Disease and Therapy

Daniel L. Clarke-Pearson, MD

Women with gynecologic cancers often suffer from complications associated with their primary disease process or from the cancer-directed treatment modalities. In addition, many women have medical comorbidities, are obese, or are elderly, all of which further complicate therapy and treatment decisions. Minimizing these problems requires the clinician to astutely evaluate the patient, be proactive in prevention strategies, and provide early intervention.

Complications of disease are, in fact, commonly the primary presenting symptom (chief complaint) of a gynecologic cancer. Common symptoms of disease include hemorrhage (cervical and endometrial cancer), urinary tract obstruction or fistulae (cervical cancer), and intestinal obstruction or weight loss (ovarian cancer). Although some complications have been discussed previously in this text, it seems appropriate to devote a chapter exclusively to complications of disease and therapy. Not all possible complications can be covered, and the reader is referred to texts that expand on them. However, the most common complications and management will be discussed.

DISEASE–ORIENTED COMPLICATIONS

Symptoms caused by cancer, such as bleeding, urinary tract obstruction, fistula, and intestinal obstruction are complications of the primary gynecologic cancer, that usually will need to be managed coincidentally with the cancer itself.

Hemorrhage

Bleeding from cervical or endometrial cancer is a common presenting symptom. Although bleeding is rarely severe, the acute management of hemorrhage may be required before cancer therapy can be undertaken. Patients who are bleeding should be initially assessed for hemodynamic stability. On rare occasions, the bleeding is so severe that the patient may be in hypovolemic shock. Immediate management should include venous access, blood volume replacement, and supportive care. When stabilized, the patient should be examined and the source of the bleeding should be determined. Most commonly, massive hemorrhage results from an exophytic cervical cancer eroding into a small cervical or vaginal artery. Prolonged slow vaginal bleeding from an endometrial cancer or sarcoma may also result in a patient presenting with profound chronic anemia. Because the bleeding has been slow over a longer period, the patient has often accommodated to the anemia and may be hemodynamically stable despite profound anemia. Biopsy should be performed to document the pathology, and the patient should be evaluated to make a clinical estimation of the extent (stage) of disease.

Control of an actively bleeding cervical lesion is usually accomplished with a vaginal pack applied firmly to the cervix, filling the entire vagina. Monsel's solution (ferric subsulfate) may be put on the portion of the pack abutting the tumor. Soaking of the entire pack with Monsel's solution should be avoided because it will desiccate the normal vaginal mucosa, making removal of the pack and subsequent pelvic examinations difficult. Application of acetone to the pack adjacent to the tumor has also been helpful, although acetone is often difficult to acquire in today's medical environment. An indwelling Foley catheter should be placed in the bladder because pressure from the pack will usually obstruct the urethra. The pack should be removed slowly 24 to 48 hours later and the patient should be observed. Removal of the pack under anesthesia may provide a level of safety if immediate cautery or repacking were necessary. This would also provide the opportunity to perform an examination under anesthesia and cystoscopy or proctoscopy if indicated. Suturing bleeding points in a cervical cancer is rarely successful because the suture will tear through the tumor.

Pelvic radiation therapy for a patient with locally advanced cervical cancer who is actively bleeding should be initiated immediately. Alternatively, if the patient's cancer is an operable lesion, surgery should be performed expeditiously. In either event, if the patient has received more than four units of packed red blood cells, it is prudent to assess coagulation factors because the patient may have developed a "dilutional" coagulopathy and require fresh-frozen plasma (FFP) or platelets.

If bleeding cannot be controlled with packing, other measures must be considered. Consultation with an interventional radiologist should be obtained to consider arteriographic embolization of the hypogastric or uterine arteries. Arteriographic evaluation will usually identify the specific bleeding vessel and selective embolization can be accomplished. Arterial access is usually obtained through the femoral artery, and the catheter is advanced to the aortic bifurcation. Using contrast injected into the artery, the arterial vascular supply of the pelvis can be investigated in order to identify the specific bleeding site. Both sides of the pelvis should be evaluated. Intravascular contrast can be nephrotoxic and therefore must be used cautiously in patients who have an element of renal failure or who are diabetic. Control of the bleeding site can be accomplished by continuous vasopressin infusion, by embolization using synthetic materials (gelfoam) or Gianturco springs imbedded with Dacron, or with a balloon catheter (Figure 16-1). Embolization is usually the procedure primarily chosen because the vasopressin infusion and balloon catheters require that the artery remain cannulated for a longer duration.

Hypogastic (internal iliac) artery ligation is usually the procedure of last resort for bleeding from a primary gynecologic cancer and is most commonly performed to control intraoperative hemorrhage. Details of hypogastric artery ligation will be discussed later in this chapter.

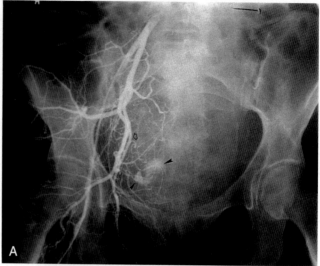

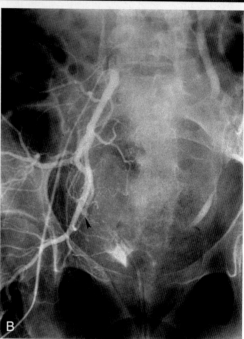

FIGURE 16-1 A patient who is postoperative from a vaginal hysterectomy with significant vaginal bleeding requiring multiple blood transfusions. The patient also has von Willebrand disease. **A,** Hemorrhage from the internal pudendal artery on the right. **B,** After embolization, no hemorrhage is seen from the internal pudendal artery. Dye in the pelvis is localized to the bladder, and the left ureter can be visualized. (*Courtesy Ivan Vujic, MD, and Keeling Warburton, MD, Medical University of South Carolina.*)

Urinary Tract Complications

Ureteral Obstruction

Ureteral obstruction may be the primary presenting symptom of a locally advanced cervical cancer and less commonly other gynecologic cancers, including endometrial and ovarian cancer. The most common evidence of ureteral obstruction is an elevated serum creatinine

TABLE 16-1 Major Causes of Acute Renal Failure in Gynecology

Disorder	Example
PRERENAL FAILURE	
Hypovolemia	Skin, gastrointestinal, or renal volume loss; hemorrhage, sequestration of extracellular fluid (pancreatitis, peritonitis)
Cardiovascular failure	Impaired cardiac output (infarction, tamponade); vascular pooling (anaphylaxis, sepsis, drugs)
POSTRENAL FAILURE	
Extrarenal obstruction	Urethral occlusion; bladder, pelvic, or retroperitoneal neoplasms surgical accident; calculi
Intrarenal obstruction	Crystals (uric acid, oxalic acid, sulfonamides, methotrexate)
Bladder rupture	Trauma
ACUTE TUBULAR NECROSIS	
Postischemic	All conditions listed above for prerenal failure
Pigment-induced	Hemolysis (transfusion reaction); rhabdomyolysis (trauma, coma, heatstroke, severe exercise, potassium or phosphate depletion)
Toxin-induced	Antibiotics; contrast material; anesthetic agents; heavy metals; organic solvents
Pregnancy-related	Septic abortion; uterine hemorrhage; eclampsia

(rather than complaints of anuria or symptoms of uremia). Of course, acute renal failure may arise from a number of causes, which should be investigated (Table 16-1). The ureters may be obstructed as a result of local extension of the cancer, by metastases to retroperitoneal lymph nodes, or by extrinsic compression of the ureter by large masses. Uremia secondary to bilateral ureteral obstruction is rarely encountered today but warrants immediate recognition and treatment. Given evidence of an elevated creatinine, evaluation of the ureters should avoid the use of nephrotoxic intravenous contrast dyes. Alternative methods may include a Lasix-renal scan or ultrasound of the kidneys. If bilateral ureteral obstruction is diagnosed, and before any intervention, the patient should be rapidly evaluated to determine the true extent of the cancer. If the cancer appears to be locally advanced and not widely metastatic, relief of the ureteral obstruction should be attempted by cystoscopy and placement of retrograde ureteral stents. If stent placement is unsuccessful, then percutaneous nephrostomy (PCN) tubes should be inserted. Dialysis may be necessary in extreme circumstances until the obstruction can be relieved. Postobstructive diuresis and correction of electrolytes should be carefully evaluated in the several days after relief of the ureteral obstruction.

Complications of PCN placement include a high frequency of urinary tract infections and pyelonephritis (70%), catheter occlusion (65%), and bleeding (28%). Seventy percent of the patients will have recovery of renal function after PCN placement (Dudley).

Comment needs to be made of two sets of circumstances in which the physician, patient, and family must seriously consider the possibility that relief of the obstruction may not be in the patient's best interest. These clinical situations include the following:

1. The patient who presents with a widely metastatic malignancy for which there is little significant opportunity to provide effective therapy.
2. The patient who has previously been treated for cervical cancer and has bilateral obstruction secondary to recurrent pelvic disease. This is a situation in which there is no therapy available that would significantly prolong the patient's life. Careful evaluation should be made to be certain that the obstruction is not a result of retroperitoneal fibrosis caused by prior radiation therapy or from a lymphocyst.

Often, patients with bilateral ureteral obstruction are uremic and comatose. Decisions regarding intervention and care then fall to the next of kin, who must make the difficult decisions regarding intervention that may reverse the uremia but cause the patient to succumb from other complications of the cancer versus allowing the patient to expire peacefully in a uremic coma. Compassionate and knowledgeable consultation and advice with an experienced gynecologic oncologist is crucial in these difficult circumstances.

Unilateral ureteral obstruction at the time of initial presentation may not require stent or PCN placement if the patient's renal function is normal and therapy (e.g., pelvic radiation therapy) is expected to control the cancer and relieve the obstruction. Placement of a PCN or stent in these circumstances must be balanced against the potential complications that might delay or interrupt therapy (Figure 16-2).

Urinary outlet obstruction (obstruction of the urethra) by a cancer that has invaded the anterior vaginal wall (vaginal, vulvar, or cervical cancers) may usually be corrected by placement of a Foley catheter. If a Foley catheter cannot be placed, either a suprapubic catheter or PCNs should be considered.

Urinary Tract Fistulas

Vesicovaginal fistula caused by a primary gynecologic cancer is relatively rare and is more commonly caused by therapy. Nonetheless, some patients will present with tumor that has eroded into the bladder and subsequent loss of integrity between the bladder and vagina results in urinary leakage. Correction of the fistula caused by a cancer cannot be considered until the cancer has been

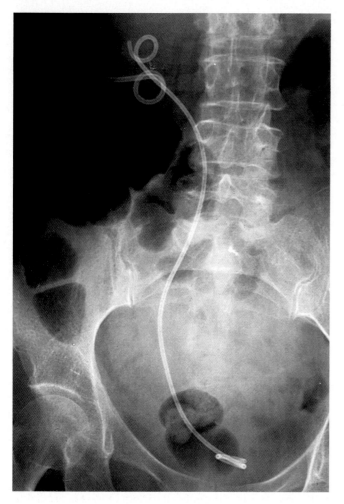

FIGURE 16-2   A double J stent has been inserted into the right kidney, ureter, and bladder through a percutaneous nephrostomy.

eradicated. In the interim, while cancer therapy is initiated, the patient may be very uncomfortable from the continued loss of urine. Attempts to diminish the leakage should be undertaken. Placement of a Foley catheter will often partially divert urine from the fistula into the catheter. Modified menstrual cups or external appliances to collect urine have been used on occasion with success. Urinary diversion (ileal or transverse colon conduit) may be the only complete solution to profuse vaginal urinary leakage. Performing this major surgery should be weighed against the delay in primary cancer therapy, which would be required while the patient recovers from surgical diversion.

Gastrointestinal Obstruction

Intestinal obstruction as a presenting symptom of a gynecologic cancer is most commonly caused by advanced ovarian cancer. In cases of small intestinal obstruction initial therapy should include correction of fluid volume and electrolytes, nutritional assessment, and nasogastric (NG) tube decompression. Assessment of intestinal patency with an upper gastrointestinal (GI) series (with small bowel follow-through) or a computed tomography (CT) scan with oral contrast should be performed to have a better understanding of the location and extent of obstruction. The colon should also be evaluated to exclude the possibility of colonic obstruction, which would need to be relieved at the same surgical procedure. In most cases, surgical exploration will be necessary in order to establish and stage the cancer diagnosis, to debulk the tumor, and to relieve the obstruction. Patients who are severely malnourished should have total parenteral nutrition (TPN) initiated perioperatively. Small bowel or colonic resection performed to relieve obstruction and to debulk primary tumor is commonly done.

Short bowel syndrome may result from extensive resection of the small bowel and/or colon. The syndrome is characterized by frequent diarrhea, fluid and electrolyte depletion, malabsorption, and weight loss. Depending on the extent and location of the intestinal segment(s) resected, malabsorption of nutrients may include copper, zinc, chromium, selenium, essential fatty acids, vitamins A and E, biotin, thiamine, and vitamin B_{12}. Over time, the remaining small bowel often adapts and fluid and nutrient absorption is improved. However, in the interim, attempts to relieve short bowel syndrome should be directed at decreasing transit time by the use of an "elemental" diet and Imodium or Lomotil, colestyramine (to decrease irritation of bile salts on the colonic mucosa), and somatostatin (to decrease intestinal digestive fluid production). In extreme cases, support with intravenous fluids and TPN may be necessary for several months.

On occasion, the preoperative assessment (usually with a CT scan) discovers far advanced disease (extensive carcinomatosis), which would be unlikely to be successfully debulked. In these patients, neoadjuvant chemotherapy, rather than surgical intervention, may be the best option. If this therapeutic strategy is taken, GI decompression (NG tube or gastrostomy) and parenteral nutritional support (TPN) will be required for several weeks while the neoadjuvant chemotherapy has the opportunity to result in a tumor response and relief of the intestinal obstruction. Fortunately, many patients with ovarian cancer will regain intestinal function after two or three cycles of chemotherapy.

Correction of a colonic obstruction is necessary to prevent colonic perforation, peritonitis, sepsis, and death. Management options include placement of an intraluminal stent or surgical intervention. Experience in deploying self-expanding metal stents to relieve colorectal obstruction shows a clinical success rate of 88% and effective palliation in 90% of patients. Advantages of stents include the avoidance of major surgery and a stoma. Risks include death (1%), perforation (4%), stent migration (10%), and reobstruction (10%). Alternatively, surgical correction of the colonic obstruction may be considered. Given that adequate mechanical bowel preparation is impossible in the face of colonic obstruction, resection and anastamosis are out of the question and a colostomy must be formed. If the patient has an excellent response to subsequent chemotherapy, colostomy take-down in the future is reasonable to consider.

Intestinal obstruction often occurs late in the course of progressive ovarian cancer. In these situations, superb clinical judgment is required to obtain an optimal palliative outcome because not all patients with recurrent ovarian cancer and intestinal obstruction will benefit from surgical intervention. It does seem intuitive that patients with colonic obstruction should be either offered a self-expanding stent or undergo surgery to create colostomy, ileostomy, or cecostomy. The patient with a small bowel obstruction requires careful thought and triage. Initially, conservative management with intravenous fluid and electrolyte replacement and NG tube decompression should be instituted. Some patients may reestablish bowel function with a few days of "bowel rest." However, if the obstruction persists, the decision to place a gastrostomy tube (which can often be placed percutaneously) or to attempt to surgically relieve the intestinal obstruction must be made. (Of course, the patient who has a small bowel obstruction caused by adhesions should undergo surgery in all cases.) The problem in decision-making comes when it is clear that the patient has recurrent ovarian cancer. Many investigators have attempted to identify factors that would predict successful outcome (often defined as surviving 30 days or being discharged from the hospital and able to take oral fluids) or postoperative complications and death. These factors include presence of ascites, poor nutritional status, amount of prior chemotherapy regimens, availability of therapy with some potential for response, prior use of radiation therapy, length of time since prior therapy, and potential for being "platin-sensitive." If surgical intervention is deemed appropriate, surgical procedures might include bypass of involved segments of small bowel (entero-enterostomy), bowel resection with anastamosis, or ileostomy. Unfortunately, in every investigator's experience there are patients who undergo laparotomy only to find such extensive carcinomatosis that they are deemed inoperable. The decision to operate, then, should be based on a clear communication between the surgeon and patient regarding expectations and definitions of "success." In our experience, which is reasonably representative of the general literature, median survival after small bowel obstruction surgery was 88 days and only 14% of patients were alive at 12 months. In addition, 49% of patients suffered at least one significant postoperative complication, including wound infections, enterocutaneous fistula, sepsis, and recurrent obstruction.

If the decision is made not to operate, further decisions regarding management are also complex, including methods to palliate vomiting (percutaneous gastrostomy is recommended) and whether to continue intravenous fluids or even consider TPN in a hospice setting.

Gastrointestinal Fistulas

Rectovaginal fistula may be discovered at the time of primary diagnosis of cervical, vaginal, or vulvar cancers. Involuntary loss of feces, flatus, and mucous discharge are the most common symptoms. If the patient has vulvar pain and excoriation, a fistula from the small intestine must be suspected. In this instance, an upper GI series (with small bowel follow-through) or a fistula-gram should be performed to define the exact anatomic structures involved. If a rectovaginal fistula is found, diversion with a loop colostomy or end-colostomy is suggested to divert the fecal stream and allow prompt treatment of the cancer (usually radiation therapy). If vulvar cancer is so advanced as to cause a rectovaginal fistula, some surgeons would manage the cancer and the fistula in the same surgical procedure (such as a posterior pelvic exenteration and modified radical vulvectomy). Others have had excellent results treating locally advanced vulvar cancer with radiation therapy and concurrent radiosensitizing chemotherapy, thereby preserving the rectal sphincter. Colostomy diversion is still suggested for patient comfort and hygiene. If the cancer treatment is successful, attempts to close the fistula are reasonable, and if successful, the colostomy may ultimately be reversed.

Enterovaginal fistulas are rare to complicate the initial cancer diagnosis and more often occur as a result of complications of therapy (radiation) or at the time of cancer recurrence. The flow of intestinal contents out of the vagina is usually liquid and caustic to vulvar skin. Thorough evaluation of the upper and lower GI tracts and the urinary tract is mandatory because many of these fistula are "complex," involving more than one viscus and more than one defect. Surgical intervention is necessary in most cases in order to either resect or isolate the involved bowel. If resection is not possible, the fistualized bowel will need to be isolated and excluded from the intestinal stream. Because the isolated bowel will continue to create succus entericus and subsequent continued vaginal drainage, resection is generally preferred.

Venous Thromboembolic Complications

Venous thromboembolic complications may precede the diagnosis of gynecologic cancer or may be the result of cancer treatments, especially surgery and chemotherapy.

Most women with gynecologic cancers have several risk factors that increase the probability of developing a venous thromboembolic event during their course of therapy.

Risk Factors

The causal factors of venous thrombosis were first proposed by Virchow in 1858 and include a hypercoagulable state, venous stasis, and vessel endothelial injury. In addition to the increased risk of venous thromboembolism (VTE) resulting from cancer, other clinical risk factors include advanced age; major surgery; nonwhite race; a history of deep venous thrombosis (DVT) or pulmonary embolism; lower-extremity edema or venous stasis changes; presence of varicose veins; being overweight; a history of radiation therapy; and hypercoagulable states, such as factor V Leiden, pregnancy, or use of oral contraceptives, estrogens, or tamoxifen. Intraoperative factors associated with postoperative DVT included increased anesthesia time, increased blood loss, and the need for transfusion in the operating room. It is important to recognize these risk factors in order to provide the appropriate level of venous thrombosis prophylaxis. A general outline of levels of thromboembolism risk can be found in Table 16-2.

Prophylactic Methods

DVT and pulmonary embolism, although largely preventable, are significant complications in women with gynecologic cancers and especially those who are postoperative. The magnitude of this problem is relevant to the gynecologic oncologist because 40% of all deaths following gynecologic surgery are directly attributed to pulmonary emboli and is the most common cause of postoperative death in patients with uterine or cervical carcinoma.

TABLE 16-2 Thromboembolism Risk Stratification

Risk	Factors
Low	Minor surgery No other risk factors*
Moderate	Age >40 years and major surgery Age <40 years with other risk factors* and major surgery
High	Age >60 years and major surgery Cancer History of deep venous thrombosis or pulmonary embolism Thrombophilias
Highest	Age >60 and cancer or history of venous thromboembolism

*Risk factors: cancer; advancing age; major surgery; obesity; varicose veins; history of deep venous thrombosis or pulmonary embolism; current estrogen, tamoxifen, or oral contraceptive use; thrombophilias.

A number of prophylactic methods have been shown to significantly reduce the incidence of DVT in women with gynecologic cancers, and a few studies have included a large enough patient population to demonstrate a reduction in fatal pulmonary emboli. The ideal prophylactic method would be effective, free of significant side effects, well accepted by the patient and nursing staff, widely applicable to most patients, and inexpensive. Available prophylactic methods may be divided into pharmacologic agents that reduce hypercoagulable states and mechanical methods that reduce stasis and may also enhance fibrinolysis. A key to the successful use of prophylactic methods is the understanding that women with gynecologic cancers are at very high risk and that more intense prophylactic measures are necessary to achieve maximal success.

LOW-DOSE HEPARIN

The use of small doses of subcutaneously administered heparin for the prevention of DVT and pulmonary embolism is the most widely studied of all prophylactic methods. More than 25 controlled trials have demonstrated that heparin given subcutaneously 2 hours preoperatively and every 8 to 12 hours postoperatively is effective in reducing the incidence of DVT. The value of low-dose heparin in preventing fatal pulmonary emboli was established by a randomized, controlled, multicenter international trial, which demonstrated a significant reduction in fatal postoperative pulmonary emboli in general surgery patients receiving low-dose heparin every 8 hours postoperatively Trials of low-dose heparin in gynecologic surgery patients with benign conditions have shown a significant reduction in postoperative DVT. However, in the patient with gynecologic cancer, the regimen that administered low-dose heparin 5000 units every 12 hours was found to be ineffective in a randomized trial.

In a subsequent trial two more intense heparin regimens were evaluated in high-risk gynecologic oncology patients. Heparin was given either in a regimen of 5000 units subcutaneously 2 hours preoperatively and every 8 hours postoperatively or 5000 units subcutaneously every 8 hours preoperatively (a minimum of three preoperative doses) and every 8 hours postoperatively. Both of these prophylaxis regimens were effective in significantly reducing the incidence of postoperative DVT in patients with gynecologic cancers. We conclude that in women undergoing surgery for gynecologic malignancy a regimen of low-dose heparin 5000 units every 8 hours is necessary to provide effective prophylaxis.

Although low-dose heparin is considered to have no measurable effect on coagulation, most large series have noted an increase in the bleeding complication rate, especially a higher incidence of wound hematoma.

Thrombocytopenia has been found to be associated with low-dose heparin use in 6% of patients after gynecologic surgery. If patients remain on low-dose heparin for more than 4 days, it would be reasonable to check a platelet count to assess the possibility of the occurrence of heparin-induced thrombocytopenia.

LOW MOLECULAR WEIGHT HEPARINS

Low molecular weight heparins (LMWHs) are fragments of heparin that vary in size from 4500 to 6500 daltons. When compared to unfractionated heparin, LMWHs have more anti-Xa and less antithrombin activity, leading to less effect on partial thromboplastin time (PTT) and possibly to fewer bleeding complications. An increased half-life of 4 hours results in increased bioavailability when compared to unfractionated heparin. The increase in half-life of LMWHs also allows the convenience of once-a-day dosing.

Randomized controlled trials have compared LMWH to unfractionated heparin in patients undergoing gynecologic surgery. In all studies, there was a similar incidence of DVT. Bleeding complications were also similar between the unfractionated heparin and LMWH groups. A metaanalysis of general surgery and gynecologic surgery patients from 32 trials likewise indicated that daily LMWH administration is as effective as unfractionated heparin in DVT prophylaxis without any difference in hemorrhagic complications. Again, based on randomized trials in other patients with cancer, it would appear that a more intense regimen of LMWH is necessary to obtain optimal prophylaxis. Finally, prolonged prophylaxis for 4 weeks postoperatively has resulted in improved outcomes. Although this is not standard of care at the moment, consideration of providing prolonged prophylaxis should be given in extremely high-risk patients.

MECHANICAL METHODS

Stasis in the veins of the legs has been clearly demonstrated while the patient is undergoing surgery and continues postoperatively for varying lengths of time. Stasis occurring in the capacitance veins of the calf during surgery plus the hypercoagulable state induced by cancer and surgery are the primary factors contributing to the development of acute postoperative DVT. Prospective studies of the natural history of postoperative venous thrombosis have shown that the calf veins are the predominant site of thrombi and that most thrombi develop within 24 hours of surgery.

Although probably of only modest benefit, reduction of stasis by short preoperative hospital stays and early postoperative ambulation should be encouraged for all patients. Elevation of the foot of the bed, raising the calf above heart level, allows gravity to drain the calf veins and should further reduce stasis.

Graduated Compression Stockings. Controlled studies of graduated pressure stockings are limited but do suggest modest benefit when they are carefully fitted. Poorly fitted stockings may be hazardous to some obese patients who develop a tourniquet effect at the knee or mid-thigh. Variations in human anatomy do not allow perfect fit of all patients to available stocking sizes. There is no therapeutic advantage of thigh-length stockings as compared with calf-length stocking. The simplicity of elastic stockings and the absence of significant side effects are probably the two most important reasons that they are often included in routine postoperative care.

External Pneumatic Compression. The largest body of literature dealing with the reduction of postoperative venous stasis deals with intermittent external compression of the leg by pneumatically inflated sleeves placed around the calf or leg during intraoperative and postoperative periods. Various pneumatic compression devices and leg-sleeve designs are available. The medical literature has not demonstrated superiority of one system over another. Calf compression during and after gynecologic surgery significantly reduces the incidence of DVT on a level similar to that of low-dose heparin. In addition to increasing venous flow and pulsatile emptying of the calf veins, external pneumatic compression also appears to augment endogenous fibrinolysis, which may result in lysis of very early thrombi before they become clinically significant.

The duration of postoperative external pneumatic compression has differed in various trials. External pneumatic compression may be effective when used in the operating room and for the first 24 hours postoperatively in patients with benign gynecologic conditions who will ambulate on the first postoperative day.

External pneumatic compression used in patients undergoing major surgery for gynecologic malignancy has been found to reduce the incidence of postoperative venous thromboembolic complications by nearly threefold, but only if calf compression is applied intraoperatively and for the first 5 postoperative days. Patients with gynecologic malignancies may remain at risk because of stasis and hypercoagulable states for a longer period than general surgical patients and therefore appear to benefit from longer use of external pneumatic compression.

External pneumatic leg compression has no significant side effects or risks and is considered slightly more cost-effective when compared with pharmacologic methods of prophylaxis. Of course, compliance to wearing the leg compression while in bed is of utmost importance and the patient and nursing staff should be educated to the proper regimen for maximum benefit. We have investigated the risk factors associated with the failure of external compression to prevent DVT in a retrospective analysis of 1862 consecutive gynecologic surgery patients who received postoperative intermittent pneumatic compression. A history of prior VTE, diagnosis of cancer, and age greater than 60 years were factors independently associated with the development of VTE despite external pneumatic compression (EPC) prophylaxis (P <0.05). Patients having two or more of these factors had a 16-fold increased risk of postoperative VTE despite prophylaxis. In these extremely high-risk patients, combined methods of prophylaxis (EPC plus low-dose unfractionated heparin [LDUH] or LMWH, for example) ought to be considered and are recommended by the guidelines written by the American College of Chest Physicians.

INTEGRATING EVIDENCE AND EXPERIENCE

Because low-dose unfractionated heparin, LMWH, and external pneumatic compression have been shown to effectively reduce the incidence of postoperative VTE in high-risk gynecologic oncology surgery patients, the question remains: Which is better?

We have undertaken two randomized clinical trials in hopes of answering this critical question. In the first trial, patients were randomly assigned to receive either LDUH (5000 units subcutaneously preoperatively and every 8 hours postoperatively until hospital discharge) or EPC (which was applied to the calf before surgery and remained on while the patient was in bed until hospital discharge). The incidence of DVT was identical in both groups of patients and none developed a pulmonary embolus within 30 days of follow-up. However, there were significantly more bleeding complications in the group who received LDUH. Specifically, nearly one fourth had activated partial thromboplastin time (APTT) levels in a "therapeutic" range and significantly more patients required blood transfusions. Following this trial, the standard of care in our institution was to use EPC because of its more favorable therapeutic ratio.

With the advent of LMWHs (which have more anti-Xa and less antithrombin activity) there was the potential that they may be associated with decreased risk of bleeding complications. We therefore undertook a second randomized trial comparing LMWH and IPC. Because higher doses of LMWH had been shown to be more effective in preventing VTE in cancer patients, we used dalteparin (Fragmin) 5000 units preoperatively and 5000 units daily postoperatively until hospital discharge. In this trial there was a similar low frequency of DVT and no PE in 30 days of follow-up. In addition, we found that LMWH was not associated with increased bleeding complications or transfusion requirements. Finally, compliance and patient satisfaction with either of these prophylaxis modalities were similar. Given the results of these two randomized clinical trials, we now feel that either LMWH or EPC are our best choices for thromboembolism prophylaxis in gynecologic oncology surgery patients.

COMBINATION PROPHYLAXIS

Combination therapy using heparin and compression stockings has been utilized in other high-risk surgical patients in an attempt to diminish both the hypercoaguability and venous stasis that can be found in postoperative patients at high risk for thromboembolism. The prophylactic use of LDH has been compared to LDH combined with graduated compression stockings (GCS) in DVT prophylaxis among general surgery patients. Willie-Jorgensen and associates in an investigation involving 245 patients undergoing acute extensive abdominal operations demonstrated that the rate of postoperative DVT was significantly lower among 79 patients receiving a combination regimen of GCS and LDH (i.e., 5000 units sq 1 hour preoperatively and q12h postoperatively) than patients receiving only the LDH regimen (P = 0.013). A statistically significant improvement (P <0.05) in postoperative DVT was similarly noted by the same investigators in the evaluation of 176 patients undergoing elective abdominal surgery. A metaanalysis of six studies involving 898 general surgery patients has shown that combination therapy with LDH and GCS provides significantly better DVT prophylaxis postoperatively than either single modality (odds ratio 0.40; 95% CI, 0.27-0.59) Recently, a multicenter prospective randomized clinical trial demonstrated that combination prophylaxis consisting of GSC and LMWH was more effective in DVT prevention than GCS alone (relative risk 0.52; 95% CI, 0.17 to 0.95, P = 0.04). "Combination" prophylaxis might be considered in the highest risk gynecologic oncology patients and is recommended by the ACCP Consensus Conference, although the efficacy, risks, and costs have not been fully evaluated in gynecologic oncology patients.

Management of Deep Venous Thrombosis and Pulmonary Embolism

DIAGNOSIS OF DEEP VENOUS THROMBOSIS

Because pulmonary embolism is the leading cause of death following gynecologic surgical procedures, identification of high-risk patients and the use of prophylactic VTE regimens is an essential part of management. In addition, the early recognition of DVT and pulmonary embolism and immediate treatment are critical. Most pulmonary emboli arise from the deep venous system of the leg, although following gynecologic surgery the pelvic veins are a known source of fatal pulmonary emboli also.

The signs and symptoms of DVT of the lower extremities include pain, edema, erythema, and prominent vascular pattern of the superficial veins. These signs and symptoms are relatively nonspecific; 50% to 80% of patients with these symptoms will not actually have DVT. Conversely, approximately 80% of patients with symptomatic pulmonary emboli have no signs or symptoms of thrombosis in the lower extremities. Because of the lack of specificity when signs and symptoms are recognized, additional diagnostic tests should be performed to establish the diagnosis of DVT.

Doppler Ultrasound. B-Mode duplex Doppler imaging is currently the most common technique for the diagnosis of symptomatic venous thrombosis, especially when it arises in the proximal lower extremity. With duplex Doppler imaging, the femoral vein can be visualized and clots may be seen directly. Compression of the vein with the ultrasound probe tip allows assessment of venous collapsibility and the presence of a thrombus diminishes vein wall collapsibility. It should be recognized that Doppler imaging is less accurate when evaluating the calf and the pelvic veins.

Venogram. Although venography has been the "gold standard" for diagnosis of DVT, other diagnostic studies are accurate when performed by a skilled technologist and, in most patients, may replace the need for routine contrast venography. Venography is moderately uncomfortable, requires the injection of a contrast material that may cause allergic reaction or renal injury, and may result in phlebitis in approximately 5% of patients. However, if noninvasive imaging is normal or inconclusive and the clinician remains concerned given clinical symptoms, venography should be obtained to obtain a definitive answer.

Magnetic Resonance Venography. Magnetic resonance venography (MRV) has a sensitivity and specificity comparable to those of venography. In addition, MRV may detect thrombi in pelvic veins that are not imaged by venography. The primary drawback to MRV is the time involved in examining the lower extremity and pelvis and the expense of this technology.

TREATMENT OF DEEP VENOUS THROMBOSIS

The treatment of postoperative DVT requires the immediate institution of anticoagulant therapy. Treatment may be with either unfractionated heparin or LMWHs, followed by 6 months of oral anticoagulant therapy with warfarin. Prolonged anticoagulation (lifetime) is recommended for women who continue to have active cancer (i.e., those not in remission after treatment) because they remain at very high risk to re-thrombose.

Unfractionated Heparin. After VTE is diagnosed, unfractionated heparin should be initiated to prevent proximal propagation of the thrombus and allow physiologic thrombolytic pathways to dissolve the clot (Table 16-3). An initial bolus of 80 units per kilogram is given intravenously, followed by a continuous infusion of 1000 to 2000 units per hour (18 units/kg/hr). Heparin dosage

TABLE 16-3 Anticoagulation Method for Deep Venous Thrombosis

Obtain a pretreatment hemoglobin level, platelet count, PT, and APTT, and repeat platelet count daily until heparin is stopped.

Administer a bolus dose of heparin: 5000 units IV.

Initiate a maintenance dose of heparin: 32,000 units IV per 24 hr by continuous infusion, or 17,000 units SC to be repeated after adjustment at 12 hr.

Adjust the dose of heparin at 6 hr according to the nomogram; maintain APTT in the therapeutic range.

Repeat APTT every 6 hr until it moves into the therapeutic range, and then daily according to the nomogram.

Start warfarin 10 mg at 24 hr and 10 mg next day.

Overlap heparin and warfarin for at least 4 days.

Perform PT daily and adjust the warfarin dose to maintain the INR at 2.0-3.0.

Continue heparin for a minimum of 5 days, then stop if the INR has been in the therapeutic range for at least 2 consecutive days.

Continue warfarin for 6 months and monitor PT daily until it is in the therapeutic range, then three times during the first week, twice a week for 2 weeks or until the dose response is stable, and then every 2 weeks.

APTT, Activated partial thromboplastin time; INR, international normalized ratio; PT, prothrombin time.

is adjusted to maintain APTT levels at a therapeutic level 1.5 to 2.5 times the control value. Initial APTT should be measured after 6 hours of heparin administration, and the dose should be adjusted as necessary. Patients having subtherapeutic APTT levels in the first 24 hours have a risk for recurrent thromboembolism 15 times the risk of patients with appropriate levels. Patients, therefore, should be managed aggressively using intravenous heparin to achieve prompt anticoagulation. A weight-based nomogram has proved helpful in achieving a therapeutic APTT (Table 16-4). Oral anticoagulant (warfarin) should be started on the first day of heparin infusion. The international normalized ratio (INR) should be monitored daily until a therapeutic level is achieved (INR 2.0-3.0). The change in INR resulting from warfarin administration often precedes the anticoagulant effect by approximately 2 days, during which time low protein C levels are associated with a transient hypercoagulable state. Therefore, heparin should be administered until the INR has been maintained in a therapeutic range for at least 2 days, confirming proper warfarin dose. Intravenous heparin may be discontinued in 5 days if an adequate INR level has been established.

Low Molecular Weight Heparin. LMWHs (exoxaparin and daltaparin) have been shown to be effective in the treatment of VTE and have a cost-effectiveness advantage over intravenous heparin in that they may be administered in the outpatient setting. The dosages used in treatment of thromboembolism are unique and weight adjusted according to each LMWH preparation. Because LMWH have a minimal effect on activated partial

TABLE 16-4   Heparin Administration for Treatment of Deep Vein Thrombosis or Pulmonary Embolism: Weight-Based Nomogram

Time of Administration	Dose
Initial dose	80-units/kg bolus, then 18 units/kg/hr
The APTT should be measured every 6 hr and the heparin dose adjusted as follows:	
APTT <35 s (<1.2 times control)	80-units/kg bolus, then 4 units/kg/hr
APTT 35-45 s (1.2-1.5 times control)	40-units/kg bolus, then 2 units/kg/hr
APTT 46-70 s (1.5-2.3 times control)	No change
APTT 71-90 s (2.3-3 times control)	Decrease infusion rate by 2 units/kg/hr
APTT > 90 s (>3 times control)	Hold infusion for 1 hr, then decrease infusion rate by 3 units/kg/hr

From Raschke RA, Reilly BM, Guidry JR et al: Ann Intern Med 119:874, 1993.
APTT, Activated partial thromboplastin time.

thromboplastin time (PTT), serial laboratory monitoring of PTT levels is not necessary. Similarly, monitoring of anti-Xa activity (except in difficult cases or those with renal impairment) has not been shown to be of significant benefit in a dose adjustment of LMWH. The increased bioavailability associated with LMWH allows for twice-a-day dosing, potentially making outpatient management for a subset of patients an option. A meta-analysis involving more than 1000 patients from 19 trials suggests that LMWH is more effective, safer, and less costly compared with unfractionated heparin in preventing recurrent thromboembolism.

ORAL ANTICOAGULANTS: WARFARIN

In most cases, the conversion from parenteral heparin or LMWH to oral warfarin may start on the initial day of therapy. Both heparin and warfarin are given and the heparin is discontinued when the warfarin has reached a therapeutic INR of 2 to 3 for 2 consecutive days. Initially, the INR should be monitored frequently to appropriately adjust the warfarin dose. Once a stable warfarin dose is established, the INR may be checked less frequently. Patients should be cautioned to avoid the use of drugs and dietary products that might alter the metabolism or absorption of warfarin. Warfarin may be a difficult drug to administer to some patients, especially if their nutrition is inadequate, their oral intake is variable, or they require prolonged use of antibiotics or other drugs that might alter the metabolism of warfarin. This is particularly common in women with advanced ovarian

cancer. Given the wide variation in the INR in many of these patients who are then predisposed to either bleeding complications or re-thrombosis, we have found that it is safer to use subcutaneous LMWH (at therapeutic doses) for prolonged therapy.

DIAGNOSIS OF PULMONARY EMBOLISM

Many of the signs and symptoms of pulmonary embolism are associated with other, more commonly occurring pulmonary complications following surgery. The classic findings of pleuritic chest pain; hemoptosis; and shortness of breath, tachycardia, and tachypnea should alert the physician to the possibility of a pulmonary embolism. Many times, however, the signs are much more subtle and may be suggested only by a persistent tachycardia or a slight elevation in the respiratory rate. Patients suspected of pulmonary embolism should be evaluated initially by chest radiograph electrocardiography, and arterial blood gas assessment. Any evidence of abnormality should be further evaluated by ventilation-perfusion lung scan or a spiral CT scan of the chest. Unfortunately, a high percentage of lung scans may be interpreted as "indeterminate." In this setting, careful clinical evaluation and judgment are required to decide whether pulmonary arteriography should be obtained to document or exclude the presence of a pulmonary embolism.

The treatment of pulmonary embolism is as follows:

1. Immediate anticoagulant therapy, identical to that outlined for the treatment of DVT, should be initiated.
2. Respiratory support, including oxygen and bronchodilators and an intensive care setting, may be necessary.
3. Although massive pulmonary emboli are usually quickly fatal, pulmonary embolectomy has been performed successfully on rare occasions.
4. Pulmonary artery catheterization with the administration of thrombolytic agents bears further evaluation and may be important in patients with massive pulmonary embolism.
5. Vena cava interruption may be necessary in situations in which anticoagulant therapy is ineffective in the prevention of re-thrombosis and repeated embolization from the lower extremities or pelvis. A vena cava umbrella or filter may be inserted percutaneously above the level of the thrombosis and caudad to the renal veins.
6. In most cases, however, anticoagulant therapy is sufficient to prevent repeat thrombosis and embolism and to allow the patient's own endogenous thrombolytic mechanisms to lyse the pulmonary embolus.

SUPERIOR VENA CAVA SYNDROME

Superior vena cava syndrome is caused by advanced cancers arising in or invading the mediastinum, subsequently obstructing the venous drainage of the head, neck, and upper thoracic regions. Primary tumors are most commonly the cause of this syndrome (bronchogenic carcinomas), although metastasis to the mediastinum from gynecologic cancers can also present in this manner. The vena cava has a low intravascular pressure and is easily compressed by adjacent masses. Most commonly the symptoms caused by venous obstruction are dramatic swelling and plethora of the head, neck, upper extremities, and chest. Pleural and pericardial effusions can occur with decreased venous return to the heart and a resultant fall in cardiac output. Patients also commonly complain of a severe headache. A similar clinical syndrome is also seen associated with thrombosis of the subclavian vein and superior vena cava, which is induced by central venous catheters. The diagnosis of the cause of superior vena cava syndrome is critical to selecting proper management. If a localized primary or metastatic neoplasm is identified, immediate radiation therapy is usually the most effective method to achieve resolution. Radiation therapy to the mediastinum in doses of 400 cGy for 3 days and then 150 to 180 cGy per day for a total dose of 3000 to 5000 cGy has been successful in relieving the vascular obstruction. Responses are commonly recognized in 3 to 4 days. Chemotherapy may also play a role, although the resolution of symptoms is usually much slower. Expandable wire stents across the constricted portion of the vena cava have also been used successfully.

In patients in whom thrombosis is the etiology of venous obstruction, immediate anticoagulant therapy should be instituted (Figure 16-3). The edema and plethora will usually diminish in 1 to 3 days. In many instances, the central venous catheter may be left in place and used. However, if the condition should persist or recur, the catheter should be removed.

Biliary Obstruction

Obstruction of the biliary tree by gynecologic cancers is rare and is usually associated with far advanced cancers and limited life expectancy. Nonetheless, the resulting jaundice and pruritus caused by the obstruction is distressing to the patient and her family. Surgical relief of the obstruction is usually impossible because of the extent of cancer involvement in the region. However, endoscopic placement of a stent in the common duct often will resolve the symptoms and provide a better quality of life. If a stent cannot be placed as a result of extreme compression or other technical reasons, percutaneous placement of a drainage tube into the dilated biliary tree will also resolve symptoms.

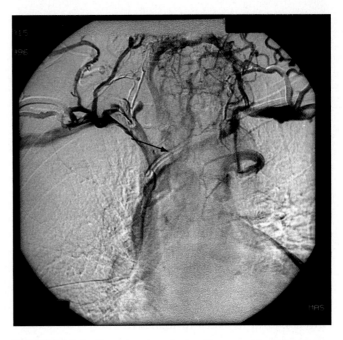

FIGURE 16-3 Extensive thrombosis of large vessels in the thorax. Multiple collaterals are present. The subclavian catheter is evident *(arrow)*.

Metastatic adenopathy high in the paraaortic chain resulting in biliary obstruction can commonly obstruct the duodenum, leading to gastric outlet obstruction. Although surgical intervention (gastrojejunostomy) or self-expanding metal stents may correct the anatomic problem, careful consideration should be given to the patient's life expectancy. These are similar considerations to those made in women with small intestinal obstruction and recurrent ovarian cancer discussed previously. In women with just days or weeks to live, placement of a gastrostomy tube may be more prudent.

TREATMENT-RELATED COMPLICATIONS

Surgical

Intraoperative and Postoperative Hemorrhage

INTRAOPERATIVE MANAGEMENT OF VASCULAR COMPLICATIONS

Surgery for gynecologic cancer often requires extensive dissection in the retroperitoneal space, which may be distorted by cancer metastatic to lymph nodes or invading adjacent structures. It is not surprising, then, that injury to pelvic veins and arteries are common and may result in significant intraoperative blood loss and hemorrhage. The surgeon must be prepared for this eventuality and have in his armamentarium the tools and skills to bring a stop to the bleeding.

Before attempting to bring final control to a significant bleeding area, a few basic principles should be used. First, the patient's blood volume and coagulation factors must be maintained at all times. Poor communication between the surgeon and the anesthesiologist can lead to significant hypovolemia and cardiovascular instability. Loss of coagulation factors during intraoperative hemorrhage results in continued bleeding that cannot be controlled by surgical means. The surgeon should pack the involved area to allow replacement of blood volume (packed red blood cells), coagulation factors (FFP and platelets), and acquisition of appropriate assistance. When the patient is stable and the team is fully prepared, the packed area should be exposed a small area at a time in order to identify the specific bleeding site.

Before attempting to control the bleeding point, the adjacent anatomy should be identified and protected. In particular, the ureter, adjacent vessels, and viscera must be recognized to avoid further injury. In most cases of arterial bleeding, the artery can be isolated and controlled with sutures. Small arteries may be best controlled by vascular clips, whereas larger arteries may require sutures with 4-0 or 5-0 vascular suture (Prolene) (Figure 16-4). This holds for injury to the aorta and common and external iliac arteries. Injury to the internal iliac (hypogastric) artery may be controlled with total ligation of the artery. Patency of distal arteries should be confirmed throughout the remainder of the procedure and postoperatively. In rare instances, arterial injuries must be managed by vascular grafting.

Venous bleeding in the pelvis is probably more common given the fragility of the thin vein wall and the extensive network of pelvic venous plexus. Often a specific bleeding point cannot be identified but, after several minutes of direct pressure on the bleeding area, a clot will form over the low-pressure veins and the bleeding will resolve. If it does not, control will have to be achieved with vascular clips, clamps, and suture ligature. Slow but persistent oozing from unidentified vessels can often be controlled by products that either serve as a matrix for clotting (Avitene, Surgicel, Gelfoam) or supply clotting factors that complete the clotting cascade (CoSeal, TISSEEL, FLOSEAL). Following application of any of these products, pressure should be applied to the site for 5 minutes and then the site should be reevaluated. If bleeding has not been controlled, it may be necessary to place a pack and transfer the patient to an intensive care unit (ICU). In all cases, it should be emphasized that prompt replacement of clotting factors provided by transfusion of FFP and platelets is critical to achieve hemostasis in the face of hemorrhage.

Replacement of platelets and clotting factors in patients with massive transfusion and microvascular bleeding is dependent on clinical and surgical assessments. Guidelines have been provided by the American Society of Anesthesiologists task force regarding replacement of these products. In general, platelet transfusion is rarely indicated for counts greater than 100,000/μL and usually indicated for counts less than 50,000/μL (with intermediate platelet counts 50,000/μL to 100,000/μL, transfusion should be based on the risk of bleeding). FFP therapy is indicated in massively transfused patients with microvascular bleeding or hemorrhage if the prothrombin (PT) or APTT values exceed 1.5 times the normal values. In cases of massive intraoperative blood loss, it may be prudent to administer FFP empirically (after 4 units of packed red blood cells). This strategy is aimed at preventing the patient from becoming hypocoagulable while awaiting the laboratory results (PT and PTT), which may take nearly an hour and another hour to thaw the FFP before it is available to be administered. Cryoprecipitate transfusions are recommended for correction of microvascular bleeding in massively transfused patients with fibrinogen concentrations less than 80 to 100 mg/dL.

Bleeding from the sacrum is usually not encountered except in the course of performing a total pelvic exenteration or rectosigmoid resection or during a sacral-colpopexy. If bleeding from the sacrum cannot be controlled by suture ligatures or vascular clips, placement of sterile thumbtacks pushed into the sacral bone will usually compress veins exiting the sacrum and achieve hemostasis.

HYPOGASTRIC (INTERNAL ILIAC) ARTERY LIGATION

In situations when the usual steps to control hemorrhage have failed, hypogastric artery ligation should be performed. Although the arterial blood supply to the pelvis is rich with anastamosis, ligation of the hypogastric

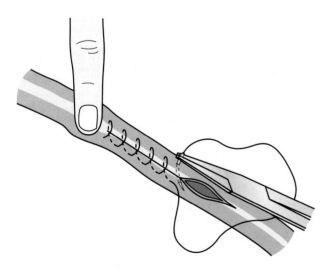

FIGURE 16-4　Laceration of a large pelvic wall vein. The operator's finger pressure on the vessel reduces flow to the site, while a continuous suture of fine silk or nylon is placed to close the defect.

arteries will usually decrease the arterial and venous pressure to the point at which (in a patient who is not hypocoagulable) venous bleeding will slow and can either be controlled by ligature or will clot with prolonged packing.

To safely perform hypogastric artery ligation, the vascular anatomy must be exposed and adjacent structures, especially the ureter, must be identified. A retroperitoneal approach should be taken. The peritoneum overlying the psoas muscle (lateral to the external iliac artery) should be incised parallel to the artery. As the peritoneum is mobilized medially, the external iliac artery will first be identified. Dissection cephalad along the external iliac artery will identify the common iliac artery and the bifurcation of the internal iliac artery. Invariably, the ureter crosses the pelvic brim at the bifurcation of the common iliac artery. At this location, the ureter will be identified attached to the medial peritoneum. Further opening of the retroperitoneal space keeping the iliac vessels lateral and the ureter medial will create the pararectal space and further expose the internal iliac artery. Be aware that the common external and internal iliac veins lie just beneath their respective arteries. Without clear identification of these veins, injury can occur, which will further complicate the procedure. The hypogastric artery bifurcates into an anterior and posterior branch 2 to 3 cm from its origin from the common iliac artery. Because most bleeding arises from the blood supply from the anterior division, the anterior branch should be ligated if at all possible. (Ligation of the posterior branch increases the risk of buttock pain and potential necrosis of the gluteus.) A right angle clamp should be carefully passed from lateral to medial beneath the hypogastric artery. A heavy suture (e.g., 0-silk) should be used to ligate the artery (Figure 16-5). There is no reason to transect the artery between two ligatures. It is usually best to perform bilateral hypogastric artery ligation as the collateral blood supply crosses over the midline.

Finally, if all methods to control hemorrhage have been unsuccessful, the bleeding site should be packed firmly and the abdomen should be closed. The patient should be taken to the surgical ICU and stabilized. Central monitoring and blood product replacement should be the primary focus of management. Once the patient is stabilized, attempts at angiographic embolization should be considered. Ultimately after 24 to 48 hours the patient should be returned to the operating room, reexplored, and the pack removed carefully. Surprisingly, many times the bleeding will have stopped as a result of compression of the injured veins and correction of the hypocoagulable state.

MANAGEMENT OF SHOCK

During and after gynecologic surgery, blood-volume deficit that results from intraoperative blood loss or

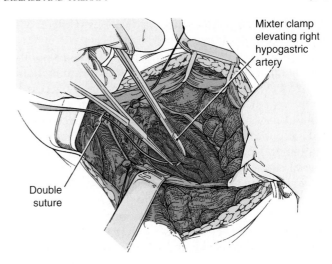

Mixter clamp elevating right hypogastric artery

Double suture

FIGURE 16-5 Technique for intraoperative ligation of the hypogastric artery. The ligature is placed 2 to 3 cm below the bifurcation so that the posterior branch will not be ligated. The clamp is passed lateral to medial to prevent trauma to the internal iliac vein. (From Nichols DH, Clarke-Pearson DL [eds]: Gynecologic, Obstetric and Related Surgery, 2nd ed. St. Louis, Mosby, 2000.)

postoperative hemorrhage is the most common cause of shock. This shock usually is manifested by arterial hypotension, tachycardia, a weak pulse, anxiety, skin pallor, diminished urinary output, and peripheral vasoconstriction. In addition to hemorrhage (hypovolemic shock), the differential diagnosis of shock must include many other causes, such as cardiogenic (myocardial infarction) and cardiac compressive conditions (cardiac tamponade or pneumothorax), sepsis, drug overdose, and pulmonary embolism. Appropriate studies are dictated by the patient's signs and symptoms.

Consideration should be given to obtaining arterial blood gas analysis, an electrocardiogram, a chest radiograph, blood chemistry studies, and blood cultures. The patient should be prepared for blood transfusion. The degree and duration of postoperative shock determine the need for resuscitation, central venous pressure monitoring, and Swan–Ganz pulmonary artery catheterization.

Resuscitation of a hemorrhaging patient during or after gynecologic surgery involves stabilization of the hemodynamic status and correction of the cause of the blood loss. When the hemorrhage is massive, fluid, electrolyte, and hemodynamic shifts are likewise massive. Central to stabilization efforts are the replacement and maintenance of adequate intravascular volume.

CENTRAL MONITORING

Invasive cardiovascular monitoring may be lifesaving for patients with massive hemorrhage or patients who are at additional risk because of preexisting cardiopulmonary disorders. The monitoring allows the rational use of fluids and cardioactive medications while avoiding their complications.

In patients with marked hemodynamic instability, peripheral artery cannulation allows continuous monitoring of systemic arterial pressure and ready access to obtain repeated analysis of arterial blood gases. The radial artery is usually chosen because of accessibility and has good collateral circulation, although the brachial and femoral arteries may be used. The complications of arterial cannulation include catheter-related septicemia (4% in one large study), local infection (as high as 18%), and arterial embolization (0.2% to 0.6%).

In patients without cardiopulmonary disease, monitoring of central venous pressure along with monitoring of the vital signs, urine output, and other clinical signs usually provide sufficient information for appropriate fluid resuscitation. In addition, central venous pressure monitoring avoids several of the complications of a pulmonary artery (Swan–Ganz) catheter.

Central venous catheter may be introduced into the great intrathoracic veins by way of the antecubital, external or internal jugular, or subclavian veins. Cannulation of the right internal jugular vein, which provides a straight course to the right atrium, has the lowest overall complication rate. In all cases, a chest radiograph should be obtained immediately after catheter insertion to confirm proper location and to assess for possible pneumothorax.

The usefulness of the Swan–Ganz catheter in critically ill patients (even those without heart disease) who do not respond to therapy based on an initial noninvasive assessment has been well documented. Additional diagnostic information may be obtained concerning unsuspected cardiac dysfunction, pulmonary artery embolization, or sepsis. Patients without primary myocardial insult, but with hypotension and evidence of inadequate perfusion of vital organs (e.g., oliguria, acidosis, mental obtundation), are better managed when data are available from central monitoring. Unnecessary fluid overload can be prevented, and the risk of congestive failure and pulmonary edema can be reduced (Table 16-5).

In patients with cardiac or pulmonary disease, cardiac output and resistance measurements allow the proper use of pressors, afterload and preload reducers, and fluids. In addition, if sepsis is part of the clinical picture, careful monitoring of pulmonary capillary wedge pressures may be necessary to prevent pulmonary edema, which is seen with even mild increases in left atrial pressures as a result of the increased permeability of the pulmonary vascular bed. This increased permeability also may be seen in patients in hypovolemic shock, again leading to pulmonary edema at relatively normal wedge pressures. Finally, invasive monitoring not only provides a direct measurement of cardiac function, but also

TABLE 16-5   Hemodynamic Calculations*

Parameter	Formula	Normal Range
MAP	⅓ (SBP − DBP) + DBP	0.70-105 mm Hg
CO	Heart rate × stroke volume	1.4-8 L/min
Cardiac index	CO/body surface area (m²)	2.5-4 L/min/m²
Systemic vascular resistance	MAP − (right arterial pressure/CO)	0.10-20 U
Pulmonary vascular resistance	PAP† − (PCWP/CO)	1.1-3 U

CO, Cardiac output; DBP, diastolic blood pressure; MAP, mean arterial pressure; PAP, mean pulmonary artery pressure; PCWP, pulmonary capillary wedge pressure; SBP, systolic blood pressure.

*Stroke volume can be derived from CO and heart rate. Resistance is derived from a relative change in pressure on each side of the circuit from which resistance is to be measured.

†PAP = [2 (pulmonary SBP) + pulmonary DBP]/3.

provides information within minutes about the effects of therapy.

These catheters may be placed from the antecubital fossa, although the percutaneous subclavian or internal or external jugular vein approaches are more commonly used. Complications of pulmonary artery catheters include pulmonary infarction distal to the catheter (1%-2% of cases), pulmonary artery rupture (0.2% of cases), balloon rupture (3% of cases), and sepsis (2% of cases), all of which are made more likely by prolonged use of the catheter.

Intraoperative Genitourinary Injuries

Given the close anatomic relationships of the gynecologic organs and the urinary tract, ureteral and bladder injury are to be anticipated, even in the hands of the most skilled surgeon. Prevention of urinary tract injury is predicated on the identification of the key urinary tract structures before embarking on radical or extended surgery for gynecologic cancers. Retroperitoneal exploration by opening the lateral retroperitoneal spaces (pararectal and paravesical spaces) allows for identification of the ureter and lateral bladder (and key vascular structures). Should the medial pelvic peritoneum require resection, the ureter must be detached from the peritoneum and mobilized laterally (ureterolysis). The ureter may be dissected throughout its entire pelvic course to the bladder, although between the uterine artery crossing the ureter and the insertion of the ureter into the bladder, techniques similar to those required for a type II or III radical hysterectomy will need to be used. Identification of the bladder is usually not a problem; however, because of anatomic distortion by advanced cancer, radiation therapy, or extensive adhesions from prior surgery, the bladder sometimes is not easily recognized. One simple method to identify the bladder is to fill it retrograde through the indwelling Foley catheter. With the bladder distended, dissection of the uterus or tumor from the bladder may be facilitated. Opening the retropubic space (space of Retzius) and the paravesical space also facilitates identification and protection of the bladder.

Injury to the bladder is usually easily corrected at the time of surgery. Incisions in the dome of the bladder should be closed in two layers with 3-0 or 2-0 delayed absorbable suture. Allow the bladder to heal by leaving the Foley catheter to dependent drainage for approximately 5 days. Cystotomies at the base of the bladder have a higher risk of fistula formation and ureteral occlusion. Further, they may be more difficult to recognize. Whenever there is concern about potential bladder injury, the bladder should be filled in a retrograde fashion with either sterile infant formula or indigo carmine dyed saline. We prefer infant formula because the formula does not stain tissues and potentially obscure the site of injury. Once the cystotomy in the base of the bladder is identified, it is important to assess the location of the ureteral orifices. This may be accomplished by cystoscopy or by opening the dome of the bladder and directly visualizing the orifices. The administration of intravenous indigo carmine may aid in the identification of the orifices. Closure of the cystotomy should again be accomplished using two layers of delayed absorbable suture. If the cystotomy is near the ureteral orifice, retrograde placement of a stent is prudent to ensure that there is no occlusion or narrowing of the ureter. If the pelvis has been previously radiated, we would recommend placement of an omental J-flap between the bladder and the vaginal cuff in order to bring a new, nonirradiated blood supply into this area. The Foley catheter should be left to drain for several weeks, and a cystogram should be obtained before the decision to remove the catheter.

Injury to the ureter as it passes through the pelvis may be managed by several methods depending on the location and extent of the injury. Ureteral injury above the pelvic brim is usually best managed by end-to-end anastamosis over a ureteral stent (Figure 16-6). Injury below the pelvic brim may be best corrected by a ureteroneocystotomy with psoas hitch or a Boari flap (Figure 16-7). In either method of repair placement, a closed suction drain in the pelvis is advised in order to prevent a urinoma from a leak of the anastamosis.

In cases of suspected injury to the ureter, intravenous indigo carmine should be injected and the pelvis should be inspected for spill of dye-colored urine. If the extent of ureteral injury is a clamp crush or ligature, placement of a ureteral double-J stent left in place for 6 weeks will usually allow the injured ureter to recover and at the same time prevent ureteral stricture.

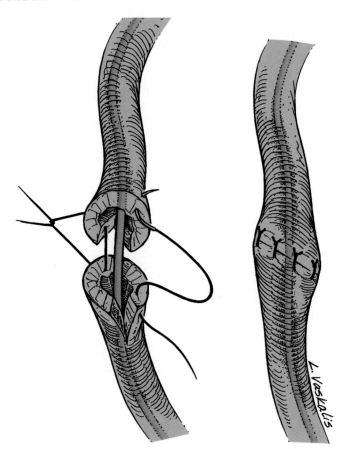

FIGURE 16-6 Ureteral injury at the pelvic brim repaired with an ureteroureterostomy using interrupted 4-0 delayed absorbance sutures. The ureter is spatulated to achieve a larger lumen at the anastomosis. The anastomosis is done over a ureteral stent, and the area is drained with a suction drain. (*From Nichols DH, Clarke-Pearson DL [eds]: Gynecologic, Obstetric and Related Surgery, 2nd ed. St. Louis, Mosby, 2000.*)

Postoperative Urinary Tract Injury

Unless bilateral ureteral obstruction has been caused by surgery, most patients with postoperative anuria or severe oliguria will have these findings secondary to prerenal hypovolemia, which will resolve with hydration and diuresis. However, unilateral ureteral injury may not be recognized until several days postoperatively; manifest by flank pain, pyelonephritis, or a slight rise in serum creatinine. The volume of urinary output is rarely altered. When postoperative ureteral obstruction is suspected, evaluation may include IVP or CT scan with contrast (in cases in which serum creatinine is normal) or with a renal ultrasound or Lasix-renal scan. If ureteral obstruction is discovered, initial management should include cystoscopy with retrograde stent placement. If successful, the obstruction is likely a result of tethering from nearby sutures or extrinsic compression from a mass (hematoma, lymphocyst, tumor). Leaving the stent in place for 6 weeks and then reevaluating with

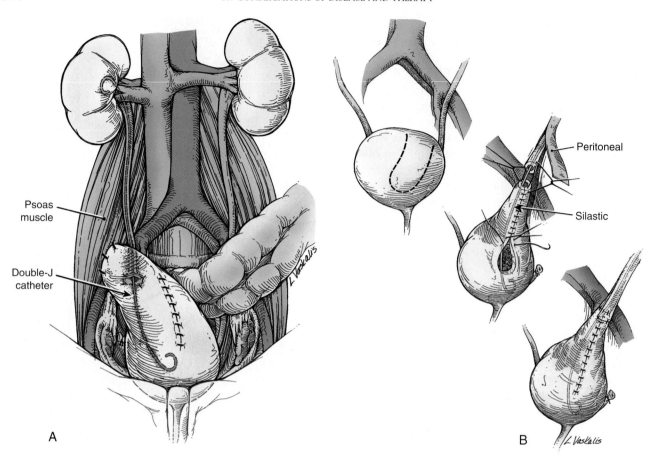

FIGURE 16-7 **A,** Ureteroneocystostomy with psoas hitch. Bladder is mobilized and sutured to the psoas muscle at the pelvic brim near the site of planned ureterovesical anastomosis. **B,** Boari flap. A flap from the dome of the bladder is created and "rolled" into a tube to substitute for the absent distal ureter and to reach the proximal ureter, which is reanastomosed. In either procedure, the area should be drained by closed suction. *(From Nichols DH, Clarke-Pearson DL [eds]: Gynecologic, Obstetric and Related Surgery, 2nd ed. St. Louis, Mosby, 2000.)*

follow-up IVP is recommended. If a stent cannot be placed, however, consideration should be given to reexploration to correct the obstruction. If reoperation is not reasonable, a PCN tube should be placed.

Urinary tract fistulae are recognized complications of radical hysterectomy for the primary treatment of cervical cancer. It is thought that the extensive dissection of the distal ureter and base of the bladder may lead to ischemic necrosis and the development of a vesicovaginal or uretrovaginal fistula. In contemporary reports these fistula occur in only 1% to 3% of cases. The risk of fistula is increased when surgery is performed after prior pelvic radiation therapy.

Vaginal leakage of fluid during the first 10 weeks postoperatively is an ominous finding and requires evaluation for a urinary tract fistula. Confirming the presence of a fistula and, if present, identifying the location are the next priorities. Initially, the bladder should be filled with dyed (indigo carmine) saline. If there is a

vesicovaginal fistula, a vaginal speculum examination should reveal dye coming from the upper vagina. If there is no leakage, then intravenous indigo carmine should be administered. If dye is then found to be draining from the vagina, a ureteral vaginal fistula must be suspected. Further investigation with IVP or CT scan with IV contrast may further delineate the location of the fistula. Acute vesicovaginal fistula should be managed by decompression of the bladder by placement of an indwelling Foley catheter to allow continuous drainage. This management will often allow the fistula to close spontaneously. If a ureterovaginal fistula is discovered, a ureteral stent should be placed across the section of ureter that is fistualized. The stent may be placed retrograde at the time of cystoscopy or antegrade via a PCN. This will usually allow the ureteral injury to heal "over" the stent. Throughout attempts at conservative management, prevention of urinary tract infection is an important priority. If after 6 weeks of conservative management the vesicovaginal or ureteral fistula has not resolved, surgical correction will be required.

Bladder Dysfunction After Radical Surgery

Voiding dysfunction following radical hysterectomy is commonly recognized and should be discussed in the preoperative informed consent. The exact frequency of occurrence depends upon how the problem is diagnosed (patient report vs prospective urodynamic testing) but occurs to a greater or lesser degree in nearly all patients. It is clear that a less radical hysterectomy (type I or II) is associated with a significantly lower incidence of bladder dysfunction as compared with the traditional radical (type III) hysterectomy.

Serial cystometric studies of patients undergoing radical hysterectomy have defined the natural history of bladder function in the perioperative period. There is a nearly uniform development of detrusor hypertonia characterized by low capacity, high resting tone, and high filling pressure in the immediate postoperative phase. Bladder insensitivity to filling is also present. The patient often has difficulty initiating her stream and may have overflow incontinence when the capacity is exceeded. Hypertonia generally subsides within 3 to 6 months, but other abnormalities often persist for years. The duration of bladder dysfunction is also variable, with extremes recognized as full recovery of bladder function to the rare patient who will require lifetime intermittent self-catheterization to achieve adequate bladder drainage. Many patients have persistent decrease in bladder sensation or prolonged urinary hesitancy.

The pathophysiologic mechanism of voiding dysfunction after radical hysterectomy is still not clearly understood. Some investigators have proposed that incomplete innervation of the bladder produced a temporary parasympathometic predominance that usually resolves with nerve regeneration. The use of parasympatholytic drugs, however, has been ineffective in altering the detrusor muscle function in this circumstance. Forney and colleagues have suggested that disruption of the sympathetic fibers that travel through the paracervical web results in loss of inhibition for the detrusor and trigone, leaving an uncoordinated parasympathetic dominance. This is supported by the observation that incomplete division of the cardinal ligament results in decreased postoperative detrusor hypertonia compared with complete division.

It also seems clear that overdistention of the bladder aggravates bladder dysfunction. Therefore a variety of techniques have been proposed to avoid overdistention, including short-term or long-term use of a uretheral Foley catheter, suprapubic catheter, or intermittent self-catheterization. All techniques have their proponents and varying degrees of success, but none have been proven to be superior.

Intraoperative Gastrointestinal Injuries

A mechanical bowel preparation should be planned for all patients undergoing major abdominal surgery. We believe that bowel preparation will reduce the risk of intestinal injury, and if injury does occur, spill of GI contents will be minimized. Further, with the bowel empty, closure is much easier and there is diminished risk of infection in the case of colonic injury. In the past, mechanical methods to prepare the bowel have included the use of cathartics such as magnesium citrate or the ingestion of 4 liters of polyethelene glycol (GoLYTELY). The use of Fleet phospha-soda, a bowel preparation method previously preferred by many, has been abandoned due to renal injury.

The use of oral antibiotics (erythromycin and neomycin) has traditionally been recommended to reduce infectious complications following colonic surgery. The data on which this recommendation has been made were developed in an era before parenteral broad-spectrum antibiotics. Today, there is little evidence that oral antibiotic bowel preparation is necessary if the patient is to receive parenteral antibiotic prophylaxis.

Prior abdominal surgery and radiation therapy increase the probability of intraoperative injury to the small intestine. Adhesions to the anterior abdominal wall or small intestines adherent to the pelvic peritoneum increase the risk of entry into the intestines as adhesions are lysed. Interruption of the serosal and superficial muscular layers should be repaired with interrupted 2-0 or 3-0 sutures. Care should be taken to avoid narrowing of the intestinal caliber (Figure 16-8). If the entire thickness of the intestine is entered, the segment of bowel must be assessed to decide whether primary closure should be undertaken or whether bowel resection and anastamosis should be performed. Primary closure is usually safely accomplished if the closure can reapproximate well-perfused bowel under no tension on the suture line and the bowel lumen is not narrowed. If these conditions cannot be met, resection and anastamosis will be necessary.

Primary closure of an enterotomy should be in two layers: the first being an interrupted layer of 2-0 or 3-0 polygycoloic acid suture incorporating the mucosa and muscularis, with the knot tied into the intestinal lumen. A second imbricating layer may be of either absorbable or nonabsorbable suture and incorporates the serosa and superficial muscularis (Figure 16-9, F). Attention to the direction of closure of the enterotomy should ensure that the lumen is not narrowed. In most cases, an NG tube is placed after closure of an enterotomy or a small bowel resection and anastamosis, although this practice is somewhat controversial.

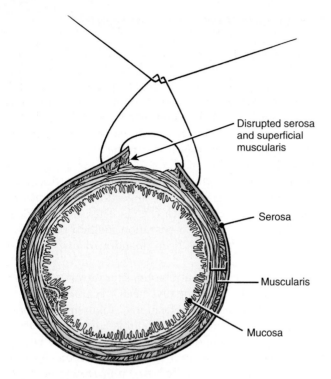

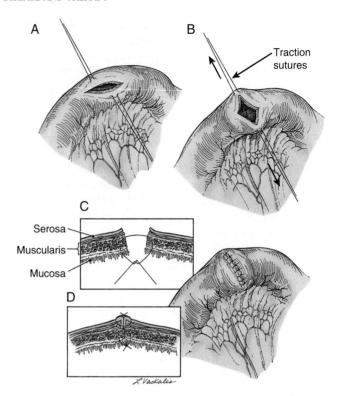

FIGURE 16-8 Repair of seromuscular injury of small or larger bowel. Interrupted imbricating sutures used to reapproximate the injured seromuscular layer. *(From Nichols DH, Clarke-Pearson DL [eds]: Gynecologic, Obstetric and Related Surgery, 2nd ed. St. Louis, Mosby, 2000.)*

FIGURE 16-9 Repair of enterotomy. **A** and **B,** The repair should be performed so that the closure is perpendicular to the axis of the small bowel. **C** and **D,** Two-layer closure incorporating the mucosa and muscularis in the inner layer and the serosa and muscularis on the outer layer. *(From Nichols DH, Clarke-Pearson DL [eds]: Gynecologic, Obstetric and Related Surgery, 2nd ed. St. Louis, Mosby, 2000.)*

Injury to the colon most commonly occurs in the pelvis and the risk is increased in the face of prior pelvic surgery, cancer involving the colon, or prior radiation therapy. If colonic injury occurs, the decision must be made as to whether a primary closure is sufficiently safe or whether the fecal stream should be temporarily diverted by performing a transverse loop colostomy or ileostomy. In most cases primary closure without diversion may be performed; especially if the patient has had a mechanical bowel preparation. The principles for closure require viable tissue and no tension on the closure. In patients who have had prior pelvic radiation, the risk of perforation of the colostomy closure is significantly increased and diversion is usually advised. Following a two-layered closure of a rectosigmoid injury, we routinely perform proctoscopy and a "bubble-test" (Figure 16-10).

Postoperative Gastrointestinal Complications

ILEUS

After abdominal or pelvic surgery, most patients will experience some degree of intestinal ileus. The exact mechanism by which this arrest and disorganization of GI motility occurs is unknown, but it appears to be associated with the opening of the peritoneal cavity and is aggravated by manipulation of the intestinal tract and prolonged surgical procedures. (Ileus is much less commonly associated with minimally invasive surgical procedures. If ileus were to occur after laparoscopy or robotic surgery, the surgeon should strongly consider a more serious bowel injury and evaluate the patient accordingly.) Infection, peritonitis, and electrolyte disturbances may also result in ileus. For most patients undergoing gynecologic cancer operations, the degree of ileus is minimal and GI function returns relatively rapidly, allowing the resumption of oral intake within a few days of surgery. Patients who have persistently diminished bowel sounds, abdominal distention, and nausea and vomiting require further evaluation and more aggressive management.

Ileus is usually manifest by abdominal distention and should be evaluated initially by physical examination assessing the quality of bowel sounds and searching for tenderness or rebound on palpation. The possibility that the patient's signs and symptoms may be associated with a more serious intestinal obstruction or other intestinal complication must be considered. Pelvic examination should be performed to evaluate the possibility of a pelvic abscess or hematoma that may contribute to the ileus. Abdominal radiograph to evaluate the abdomen

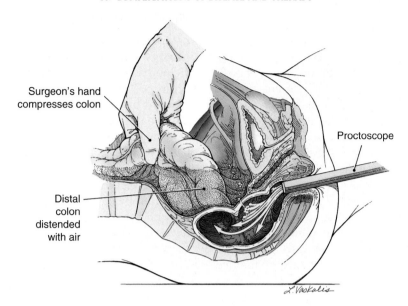

Surgeon's hand compresses colon

Proctoscope

Distal colon distended with air

L. Vaskalis

FIGURE 16-10   "Bubble test" to evaluate for rectosigmoid injury and to ensure a "watertight" closure of a colostomy or rectosigmoid anastomosis. The pelvis is filled with saline, and the proximal sigmoid or descending colon is occluded above the segment to be tested. Insert a proctoscope into the anus and inflate with air. Distend the occluded rectosigmoid colon with air and observe for bubbles, which would indicate a bowel defect. *(From Nichols DH, Clarke-Pearson DL [eds]: Gynecologic, Obstetric and Related Surgery, 2nd ed. St. Louis, Mosby, 2000.)*

in the supine position and in the upright position usually will aid in the diagnosis of an ileus. The most common radiographic findings include dilated loops of small and large bowel and air–fluid levels in the upright position. In the postoperative patient, especially in the upright position, the flat plate of the abdomen may also show evidence of free air. This is a common finding following surgery, which lasts 7 to 10 days in some instances and is not indicative of a perforated viscus in most patients. The remote possibility of distal colonic obstruction or pseudoobstruction (Ogilvie syndrome) suggested by a dilated cecum should be excluded by rectal examination, proctosigmoidoscopy, or barium enema.

The initial management of a postoperative ileus is aimed at GI tract decompression and maintenance of appropriate intravenous replacement fluids and electrolytes.

1. An NG tube should evacuate the stomach of its fluid and gaseous contents. Prolonged NG suction continues to remove swallowed air, which is the most common source of air in the small bowel.
2. Fluid and electrolyte replacement must be adequate to keep the patient well perfused. Significant amounts of third-space fluid loss occur in the bowel wall, the bowel lumen, and the peritoneal cavity during the acute episode. GI fluid losses from the stomach may lead to a metabolic alkalosis and depletion of other electrolytes also. Careful monitoring of serum chemistries and appropriate replacement are necessary.

3. Most cases of severe ileus will begin to improve over a period of several days. In general, this is recognized by reduction in the abdominal distention, return of normal bowel sounds, and passage of flatus or stool. Follow-up abdominal radiographs should be obtained as necessary for further monitoring.
4. When the GI tract function appears to have returned to normal, the NG tube may be removed and a liquid diet may be instituted.
5. If a patient shows no evidence of improvement during the first 48 to 72 hours of medical management, other causes of ileus should be sought. Such cases may include ureteral injury, peritonitis from pelvic infection, unrecognized GI tract injury with peritoneal spill, or fluid and electrolyte abnormalities such as hypokalemia. In the evaluation of persistent ileus, the use of water-soluble upper GI contrast studies may assist in the resolution of the ileus, the recognition of a small bowel obstruction, or injury (leak) of the GI tract.

SMALL BOWEL OBSTRUCTION

Obstruction of the small bowel following abdominal surgery occurs in approximately 1% to 2% of patients, but it may be more common after radical gynecologic oncology procedures as a result the extensive dissection and sometimes extensive manipulation of the small bowel. (Again, this complication is less common in patients who have undergone minimally invasive surgery.) The most common cause of small bowel obstruction is adhesions to the operative site. If the small bowel becomes adherent in a twisted position, partial or complete obstruction may result from distention, ileus, or bowel wall edema. Less common causes of postoperative small bowel obstruction include entrapment of the small bowel into an incisional hernia and an unrecognized defect in the small bowel or large bowel mesentery. Early in its clinical course, a postoperative small bowel obstruction may exhibit signs and symptoms identical to those of ileus. Initial conservative management as outlined for the treatment of ileus is appropriate. Because of the potential for mesenteric vascular occlusion and resulting ischemia or perforation, worsening symptoms of abdominal pain, progressive distention, fever, leukocytosis, or acidosis should be evaluated carefully because immediate surgery may be required.

However, in most cases of postoperative small bowel obstruction, the obstruction is only partial and the problem usually resolves with conservative management.

1. After several days of conservative management (NG tube drainage, fluid and electrolyte replacement) further investigation may be necessary. Evaluation of the GI tract with barium enema and an upper GI series with small bowel follow-through are appropriate. Alternatively, an abdominal and pelvic CT scan with GI contrast may be useful in identifying the location of obstruction ("transition point") and also evaluates for the presence of an abscess, lymphocele, or ureteral injury. In most cases, complete obstruction is not documented, although a narrowing or tethering of the segment of small bowel may indicate the site of the problem.
2. Further conservative management with NG decompression and intravenous fluid replacement may allow time for bowel wall edema or torsion of the mesentery to resolve.
3. If resolution is prolonged and the patient's nutritional status is marginal, the use of TPN may be necessary.
4. Conservative medical management of postoperative small bowel obstruction usually results in complete resolution. However, if persistent evidence of small bowel obstruction remains after full evaluation and an adequate trial of medical management, exploratory laparotomy may be necessary to surgically evaluate and manage the obstruction. In most cases, lysis of adhesions is all that is required, although a segment of small bowel that is badly damaged or extensively sclerosed from adhesions may require resection and reanastomosis.

COLONIC OBSTRUCTION

Postoperative colonic obstruction following gynecologic oncology surgery is exceedingly rare. Advanced ovarian carcinoma is the most common cause of colonic obstruction in postoperative gynecologic surgery patients and is caused by extrinsic impingement on the colon by the pelvic malignancy. Occult intrinsic colonic lesions (e.g., colon cancer) also may cause obstruction. When colonic obstruction is manifest by abdominal distention and abdominal radiographs reveal a dilated colon and enlarging cecum, further evaluation of the large bowel is required by barium enema or colonoscopy. Dilation of the cecum to more than 10 to 12 cm in diameter as viewed by abdominal radiograph requires immediate evaluation because there is a higher probability of colonic perforation. When there is no logical cause for a mechanical obstruction, Ogilvie syndrome should be considered. Colonoscopy should be performed, and the colonic gas should be evacuated. If a true mechanical obstruction is documented, surgical decompression by performing a colectomy, colostomy, or cecostomy may be required on an urgent basis. In some circumstances an intraluminal stent may be placed endoscopically. Surgery should be performed as soon as the obstruction is documented. Conservative management of colonic obstruction is not appropriate because the complication of colonic perforation has an exceedingly high mortality rate.

DIARRHEA

Episodes of diarrhea often occur after abdominal and pelvic surgery as the GI tract returns to its normal function and motility. However, prolonged and multiple episodes may represent a pathologic process such as impending small bowel obstruction, colonic obstruction, or pseudomembranous colitis. Excessive amounts of diarrhea should be evaluated by abdominal radiographs and stool samples tested for the presence of ova and parasites, bacterial culture, and *Clostridium difficile* toxin. Proctoscopy and colonoscopy may also be advisable in severe cases. Evidence of intestinal obstruction should be managed as outlined previously. Infectious causes of diarrhea should be managed with the appropriate antibiotics and fluid and electrolyte replacement. *C. difficile*–associated pseudomembranous colitis may result from recent exposure to any antibiotic. Discontinuation of these antibiotics (unless they are needed for another severe infection) is advisable, along with the institution of appropriate therapy. Because of the expense of vancomycin, we usually institute therapy with oral metronidazole. Therapy should be continued until the diarrhea abates, and several weeks of oral therapy may be required in order to obtain complete resolution of the pseudomembranous colitis.

FISTULA

GI fistulas are relatively rare after gynecologic surgery. They are most often associated with malignancy, prior radiation therapy, or surgical injury to the large or small bowel that was unrecognized or a leak from an anastamosis. Signs and symptoms of GI fistula are often similar to those of small bowel obstruction or ileus, except that a fever is usually a more prominent component of the patient's symptoms. When fever is associated with GI dysfunction postoperatively, evaluation should include early assessment of the GI tract for its continuity. When fistula is suspected, the use of water-soluble GI contrast material is advised to avoid the complication of barium peritonitis. Evaluation with abdominal pelvic CT scan may also assist in identification of a fistula and associated abscess. Recognition of an intraperitoneal GI leak or fistula formation usually requires immediate surgery unless the fistula has drained spontaneously through the abdominal wall or vaginal cuff.

An enterocutaneous fistula arising from the small bowel and draining spontaneously through the abdominal incision may be managed successfully with medical therapy. Therapy should include NG decompression, replacement of intravenous fluids, TPN, and appropriate antibiotics to treat an associated mixed bacterial infection. If the infection is under control and there are no other signs of peritonitis, the surgeon may consider allowing potential resolution of the fistula over a period of up to 6 weeks. Some authors have suggested the use of somatostatin to decrease intestinal tract secretion and allow earlier healing of the fistula. In many cases, especially if the bowel was not radiated, the fistula will close spontaneously with this mode of management. If the enterocutaneous fistula does not close with conservative medical management, surgical correction with resection, bypass, or reanastomosis will be necessary in most cases.

A rectovaginal fistula that occurs following gynecologic surgery is usually the result of surgical trauma that may have been aggravated by the presence of extensive adhesions or tumor involvement of the rectosigmoid colon and cul de sac. Low rectal anastamoses are also at risk to breakdown and lead to a rectovaginal fistula. Perforation of a colonic diverticulum is another possible cause for a colovaginal fistula. A small rectovaginal fistula may be managed with a conservative medical approach, in the hope that decreasing the fecal stream will allow closure of the fistula. A small fistula that allows continence except for an occasional leak of flatus may be managed conservatively until the inflammatory process in the pelvis resolves. At that point, usually several months later, correction of the fistula is appropriate. Larger rectovaginal fistulas that have no hope of closing spontaneously are best managed by performing an initial diverting colostomy followed by repair of the fistula after inflammation has resolved. After the fistula closure is healed and deemed successful, the colostomy may be taken down and closed.

Lymphocysts

The occurrence of lymphocysts after pelvic and paraaortic lymphadenectomy is recognized in approximately 2% of cases. It has been suggested that prevention requires the ligation of the ascending lymphatics at the time of lymphadenectomy. Further, there is evidence that the use of low-dose heparin increases lymphatic drainage and lymphocyst formation. In years past, the parietal peritoneum was closed after lymphadenectomy and a closed suction drain was placed in the retroperitoneal space in order to aspirate any lymphatic fluid. Certainly a suction drain is reasonable and likely does prevent lymphocysts whenever the retroperitoneum is closed. Currently, most gynecologic oncologists do not close the peritoneum, allowing the lymphatic fluid to drain into the peritoneal cavity and be reabsorbed. Retrospective reports indicate that there is no increase in lymphocyst formation using this strategy. However, the problem of lymphocyst formation has not been entirely eliminated.

Lymphocysts may be recognized clinically by palpation of a mass along the pelvic sidewall or in the iliac fossa on abdominal examination. Most will be asymptomatic. However, when a lymphocyst is found, investigation should be undertaken to evaluate for the possibility of ureteral or venous obstruction. If hydroureter is found, the lymphocyst should be drained. This may usually be accomplished by an interventional radiologist who can place a percutaneous drain in the lymphocyst. Suction drainage will collapse the lymphocyst and allow the cyst walls to sclerose together. If percutaneous drainage is not feasible or is unsuccessful, surgical exploration may be required to excise a wall of the lymphocyst and allow the lymphatic fluid to drain into the peritoneal cavity. There are reports of successfully performing this surgery laparoscopically. Placing an omental J flap into the cavity of the lymphocyst has been suggested to provide additional routes of lymphatic drainage. When extrinsic venous compression is discovered to be associated with a lymphocyst, the patient should be evaluated for the possibility of a venous thrombosis. If a venous thrombosis is found, we would advise anticoagulation in order to stop propagation and allow stabilization of the thrombus. Thereafter the lymphocyst should be drained. Drainage of the lymphocyst before anticoagulation may result in venous decompression and subsequent embolization of the thrombus. Rarely, lymphocysts will become infected and require drainage and antibiotic therapy.

Lymphocysts can also occur in the inguinal region after inguinofemoral lymphadenectomy performed as part of the staging and treatment of vulvar carcinoma.

Small, asymptomatic lymphocysts may be managed by observation. However, larger lymphocysts usually cause pain or lymphedema and will require drainage with placement of a closed suction drain. If repeated aspiration is required, sclerotherapy should be considered.

Postoperative Infections

Infections are a major source of morbidity in the postoperative period. Risk factors for infectious morbidity in the gynecologic oncology patient include a lack of perioperative antibiotic prophylaxis, contamination of the surgical field from infected tissues or from spillage of large bowel contents, an immunocompromised host, diabetes, poor nutrition, chronic and debilitating severe illness, poor surgical technique, and preexisting focal or systemic infection. Sources of postoperative infection can include the lung, urinary tract, surgical site, pelvic sidewall, vaginal cuff, abdominal wound, and sites of indwelling intravenous catheters. Early identification and treatment of any infections will result in the best outcome from these potentially serious complications.

Although infectious morbidity is an inevitable complication of surgery, the incidence of infections can be decreased by the appropriate use of simple preventive measures. In cases that involve transection of the large bowel, spillage of fecal contents also inevitably occurs. Preoperative mechanical preparation in combination with systemic antibiotic prophylaxis will help decrease the incidence of postoperative pelvic and abdominal infections in these patients. The surgeon can further decrease the risk of postoperative infections by using meticulous surgical technique. Blood and necrotic tissue are excellent media for the growth of aerobic and anaerobic organisms. In cases in which there is higher-than-usual potential for serum and blood to collect in spaces that have been contaminated by bacterial spill, closed-suction drainage may reduce the risk of infection. Elective surgical procedures should be postponed in patients who have an infection preoperatively.

Historically, the standard definition of febrile morbidity for surgical patients has been the presence of a temperatures of 100.4° F (38° C) or higher on two occasions at least 4 hours apart in the postoperative period, excluding the first 24 hours. However, other sources have defined fever as two consecutive temperature elevations greater than 101.0° F (38.3° C). Febrile morbidity has been estimated to occur in as many as half of patients; however, it is often self-limited, resolves without therapy, and is usually noninfectious in origin.

The assessment of febrile surgical patients should include a review of the patient's history with regard to risk factors. Both the history and the physical examination should focus on the potential sites of infection. The examination should include inspection of the pharynx, a thorough pulmonary examination, percussion of the kidneys to assess for costovertebral angle tenderness, inspection and palpation of the abdominal incision, examination of sites of intravenous catheters, and an examination of the extremities for evidence of DVT or thrombophlebitis. In gynecologic surgery patients, an appropriate workup may also include inspection and palpation of the vaginal cuff for signs of induration, tenderness, or purulent drainage. A pelvic examination should also be performed to identify a mass suggesting a pelvic hematoma or abscess and to recognize signs of pelvic cellulitis.

Patients with a fever in the early postoperative period should have an aggressive pulmonary toilet, including incentive spirometry. If the fever persists beyond 72 hours postoperatively, additional laboratory and radiologic data may be obtained. The evaluation may include complete and differential white blood cell counts and a urinalysis. A routine urine culture has a yield of only 9%; therefore one should not be sent unless indicated by the urinalysis results or symptoms. Routine chest radiographs have a yield of 12.5% and should be obtained in patients with and without signs and symptoms localizing to the lung. Blood cultures can also be obtained but will most likely be of little benefit unless the patient has a high fever (102° F). In patients with costovertebral angle tenderness, CT scan, renal ultrasound, or IVP may be indicated to rule out the presence of ureteral damage or obstruction from surgery, particularly in the absence of laboratory evidence of urinary tract infection. Patients who have persistent fevers without a clear localizing source should undergo CT scanning of the abdomen and pelvis to rule out the presence of an intraabdominal abscess. Finally, in patients who have had GI surgery, a CT scan with oral contrast, a barium enema, or an upper GI series with small bowel follow-through may be indicated late in the course of the first postoperative week if fever persists to rule out an anastomotic leak or fistula.

URINARY TRACT INFECTIONS

Historically, the urinary tract has been the most common site of infection in surgical patients. However, the incidence reported in the more recent gynecologic literature has been less than 4%. This decrease in urinary tract infections is most likely the result of increased perioperative use of prophylactic antibiotics.

Symptoms of a urinary tract infection may include urinary frequency, urgency, and dysuria. In patients with pyelonephritis, other symptoms include flank pain, headache, malaise, nausea, and vomiting. A urinary tract infection is diagnosed on the basis of microbiology and has been defined as the growth of 10^5 organisms/mL urine cultured. Most infections are caused by coliform bacteria, with *Escherichia coli* being the most common pathogen. Other pathogens include *Klebsiella, Proteus, and Enterobacter* species. *Staphylococcus* organisms are the causative bacteria in fewer than 10% of cases.

Despite the high incidence of urinary tract infections in the postoperative period, few of these infections are serious. Most are confined to the lower urinary tract, and pyelonephritis is a rare complication. Catheterization of the urinary tract, either intermittently or continuously with the use of an indwelling catheter, has been implicated as a main cause of urinary tract contamination.

The treatment of urinary tract infection includes hydration and antibiotic therapy. Commonly prescribed and effective antibiotics include sulfonamide, cephalosporins, fluoroquinolones, and nitrofurantoin. The choice of antibiotic should be based on knowledge of the susceptibility of organisms cultured at a particular institution. In some institutions, for example, more than 40% of *E. coli* strains are resistant to ampicillin. For uncomplicated urinary tract infections, an antibiotic that has good activity against *E. coli* should be given in the interim while awaiting the urine culture and sensitivity data.

Patients who have a history of recurrent urinary tract infections, those with chronic indwelling catheters (Foley catheters or ureteral stents), and those who have urinary conduits should be treated with antibiotics that will be effective against the less common urinary pathogens such as *Klebsiella* and *Pseudomonas*. Chronic use of the fluoroquinolones for prophylaxis is not advised because these agents are notorious for inducing antibiotic-resistant strains of bacteria.

PULMONARY INFECTIONS

The respiratory tract is a relatively common site for complications following surgery for gynecologic cancer. Risk factors include extensive or prolonged atelectasis, preexistent chronic obstructive pulmonary disease, severe or debilitating illness, central neurologic disease causing an inability to clear oropharyngeal secretions effectively, and NG suction. In surgical patients, early ambulation and aggressive management of atelectasis are the most important preventive measures.

A significant proportion (40% to 50%) of hospital-acquired pneumonias are caused by gram-negative organisms. These organisms gain access to the respiratory tract from the oral pharynx. Gram-negative colonization of the oral pharynx has been shown to be increased in patients in acute care facilities and has been associated with the presence of NG tubes, preexisting respiratory disease, mechanical ventilation, tracheal intubation, and paralytic ileus, which is associated with microbial overgrowth in the stomach.

A thorough lung examination should be included in the assessment of all febrile surgical patients. In the absence of significant lung findings, a chest radiograph should nonetheless be obtained in patients at high risk for pulmonary complications. A sputum sample should also be obtained for Gram stain and culture. The treatment should include postural drainage, aggressive pulmonary toilet, and antibiotics. The antibiotic chosen should be effective against both gram-positive and gram-negative organisms, and in patients who are receiving assisted ventilation, the antibiotic spectrum should include drugs that are active against *Pseudomonas* organisms.

WOUND INFECTIONS

The results of a prospective study of more than 62,000 wounds are revealing in regard to the epidemiology of wound infections. The wound infection rate varied markedly, depending on the extent of contamination of the surgical field. The wound infection rate for clean surgical cases (infection not present in the surgical field, no break in aseptic technique, no viscus entered) was lower than 2%, whereas the incidence of wound infections with dirty, infected cases was 40% or higher. Preoperative showers with hexachlorophene slightly lowered the infection rate for clean wounds, whereas preoperative shaving of the wound site with a razor (but not clippers) increased the infection rate. A 5-minute wound preparation immediately before surgery was as effective as preparation 10 minutes before surgery. The wound infection rate increased with the duration of the preoperative hospital stay and with the duration of the surgical procedure. (Prophylactic antibiotics should be readministered if the surgical procedure lasts longer than 4 hours.) In addition, incidental appendectomy increased the risk of wound infection in patients undergoing clean surgical procedures. The study concluded that the incidence of wound infections could be decreased by short preoperative hospital stays, hexachlorophene showers before surgery, clipping hair (not shaving) of the wound site immediately before incision, use of meticulous surgical technique, decreasing operative time as much as possible, bringing drains out through sites other than the wound, and dissemination of information to surgeons regarding their wound infection rates. A program instituting these conclusions led to a fall in the clean wound infection rate from 2.5% to 0.6% over an 8-year period. Although the wound infection rate in most gynecologic services has been lower than 5%, reflective of the "clean" nature of most gynecologic operations, it is higher in the gynecologic oncology patient.

The symptoms of wound infection often occur late in the postoperative period, usually after the fourth postoperative day, and may include the presence of fever, erythema, tenderness, induration, and purulent wound drainage. Wound infections that occur on postoperative days 1 through 3 are generally caused by streptococcal and clostridial infections. The management of wound infections is mostly mechanical and involves opening the infected portion of the wound above the fascia, with cleansing and debridement of the wound edges as necessary. Wound care, consisting of débridement and dressing changes 2 to 3 times daily with mesh gauze, will promote growth of granulation tissue, with gradual filling in of the wound defect by secondary intention. The application of a Wound-Vac to larger wounds speeds recovery and minimizes dressing changes. Clean, granulating wounds can often be secondarily closed with good success, shortening the time required for complete wound healing.

The technique of delayed primary wound closure can be used in contaminated surgical cases to reduce the incidence of wound infection. Briefly, this technique involves leaving the wound open above the fascia at the time of the initial surgical procedure. Vertical interrupted mattress sutures though the skin and subcutaneous layers are placed 3 cm apart but are not tied. Wound care is instituted immediately after surgery and continued until the wound is noted to be granulating well. Sutures may then be tied and the skin edges can be further approximated using sutures or staples. Using this technique of delayed primary wound closure, the overall wound infection rate has been shown to be decreased from 23% to 2.1% in high-risk patients.

Vaginal cuff infection following hysterectomy is characterized by erythema, induration, and tenderness at the vaginal cuff. Occasionally, a purulent discharge from the apex of the vagina may also be present. The cellulitis is often self-limited and does not require any treatment. Fever, leukocytosis, and pain localized to the pelvis may accompany severe cuff cellulitis and most often signifies extension of the cellulitis to adjacent pelvic tissues. In such cases, broad-spectrum antibiotic therapy should be instituted with coverage for gramnegative, gram-positive, and anaerobic organisms. If purulence at the vaginal cuff is excessive or if there is a fluctuant mass noted at the vaginal cuff, the vaginal cuff should be gently probed and opened with a blunt instrument. The cuff can then be left open for dependent drainage.

INTRAABDOMINAL AND PELVIC ABSCESS

The development of an abscess in the surgical field or elsewhere in the abdominal cavity is most likely to occur in contaminated cases in which the surgical site is not adequately drained or as a secondary complication of hematoma that becomes infected. The causative pathogens in patients who have intraabdominal abscess are usually polymicrobial in nature. The aerobes most commonly identified include *E. coli*, *Klebsiella*, *Streptococcus*, *Proteus*, and *Enterobacter*. Anaerobic isolates are also common, usually from the *Bacteroides* group. These pathogens are mainly from the vagina but also can be derived from the GI tract, particularly when the colon has been entered at the time of surgery.

An intraabdominal abscess is sometimes difficult to diagnose. The evolving clinical picture is often one of persistent febrile episodes with a rising white blood cell count. Findings on abdominal examination may be equivocal. If an abscess is located deep in the pelvis, it may be palpable by pelvic or rectal examination. For abscesses above the pelvis, diagnosis will depend on radiologic confirmation.

Ultrasound can occasionally delineate fluid collections in the upper abdomen and the pelvis. However, bowel gas interference makes visualization of fluid collections or abscesses in the mid-abdomen difficult to distinguish. CT scanning with oral and intravenous contrast is much more sensitive and specific for diagnosing intraabdominal abscesses and is the radiologic procedure of choice.

Standard therapy for an intraabdominal abscess is drainage combined with appropriate parenteral administration of antibiotics. Abscesses located low in the pelvis, particularly in the area of the vaginal cuff, can often be reached through a vaginal approach. In many patients, the ability to drain an abscess by placement of a drain percutaneously under CT guidance has obviated the need for surgical exploration. With CT guidance, a pigtail catheter is placed into an abscess cavity via percutaneous, transperineal, transrectal, or transvaginal approaches. The catheter is left in place and irrigated daily until drainage decreases. Transperineal and transrectal drainage of deep pelvic abscesses has been successful in 90% to 93% of patients, obviating the need for surgical management. However, for those patients in whom radiologic drainage is not successful, surgical exploration and evacuation are indicated. The gold standard of initial antibiotic therapy has been the combination of ampicillin, gentamycin, and clindamycin. Adequate treatment can also be achieved with currently available broad-spectrum single agents (including the broad-spectrum penicillin), second- and third-generation cephalosporins, levofloxacin and metronidazole, and the sulbactam/clavulanic acid–containing preparations.

NECROTIZING FASCIITIS

Necrotizing fasciitis is an uncommon infectious disorder; approximately 1000 cases occur annually in the United States. The disorder is characterized by a rapidly progressive bacterial infection involving the subcutaneous tissues and fascia while characteristically sparing underlying muscle. Systemic toxicity is a common feature of this disease, as manifested by the presence of dehydration, septic shock, disseminated intravascular coagulation, and multiorgan system failure.

The pathogenesis of necrotizing fasciitis involves a polymicrobial infection of the dermis and subcutaneous tissue. Historically, hemolytic streptococcus was believed to be the primary pathogen responsible for necrotizing fasciitis. However, it is now evident that numerous other organisms are present in addition to streptococcus, including other gram-positive organisms, coliforms, and anaerobes. Bacterial enzymes such as hyaluronidase and lipase released in the subcutaneous space destroy the fascia and adipose tissue and induce a liquefactive necrosis. In addition, noninflammatory intravascular coagulation or thrombosis subsequently occurs. Intravascular coagulation results in ischemia and necrosis of the subcutaneous tissues and skin. Late in the course of the infection, destruction of the superficial nerves produces anesthesia in the involved skin. The release of bacteria and bacterial toxins into the systemic circulation results in septic shock, acid–base disturbances, and multiorgan impairment.

The diagnostic criteria for necrotizing fasciitis include extensive necrosis of the superficial fascia and subcutaneous tissue with peripheral undermining of the normal skin, a moderate to severe systemic toxic reaction, the absence of muscle involvement, the absence of clostridia in wound and blood culture, the absence of major vascular occlusion, intensive leukocytic infiltration, and necrosis of subcutaneous tissue.

Most patients with necrotizing fasciitis suffer pain, which in the early stages of the disease is often disproportionately greater than that expected from the degree of cellulitis present. Late in the course of the infection, the involved skin may actually be anesthetized secondary to necrosis of superficial nerves. Temperature abnormalities, both hyperthermia and hypothermia, are concomitant with the release of bacterial toxins and with bacterial sepsis, which is present in up to 40% of patients. The involved skin is initially tender, erythematous, and warm. Edema develops and the erythema spreads diffusely, fading into normal skin, characteristically without distinct margins or induration. Subcutaneous microvascular thrombosis induces ischemia in the skin, which becomes cyanotic and blistered. As necrosis progresses, the skin becomes gangrenous and may slough spontaneously. Most patients will have leukocytosis and acid–base abnormalities. Finally, subcutaneous gas may develop, which can be identified by palpation (crepitus) and by radiograph. The finding of subcutaneous gas by radiograph is often indicative of clostridial infection, although it is not a specific finding and may be caused by other organisms. These organisms include *Enterobacter, Pseudomonas,* anaerobic streptococci, and *Bacteroides,* which, unlike clostridial infections, spare the muscles underlying the affected area. A tissue biopsy specimen for Gram stain and aerobic and anaerobic culture should be obtained from the necrotic center of the lesion in order to identify the causative organisms.

Predisposing risk factors for necrotizing fasciitis include diabetes mellitus, alcoholism, an immunocompromised state, hypertension, peripheral vascular disease, intravenous drug abuse, and obesity. Increased age, delay in diagnosis, inadequate debridement during initial surgery, extent of disease on initial presentation, and the presence of diabetes mellitus are all factors that have been associated with an increased likelihood of mortality from necrotizing fasciitis.

Early diagnosis and aggressive management of this lethal disease have led to improved survival. In an earlier series, the mortality rate was consistently higher than 30%, but in more recent series the mortality rate has decreased to less than 10%.

Successful management of necrotizing fasciitis involves early recognition, immediate initiation of resuscitative measures (including correction of fluid, acid–base, electrolyte, and hematologic abnormalities), aggressive surgical debridement (and redebridement as necessary), and broad-spectrum antibiotic therapy. Many patients will benefit from central venous monitoring and high caloric nutritional support.

During surgery, the incision should be made through the infected tissue down to the fascia. An ability to undermine the skin and subcutaneous tissues with digital palpation often will confirm the diagnosis. Multiple incisions can be made sequentially toward the periphery of the affected tissue until well-vascularized, healthy, resistant tissue is reached at all margins. The remaining affected tissue must be excised. The wound can then be packed and sequentially debrided on a daily basis as necessary until healthy tissue is displayed at all margins.

Hyperbaric oxygen therapy may be of some benefit, particularly in patients for whom culture results are positive for anaerobic organisms. Retrospective studies have demonstrated that the addition of hyperbaric oxygen therapy to surgical debridement and antimicrobial therapy appear to significantly decrease both wound morbidity and overall mortality in patients with necrotizing fasciitis.

After the initial resuscitative efforts and surgical debridement, the primary concern is the management of the open wound. Allograft and xenograft skin can be used to cover open wounds, thus decreasing heat and evaporative water loss. Interestingly, temporary biologic closure of open wounds also seems to decrease bacterial growth. Application of a wound vacuum-assisted closure (VAC) device will also promote wound healing. In situations in which spontaneous closure is not likely, the VAC device may allow for the development of a suitable granulation bed and prepare the tissue for graft placement, thereby increasing the probability of graft survival. Finally, skin flaps can be mobilized to help cover open wounds once the wound infections have resolved and granulation has begun.

Obesity

INCIDENCE AND DEFINITION

Obesity is an increasing problem in the United States and is more commonly encountered as a risk factor for complications associated with gynecologic oncology surgery. Centers for Disease Control and Prevention (CDC) statistics from the year 2008 indicate that 33.8% of U.S. adults (and 35.5% of women) older than age 20 years are obese. If these statistics are expanded to include overweight and obese persons, 68% of the U.S. adult population is facing a significant medical problem.

Obesity is defined by body mass index (BMI), which is calculated by dividing weight in kilograms by the height in centimeters squared. Alternatively, body weight in pounds is multiplied by 704 and then divided by the height in inches squared. Current American Gastroenterology Association Guidelines use BMI to define classes of obesity. A BMI of 25 to 29.9 is defined as overweight; BMI 30 to 34.9, class I obesity; BMI 35 to 39.9, class II obesity; and BMI greater than 40 extreme class III obesity. In practical terms, a 5′4″ American woman who is 30 pounds overweight will have a BMI greater than 30, classifying her in obesity class I.

POSTOPERATIVE COMPLICATIONS AND MANAGEMENT

Obese patients are at much higher risk for postoperative complications because of the more common occurrence of comorbidities including diabetes, hypertension, coronary artery disease, sleep apnea, obesity hypoventilation syndrome (OHS), and osteoarthritis of the knees and hips. These underlying alterations in physiology result in increased surgical risks and complications, including respiratory failure, cardiac failure, DVT and pulmonary embolism, aspiration, wound infection and dehiscence, postoperative asphyxia, and misdiagnosed intraabdominal catastrophe.

Control of the airway is critical in the immediate postoperative period. Extubation may not be prudent or possible at the end of the case as a result of tracheal edema resulting from a difficult intubation. Alternatively, the patient may not have the physical capacity to adequately ventilate as a result of suppression of the respiratory drive from anesthetics and excess chest wall weight. Many obese patients suffer from OHS, which increases their baseline hypercarbia and may also delay extubation. It is often prudent to plan immediate postoperative admission to a surgical ICU with mechanical ventilation and serial arterial blood sampling to aid in the proper timing for extubation.

After extubation, ventilation of the obese patient during sleep may be aided by the use of noninvasive positive pressure ventilation units, particularly if the patient has a history of sleep apnea and uses a continuous positive airway pressure (CPAP) machine at home. Respiratory therapists can be of assistance in patient instruction and management of CPAP machinery, in addition to other respiratory toilet. Monitoring with continuous pulse oximetry will assist the detection of impending respiratory failure.

There is a higher risk of aspiration in obese patients due to increased gastric residual volumes, a higher rate of gastroesophageal reflux disease (GERD), and increased intraabdominal pressure from mass effect. Neutralization of the stomach contents with a proton pump inhibitor can minimize the chemical burn potential of aspirated stomach contents. GI motility agents such as metaclopromide may decrease residual volume by increasing intestinal transit. It is also prudent to raise the head of the bed to prevent aspiration.

Prophylaxis for postoperative venous thrombosis and pulmonary embolism (as detailed earlier) should be ordered for obese patients because they are at higher risk for these complications.

Venous access poses another problem. Extreme obesity obliterates anatomic landmarks and makes insertion of peripheral lines and central lines problematic. Adjunctive visualization technology such as Doppler ultrasound or fluoroscopy should increase the accuracy and safety of line placement. Arterial line placement facilitates monitoring of pressures and blood gas parameters. Ideally, central venous lines and arterial lines should be placed intraoperatively by the anesthesia team to ensure adequate access in the postoperative period. The intraoperative placement of central lines should be verified for position postoperatively by chest radiograph in the postanesthesia care unit.

Medication administration must consider the concepts of total body weight and ideal body weight. Certain medications are dosed on ideal body weight (corticosteroids, penicillin, cephalosporins, beta blockers). Others are dosed on total body weight (heparin), and still others are based on a calculated "dosing weight" (aminoglycosides, fluoroquinolones, vancomycin). An inpatient pharmacist should be consulted for assistance with proper dosing and monitoring of pharmacotherapy.

Minimally invasive surgical techniques are reported to decrease the morbidity of surgery in obese patients. In particular, wound complications are greatly reduced, and patients are usually able to ambulate sooner and have a faster return to full levels of activity. The advantages of minimally invasive surgery may be negated by longer operating times and the patient's inability to tolerate steep Trendelenberg positioning (difficulty in ventilating the patient).

The Elderly Patient

The life expectancy of American women continues to increase. In addition, as the "baby-boomer" generation ages we will see an increasingly larger population of older women who will develop gynecologic cancers. The elderly woman is at higher risk of developing gynecologic cancer in that 65% of vulvar cancers, 43% of epithelial ovarian cancers, 45% of endometrial cancers, and 27% of cervical cancers occur in women older than 65 years of age. Although many of these cancers are managed with radical surgery, careful consideration must be given in selection of surgical procedures in women who may be at high risk for surgical complications. In fact, complications of radiation therapy and chemotherapy are more likely to occur in older patients, so selection of any therapy requires consideration of patient tolerance. In past years, radical surgery was avoided in elderly women. We now know that surgery can be safely and successfully accomplished, despite a patient's age, if the patient is fully evaluated and determined to be a surgical candidate. There is no doubt that older patients present with more advanced disease and have poorer presurgical performance status and more intercurrent medical problems than younger patients. Retrospective review of elderly patients with gynecologic cancers demonstrates that 90% of women older than age 65 years can undergo radical surgery as definitive therapy for their gynecologic cancer. When compared with women younger than 65 years, the postoperative mortality was 1.5%, and the minor complications and length of stay were similar in the two groups. In women older than 65 years of age who underwent radical hysterectomy for early-stage cervical cancer, there was no perioperative mortality or ureteral fistula. Transfusion requirements and lymphedema were also similar. Febrile morbidity was less common in the older patients, although postoperative small bowel obstruction, bladder dysfunction, and pulmonary emboli were more commonly encountered in the older patients.

Perioperative management is the key to success when managing the elderly woman. Cardiac and pulmonary complications are the two most common serious problems encountered postoperatively. Careful preoperative assessment of cardiac status should include assessment for underlying coronary artery disease, valvular heart disease, and chronic congestive heart failure. There are several risk-assessment algorithms that may be applied to estimate risk of major surgery. Because more than 40% of elderly women have hypertension, optimal blood pressure control should be achieved preoperatively; intraoperative hypotension is one of the most common causes of myocardial ischemia and infarction. Pulmonary complications occur in nearly 40% of elderly women following major abdominal surgery. Because physiologic changes of aging diminish vital capacity, lung compliance, reduced expiratory flow rates, and increased residual volume, the elderly patient is more likely to suffer pulmonary complications following general anesthesia.

These women may be at even higher risk if they have chronic obstructive pulmonary disease (COPD) or asthma. Preoperative assessment may include assessment of pulmonary function by performing spirometry and obtaining an arterial blood gas measurement. Patients with underlying pulmonary disease should have their medical regimen maximized preoperatively including the use of bronchodilators and corticosteroids. Conduction anesthesia should be strongly considered in consultation with the anesthesiologist in order to avoid the pulmonary complications more often encountered with general anesthesia.

Avoiding perioperative hypothermia and hypoxemia are extremely important to avoid additional cardiac oxygen consumption. Invasive monitoring and planned ICU admission should be considered in any circumstance in which there is an increased risk of cardiac or pulmonary complications. Care must also be taken when ordering pharmacologic agents because the elderly may have altered GI absorption and decreased renal or hepatic clearance of specific drugs. Consultation with a clinical pharmacist is advised to establish the correct dose of drug for patients with altered renal or hepatic function.

Radiation complications in the elderly patient are also increased. The thin, hypertensive patient appears to be at greater risk for radiation therapy complications to both the GI and genitourinary tracts. It appears that elderly women tolerate initial therapy poorly and often require delays in treatment or discontinuation of treatment because of acute toxicity such as diarrhea, dehydration, or neutropenia. This observation, then, requires carefully planned treatment decisions as to whether the patient would be best treated with surgery or radiation therapy. Neither is without risk, and it cannot be assumed that radiation therapy is necessarily less toxic.

Radiation Therapy

Radiation therapy serves as a primary treatment modality for cervical and vaginal cancers (and occasionally advanced vulvar cancers) and as an adjuvant therapy for patients with high-risk endometrial cancers. Further, individualized radiation therapy may be used in nearly all gynecologic cancers to achieve palliation under specific circumstances. Morbidity resulting from properly conducted radiation therapy in patients with carcinoma of the cervix and vagina is usually minimal. However, there are unfortunate misconceptions about the magnitude of radiation morbidity in both the medical and lay community. We believe that these misconceptions have several origins.

First, many investigators fail to distinguish that unnecessary adverse effects result from poor techniques and should not be extrapolated to the use of proper techniques. Second, there has been a failure to recognize that a great deal of radiation morbidity is usually related to compromised treatment of patients with extensive tumors in whom surgery is not applicable. Results in these patients cannot be extrapolated to the use of optimal techniques in the treatment of patients with limited malignancy. Finally, it is an often unrecognized fact that a great deal of morbidity attributed to irradiation actually results from uncontrolled tumor (i.e., rectovaginal and vesicovaginal fistulas). As in the case of surgery, the treatment-related morbidity can be minimized by good application, but it cannot be eliminated.

Because the small bowel, bladder, and rectum are adjacent to the female genital tract, most of the side effects and complications of radiation involve these adjacent organs. Radiation complications are related to the dose, field size, and type of radiation equipment used. The larger the field, the greater the risk of problems if the dose remains constant. Usually, as the fields enlarge, the dose must be decreased. Conversely, as the fields become smaller, a larger dose can be tolerated. The use of brachytherapy also increases the risk of local complications. Finally, the use of combined chemoradiation therapy seems to increase slightly some complications during therapy (e.g., neutropenia) but does not seem to lead to serious long-term sequelae.

The pathogenesis of radiation-induced injury may be divided into acute and delayed complications. Complications during therapy are caused by ionizing radiation injury to cells that are mitotically active such as GI epithelium. Damage of the mucosal cells results in mucosal thinning and denudation followed by malabsorption and fluid and electrolyte loss (resulting from diarrhea). The GI mucosal stem cells generally recover totally and the acute symptoms resolve. Late complications involve a different mechanism of tissue injury based on vascular endothelial damage. Radiation results in an endarteritis and the gradual occlusion of small vessels. Subsequent tissue hypoxia leads to fibrosis of the affected tissue. These changes are progressive and may be aggravated further by other vascular compromise such as diabetes, hypertension, and aging. In severe cases, ulceration, stricture, perforation, and fistula formation may occur.

Gastrointestinal Complications

ACUTE COMPLICATIONS

Nearly all patients receiving external radiation to the pelvis will develop radiation proctitis or enteritis with associated diarrhea. This problem commonly begins after 2 weeks of radiation therapy and is usually easily managed by dietary modification and antidiarrheal medications (diphenoxylate; Lomotil). As a rule, the diarrhea resolves within 7 to 10 days of completing radiation. Some of the transitory symptoms are tenesmus and the passage of mucus and even blood per the rectum. Diarrhea and abdominal cramping characterize small intestinal irritation (radiation enteritis). This problem is more common and more severe when a portion of the small intestine is fixed in the pelvis as a result of adhesions or other pathologic conditions. Anorexia may also occur during radiation therapy. If nausea and vomiting occur, the patient should be evaluated for dehydration. This is more common when concurrent chemotherapy is being given along with the radiation. Intravenous hydration and correction of electrolytes is occasionally required. If dehydration is severe, radiation should be interrupted until these acute side effects are corrected.

The patient should have a complete blood count weekly during radiation therapy. If the hemoglobin decreases below 10 g/dL, packed red cell transfusion is advised in order to achieve improved tumor kill. Occasionally, radiation of the pelvic bone marrow will result in neutropenia or thrombocytopenia. In severe cases, radiation will need to be temporarily interrupted. In nearly all cases the acute side effects of radiation therapy will resolve once the radiation course is completed.

CHRONIC CONDITIONS

Radiation injury to the small intestine may manifest itself at any time following therapy and may vary from chronic diarrhea to small bowel obstruction or fistula. A typical patient with small bowel injury will initially present with postprandial abdominal cramps and pain, anorexia and diarrhea. About half of small bowel injuries occur within 1 year after radiation, and three fourths occur within 2 years. These symptoms are more common in patients who have had a prior laparotomy. Initial conservative management focuses on dietary modification (avoiding green leafy vegetables, milk products, and fried foods). Antidiarrheal drugs and oral cholestyramine (which binds bile salts) are often useful in managing symptoms.

As small bowel injury progresses, fibrosis of the injured bowel wall develops, leading to stricture and partial or complete obstruction. Patients usually present with worsening abdominal pain, cramps, diarrhea, and vomiting. Sometimes, the intermittent obstruction goes unrecognized until a significant weight loss is recorded. If medical management of a partial small bowel obstruction fails, surgical intervention is the course of last resort. The decision to proceed with surgical intervention in cases of intermittent obstruction is a difficult one and should be undertaken with proper preoperative preparation. Often, patients have developed a significant degree of malnutrition and should have their nutritional status corrected with preoperative TPN. Mechanical bowel preparation is mandatory, although sometimes it must be limited to enemas because the patient's small bowel obstruction will not allow the ingestion of oral cathartics. Dilated loops of bowel should be decompressed preoperatively with NG suction. Surgical correction depends upon the situation encountered at the time of surgical exploration. The obstruction is usually found to be bowel adherent in the pelvis that has been radiated. The bowel usually is thickened, edematous, and fibrotic. The two primary surgical options are resection of the obstructed loops with either reanastamosis or small bowel bypass. In either event, it is preferable to make anastamoses to intestinal segments that have not been radiated in order to have maximum opportunity for healing. Care should be taken to have adequate perfusion and no tension on the anastamosis. Perforation or fistula, if present, must be isolated and diverted; more extensive surgery (resection and anastamosis) must be done only if it is technically feasible (Figure 16-11).

Radiation injury to the rectum is more common after treatment for cervical cancer because of the high rectal doses from the intracavitary brachytherapy. Injury to the rectum may manifest as proctitis, rectal ulcer, stricture, or fistula. Complete colonic obstruction from radiation injury is extremely rare. The symptoms of radiation proctitis may develop after an asymptomatic interval of many months to years after radiation therapy is completed. Diarrhea with or without rectal bleeding is the most common presenting symptom. Cramping abdominal pain maybe associated with the diarrhea. The injury is most often located on the anterior rectal wall that received the maximal dose from the brachytherapy

application and range from thickened, fragile mucosa to thin, atrophic mucosa or mucosal ulceration. These changes usually heal with conservative measures including low-residue diet, anticolinergic drugs, stool softeners, and corticosteroid enemas. Hyperbaric oxygen treatments also appear to enhance healing of a rectal ulcer. If there is excessive bleeding from the rectal ulcer or proctitis, diversion of the fecal stream (colostomy) may be necessary to allow healing. Obviously, when bleeding is encountered, full evaluation of the rectosigmoid colon with flexible sigmoidoscopy is mandatory to exclude recurrent cancer, rectal cancer, polyps, diverticulae, or hemorrhoids as the cause for bleeding.

Rectovaginal fistula is the most common significant radiation injury to the large bowel and is often preceded by radiation proctitis and rectal ulceration. All patients with rectovaginal fistulas should have a diverting colostomy. It is rare that diversion will result in spontaneous healing of radiated colon, and it is often necessary to decide as to whether repair of the fistula may be subsequently undertaken. Whenever surgical correction is considered, endovascular flaps are used to bring a new blood supply to the repair (Figure 16-12). Only after the fistula repair has completely healed and absence of obstruction of the bowel has been documented should the colostomy be reversed.

Radiation-induced strictures or obstruction of the rectosigmoid colon appear at approximately 24 months from the completion of the radiation therapy. Again, the initial step in management is a diverting colostomy.

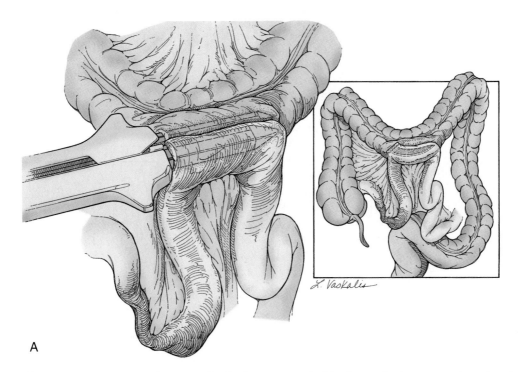

FIGURE 16-11 **A,** Small bowel obstruction that has been managed with a bypass ileotransverse enteroenterostomy.

FIGURE 16-11, cont'd   **B,** Resection of the involved bowel has been done with reanastomosis of the small bowel. Sufficient terminal ileum must be present for this procedure to be accomplished. **C,** The obstructed bowel has been isolated with formation of a mucous fistula. An end to side anastomosis has also been done. *(From Nichols DH, Clarke-Pearson DL [eds]: Gynecologic, Obstetric and Related Surgery, 2nd ed. St. Louis, Mosby, 2000.)*

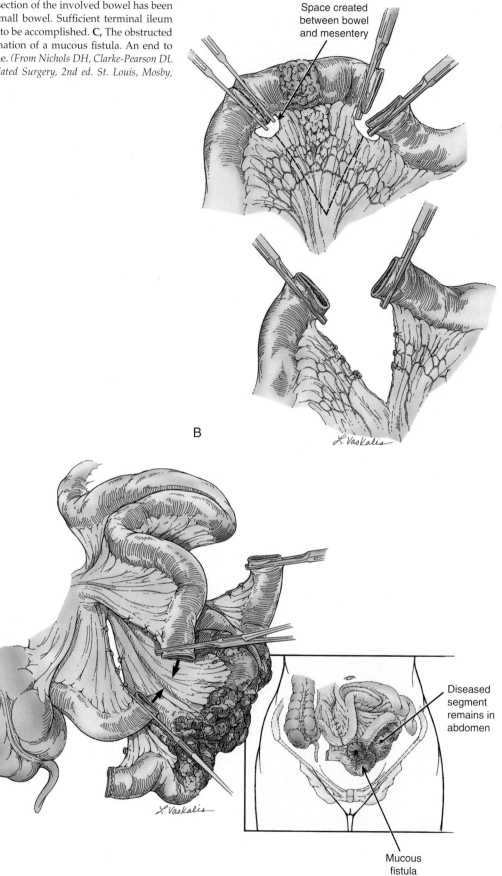

Space created between bowel and mesentery

B

Diseased segment remains in abdomen

Mucous fistula

C

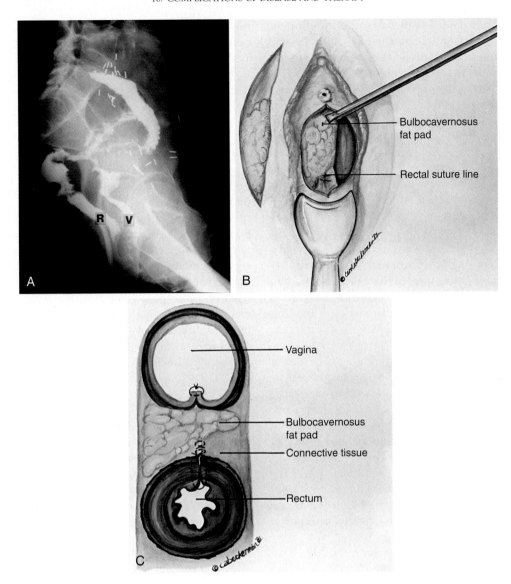

FIGURE 16-12 **A,** Barium enema demonstrating a rectovaginal fistula after irradiation. **B,** Repair of the rectovaginal fistula has been strengthened by interposition of the bulbocavernosus fat pad. **C,** The cross section shows placement of the neovascular fat pad.

Correction will require a rectosigmoid resection with low rectal anastamosis. Harris and Wheeless reported their experience with the end-to-end stapler device in low colorectal anastamosis associated with rectal injury. This was accomplished in 49 patients, 17 of whom had prior radiation therapy. All five postoperative complications (two strictures, two anastamosis breakdowns, and one fecal incontinence after colostomy closure) occurred in the patients who had prior radiation.

Complex fistulas may include a variety of communications between small bowel, colon, vagina, bladder, and skin. Thorough evaluation of the anatomy involved is mandatory and should include all organ systems that are possibly involved. The evaluation may include barium enema, proctosigmoidoscopy, upper GI series with small bowel follow-through, IVP, cystogram, cystoscopy, and

a "fistulogram" (injection of contrast directly into the fistula and imaging the retrograde flow of the contrast dye). These complex fistulas are often very difficult to repair, and the patients should be in optimal medical condition before surgery is performed. This usually includes antibiotics to control infection, TPN, and mechanical bowel preparation. If a fistula can be resected, it should be; however, many times the fistula must be isolated and the intestinal stream diverted around the lesion.

Prior pelvic radiation to the ileum (or resection or bypass surgery of the ileum) may lead to the malabsorption of vitamin B_{12} and result in a megaloblastic anemia. Because the liver usually has significant stores of B_{12}, it may be several years after radiation or surgery before the anemia is recognized. It is therefore advised that patients have annual complete blood counts indefinitely. A Shilling test can differentiate between B_{12} and folic acid deficiency. Treatment of B_{12} deficiency requires weekly B_{12} injections until the hemoglobin level returns to normal (usually 4-6 weeks) and then monthly injections to prevent recurrent anemia.

Urologic Complications

Acute radiation cystitis is occasionally encountered during radiation therapy or in the period immediately after completion of therapy. Typical symptoms of cystitis are usually present but urine cultures show no significant bacterial growth. Management includes increased oral liquid intake and urinary analgesics and anticholinergics to relieve symptoms. Chronic radiation cystitis commonly presents with symptoms of urinary frequency, suprapubic pain, and hematuria. The patient should have an immediate urine culture because a urinary tract infection further aggravates bladder mucosa damaged by radiation therapy. Gross hematuria (rather than microscopic hematuria) usually can be relieved by continuous bladder irrigation using either 0.5% or 1% acetic acid or a 1:1000 potassium permanganate or an alum solution. Clots may need to be evacuated by cystoscopic irrigation to relieve bladder spasms. Cystoscopy may also be needed to identify bleeding points that may be fulgurated. An experienced urologist should be consulted because excessive fulguration or unnecessary biopsies may lead to an iatrogenic vesicovaginal fistula. As a last resort, the bladder may be sclerosed with formaldehyde irrigation. In the most extreme cases, cystectomy and urinary diversion may be required to control bleeding.

Vesicovaginal fistulas are more common when the patient has had intensive radiation therapy and are increased by brachytherapy. Improper placement of the tandem and ovoids may result in an excessive dose to the base of the bladder and speaks to the importance of careful placement of intracavitary devices and attention to bladder doses delivered. Surgery following radiation therapy, such as a "completion" hysterectomy for bulky stage IB2 or "barrel" lesions of the cervix, further increases the risk of vesicovaginal fistula. In many cases, upper vaginal radiation necrosis is recognized months before the occurrence of the fistula. Treatment of the necrosis may prevent the progression to a fistula. Therapy includes half-strength hydrogen peroxide douches, intravaginal estrogen, and hyperbaric oxygen therapy.

Evaluation of an apparent vesicovaginal fistula should include a complete evaluation of the bladder and the upper tracts. It is not uncommon to discover an associated ureterovaginal fistula or ureteral stricture/stenosis, which must be addressed at the time of fistula repair. Further, given the proximity of the upper vagina to the bladder and rectum, proctosigmoidoscopy is advised because the rectosigmoid colon may also communicate with the fistula.

Repair of a radiation-induced vesicovaginal fistula is difficult and less successful than fistula repair in nonirradiated areas. The primary complicating matter is diminished blood supply to the radiated tissues. Therefore techniques of repair often utilize the mobilization of a nonirradiated tissue with a good blood supply into the surgical repair. If an intraabdominal, transvesical approach is taken to repair of a vesicovaginal fistula, the omentum and its blood supply may be mobilized and used to cover the repair of the fistula, often being interposed between the closed bladder and vagina. Vaginal approaches to vesicovaginal fistula repair may include repair combined with colpocleisis or the use of the bulbocavernosis labial flap (Martius flap), which is mobilized and interposed between the repaired bladder and vagina (Figures 16-13 and 16-14). Ureteral injury following radiation therapy may require reimplantation of the distal ureter into the bladder (ureteroneocystostomy) or permanent diversion (urinary conduit).

Chemotherapy

Chemotherapy is widely used in the initial treatment of many gynecologic malignancies. In some instances, such as gestational trophoblastic disease, ovarian germ cell malignancies, and some patients with epithelial ovarian cancer, chemotherapy can result in a cure. In many other instances, chemotherapy is palliative but can relieve symptoms and prolong meaningful life. There are numerous acute and chronic toxicities associated with chemotherapy and the reader is referred to more comprehensive discussions in Chapter 17.

Myelodysplastic Syndrome and Acute Nonlymphocytic Leukemia

Myelodysplastic syndrome and acute nonlymphocytic leukemia—serious and usually fatal complications of chemotherapy—were initially recognized in women receiving alkylating agents and are more likely to occur after chronic administration. The risk of secondary leukemia peaks 4 to 5 years after completing chemotherapy. These leukemias often go through the myelodysplasia or preleukemic stage. Unfortunately, the response to leukemia therapy is poor. Modern chemotherapy for ovarian cancer, which is platin based, has eliminated the exposure to alkylators (Taxol has been substituted for cyclophosphamide). Further, current primary therapy has reduced the number of cycles of therapy to six, avoiding chronic exposure to cytotoxic agents. The association of leukemia and the administration of cisplatin or carboplatin is uncertain. One report suggests that there is a fourfold increased risk of leukemia in women with

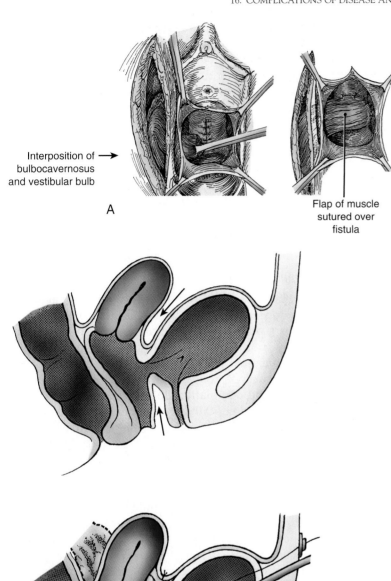

Interposition of →
bulbocavernosus
and vestibular bulb

A

Flap of muscle
sutured over
fistula

B

FIGURE 16-13 **A,** Vesicovaginal fistula repair using the bulbocavernosus fat pad as a source of neovascularization. **B,** Repair using an omental J flap for neovascularization. *(From Nichols DH, Clarke-Pearson DL [eds]: Gynecologic, Obstetric and Related Surgery, 2nd ed. St. Louis, Mosby, 2000.)*

ovarian cancer treated with platin-containing regimens. However, this conclusion is uncertain in that most of these patients also received cytoxan (an alkylator) in combination with cisplatin.

Etoposide (usually administered in the treatment of gestational trophoblastic disease or for ovarian germ cell tumors) is also associated with an increased risk of acute myeloid leukemia. The risk seems to be associated with the total cumulative dose of drug administered over time. Therefore, especially in young women who are likely to be cured, attention should be paid to minimizing the dose and duration of etoposide therapy. Leukemia following etoposide therapy usually occurs earlier than alkylator-induced leukemias (35 months versus 4-5 years) and has a good response to chemotherapy (complete response of 50%-60%). During postchemotherapy

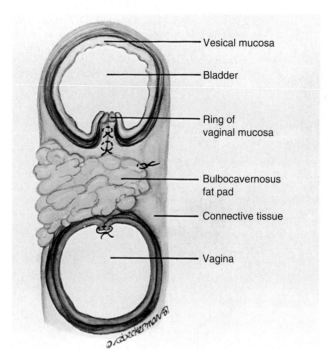

FIGURE 16-14   Cross section of the vesicovaginal repair using the bulbocavernosus fat pad as a source of neovascularization.

follow-up, women who have been treated with alkylating agents or etoposide should have periodic determination of complete blood counts.

Neurotoxicity

Some degree of neurotoxicity is commonly encountered with the use of cisplatin (or carboplatin) and/or paclitaxel. The most common neurologic effects of cisplatin include peripheral sensory neuropathy and ototoxicity, whereas paclitaxel commonly causes peripheral sensory toxicity in the hands and feet. These toxicities are often the dose-limiting side effect and are more common with cumulatively increasing doses of the drug or if the drugs are used in combination. The literature reports an incidence of neuropathy of approximately 15% if the cumulative cisplatin dose is less than 300 mg/m^2 but may be as much as 85% with doses of more than 300 mg/m^2. The combination of paclitaxel and cisplatin has even a higher incidence of neuropathy and is particularly severe with the combination of cisplatin (75 mg/m^2) and paclitaxel (175 mg/m^2 administered over 3 hours). Although carboplatin causes much less neurotoxicity than cisplatin, the combination of carboplatin and paclitaxel may still cause significant sensory neuropathy.

The most common neurologic side effects are due to toxicity to the peripheral sensory nerves, which results in numbness, tingling, and parasthesias of the feet and hands. Neurologic testing documents loss of ankle and knee reflexes and diminished vibratory sensation. In extreme cases the neuropathy may progress proximally to the arms and legs and patients may have difficulty walking and using their hands for fine motion (e.g., buttoning clothing, writing). Recovery following the onset of peripheral sensory neuropathy is common but may take several months to notice improvement, and the improvement may never be complete. Some authors have recommended the use of vitamin B$_6$ (pyridoxine), amitriptyline (Elavil), and neurontin to reduce symptoms.

Cisplatin may also cause tinnitus and high-frequency hearing loss, and this is more common with high-dose regimens. In most cases, the hearing loss is not perceptible to the patient but is readily documented with audiology testing.

Cardiac Toxicity

Doxorubicin, which is commonly used to treat metastatic endometrial adenocarcinoma and leiomyosarcomas, has a potential life-threatening toxicity of causing cardiomyopathy and resultant congestive heart failure. Arrhythmias and pericarditis have also been reported. The incidence of congestive heart failure is directly related to the cumulative does of doxorubicin and is rarely encountered with a dose of less than 350 mg/m^2. Cumulative doses of greater than 550 mg/m^2 are associated with up to a 10% incidence of cardiomyopathy. Age older than 70 years, hypertension, preexisting cardiac disease, and prior mediastinal radiation are factors that significantly increase the risk of cardiomyopathy, and a lower dose of doxorubicin should be considered in these circumstances. Before treatment, a cardiac ejection fraction should be evaluated (MUGA [multigated acquisition] scan). Because a significant drop in cardiac ejection fraction precedes the onset of clinical symptoms, subsequent scans (especially as the dose exceeds 350 mg/m^2) may allow discontinuation of doxorubicin before serious myocardial damage occurs. Cardiotoxicity is usually irreversible, but treatment of doxorubicin-induced heart failure may reduce symptoms of congestive heart failure by improving myocardial contractility with the administration of digitalis, diuretics, and afterload reduction. In contrast, pegylated liposomal doxorubicin is associated with minimal cardiotoxicity.

Pulmonary Toxicity

Bleomycin is commonly used in a regimen of multiagent chemotherapy for the treatment of ovarian germ cell malignancies. Subacute and chronic interstitial pneumonitis is a serious, life-threatening side effect of bleomycin. This inflammatory process may progress to pulmonary fibrosis, respiratory failure, and death. Before the onset of fibrosis, the patient may complain of shortness of breath and cough. Risk factors for bleomycin pulmonary toxicity include age greater than 70 years, preexisting

COPD, higher doses of bleomycin, bolus infusion, and prior chest irradiation. Whereas toxicity has been reported at doses of less than 100 mg, the incidence rises to 10% in patients receiving a dose in excess of 450 mg/ m². In addition, general anesthesia following the use of bleomycin may be complicated by postoperative respiratory failure possibly secondary to a bleomycin-induced sensitivity of oxygen.

Pulmonary toxicity may be predicted from deteriorating pulmonary function testing; particularly the carbon monoxide–diffusion capacity. When deterioration is discovered, bleomycin therapy should be discontinued. There is no specific treatment of bleomycin pulmonary toxicity. Steroid therapy may reduce inflammation and improve symptoms, but it will not reverse pulmonary fibrosis.

For full reference list, log onto www.expertconsult.com ⟨http://www.expertconsult.com⟩.

Basic Principles of Chemotherapy

Christina S. Chu, MD, and Stephen C. Rubin, MD

HISTORICAL OVERVIEW

The era of modern chemotherapy began in the 1940s with the Nobel Prize–winning work of Huggins and Hodges on the antitumor effect of estrogens in prostate cancer. This observation was followed in the mid-1940s by the investigation of nitrogen mustard, a by-product of nitrogen gas used in World War I, for its effects against lymphomas and solid tumors. Between 1945 and 1965, a wide variety of chemotherapeutic agents was identified and studied, including actinomycin D, cyclophosphamide, the vinca alkaloids, 5-fluorouracil, and the progesterones. In the 1970s, cisplatin was noted to exert significant antitumor effects against ovarian and testicular cancers, and tamoxifen was found to have activity against breast cancer for both adjuvant therapy

and treatment of advanced disease. In the same decade, bleomycin, etoposide, and doxorubicin came into clinical use, and derivative compounds such as carboplatin, vinorelbine, and idarubicin were developed for their ability to achieve similar antitumor effects but with less hematologic toxicity. The 1980s and 1990s have led to the widespread use of a host of new drugs, such as the taxanes (paclitaxel and docetaxel), ifosfamide, the topoisomerase inhibitors (topotecan and irinotecan), and nucleoside analogs (gemcitabine and capecitabine).

The growing number of agents in the chemotherapeutic armamentarium has been accompanied by advances in alternative dosing regimens; differing formulations using liposomal or polymer-based encapsulation; and varying schedules, sequences, and routes of administration. Fortunately, supportive therapies for gastrointestinal and hematologic toxicities have also evolved to include routine usage of 5-HT3 receptor antagonists (such as ondansetron and granisetron) for antiemetic prophylaxis and hematopoietic growth factors (such as epoetin) and colony-stimulating factors (such as sargramostim and filgrastim) to allow for greater chemotherapeutic dose intensity.

GENERAL PRINCIPLES

Chemotherapeutic agents are a crucial part of the physician's armamentarium in the ever-broadening fight against cancer. The physician can, with use of these drugs, ameliorate and sometimes even cure diseases that were usually fatal in the past. Until recently, in most cases chemotherapy has been reserved for relatively late stages of the disease, but its increasingly successful use, particularly in the treatment of hematologic malignancies, suggests that chemotherapy should be administered earlier. All physicians and surgeons must understand the nature and use of cancer chemotherapy so that they can make rational decisions about when it may be indicated. The outcome of cancer chemotherapy is not fully predictable, but the chances of remission can be improved by judicious selection of patients, careful assessment of the tumor's growth pattern, and treatment of the neoplasm with the drug or drugs most likely to be effective. The clinical response to chemotherapy may be assessed utilizing standard Response Evaluation Criteria in Solid Tumors defined by the National Cancer Institute (Table 17-1).

Unfortunately, not all patients with cancer are amenable to chemotherapy. The suitability of a patient for treatment depends on at least three critical criteria:

1. The nature of the neoplasm
2. Its extent of spread or stage
3. The patient's clinical condition

Not all cancers are equally sensitive to drugs. Factors that determine a given tumor's susceptibility include how the drug is distributed to the tumor, drug transport into the cell, whether a drug-sensitive biochemical pathway is present in the tumor cell, and the relative rates of intracellular activation and inactivation of the drug. A thorough knowledge of the cell cycle and growth kinetics is fundamental to understanding of the appropriate uses of chemotherapy.

CELL CYCLE CONTROL AND GROWTH KINETICS

All living things have an inherent capacity to multiply, and they cease multiplication for various reasons. Control appears to be mediated by an unknown feedback mechanism, probably resulting from contact phenomena when cells are crowded together. Knowledge of growth patterns has aided in the derivation of chemotherapeutic principles. Strategies for therapy have evolved to take advantage of these differences in growth characteristics between normal and malignant tissues.

Normal tissues fall into three predominant categories: static, expanding, and renewing. Static populations of cells are generally well differentiated and after a period of proliferation in fetal life rarely undergo division during adult life. Examples of static tissues include neurons and skeletal muscle. Because of the rare incidence of cell division, these cells are unlikely to be injured by chemotherapies that target rapidly dividing

TABLE 17-1 National Cancer Institute Response Evaluation Criteria in Solid Tumors

	Evaluation
TARGET LESIONS	
Complete response	Disappearance of all target lesions
Partial response	At least a 30% decrease in the sum of the longest diameter of target lesions, taking as reference the baseline sum longest diameter
Progressive disease	At least a 20% increase in the sum of the longest diameter of target lesions, taking as reference the smallest sum longest diameter recorded since the treatment started or the appearance of one or more new lesions
Stable disease	Neither sufficient shrinkage to qualify for partial response nor sufficient increase to qualify for progressive disease, taking as reference the smallest sum longest diameter since the treatment started
NONTARGET LESIONS	
Complete response	Disappearance of all nontarget lesions and normalization of tumor marker level
Incomplete response/ stable disease	Persistence of one or more nontarget lesion(s) or/and maintenance of tumor marker level above the normal limits
Progressive disease	Appearance of one or more new lesions and/or unequivocal progression of existing nontarget lesions*

Although a clear progression of "nontarget" lesions only is exceptional, in such circumstances the opinion of the treating physician should prevail and the progression status should be confirmed later on by the review panel (or study chair).

cells. Expanding tissue populations are also usually inactive in adult life, but unlike static populations they retain the ability to proliferate rapidly in response to stress or injury. Typical examples of expanding cells include hepatocytes and vascular endothelium. Last, the renewing cell populations are those that are constantly undergoing division, such as bone marrow and gastrointestinal epithelium. Renewing tissues are most sensitive to injury by chemotherapeutic agents (Table 17-2).

In the malignant growth, cells do not cease multiplying when they reach a critical mass. This unregulated growth appears to result from a combination of loss of normal cell cycle controls and a failure of normal apoptotic mechanisms. Despite uncontrolled growth, malignant cell division does not appear to be more rapid than normal cell division.

In general, as tumors grow they display gompertzian growth characteristics (Figure 17-1): As the tumor mass increases in size, the time necessary to double its size also becomes progressively longer. Thus, in the early phases of growth, tumor cells appear to grow exponentially, but as tumor mass increases there is a progressive increase in the doubling time, although doubling times in humans may vary greatly. For example, embryonal tumors and some lymphomas have relatively short doubling times (20-40 days), whereas adenocarcinomas and squamous cell carcinomas have relatively long doubling times (50-150 days). Three explanations have been given for this prolonged volume-doubling time:

1. An increase in cell cycle time (the time from one mitosis to the next)
2. A decrease in the growth fraction (cells participating in cell division in the tumor)
3. An increase in cell loss from tumor cells with insufficient nutrients and vascular supply

The gompertzian model has several important implications for cancer progression. First, metastases generally have a shorter doubling time than the primary lesion. If it is assumed that an exponential growth occurs early in the malignancy's history and that the malignancy starts from a single cell, then a 1-mm mass will have undergone approximately 20 tumor doublings. A 5-mm mass (a size that is first recognizable on a radiograph) may have undergone 27 doublings. It follows that a 1-cm mass will have undergone 30 doublings, and a clinician will be pleased to have detected such an "early" lesion. Unfortunately, this "early" lesion has already undergone 30 doublings, with significant DNA change being possible. Using this rationale, clinical techniques that are currently available tend to recognize malignancies late in their growth, and metastatic disease may well have occurred long before there was obvious clinical manifestation of the primary lesion. Another implication from this kinetic information is that in late stages of tumor growth a few doublings in tumor mass make a dramatic impact on the size of the tumor and the status of the patient. Once a tumor becomes palpable (1 cm in diameter—30 doublings), only three more doublings will produce a very large tumor mass (8 cm in diameter).

The gompertzian model also has clinical implications that have guided a good deal of clinical chemotherapy research. As a mass responds to treatment (i.e., gets smaller), the doubling time has been assumed to decrease as a consequence of a greater number of cells moving into cycle. This larger percentage of metabolically active cells would therefore increase the sensitivity of the neoplastic population of cell cycle–specific agents. This has led to the sequential use of cell cycle–nonspecific agents (e.g., cyclophosphamide) to bring down the mass, to be followed by cell cycle–specific agents (e.g., methotrexate). Although these sequential combinations have been theoretically attractive, none has shown clear superiority in clinical trials. Another implication of the gompertzian growth concept is that metastases can be expected to be

TABLE 17-2   Classification of Normal Tissues by Rate of Proliferation

Renewing (rapid proliferation)	Expanding (slow proliferation)	Static (rare proliferation)
Bone marrow	Lung	Muscle
Gastrointestinal mucosa	Liver	Bone
Ovary	Kidney	Cartilage
Testis	Endocrine glands	Nerve
Hair follicles	Vascular endothelium	

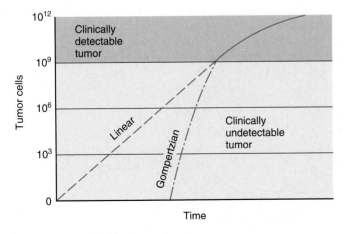

FIGURE 17-1   Tumor growth. As tumors grow, they display gompertzian characteristics. As tumor mass increases, doubling time becomes longer. However, a palpable tumor needs relatively few doublings to achieve a large mass.

more sensitive to chemotherapy in general, and to cell cycle–specific agents in particular, than the primary tumor from which they arise. The smaller the size of the metastatic focus, the greater is the differential sensitivity. Therefore the insensitivity of a primary tumor to a given drug regimen might not necessarily predict the response of metastasis to the same regimen.

The rationale for the use of drugs in the treatment of cancer is to achieve the selective killing of tumor cells. Underlying this rationale are the basic principles of the "cell kill" hypothesis first described by Skipper and associates. The following four principles were worked out in the L1210 leukemia model.

1. The survival of an animal with cancer is inversely related to the number of cancer cells.
2. A single cell is capable of multiplying and eventually killing the host.
3. For most drugs, a clear relationship exists between the dose of the drug and its ability to eradicate tumor cells.
4. A given dose of a drug kills a constant fraction of cells, not a constant number, regardless of the cell numbers present.

This fourth and most important principle implies that chemotherapeutic agents work by first-order kinetics—that is, they kill a constant fraction of cells rather than a constant number. This concept has important implications in cancer treatment. A single exposure of tumor cells to an antineoplastic drug may be capable of producing two to four logs of cell kill. With a common tumor burden of 1012 cells (1 kg), a single dose of chemotherapy will destroy a large number of cells but not be curative. Thus there is a need for intermittent courses of chemotherapy to achieve the magnitude of cell kill necessary to eradicate the lesion. Clinically, first-order cell kinetics dictate that to eradicate a tumor population effectively it is necessary to either:

- Increase the total dose of the drug or drugs to the maximal limits tolerated by the host, or
- Start treatment when the number of cells is small enough to allow the destruction of the tumor at total doses of the drug that are reasonably tolerated.

The logical conclusion derived from this hypothesis is that the maximal opportunity for achieving cure exists during the early stage of disease. In the past, chemotherapy was generally reserved for the treatment of disseminated cancer; surgery and/or radiotherapy were treatments of choice for localized disease. However, this concept of "log kill hypothesis" provides a rationale for the philosophy of adjuvant chemotherapy, which assumes the presence of undetectable cell masses of 101-104 cells after the initial surgical therapy that are capable of producing tumor relapse. This small tumor burden is particularly vulnerable to effective chemotherapy.

To better understand cell kinetics, it is imperative to visualize cell cycling. All dividing cells follow a predictable pattern for replication. The time that it takes a cell to complete one cycle of growth and division is termed its generation time. There are five basic phases (Fig. 17-2). The G1 phase (G stands for gap and uncertainty as to purpose) lasts for a variable amount of time—usually between 4 and 24 hours. If this phase is prolonged, the cell is usually referred to as being in the G0, or resting, phase. The S phase is the phase of DNA synthesis and usually lasts between 10 and 20 hours. The G2 phase is a premitotic phase that lasts from 2 to 10 hours, and the M phase, when actual mitosis takes place, lasts between 0.5 and 1 h. Tumors do not have faster generation times but

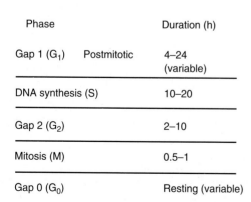

Phase		Duration (h)
Gap 1 (G_1)	Postmitotic	4–24 (variable)
DNA synthesis (S)		10–20
Gap 2 (G_2)		2–10
Mitosis (M)		0.5–1
Gap 0 (G_0)		Resting (variable)

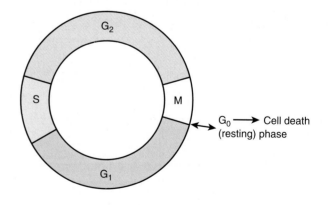

FIGURE 17-2   Cell generation time and sequence are similar for all mammalian cells. Tumor cells do not have faster generation times but do have more cells in the active phases of replication.

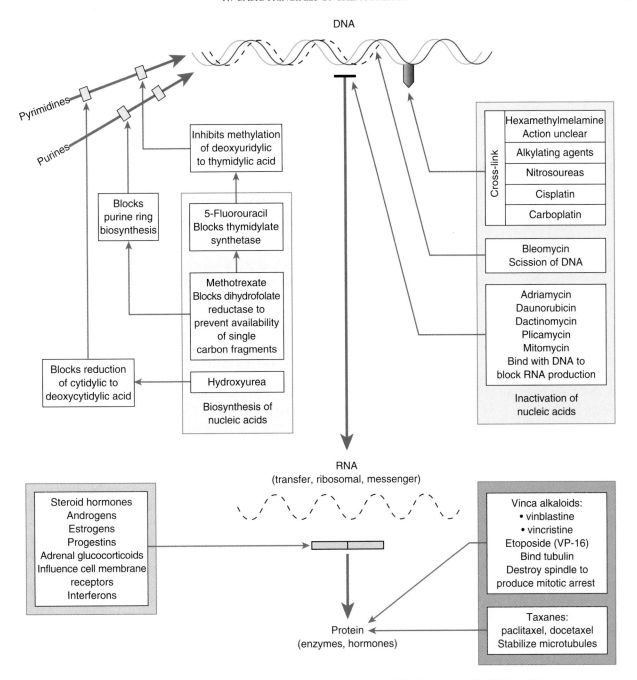

FIGURE 17-3   Cancer chemotherapeutic agents. (*After Krakoff IH: CA Cancer J Clin 37:93, 1987.*)

have more cells in the active phases of replication than normal tissues. Normal tissues have a large number of cells in the G0 phase, wherein the cell is not actively committed to division or is "out of cycle."

Some chemotherapeutic agents appear to act at several phases of the cell cycle (Fig. 17-3). Alkylating agents appear to act in all phases from G0 to mitosis. They are called cycle-nonspecific agents. Drugs such as hydroxyurea, doxorubicin (Adriamycin), and methotrexate appear to act primarily in the S phase. Bleomycin appears

to act in the G2 phase, and vincristine appears to act in the M phase. These drugs are called cycle-specific agents (Table 17-3) because they act chemotherapeutically only on cells that are in a specific phase of a cell generation cycle. Steroids, 5-fluorouracil, and cisplatin have rather uniform activity around the cell generation cycle. In theory, if certain cancer therapeutic agents attack only cells that are dividing and more tumor cells are dividing than normal tissue cells, then by properly spacing the chemotherapeutic agent and combining agents that act

TABLE 17-3   Cell Cycle (Phase)–Specific Drugs

Phase Dependence	Type	Drugs
S phase-dependent	Antimetabolite	Cytarabine
		Doxorubicin
		5-Fluorouracil
		6-Mercaptopurine
		Methotrexate
		Hydroxyurea
		Prednisone
M phase-dependent	Vinca alkaloids	Vincristine
		Vinblastine
	Taxanes	Paclitaxel
		Docetaxel
	Podophyllotoxins	Etoposide
		Teniposide
	Epothilones	Ixabepilone
G2 phase-dependent	—	Bleomycin
G1 phase-dependent	—	Corticosteroids

in different phases of the cell cycle one should be able to kill tumor cells in much greater numbers than normal cells. Kinetic studies in humans and animals suggest that tumors that have been cured by chemotherapy are those with large fractions of cells in the proliferative phase (e.g., gestational choriocarcinoma and Burkitt lymphoma). The extent of the disease rather than the total mass of tumor is the most important factor when considering curative radiation or surgery, but in using chemotherapy the total mass is most important. When tumor volume is reduced, the remaining tumor cells can begin to divide actively (they are propelled from the G0 phase into the more vulnerable cell generation cycle), thus rendering them susceptible to chemotherapy. These chemotherapeutic agents, as in radiation therapy, kill by first-order kinetics—that is, there is a reduction of the tumor population by a characteristic percentage, regardless of the actual number of tumor cells initially present (Fig. 17-4). If the tumor burden is small, fewer cycles of chemotherapy may be necessary. One milligram of tumor usually consists of 106 cells. One cubic centimeter of tumor usually consists of 109 cells. Patient death usually occurs at 1012 cells.

DYNAMICS OF CHEMOTHERAPY

The doubling time of a tumor depends on both generation time and cell death rate (Fig. 17-5). One cannot assume a long generation time simply because a tumor enlarges slowly. Slow tumor growth can result from rapid generation time combined with a high cell death rate. For similar reasons, a small tumor discovered on radiographic or physical examination is not necessarily an early tumor; only serial studies to judge its growth

rate will help establish its age. Bulky tumors (diameters >2-3 cm) enlarge more slowly than small ones because their cells, especially those of the inner core (farthest from the blood supply), have a long generation time. Competition for nutrients and other less-defined competitive pressures reduce the activity of the entire mass.

Successful chemotherapy of cancer requires a physiologic edge that can be exploited to differentially kill cancer cells but spare normal cells as much as possible. The more rapid growth rate of tumors and the increased synchronicity of tumor cells compared with normal tissues may be taken advantage of when designing therapeutic regimens. At any given time, comparatively large numbers of cancer cells will be in the DNA synthesis phase (S phase) of the cell cycle, the only time during which cycle-dependent agents (those inhibiting DNA synthesis) can act. Thus short-term high-dose chemotherapy with agents affecting DNA synthesis, such as methotrexate, is most effective in killing rapidly dividing tumor cells with relative sparing of normal bone marrow elements. Unfortunately, bone marrow cells, the epithelial cells that line the gastrointestinal tract, and hair follicles all have generation times comparable with those of tumors, and they are therefore vulnerable to compounds that inhibit DNA synthesis (Table 17-2). However, compared with the more synchronously growing tumor cell population, only a few of the bone marrow cells are in their S phase at any given time, and this accounts for the selective toxicity of phase-dependent compounds. A course of therapy extending over a period of several days, or even weeks, may be required to kill a slow-growing tumor in which only a few cells are in the stage of DNA synthesis at any one time. Agents that do not depend on DNA synthesis for their effects (i.e., cycle-nonspecific agents), such as alkylating agents, are most effective against bulky, slow-growing tumors. The cells remaining after treatment tend to divide more rapidly and are more susceptible to attack by cycle-specific agents. Thus there is some flexibility in the interplay of chemotherapeutic agents.

The phenomenon of increased susceptibility of tumor cells during recovery from alkylating agents is the rationale for sequentially combining cycle-nonspecific and cycle-specific agents in many new regimens. If, in addition, drugs with different mechanisms of toxicity are combined, each drug can be given safely in the dose used when it is given alone. Each drug chosen for combination therapy should have antitumor activity when used alone. Whenever possible, intermittent courses of chemotherapy are used to allow restoration of normal cells if they were reduced in number by treatment. In cases in which an antidote to the chemotherapeutic agent is known, for example leucovorin (citrovorum factor, folinic acid) for methotrexate, this antidote can also be given to hasten normal cell recovery. Of course,

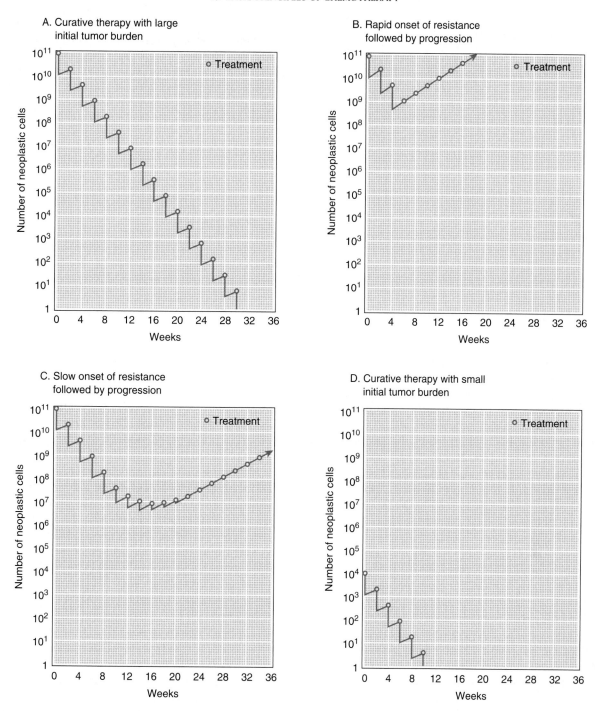

A. Curative therapy with large initial tumor burden

B. Rapid onset of resistance followed by progression

C. Slow onset of resistance followed by progression

D. Curative therapy with small initial tumor burden

FIGURE 17-4   Efficacy of chemotherapy related to tumor kinetics. *(After Bodye GB Sr, Frei E III, Luce JK: Hosp Pract 2(10):42, 1967.)*

the danger of revitalizing sublethally injured tumor cells also exists and must be evaluated with each new treatment regimen. Although careful studies are needed to compare each new combination with the single agents concerned, the trend in chemotherapy is unquestionably toward exploitation of drug combinations used simultaneously and sequentially.

PHARMACOLOGIC PRINCIPLES

Several general pharmacologic factors significantly affect the appropriate use of chemotherapeutic agents, including drug absorption, distribution, transport, metabolism, and excretion. These principles not only impinge on drug effectiveness, but also dictate drug

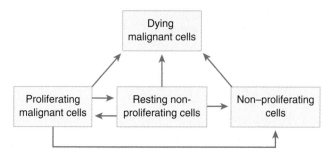

FIGURE 17-5 Dynamics of tumor growth, showing interrelationship of cell compartments contributing to clinical presence of tumor.

dose and schedule and how drugs are selected for use in combination. The effectiveness of a given regimen depends on optimizing the *concentration x time* (also known as the area under the curve, AUC) at the site of tumor. Drug absorption influences route of administration, which in turn affects the AUC. Whether a drug is given orally, intravenously, intra-arterially, intramuscularly, or intraperitoneally is also determined by patient acceptance, feasibility, and toxicity. Drug distribution and delivery to the tumor site also affects AUC. Factors such as drug binding (to albumin or to plastic catheters), lipid solubility, and membrane transport are critical in determining effectiveness of a given agent. Certain sites in the body, such as the brain and testes, represent pharmacologic sanctuaries where drug delivery is limited. Similarly, poor tumor perfusion due to necrosis or hypoxia may also impair drug delivery and concentration. Understanding of membrane transport mechanisms is also key: certain drugs, such as 5-fluorouracil or mitomycin C, may enter cells through passive diffusion, whereas others, such as cisplatin and melphalan, require active transport.

Drug metabolism is often necessary to convert an inactive prodrug into the active form. One example is cyclophosphamide, which requires cytochrome P-450 activation before antitumor effects are possible. Agents requiring hepatic metabolism to active forms are not amenable to intraperitoneal or intra-arterial administration. Conversely, metabolism and excretion of the active drug also affects AUC. The liver and the kidneys are responsible for the majority of drug elimination, although excretion in bile, stool, and respiration may also contribute in some cases. Organ dysfunction may result in increased drug toxicity and may require dose modification.

Drug Interactions

Although patients undergoing chemotherapy treatment may also receive a variety of other drugs for treatment of acute side effects or chronic medical conditions, few drug interactions are clinically significant. However, a few interactions are noteworthy. In particular, doxorubicin and taxane agents are known to exert increased toxicity in the setting of impaired biliary excretion, whereas the platinums and methotrexate may cause increased toxicity in the setting of decreased renal function. Aspirin and sulfonamides are known to displace methotrexate from plasma proteins, and direct chemical interactions are noted between cisplatin and mannitol, and mitoxantrone and heparin.

Drug Resistance

The effectiveness of any cancer treatment is limited by drug resistance, which may be intrinsic or acquired and may develop to one drug or to multiple drugs (pleiotropic resistance). It has been suggested that spontaneous mutation is a basis for drug resistance. This spontaneous mutation occurs rapidly in malignant tumors. This concept, the Goldie–Coldman hypothesis, has been applied to the growth of malignant tumors and has important clinical implications. The theory suggests that most malignant cells begin with intrinsic sensitivity to chemotherapeutic agents but develop spontaneous resistance at variable rates. Goldie and Coldman have developed a mathematic model that relates curability to the time of recurrence of the singly or doubly resistant cells. Assuming that there is a natural mutation rate, the model predicts a variation in the size of the resistant fraction in tumors of the same size and type, which depends on that mutation rate and the point at which the mutation develops. Thus the proportion of resistant cells in any untreated tumor is likely to be small, and the initial response to treatment would not be influenced by the number of resistant cells. In clinical practice, this means that a complete remission could be obtained even if the resistant cell line were present. The failure to cure such a patient, however, would depend directly on the presence of these resistant cells. This model of spontaneous drug resistance implies that minimizing the emergence of drug-resistant clones requires that multiple effective drugs or therapies be applied as early as possible in the course of the patient's malignant disease process.

In cell lines and animal models, resistance to specific drugs likely occurs via a wide variety of mechanisms, although only a few have been confirmed to be of clinical significance in human cancers. These include increase in proficiency of DNA repair, decrease in drug uptake or increase in efflux by cells, increased levels of or alterations in target enzymes, alterations in drug activation/degradation, gene amplification, and defective drug metabolism. These mechanisms are reviewed in Table 17-4.

TABLE 17-4   Probable Mechanisms Associated with Resistance to Some Commonly Used Anticancer Drugs

Mechanism	Drugs
Increase in proficiency of repair of DNA	Alkylating agents, cisplatin
Decrease in cellular uptake or increase in efflux of drugs	Cisplatin, doxorubicin, etoposide, melphalan, 6-mercaptopurine, methotrexate, nitrogen mustard, vinblastine, vincristine
Increase in levels of "target" enzyme	Methotrexate
Alterations in target enzyme	5-Fluorouracil, 6-mercaptopurine, methotrexate, 6-thioguanine
Decrease in drug activation	Cytosine arabinoside, doxorubicin, 5-fluorouracil, 6-mercaptopurine, 6-thioguanine
Increase in drug degradation	Bleomycin, cytosine arabinoside, 6-mercaptopurine
Alternative biochemical pathways	Cytosine arabinoside
Inactivation of active metabolites by binding to	Alkylating agents, cisplatin, doxorubicin sulfhydryl compounds
Decreased activity of topoisomerase	Camptothecins, doxorubicin, etoposide
Alteration of tubulin-binding sites	Vincristine, paclitaxel, ixabepilone
Increased damage tolerance	Alkylating agents, cisplatin

(After Tannock IF, Hill RT [eds]: The Basic Science of Oncology, 3rd ed., 1988. Reproduced by permission of The McGraw-Hill Companies.)

Multidrug resistance also occurs via various mechanisms. Some experimental evidence in murine tumors suggests that one form of multiple-drug resistance relates to the ability of drug-resistant tumor cells to limit drug accumulation of structurally unrelated agents. This cross-resistance is seen most often with natural products (e.g., doxorubicin, etoposide, paclitaxel, and vinca alkaloids); resistance to a single drug may confer a cross-resistance to structurally dissimilar drugs with different modes of action. This is the best studied mechanism for multidrug resistance and has been characterized involving the p-170 glycoprotein and its gene MDR1. Ling's coworkers initially demonstrated the appearance of a P-glycoprotein with a molecular weight of 170 kD on the cell membrane. The appearance of pleiotropic drug resistance is associated with permeability of the cell to accumulate and retain antineoplastic drugs. It has been demonstrated that this P-glycoprotein is directly related to the expression of resistance, and cells that revert to the drug-sensitive state lose this membrane glycoprotein. DNA can be transferred from resistant cells to the sensitive cells, producing a transfer of pleiotropic resistance to unexposed cells.

Although best characterized, MDR1 is unlikely to be the most common mechanism for chemotherapy resistance among ovarian cancers, given that most do not express the MDR1 gene. Another mechanism for the multiple-drug resistance phenotype is seen among alkylating agents, cisplatin, and irradiation. Resistance in this group of agents has been linked to elevations in intracellular glutathione levels and is not associated with an overall measurable decrease in drug accumulation. Other transport proteins, including multidrug resistance–associated protein, have been identified that do not involve the p-170 glycoprotein pump. Furthermore, alterations in genes controlling apoptosis and growth arrest have also been cited. Although the relative importance of these separate mechanisms in ovarian cancer

TABLE 17-5   Equations for Calculation of Body Surface Area

	Equation*
Mostellar (m^2)	$\sqrt{Weight \times height / 3600}$
DuBois and DuBois (m^2)	$(Weight^{0.425}) \times (height^{0.725}) \times 71.84$
Haycock (m^2)	$(Weight^{0.5378}) \times (height^{0.3964}) \times 0.024265$

*Weight in kg, height in cm.

remains to be established, it seems most likely that in clinical situations various combinations of mechanisms are at work.

Calculation of Dosage

Dosages of chemotherapeutic agents are usually discussed in terms of mg/kg of body weight or mg/m^2 of total body surface area (Table 17-5). Dosage based on surface area is preferable to that based on weight, because surface area changes much less during the course of therapy, allowing a more consistent absolute amount of drug to be given throughout therapy. Dosages per unit are also more comparable in adults and children (Figs. 17-6 and 17-7), and the variation in total dose between very obese and very thin people is minimized. Dosage in experimental animals expressed as mg/m^2 is more easily related to that in humans. In adults, mg/kg can be converted with reasonable accuracy to mg/m^2 by multiplying by 40.

Dose adjustments should be made for patients who are likely to have a compromised bone marrow reserve—that is, those older than 70 years of age, those who have received previous pelvic or abdominal irradiation, and those who have had previous chemotherapy. In these subsets of patients, the physician should consider beginning with a dose reduced by 35% to 50% and escalate up to a full dose with subsequent courses if initial doses are

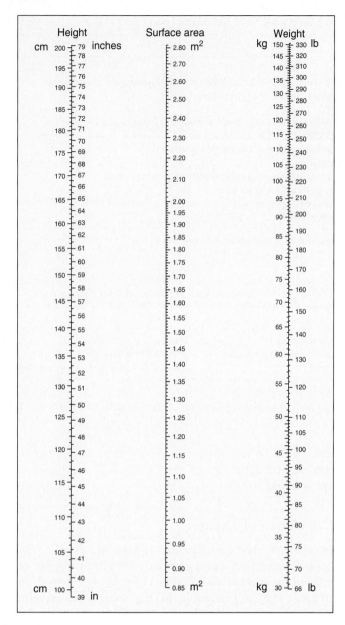

FIGURE 17-6   Nomogram for calculating the body surface area of adults.

TABLE 17-6   Recommended Individualized Dosing of Carboplatin

Carboplatin dose (mg) = target AUC × (glomerular filtration rate + 25)
AUC is selected for appropriate clinical situation:
AUC 6 in untreated patients, when used in combination with taxanes
AUC 5 in previously treated patients
AUC 7 in previously untreated patients

Glomerular filtration rate is equivalent to creatinine clearance, which can be measured or can be estimated from patient's age, weight, and serum creatinine.
AUC, Area under the curve.

(glomerular filtration rate, GFR) in individuals with cancer. The calculated creatinine clearance (Cr Cl) using serum creatinine is the most commonly used. The elimination of creatinine is primarily via glomerular filtration, although a small amount may be secreted in the renal tubules. Several studies have compared the different methods of estimating Cr Cl using a serum creatinine value. These methods are based on correlations of Cr Cl with age, body weight, serum creatinine, and creatinine metabolism. The most utilized methods follow.

Jelliffe Method

The Jelliffe method was used originally as a simple estimate of Cr Cl using serum creatinine, making minor adjustments in the calculation for female patients. The current Jelliffe formula takes into consideration age and renal function, and is as follows:

$$Cr\ Cl\ (mL/min) = 1.73[(100/serum\ creatinine) - 2].$$

(For female patients, use 90% of predicted Cr Cl.)

Cockroft–Gault Method

This equation includes factors for lean body weight, which is especially important for obese patients, and correlation for female patients (the obtained value is multiplied by 0.85 for women). This method is similar to the Jelliffe calculation and is as follows:

$$Cr\ Cl = (140 - age) \times$$
$$(lean\ body\ weight\ in\ kg)/(serum\ creatinine) \times 72.$$

Calvert Formula

The use of the Cr Cl has also been incorporated into the so-called Calvert formula. Based on good data, there is evidence showing that there is an inverse linear correlation between the GFR and the AUC of drugs such as carboplatin (Table 17-6). This finding suggests that in order to obtain the desired AUC, the dose must not only

well tolerated. In a similar manner, any moderate to severe toxicity during the patient's course of therapy should direct a reduction in future doses. Many clinicians favor limiting body surface area to 2 mg/m² in calculation of dosage. The adverse effects criteria table used by the Gynecologic Oncology Group is included as Appendix B.

Dose adjustments are often required in patients receiving anticancer agents that are eliminated by the kidneys. These adjustments reduce the likelihood of overly high plasma drug concentrations and the attendant risk of serious renal toxicity. Several techniques have been used to assess renal function

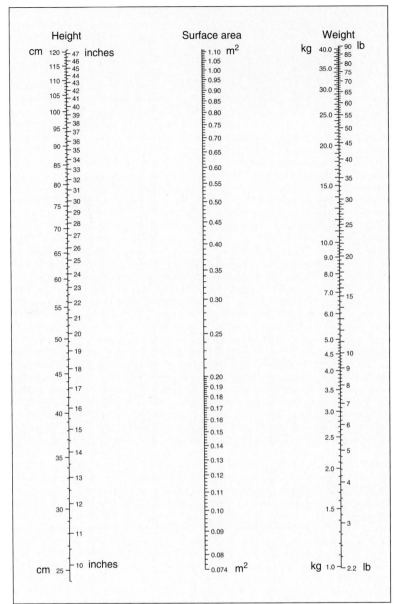

FIGURE 17-7 Nomogram for calculating body surface area of children.

be decreased in patients with low renal function, but also higher than standard doses may be required for patients with high renal clearance values. The Calvert formula is as follows:

$$dose\ (mg) = target\ AUC \times (GFR + 25).$$

The original Calvert calculations were derived from GFR as measured by the chromium-51–EDTA method. Although calculated GFR is not the same as one that is measured, and Cr Cl can exceed GFR by 10% to 40%, the majority of physicians calculate rather than measure the GFR by using formulas such as Jelliffe or Cockcroft–Gault and then insert these numbers into the Calvert formula.

CATEGORIES OF DRUGS IN CURRENT USE (TABLE 17-7)

Alkylating Agents

Alkylating agents prevent cell division primarily by cross-linking strands of DNA. Because of continued synthesis of other cell constituents, such as RNA and protein, growth is unbalanced and the cell dies. Activity of

TABLE 17-7 Chemotherapy Agents Used in the Treatment of Gynecologic Cancer

Drug	Dosage and Route of Administration	Acute Side Effects	Toxicity	Precautions	Major Indications
ALKYLATING AGENTS					
Cisplatin (CDDP or Platinol)	50-100 mg/m² IV every 3 weeks; 40 mg/m² IV every week with radiation therapy; 50-100 mg/m² i.p. in 2 L over 30 min every 3 weeks	Nausea and vomiting, often severe	Renal damage, moderate myelosuppression, neurotoxicity; severe renal damage can be minimized by not exceeding a total dose of 500 mg/m² in any treatment course	Infuse at a rate not to exceed 1 mg/min and only after 10-12 h of hydration; avoid nephrotoxic antibodies; watch renal function and discontinue if blood urea nitrogen exceeds 30 or creatinine exceeds 2	Carcinoma of the ovary, endometrium, or cervix
Carboplatin (Paraplatin)	250-400 mg/m² IV bolus or by 24-h continuous infusion every 2-4 weeks (most authorities recommend dosing to area under the curve values of 5.0-8.0)	Mild nausea and vomiting	Bone marrow suppression, especially thrombocytopenia	Decreased dose in patients who have had previous chemotherapy	Carcinoma of the cervix, ovary, and endometrium
Cyclophosphamide (Cytoxan)	50-1500 mg/m² as a single dose IV or **1-5 mg/kg/day** (usually 50 mg PO per day); dose decreased if severe leukopenia develops	Nausea and vomiting	Bone marrow depression, alopecia, cystitis	Maintain adequate fluid intake to avoid cystitis	Carcinoma of the cervix, ovary, endometrium, and fallopian tube
Chlorambucil (Leukeran)	0.1-0.2 mg/kg per day PO; dose decreased if severe bone marrow depression develops	Nausea, vomiting (with high doses)	Bone marrow depression	None	—
Melphalan (Alkeran)	0.2 mg/kg per day PO for 4 days every 4-6 weeks	Nausea, vomiting (with high doses)	Bone marrow depression	None	—
Triethylenethio-phosphoramide (thiotepa)	0.2 mg/kg per day IV for 5 days	None	Bone marrow depression	None	—
Ifosfamide (Ifex)	7-10 g/m² IV over 3-5 days every 3-4 weeks	Nausea, vomiting	Bone marrow depression, alopecia, cystitis	Uroprotectant to prevent hemorrhagic cystitis	Carcinoma and sarcoma of ovary, cervix, and endometrium
Oxaliplatin	59-130 mg/m² IV as a 20-min or 2-h infusion every 3 weeks	Nausea, vomiting, diarrhea, mucositis	Mild to moderate myelosuppression; transaminase elevation; peripheral neuropathy	Should not be given to patient with significant renal or hepatic dysfunction	Ovarian carcinoma
Altretamine (Hexalen)	4-12 mg/kg per day PO in divided doses for 14-21 days, repeated every 6 weeks	Nausea and vomiting	Bone marrow depression; neurotoxicity, both central and peripheral	None	Ovarian carcinoma

ANTIMETABOLITES

Drug	Dosage	Acute toxicity	Delayed toxicity	Precautions	Indications
5-Fluorouracil (5-FU)	12 mg/kg per day IV for 4 days, then alternate days at 6 mg/kg for 4 days or until toxicity; repeat course monthly or give weekly IV dose of 12-15 mg/kg; maximal dose 1 g for either regimen; often used in combination regimens at a dose of 500 mg/m² IV	Bone marrow depression, diarrhea, stomatitis, alopecia	Occasional nausea and vomiting	Decrease dose in patients with diminished liver, renal, or bone marrow function or after adrenalectomy	Carcinoma of the ovary and endometrium
Methotrexate	Choriocarcinoma: 10-30 mg/day IV for 5 days; Ovarian or cervical carcinoma: 200-2000 mg/m² IV with concomitant or sequential systematic antidote ("leucovorin rescue")	None	Bone marrow depression, megaloblastic anemia, diarrhea, stomatitis, vomiting; alopecia less common; occasional hepatic fibroids, vasculitis, pulmonary fibrosis	Adequate renal function must be present, and urine output must be maintained	Choriocarcinoma, carcinoma of the ovary and cervix
Cytarabine (Ara-C, Cytosar-U) (2′,2′-difluorodeoxy cytarabine)	200 mg/m² daily for 5 days by continuous infusion	Nausea and vomiting	Bone marrow depression, megaloblastosis, leukopenia, thrombocytopenia	None	Carcinoma of the ovary (intraperitoneal use)
Gemcitabine (Gemzar)	800-1000 mg/m² IV days 1, 8, 15 every 28 days; 800-1000 mg/m² IV days 1, 8 every 21 days; 900 mg/m² IV days 1, 8 every 21 days for patients with leiomyosarcoma	Mild nausea, vomiting, malaise (usually mild), transient febrile episodes, maculopapular rash	Bone marrow suppression	None	Carcinoma of the breast and ovary; leiomyosarcoma of the uterus
Capecitabine (Xeloda)	1500-2000 mg/m² PO daily in two divided doses for 2 weeks with a 1-week rest period, repeat every 3 weeks	Hand and foot syndrome (palmar–plantar syndrome); nausea, vomiting, diarrhea; abdominal pain; constipation	Myelosuppression; hyperbilirubinemia	Should be taken in divided doses 12 h apart, administered with water 30 min after a meal	Ovarian carcinoma

Continued

TABLE 17-7   Chemotherapy Agents Used in the Treatment of Gynecologic Cancer—cont'd

Drug	Dosage and Route of Administration	Acute Side Effects	Toxicity	Precautions	Major Indications
ANTITUMOR ANTIBIOTICS					
Dactinomycin (actinomycin D, Cosmegen)	15 µg/kg per day IV or 0.5 mg/day for 5 days	Pain on local infiltration with skin necrosis; nausea and vomiting in many patients 2 h after the dose; occasional cramps and diarrhea	Bone marrow depression, stomatitis, diarrhea, erythema, hyperpigmentation with occasional desquamation in areas of previous irradiation	Administer through running IV infusion; use with care in patients with liver disease and in the presence of inadequate marrow function; prophylactic antiemetics are helpful;	Embryonal rhabdomyosarcoma, choriocarcinoma, ovarian germ cell tumors
Mitomycin C (Mutamycin)	0.05 mg/kg per day IV for 6 days, then alternate days until a 50-mg total dose	Nausea, vomiting, local inflammation and ulceration if extravasated	Neutropenia, thrombocytopenia, oral ulceration, nausea, vomiting, diarrhea	Administer through running IV infusion or inject with great care to prevent extravasation	Carcinoma of the cervix
Bleomycin	10-20 mg/m² IV or IM one or two times a week	Fever, chills, nausea, vomiting; local pain and phlebitis less frequent	Skin: hyperpigmentation, thickening, nail changes, ulceration, rash, peeling, alopecia; Pulmonary: pneumonitis with dyspnea, rales, infiltrate can progress to fibrosis; more common in patients older than 70 years of age and with more than a 400-mg total dose, but unpredictable	Watch for hypersensitivity in lymphoma with first one or two doses; use with extreme caution in presence of renal or pulmonary disease; start in hospital under observation; do not exceed a total dose of 400 mg	Squamous cell carcinoma of the skin, vulva, and cervix; choriocarcinoma; germ cell and sex cord–stromal tumors
Doxorubicin (Adriamycin)	60-100 mg/m² IV every 3 weeks	Nausea, vomiting, fever, local phlebitis, necrosis if extravasated, red urine (not blood)	Bone marrow depression, alopecia, cardiac toxicity related to the cumulative dose, stomatitis; atrophy of the myocardia can occur, especially if a total dose of 450-500 mg/m² is exceeded	Administer through running IV infusion; avoid giving to patients with significant heart disease; observe for electrocardiogram abnormalities and signs of heart failure	Adenocarcinoma of the endometrium, fallopian tube, ovary, and vagina; uterine sarcoma
Mitoxantrone		—		—	
Liposomal doxorubicin hydrochloride (Doxil)	40-50 mg/m² IV every 4 weeks	Hand and foot syndrome (palmar–plantar erythrodysesthesia syndrome); mild nausea/vomiting, mucositis, stomatitis	Mild myelosuppression; cardiomyopathy is less common compared with standard doxorubicin	Hypersensitivity reported in approximately seven patients	Ovarian carcinoma

Drug	Dose and Schedule	Acute Toxicity	Delayed Toxicity	Special Precautions	Major Indications
Vinca Alkaloids					
Vinblastine (Velban)	0.10-0.15 mg/kg per week IV	Severe, prolonged inflammation if extravasated; occasional nausea, vomiting, headache, and paresthesias	Bone marrow depression, particularly neutropenia; alopecia, muscle weakness, occasional mild peripheral neuropathy, mental depression 2-3 days after treatment, rarely stomatitis	Administer through running IV infusion or inject with great care to prevent extravasation; decrease dose in liver disease	Choriocarcinoma
Vincristine (Oncovin)	0.4-1.4 mg/m² IV weekly in adults; 2 mg/m² weekly in children	Local inflammation if extravasated	Paresthesias, weakness, loss of reflexes, constipation; abdominal, chest, and jaw pain; hoarseness, foot drop; mental depression; marrow toxicity generally mild, anemia and reticulocytopenia most prominent; alopecia	Administer through running IV infusion or inject with great care to prevent extravasation; decrease dose in patients with liver disease; patients with underlying neurologic problems may be more susceptible to neurotoxicity; alopecia may be prevented by use of a scalp tourniquet for 5 min during and after administration	Uterine sarcoma, germ cell tumor of the ovary
Vinorelbine (Navelbine)	30 mg/m² weekly IV	Mild nausea, 10% alopecia	Bone marrow depression, mild to moderate peripheral neuropathy	Local irritant, dose modification with hepatic dysfunction	Ovarian carcinoma
Epipodophyllotoxins					
Etoposide (VP-16)	100 mg/m² IV days 1, 3, and 5; repeat in 4 weeks	Nausea and vomiting	Leukopenia, thrombocytopenia, alopecia, headache, fever, occasional hypotension	Reduce dose by 25% to 50% for hematologic toxicity	Trophoblastic disease, germ cell tumors
Taxanes					
Paclitaxel (Taxol)	135-175 mg/m² IV over 3 h every 3 weeks	Allergic reaction, nausea, vomiting	Bone marrow depression, severe allergic-like reactions with facial erythema, dyspnea, tachycardia, and hypotension cardiotoxicity with bradycardia, alopecia, stomatitis, fatigue	Cardiac monitoring may be necessary	Ovarian carcinoma; endometrial cancer; cervical cancer
Protein-bound paclitaxel (Abraxane)	80-200 mg/m² IV over 30 min weekly; 175-260 mg/m² IV over 30 min every 3 weeks	Nausea, vomiting, diarrhea	Bone marrow depression, 1% hypersensitivity; abnormal EKG; neuropathy	Dose adjustment in hepatic impairment	Ovarian carcinoma
Docetaxel (Taxotere)	60-100 mg/m² IV over 1 h every 3 weeks	Hypersensitivity	Myelosuppression; mucositis; alopecia; fluid retention	Requires premedication with steroids	Ovarian carcinoma

Continued

TABLE 17-7 Chemotherapy Agents Used in the Treatment of Gynecologic Cancer—cont'd

Drug	Dosage and Route of Administration	Acute Side Effects	Toxicity	Precautions	Major Indications
EPOTHILONES					
Ixabepilone	20 mg/m² IV day 1, 8, 15 of 28-day cycle	Nausea, vomiting, diarrhea	Myelosuppression; neuropathy; fatigue; mucositis	Avoid concomitant use of CYP3A4 inhibitors; avoid grapefruit juice	Ovarian carcinoma
Camptothecin Analogs					
Topotecan	1.5 mg/m² daily for 5 days; 4 mg/m² IV day 1 and day 8, repeat every 21 days	Maculopapular pruritic exanthema	Bone marrow depression	Watch for neutropenic fever	Ovarian carcinoma, cervical carcinoma
Irinotecan (CPT-11)	300 mg/m² IV every 3 weeks; 100 mg/m² IV weekly for 4 weeks every 6 weeks	Nausea and vomiting, diarrhea	Myelosuppression, alopecia, rash	None	Ovarian carcinoma
HORMONAL AGENTS					
Progestational Agents					
Medroxyprogesterone acetate	400-800 mg/week IM or PO	None	Occasional liver function abnormalities, occasional alopecia and hypersensitivity reactions	Use with care when liver dysfunction present	Carcinoma of the endometrium
Hydroxyprogesterone caproate	1000 mg IM twice weekly				
Megestrol acetate (Megace)	20-80 mg PO twice a day				
Antiestrogens					
Tamoxifen	10-20 mg PO twice daily	Nausea, usually mild	Caused by antiestrogenic action (e.g., hot flashes, pruritus vulvae, and occasionally vaginal bleeding)	None	Breast cancer, possibly useful in endometrial carcinoma (metastatic)
Miscellaneous					
Hydroxyurea (Hydrea)	80 mg/kg PO every 3 days or 20-30 mg/kg per day	Anorexia and nausea	Bone marrow depression, megaloblastic anemia; stomatitis, diarrhea, and alopecia less common	Decrease dose in patients with marrow and renal dysfunction	Carcinoma of the cervix (with radiotherapy)

alkylating agents does not depend on DNA synthesis in the target cells. Cyclophosphamide, however, also inhibits DNA synthesis, which makes it distinctive among the alkylating agents in its mode and spectrum of activity. Alkylating agents now used in gynecologic oncology are as follows:

- Carboplatin
- Cisplatin
- Oxaliplatin
- Cyclophosphamide
- Chlorambucil
- Melphalan
- Triethylenethiophosphoramide
- Ifosfamide
- Altretamine (hexmethylmelamine)

Antimetabolites

Antimetabolites act by inhibiting essential metabolic processes that are required for synthesis of purines, pyrimidines, and nucleic acids. These agents are typically S phase-specific. The currently used drugs in this category are as follows:

- 5-fluorouracil
- Methotrexate
- Cytarabine
- Capecitabine
- Gemcitabine
- Pemetrexed

Antitumor Antibiotics

Antitumor antibiotics have generally been derived from fermentation products of various fungi, and most work via DNA intercalation. Several cytotoxic antibiotics have come into use for chemotherapy of certain neoplasms. Those used in gynecologic oncology are as follows:

- Dactinomycin (actinomycin D)
- Bleomycin
- Doxorubicin and liposomal doxorubicin hydrochloride
- Mitomycin C
- Mitoxantrone

Agents Derived from Plants

Several chemotherapeutic agents have been developed from plants. The vinca alkaloids, the epipodophyllotoxins, the epothilones, and the taxanes act to disturb the normal assembly, disassembly, and stabilization of microtubules. The camptothecin analogs serve to inhibit topoisomerase I, thereby inducing single-stranded DNA breaks. Inhibitors of topoisomerase II include etoposide (VP16) and mitoxantrone. These drugs are as follows:

- Vinca alkaloids:
  - Vinblastine
  - Vincristine
  - Vinorelbine
- Taxanes:
  - Paclitaxel
  - Protein-bound paclitaxel
  - Docetaxel
- Epipodophyllotoxins:
  - Etoposide
- Camptothecin analogs:
  - Topotecan
  - Irinotecan
- Epothilones:
  - Ixabepilone

Hormonal Agents

These agents are often utilized in the treatment of endometrial, breast, and ovarian cancers and are classified in two broad categories: antiestrogens and progestational agents. Megestrol acetate may both downregulate estrogen-responsive genes and reduce the number of available cell surface estrogen receptors. Examples of these agents are as follows:

- Antiestrogens:
  - Tamoxifen
- Progestational agents:
  - Megestrol acetate
  - Medroxyprogesterone acetate
  - Hydroxyprogesterone
- Aromatase inhibitors:
  - Anastrazole
  - Letrozole
  - Exemestane

Targeted Therapies/Immunotherapy

To date, traditional chemotherapy has predominantly focused on killing rapidly dividing cells. Unfortunately, normal cells may also be affected, causing significant toxicity. Targeted therapies have attempted to focus anticancer treatment on particular pathways and mechanisms that cause cancer to both increase efficacy and decrease toxicity in comparison with traditional chemotherapies. These therapies may aim to affect pathways for angiogenesis, cell cycle, and apoptosis in tumor cells. Several broad categories of targeted therapies exist. Monoclonal antibodies target receptors on the surface of tumor cells. As part of anticancer therapy, monoclonal antibodies have been used in two fashions. First, infusion of the antibody has allowed binding to target cells, which in turn triggers normal effector mechanisms of the body. Second, monoclonal antibodies have been conjugated to a strongly radioactive atom, such as iodine-131, to aid in killing the target. Other targeted therapies focus on the internal components and function of the cancer cell, using small molecules to disrupt the function of the cells, triggering apoptosis. There are several types of targeted therapy that focus on the inner parts of the cells. Other immunomodulators are nonspecific in their action. Another class of immune therapies includes vaccines (which may be dendritic cell, protein/peptide, DNA, or RNA based) and adoptive immunotherapy. Although many agents are in clinical trial, none are currently FDA approved. Collectively, these therapies cannot currently be considered replacement for traditional cytotoxics but may be best used in combination with chemotherapeutic agents. Some examples, along with their targets, are as follows:

- Monoclonal antibodies:
  - Oregovamab (CA-125)
  - Cetuximab (EGFR)
  - Bevacizumab (VEGF)
  - Trastuzumab (HER-2/neu)
- Small molecules:
  - Gefitinib (EGFR)
  - Erlotonib (EGFR)
  - OSI-774 (EGFR-TK)
  - Bortezomib (proteosome)
  - Imatinib (Bcr-Abl protein tyrosine kinase, c-kit receptor tyrosine kinase)
  - Sorafenib (Raf/Mek/Erk)
  - Sunitinib (multiple receptor tyrosine kinases)
- Nonspecific:
  - BCG
  - IL-2
  - IFN-alpha
  - Thalidomide

DRUG TOXICITY

Unfortunately, traditional chemotherapeutic agents are indiscriminate in their effects: Both malignant and normal tissues are affected. Although their goal is to kill more cancerous than normal cells, many side effects, particularly those to organ systems with rapidly proliferating cell populations, are inevitable. Usually, the mechanism of toxicity is similar to the one producing the desired cytotoxic effect. Even organs with limited cell proliferation can be damaged by chemotherapeutic agents, especially if the agents are utilized at high doses. Chemotherapeutic agents must be used at doses that produce some degree of toxicity to normal tissue in

TABLE 17-8 Drug Dose Modification Based on Common Hematologic Toxicity

Count Before Next Course (per mm^3)	Dose Modification*
Leukocytes	
>4000	100% of dose
3000-3999	100% of nonmyelotoxic agents 50% of myelotoxic agents
2000-2999	100% of nonmyelotoxic agents 25% of myelotoxic agents
1000-1999	25% of myelotoxic agents
≤999	No drug
PLATELETS	
>100,000	100% of dose
50,000-100,000	100% of nonmyelotoxic agents
<50,000	No drug

Based on myelosuppression.

order to be effective. The incidence of severe side effects of chemotherapeutic agents is greatly influenced by states such as severe disability, advancing age, poor nutrition, or direct organ involvement by primary or metastatic lesions. The physician must monitor these patients with extreme care, and appropriate dose modifications must be made (Table 17-8).

Hematologic Toxicity

Hematologic toxicity is the most frequently seen side effect. Acute granulocytopenia occurs 6-12 days after the administration of most myelosuppressive chemotherapeutic agents. Recovery occurs in 10-14 days. The megakaryocyte series is affected later, such that platelet suppression usually occurs 4 or 5 days after granulocytopenia and recovers several days after the white blood cell count. Mitomycin C and nitrosourea are particularly unique in their ability to produce delayed bone marrow suppression. Myelosuppression with these two drugs commonly occurs within 28-42 days, with recovery 40-60 days after treatment.

Most clinicians consider patients with absolute granulocyte counts less than 500/mm^3 for 5 days or longer to be at a higher risk for sepsis. The practice of utilizing prophylactic broad-spectrum antibiotics in febrile granulocytopenic cancer patients has significantly decreased the incidence of life-threatening infections in this group of patients. Granulocytopenic patients should have their temperature checked every 4 hours, and they should be examined frequently for evidence of infection. Thrombocytopenic patients with platelet counts less than 20,000/mm^3 are at increased risk for spontaneous hemorrhage, particularly from the gastrointestinal tract. Routine platelet transfusions for platelets under 10-20,000/mm^3 have been utilized by some clinicians.

Others wait and watch until patients manifest some evidence of bleeding. Repeat transfusions of platelets at 2- to 3-day intervals may be necessary in patients with severe thrombocytopenia. Patients with active peptic ulcer disease and patients needing surgical procedures need to be transfused with counts lower than 50,000/mm³.

Growth Factor Therapy

GRANULOCYTE STIMULATING THERAPY

The application of hematopoietic factors to supportive care has been dramatic. Rapid advances in unraveling the molecular biology and biochemistry of these glycoprotein hormones that regulate hematopoiesis have led to their routine clinical use. Since their emergence in 1989, their use has allowed amelioration of therapy-related myelosuppression, modulation of disease-related myelosuppression, and enhanced host defense to infection. This class of agents includes molecules such as granulocyte-colony stimulating factor (G-CSF) and granulocyte macrophage colony–stimulating factor (GM-CSF). The biologic activities of these proteins are complex and multifunctional, stimulating potent changes in the growth, differentiation, distribution, and functional status of mature cells and their precursors (Table 17-9).

Initial studies with G-CSF and GM-CSF focused on their administration via the intravenous route. Since then, numerous studies have shown that subcutaneous administration once or twice a day is even more myelostimulatory than 2- to 4-hour intravenous infusions. The recommended dose of GM-CSF is 250 µg/m² or 3-5 µg/kg. It is interesting that, at least in some cases, a fairly low dose of GM-CSF may be more myelostimulatory than a higher dose. The enhancement of neutrophil function in terms of adherence, phagocytosis, and chemotaxis has also been noted in clinical studies, and GM-CSF may also function to activate lymphocytes. Two types of G-CSF are available: filgrastim and a long-acting pegfilgrastim. The recommended dose of filgrastim is 5 µg/kg, given subcutaneously. Treatment should begin at least 24 hours after completion of chemotherapy, and should continue daily until the absolute neutrophil count exceeds 10,000/mm³. Subsequent chemotherapy should not begin until at least 48 hours have elapsed since the last dose. The recommended dose of pegfilgrastim is 6 mg. A subcutaneous injection is recommended at least 24 hours after the completion of chemotherapy infusion, and should not be given within 14 days of any subsequent chemotherapy. Bone pain is the most common side effect of G-CSF. Other more rare effects include the following:

- A cutaneous eruption of macules and papules
- Exacerbation of underlying autoimmune disease
- Anaphylaxis, which is rare
- Mild increased risk of thrombosis
- A theoretic possibility of the exacerbation of the underlying malignancy

Unquestionably, the administration of G-CSF or GM-CSF accelerates neutrophil recovery to a significant degree after standard-dose chemotherapy. G-CSF is indicated to decrease the incidence of febrile neutropenia with regimens associated with a significant incidence of neutropenia with fever.

ERYTHROCYTE STIMULATING THERAPY

The existence of a hormone that regulates erythropoiesis (Epo) has been proposed for 100 years. In 1985 two independent groups cloned the gene responsible for this growth factor. This gene was labeled the Epo gene. The kidney appears to be the major site of production of erythropoietin. Apparently, the site of production in the fetus is the liver, and in the last third of the gestational period the responsibility is gradually transferred to the kidney. Erythropoietin stimulates the division and differentiation of committed erythroid progenitors in the bone marrow. Epoetin alpha is a glycoprotein manufactured

TABLE 17-9   Characteristics of the Hematopoietic Growth Factor Family of Cytokines

Cytokine	Source	Function
Granulocyte-macrophage colony stimulating factor (GM-CSF)	T cells, endothelial cells, stromal cells	Stimulates hematopoiesis of granulocyte and macrophage lineage; activates granulocytes and macrophages
Granulocyte-colony stimulating factor (G-CSF)	Endothelial cells, monocytes, stromal cells	Stimulates hematopoiesis of granulocyte lineage; activates granulocytes
Erythropoietin	Kidney	Stimulates erythroid growth and development
Interleukin-1	Monocytes/macrophages, B and T cells, endothelial cells	Costimulates early stages of hematopoiesis; T- and B-cell activation
Interleukin-3	T cells	Stimulates early stages of hematopoiesis
Interleukin-6	T cells, monocytes/macrophages, fibroblasts	Costimulates early stages of hematopoiesis; T- and B-cell activation

(After Kouides PA: The hematopoietic growth factors. In Haskell CM [ed]: Principles of Cancer Treatment, 4th ed. Philadelphia, Saunders, 1995.)

by recombinant DNA technology. It is produced by mammalian cells into which the human Epo gene has been introduced. The product contains the exact amino acid sequence of natural Epo. Tissue hypoxia is the chief stimulus for the production of Epo. Relatively small blood losses (e.g., 1 U of blood) only modestly stimulate Epo production. Most patients on chemotherapy develop anemia at some point during the course of their illness. The hemoglobin concentration of these patients usually ranges from 7 to 12 g/dL, and the hematocrit is somewhere between 25% and 38%. This is sufficient to stimulate the production of Epo endogenously. However, there appears to be a large blunting of response to Epo in patients who have undergone chemotherapy.

Epoetin reduces the transfusion requirement in anemic patients and may enhance overall quality of life, and administration is indicated when hemoglobin levels have decreased below 10 mg/dL during chemotherapy treatment, or when a significant chance for blood transfusion exists. However, iron deficiency must be corrected before starting epoetin. Epoetin injected at a dose of 150 U/kg subcutaneously three times a week for 12 weeks has been used by many clinicians. The dose may be increased up to 300 U/kg. Others utilize a daily dose of 60 U/kg, progressing to a maximum dose of 90 U/kg per day. Another commonly used approach is to inject 40,000 U/week, with escalation to 60,000 U for nonresponders. Darbepoetin alfa is a long-acting form that may be administered at doses of 3.0 µg/kg every 3 weeks. Adverse effects are uncommon but include worsening hypertension in patients with end-stage renal disease. Other effects include edema and diarrhea.

Erythropoesis-stimulating agents must be used with caution. In 2007 the U.S. Food and Drug Administration issued a black box warning regarding the use of both epoetin alfa and darbepoetin alfa. Indeed, two large randomized trials have reported significantly worse tumor control and survival rates in patients receiving epoetin. Research also indicates that the erythropoietin receptor is expressed in several cancer cell lines, raising the concern of possible stimulation of tumor cell growth by these drugs. Epoetin has also been implicated in possible thromboembolic complications, possibly related to elevated hemoglobin levels. Currently, physicians who wish to utilize these agents for chemotherapy-related anemia must register with the Risk Evaluation and Mitigation Strategy (REMS) program. Physicians must complete a 15-minute online education course and document informed consent from the patient prior to administration.

Platelet Stimulating Therapy

Oprelvekin is produced in E. coli by recombinant DNA methods. The protein is very similar to interleukin (IL)-11, which is a thrombopoietic growth factor that directly stimulates the proliferation of hematopoietic stem cells and megakaryocyte maturation, which in turn increase platelet production. IL-11 is produced by bone marrow stromal cells and is part of the cytokine family. The usual dose is 50 µg/kg, which is given once daily subcutaneously as a single injection in the abdomen, thigh, or hip. Treatment should begin 6-24 hours after completion of chemotherapy and continued until the nadir platelet count is 50,000 cells/µL. Potential side effects include mild to moderate fluid retention, and IL-11 should be used with caution in patients with a history of atrial arrhythmia, transient mild visual blurring, and transient rashes at the injection site. Anaphylactic reactions have been reported.

Gastrointestinal Toxicity

Gastrointestinal toxicity is another frequent manifestation of chemotherapeutic agents. Mucositis may be caused by direct effects on the rapidly dividing epithelial mucosa. Concomitant granulocytopenia allows the injured mucosa to become infected and serve as a portal of entry for bacteria and fungi. The onset of mucositis is frequently 3-5 days earlier than myelosuppression. The nasopharyngeal lesions are difficult to distinguish from viral lesions. Candidiasis is often seen and is difficult to distinguish from stomatitis secondary to chemotherapy; antifungal agents have been very effective in treating this condition. Necrotizing enterocolitis is another condition that is seen in patients receiving chemotherapy. Symptoms of this condition are watery or bloody diarrhea, abdominal pain, nausea, vomiting, and fever. Patients usually have abdominal tenderness and distension. They also have a history of broad-spectrum antibiotic use. Most necrotizing enterocolitis is caused by anaerobic bacteria such as Clostridium difficile. The treatment of choice for C. difficile infection is oral vancomycin, 125 mg four times daily for 10-14 days.

The most common side effect of chemotherapy is nausea and vomiting. Although the exact mechanisms are not clearly defined, most agents appear to stimulate the chemoreceptor trigger zone in the area postrema of the brain to secrete neurotransmitters such as dopamine, serotonin, and histamine. These neurotransmitters may activate the neighboring vomiting center to induce nausea and emesis. Direct stimulation of serotonin receptors in the gastrointestinal tract, direct cerebral action, and psychogenic effects may also play a role. Different patterns of emesis include acute emesis (within 24 hours of chemotherapy infusion), delayed emesis (typically beginning 16-24 hours after chemotherapy but persisting up to 72-96 h), and anticipatory emesis. Common antiemetic regimens are detailed in Table 17-10. Choice of agents should be governed by knowledge of the emetogenic potential of the chemotherapies administered (Table 17-11).

TABLE 17-10   Common Antiemetic Regimens

	Drug(s)	Dosage
PREMEDICATION		
5-HT3 receptor antagonists	Ondansetron	8-24 mg IV/PO
	Granisetron	10 µg/kg IV; 2 mg PO
	Dolasetron	1.8 mg/kg IV; 100 mg IV; 100 mg PO
Substance P/NK1 receptor antagonist	Aprepitant	125 mg PO
Motility agent	Metoclopramide	2-3 mg/kg IV; 20-40 mg PO
Phenothiazine	Prochlorperazine	10 mg IV/IM/PO; 25 mg PR; 15 mg spansule
Benzodiazepine	Lorazepam	0.5-2 mg IV/PO/SL
Corticosteroid	Dexamethasone	8-20 mg IV/PO
Acute-phase emesis	Dexamethasone	20 mg IV
	Ondansetron	8-24 mg IV
	Metoclopramide	3 mg/kg IV (repeat q2h prn)
	Diphenhydramine	25-50 mg IV (repeat q2h prn)
	Lorazepam	1-2 mg IV
Prophylaxis of delayed emesis	Dexamethasone	8 mg PO b.i.d. × 2 days, then 4 mg PO b.i.d. × 2 days
	plus metoclopramide	40 mg PO q.i.d. × 2-3 days*
	or 5-HT3 antagonist	ondansetron 8 mg PO b.i.d. or t.i.d. × 2-3 days, or granisetron 1 mg PO b.i.d. or 2 mg PO q.i.d. × 2-3 days)
	5-HT3 antagonist	PO × 2-3 days alone, or plus aprepitant 80 mg PO and dexamethasone 8 mg PO q.i.d. × 3 days

Patients should be advised to take 50 mg of diphenhydramine PO at the first sign of dystonic reaction.

TABLE 17-11   Emetogenic Potential of Cancer Chemotherapeutic Agents Used in Gynecologic Oncology

Emetogenic potential (frequency, %)	Agent
<10	Bleomycin
	Hydroxyurea
	Melphalan (PO)
	Methotrexate (<50 mg/m^2)
10-30	Docetaxel
	Doxorubicin (<20 mg/m^2)
	Etoposide
	Fluorouracil (<1000 mg/m^2)
	Gemcitabine
	Methotrexate (50-250 mg/m^2)
	Paclitaxel
	Topotecan
30-60	Cyclophosphamide (<750 mg/m^2)
	Dactinomycin (<1.5 mg/m^2)
	Doxorubicin (20-60 mg/m^2)
	Ifosfamide
	Methotrexate (250-1000 mg/m^2)
60-90	Carboplatin
	Cisplatin (<50 mg/m^2)
	Cyclophosphamide (750-1500 mg/m^2)
	Dactinomycin (>1.5 mg/m^2)
	Doxorubicin (>60 mg/m^2)
	Irinotecan
	Melphalan (IV)
	Methotrexate (>1000 mg/m^2)
> 90	Cisplatin (>50 mg/m^2)
	Cyclophosphamide (>1500 mg/m^2)

(After Hesketh PJ, Kris MG, Grunberg SM et al: J Clin Oncol 15:103-109, 1997.)

Highly emetogenic chemotherapies include cisplatin (>50 mg/m^2) and high-dose cyclophosphamide (>1500 mg/m^2). Cisplatin may induce both acute and delayed vomiting. A premedication regimen should consist of a combination of antiemetics given 30 minutes prior to chemotherapy infusion. Common regimens include use of a 5-HT3 receptor antagonist with dexamethasone. Lorazepam and oral aprepitant may also be utilized. Moderately emetogenic chemotherapies include lower doses of cisplatin (<50 mg/m^2) and cyclophosphamide (750-1500 mg/m^2) and carboplatin, doxorubicin, methotrexate (>1000 mg/m^2), ifosfamide, and high-dose 5-fluorouracil. These agents may be premedicated with 5-HT3 receptor antagonists in combination with dexamethasone. Mildly emetogenic chemotherapies include methotrexate, paclitaxel, docetaxel, liposomal doxorubicin, gemcitabine, bleomycin, and etoposide. These agents may be premedicated with single-agent antiemetics. Delayed emesis requires special consideration. Prophylaxis may include use of single-agent 5-HT3 receptor antagonist therapy or a brief pulse of dexamethasone in combination with metoclopramide, a 5-HT3 receptor antagonist, or aprepitant, a substance P/NK1 antagonist.

Skin Reactions

Skin reactions, including alopecia and allergic hypersensitivity reactions, are also often seen with chemotherapeutic agents. Skin necrosis and sloughing at the site of intravenous extravasation is associated particularly with agents such as doxorubicin, actinomycin D, mitomycin C, vinblastine, vincristine, and nitrogen mustard. The extent of the necrosis is determined by the amount of extravasated drug. Management includes removal of the intravenous line and local infiltration of the area with corticosteroidsand ice pack therapy four or five times a day for 3 days. Long-term monitoring of these patients is essential. Palmar–plantar erthrodysesthesia, or hand and foot syndrome, may be a dose-limiting toxicity of liposomal doxorubicin and is characterized by painful edema and erythema. Alopecia is a common side effect of many chemotherapeutic agents. Therapies designed to reduce alopecia have not been successful. Hair growth resumes 10-20 days after treatment is completed.

Hypersensitivity

Many chemotherapeutic agents may be associated with hypersensitivity reactions, although only a few agents elicit these responses in more than 5% of patients. Of the agents commonly used in gynecologic oncology, the taxanes and platinum compounds are the most likely culprits, although occasional reactions may also be seen with bleomycin, doxorubicin, etoposide, cyclophosphamide, ifosfamide, and methotrexate.

In phase I trials, the incidence of severe hypersensitivity to paclitaxel was approximately 30%; however, with adequate prophylaxis (Table 17-12) the incidence is now less than 10%. Although hypersensitivity associated with paclitaxel is often attributed to its formulation in Cremophor EL, a polyoxyethylated castor oil, docetaxel has also been associated with a similar incidence of hypersensitivity despite its formulation in Tween 80. With appropriate premedication, hypersensitivity to docetaxel has been reduced to 2% to 3%. The occurrence of hypersensitivity does not preclude further treatment with the drug. If additional diphenhydramine or corticosteroids do not allow the infusion to be completed after a delay, patients may undergo successful systematic desensitization.

TABLE 17-12   Prophylaxis for Taxane Hypersensitivity

Agent	Prophylaxis Regimen
Docetaxel	Starting 1 day prior to infusion: dexamethasone 8 mg PO b.i.d. × 3 days
Paclitaxel	Night before and morning of infusion: dexamethasone 20 mg PO*
	30 min prior to infusion[†]: diphenhydramine 25-50 mg IV *plus* H2 antagonist IV(cimetidine 300 mg or ranitidine 50 mg)

May be repeated PO or IV 30 min prior to infusion.
[†]*If the first cycle of treatment is well tolerated, subsequent cycles may be premedicated using oral doses.*

The incidence of hypersensitivity to platinum analogs varies from 5% to 20%. Unlike reactions to taxanes, which typically occur within minutes of starting the initial dose, reactions to platinum agents typically do not manifest until several cycles have already been administered. In one series, a median of eight platinum courses were administered before hypersensitivity occurred. Routine premedication for hypersensitivity is not recommended, and patients who experience mild reactions may respond well to the addition of appropriate premedications. Patients with severe reactions may attempt systematic desensitization if indicated, although success is variable.

Hepatic Toxicity

Hepatic toxicity is uncommon. Mild elevations in transaminase, alkaline phosphatase, and bilirubin are seen with many agents, but rarely is the condition severe. Psoriasis and drug-induced hepatitis can affect the amount of the chemotherapeutic agent given, as can preexisting liver disease or exposure to other hepatic toxins.

Pulmonary Toxicity

Interstitial pneumonitis with pulmonary fibrosis is seen with certain chemotherapeutic agents. The agents most likely to produce this are doxorubicin, alkylating agents, and nitrosoureas. Treatment of patients with drug-induced interstitial pneumonitis involves discontinuation of the cytotoxic agent and supportive care. Steroids may be of some benefit.

Cardiac Toxicity

The risk of cardiac toxicity is seen primarily with doxorubicin. The risk increases dramatically when the cumulative dose exceeds 500 mg/m^2 of ideal body surface area. In recent years, this limit has rarely been exceeded; thus cardiomyopathy has diminished greatly in incidence. Acute arrhythmias may often be seen, but these disappear with a few days of supportive care. On rare occasions, cyclophosphamide has been reported to produce cardiotoxicity, particularly when it is used in massive doses. Mitomycin C has been reported to cause endocardial fibrosis and myocardial fibrosis, but again these events occur rarely.

Renal Toxicity

Nephrotoxicity may be dose-limiting in up to 35% of patients receiving cisplatin. Proximal and distal tubule damage leads to electrolyte wasting and increase in serum creatinine with concomitant decrease in Cr Cl. Renal toxicity may be reduced with adequate intravenous hydration and mannitol and/or furosemide-induced diuresis. Antibiotic therapy with aminoglycosides potentiates the nephrotoxicity of drugs such as cisplatin and should be avoided if possible.

Genitourinary Toxicity

Metabolites of cyclophosphamide are irritants to the bladder mucosa and can cause chronic hemorrhagic cystitis. The toxic metabolite of cyclophosphamide that causes bladder toxicity is known as acrolein. Vigorous hydration and diuresis during administration of cyclophosphamide are essential. Cisplatin produces renal tubular toxicity associated with azotemia and magnesium wasting. Again, this complication can be minimized with diuresis during administration of cisplatin. Other agents known to cause genitourinary toxicity are methotrexate, nitrosoureas, and mitomycin C. Mesna or N-acetylcysteine has been used in recent times in conjunction with cyclophosphamide to prevent bladder toxicity. This agent acts by inactivating the toxic metabolite acrolein.

Neurologic Toxicity

In general, most antineoplastic drugs are associated with mild neurologic side effects. There are some exceptions, however. Vinca alkaloids are commonly associated with peripheral motor sensory and autonomic neuropathies. Agents such as vincristine, vinblastine, paclitaxel, and vinorelbine can produce loss of deep tendon reflexes with distal paresthesias. Paclitaxel may also cause peripheral neuropathy. In most cases, these neurologic toxicities are reversible following cessation of the drug. Cisplatin produces ototoxicity and peripheral neuropathy, and occasionally retrobulbar neuritis. High doses of cisplatin, which are often used in ovarian cancer therapy, are particularly likely to produce progressive and somewhat delayed peripheral neuropathy. 5-Fluorouracil has been associated with acute cerebellar toxicity. Hexamethylmelamine is reported to produce peripheral neuropathy and encephalopathy. Ifosfamide has also been associated with encephalopathy, particularly in patients with low serum albumin.

Gonadal Dysfunction

Many chemotherapeutic agents have lasting effects on testicular and ovarian functions. This is particularly true of alkylating agents, which can cause azoospermia and amenorrhea. The onset of amenorrhea and ovarian failure is accompanied by an elevation of the serum follicle stimulating hormone and a fall in serum estradiol. Indeed, these patients often end up with premature menopause. The younger the patient at the onset of therapy, the less likely it is that chemotherapy would eventuate in permanent gonadal dysfunction. In women older than 30 years of age, most chemotherapeutic regimens are associated with a high incidence of premature ovarian failure.

Supportive Care

Supportive social workers, chaplains, and psychiatrists in a concentrated total care setting are of great value in enabling a patient to cope with the emotionally and financially shattering experience of having cancer. Home healthcare services have improved in most areas of the United States, so that intravenous fluids, antibiotics, intravenous alimentation, and even chemotherapy can be administered in the home if the situation allows. Although treatment of many patients must be conducted at large medical centers where new agents and multidisciplinary facilities are available, continuing collaboration between the medical center and the patient's primary physician is essential. Problems caused by the disease or its treatment often arise when the patient returns to her community. An informed local physician can rapidly evaluate these crises and take appropriate action. The performance status of the patient should be watched carefully (Table 17-13).

EVALUATION OF NEW AGENTS

The development of new, promising agents is a long, complicated, and expensive process. After identification of potential drugs in in vitro and animal models, all anticancer therapeutic agents must undergo rigorous clinical testing. Several levels of clinical trials are necessary to demonstrate that a newly developed agent should be allowed in regular medical practice. Such trials have been defined as follows.

Phase I

These initial trials are designed to test new drugs at various doses to evaluate toxicity and determine the tolerance to a particular agent. The primary endpoint to these trials is safety evaluation. A dose escalation design is often used in order to define the maximum tolerated dose and to characterize the dose-limiting toxicities of the drug. Some therapeutic effects may be observed, even though the intent of these trials is not response measurement.

Phase II

Phase II studies attempt to determine the response rate of the particular agent at the dose and schedule defined by phase I trials. Secondary endpoints include

TABLE 17-13   Performance Status

GOG/ECOG Group score	Zubrod Description	Scale (%)	Karnofsky Description	Scale (%)
0	Fully active, able to carry on all predisease performance without restriction.	90-100	Normal, no complaints, no evidence of disease.	100
			Able to carry on normal activity, minor symptoms or signs of disease.	90
1	Restricted in physically strenuous activity but ambulatory and able to carry out work of a light or sedentary nature (e.g. light housework, office work).	70-80	Normal activity with effort; some signs and symptoms of disease.	80
			Cares for self, unable to perform normal activity or to do active work.	70
2	Ambulatory and capable of all self-care but unable to carry out any work activities. Up and about more than 50% of waking hours.	50-60	Requires occasional assistance but is able to care for most of own needs.	60
			Requires considerable assistance and frequent medical care.	60
3	Capable of only limited self-care, confined to bed or chair more than 50% of waking hours.	30-40	Requires special care and assistance; disabled.	40
			Severely disabled, hospitalization indicated, although death not imminent.	30
4	Completely disabled. Cannot carry on any self-care. Totally confined to bed or chair.	10-20	Very sick, hospitalization indicated.	20
			Fatal processes progressing rapidly; moribund.	10
5	Dead.	0	Dead.	0

GOG/ECOG, Gynecologic Oncology Group, European Cooperative Oncology.

determination of progression-free interval, determination of toxicity, and overall survival. Most phase II trials are single-arm nonrandomized studies.

Phase III

Phase III trials are designed to compare a drug identified as promising in phase II trials to current standard treatment regimens. Commonly, a new drug is tested against the accepted gold standard drug therapy for a particular disease site and histology. These trials are typically large in order to provide sufficient power to detect a difference between the treatment arms. The primary endpoint in phase III trials is usually progression-free survival, while secondary endpoints usually include response rate and overall survival.

For full reference list, log onto www.expertconsult.com
⟨http://www.expertconsult.com⟩.

Targeted Therapy and Molecular Genetics

*Shannon N. Westin, MD, MPH, Anil K. Sood, MD,
and Robert L. Coleman, MD*

TARGETED THERAPY

The use of site-specific combinations of surgery, chemotherapy, and radiation therapy in gynecologic malignancies has led to marked initial improvements in patient survival. Unfortunately, over the past 30 years, there has been little improvement in disease-specific mortality from the three major gynecologic malignancies (Table 18-1). The addition of further traditional cytotoxic chemotherapies to current treatment regimens is likely to offer only increased toxicities in the absence of further survival benefit. To critically affect patient outcome and improve quality of life, the therapeutic armamentarium of the modern oncologist must be expanded. The search for novel therapeutic options has led to an exploration of therapies targeting molecular pathways, which may confer a survival advantage to cancer cells.

FOUNDATION OF TARGETED THERAPY

The development of new and effective therapies should be rooted in a clear understanding of tumor biology. In a seminal paper, Hanahan and Weinberg described the key capabilities acquired by normal cells that lead to the development of cancer. Figure 18-1 represents the six "hallmarks of cancer" implicated in the tumorigenic process. Self-sufficiency in growth signals and insensitivity to antigrowth signals relate to the development of cellular autonomy, which is essential to uncontrolled proliferation. Limitless replicative potential indicates that the cell is unencumbered by the typical process of senescence, the cessation of growth upon reaching a set number of cellular doublings. The evasion of apoptosis is a feature seen in most cancer types, allowing the cells to continue to grow and replicate in the setting of damage that would lead to attrition in a normal cell. The ability to invade tissues and metastasize is crucial to the continued expansion of tumor when space and nutrients become limited. The final characteristic, sustained angiogenesis, describes uncontrolled growth of new blood vessels, which supply oxygen and nutrients to the tumor.

Acquisition of survival capabilities by cancer cells is theorized to be directly related to dysfunction of the normal molecular mechanisms and pathways within the cell and surrounding microenvironment. As these pathways are driving the progression of cancer, identifying and targeting the changes in the pathways to treat malignancy is a rational strategy. Thus the field of targeted therapy has flourished in modern cancer treatment, especially among common gynecologic malignancies.

Cytotoxic chemotherapy typically acts primarily on any rapidly dividing cells. Although this may have the desired effects on tumor cells, these drugs do not discriminate between tumor cells and normal host cells, resulting in undesirable side effects in the gastrointestinal tract, bone marrow, and integumentary and other systems. Ideal targeted therapies provide a more directed approach by acting on targets selectively expressed or overexpressed on the tumor cells or in the tumor microenvironment. These targets are typically members of the pathways involved in tumorigenesis, supporting growth, proliferation, metastasis, and angiogenesis. By honing in on those pathways rather than broad-based activity, normal tissues are spared and adverse events are minimized.

These therapies hold potential to reduce mortality from gynecologic malignancy, while concurrently reducing the morbidity associated with cancer treatment by targeting abnormal rather than normal tissue. This chapter will provide a broad overview of the pertinent molecular pathways in gynecologic cancer and the targeted agents that are currently being explored as treatment options. In addition, the unique toxicities of these targeted agents will be reviewed. As our knowledge continues to expand, there will no doubt be a myriad other pathways to exploit and agents used to treat gynecologic malignancies.

TABLE 18-1   Mortality Rates* of Major Gynecologic Malignancies over 25 Years

	1975	1985	1995	2003-2007
Cervical	5.5	3.82	3.24	2.4
Endometrial	5.28	4.61	4.15	4.1
Ovarian	9.84	9.08	9.12	8.6

*Mortality rates presented as per 100,000 women.

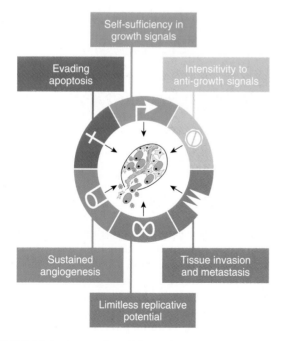

FIGURE 18-1   Acquired capabilities of cancer. (*Used with permission from Hanahan D, Weinberg RA: Cell 100:57, 2000.*)

TARGETED AGENTS

Targeting molecular pathways that drive tumor progression can be accomplished through a variety of mechanisms. The first is a humanized monoclonal antibody, which is created to bind cancer-associated antigens or molecules for cancer therapy. Monoclonal antibodies may be directed toward ligands or cell-surface molecules that participate in pathways of tumorigenesis. Table 18-2 describes standard nomenclature of the monoclonal antibody classes. These agents are classified based on the origin of the antibody. By definition, monoclonal antibodies have affinity for a single target, which allows for minimal non–tumor-related effects. These agents are administered systemically and have long clearance times allowing biweekly and monthly administration. One such agent is bevacizumab, which is a monoclonal antibody to a vascular endothelial growth factor A (VEGF-A), a key active ligand in angiogenesis, to be discussed later in the chapter.

Small molecule inhibitors are primarily oral agents that inhibit the function of molecular receptors through the blockage tyrosine kinase activity. Tyrosine kinases are enzymes involved in an array of normal and abnormal cellular functions. Their activity causes the transfer of a phosphate group from adenosine triphosphate (ATP) to a downstream protein tyrosine residue resulting in changes in protein conformation and association affecting innumerable biologic processes. Two types of tyrosine kinases exist: receptor and nonreceptor tyrosine kinases. Figure 18-2 demonstrates the typical structure of a receptor tyrosine kinase, exhibiting three major domains: extracellular ligand binding, transmembrane, and cytoplasmic. Currently, approximately 60 receptor tyrosine kinases have been identified and classified.

Nonreceptor tyrosine kinases are typically present in the cytoplasm or nucleus and interact with transmembrane receptors to phosphorylate downstream substrates. They may also be activated through signals derived from extracellular processes such as ion exchange. Erlotinib is one small molecule inhibitor that targets the epidermal growth factor receptor (EGFR) pathway affecting cellular division and proliferation.

Small molecule inhibitors typically block tyrosine kinase phosphorylation through interaction with the ATP-binding site on the intracellular domain of the tyrosine kinase. Binding to this site may be reversible or irreversible, depending on the agent. These molecules often have short half-lives, which necessitate frequent administration. Secondary to the high degree of homology found at the ATP-binding domain of the various tyrosine kinases, many of these molecules may inhibit one or more receptors within the cellular mechanism. Depending on the pathways affected, this can improve antitumor activity or lead to undesired adverse effects related to "off target" inhibition.

To reduce off-target associations, unique structural features of a given target are being identified. Then, agents that are chemically altered to maximize interaction with these specific components can be introduced. One example is the development of wrapping technology. This involves targeting a defect that is inherently specific to a given region in a protein called a dehydron. Dehydrons are hydrogen bonds of the protein that are poorly protected from water. Drugs designed to

TABLE 18-2 Biologically Targeted Monoclonal Antibody Class and Nomenclature

Suffix	Antibody Class	HAMA Potential	Example
"-omab"	Murine	+++	
"-ximab"	Chimeric	+/++	Cetuximab
"-zumab"	Humanized	+	Bevacizumab
"-mumab"	Fully human	−	Panitumumab

HAMA, Human anti-mouse antibody.

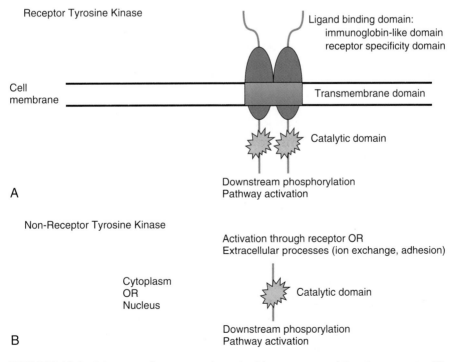

FIGURE 18-2 Schematic of two types of tyrosine kinases: receptor *(A)* and nonreceptor *(B)*.

protect a given dehydron from water will selectively direct ligands to the receptor with that specific defect. Additional methods of introducing selectivity are being explored, including the disruption of protein–protein interactions.

The use of RNA interference technology has great promise for expanding targeted therapy through knock down of expression of specific genes involved in tumorigenesis. RNA silencing pathways are mechanisms within the cell that directly control gene expression. In general, short interfering RNAs (siRNAs) are generated from double-stranded RNA (dsRNA) within the cell by an endonuclease called Dicer. The antisense strands of the siRNA then associate with an RNA-induced silencing complex (RISC) that targets a specific messenger ribonucleic acid (mRNA) for cleavage by Argonaute 2. Cleavage of the mRNA can silence genes involved in cellular survival, proliferation, invasion, and metastasis. Of note, the level of expression of the components of RNA silencing pathways correlates with survival in a variety of cancers.

The delivery of siRNA in vivo has been challenging. However, local delivery (intranasal or intravitreal) approaches have been advanced into clinical trials in nonmalignant diseases such as macular degeneration. Recent methods of delivery utilizing biodegradable lipids and polymers have shown safety and efficacy in cancer models. Furthermore, an ongoing first-in-human phase I trial has demonstrated successful delivery of siRNA through nanoparticles. Early results from this trial revealed induction of RNA interference mechanisms at specifically targeted sites. This mechanism of targeted therapy has the potential to greatly expand the possible targets while reducing undesirable adverse effects.

Other unique agents have also been explored as prospective biologic options to disrupt carcinogenic pathways. Decoy receptors that bind key ligands of carcinogenic pathways have been developed. An example of this is VEGF-Trap (aflibercept), which binds VEGF to negatively affect angiogenesis. There is no doubt that as our knowledge of cellular signaling mechanisms grows, so will the variety of agents for targeted therapy.

ANGIOGENESIS

To date, the most successful examples of targeted therapy in gynecologic cancer are found in the arena of angiogenesis. Angiogenesis is a key process for the supply of nutrients, oxygen, growth factors, and dissemination of a tumor. Thus the development of new vasculature is an essential process for a tumor to grow beyond 1 mm in size. There are two primary mechanisms for the growth of new blood vessels in both the normal and tumor microenvironment. Sprouting, the dominant means of vessel formation, is the branching of a new vessel from an established blood vessel. The other major mechanism is nonsprouting, which occurs when an existing blood vessel enlarges and splits into two separate vessels. Aggressive tumor cells may also develop microvascular channels to support neovascularization in a process known as vasculogenic mimicry. Finally, existing vasculature in the host tissue may be coopted by the tumors to increase vascular supply.

In normal tissues, the vasculature is organized and uniform in size and shape. Angiogenesis in the tumor microenvironment results in vessels that are more irregular, appearing tortuous, dilated, and leaky. The regulation of angiogenic mechanisms is provided by a complex set of growth factors that stimulate and inhibit vascular growth in response to internal and external stimuli. In general, these factors act on the cells lining the blood vessel (the endothelial cells) to regulate activity within the cellular microenvironment. In the normal cellular microenvironment, the endothelial cells are stable, dividing rarely. Pathologic angiogenesis secondary to an increase in pro-angiogenic factors results in endothelial cells that demonstrate unregulated division and growth. In fact, high expression of pro-angiogenic molecules and increased microvessel density (a marker of increased tumor vascularization) are poor prognostic factors in many solid malignancies.

VEGFS AND VEGF RECEPTORS

Figure 18-3 demonstrates a schematic of the VEGF pathway, a key contributor to the regulation of angiogenesis. Activation of this pathway promotes the proliferation, survival, and migration of endothelial cells leading to vascular growth. In addition, VEGF stimulation increases cell fenestration and vascular permeability, which has been associated with the development of malignant effusions in the lungs and peritoneal cavity. VEGF overexpression has been found in a majority of solid tumors, including ovarian and endometrial cancers, and is associated with poor prognosis and tumor progression.

As demonstrated in Figure 18-3, the VEGF pathway includes seven different ligands: VEGF-A, VEGF-B, VEGF-C, VEGF-D, VEGF-E, placental growth factor (PlGF)-1, and PlGF-2. The mediation of the angiogenic effects for each VEGF ligand is accomplished through one of three receptors (VEGFRs), including VEGFR-1, VEGFR-2, and VEGFR-3. These receptors belong to the class III family of tyrosine kinase receptors and are typically expressed on the vascular and lymphatic endothelium. However, these receptors may also be expressed by tumor tissue. The overexpression of VEGF in tumor cells is associated with increased tumor growth and metastasis in several solid malignancies, including ovarian and endometrial cancer. Recent studies revealed

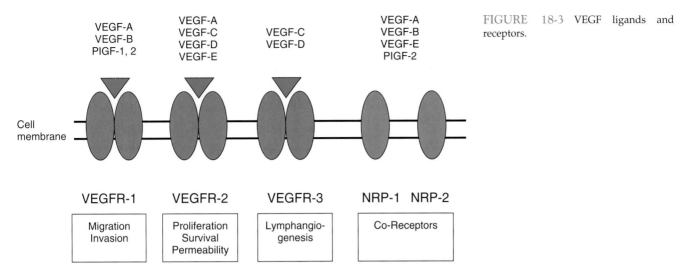

FIGURE 18-3 VEGF ligands and receptors.

that ovarian cancers expressing VEGF receptors have higher mortality rates compared to tumors lacking VEGF receptor expression.

Activation of a given VEGFR results in subsequent downstream activation of a variety of known survival, proliferation, and migration pathways in the cell. These downstream pathways include phosphoinositide-3-kinase/akt (PI3K-AKT), Ras and Raf superfamily-MAPK (Ras-Raf-MAPK), focal adhesion kinase (FAK), and v-src sarcoma viral oncogene homolog (SRC). The activity of the VEGFR2 appears to be potentiated by the binding of co-receptors, neuropilin-1 (NRP-1) on arteries, and NRP-2 on venous and lymphatic vessels. NRP-1 and NRP-2 may have intrinsic activity through the binding of small G proteins and regulation of the cytoskeleton also.

Given the importance of the VEGF pathway, the majority of angiogenesis-related targeted therapies are focused on the VEGF family of ligands and receptors. Current options for therapy summarized in Table 18-3 include drugs that directly target VEGF and its receptors and vascular disrupting agents that damage existing tumor related blood vessels.

Agents Targeting VEGF

Bevacizumab

OVARIAN CANCER

Bevacizumab, a humanized monoclonal antibody to human VEGF, was the first U.S. Food and Drug Administration (FDA)-approved drug targeting angiogenesis. In ovarian cancer, bevacizumab has been evaluated both as a single agent and in combination therapy for primary and recurrent disease. After encouraging preclinical studies and multiple case studies, the Gynecologic Oncology Group (GOG) instituted a phase II trial of single-agent bevacizumab (15 mg/kg every 3 weeks) in persistent or recurrent refractory epithelial ovarian

TABLE 18-3 Anti-Antigenic Therapies for Gynecologic Cancer

Drug	Class	Target
Bevacizumab	Mab	VEGF
VEGF-Trap	Receptor	VEGF
IMC-1121B	Mab	VEGFR-2
Cediranib	SMI	VEGFR
Sunitinib	SMI	VEGFR, PDGFR, EGF, KIT
Pazopanib	SMI	VEGFR1, VEGFR2, VEGFR3, PDGFR, KIT
Vatalanib	SMI	VEGFR1, VEGFR2, VEGFR3, PDGFR, KIT
Brivanib	SMI	VEGFR2, FGFR
Intedanib	SMI	VEGFR, PDGFR, FGFR
Vadimezan	VDA	Endothelial cell
Fosbretabulin	VDA	Endothelial cell

Mab, Monoclonal antibody; SMI, small molecule inhibitor; VDA, vascular disrupting agent.

cancer. Despite a heavily pretreated cohort, the authors reported 13 of 62 patients (21%) experienced a clinical response, including 11 patients with partial response (PR) and 2 patients with a complete response (CR). The median number of cycles was 7 and 25 patients (40.3%) had a progression-free survival of at least 6 months. Overall, toxicity was low and there were no reports of bowel perforation. Another phase II trial of bevacizumab (15 mg/kg every 3 weeks) in 44 ovarian cancer patients receiving third- or fourth-line chemotherapy demonstrated a partial response rate of 16%. Median progression-free survival was 4.4 months and median overall survival was 10.7 months at study closure. This study was terminated early secondary to 5 patients (11.4%) experiencing spontaneous bowel perforation. The risk of bowel perforation appeared to be higher in those patients with a higher median number of prior treatments and in whom impending bowel obstruction was suspected. Further studies are ongoing to elucidate a clear list of risk factors for perforation in the setting of bevacizumab therapy.

In the recurrent setting, bevacizumab has been evaluated in combination with both cytotoxic and biologic therapies. A phase II study of bevacizumab (10 mg/kg every 2 weeks) combined with oral cyclophosphamide (50 mg daily) demonstrated a partial response rate of 24% (17 of 70 patients) at a median follow-up of 23.2 months. Probability of being progression free at 6 months was 56% in this study. Overall toxicity was acceptable in this study. This combination has also been evaluated retrospectively at several institutions with similar encouraging results (objective response rate 44% to 53.3%). A phase II trial combining bevacizumab (15 mg/kg every 21 days) and oral erlotinib (150 mg daily) in 13 patients with recurrent müllerian cancer showed an objective response rate of 15% and a stable disease rate of 54%. However, this trial was stopped early secondary to lack of clear benefit of the combination over single-agent bevacizumab and a higher than expected rate of bowel perforation (15%).

Two phase II studies have been performed to evaluate the addition of bevacizumab (15 mg/kg every 21 days) to standard carboplatin (AUC 5) and paclitaxel (175 mg/m²) chemotherapy in the adjuvant setting for advanced müllerian cancer. Micha and colleagues noted an objective response rate of 80% among 21 patients with acceptable toxicity. An additional study of this regimen in 62 women after debulking surgery found a comparable response rate of 76% and a progression-free survival rate of 58% at 36 months. This study included 1 year of maintenance bevacizumab (15 mg/kg every 21 days), which resulted in mild toxicity over a median of 17 maintenance bevacizumab cycles. The National Cancer Institute (NCI) currently lists multiple phase I and II trials, which include bevacizumab for the treatment of primary or recurrent ovarian cancer.

Five major phase III trials have been initiated in ovarian cancer. In the upfront setting, GOG 218 and International Collaborative Ovarian Neoplasm (ICON) 7 both include bevacizumab in combination with standard cytotoxics followed by maintenance bevacizumab. Key characteristics of these studies are summarized in Table 18-4. Preliminary data from GOG 218 revealed a progression-free survival benefit of 3 months in the arm that included bevacizumab treatment up front and continued as single-agent maintenance. It is interesting that there was no progression-free survival benefit in the patients who only received adjuvant bevacizumab compared to standard therapy alone. Although different in design, ICON7 reached similar conclusions. In the arm receiving paclitaxel, carboplatin, and bevacizumab followed by bevacizumab maintenance, the progression-free survival was improved by 1.7 months (19.0 vs 17.3 months, HR 0.81, $P = 0.004$). Overall survival, albeit immature, was similar between the arms.

TABLE 18-4   Comparison of Trial Design of GOG 218 and ICON 7

	GOG 218	ICON 7
n	2000	1520
Type	Randomized Placebo-controlled	Randomized Open Label
Primary end points	Overall survival Progression-free survival	Progression-free survival
Secondary end points	Toxicity Quality of life Translational research	Overall survival Response rate Biologic progression-free survival Toxicity Quality of life Economics
Strata	Stage (III ≤1 cm vs >1 cm vs IV) PS: (0 vs 1-2)	Stage (I-III ≤1cm vs >1 cm vs IV) Chemo start (≤4 wk vs > 4) Enrolling center
Sites	490	142
Opened	September 2005	April 2006
Closed	June 2009	February 2009

GOG 213 is a bifactorial randomized study to evaluate the effect of the addition of bevacizumab to standard paclitaxel and carboplatin on overall survival in platinum-sensitive patients. This study is also addressing the benefit of secondary cytoreductive surgery by randomly assigning a subset of patients who meet criteria for cytoreduction to surgery versus no surgery before initiation of chemotherapy (Figure 18-4). In the OCEANS trial, patients with platinum-sensitive ovarian cancer are treated with gemcitabine and carboplatin with or without bevacizumab. This trial aims to evaluate progression-free survival and potential gastrointestinal toxicity of this combination. In the platinum-resistant setting, the AURELIA trial design compares bevacizumab with a standard agent, including paclitaxel, liposomal doxorubicin, or topotecan, to the standard agent alone.

The use of bevacizumab is also being explored in mucinous ovarian cancer. The Gynecologic Cancer Intergroup (GCIG) recently began accruing to a trial comparing two cytotoxic regimens, carboplatin and paclitaxel versus oxaliplatin and capecitabine, for the treatment of primary advanced or recurrent stage I mucinous ovarian cancer. Each arm undergoes an additional randomization for possible addition of bevacizumab to the regimen. The primary end point of this trial is overall survival.

Bevacizumab has also shown promise in nonepithelial ovarian cancer. A retrospective review of eight patients with recurrent granulosa cell tumors demonstrated a partial response rate of 38% and stable disease rate of 25%. These tumors are notoriously chemoresistant, and this study has encouraged the development of

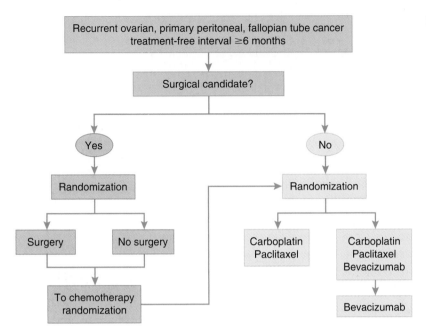

FIGURE 18-4   GOG 213 schema.

a phase II trial by the GOG evaluating bevacizumab for recurrent ovarian sex cord–stromal tumors.

UTERINE CANCER

VEGF expression has been correlated with adverse outcomes in endometrial cancer, and bevacizumab has demonstrated encouraging results in the preclinical setting. Thus far, results of the use of bevacizumab in uterine cancer are limited. A retrospective review of 11 patients with uterine cancer treated with bevacizumab combination therapy revealed two partial responses and three patients with stable disease. There were no major adverse reactions in this study. The GOG initiated a phase II study of single-agent bevacizumab (15 mg/kg every 21 days) for advanced endometrial cancer with preliminary results demonstrating a 15.1% response rate and median overall survival of 10.5 months. Multiple trials are currently under way to evaluate bevacizumab alone and in combination for the treatment of uterine cancer. Of note, the combination of bevacizumab and radiation therapy is also under evaluation in this disease site.

CERVICAL CANCER

Bevacizumab is the first targeted agent that has demonstrated activity in recurrent cervical cancer. A phase II trial of single-agent bevacizumab (15 mg/kg every 21 days) had promising results in a cohort of patient with fewer than three prior regimens, achieving a median overall survival of 7.29 months and acceptable toxicity. Five patients (10.9%) had a partial response and an additional 11 patients were progression free for a minimum of 6 months. Furthermore, an analysis of 6 patients treated with bevacizumab in combination with 5-fluorouracil or capecitabine demonstrated a clinical

benefit rate of 67%. There are several trials with bevacizumab in cervical cancer actively accruing in the upfront and recurrent settings. GOG 240 combines bevacizumab with standard chemotherapy in four regimens, described in Figure 18-5. The planned enrollment is 450 patients with primary stage IVB or recurrent cervical carcinoma and will evaluate overall survival, toxicity, and progression-free survival.

VEGF-Trap (Aflibercept)

VEGF-Trap is manufactured protein that acts as a decoy receptor for all VEGF-A isoforms and placental growth factor. This agent was engineered through fusion of the ligand-binding domains from two VEGF receptors with the constant region of IgG1, resulting in high-affinity VEGF binding and prevention of VEGF pathway activation. In the in vivo setting, VEGF-Trap was found to improve ascites and reduce tumor growth.

Initial phase I trials of VEGF-Trap for advanced solid malignancy demonstrated acceptable toxicity with clinical benefit approaching 50%. Several partial responses were observed in ovarian cancer. This led to a randomized phase II trial of VEGF-Trap (2 mg/kg vs 4 mg/kg) in platinum-resistant recurrent ovarian cancer. A response rate of 11% was reported with five partial responses and no mention of stable disease. VEGF-Trap has also been studied for the treatment of malignant ascites in ovarian cancer. Columbo and colleagues treated 12 patients with aflibercept (4 mg/kg) every 2 weeks and found successful prolongation in time to repeat paracentesis with minimal adverse advents. A recently published phase I/II, multi-institutional trial reported the activity and toxicity of aflibercept in combination with docetaxel in women with recurrent

FIGURE 18-5   GOG 240 schema.

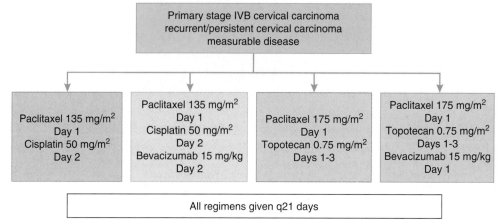

FIGURE 18-6   ICON 6 schema. Randomization is 2:3:3 in this trial.

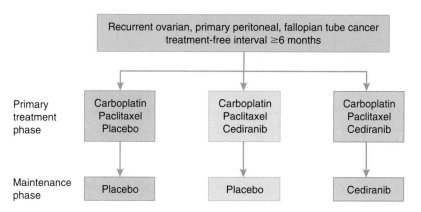

ovarian cancer. Overall response in the Phase II component was 54%, including 11 of 25 responders being complete. Median PFS and OS were 6.4 and 26.6 month, respectively. As expected, the most frequent aflibercept-associated toxicity was hypertension (11% grade 1 or 2). The GOG has also completed a single agent study of aflibercept in endometrial cancer.

Agents Targeting VEGF Receptors

IMC-1121B (Ramucirumab)

IMC-1121B is the most developed fully humanized monoclonal antibody to VEGFR-2. A phase I trial in 12 patients with advanced solid malignancy demonstrated a clinical benefit in 9 patients (2 partial responses, 7 with stable disease). These promising results have led to a phase II trial of IMC-1121B in recurrent ovarian cancer. Several other monoclonal antibodies to VEGF receptors are still in development, including IMC-18F1 and IMC-1C11.

AZD2171 (Cediranib)

Cediranib is a small molecule inhibitor of VEGFR-2, platelet-derived growth factor receptor (PDGFR), and c-kit, which has shown promise in several phase II trials.

In a study of 46 patients with recurrent ovarian cancer, the clinical benefit rate of single-agent cediranib was 30%. Eight patients achieved partial response and 6 patients had stable disease, and median progression-free survival for the group was 5.2 months. Hirte and colleagues reported a response rate of 41% in platinum-sensitive and 29% in platinum-resistant ovarian malignancy. Toxicities in both studies included diarrhea, hypertension, mucositis, fatigue, and anorexia. Cediranib is currently being evaluated in the upfront setting in combination with standard paclitaxel and carboplatin as part of ICON6 (Figure 18-6). In addition, the use of single-agent cediranib will be studied by the GOG for the treatment of recurrent endometrial cancer.

Agents Targeting Multiple VEGF-Related Molecules

Sunitinib

Sunitinib is an oral receptor tyrosine kinase inhibitor whose targets include VEGFR, PDGFR, epidermal growth factor (EGF), and the stem cell factor (KIT) receptor. This drug is currently being evaluated in the treatment of recurrent ovarian cancer in several phase II trials and one phase III trial. An interim report of a phase II trial of sunitinib (50 mg daily) in recurrent ovarian

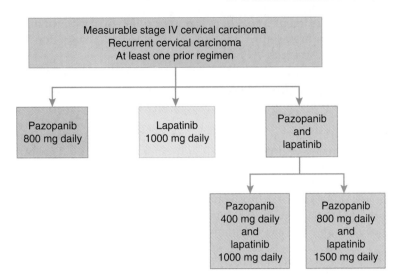

FIGURE 18-7 Schema of trial of pazopanib and lapatinib for advanced cervical cancer.

cancer demonstrated a 70% clinical benefit with partial response in 2 patients and stable disease in 10 patients. Common side effects were hand and foot reaction, fatigue, hypertension, and mucositis. Mackay and colleagues reported the results from a phase II trial of sunitinib (50 mg daily) in 19 patients with advanced or metastatic cervical cancer. Although they achieved no objective responses, 16 patients achieved stable disease with a median duration of 4.4 months. There are several ongoing active phase II trials of single-agent sunitinib in endometrial and cervical cancer and clear cell ovarian cancer (GOG 254).

Pazopanib

Pazopanib inhibits all of the VEGF receptors (VEGFR1, VEGFR2, and VEGFR3) and PDGFR-α and -β and the KIT receptor. This small molecule inhibitor (800 mg daily) has been evaluated in a phase II study of 36 patients with recurrent ovarian cancer by CA-125 and nonbulky disease. This study revealed a 31% response by CA-125 level and a 56% stable disease rate. Among the 17 patients with measurable disease, 18% had a partial response. Ongoing ovarian cancer studies of pazopanib include combination with liposomal doxorubicin in the recurrent setting and in combination with paclitaxel/carboplatin in the upfront setting. A phase III, placebo-controlled study of pazopanib for consolidation after completion of primary chemotherapy in ovarian cancer has recently completed enrollment. In cervical cancer, pazopanib was explored alone and in combination with lapatinib (a small molecule EGFR inhibitor to be discussed later) in the treatment of advanced and recurrent disease (Figure 18-7). The combination pazopanib and lapatinib arm was closed early following a futility analysis, leaving the randomized phase II trial to compare pazopanib to single-agent lapatinib. Both progression-free (HR, 0.66, 90% CI, 0.48-0.91) and overall survival (HR, 0.67, 90% CI,

0.49-0.99) were superior in the monotherapy pazopanib arm. Median OS was 50.7 weeks versus 39.1 weeks for pazopanib and lapatinib, respectively.

Vatalanib (PTK787)

This tyrosine kinase inhibitor acts on all of the VEGFRs, PDGFR, and KIT receptor. Activity against ovarian cancer is being actively explored and has been promising in a front-line phase I trial in advanced disease in combination with paclitaxel and carboplatin.

Brivanib

Brivanib alaninate is a prodrug of brivanib, a dual inhibitor of VEGFR2 and FGFR. This compound has demonstrated acceptable toxicity and activity when given alone or in combination, in multiple solid tumors, including hepatocellular carcinoma refractory to other antiangiogenic therapies. Brivanib is under evaluation for advanced or recurrent endometrial cancer as part of the GOG 229 queue.

BIBF-1120 (Intedanib)

BIBF-1120 is a multikinase inhibitor targeting three key angiogenic receptors: VEGFR, PDGFR, and FGFR. A phase I trial of this agent in patients with gynecologic malignancies revealed a promising response rate, with five of seven patients with measurable disease demonstrating response and two achieving stable disease. BIBF-1120 (250 mg daily) was evaluated as a maintenance therapy compared to placebo in recurrent ovarian cancer after response to standard therapy. Although the trial was not powered to compare the two arms, PFS was less in the placebo arm (2.8 mo) compared to the BIBF-1120 arm (4.8 mo). This agent is currently under investigation in a randomized control trial combined with standard paclitaxel and carboplatin in previously untreated primary ovarian cancer patients.

Vascular Disrupting Agents

This broad group of anti-angiogenic drugs acts to occlude preexisting vasculature in the tumor rather than prevent neovascularization. The disturbance of existing vessels leads to ischemia, hemorrhagic necrosis, and ultimately cellular death. Of note, these agents are able to selectively target tumor blood vessels by taking advantage of the differences between normal and tumor endothelial cells. Figure 18-8 demonstrates the necrosis caused by treatment with a vascular disrupting agent. Two major types of vascular disrupting agents exist: small molecule–based and ligand-based. The majority of vascular disrupting agents under evaluation in gynecologic cancers target small molecules.

Vadimezan (ASA404/DMXAA)

Vadimezan, 5,6-dimethylxanthenone-4-acetic acid, is a flavone acetic acid analog that increases production and release of tumor necrosis factor α. This leads to endothelial cell apoptosis and decreased perfusion of the tumor. Gabra and colleagues evaluated this drug in combination with paclitaxel and carboplatin for the treatment of recurrent ovarian cancer. The arm that received vadimezan conferred significant improvement in response rate when compared to the control arm (64% vs 49%) without additional adverse effects.

Fosbretabulin (Combretastatin A4); Ombrabulin (AVE8062)

Fosbretablin is a tubulin-binding agent that causes vascular congestion and decreased tumor blood flow by changing endothelial cell shape. This effect is very rapid, occurring within 1 hour of drug administration. This agent has been evaluated primarily for the treatment of platinum-resistant ovarian cancer. Treatment with combretastatin A4 (63 mg/m²) in addition to paclitaxel (175 mg/m²) and carboplatin (AUC 5) resulted in a 32% response rate without additional observed toxicity. A randomized phase II trial of bevacizumab with or without fosbretabulin is under development at the GOG. Ombrabulin is a combrestatin derivative that has shown excellent efficacy in preclinical ovarian cancer models.

This agent appears to have a similar toxicity profile to combretastatin A4 and is undergoing evaluation in phase I trials.

Other Anti-Angiogenic Agents

Thalidomide

Thalidomide is a legacy agent that has found recent renewed interest as an anti-angiogenic agent. Thalidomide inhibits FGF-2 by interacting with the FGF-2 receptor. In addition, this agent acts as an immune modulator by inducing production of interferon γ, IL-2, and IL-10. Thalidomide (200 mg daily) added 4 months to overall survival when added to topotecan (1.25 mg/m²) for the treatment of recurrent ovarian cancer. A phase II of thalidomide (200-1000 mg daily) in persistent or recurrent endometrial cancer demonstrated a 25% clinical benefit with two partial responses and four patients with disease stabilization. The GOG recently reported randomized phase III trial results comparing thalidomide (200 mg daily) to tamoxifen (20 mg daily) for biochemically recurrent ovarian carcinoma. In this study, there was essentially no difference in progression-free survival, with thalidomide achieving 3.2 months compared to 4.5 months for tamoxifen. Furthermore, patients receiving thalidomide had a higher incidence of grade III and IV toxicity. Common toxicities of thalidomide include hematologic, gastrointestinal, and cardiovascular complications. Thalidomide is currently under evaluation in ovarian cancer as a possible consolidation agent and in combination with carboplatin in the recurrent setting. Lenalidomide (Revlimid) is a thalidomide derivative currently under analysis in combination with traditional cytotoxic agents for recurrent ovarian cancer.

PHOSPHATIDYLINOSITOL-3-KINASE/ AKT PATHWAY

The PI3K/AKT pathway plays a central role in cell survival, growth, and avoidance of apoptosis. Figure 18-9 demonstrates a simple schematic of this complex pathway that is known to interact with many other

FIGURE 18-8 Antitumor effects of vascular disrupting agent, AVE8062. *(Used with permission from Kim et al: Cancer Research 67:9337, 2007.)*

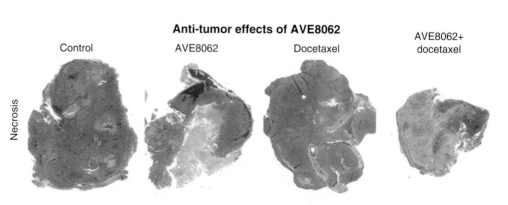

Anti-tumor effects of AVE8062

Control   AVE8062   Docetaxel   AVE8062+ docetaxel

Necrosis

cellular growth and survival pathways. This pathway may be activated by a large number of receptor tyrosine kinases, including the EGFR family and the insulin-like growth factor receptors (IGFRs). Thus a variety of mitogenic substances are involved in its activation.

Activation of the pathway starts with the PI3K family, which are lipid and serine/threonine kinases composed of heterodimers including a catalytic and regulatory subunit. Activation of PI3K leads to phosphorylation of phosphatidylionositol-4,5-bisphospate (PIP2) to phosphatidylinositol-3,4,5-triphosphate (PIP3). PIP3 acts as a second messenger to bind a variety of targets and recruit them to the plasma membrane, leading to their activation. One critical downstream mediator of PIP3 is AKT, which on activation acts on a number of different targets that directly affect cellular survival, proliferation through activation of transcription/translation, evasion of apoptosis, and resistance to chemotherapy. One key downstream target of AKT is the mammalian target of rapamycin (mTOR), a serine/threonine kinase. The upregulation of mTOR by AKT leads to activation of downstream regulator protein S6 kinase, which directly affects protein translation and the progression of growth through the cell cycle.

The PI3K/AKT pathway is known to be activated in a variety of cancers, especially in gynecologic malignancies. The phosphatase and tensin homolog on chromosome 10 (PTEN) is a tumor suppressor that encodes for a serine/threonine kinase, which acts directly to dephosphorylate PIP3 to PIP2. In patients with PTEN mutation and loss of function, there is an overaccumulation of PIP3, leading to constitutive activation of the AKT pathway. The PI3K/AKT pathway is also frequently activated through mutations in PIK3CA, which encodes for the activating subunit (110α) of PI3K or through mutations in AKT.

As described in Chapter 19, the aforementioned mutations are commonly found in endometrial cancer and less frequently in the other gynecologic malignancies. Furthermore, this pathway is thought to be targeted more frequently in cancer than any other pathway aside from p53. Thus PI3K/AKT signaling provides a promising target for the treatment of malignancy and is under active exploration. Currently, the drugs targeting this pathway consist primarily of small-molecule inhibitors of key pathway components. The inhibition of only one member of the pathway may not be sufficient to affect tumor growth given the significant pathway cross-talk and feedback loops. For example, mTOR is known to regulate cellular growth and proliferation through activation of several downstream proteins. These proteins also participate in a feedback loop that can lead to subsequent upregulation of AKT phosphorylation. Thus the exploration of combination therapies in this pathway is paramount.

Agents Targeting mTOR (Rapalogues)

Temsirolimus (CC1-779)

To date, the mTOR inhibitor with the most promise in gynecologic cancers is temsirolimus, a water-soluble

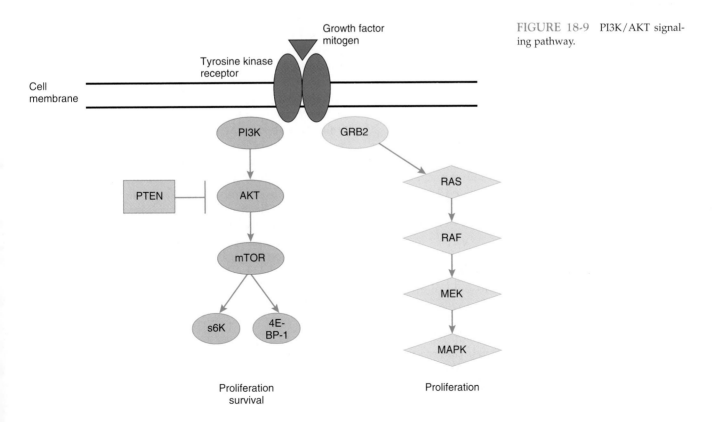

FIGURE 18-9 PI3K/AKT signaling pathway.

ester of rapamycin given parenterally. Temsirolimus (25 mg weekly) had favorable response rate in a phase II trial of patients with recurrent or metastatic endometrial cancer treated with a maximum of one prior regimen. Twenty-five percent of 19 evaluable patients had a partial response and an additional 63% achieved stable disease. A study of temsirolimus (25 mg IV weekly) in 27 heavily pretreated patients with recurrent endometrial cancer achieved partial response in 2 patients and stable disease in 12 patients. Temkin and colleagues reported on a phase I trial of temsirolimus combined with topotecan to treat a variety of advanced and recurrent gynecologic malignancies. The drug combination was well tolerated in patients without a history of radiotherapy and achieved stable disease in 9 of 11 patients at 8 weeks. Trials incorporating temsirolimus have shown manageable toxicities including hypertriglyceridemia, hyperglycemia, electrolyte abnormalities, and rash.

Ongoing studies of this drug in endometrial cancer include combination regimens of temsirolimus and a variety of cytotoxic and hormone therapies. The GOG has recently opened a randomized phase II trial of a variety of combination therapies for endometrial cancer (GOG0086P; NCT:00977574). There are three arms in this trial, including temsirolimus in combination with paclitaxel and carboplatin; compared to bevacizumab, paclitaxel, carboplatin; and ixabepilone, paclitaxel, carboplatin. Other studies combining temsirolimus with bevacizumab in ovarian cancer and temsirolimus as a single-agent therapy in advanced or recurrent cervical cancer are ongoing.

Everolimus (RAD001)

Everolimus is an orally bioavailable ester that is a potent inhibitor of mTOR. The largest phase II study of everolimus (10 mg daily) as a single agent in recurrent endometrial cancer demonstrated an encouraging short- and long-term clinical benefit rate with 43% and 21% of patients achieving stable disease at 8 weeks and 20 weeks, respectively. Given these results, current studies of this drug are in combination with other targeted agents, traditional cytotoxic chemotherapy, and hormones. The latter combination has gained keen interest in breast and endometrial cancers as endocrine resistance may be mediated by activation of the PI3K pathway.

Ridaforolimus (AP23573; MK-8669)

Ridaforolimus, previously known as deforolimus, is an mTOR inhibitor that may be given orally or intravenously. In a phase II study of ridaforolimus (12.5 mg daily × 5 days every other week) for patients with advanced or recurrent endometrial cancer, 9 of 27 patients achieved clinical benefit, including 2 with partial response. A recent multi-institutional randomized phase II trial of ridaforolimus (40 mg orally for 5 days every 28 days) in women with recurrent, previously treated endometrial cancer has been reported. The control arm of the trial was the physician's choice of either hormones or chemotherapy. Overall, 150 patients (114 evaluable) were enrolled; 64 to ridaforolimus, 53 to hormonal therapy, and 13 to chemotherapy. The response rates in each arm were similar (8% vs 4% for ridaforolimus and control, respectively). However, PFS was significantly longer in the ridaforolimus arm when assessed by either the investigators or by independent radiological review. Overall survival is maturing.

Agents Targeting AKT

Perifosine is an alkylphospholipid with oral bioavailability that is thought to have multiple mechanisms of antitumor activity. One relevant mechanism is the inhibition of AKT by prevention of its recruitment to the cell membrane. Perifosine has shown response in phase I trials for advanced solid tumors. A trial combining this drug with docetaxel in recurrent ovarian cancer is currently ongoing. MKC-1 is a cell cycle inhibitor shown to reduce the levels of phosphorylated AKT in cell lines. A phase II trial of MKC-1 (125 mg/m^2 orally bid) in advanced endometrial and ovarian cancer demonstrated promising results. This included 37% of ovarian and 44% of endometrial cancer patients with stable disease. Most common toxicities were fatigue, elevated liver transaminases, and gastrointestinal disorders. Many other AKT-inhibiting agents are currently in preclinical development and undergoing evaluation in phase I trials for solid tumors.

MK-2206 is a highly selective non-ATP competitive allosteric Akt inhibitor that is equally potent against Akt1 and Akt2 and demonstrated efficacy in vitro and in vivo in several tumor models. A phase I dose escalation study in patients with solid tumors has been completed to identify tolerance of the compound at 60 mg orally every other day. Dose-limiting toxicities were skin rash, mucosal inflammation, and hyperglycemia. Three ovarian cancer patients treated in this study had reducing CA-125 values. Although the ras/raf/MEK pathway activation can promote cell survival in the presence of Akt blockade, interest in this agent in ovarian and endometrial cancer is actively being sought, both as a single agent and in combination with ras/raf/MEK blockade.

Agents Targeting PI3K

Although there are several companies exploring the inhibition of PI3Kinase in solid tumors, there are only two PI3K inhibitors in Phase II trials. XL147 (SAR245408) is a highly selective oral inhibitor of PI3K and successfully inhibits tumor growth in vivo. A phase I trial of

XL147 revealed acceptable toxicity and durable clinical benefit. A phase I trial combining XL147 with carboplatin and paclitaxel is currently in dose expansion for ovarian and endometrial cancer patients secondary to favorable responses in those tumor types. XL147 is also under phase II evaluation for the treatment of advanced and recurrent endometrial cancer.

Enzastaurin is an oral multikinase inhibitor that primarily acts to suppress tumor growth through the inhibition of PI3K. A phase I study of enzastaurin combined with bevacizumab revealed promising responses in advanced solid tumors, especially among ovarian cancer (29% PR/CR). Furthermore, 51% of 21 ovarian cancer patients remained in the study for greater than 6 months. A phase II study of enzastaurin alone in recurrent ovarian cancer had limited activity, with a response rate of only 7.4% (D. Armstrong, personal communication). These results have led to the development of several phase II trials of enzastaurin in combination with standard chemotherapy for advanced or ovarian cancer.

Combination Agents

In addition to the agents targeting specific aspects of the PI3K/AKT pathway noted previously, there are a large number of combination drugs in development and in early clinical trials. These include combination PI3K/mTOR, PI3K/AKT, and PI3K/MEK inhibitors. As already noted, given the extensive cross-talk and feedback loops involved in this pathway, the inhibition of two major nodes in the pathway is rational and will likely lead to improved outcomes.

EPIDERMAL GROWTH FACTOR RECEPTOR PATHWAY

The EGFR pathway was identified as an anticancer therapy target secondary to myriad genetic alterations found in a variety of solid tumor types, including ovarian, endometrial, and cervical carcinomas. The pathway consists of four tyrosine kinase cell-surface receptors including EGFR (ErbB-1), HER2/neu (ErbB-2), Her-3 (ErbB-3), and Her-4 (ErbB-4). Each receptor is specific for a variety of ligands, including epidermal growth factor (EGF), transforming growth factor α (TGF-α), and neuregulins (NRGs) (Table 18-5). Although the receptors are activated through a traditional tyrosine kinase receptor mechanism, they also require the union between two identical receptors (homodimerization) or two different receptors within the same family (heterodimerization) for downstream activation.

Upon activation, the EGFRs induce activation of a variety of cell survival pathways including the ras/raf/MEK and PI3K pathways (Figure 18-10). In addition,

TABLE 18-5 EGF Ligands and Receptor

EGF Receptor	Ligands
EGFR (ErbB-1)	Epidermal growth factor (EGF)
	Transforming growth factor α
	Amphiregulin
	Epigen
	Betacellulin
	Heparin-binding growth factor
	Epiregulin
HER2/neu (ErbB-2)	None
HER-3 (ErbB-3)	Neuregulin 1
	Neuregulin 2
HER-4 (ErbB-4)	Betacellulin
	Heparin-binding growth factor
	Epiregulin
	Neuregulin 1
	Neuregulin 2
	Neuregulin 3
	Neuregulin 4
	Tomoregulin

EGFRs are known to negatively affect apoptosis and induce invasion. EGFRs are also present on endothelial cells within the tumor microenvironment. EGF ligands demonstrate a direct effect on the endothelial cells, leading to increase in endothelial cell proliferation and angiogenesis. Thus targeting this pathway has been an area of significant research for the treatment of gynecologic malignancies. Unfortunately, recent studies of drugs affecting the EGFR pathway have only demonstrated modest success in gynecologic cancer. This may be explained in part by research that demonstrates that EGFR has a role in glucose transport in cancer cells. EGFR associates with the sodium/glucose cotransporter (SGLT1) to promote the uptake of glucose into cancer cells. Of note, the action appears to be kinase independent. Thus the blockage of kinase activity with antibodies or small molecules may not be sufficient to make a significant impact on tumorigenesis. Furthermore, based on data in multiple tumor types response to EGFR inhibitors appears to be correlated with mutation status rather than expression. The rate of EGFR mutations in gynecologic malignancies is quite low; thus potential for success of these compounds as a single agent is unclear.

Small Molecule Inhibitors Targeting EGFR

Gefitinib

Gefitinib is a small molecule inhibitor that prevents EGFR activation through binding the ATP-binding site of the receptor. This agent has been evaluated extensively in ovarian cancer with unsatisfactory results. Gefitinib (500 mg daily) was evaluated in a phase II trial in 30 patients with recurrent or persistent ovarian cancer treated with up to two prior regimens. Of 27 evaluable patients, 4 had stable disease for more than 6 months and

FIGURE 18-10   EGFR signaling pathway.

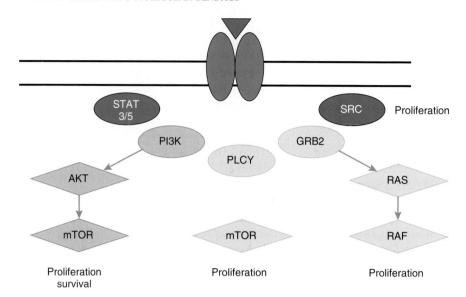

only 1 patient had an objective response. Of note, patients with EGFR expression in their tumor had longer median progression-free survival and the one objective response was found in a patient with a mutation in EGFR. This suggests that the use of mutation status to guide targeted therapies may provide better response rates.

Gefitinib (500 mg daily) has also been evaluated in combination with carboplatin (AUC 5) and paclitaxel (175 mg/m²) for platinum-sensitive and platinum-resistant recurrent ovarian cancer. Nineteen percent of platinum-resistant and 62% of platinum-sensitive patients had response to this combination therapy. Overall survival was also acceptable, reaching 17 months for the resistant group and 26 months for the sensitive group. However, there appeared to be more hematologic toxicity when compared to the standard regimen. The combination of gefitinib (500 mg daily) with tamoxifen (40 mg daily) in recurrent ovarian cancer required dose reduction secondary to diarrhea in 10 of 56 patients and resulted in no objective responses. However, 16 patients achieved stable disease and median survival was 253 days.

The only published trial of gefitinib (500 mg daily) in cervical cancer reported minimal activity. Of 28 evaluable patients, there were no objective responses and 20% achieved stable disease for a median duration of 112 days. It is interesting that disease control was not associated with the expression of EGFR in tumor specimens. Additional trials of gefitinib monotherapy in recurrent cervical, endometrial, and ovarian cancer are ongoing. Furthermore, gefitinib is under evaluation for treatment of recurrent ovarian cancer in combination with topotecan and anastrazole.

Erlotinib

Erlotinib (150 mg daily) is reversible inhibitor of EGFR, acting to block autophosphorylation of the tyrosine kinase portion of the receptor. Preliminary results of a trial of erlotinib in combination with standard paclitaxel (175 mg/m²) and carboplatin (AUC 6) for first-line treatment in ovarian cancer are promising, and the trial is continuing accrual into the second stage.

In the setting of recurrent ovarian cancer, erlotinib has been primarily evaluated in combination with other therapies, although a solo trial is ongoing. Erlotinib in combination with carboplatin (AUC 5) achieved a response rate of 57% in the platinum-sensitive arm and 7% in the platinum-resistant arm with no unexpected toxicities. As noted previously, a trial of erlotinib with bevacizumab (15 mg/kg) was terminated early secondary to a high level of bowel perforation. The use of erlotinib as a single agent in chemotherapy-naïve endometrial cancer was well tolerated and 4 of 32 patients had an objective response. In addition, 15 patients had stable disease lasting a median of 4 months. EGFR mutations were evaluated and did not correlate with response.

Schilder and colleagues reported disappointing results of erlotinib as a single agent in cervical cancer, with only 1 of 25 patients achieving objective response and 4 with stable disease. Only 1 patient in this trial had progression-free survival greater than 6 months. The combination of erlotinib with cisplatin (40 mg/m² weekly) with radiotherapy in locally advanced cervical cancer was found to be feasible, with acceptable toxicity and a complete response rate of 91%. Further studies of this drug as a single agent in cervical cancer and as a consolidation therapy in ovarian cancer are ongoing.

Monoclonal Antibodies Targeting EGFR

Cetuximab

Cetuximab (250 mg/m²) is a chimerized monoclonal antibody to the ligand-binding domain EGFR, which has been evaluated as a treatment for primary and recurrent ovarian cancer as a single agent and in combination with traditional cytotoxics. As a single agent in 25 patients, cetuximab achieved only 1 partial response and 9 patients with stable disease. Median progression-free survival was only 2.1 months. Cetuximab in combination with carboplatin (AUC 6) in 28 patients with recurrent platinum-sensitive ovarian cancer also had disappointing results, with only 9 objective responses and 8 patients with stable disease. Although cetuximab in combination with paclitaxel (175 mg/m^2) and carboplatin (AUC 6) was well tolerated, it offered no increased benefit in terms of progression-free survival when compared to traditional cytotoxic agents alone.

The combination of cetuximab with topotecan (0.75 mg/m^2) and cisplatin (50 mg/m^2) for advanced cervical cancer induced a high rate of serious adverse events including myelosuppression, infection, and skin reaction. Furthermore, five patients died, with three deaths attributable to toxicity. Cetuximab and cisplatin (30 mg/m^2) for recurrent cervical cancer was better tolerated but did not show any additional benefit compared to historical rates of cisplatin alone. A recent GOG study of single-agent cetuximab for recurrent endometrial cancer has completed accrual and preliminary results are pending.

Trastuzumab

The overexpression of HER2 in gynecologic cancers has been associated with prognosis in endometrial cancer and other gynecologic malignancies. Trastuzumab is a humanized monoclonal antibody to the extracellular domain of HER2, which prevents ligand binding. Although this drug has found great success in the treatment of Her-2/neu–positive breast cancer, its use in gynecologic oncology has been limited. A phase II trial of trastuzumab (2 mg/kg) for patients with advanced or recurrent HER2-positive endometrial cancer demonstrated no responses. Of 30 patients, 12 had stable disease, and the trial was closed early secondary to poor accrual. This drug is not currently under investigation in any gynecologic cancer.

Pertuzumab

The humanized monoclonal antibody pertuzumab prevents the linkage of HER2 to other receptors by binding a protein site in the dimerization domain. To date, pertuzumab has only been evaluated in recurrent ovarian cancer. In a trial of two dosing regimens of pertuzumab (840 mg loading with 420 mg every 21 days vs 1050 mg every 21 days), five patients achieved partial response and eight patients had stable disease. This study found a trend toward improved median progression-free survival and expression of phospho-HER2. The GOG evaluated pertuzumab as a monotherapy in recurrent ovarian cancer and achieved an overall response rate of 4.3%. An additional 6.8% of patients had stable disease for greater than 6 months. A large randomized trial comparing gemcitabine (800 mg/m^2) alone to gemcitabine with pertuzumab (420 mg every 21 days) found that the addition of pertuzumab resulted in improved response rates (4.6% vs 13.8%, respectively) and a trend toward improved progression-free survival. The greatest treatment benefit was found in patients with low HER3 mRNA expression. Further studies of pertuzumab for the treatment of recurrent ovarian cancer are accruing.

Matuzumab

Matuzumab is a humanized monoclonal antibody that binds to the ligand-binding domain of EGFR with higher affinity than natural EGFR ligands. This agent was evaluated in a group of 37 heavily pretreated patients with EGFR-positive recurrent ovarian cancer. Although no clinical responses were observed, 21% of patients achieved stable disease for more than 3 months with acceptable toxicity.

Combination Agents

Lapatinib

Lapatinib is an oral tyrosine kinase inhibitor of EGFR and HER2. It acts through binding of the ATP-binding domain and prevents pathway activation downstream. The evaluation of lapatinib has primarily been in combination with other agents. In recurrent ovarian cancer, lapatinib (1000 mg daily) with metronomic carboplatin (AUC 2 weekly) and paclitaxel (60 mg/m^2 weekly) achieved response rates of 50% and stable disease in 30% of patients. These results are especially encouraging given the high number of median prior therapies in this group of patients. Other combinations with lapatinib including carboplatin and topotecan have not been as successful and have demonstrated unacceptable toxicity.

The use of lapatinib in combination with pazopanib in cervical cancer was discussed earlier in the chapter. The GOG also recently completed first-stage accrual for a trial of lapatinib as monotherapy in recurrent or advanced endometrial cancer. Results are currently unavailable; however, this trial did not enter the second stage of accrual, indicating probable low levels of response.

POLY-ADP-RIBOSE POLYMERASE PATHWAY

DNA damage can be repaired through a variety of pathways in the cell including base excision, direct repair, mismatch repair, and nucleotide excision repair. High activity of DNA damage repair pathways is a known mechanism of resistance to cytotoxic chemotherapy. Poly-ADP-ribose polymerase (PARP) is a nuclear enzyme that contributes to the repair of single-stranded breaks in DNA along the base excision repair pathway (Figure 18-11). When PARP is inhibited, accumulation of

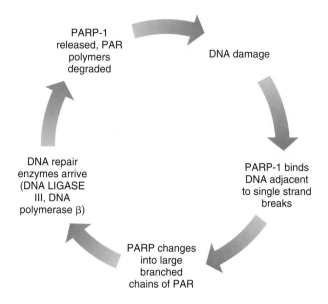

FIGURE 18-11   Function of PARP in DNA repair.

single-stranded breaks can lead to double-stranded breaks and cellular death. The use of PARP inhibitors in carriers of *BRCA* mutations is promising because tumor cells in these patients have impaired double-stranded break repair mechanisms. These drugs have been primarily explored in ovarian cancer given the strong correlation between *BRCA* mutations and this disease.

Olaparib

Olaparib is the most studied PARP inhibitor to date in ovarian cancer. Preclinically, this orally active PARP inhibitor induces synthetic lethality in cells deficient in *BRCA*. In an ongoing study of two doses of olaparib in *BRCA*-mutant patients with advanced ovarian cancer, both doses were well tolerated and demonstrated modest effect. Olaparib at 100 mg bid achieved a response rate of 12.5% and a clinical benefit rate of 16.7% among 24 patients. The 400-mg bid dose had higher levels of response and clinical benefit among 33 patients, 33% and 57.6%, respectively. Additional phase II studies of olaparib in recurrent serous ovarian cancer have confirmed favorable response in patients with and without *BRCA* mutations. Olaparib also appears to reintroduce chemosensitivity to carboplatin and paclitaxel in heavily pretreated patients. Of note, some mutation carriers appear resistant to this therapy. Proposed mechanisms of PARP inhibitor resistance include the presence of secondary *BRCA2* mutations that restore *BRCA* function.

Overall, PARP inhibitors are well tolerated. Fatigue, nausea, and vomiting are the most common toxicities. In addition, cognitive dysfunction, consisting of mood alterations, has been described as a dose-limiting toxicity. Early studies have also indicated there may be increased toxicity when combing PARP inhibitors with traditional cytotoxic chemotherapy, necessitating dose reduction. Whether this class of compound outperforms chemotherapy in selected germline *BRCA* mutation carries is debatable. A recent randomized phase II trial compared olaparib (200 mg bid and 400 mg bid) to pegylated liposomal doxorubicin (50 mg/m^2) in *BRCA* patients progressing within 12 months of platinum. The primary end point was progression-free survival. Although response rates were numerically higher for the olaparib arms, PFS was no different between the arms. Nevertheless, several additional PARP inhibitors (e.g., iniparib, veliparib, MK-4827, etc.) are currently under study in mutation carriers and sporadic ovarian cancer.

MULTIPATHWAY TARGETED AGENTS

Sorafenib

Sorafenib is an interesting small molecule inhibitor that effectively blocks several angiogenesis-related receptors (VEGFR, PDGFR, and KIT) and raf, a key component of the Raf-MAPK kinase (MEK)-MAPK proliferation pathway. Sorafenib is of considerable interest in ovarian cancer that has been shown to harbor alterations in this pathway. Consequently, several trials are ongoing to evaluate the efficacy of sorafenib in the upfront, recurrent, and consolidation setting. Matei and colleagues reported the results of a phase II trial of sorafenib (400 mg bid) in recurrent ovarian cancer treated with fewer than two prior therapies. Of 73 patients, 22 achieved partial response or stable disease with toxicities including rash and metabolic abnormalities. Of note, among the 59 patients with measurable disease, 12 were progression free for at least 6 months. The combination of sorafenib (200 mg twice daily) with bevacizumab (5 mg/kg) for the treatment of solid tumors was explored in a phase I study. Although the combination appeared to have significant activity in 13 patients with ovarian cancer (43% response rate), toxicity was common, leading to sorafenib dose reductions in 74% of patients. The most prevalent toxicities were diarrhea, elevated liver transaminases, hypertension, hand and foot syndrome, and fatigue.

In combination with traditional cytotoxic chemotherapy, including topotecan and gemcitabine, sorafenib has shown similar clinical benefit rates in recurrent ovarian cancer with minimal additional toxicity. A current phase III trial in newly diagnosed ovarian cancer after cytoreductive surgery seeks to determine if the addition of sorafenib (400 mg bid) to standard paclitaxel (175 mg/m^2) and carboplatin (AUC 6) provides any additional progression-free survival benefit. Sorafenib is also being explored as a maintenance agent in ovarian cancer and an additional chemosensitizer in the upfront treatment of advanced cervical cancer with radiotherapy.

Vandetanib

Vandetanib inhibits the tyrosine kinase activity of two parallel pathways through action on VEGFR-2 and EGFR. This leads to suppression of angiogenesis, cell proliferation, migration, and survival mechanisms. A phase II trial of vandetanib alone to treat recurrent ovarian cancer was terminated after the first stage of accrual because no patients achieved response or stable disease. Of note, molecular testing in this study revealed evidence of blockage of the EGFR pathway but no activity against VEGFR. Although single-agent activity has been disappointing, this agent is currently under exploration in combination with docetaxel and liposomal doxorubicin for the treatment of ovarian cancer.

Imatinib

Imatinib mesylate is an example of a small molecule that inhibits multiple pathways, including c-kit, bcr-abl, and PDGFR. Although imatinib has been quite successful for the treatment of chronic myelogenous leukemia, in which the tyrosine kinase bcr-abl is constitutively activated, the success in gynecologic malignancies as a single agent has been limited. This may result in part from the impact of the PDGF axis on pericytes, which are mesenchymal cells that support endothelial cells and newly developing blood vessels. PDGF activity recruits pericytes, which produce VEGF to stimulate angiogenesis and survival. Research on pericytes has indicated that blocking the PDGF axis in addition to the VEGF axis may be necessary to achieve improved response rates. Thus far, imatinib has only been explored as a single agent or in combination with cytotoxic chemotherapy for gynecologic malignancies.

Several phase II trials for recurrent ovarian cancer have been performed utilizing imatinib (400 mg daily) as a single agent. Unfortunately, rates of response have been low, with only one objective responder in all three trials. Rates of stable disease ranged from 14% to 33%. Similar disappointing results have been seen in cervical cancer. In a trial of 12 patients with recurrent cervical cancer treated with imatinib, there were no responses and only 1 patient with stable disease. In all trials, expression of drug-related targets has not been associated with response. The use of imatinib in combination with docetaxel (30 mg/m^2 weekly) in 23 patients with recurrent ovarian cancer achieved 5 responses, including 1 complete response. Three additional patients had stable disease lasting greater than 4 months. Further evaluations of this drug in combination with other cytotoxic chemotherapy for recurrent ovarian cancer are ongoing.

Dasatinib

Dasatinib is a strong inhibitor of the Src family of kinases, which participate in the regulation of cellular growth, adhesion, invasion, and migration. At higher concentrations, dasatinib has effects on a variety of different targets relevant to tumor progression including bcr-abl, c-kit, and PDGF. In addition, dasatinib targets the EphA2 receptor, which modulates cell migration, survival, proliferation, and angiogenesis. EphA2 overexpression correlates with poor outcome in ovarian cancer. Dasatinib (70 mg bid or 100 mg daily) has been explored in multiple solid tumors in early phase trials with promising response rates. Current trials of single-agent dasatinib and in combination with paclitaxel and carboplatin in recurrent ovarian cancer are ongoing.

Cabozantinib (XL-184)

Exploration into mechanisms of resistance to anti-VEGF therapies has suggested pathways responsive to the observed upregulation of HIF-1alpha. One pathway of interest is c-Met which is also implicated in tumor growth, survival and metastases. Cabozantinib is a small molecule inhibitor of VEGFR-2 and c-Met, which has been evaluated in a number of solid tumors including, recently, ovarian cancer. In this latter phase II trial, cabozantinib was administered to 68, platinum sensitive and resistant patients. Overall response was 24% with 35% of patients also exhibiting prolonged stable disease. Response rates were similar between the platinum-sensitive and resistant cohorts. Because of better-than-expected results, the trial was terminated early; further development plans are underway.

OTHER TARGETS OF INTEREST

Angiopoietin (Ang)/Tie-2

In addition to the classic VEGF pathways of angiogenesis, other pathways involved in later stages of neovascularization hold promise for targeted therapy. Ang-1 and Ang-2 bind the receptor Tie-2 to activate pathways that stimulate endothelial cell proliferation, motility, and survival. In addition, the angiopoeitins recruit pericytes to support vascular maturation. AMG-386 is a peptibody, a peptide fusion protein, that selectively binds Ang-1 and Ang-2, preventing interaction with Tie-2. In phase I studies of solid tumors, this compound was well tolerated, without many of the classic toxicities associated with anti-angiogenic agents. A phase II study comparing two different dose levels of AMG-386 (3 mg/kg, 10 mg/kg) versus placebo in combination with weekly paclitaxel (80 mg/m^2) demonstrated a trend toward improved progression-free survival in patients who achieved higher steady-state concentrations of AMG-386. These results lead to the dose selection for TRINOVA-1, which is a study comparing AMG-386 versus placebo plus weekly paclitaxel in recurrent ovarian cancer. AMG-386 (10 mg/kg) is also being explored in combination with liposomal doxorubicin (50 mg/m^2) or topotecan (4 mg/m^2) for recurrent ovarian cancer in a Phase Ib trial. Interim results have demonstrated acceptable toxicity; however, efficacy data are not yet mature. AMG-386 is also to be evaluated as a single-agent treatment for recurrent uterine cancer as part of a GOG study.

Aurora Kinase

Three members of the aurora kinase family (Aurora kinase, A, B, and C) play large roles in the phases of mitosis. These proteins are serine/threonine kinases that act to control cell division through regulation of spindle assembly, chromosome separation, and centrosome maturation. Overexpression of Aurora A and aurora B is associated with tumorigenesis in multiple solid tumor types. Currently, there are 14 agents targeting aurora kinase activity, which are under investigation in phase I and II trials. One agent targeting Aurora kinase A, MLN 8237, has demonstrated significant activity in recurrent ovarian cancer and is proceeding to phase II trial as a single agent. Additional phase II trials of this agent in combination with cytotoxic chemotherapy are ongoing. An interesting new Aurora kinase A inhibitor, ENMD-2076, has additional activity against VEGFR, Flt-3, and FGFR3 kinases and has demonstrated activity in a phase I expansion cohort study of refractory ovarian cancer patients. Based on Response Evaluation Criteria for Solid Tumors (RECIST, defined later) or GCIG CA-125 response criteria, 2 of 20 patients and 6 of 20 patients, respectively, responded to single-agent therapy. This has encouraged pursuit of additional phase II studies in ovarian cancer patients, which are ongoing.

Delta-Like 4 (DII4)/Notch

The Notch signaling pathway participates in the regulation of angiogenesis, proliferation, and apoptosis, making it an attractive potential target for anticancer therapy. One major avenue of Notch activation is through one of its ligands, Dll4, which creates a negative feedback loop to block cellular proliferation stimulated through VEGFR2. In addition, Notch signaling through Dll4 appears to activate cell cycle arrest through a variety of mechanisms. Notch overexpression has been demonstrated in multiple tumor types, including ovarian carcinoma. Two major therapeutic avenues exist that block signaling through the Notch pathway. The gamma secretase complex acts as a mediator of Notch signaling. Gamma secretase inhibitors are nonspecific agents that are currently in multiple phase I trials for solid tumors.

Their lack of specificity has led to significant toxicity in the gastrointestinal tract. Thus antibodies that target the Dll4 ligand have been developed to reduce toxicity. These compounds have demonstrated significant activity in in vivo models and are entering clinical trials.

Folate Receptor Alpha

Folate receptor alpha binds folic acid with high affinity and is involved in folate transport. This is quite relevant in gynecologic malignancy because this receptor is overexpressed in greater than 90% of ovarian cancers. Furthermore, there is minimal expression of this target in normal tissues, making this an attractive target for anticancer therapy. Farletuzumab (MORAb-003), a humanized monoclonal antibody to folate receptor alpha, demonstrated inhibition of cellular proliferation and stimulation of cell death in preclinical models. A phase II trial of this agent (100 mg/m^2) in platinum-sensitive ovarian cancer was designed as a single-agent study with subsequent addition of traditional chemotherapy (carboplatin and paclitaxel) at the time of disease progression. In the single-agent arm, 24 of 28 patients remained on therapy at least 9 weeks. With combination therapy, 90% of patients achieved normalization of their CA-125 and 70% had complete or partial response. This drug is now under further exploration in combination with a variety of cytotoxic chemotherapies and as a single agent in ovarian cancer.

EC-145

Another agent leveraging the folate receptor alpha is EC-145. This novel ligand drug conjugate combines folic acid with desacetylvinblastine hydrazide, a chemotherapeutic agent difficult to deliver systemically. In a recently reported randomized phase II trial, EC-145 combined with pegylated liposomal doxorubicin (PLD) was associated with a significantly longer PFS than PLD alone (21.7 weeks vs 11.7 weeks, HR: 0.63, P <0.031). Of interest, and in support of the target selectivity, there were few differences in the observed toxicities between the two arms. Further, patients with global tumor expression of folate receptor alpha as measured by EC-20, a tracer conjugated to folic acid, had a PFS that was similar to that of the overall population, but substantially better than the control arm, suggesting high receptor expression is associated with poor prognosis.

Histone Acetyltransferases and Histone Deacetylases

The epigenetic modulation of gene expression is a promising target for the treatment of gynecologic malignancies. The post-translational modification of histones is a key mechanism to regulate the expression of certain genes and has been implicated in tumorigenesis. Histones may be modified through acetylation, methylation, phosphorylation, and ubiquitination. Two enzymes, histone acetyltransferase and histone deacetylases (HDAC), mediate the addition and removal of acetyl groups, respectively. HDAC activity leads to a change in the histone structure, which leads to a change in transcription activity. Through activation of oncogenes or inactivation of tumor suppressors, cell growth, proliferation, and evasion of apoptosis may occur. HDAC inhibitors have been explored in a variety of solid tumor types. Suberoylanilide hydroxamic acid (Vorinostat) is FDA approved for the treatment of refractory cutaneous T-cell lymphoma and has been explored in recurrent ovarian cancer. A phase II study of single-agent vorinostat (400 mg daily) in 27 patients had limited success with only 1 PR (4%) and 2 patients with SD for 6 months (7%). There is evidence to suggest that the combination of HDAC inhibitors with traditional cytotoxic chemotherapy may yield improved results; thus this agent is being explored in combination with paclitaxel/carboplatin and gemcitabine/carboplatin in recurrent ovarian cancer. In addition to vorinostat, there are multiple other HDAC inhibitors undergoing evaluation in phase I and II trials for solid tumors.

Platelet-Derived Growth Factor

In addition to the combination agents noted previously, there are agents in development that solely target the PDGF-receptor. This is supported by recent research indicating that the v-sis oncogene is derived from the PDGF gene. Furthermore, the PDGF pathway is involved not only in angiogenesis, but also in stimulation of cancer growth and regulation of fibroblasts. The use of a monoclonal antibody to target this pathway promises to improve efficacy and reduce off-target effects. IMG-3G3 is a monoclonal antibody to PDGFR α that has demonstrated significant antitumor activity in preclinical studies in ovarian cancer cell lines. Phase I trials in advanced solid malignancy toxicity have led to the development of a current phase II study of this agent (20 mg/kg) in combination with liposomal doxorubicin (40 mg/m^2) for platinum-resistant recurrent ovarian cancer. As noted previously, as a result of the effects on pericytes, the use of this agent in combination with other therapies promises to improve efficacy over it as a single agent.

UNIQUE TOXICITIES OF TARGETED THERAPY

In addition to survival benefit, a major goal of targeting tumor-specific pathways is to reduce the incidence of adverse events caused by "nonspecific" cytotoxic agents. Targeted agents may have similar toxicities to the traditional agents such as myelosuppression, fatigue, and diarrhea. As our experience with novel targeted agents grows, it is apparent that there exist toxicities unique to these compounds. Side effects may be secondary to the inherent mechanism of the agent or unintended "off-target" effects. This section of the chapter will serve as a brief review of the most commonly encountered toxicities and methods of prevention and treatment.

Hypertension

Hypertension is one of the most commonly experienced side effects related to targeted agents, with a prevalence that approaches 40%. This adverse event is most commonly related to the use of anti-angiogenic agents, including bevacizumab, and combination agents such as sorafenib. The mechanism of hypertension is currently hypothesized to be twofold. First, the inhibition of VEGF results in the reduction of production of nitric oxide by endothelial cells. Resultant vasoconstriction and endothelial cell dysfunction are compounded by the occurrence of microvascular rarefaction. Microvascular rarefaction is a process found in a majority of patients with hypertension, regardless of etiology, and consists of the loss of the arterioles and capillaries that make up the microcirculation. Vasoconstriction from loss of nitric oxide serves to exacerbate nonperfusion and elevate peripheral vascular resistance, which can result in permanent microvessel extinction.

Hypertension appears to be dose-dependent for several of the anti-angiogenic agents. Bevacizumab at the typical doses given for gynecologic malignancies (10-15 mg/kg) has an incidence of hypertension between 18% and 36% compared to an incidence of 3% to 30% in patients treated with low-dose bevacizumab (3-7.5 mg/kg). This incidence may be further increased when bevacizumab is combined with cytotoxic agents known to have anti-angiogenic activity such as topotecan or paclitaxel. Agents affecting the hypoxia-inducing factor-1 alpha (HIF-1α) pathway reduce nitric acid synthesis and metabolism, leading to exacerbation of anti-angiogenic drug-induced hypertension. Of note, small molecular inhibitors to VEGF have reduced incidence and severity of hypertension when compared to monoclonal antibodies targeting the receptor.

Hypertension induced by anti-angiogenic agents is most commonly found in patients with preexisting hypertension. Thus, active management of blood pressure and cardiac risk factors such as elevated lipids is paramount. The use of several antihypertensive agents is often necessary to control hypertension in this setting. Acceptable treatments for angiogenesis inhibitor–induced hypertension include angiotensin-converting enzyme (ACE) inhibitors, beta-blockers, and dihydropyridine calcium-channel blockers (amlodipine, felodipine). Nondihydropyridine calcium-channel blockers should be avoided given their inhibition of the P450 CYP3A4, which can affect the metabolism of tyrosine kinase inhibitors. Nifedipine is also not an optimal therapeutic choice secondary to the increase in VEGF levels associated with chronic use.

Reverse Protein Leukoencephalopathy (RPLS)

Reverse protein leukoencephalopathy (RPLS) is a rare complication of anti-angiogenic agents including bevacizumab, sorafenib, and sunitinib. Occurring in less than 1% of all patients treated with these agents, this syndrome is characterized by finding of diffuse, hyperintense T2-weighted signaling secondary to leaking of the capillaries in the brain. Symptoms of RPLS include change in mental status, headache, seizures, and lethargy. Aggressive antihypertensive management and supportive care will typically lead to full recovery; however, in rare cases this syndrome may be fatal. Typically, further use of anti-VEGF therapy in these patients is contraindicated.

Cardiotoxicity

Other effects of targeted agents on the cardiovascular system can include left ventricular dysfunction, congestive heart failure, and myocardial infarction. Uncontrolled hypertension can lead to left ventricular hypertrophy and cardiac musculature that outgrows its vascular supply. This results in traumatic cardiovascular events, which may be seen in any of the anti-VEGF agents. Furthermore, any tyrosine kinase inhibitor may have off-target effects that damage cardiac muscle cells and impair their survival. For example, sorafenib and sunitinib have been associated with decreased left ventricular ejection fraction in up to 30% of patients. Of note, this damage appears to be reversible secondary to mitochondrial dysfunction rather than the permanent free radical–induced cardiac damage found after anthracycline cardiac toxicity.

Thus far, prediction of the development of cardiac toxicity from targeted agents has been difficult. It does appear more common in those patients with preexisting cardiac disease and prior treatment with anthracyclines. Again, aggressive medical management of preexisting conditions and careful monitoring of cardiac function are essential to maximize outcomes.

Renal Toxicity

Renal adverse effects may be found in response to a variety of targeted agents as a result of the expression of key targets along the nephron. The most common toxicity is proteinuria, especially among the anti-angiogenic agents. This is thought to originate secondary to damage of endothelial cells, which depend on VEGF for integrity and regulation of permeability. In addition, thrombotic microangiopathy that leads to further damage of the glomerular capillaries may compound the loss of protein from the vasculature. Proteinuria is typically low grade, is asymptomatic, and may be monitored through assessment of albumin levels by urine dipstick. If protein readings exceed 2+ protein, collection of 24-hour urine protein is indicated for treatment decision-making. Urine protein levels exceeding 2 g require treatment interruption and possible dose reduction depending on protocol requirements. Spot urine protein to creatinine ratios may also be used to monitor renal effect of targeted agents. Renal failure caused by targeted agents is rare and appears to be primarily related to glomerulonephritis, interstitial nephritis, and acute tubular necrosis. Prevention and management of renal toxicity is based on thorough assessment of renal risk factors before therapy institution and optimization of any preexisting conditions.

Thromboembolic Events

The risk of venous thromboembolism (VTE) is increased at baseline among patients with active malignancy receiving chemotherapy. Anti-angiogenic agents also appear to increase the propensity for thrombosis, especially arterial thromboembolism (ATE), including myocardial, cardiovascular, cerebral, and peripheral vascular events. In a large meta-analysis of patients treated as part of a randomized trial for a variety of solid tumors, patients treated with bevacizumab in addition to chemotherapy had two times greater incidence of ATE. Multivariate analysis revealed that bevacizumab remained a significant risk factor for ATE, in addition to age 65 years or older and prior history of ATE. Of note, the rate of thromboembolic complications appears low for VEGF-Trap and VEGF tyrosine kinase inhibitors. This may be secondary to formation of complexes by anti-VEGF antibodies that create a nidus for the formation of thromboses in the vasculature. Further study of this complication in large randomized control trials is necessary to determine the true incidence rates. At this point, patients with a history of VTE warrant the careful assessment and aggressive use of anticoagulation therapy. Anti-VEGF therapy should be avoided in patients with a history of prior ATE. Support for the use of routine thromboprophylaxis has not been established.

Gastrointestinal Perforation and Fistula

Gastrointestinal toxicity is a life-threatening complication that has been primarily associated with anti-VEGF therapy. Risk of intestinal perforation or fistula in any tumor type is associated with prior gastrointestinal surgery, acute diverticulitis or active abdominal infection, obstruction, carcinomatosis, or history of prior radiotherapy. Rates of bowel perforation are highest among patients with ovarian cancer, ranging as high as 11% in one study of bevacizumab in the recurrent setting. In this study, higher risk of perforation was associated with a history of more than two prior chemotherapy regimens. Furthermore, the high perforation rate in a trial combining bevacizumab and erlotinib in ovarian cancer led to early closure. Of note, frontline treatment does not appear to lead to increased gastrointestinal toxicities, as evidenced by equivalent rates of perforation in the control and experimental arms of GOG 218 (reviewed in Table 18-4). Proposed mechanisms for bowel injury include the negative effect on wound healing secondary to damage of normal endothelial cells. Anti-VEGF therapies may induce microangiopathic events in the intestinal lining that cause edema and hemorrhage, making the wall more susceptible to bacterial dissemination and infection. In addition, rapid tumor shrinkage may cause the bowel wall to become weak, leading to perforation.

The management of anti-VEGF therapy-induced gastrointestinal perforation must be individualized based on patient history, amount of disease, and status. In general, surgical exploration with intestinal diversion is the standard of care for patients with acceptable performance status; however, consideration should be made for risk of further poor wound healing. If a patient cannot undergo surgical exploration, conservative management with decompression, bowel rest, drainage, antibiotics, and nutritional support may be indicated.

Diarrhea and mucositis are not uncommon among patients treated with a majority of the small molecule inhibitors regardless of target. These adverse events may be the dose-limiting toxicity for a patient, requiring admission for intravenous hydration and drug discontinuation. Prevention with antimotility agents or neutralizing mouthwashes may be helpful to reduce incidence of these off-target effects. Esophagitis or gastritis may be an issue in patients treated with sorafenib or sunitinib; therefore prevention with a proton-pump inhibitor is reasonable.

Cutaneous Complications

Skin toxicities are quite common in patients treated with anti-EGFR agents (50%-100%), are dose dependent, and appear to be indicative of drug efficacy. Typically, an acneiform rash consisting of pruritic papules and pustules presents within 3 weeks of treatment on skin areas that have sebaceous glands. A similar rash may be seen in patients treated with mTOR inhibitors. The mechanism is thought to be related to follicular hyperkeratosis that causes glands blockage and inflammatory eruption.

This rash may be managed with topical antiseptics and anti-inflammatory agents. Oral antibiotics such as doxycycline or minocycline may be used daily for a short course to improve rash severity and symptoms. In addition to this rash, patients may experience significant xerosis, which may be managed with over-the-counter emollients. Changes to the nail bed may be seen, including fragility, paronychia (inflammation of nail folds), and fissures. The hair may also be affected by the use of these agents. Most commonly, hypertrichosis, including growth of the eyelashes and scalp hair, has been reported.

Hand and foot skin reaction or acral erythema is a classic skin toxicity of sorafenib and sunitinib. Occurring in 20% to 25% of patients, it may consist of erythema, hyperkeratosis, xerosis, and dysaesthesias and parasthesia in the bilateral hands and/or feet. Patients can develop callous-like blisters and desquamation in both pressure- and non–pressure-bearing areas. Treatment for hand and foot skin reaction is primarily supportive, consisting of elevation, compresses, avoidance of trauma, and topical application of corticosteroid cream. Symptoms usually resolve during the course of therapy, but some patients may require dose reduction or complete cessation of therapy. In addition to hand and foot skin reaction, patients treated with sorafenib or sunitinib can develop stomatitis, scalp dysaesthesias, perianal rash, and a skin rash that resembles seborrheic dermatitis.

Metabolic Abnormalities

The nonspecific nature of some of the targeted agents has led to a variety of unique metabolic side effects, requiring careful monitoring and action. Endocrine effects of tyrosine kinase inhibitors may include altered thyroid function, glucose metabolism, and bone metabolism. For example, sunitinib and sorafenib have been associated with onset of hypothyroidism in previous euthyroid patients. mTOR inhibitors, including temsirolimus and everolimus, have been associated with incidence of any hyperglycemia as high as 50%. Of note, alterations in glucose metabolism can occur in either direction in patients treated with sunitinib or imatinib. Glucose levels must be monitored closely because these changes may necessitate change in dosing of antihyperglycemic agents among patients with diabetes. Glycemic control should be maximized before treatment with these agents. Lipid abnormalities, including elevated triglycerides and cholesterol, are common toxicities experienced by patients treated with mTOR inhibitors. These levels should be followed during treatment and, depending on patient cardiac risk factors, lipid-lowering agents may be instituted. Electrolytes should be monitored during treatment with targeted agents because many tyrosine kinase inhibitors have caused profound hypophosphatemia manifested as muscle weakness and fatigue.

TABLE 18-6   Recist Response Definitions

Response	Definition
Complete response (CR)	Disappearance of all target and nontarget lesions
Partial response (PR)	30% decrease in the sum of the diameters of the target lesions; stable nontarget lesions
Stable disease (SD)	Neither sufficient decrease or increase in the sum of the diameters of target lesions to qualify for CR or PD
Progressive disease (PD)	20% increase in sum of the diameters of the target lesions; progressive nontarget lesions; new lesions

RECIST, *Response Evaluation Criteria in Solid Tumors.*

SPECIAL CONSIDERATIONS FOR TARGETED THERAPIES

The unique nature of the targeted agents has led to several areas of controversy in the clinical management of patients receiving these drugs. Specifically, the design of clinical trials incorporating such agents is receiving scrutiny. The traditional method of determining the efficacy of a given drug by RECIST is based on the mechanism of action of cytotoxic chemotherapy (Table 18-6). These drugs are expected to shrink tumor cells, and thus a "successful" response as defined by RECIST would include a complete response or partial response. Typically, stable disease would be considered a failure of the agent. However, as noted earlier, targeted agents are generally cytostatic. Given that these agents may simply inhibit tumor growth, SD may actually indicate an efficacious targeted agent. In fact, some authors have advocated the inclusion of SD into the end points of early clinical trials of targeted agents to ensure that potentially beneficial treatments are not eliminated from further study.

For patients with ovarian cancer, response to treatment may be monitored using CA-125 levels. However, it is unclear if this method is reliable for patients being treated with a targeted agent. In the aforementioned study of patients with recurrent ovarian cancer treated with bevacizumab and sorafenib, Azad and colleagues noted that changes in the concentration of CA-125 did not correspond to response based on RECIST measurements in all patients. Of note, three patients with PR by RECIST had elevations in their CA-125 level that would have required removal from the study if strict CA-125 criteria had been utilized. Conversely, of eight patients with response by CA-125, only five had response confirmed by computed tomography (CT) results.

It is clear that the expression of the receptors and proteins targeted by these agents varies across each tumor and histology type. The use of a targeted agent in an unselected patient population may lead to lower response rates and lack of further exploration of a potentially useful drug. It is clear that determination of which patients are more likely to benefit from a given targeted therapy is necessary. As molecular testing continues to advance, we anticipate that pretreatment determination of mutation status, gene and protein expression levels, or target function will result in a patient being treated with an appropriately selected targeted agent.

The cytostatic nature of the targeted agents may also limit their effectiveness as a single-agent therapy. As seen in the text, many of these agents may control disease but not eliminate the disease entirely. Thus the combination of targeted agents with other treatment modalities such as cytotoxic chemotherapy, surgery, and radiation is rational and currently being explored. As the use of targeted agents continues to increase, the considerations noted previously will need to be addressed and consensus achieved to ensure appropriate trial design and patient management.

CONCLUSIONS

As knowledge regarding tumor biology and pathogenesis continues to expand, the number of targeted agents will no doubt increase exponentially. These agents have the potential to have a profound impact on the treatment of patients with gynecologic malignancies. Future considerations will include determining the appropriate combination of targeted agents with other modalities to optimize survival outcomes and quality of life. Furthermore, directly targeting genes with RNA interference technology and assigning therapies based on the molecular profile of the tumor hold the promise to personalize the care of each gynecologic cancer patient.

Acknowledgments

The authors would like to acknowledge support from the NIH (CA 110793, CA 109298, P50 CA083639, P50 CA098258, CA128797, RC2GM092599, U54 CA151668), the Ovarian Cancer Research Fund, Inc. (Program Project Development Grant), the DOD (OC073399, W81XWH-10-1-0158, BC085265), the Marcus Foundation, the Betty Anne Asche Murray Distinguished Professorship, the Anne Rife Cox Chair in Gynecology, the Gynecologic Cancer Foundation, and the Meyer and Ida Gordon Foundation.

For full reference list, log onto www.expertconsult.com
⟨http://www.expertconsult.com⟩.

Genes and Cancer: Genetic Counseling and Clinical Management

David G. Mutch, MD, and Philip J. Di Saia, MD

Cancer is a genetic disease that is the result of alterations in DNA; these alterations are called mutations. Mutations, if they occur in a gene or genes critical for cell growth, may allow a cell to reproduce in an uncontrolled fashion. This uncontrolled growth of a cell or tissue is known as a cancer. Cancer is seldom the result of a single mutation but usually requires several different mutations in many different genes to allow this irreversible and uncontrolled change in cell function. The concept that cancer is the result solely of genetic mutations is relatively new and comes from the past four decades of cancer research. Before the 1970s, the cause of cancer was essentially a black box and its etiology largely unknown. To some extent, it is still unclear, but we no longer believe that defective immunity, viruses, or metabolic errors directly cause cancer. These factors may contribute to the development of this disease, but the basis of cancer lies in an individual organism's DNA and in that individual organism's ability to express the genetic material in a normal fashion. This is simply related to the DNA sequences that make up that individual's genome that has been inherited and altered through the course of normal living. Thus cancer is a disease of abnormal DNA expression. Alterations or differences in the DNA sequences are known as mutations, a change in DNA such that a protein alteration occurs, or polymorphisms, a change in DNA that results in a more subtle change in gene function and protein structure. Polymorphisms are

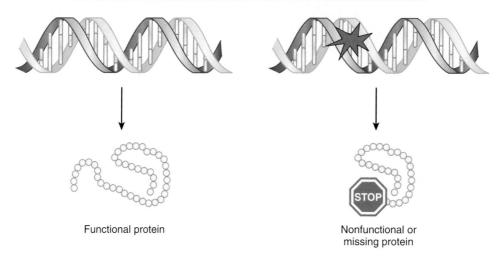

FIGURE 19-1   Disease-associated mutations alter protein function.

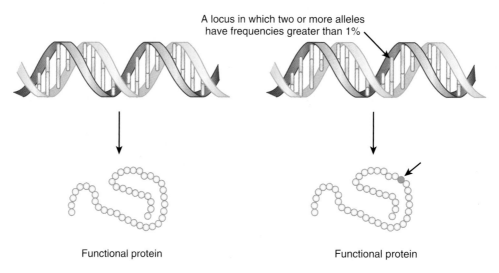

FIGURE 19-2   A depiction of a polymorphism.

one of the factors responsible for normal population differences. There is a fine line between a mutation and polymorphism (Figures 19-1 and 19-2).

There is a genetic component to most diseases. Heart disease is known to have an inherited component. Individuals can inherit defective genes that alter lipid metabolism, and therefore those people are at risk for development of atherosclerosis and thus have an increased risk of dying of a fatal myocardial infarction or stroke. We also know that these individuals may alter the natural history of their disease, to a great extent, by changing their environment. For example, an individual prone to heart disease may decrease the risk of dying by increasing the level of exercise, avoiding obesity, or eating a low-fat diet. Cancer is similar to this example of atherosclerosis in that an individual may inherit a genetic

mutation or may be exposed to an environmental insult that predisposes to the development of a cancer. Such insults can occur from everyday living or as the result of repetitive exposure to smoke, other substances, and other environmental factors that cause DNA damage. In addition, any process that causes cells to divide, such as ovulation, can allow an opportunity for an error in DNA replication to be made. Similar to the example of heart disease, an individual prone to the development of ovarian cancer can reduce her risk of developing this disease by taking oral contraceptives. This will inhibit ovulation and decrease the damage to the surface of the ovary that could allow a mutation to occur. Cancers, unlike many other inherited diseases, become apparent after there is an accumulation of several genetic injuries or mutations. In this respect, cancer is different from

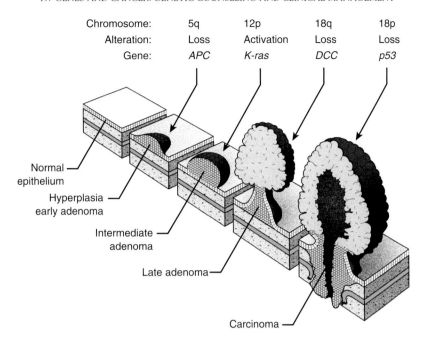

Chromosome:	5q	12p	18q	18p
Alteration:	Loss	Activation	Loss	Loss
Gene:	*APC*	*K-ras*	*DCC*	*p53*

Normal epithelium

Hyperplasia early adenoma

Intermediate adenoma

Late adenoma

Carcinoma

FIGURE 19-3   A model for colorectal tumorigenesis. This shows the molecular progression of normal colon epithelium to frank cancer.

most inborn errors of metabolism because more than one genetic event is required to allow expression of the disease. One does not inherit cancers as one would inherit cystic fibrosis or sickle cell disease. One may inherit a mutation in a gene that predisposes one to the development of cancer, but most cancers are the result of the accumulation of somatic mutations that result from the process of normal living. Viruses, smoking, eating charcoal-broiled steak, or simply random mistakes made during DNA replication may cause these mutations. After all, a replicating cell must copy 3 billion base pairs—with each division, mistakes will occur.

That progression from a normal to a malignant cell is the result of the accumulation of a series of mutations has probably best been demonstrated in colon cancer by Burt Vogelstein and colleagues (Figure 19-3). In this model, a series of mutations must occur that involve tumor suppressor genes and oncogenes; a benign tumor progresses to a malignant tumor as the necessary mutations occur during a prolonged and somewhat erratic interval.

In general, three broad classes of genes are involved in the development of cancer. These are tumor suppressor genes, oncogenes, and mismatch repair (MMR) genes. Tumor suppressor genes are responsible for making a product that inhibits cell growth. These types of genes are expressed in a recessive manner, and therefore both alleles need to be lost before the phenotype becomes apparent. Oncogenes are expressed dominantly and are usually responsible for a product that promotes cell growth. If they express their protein in an uncontrolled manner, uncontrolled growth occurs. MMR genes are responsible for repairing DNA damage that results from loss of fidelity in normal DNA replication. If one of these genes does not function properly, errors in DNA can accumulate, and ultimately some of these errors will occur in genes critical for cell control, resulting in uncontrolled cell growth. The development of cancers is therefore not the result of a single error or insult but rather the accumulation of errors over time.

One thing to bear in mind is that mutations are a means of evolution. The paradox of life is that the same mutations responsible for an individual organism's death in the form of cancer or metabolic error also can account for the evolution of the species. Mutations can be good, bad, or even neutral.

GENETIC ALTERATIONS IN CANCER

Genetics is not a new field and has been a study for several centuries from Mendel in 1865 to the present. Johannsen first coined the term *gene* in 1911 as it applied to the unit of a hereditary characteristic. This was further refined to the one gene–one enzyme concept in the 1940s and put forth by Tatum and Beadle. These concepts have been clearly defined in *Drosophila* but apply equally to humans and other organisms; after all, all living things are defined by their DNA. Humans have more DNA

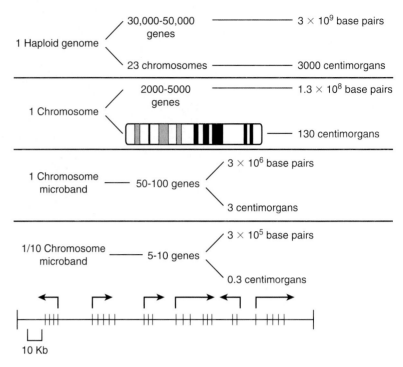

FIGURE 19-4 The structure of the human chromosome demonstrated in terms of functional units (centimorgans) and physical units (base pairs).

than other organisms and are therefore more complex, but the DNA behaves the same way in all organisms.

The one gene–one enzyme concept that developed from the ideas expressed by Tatum and Beadle can be summarized as follows:

1. All biologic processes are under genetic control.
2. These biochemical processes are expressed as a series of stepwise reactions.
3. Each biochemical reaction is ultimately under the control of different single genes.
4. Mutation of a single gene results in an alteration of the cell to carry out a single chemical reaction.

The one gene–one enzyme concept has since been refined and extended to cover proteins that are not enzymes. Now further information suggests that some genes combine with others to form unique proteins, indicating that a few genes may interact to form more than one protein per gene. The human genome is estimated to contain about 3 billion base pairs and was thought to have between 50,000 and 100,000 genes. Now that the human genome has been sequenced we have discovered that there are only about 30,000 genes. These genes interact much more than we previously believed and are stored on linear strands of DNA, which are combined with certain nuclear proteins and form chromosomes. The genes are not continuous sequences of DNA but consist of coding sequences called exons interrupted by noncoding sequences called introns. Most of the DNA is not made of exons or "expressed DNA";

rather, it is composed of intronic DNA that is usually not expressed in any form and is just filler DNA. An approximation of the size of the human genome and its organization can be seen in Figure 19-4. The functional length of the human chromosome is expressed in centimorgans (cM). A cM is the distance over which there is a 1% chance of crossover during meiosis. Linkage studies indicate that the human genome is about 3000 cM. The average chromosome contains about 1500 genes in 130 million base pairs. Figure 19-4 shows the estimated physical and functional size of the genome. The physical size is estimated in base pairs, whereas the functional size is estimated in centimorgans. Much of the human genome is not composed of coded DNA and is therefore not expressed.

DNA is transcribed into RNA that is translated into protein. Therefore the sequence of DNA base pairs ultimately determines the sequence of the functional proteins within the cell. All cellular functions are expressed in this manner (Figure 19-5):

$$DNA \rightarrow RNA \rightarrow Protein$$

Humans and other mammals may be more complex than some other organisms in that pieces of genes may combine with parts of other genes to make a totally new protein. Hence, we may essentially increase the number of genes expressed without really increasing the amount of functional DNA or the number of actual genes. Overall, only about 30% of the genetic material is expressed and 70% is not.

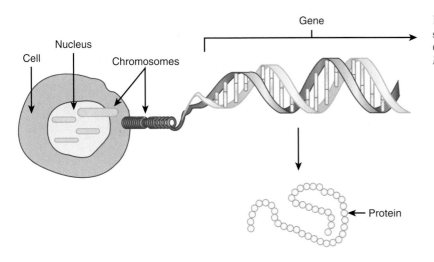

FIGURE 19-5   The progression of protein synthesis from DNA to RNA to protein. *(From National Cancer Institute. Understanding Gene Testing. Rockville: National Cancer Institute; 1995.)*

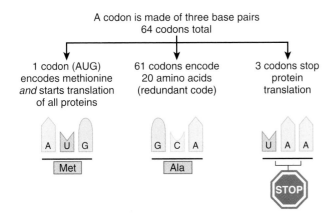

FIGURE 19-6   Stop codons. *(Reprinted with permission from ASCO Curriculum: Cancer Genetics and Cancer Predisposition Testing 2nd Edition.)*

TABLE 19-1   Categories of Human Mutations Identified in Cancers

Single base pair substitutions
    Types of nucleotide substitution and hypermutable nucleotides
    mRNA splice junction mutations
    mRNA processing and translation mutations
    Regulatory mutations
Deletions
Insertions
Duplications
Inversions
Expansion or contraction of unstable repeat

MECHANISMS OF HUMAN GENE MUTATION

All cancers result from alterations in DNA structure leading to changes in the proteins responsible for cellular function. All living organisms use the same 20 amino acids as building blocks for proteins. The translation of a nucleotide sequence from DNA to protein is dependent on a triplet code of nucleotides. Each of these triplet codes is called a *codon.* Some codons have very special functions. The code AUG codes for methionine and this starts the initiation of synthesis (translation) of every protein. The code UAA is a stop codon and ends translation of a protein (Figure 19-6). Much of the data available about genetic alterations in cancers come from studies other than of gynecologic malignant neoplasms. These studies often involve hematologic malignant neoplasms such as lymphomas and leukemia because pure subsets of cells are easily obtained. More recently, we have been able to improve our study of solid carcinomas because of our ability to study pure tumor preparations, single out cells, and isolate the DNA with microdissection and laser capture techniques. Using this technique and techniques like it, we can dissect out a single cancer cell, replicate its DNA, and evaluate the mutations that occur in this single cell or group of cells. Figure 19-7 demonstrates the heterogeneity of cancer and why there is a need for these special techniques. Cancer is the result of clonal expansion, but as the various cells replicate in an uncontrolled manner they continue to mutate. Initially, cancers usually have a single clonal origin. As the cancer progresses mutations occur, and therefore some cells may become genetically different from the original cancer. Hence, the term *mutator phenotype* is often applied to cancers.

A wide number of and various types of mutations have been described. These mutations are fundamental to the understanding of cancer and of human evolution. Although many types of mutations can occur, some common ones are listed in Table 19-1. A more comprehensive listing of the specific different mutations found

FIGURE 19-7 Heterogeneity within tumors often prevents accurate evaluation of tumor because of normal contamination.

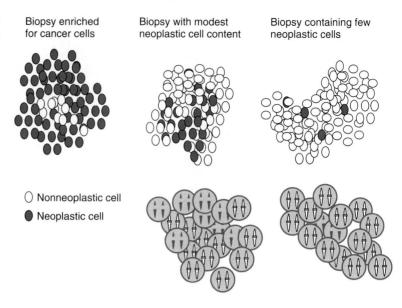

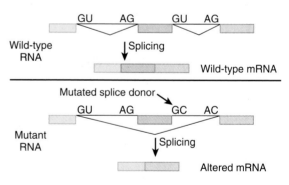

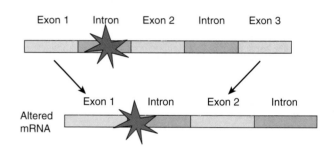

Normal	THE BIG RED DOG RAN OUT.
Missense	THE BIG RAD DOG RAN OUT.
Nonsense	THE BIG RED.
Frameshift (deletion)	THE BRE DDO GRA.
Frameshift (insertion)	THE BIG RED ZDO GRA.

FIGURE 19-8 Example of how a point mutation (a change in a single base pair) can result in changing the meaning of a gene sequence using a common phrase.

FIGURE 19-9 Cryptic splice site mutations. Splice site mutation, a change that results in altered RNA sequence.

FIGURE 19-10 Exon skipping splice site mutations. Splice site mutation, a change that results in altered RNA sequence.

in cancers can be viewed on the Human Gene Mutation Database (HGMD) (http://www.hgmd.cf.ac.uk/ac/index.php). These mutations are periodically updated. Cartoons of some common mutations can be seen in Figures 19-8 to 19-13.

Single Base Pair Substitutions and Point Mutations

DNA replication is the result of an accurate yet accident-prone process. The final accuracy of DNA replication depends on the fidelity of the initial process and the ability of subsequent repair processes to correct any mistakes. Point mutations lead to single changes in the DNA sequence. These single mutations can have very different effects on the reading of a protein, as demonstrated in Figures 19-10 and 19-11. If this mutation is in a regulatory portion of a gene, loss or alteration of

regulation of gene expression can occur. If the mutation is in a coding portion of the gene, an altered protein can be formed. HGMD is one of several catalogs of reported point mutations that can be obtained from the Internet.

The most common mutation as the result of substitution occurs in CpG dinucleotides (3′ cytosine-guanine 5′). Data show that these transversions account for about

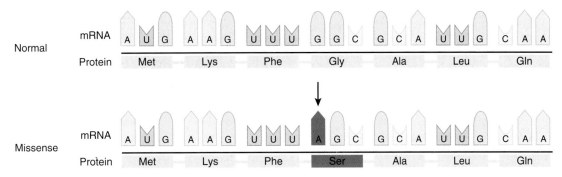

FIGURE 19-11 Missense mutation, changes to a codon for another amino acid (can be a harmful mutation or neutral polymorphism). *(Reprinted with permission from ASCO Curriculum: Cancer Genetics and Cancer Predisposition Testing, 2nd ed.)*

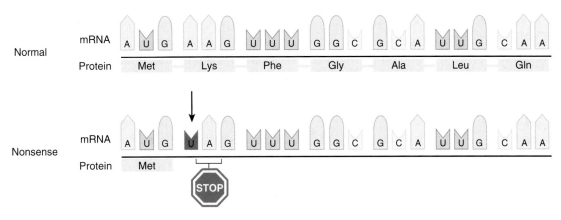

FIGURE 19-12 Nonsense mutation, change from an amino acid codon to a stop codon, producing a shortened protein. *(Reprinted with permission from ASCO Curriculum: Cancer Genetics and Cancer Predisposition Testing, 2nd ed.)*

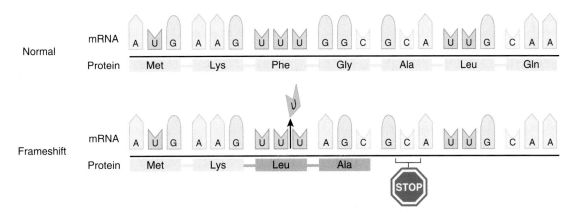

FIGURE 19-13 Frame shift mutation in which insertion or deletion of base pairs produces a stop codon downstream and (usually) a shortened protein. *(Reprinted with permission from ASCO Curriculum: Cancer Genetics and Cancer Predisposition Testing, 2nd ed.)*

30% of point mutations. Therefore they represent the most common substitution mutation. The fidelity of this process is related to the efficiency and accuracy of the DNA polymerase responsible for replication. Other types of these small nucleotide substitutions that can also occur are messenger ribonucleic acid (mRNA) splice junction mutations, translational mutations, and single

deletions. Alternatively, mismatches can occur by slipped mispairing, which leads to single base pair mutagenesis and deletion.

Deletion or insertion of a single nucleotide may be secondary to DNA mispairing during replication. This type of mutation often occurs in runs of identical base pairs and is the result of slippage of a single base pair

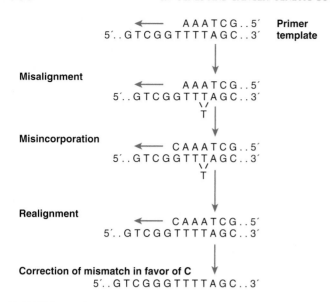

Misalignment

Misincorporation

Realignment

Correction of mismatch in favor of C

FIGURE 19-14   DNA mispairing that results in a single base deletion of a T. This causes a complete change of sequence. Attempt at correction adds a G or C to the sequence.

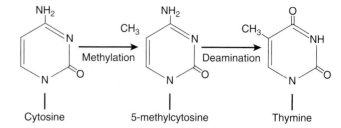

FIGURE 19-15   Cytosine to thymine transition from methylation. *(From Korf B [ed]. Human Genetics: A Problem-Based Approach, 2nd ed. Blackwell Publishers, 2000.)*

(Figure 19-14). This mechanism is similar to larger deletions caused by this same mechanism. The significance of this type of mutation to human malignant neoplasia is as yet undefined. As more information becomes available about mismatch repair, we should have a better estimate of the significance of this type of mutation to cancer formation. However, this slippage is common and similar to the errors found in individuals who have an inherited cancer syndrome, hereditary nonpolyposis colon cancer (HNPCC), or Lynch syndrome.

CpG dinucleotides are very susceptible to mutations. Methylation of cytosine results in a high level of mutation because of its propensity to undergo deamination. This then forms thymidine and therefore can result in a change of gene expression. The evolution of the human genome seems to indicate a progressive loss of CpG islands because of this transition. The frequency of these islands is about 20% to 30% of the predicted frequency, probably because of the progressive loss of CpG dinucleotides. This excess of transition from cytosine to thymine (C to T) transitions was first reported by Vogel and Rohrborn in a study of the mutations responsible for variants of hemoglobin. Others now also have shown that CpG islands are associated with a high rate of transition, supporting the thought that these mutations play a significant role in human disease (Figure 19-15).

Larger Deletions

Gene deletions are responsible for more than 150 inherited diseases. Deletions can range from a few base pairs to several hundred kilobases and are usually classified by size. These are also nonrandom in that certain sequences appear to be more prone to deletion than others are. This nonrandomness is apparent when one evaluates genetic disease. Spontaneous deletions often occur in the same sequences of various genes, indicating that some sequences of DNA are more prone to deletion than others are.

Deletions occur when there is homologous but unequal recombination between gene sequences. Similar sequences in the human genome can cross over during mitosis or meiosis, resulting in a shortened portion of the gene sequence. Long areas of homology (homology boxes) are thought to be the most likely to have this type of mutation. Repetitive DNA sequences are particularly susceptible to deletions because this can allow slippage. This mechanism is called homolog or unequal recombination between repetitive sequence elements. The most common repetitive sequence is the Alu repeat (up to 106 Alu sequences are in the human genome). Alu repeats are characterized by an average spacing of 4 kilobases and 300–base pair length separated by a short A-rich region. The Alu element is 70% to 90% homologous to the consensus sequence. The 3′ homology (homology boxes) is thought to be the most likely to have this type of mutation. Repetitive DNA sequences are particularly prone to mutation.

There are more than 400 gross gene deletions recorded in the HGMD and 3000 or so smaller gene deletions. Almost 2500 gene deletions of 20 base pairs or fewer have been identified. These can be the result of deletion of repeats or a part of the excision repair process. Deletion is not random; particular sequences are more prone to deletion and often contain regions involving guanine or other repeats. The application of the techniques of molecular biology, such as gene cloning, in situ hybridization, restriction endonuclease mapping of genetic sequences, and polymerase chain reaction analysis of gene transcription, has led to the conclusion that a given chromosome abnormality may be associated with a variety of neoplasms and that a given oncogene may be activated in a variety of human cancers. The most common defects in solid tumors are deletions in specific

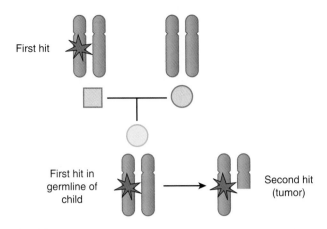

FIGURE 19-16 Knudsen's two-hit theory that is essential to the concept of tumor suppressor genes. *(Reprinted with permission from ASCO Curriculum: Cancer Genetics and Cancer Predisposition Testing, 2nd ed.)*

gene sequences, observed as a loss of part of a banding region or the loss of heterozygosity of a specific genetic allele. Deletion of genetic material in a cancer cell suggests loss of function that regulates cell proliferation and differentiation. Many human solid tumors have been shown to have some type of chromosome deletion. The Tp53 tumor suppressor gene–containing region of chromosome 17p is deleted or mutated in a wide variety of human cancers. The fact that there is such commonality among cancer cell types in the loss of chromosome material suggests that these regions contain genes coding for regulating functions of a wide variety of cell types. Induction of the malignant neoplastic process must involve at least two hits when a tumor suppressor gene is involved. This implies that two mutations or deletions in each of the two alleles are necessary before the effect can be expressed. This is the two-hit theory proposed by Knudson. The possibilities for the two hits necessary to express a recessive gene can be seen in Figure 19-16. This explained why some people could inherit a predisposition for a malignant disease and also raised the question of whether sporadic cancers could have a genetic basis. In a genetically predisposed cell, the remaining single normal allele may be sufficient to maintain normal growth and regulation; a second deletion or mutation is required to inactivate the remaining normal allele.

Insertions

Most insertions appear to be small, between one and a few base pairs. This phenomenon has been studied extensively, and these insertions often appear to be non-random in character. Predisposing factors lead to these insertions. These insertions can be due to slipped mispairings, or they may be mediated by inverted repeat sequences or by symmetric elements. These sorts of DNA sequences are particularly prone to mutation.

Less common are large insertions. The largest insertion known is the 220-kilobase segment inserted into the DMD gene. Alu and LINE (long interspersed nucleotide elements) sequences are especially susceptible to insertion and deletion. Mutations are nonrandom, and some DNA segments are more susceptible to mutation than others are. For example, the myc gene is especially susceptible to insertions; a 50-base pair LINE element has been noted to be inserted in this gene in breast cancer cell lines. The fact that insertional mutations may not be random is underscored by the finding of Fearon, who reported 10 independent examples of insertions within the same 170-bp intronic region of the DCC gene involved in the progression of colorectal cancers.

Duplications

Duplication of small parts of whole exons, or even of whole chromosomes, has played a large part in the development of cancer. This phenomenon also has a large role in the evolution of the human genome. Again, the paradox is that mutations are sometimes good and sometimes bad. Duplication of larger segments of DNA may lead to gene amplification. Gene amplifications can occur in many ways. A gene that is usually present in a single copy in the normal cell may be duplicated or may undergo a small increase in the copy number. Another type of amplification may involve a 10-fold to 100-fold increase in copies of a genetic locus containing key regulatory genes. A third type of amplification can result in the duplication of whole chromosomes. One can envision how amplification has been important over the course of evolution. We have 23 pairs of chromosomes, and all other organisms have fewer chromosomes. This is due to millions of years of evolution resulting from innumerable insertions and duplications.

Inversions

Inversions are perhaps the least common type of mutation. In this mutation, a long segment of DNA forms a loop and alters its direction; the 3' end now becomes the 5' end. These segments can obviously be large or quite small. The most important inversion event in human disease involves the factor VIII gene, causing severe hemophilia A. There are to date no cancers known to have resulted from a significant inversion.

Translocations

More than 100 common translocations have been observed in malignant cells. Many of these occur consistently in certain specific cancer types, which argues that these areas are involved in the malignant process of the cell. Some of the translocations may be secondary events in the evolution of more aggressive phenotypic changes. The inherent genetic instability of malignant cells leads to further karyotypic abnormalities as the disease progresses, reflecting additional genetic alterations that increase growth potential. Evidence that malignant transformation does not usually result from a single translocation event comes from the study of patients with ataxia-telangiectasia who are at high risk for leukemia. These patients have lymphocytes with a characteristic translocation present for many years before a malignant change develops.

A common finding in cancers is some form of genetic instability. This is most clearly manifested in the disease called hereditary nonpolyposis colon cancer, also known as Lynch II syndrome. This disease is characterized by genetic instability at microsatellite sequences and has been linked to several MMR genes. Mutation rates in cells that are positive for MMR defects are orders of magnitude higher than MMR intact cells. Cancers in patients with this hereditary disease may serve as a model for sporadic disease because mutations that occur in the sporadic tumors are often very similar. The same genes and sequences seem to be targeted. For instance, Krawczak demonstrated that the bulk of single base substitutions in the Tp53 gene in sporadic cancers strongly resemble those found in inherited cancers.

CANCER EPIGENETICS

Epigenetics refers to alternative types of gene expression that are not specifically related to differences in the genotype. This is a concept of differential expression of the genotype based on factors outside of the genome. It is interesting that these differences can be inherited and appear to be quite stable. Epigenetic changes basically refer to alterations in DNA expression not related to the actual sequence and can involve chromatin structure; histone modification; changes in transcriptional activity; and, most easily measured in mammals, changes in methylation of CpG loci.

Methylation is the only known covalent modification of DNA in normal mammalian cells. This change occurs at the fifth position of cytosine at 5CG-3′ dinucleotides. About 80% of these types of dinucleotides are methylated and therefore are probably important in cell control and gene expression. Generalized hypomethylation is present in colorectal cancers and endometrial cancers early on in the development of these diseases, but the exact cause and effect of this observation is unclear. Presumably, hypomethylation allows some genes to be overexpressed. Alternatively, some regions on some genes, particularly the promoter region of MMR genes,

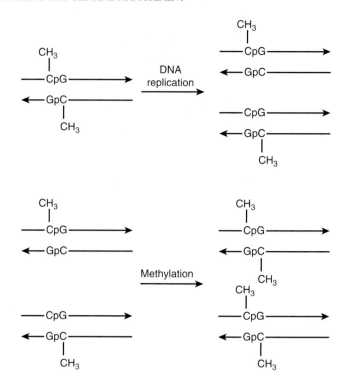

FIGURE 19-17   Methylation can cause gene silencing. *(From Korf B [ed]. Human Genetics: A Problem-Based Approach, 2nd ed. Blackwell Publishers, 2000.)*

can cause gene silencing (Figure 19-17). This allows a tumor suppressor gene to be silenced, thus promoting the development of that cancer. Changes in methylation status are not clonal. Hence, some cancers can have different gene expression in the same cancer because of differential methylation. Changes in methylation status could also cause aberrant chromosome condensation during division and result in abnormal chromosome segregation. Therefore epigenetics can affect tumor behavior in several ways.

GENOMIC IMPRINTING AND CANCER

Genomic imprinting is a modification of DNA away from the physical gene (epigenetic modification), which alters the expression of that gene. These alterations often lead to a different expression of the gene and may be passed from generation to generation. However, the specific expression of these modifications may change from generation to generation (Figure 19-18). These epigenetic alterations appear to occur commonly in human malignancies and because of their unique properties may lead to novel forms of therapy.

Assumptions made in the Mendelian genetics we apply to human cancers are that the maternal and paternal alleles are equivalent. We also assume that both

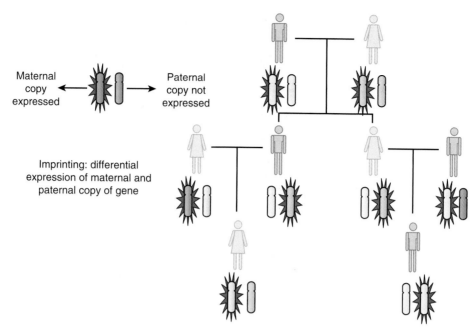

Maternal copy expressed ← → Paternal copy not expressed

Imprinting: differential expression of maternal and paternal copy of gene

FIGURE 19-18   Significance and mechanism of imprinting. *(From Korf B [ed]. Human Genetics: A Problem-Based Approach, 2nd ed. Blackwell Publishers, 2000.)*

copies of the gene are necessary for normal function. This is not true with respect to imprinting. An example of imprinting is the differences noted between the mule and the hinny. The mule is the cross between the maternal horse and paternal donkey. It is much larger than the hinny, which is a cross between the maternal mule and paternal horse. Although these two have the same genomic equivalent, they are distinctly different, indicating differential expression of maternal and paternal genes.

Examples of genomic imprinting and cancer are the hydatidiform mole and the teratoma. The hydatidiform mole is composed of paternal chromosomes, and the teratoma is composed of only maternal chromosomes. These examples demonstrate that not only does it take 46 chromosomes to make a human being, but there must also be a balance between maternal and paternal elements.

GENETIC ALTERATIONS THAT CAUSE CANCER

Oncogenes

The past 25 years have contributed significantly to our understanding of the molecular mechanism of cancer and have identified three types of molecular aberrations that can lead to cancer: dominant transforming genes called oncogenes, recessive transforming genes called

tumor suppressor genes, and genes responsible for repairing DNA errors (MMR repair genes). Many oncogenes have been isolated as forms of protooncogenes acquired by RNA tumor viruses. We have known for many years that viruses can cause malignant tumors in animals. The link noted in animals spurred a great deal of research aimed at identifying the cancer-causing genes carried by the viruses and finding the human genes that were affected. These investigations surprisingly revealed that the genes implicated in malignant disease were often altered forms of viral genes. These were probably acquired when the virus infected the animal and then moved on to other animals. At other times, the viruses activated host genes that were normally quiescent. The normal versions of these pirated and activated genes, now termed protooncogenes, carried codes specifying the composition of proteins that encourage and stimulate cell replication. These growth-promoting genes come in various forms. Some specify the amino acid sequences of receptors that are found on the cell surface and bind to molecules known as growth factors. When bound by such factors, the receptor issues an intracellular signal that ultimately causes cells to replicate. Other growth-promoting genes code for proteins that lie inside the cell and govern the propagation of intracellular growth signals. A third group encodes proteins that control cell division and are under nuclear control. These oncogenes can be activated via several mechanisms. The oncogene can be amplified and many copies of the gene can become activated. Occasionally,

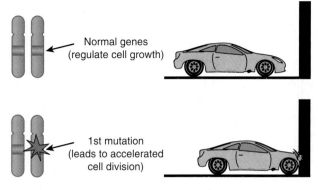

FIGURE 19-19   Schematic of oncogene function.

the gene may be translocated to another chromosome, where, under the influence of another promoter, it promotes uncontrolled growth.

The three classes of oncogenes are controlled differently. The first comprises a group of peptide growth factors and their receptors. Included in this group would be the peptide growth factors and their receptors such as epidermal growth factor receptor (EDGFR) or platelet-derived growth factor (PDGFR). These peptide growth factor receptors likely serve as stimulatory cofactors rather than the actual force that drives the malignant process. Targeted therapy is becoming a reality as our understanding of these cancer-promoting entities increases. There are unique molecules that are aimed at gene products or proteins activated by these factors. Another class of oncogenes comes from non–membrane–traversing extranuclear growth factors. These would include G-proteins and the ras gene family. Finally, there are oncogenes of the nuclear regulatory variety such as myc. A schematic of oncogenes representing their function can be seen in Figure 19-19. A more detailed description of targeted therapy can be found in Chapter 18.

The discovery that viral genes had human counterparts introduced the intriguing possibility that human cancers, including the majority not caused by viruses, might originate from mutations that convert useful protooncogenes into harmful genes—that is, oncogenes. Consistent with this notion, studies indicated that alteration of just one copy, or allele, of these protooncogenes was enough to transform and render cancerous some types of cells growing in culture. Such dominant mutations cause cells to overproduce a normal protein or make an aberrant form that is overactive. In either case, the result is that stimulatory signals increase within the cell even when no such signals come from the outside.

It is ironic that research on animal RNA tumor viruses (retroviruses) having no ability to cause human cancer provided the first key to uncovering the identity of some oncogenes and the verification that they actually exist. These retroviruses, which infected chickens, rodents, cats, and monkeys, were extremely tumorigenic in that infected animals often showed tumors on initial exposure to the virus. One of these viruses, the Rous sarcoma virus of a chicken, was found to carry a specific gene that it used to transform infected cells to a malignant state. This type of transforming oncogene was termed a viral oncogene. A single oncogene carried onto a chicken cell by a Rous sarcoma virus was able to derail and redirect the entire metabolism of the cell, forcing it to grow in a malignant fashion.

In 1976 Varmus and Bishop found that the oncogene in the Rous sarcoma virus was not a viral gene at all; instead, it rose directly from a preexisting cellular gene that had been captured by an ancestor of the Rous sarcoma virus. Once captured, this gene was used by the Rous sarcoma virus to transform mammalian cells. The early ancestor of the Rous sarcoma virus was capable of replicating in infected cells but was unable to transform them; it instantly gained tumorigenic potency by kidnapping this normal cellular gene, the protooncogene. In the end, this work by Varmus and Bishop revealed much more about the cell than it did about the Rous sarcoma virus because it pointed to the existence of a gene residing in a normal mammalian genome that possessed potent transforming ability when appropriately activated, in this case by a retrovirus. Here was clear proof of the presence of at least one gene in the normal cellular DNA that might serve as one of the target genes activated by nonviral carcinogens of the retrovirus; such nonviral agents might also activate this protooncogene, converting it to a powerful oncogene. A cell carrying such a mutant gene might, in turn, respond to this damage by launching a program of deregulated growth and thus become a cancer cell.

The information uncovered concerning retroviruses and oncogenes provided little immediate comfort to investigators interested in the origins of human cancer. Retroviruses, like Rous sarcoma virus, never infected humans and therefore could not act to mobilize human protooncogenes. The possible connection came from a notion that many such protooncogenes could be activated through an alternative route. Changes in the DNA sequence created by chemical or physical rearrangement might substitute for the virus. Mutations induced by these chemical or physical conditions in the genomes of target cells in one or another tissue might be as effective as retroviruses in activating latent carcinogenic potential in the protooncogenes. By the early 1980s, these suspicions were validated: mutated genes (protooncogenes) were found in human tumor genomes. In each case, a change in the sequence of the gene was identified as being responsible for converting a protooncogene into an active oncogene. For example, a ras oncogene in one human bladder carcinoma was found to have arisen through a single base change that altered the DNA sequence of a precursor protooncogene; myc oncogenes arose through gene amplification in various malignant neoplasms.

Next, researchers tried to ascertain how these genes succeeded in transforming cells. A simple theme emerged that makes it possible to understand and explain the mechanism of action of most if not all of the oncogenes. This comes through the understanding of how cells regulate their own growth. The growth and division of a normal cell residing in a particular tissue is controlled largely by its surroundings. A normal cell rarely if ever decides its own rate of proliferation; rather, it responds to the signals or messages from surrounding cells. These messages, which may carry growth-stimulatory or growth-inhibitory information, are conveyed by growth factors released by surrounding cells, traverse the intercellular space, and bind to the cell surfaces. These cells then respond to these growth signals by activating their synthetic machinery, copying their DNA, and dividing. A normal cell will never commit itself to such a growth program without having been simulated by these external signals. Each cell possesses complex machinery that enables it to receive these signals, process them, and launch a growth program. The machinery consists of an array of proteins that function to acquire growth-activating signals and transmit them throughout the cell. These proteins include the following:

1. Cell surface receptors that recognize the presence of growth factors in the extracellular space and transmit signals into the cell's interior
2. Cytoplasmic signal transducers that become activated by these receptors and then pass signals farther into the cell
3. Nuclear transcription factors that are activated by the cytoplasmic signal transducers and in turn respond by activating entire banks of cellular genes

These activated gene banks together orchestrate the cell's growth program; they detail events that, acting in concert, enable the cell to grow and divide. Protooncogenes encode many of the proteins in this complex signaling circuitry that enable a normal cell to respond to exogenous growth factors. Oncogenes participate in this signaling circuitry by selecting aberrantly functioning versions of the components of this circuitry. Oncogene proteins succeed in activating these signal circuits even in the absence of stimulation by extracellular growth factors. In doing so, they force a cell to grow even when its surroundings do not contain some of the clues that are normally required to provoke growth.

Other researchers suggest that mutations in at least two protooncogenes have to be present and that

TABLE 19-2 Functional Classification of Selected Oncogenes and Associated Human Tumors

Function	Oncogene	Associated Tumors
Growth factor	hst	Gastric cancer
	KS3	Kaposi's sarcoma
Growth factor receptor	Neu-erB-B2	Breast, ovary, gastric cancers
	erb-B	Breast cancer, glioblastoma
	trk	Papillary thyroid, colon cancers
Signal transducing (GTP-binding) proteins	Ha-ras	Bladder cancer
	Ki-ras	Lung, colon cancers
	N-ras	Leukemias
	gsp	Pituitary tumors
Protein kinases	raf	Gastric cancer
	met	Osteosarcoma
	abl	Leukemia/lymphoma
Nuclear transcription factor	myc	Lymphomas, carcinomas
	N-myc	Neuroblastoma
	L-myc	Small cell lung cancer
Membrane protein	bcl-2	Follicular, undifferentiated lymphoma
	mas	Breast cancer
	ret	Papillary thyroid cancer

From Mastrangelo MJ et al: Semin Oncol 23:4, 1996.

only certain combinations of mutations lead to malignant change. These findings suggest that individual oncogenes, although powerful controllers of cell metabolism, are not capable of causing malignant neoplasms by themselves. Thus oncogenes cannot explain most cancers by themselves. This view was strengthened by the discovery of more than a dozen different oncogenes in human tumors (Table 19-2). However, on careful evaluation, only about 20% of tumors turned out to carry expected alterations. None of the tumors had pairs of cooperative alterations sometimes found in cultured cells. It also appeared that the inherited mutations responsible for predisposing people to cancer were not oncogenes. The concept of a recessive-type anti-oncogene was conceived. This type of gene is called a tumor suppressor gene. This class of gene appears to be equally important in the development of cancer.

Tumor Suppressor Genes

The direct identification of tumor suppressor genes has been more difficult than the identification of oncogenes. Tumor suppressor genes were first conceived of in a theoretical sense long before any were actually identified. Harris was the first to demonstrate that the malignant characteristics of a cell could be suppressed when malignant cells were fused with nonmalignant cells. Furthermore, loss of portions of chromosomes can be

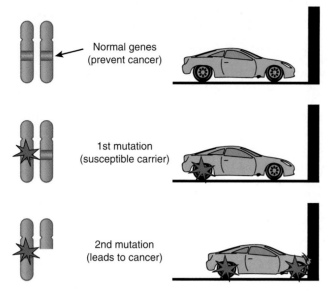

FIGURE 19-20 Schematic of tumor suppressor gene function. *(Reprinted with permission from ASCO Curriculum: Cancer Genetics and Cancer Predisposition Testing. 2nd Edition. Schematic of tumor suppressor gene function.)*

associated with malignant transformation, and transfer of a normal chromosome can reverse these traits into the malignant cells. These data suggested a recessive type of control in normal cells. A schematic of a tumor suppressor gene can be seen in Figure 19-20.

The first tumor suppressor gene cloned was the Rb gene; it is the defective gene in retinoblastoma. Knudson extensively studied the epidemiology of retinoblastoma. Most cases of retinoblastoma are sporadic, but some cases appear to be clustered around families. He noted that cases of familial retinoblastoma were more likely to be bilateral or multifocal. On the basis of these data, he developed the two-hit hypothesis that bears his name (see Figure 19-16). That is to say that two mutagenic events are required for retinoblastoma to develop. In patients with inherited disease, the first hit was inherited in one allele of the Rb gene in the germline. Although one abnormality was not enough for development of the disease, there was an increased likelihood that the second allele would be damaged during eye development. The hypothesis of two mutational events developed by Knudson applies specifically to tumor suppressor genes. This is the basis of most inherited gene models.

Tumor suppressor genes have proved difficult to identify, and many techniques have been used to locate such genes within the human genome. Cytogenetic studies provide some clues to the location of tumor suppressor genes. A significant percentage of patients with retinoblastoma or some patients with Wilms' tumor have large deletions in 13q14 or 11p13, respectively. These are the regions of the respective tumor suppressor

genes responsible for each malignant neoplasm. Significant loss on 5q is associated with adenomatous polyps of the colon. This can be measured on a gel during electrophoresis and is called loss of heterozygosity. Although recurrent loss of a chromosome region associated with a specific malignant neoplasm is highly suggestive that this region is important in the development of the cancer, it is not sufficient to prove that there is a tumor suppressor gene in this region. Figure 19-16 shows the possible combinations of loss that would lead to the expression of a tumor suppressor gene. Use of genome-wide linkage scans can further localize the presence of such a gene. Much smaller areas of deletion can be detected by molecular techniques such as pulsed-field electrophoresis. Now we can also easily and cheaply sequence long segments of the genome as these technologies improve.

When scientists were first trying to identify the regions of loss, they used DNA probes for specific regions of chromosomes. If allelic loss is noted, this is called loss of heterozygosity; if this loss is disproportionate relative to the general population, this suggests a tumor suppressor gene in the region specific for the probe. An example of loss of heterozygosity can be seen in Figure 19-6. Here, a region on 10q in endometrial cancers indicates the existence of a possible tumor suppressor gene. By use of various markers, a precise location of the tumor suppressor gene can be identified. A contig of the region must then be built and the region sequenced to look for specific genes. Many regions of loss have been identified by this technique. There are many more candidate regions than actual tumor suppressor genes.

The tumor suppressor gene Tp53 is a gene associated with many cancers that was identified by searching for loss of heterozygosity. Several other tumor suppressor genes have been identified since. This is almost certainly only the tip of the iceberg, and many more tumor suppressor genes are likely to be discovered as investigators learn more about cancer cell genetics and as the Human Genome Project continues and reaches completion. Several generalizations can be made, and a comparison with the activation of oncogenes is constructive. Mutations in oncogenes are gain of function events and lead to increased cell proliferation and decreased cell differentiation. Oncogene mutations do not appear to be inherited through the germline. In contrast, tumor suppressor gene inactivations are loss of function events, usually requiring a mutational event in one allele followed by a loss or inactivation of the other allele. This loss of gene function leads to loss of cellular control and unchecked growth. Tumor suppressor genes are recessive, and mutations may be inherited as a germline mutation. Somatic mutations may occur in both types of genes and accumulate throughout life. Comparison of oncogenes and tumor suppressor genes is made in

TABLE 19-3   Comparison of Oncogenes and Tumor Suppressor Genes

Characteristic	Oncogene	Tumor Suppressor Gene
Number of mutational events in cancer	One	Two
Role of mutation	Gain of function ("dominant")	Loss of function ("recessive")
Germline inheritance	No	Yes
Somatic mutations	Yes	Yes
Genetic alterations	Point mutations, amplifications, gene rearrangements	Point mutations, deletions
Effect on growth control	Activates cell proliferation	Negatively regulates growth-promoting genes
Result of gene transfection	Transforms cells to a partly malignant behavior	Suppresses malignant phenotype

TABLE 19-4   Tumor Suppressor Genes

Gene	Gene Product	Tumor Associations
RB1 (13q)*	110-kDa nuclear hypophosphorylated protein, negative cell cycle regulator	Retinoblastoma Osteosarcoma Small cell lung cancer Soft tissue sarcoma Breast cancer Bladder cancer
p53 (17p)	53-kDa sequence-specific DNA-binding protein and transcriptional activator	Li-Fraumeni syndrome Most common alteration in human cancer
DCC (18q)	1447-Amino acid transmembrane protein with homology to known adhesion molecules; role in terminal cell differentiation	Colorectal cancer
APC (5q21)	2843-Amino acid protein that interacts with membrane-associated cadherin-catenin complexes and with microtubules	Familial adenomatous polyposis Gardner's syndrome
MTSI (9q21)	148-amino acid protein inhibitor of cyclin-dependent kinase-4	Familial melanoma Bladder cancer
BRCA1 (17q)	1863-Amino acid protein with zinc finger–like domains suggesting function as a transcriptional factor	Breast cancer Ovarian cancer
BRCA2 (13q)	Possibly BRUSH I	Familial breast cancer
VHL (3p)	Protein with short homology to a glycan-anchored membrane protein of *Trypanosoma brucei*, no function assigned	Pheochromocytoma Renal cell cancer Pancreatic cancer Hemangioblastomas of CNS and retina
WT1 (11q)	50-kDa gene, related to the early growth response gene, encodes four 46- to 49-kDa proteins, which appear to function as DNA-binding transcriptional repressors	Wilms' tumor
NF1 (17q11.2)	Neurofibromin (about 2500 amino acids), probably negative regulator for p21 ras	von Recklinghausen's neurofibromatosis
NF2 (22q12)	Schwannomin (~600 amino acids), regulator of cellular response to external environment	Neurofibromatosis type 2

Chromosome location. From Mastrangelo MJ et al: Semin Oncol 23:4, 1996.

Table 19-3. Common tumor suppressor genes are listed in Table 19-4.

Apoptosis

Apoptosis means programmed cell death and refers to the intentional induction of cell death. Apoptosis is important in the growth and development of an organism because as an organism matures and differentiates, cells must die to give way to more differentiated and specialized cells. If a cell does not die and becomes immortal, a cancer can result. Apoptosis was first described in the 1970s, but only recently have scientists begun to realize the importance of this phenomenon in organism development, differentiation, and cancer formation. Excitement about this process has been driven by the finding that apoptosis is controlled at the molecular level by genes associated with malignant change (i.e., oncogenes, protooncogenes, and tumor suppressor genes). It is also clear that many of these same controlling elements and pathways are active during development. Many believe that understanding the control of the apoptotic process is essential to understanding the control of the developing organism and control of senescence. Loss of these aspects of cellular control could lead to cancer.

Apoptosis is a distinct mode of cell death that is responsible for the deletion of cells in normal tissues; of note, it also occurs in pathologic conditions. The process of apoptosis is characterized histologically by cell contraction, blebbing of the cell membrane, and condensation of the nucleus. Apoptotic bodies are formed that contain intact organelles; surrounding cells eventually phagocytose these. There is no associated inflammatory response. Cell swelling and disintegration of the cell components characterize necrotic cell death, and there is a marked inflammatory response. On a molecular level, apoptotic death causes cellular enzymes to autodigest the genome into little fragments, and this can be identified on polyacrylamide gels by multiple regular fragments seen as a DNA ladder.

Apoptosis is important in the development of the normal organism, and it is important in the development and growth of cancers. It occurs spontaneously in malignant tumors, often markedly retarding their growth, and it is increased in tumors responding to radiation, chemotherapy, heat, and hormone damage. In cancer, apoptosis appears to be a mechanism for deleting cells from the population that have sustained carcinogenic DNA damage; however, when apoptosis of such cells is blocked or inhibited by mutations in genes that help control this process, such as *BCL2* or *Tp53*, these cells are suddenly free to continue replicating and propagating their mutations. This genetic instability may be an early

step in the development of cancers. Many of the current cancer treatments, such as radiotherapy and chemotherapy, kill cells by the production of DNA damage. Mutations in BCL2 and Tp53 may then influence the effectiveness of these therapies through their ability to inhibit cell death.

The primary importance of apoptosis related to cancer and cancer treatment lies in its being a regulated phenomenon subject to stimulation and inhibition. Although little is known about how to establish therapeutic agents to affect its initiation, it seems reasonable to suggest that greater understanding of the process of apoptosis might lead to the development of improved treatment possibilities. Inhibitory mechanisms such as *BCL2* protooncogene expression may be implicated in the development of resistance to therapeutic agents and may contribute to tumor growth and perhaps to oncogenesis by allowing the inappropriate survival of cells with DNA abnormalities. It is likely that other inhibitory mechanisms will be identified, and a better understanding of the apoptotic process may lead to novel treatment regimens by allowing us to control cell death. Apoptosis is not simply a description of cell death, nor is it a spurious trend in the biology literature. It is a fundamental process and is controlled at the molecular level; as such, it can be understood and manipulated. Figure 19-21 demonstrates how apoptosis may occur.

Mismatch Repair Defects

A number of mechanisms are involved in the correction of DNA changes that result from exogenous or endogenous mutagenic agents. These mechanisms include base excision repair, nucleotide excision repair, and DNA

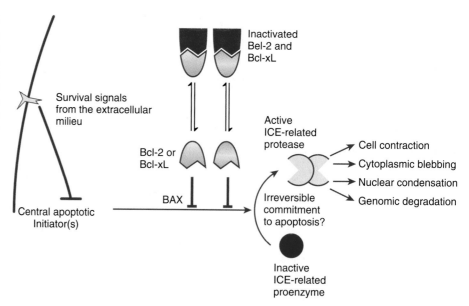

FIGURE 19-21 Possible pathways and possible factors controlling apoptosis. A signal from outside the cell initiates a cascade of events involving *BCL2, BCL-xL,* and *BAX*. This results in the programmed death of the cell. This pathway can be blocked at a number of points, resulting in cell immortality. (*ICE,* Interleukin-1βA signal fleukin-1id.) (*From Rudin CM, Thompson CB: Annu Rev Med 48:267, 1997.*)

mismatch repair. The MMR system repairs mistakes that are made in the course of normal division. These mutations often occur in regions of multiple repeats because these regions appear to be particularly prone to DNA slippage. One can intuitively see how this can happen by looking at Figure 19-22. There are six genes that must work in concert to repair DNA damage. These genes and an example of how we think they work can be seen in Figure 19-23.

A paradox of human tumor genesis is that the rates of mutation in normal cells are too low to account for the transformation of benign to malignant. The instability of some colon cancers was the first strong evidence for the so-called mutator phenotype. If a cell cannot repair DNA damage that occurs during the course of normal cell division, mutations can continue to accumulate; eventually enough mutations occur in genes critical for cell control, and cancer results. This is how absence of DNA repair can lead to cancer. Many studies have shown that tumors, which have microsatellite instability, have defects in mismatch repair. Key metabolic genes usually do not have large areas of microsatellite repeats that are particularly prone to mismatch problems. The mutation rate in nonrepetitive sequences is also elevated 100 to 10,000 times above that in normal cells with normal mismatch repair. Although microsatellite sequences are largely absent from functional genes, mononuclear repeats in some key genes can lead to their inactivation. Examples of such genes include $TGF-BR2H$ (A_{10}), $hMSH3$ (A_8), $hMSH6/GTBP$ (C_8), $IGF2R$ (G_8), and BAX (G_8). Paradoxically, instability of chromosome numbers is often observed in tumors without MMR defects; tumors with MMR defects often have stability of chromosome number.

Germline mutations in MMR genes are present in many families with hereditary cancers. These include some colon cancers (HNPCC), endometrial cancers, stomach cancers, and several other cancers. This hereditary cancer syndrome is called Lynch syndrome or hereditary nonpolyposis colon cancer syndrome; other cancer syndromes associated with mismatch repair are Muir–Torre and Turcot's syndromes. Lynch syndrome or HNPCC accounts for about 5% of all colon cancers and is a syndrome that can be defined by three criteria:

1. An individual must have three relatives with colon cancer, with at least two being first-degree relatives
2. At least two successive generations must be involved
3. At least one of the cancers must have been diagnosed before the age of 50 years.

Seventy percent of patients with HNPCC have a germline mutation segregated around an MMR gene: $hMLH1$ (49%), $hMLH2$ (45%), and $hPMS2$ (6%). Endometrial cancers have about a 25% incidence of MMR defects; approximately one fourth of these are germline mutations, and the rest are largely the result of $MLH1$ inactivation resulting from hypermethylation of the promoter region. Mismatch repair will be increasingly investigated and more clearly defined during the next decade.

Telomerase

Normal cells divide; this process is repeated many times as an organism grows and matures. Normal cells stop dividing and terminally differentiate, but cancer cells continue to divide. Cells from younger animals divide more times than do cells from older animals. One difference between normal cells and tumor cells is at the end of their chromosomes. Telomeres, specialized structures at the ends of chromosomes, act as protective caps. In humans, telomeres are made up of 5000 to 15,000 base pairs of TTAGGG repeats. These terminal structures protect the chromosome ends from exonuclease digestion, prevent aberrant chromosome recombination, and form specific complexes that bind proteins.

Normal cells lose about 50 to 100 base pairs from the end of each chromosome every time the cell divides. When a telomere loses a critical number of base pairs, it triggers a signal for the cell to stop dividing and for senescence. Cells have developed several mechanisms to get around this terminal trigger. Some of these are uncommon, such as complex recombination and retrotransport techniques. The most common mechanism is the development of an enzyme complex called telomerase, which adds back telomere sequences lost during replication. Cells that have significant telomerase activity are immortal cells like cancer cells or germ cells.

1. 5′AGCTTGGCTGCAGGTG **CACA** GTGTCACGGTCAGGTAC3′
   TCGAACCGACGTCCAC **GTGT** CACAGTGCCAGTCCATG

Replication

2. 5′AGCTTGGCTGCAGGTG **CACA** GTGTCACGGTCAGGTAC3′
   GT CACAGTGCCAGTCCATG

Mismatch Repair
susceptible intermediate   CA   Slippage
3. 5′AGCTTGGCTGCAGGTG   CA GTGTCACGGTCAGGTAC3′
   C   GT CACAGTGCCAGTCCATG

−2Frameshift   Replication
4. 5′AGCTTGGCTGCAGGTG **CA** GTGTCACGGTCAGGTAC3′
   TCGAACCGACGTCCAC **GT** CACAGTGCCAGTCCATG

FIGURE 19-22 Mismatch repair occurs by slippage of CA within a CA repeat. This results in the deletion of a CA. This is the exact kind of deletion that the MMR system is designed to correct. If the MMR system is not working properly, errors cannot be corrected and mutations accumulate.

Normal cells lack telomerase activity. Telomerase becomes reactivated in most cancer cells. It is the most prevalent cancer marker known. Therefore telomerase may be used as a generic cancer marker and as a possible treatment.

CLINICALLY RELEVANT HEREDITARY SYNDROMES

The advent of linkage analysis and the rapidity of DNA sequencing with other molecular technologies have made it possible to identify many inherited disorders that we could not identify a few short decades ago. Cancers with a hereditary component that are relevant to gynecologist and other health care professionals caring for women that have been identified thus far are as follows:

Disease	Genetic Abnormality
Hereditary breast–ovarian	BRCA1/BRCA2
Hereditary nonpolyposis colon cancer or Lynch syndrome	MLH1, MSH2, MSH6, PMS1, PMS2
Cowden syndrome	PTEN
Familial adenomatous polyposis (FAP)	APC (dominant)
	MYH (recessive)
Li-Fraumeni syndrome	p53
Von Hippel-Lindau syndrome	VHL

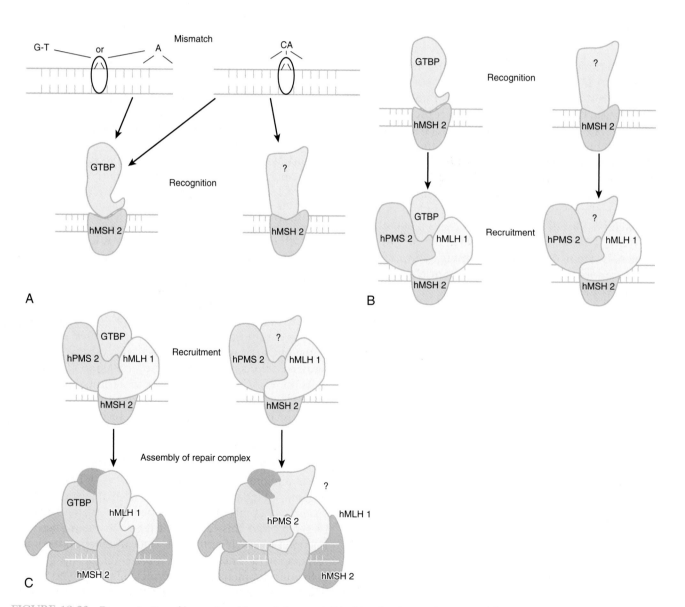

FIGURE 19-23   Demonstration of how mismatch repair is accomplished by the six proteins required for correction. There must be the following: **A,** recognition of slippage; **B,** recruitment of repair complex; and, finally, **C,** repair. *(From Karran P: Semin Cancer Biol 7:15, 1996.)*

These syndromes can now be tested for on a commercial basis. The cost of testing varies from a few hundred dollars for site-specific testing to $1000 or $2000 to sequence a single whole gene. The disease about which we know the most is hereditary breast and ovarian cancer syndrome and is associated with mutations in the *BRCA1* and *BRCA2* genes. Genetic testing for the predisposition to ovarian cancer by testing for mutations in the *BRCA1* or *BRCA2* genes became available in 1996, and this technology is now well established. Mutations in these two genes are associated with up to 13% of all epithelial ovarian cancers. Other genes that are associated with hereditary ovarian cancer or other gynecologic cancers are the MMR genes (*MLH1*, *MSH2*, and *MSH6*) and are associated with Lynch syndrome or HNPCC. They account for 2% to 3% of ovarian cancer cases. Defects in the MMR genes are more commonly associated with endometrial cancer and are associated with up to 5% of all of these cancers. The ability to identify populations of patients at risk for developing cancers has led to a whole new field of preventive oncology. An increasing number of patients are seeking the advice of physicians and specifically gynecologic oncologists for advice regarding hereditary disease. Tools in these physicians' armamentarium include counseling, genetic testing, and preventive medicines such as oral contraceptives and prophylactic surgery. More frequent screening has not yet been shown to decrease the incidence or improve survival of these diseases except in the case of colon cancer. However, prophylactic surgery has been shown to decrease the incidence of many of these diseases— specifically, breast, ovarian and endometrial cancers.

Familial Breast and Ovarian Cancer (BRCA1 and BRCA2)

Familial breast and ovarian cancer syndrome is the best known and most well characterized of the hereditary cancer syndromes. The two genes most commonly responsible for this syndrome are *BRCA1* and *BRCA2* and were identified in the early 1990s (1994 for *BRCA1* and 1995 for *BRCA2*). Since that time the field of clinical genetics has grown at an ever-increasing rate such that we can now identify mutations by sequencing these genes in patients who are at risk for inherited breast or ovarian cancer. *BRCA1* and *BRCA2* genes are located on chromosomes 17q and 13q, respectively (Figure 19-24). Both of these genes are quite large, containing at least 20 exons (coding regions) and are of at least 7000 base pairs (Figure 19-25). Many inactivating mutations have been identified and span the entire coding sequences of both genes. An individual carrying a *BRCA1* germline mutation will have about a 70% chance of developing breast cancer and around a 45% chance of developing ovarian cancer by the age of 70. The overall contribution of each gene to the risk of ovarian cancer can be seen in Figure 19-26. Both of these genes are important in the general DNA repair process; therefore if they are defective,

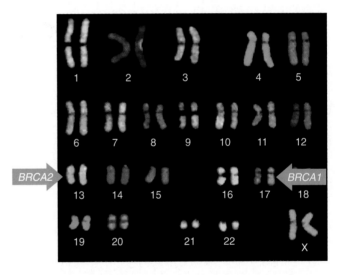

FIGURE 19-24 Karyotype of the human genome showing location of the *BRCA* and *BRCA2* genes.

FIGURE 19-25 Representation of the *BRCA1* and *BRCA2* genes with characteristics of each.

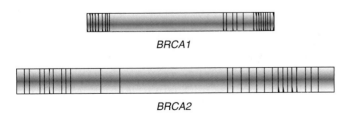

BRCA1

BRCA2

BRCA1
- Tumor suppressor gene on chromosome 17
- Coding region — 5589 nucleotides
- Span 81 KB Genomic DNA
- ~1200 different mutations reported

BRCA2
- Tumor suppressor gene on chromosome 13
- Coding region — 10,254 nucleotides
- Span 84 KB Genomic DNA
- ~1380 different mutations reported

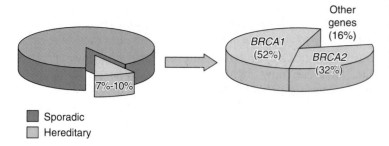

FIGURE 19-26 Hereditary breast and ovarian cancer. Representation of the percent contribution of inherited disease and the percent contribution by each of the known genes predisposing patients to cancer. *(Modified from Ford D et al: Am J Hum Genet 1998; 62:676.)*

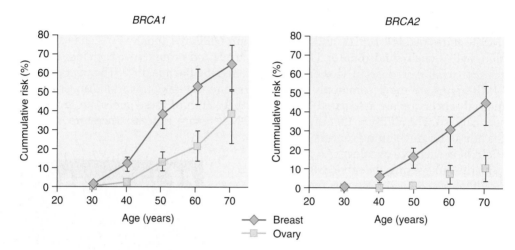

FIGURE 19-27 Cumulative incidence of cancer over time in individuals with *BRCA* mutations. (Summary analysis of 22 studies). *(Modified from Antoniou A et al: Am J Hum Genet 2003; 72:1117.)*

TABLE 19-5   Factors That Should be Considered When Considering Referring a Patient for Genetic Counseling for Risk Assessment of Familial Breast or Ovarian Cancer

Breast Cancer at younger than 40
Family member with a male breast cancer
Premenopausal breast cancer and a first- or second-degree relative with breast or ovarian cancer or two relatives of any degree or age
Breast cancer or ovarian cancer in a family of Ashkenazi Jewish heritage
High-grade papillary serous carcinoma of the ovary, fallopian tube or primary peritoneal cancer at any age
Two primary cancers of the breast or breast and ovary at any age
A known mutation within the family
Bilateral breast cancer

mistakes that occur within DNA as the result of normal injury cannot be repaired. Thus the concept of cumulative risk is important—that is, the longer one is alive, the more likely an abnormality or series of abnormalities in the DNA will develop that will lead to a cancers (Figure 19-27 and Table 19-5).

BRCA1 mutations are responsible for 60% to 89% of inherited ovarian cancers. Of inherited ovarian cancers, 60% to 80% are of papillary serous histology. However,

there is no appreciable difference in the histologic types of cancers that result from *BRCA1* or *BRCA2* mutations and most are of high-grade papillary serous histology. Of note, patients with *BRCA1* or 2 mutation-associated cancers tend to have longer survival when compared to patients with sporadic disease. This may be because cancers with DNA repair problems as occur with a *BRCA1* or 2 mutations are more susceptible to chemotherapeutic agents that cause DNA damage. Furthermore, more than 13% of all patients with epithelial ovarian cancer of high-grade papillary serous type will have a *BRCA* mutation. Therefore it is reasonable to assess all patients with this histologic type for inherited disease.

Generally, the affected individual, known as the proband, is counseled and tested first. Then testing is offered to the other family members who are at risk. This testing can then be for the already known mutation in that family group. Testing for a specific mutation is much cheaper for the family than sequencing the whole gene—a few hundred dollars compared to $3500 for the whole gene.

Many factors are involved with a patient's risk of developing an ovarian cancer, but there are easily

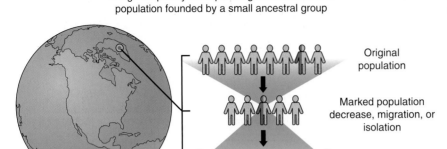

Founder Effect
A high frequency of a specific gene mutation in a population founded by a small ancestral group

Original population

Marked population decrease, migration, or isolation

Generations later

FIGURE 19-28 Representation of founder mutations and how the prevalence can increase in a population over time.

TABLE 19-6 Criteria for Referral to a Genetic Counselor for Suspected Lynch Syndrome

Bethesda guidelines
Amsterdam Criteria fulfilled
Persons with two relatives with Lynch syndrome
Colorectal cancer and first-degree relative with a Lynch cancer <45 years or a first-degree relative with an adenoma <40 years
Colorectal cancer or endometrial cancer <45 years
Right-sided, undifferentiated colon cancer <45 years
Signet ring colon cancer <45 years
Adenoma <40 years

Populations with *BRCA* Founder Mutations

- Ashkenazim
- Icelanders
- Finns
- Norwegians
- Swedish
- Dutch
- French-Canadians
- Hungarians
- Poles
- Baltics/Russians

FIGURE 19-29 Populations that have known founder mutations.

ascertainable features that can help predict those at risk for hereditary disease. Family history is one of these, with the number of relatives with ovarian or breast cancer, the proximity of relationship to the proband or affected individual, and the age of onset of the disease of utmost importance. Early onset of the cancers may be the most predictable feature of inherited disease. Features in the history in families that should be considered when deciding when to patients for genetic counseling are listed in Table 19-6.

Another important concept is the idea of a founder mutation. These are mutations that are common or even unique to a specific patient population and occur in populations of patients who have been genetically isolated for many generations. The population may have shrunk as a result of a disaster, but the mutation was preserved in a few individuals. When the population reexpands, the frequency of that specific mutation can be quite high within a population (Figure 19-28). There are many specific known DNA differences in various groups of similar heredity. These specific mutations are called founder mutations and can be tested for in patients of a specific heritage (Figure 19-29). It is often worth testing for these specific mutations in these groups of patients first because it is much less expensive than sequencing the whole gene.

Lynch Syndrome or Hereditary Nonpolyposis Colon Cancer

In 1895 a pathologist at the University of Michigan, Aldred Scott Warthin, had a seamstress who had a family with a preponderance of gastric and endometrial cancers. This family became known as family G and is part of the basis for the discovery of Lynch syndrome or HNPCC. Warthin described this family in a report in the *Archives of Internal Medicine* in 1913 (Figure 19-30). The family pedigree was updated in 1925 but was largely forgotten until Henry Lynch and colleagues discovered two other families with similar pedigrees in Iowa and Nebraska, which they reported in the 1970s. This was proposed as the cancer family syndrome in 1971 and is now known as Lynch syndrome or HNPCC. There has now been a shift of the frequency of stomach cancers seen within family G to a preponderance of colon cancers similar to the shift noted in society at large as we made the shift from preserved to frozen foods. Furthermore, this syndrome is associated with a wide range of cancers (Figure 19-31).

Hereditary nonpolyposis colorectal cancer is an autosomal dominantly inherited disease of the DNA MMR system. Lynch syndrome results in genetic susceptibility to many types of malignancies, but the two most common

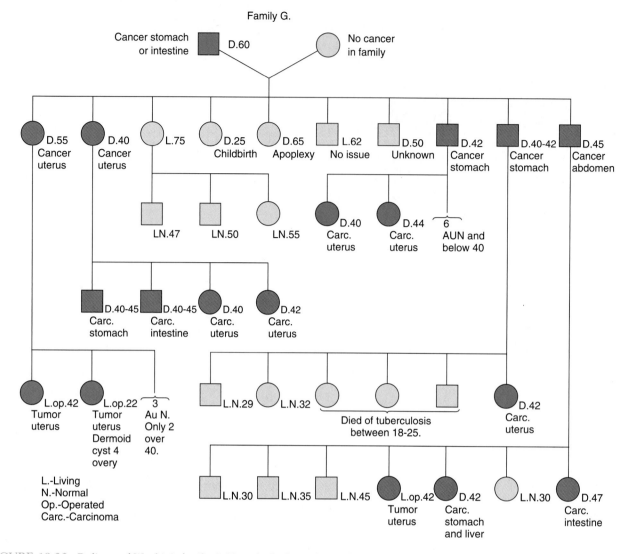

FIGURE 19-30   Pedigree of Warthin's family G. Note the high incidence of stomach cancer. This transitioned to colon cancer through the 1900s.

FIGURE 19-31   Various cancers associated with Lynch Syndrome and their frequencies.

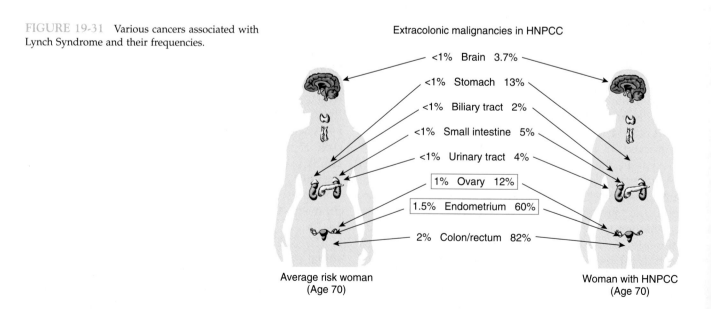

Extracolonic malignancies in HNPCC

<1% Brain 3.7%
<1% Stomach 13%
<1% Biliary tract 2%
<1% Small intestine 5%
<1% Urinary tract 4%
1% Ovary 12%
1.5% Endometrium 60%
2% Colon/rectum 82%

Average risk woman
(Age 70)

Woman with HNPCC
(Age 70)

Genetic Heterogeneity
in HNPCC

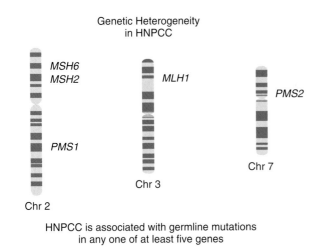

HNPCC is associated with germline mutations
in any one of at least five genes

FIGURE 19-32 Location of the MMR genes within the human genome.

Mismatch repair failure leads
to microsatellite instability (MSI)

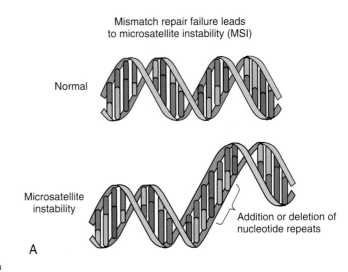

A

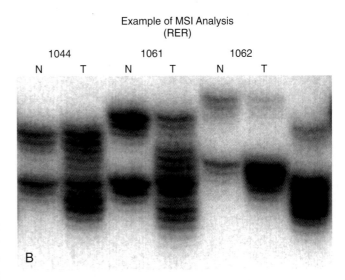

B

FIGURE 19-33 **A**, Representation of how mismatch repair occurs and how a DNA segment is lengthened or shortened. **B**, Gel showing microsatellite instability. N stands for normal tissue. Note two bands. T stands for tumor and not the smearing of the bands, indicating that there are fragments of different sizes of that DNA segment.

are colorectal and endometrial cancers, followed by ovarian cancer. Many authorities refer to HNPCC as the Lynch syndrome, believing that HNPCC fails to adequately acknowledge the importance of extracolonic malignancies such as endometrial, ovarian, upper gastrointestinal tract, and urinary tract cancers. This syndrome accounts for 5% to 10% of all colon and endometrial cancers.

Linkage analysis of high-risk families led to the discovery that Lynch syndrome is caused by germline mutations MMR genes, which give rise to proteins that proofread DNA and correct mistakes that are made during the normal process of replication. *MSH2* (MutS homolog 2) and *MLH1* (MutL L homolog 1) are the most commonly mutated MMR genes in this syndrome. *MSH2* and *MLH1* are located on chromosomes 2p16 and 3p21, respectively. Germline mutations in other MMR genes (*MSH6, PMS1,* and *PMS2*) have been identified but at a lower frequency (Figure 19-32). MMR proteins interact to form complexes that recognize mismatched DNA base pairs and abnormal loops of DNA. The repair complexes initiated by MMR genes trigger excision and repair of DNA mutations. This system is critically important in ensuring the fidelity of the replicative process and is highly conserved throughout all living organisms. Areas in the genome that contain simple repetitive DNA base sequences called microsatellites (e.g., CACACACA or AAAAAAA) are especially prone to mutation. If the MMR system does not function normally, these errors will go unrecognized and continue to accumulate. Cells in which both copies of one of the MMR genes have been inactivated exhibit the so-called mutator phenotype; this allows cells to accumulate mutations as they divide. These random mutations eventually accumulate in a series of genes that are important in controlling cellular growth; the result is loss of growth control and transformation to cancer.

Cells with a defective MMR system exhibit a phenomenon called microsatellite instability (MSI). This phenomenon occurs as DNA mismatches cause shortening or lengthening of repetitive DNA sequences and these mismatches go unchecked. This results in generation of alleles in the cancer that contain a greater or lesser number of repeats than are present in normal cells from that individual. Laboratory testing for MSI uses an established consensus panel of five microsatellite markers (D2S123, D5S346, D17S250, Bat 25, and Bat 26). Figure 19-33 shows an example of MSI detection when mismatch prone regions are compared in blood and

TABLE 19-7   Amsterdam Criteria: Three Two One Rule

Three or more relatives with verified Lynch-associated cancer within
  the family
    Colorectal, endometrial, small bowel, ureter, or renal pelvis
    Any combination of histologies in three different generations
    One case is a first-degree relative of the other two
At least two successive generations affected
One or more cases by the age of 50
Exclude familial adenomatous polyposis

TABLE 19-8   Criteria for Consideration of Referral to a Genetic
Counselor for Possible Cowden Syndrome

Pathognomonic criteria	Adult Lhermitte-Duclos disease
	Mucocutaneous lesions
	Trichilemmonas
	Acral keratoses
	Papillomatous papules
Major criteria	Breast cancer
	Thyroid cancer
	Macrocephaly
	Endometrial cancer
Minor criteria	Thyroid lesions adenomas or goiter
	Mental retardation
	Gastrointestinal hamartomas
	Breast fibrocystic disease
	Lipomas
	Fibromas
Genitourinary tumors (specifically renal cell carcinoma) and structural abnormalities	Uterine fibroids
Diagnosis in an individual	Any single pathognomonic criterion, but mucocutaneous lesions if meeting specific criteria one major and at least three criteria or at least four minor criteria alone
Diagnosis in a family where one individual has characteristics diagnostic for Cowden	Individuals must have at least one of the following
	A pathognomonic criteria
	Any one major criteria with or without minor criteria
Two minor criteria or history of Bannayan-Riley-Ruvalcaba syndrome	

tumor. Nearly all HNPCC-related colorectal cancers and endometrial cancers demonstrate MSI, whereas this is a much less common finding in sporadic colorectal and endometrial cancers. Some centers advocate MSI testing of all colon and endometrial cancers, especially those occurring in patients younger than age 50. It is noteworthy that about 25% of sporadic endometrial cancers exhibit MSI as a result of epigenetic inactivation of MMR genes, particularly *MLH1,* owing to gene silencing by way of promoter methylation. This finding makes Lynch syndrome screening by MSI testing somewhat less specific in cases of endometrial cancer. Evaluation of hereditary endometrial cancers is more complicated than for colon cancers because MSI from promoter methylation must be distinguished from MSI because of an inherited MMR defect.

Family history is the first step in determining whether a patient is at increased risk for an inherited disease. Several relatively stringent criteria have been developed to identify individuals at high risk for Lynch syndrome. The Bethesda criteria seem to be the most sensitive in predicting MMR mutations in HNPCC families, but the Amsterdam II criteria is more specific (Tables 19-7 and 19-8). About 30% of families fulfilling the Bethesda criteria and 50% to 92% of families fulfilling the Amsterdam criteria will have a germline DNA MMR gene mutation. Many of the families fulfilling the Bethesda criteria with a preponderance of endometrial cancers will have *MSH6* mutations, because the incidence of colorectal cancers is quite low in individuals carrying this mutation. A typical pedigree of a family meeting the criteria for a Lynch syndrome family can be seen in Figure 19-34.

All patients should be asked about their family history of cancer. If it appears there could be a genetic predisposition based on the presence of excessive cancer cases, with some occurring at an early age, a family pedigree should be drawn. This allows for a rapid assessment of whether the women should be suspected of having a hereditary cancer syndrome and be referred for genetic counseling. Individuals with Lynch syndrome have an increased risk of a variety of different cancers. When evaluating a family pedigree, it is important to consider the size of the family. A small family often makes it

difficult to determine the exact risk of a mutation, and for this reason family history may not be as reassuring in these families. Furthermore, in contrast to breast–ovarian cancer families, cancer in male probands may significantly contribute to the assignment of risk. It is important to understand that the accuracy of a family history can be variable and depends on a number of factors, including the woman's closeness to her relatives and her understanding of the family's medical histories. As an example, one study compared patient-reported family history with cancer registry data and found that one third of the colorectal cancers in first-degree relatives and two thirds of cases in second-degree relatives were not reported by the family member. This was especially true in older family members. Stomach, gynecologic, and second primary cancers were also all underreported.

Patients meeting the Bethesda or Amsterdam criteria should be referred for genetic counseling and possible genetic testing. The criteria for referral to a genetic counselor should be liberal because some families with MMR

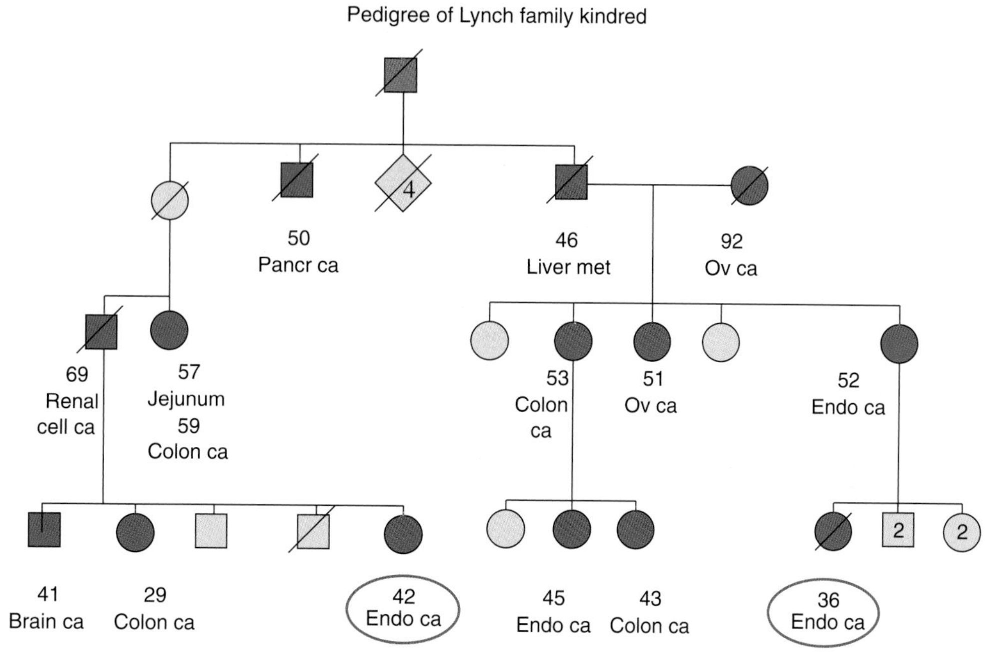

Pedigree of Lynch family kindred

FIGURE 19-34   Typical pedigree of a family with Lynch syndrome.

mutations may not completely fulfill either the Bethesda or Amsterdam criteria. Often, it is not clear if these diagnostic criteria are met until the patient and her family meet with the genetic counselor and their medical and family histories are analyzed in detail. The American Gastrointestinal Association, the American Society of Clinical Oncology, and the U.S. Multi-Society Task Force have advanced clinical cancer screening recommendations on colorectal cancer. These organizations suggest that colonoscopy be performed every 1 to 2 years from age 25 to 30, or 10 years before the earliest relative with a Lynch-related cancer.

In families that fulfill the Amsterdam criteria, the likelihood that a mutation will be found is quite high; the chance of identifying a mutation in one of the MMR genes is between 50% and 92%. If a family meets the Bethesda or Amsterdam criteria, examination of tumor tissue is indicated. MSI testing followed by immunohistochemical staining for the MMR genes is quite accurate in detecting patients with colon cancer who have germline mutations. This approach is less accurate in patients with endometrial cancer because epigenetic silencing by promoter methylation of the MMR genes can lead to MSI in the absence of a germline MMR gene mutation. Nonetheless, these tumor tissue tests can help determine which patients are the best candidates for gene sequencing because this analysis can be both expensive and time consuming. Some recent data suggest that as many as 7 of 10 individuals with Lynch syndrome who develop endometrial cancer do not meet any published criteria for Lynch syndrome and many of these cancers are

diagnosed after age 50. Therefore some investigators suggest screening all endometrial cancers with a combination of immunohistochemistry (IHC) and MSI. This more intensive evaluation of all patients certainly would pick up more patients with an inherited defect. This screening algorithm suggested by the Ohio State team can be seen in Figure 19-35. The authors and others are currently planning a trial that would determine the efficacy and cost effectiveness of this screening pathway but do not currently endorse it on every patient.

If there is no tumor tissue available, then a three-generation family history is the most powerful means of determining if genetic testing will be helpful. The American Gastroenterological Association (AGA) recommends considering germline genetic screening when any one of the following criteria are met: the patient or her family members meet any of the first three modified Bethesda criteria outlined or a family member has a known Lynch germline mutation already detected by prior genetic testing. Approximately 40% of patients fulfilling these criteria will have an *MLH1* or *MSH2* mutation. Patients who do not meet the AGA guidelines but are still felt to be at risk for Lynch syndrome can undergo testing of tumor tissue to determine MSI status, or the tumors can be evaluated for the loss of MMR protein expression by IHC. If either of these is positive, then germline testing should be performed. As stated previously, as many as 75% of endometrial cancers do not meet any published criteria for Lynch.

Commercial testing for the genetic defects associated with mismatch repair is currently available. Several

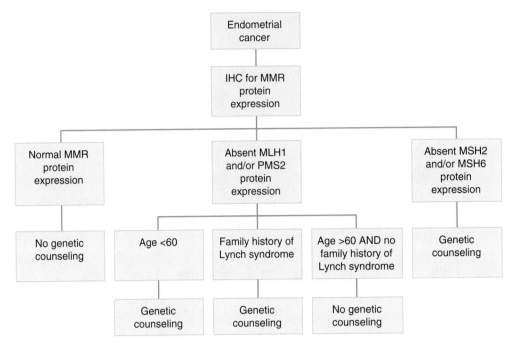

FIGURE 19-35   Screening algorithm used by the Ohio State group. *(From Backes et al: Gyn Onc 114:486, 2009.)*

methods are used, but most authorities recommend complete gene sequencing of *MLH1*, *MSH2*, and *MSH6*, the three most commonly affected genes. Usually a family member with the Lynch-associated malignancy should be tested first. Once the mutation is identified, a simpler and less costly genetic analysis can be performed on other family members. Extensive counseling is recommended before and after the testing. A formally trained genetic counselor should perform this portion of the evaluation. The entire process of obtaining a complete family history, obtaining the records for verification, explaining the testing options, and discussing the pros and cons of genetic testing can be complicated and time consuming.

Results can return as positive, negative, or indeterminate. Patients who test negative in a family with a known mutation can be reassured that their risk of developing a Lynch-related malignancy is that of the general population and they should follow American Cancer Society screening recommendations for these cancers. A negative test in a family at risk but without a known mutation can be difficult to interpret. This is because not all mutations have been identified and there may be other unrecognized deleterious genes and genetic abnormalities. These patients probably should be followed in a manner similar to those who test positive until more information is available. Indeterminant results are reported when a DNA variant of uncertain significance is detected. If the variant is consistently present in individuals with Lynch-related malignancies, the abnormality should be considered positive for a disease-causing mutation. Over time,

as more individuals are tested, the incidence of indeterminant results should diminish.

Once the genetic testing process has been completed, cancer risk can be assigned for the patient and her family. When a mutation has been identified, genetic testing should be offered to all family members. These individuals should each undergo genetic counseling so that pros and cons of testing can be explained. Carriers of a mutation are offered more intensive surveillance than the general population, as outlined in Figure 19-36. If no mutation is identified in the patient but the family meets Amsterdam criteria, the protocol for Lynch syndrome surveillance should be observed. Incidence of and mortality from colorectal cancers in this group have been shown to be reduced by colonoscopy screening (Figures 19-37 and 19-38). The International Collaborative Group on Hereditary Nonpolyposis Colorectal Cancer and the Cancer Genetics Study Consortium recommends screening based on the currently available data. Prospective data do not exist to validate the utility of endometrial cancer screening utilizing ultrasound and endometrial biopsy as a tool. Most authorities believe that risk-reducing hysterectomy with bilateral salpingo-oophorectomy has a role in the management of these patients. One study demonstrated that there were no cases of endometrial cancer in 61 patients with a mutation who underwent risk-reducing hysterectomy, but endometrial cancer developed in 69 of 210 who did not undergo surgery. Although not evidence-based and the penetrance of ovarian cancer in the Lynch syndrome is much less than that of BRCA mutation carriers, the

Surveillance Options for Carriers of HNPCC-Associated Mutations		
Malignancy	Intervention	Recommendation
Colorectal cancer	Colonoscopy	Begin at age 20-25, repeat every 1-2 years
Endometrial cancer	• Transvaginal ultrasound • Endometrial aspirate	Annually, starting at age 25-35

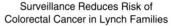

FIGURE 19-36   Recommended screening in families with Lynch syndrome. *(From Cancer Genetics Studies Consortium Task Force Recommendations. Modified from Burke W et al: JAMA 277:915, 1997.)*

guidelines for ovarian cancer screening using ultrasound and CA-125 are similar.

Colorectal cancers in Lynch syndrome have a propensity to occur in the proximal colon, relative to sporadic cases, which are more often distal. Prophylactic colectomy is recommended to patients with a MMR mutation in whom polyps are identified at a young age and also to patients who have polyps that are MSI positive or those individuals who are unable to undergo regular surveillance. Chemoprevention using nonsteroidal anti-inflammatory agents in this group of patients to prevent colon polyps is currently under study and data should be forthcoming. Prophylactic total hysterectomy with bilateral salpingo-oophorectomy should also be considered, recognizing that prospective data documenting its benefit are currently lacking. However, one must take into account that endometrial cancer is the most common extracolonic cancer in this syndrome and ovarian cancer risk also is elevated. The cumulative lifetime risk of endometrial cancer is between 40% and 60%, and the ovarian cancer risk is approximately 12%. If the patient is being explored for another reason, consideration should be given to counseling regarding possible risks and benefits of a total hysterectomy with bilateral salpingo-oophorectomy.

Other Inherited Diseases Relevant to Gynecology

Three other inherited diseases related to gynecologic diseases are Peutz-Jeghers syndrome (PJS), Cowden syndrome, and Li-Fraumeni syndrome. These all have gynecologic manifestations.

Peutz-Jeghers Syndrome

Patients with PJS are usually characterized by having pigmented lesions on visible mucosal surfaces; most easily seen are those on the lips and buccal mucosa. This syndrome was first identified in 1921 by Peutz and then subsequently described again in 1949 by Jehgers. Shortly thereafter it became known as Peutz-Jeghers syndrome.

The PJS susceptibility gene was not identified until 1998. This susceptibility gene is known as *STK11* or *LKB1*,

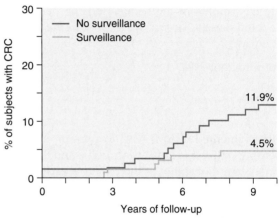

FIGURE 19-37   Effect of recommended colon screening on incidence of colon cancer in Lynch families. Regular recommended screening decreases the incidence. *(Modified from Jarvinen HJ et al: Gastroenterology 108:1405, 1995.)*

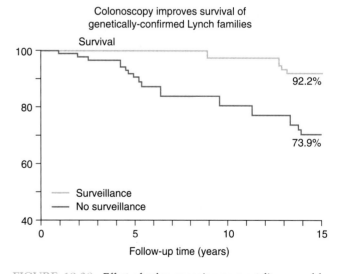

FIGURE 19-38   Effect of colon screening on mortality caused by colon cancer in families with Lynch syndrome. Regular recommended screening decreases mortality. *(From Jarvinen HJ et al: Gastroenterology 2000;118:829.)*

and its function has not been entirely elucidated. However, it appears to be a serine/threonine kinase type gene that is recessively expressed and therefore should be considered a tumor suppressor gene. It is also involved with determining and possibly controlling cellular polarity. The gene maps to chromosome 19p. However, only about 60% of patients with PJS have an *SKT11* mutation, suggesting that there are other heretofore unrecognized genes associated with this syndrome.

Flat pigmented lesions that look like dark-bluish freckles characterize this syndrome. They occur in about 95% of cases and are seen on very characteristic surfaces such as around the mouth and lips, buccal mucosa, soles of the feet, palms of the hands, and the perianal area. Pigmented areas occur with about the following frequencies:

Perioral region: 94%
Hands: 74%
Buccal mucosa: 66%
Feet: 62%

The pigmented lesions tend to present early in life, presenting within the first 2 years of life and then becoming more pronounced over the patient's early life. After puberty the external lesions can fade, often making the diagnosis difficult later in life. However, the buccal lesions tend to persist, so this is always an important area to examine.

Manifestations of this syndrome are gastrointestinal polyps that can cause gastrointestinal bleeding and even intussusception or obstruction. About half of the patients will undergo surgery during their lifetime for these issues. It is also associated with many tumors of the ovary, testicles, and cervix. Women with PJS can develop a very unusual ovarian stoma tumor known as sex cord–stromal tumors with annular tubules. These tumors have the distinction of almost always being associated with PJS and are fortunately usually benign and are usually found incidentally. Ovarian tumors that are associated with PJS are tumors of low malignant potential, granulosa cell tumors, Sertoli–Leydig cell tumors, and mucinous tumors. Another gynecologic tumor associated with PJS is a rare cervical cancer known as adenoma malignum. This tumor appears to be histologically benign but can behave quite aggressively. Therefore, patients with PJS should have an annual cervical examination with this in mind and any abnormality should be evaluated aggressively.

Patients with PJS have a significantly elevated risk of developing a malignancy. One meta-analysis suggested that the risk could be as high as 93%. However, most studies put the risk below 50%. Sadly, in the original Dutch report by Peutz, only 17 of 22 affected family members survived into adulthood, with the average individual dying by age 38.

TABLE 19-9   Diagnostic Criteria for Li-Fraumeni Syndrome

Proband of less than 45 years of age with a sarcoma
Plus
First-degree relative of less than 45 with any cancer
Plus
Additional first- or second-degree relative in the same lineage with any cancer or sarcoma

Surveillance for cancers associated with PJS is by expert opinion only and therefore needs to be validated by population-based studies. Unfortunately, the incidence of the disease is so low that these studies are not likely to be forthcoming. Therefore screening and care should be performed by being cognizant of the cancers and other problems associated with this disease. Follow-up should include a regular detailed physical examination with pelvic examination. Endoscopy should be considered starting in the late teens and continued every year or two. Mammograms starting at age 25 and yearly Pap smears should be considered. Regular ultrasounds or computed tomography (CT) of the pancreas beginning at age 25 may also be helpful. The greatest morbidity from the gastrointestinal tract occurs in the 20s from large gastrointestinal hamartomas; endoscopic resection of these may be helpful early in life. Finally, genetic counseling is critically important to help the patient and family assess risks of this disease, make future reproductive choices, and undergo testing.

Cowden Syndrome

Cowden syndrome was first described in the family of Rachel Cowden in 1963. This is a multiple hamartoma syndrome and is characterized by individuals with multiple hamartomas and a predisposition to a variety of cancers. A variety of mucocutaneous lesions usually develop by the age of 29. The cancers associated with this disease are endometrial, thyroid, and breast cancer.

The gene associated with Cowden syndrome is *PTEN*. This is a tumor suppressor gene located on chromosome 10q. Thus far, about 80% of patients with Cowden syndrome have an identifiable mutation within this gene. *PTEN* codes for a multifunctional phosphatase that inhibits the P13-AKT pathway. *PTEN* mutations can be found in many sporadic cancers including thyroid, endometrial, breast, and neural.

The diagnostic criteria for Cowden can be seen in Table 19-9 and can be found in the NCCN website for Cowden syndrome. Patients who meet criteria of Cowden syndrome should be offered counseling and, if indicated, subsequent genetic testing. *PTEN* mutational analysis has become available. Diagnosis of Cowden syndrome allows for increased surveillance for associated cancers. Yearly endometrial biopsy should be considered in these individuals.

TABLE 19-10 Risk of Lynch Syndrome if the Patient Has the Following:

Endometrial cancer at any age	1.8%
Endometrial cancer diagnosed under the age of 50	9%
Endometrial and colon cancer at any age	18%
Endometrial and colon cancer under the age of 50	43%
Endometrial and ovarian cancer	7%

Li-Fraumini Syndrome

Li-Fraumini syndrome was first described in 1969. This was noted as a familial clustering of soft tissue sarcomas and a clustering of diverse neoplasms including early-onset breast cancer. In 1988 Li-Fraumini published the follow-up of 24 families. This established the criteria for diagnosing this syndrome (Table 19-10). Subsequently, in 1990 deleterious germline mutations were discovered in the tumor suppressor gene p53. Thus the molecular basis for this inherited disease was established.

Gynecologic cancers are not a diagnostic criteria for the diagnosis of Li-Fraumini syndrome; however, many gynecologic cancers commonly have a p53 mutation. Examples include ovarian and papillary serous of the endometrium. It is therefore not surprising that gynecologic cancers are reported in individuals with this syndrome. These patients may be confused with patients who are thought to have hereditary breast ovarian syndrome because of the high frequency of breast cancer. Physicians should always bear this in mind when evaluating patients for hereditary disease that just does not quite fit the BRCA1 or BRCA2 type pedigree. There are no specific criteria for screening recommendations for gynecologic cancers. However, NCCN does make a recommendation for screening with magnetic resonance imaging (MRI) in addition to mammography for high-risk women.

COUNSELING, TESTING, AND RISK ASSESSMENT FOR HEREDITARY CANCERS

Genetic counseling is a service designed to help patients and their families understand the medical, familial, and psychological aspects of how an inherited genetic problem may affect their lives and the lives of their families. The process of counseling is time consuming and involved but is very important in helping the patient understand all of the implications of the testing and results of that testing. These issues include interpretation of family history, education about inheritance, disease occurrence, testing and its limitations, disease management, prevention, screening, and potential future issues based on current research. This counseling process should be designed to help patients and their families make informed decisions. It is critically important in the management of patients with the possibility of inherited disease.

Ovarian Cancer (BRCA1 and BRCA2)

Referral for genetic risk assessment has been suggested and should be a consideration for all women with ovarian cancer. Criteria that may be useful in deciding on genetic counseling and possible BRCA1 or BRCA2 testing are the following SGO guidelines:

- Women with a personal history of breast cancer and ovarian cancer at any age
- Women with a personal history of ovarian cancer and a close relative with breast cancer at less than 50 years of age or ovarian cancer at any age
- Women with ovarian cancer and Ashkenazi Jewish ancestry
- Women with breast cancer at an age less than 50 and a close relative with ovarian cancer or a male breast cancer at any age
- Women of Ashkenazi Jewish ancestry and breast cancer under the age of 40
- Women with a close relative with a known BRCA1 or BRCA2 mutation

Given the stringency of these criteria, many inherited cancers may be missed. Other features that may be useful in deciding whether a patient should be referred to a genetic counselor for counseling and possible testing are as follows:

- Women with breast cancer younger than age 40
- Women with a high-grade papillary serous ovarian cancer
- Women with bilateral breast cancer
- Women of Ashkenazi Jewish heritage and a breast cancer
- Women with a breast cancer or an ovarian cancer at any age with two or more close relatives close relatives with breast or ovarian cancer at any age
- Unaffected women with a first or second-degree relative who meet any of the aforementioned criteria

Referral to a genetic counselor for risk counseling and possible testing should not be limited to those with high-risk criteria. Some features may not be apparent at first glance in the patient's history. Inaccurate histories are common; furthermore, as families become smaller the accuracy of family history in predicting inherited disease becomes less. Referral to a counselor can occur at any time, but immediately after or during treatment seems like the most practical and common.

The counseling and testing at this point may not help the individual, but many women with ovarian cancer often express concern over their relative's risk of developing ovarian cancer. It is always preferable to test an affected individual. Then site-specific testing can be performed on the other family members at risk who wish to be counseled and tested. This allows those individuals to undergo more intensive screening, chemoprevention with something like oral contraceptives, and possible surgical prophylaxis.

The overall survival of patients with ovarian cancer is less that 50%, so it is important for women and relatives with the potential to develop breast or ovarian cancer to know their risk so they can institute some preventive measures. Hence, referral immediately after diagnosis will alert the patient and other family members of possible increased risk. Unfortunately, many individuals are not referred until after the affected individual has passed away. This means that this individual cannot be tested. Initiating counseling and possibly testing in unaffected probands is not ideal but is sometimes unavoidable. The affected person may be dead or not available for testing for other reasons. In these cases testing and subsequent follow-up can be problematic because a negative test in the absence of a known mutation does not completely free the patient from inherited risk. Recommendations may need to be given based solely on family history in these cases.

Important areas to cover and questions that should be asked during counseling are as follows:

- Age and if there is a cancer age at diagnosis
- Personal history of any tumors and where those tumors or cancers developed. Also, grade, histologic type, and stage of the tumor should be noted
- Treatment of any cancers should be noted
- Major illnesses, hospitalizations, surgeries, biopsy history, and reproductive history should be noted
- Previous cancer surveillance and environmental exposures
- Informed consent

Genetic counselors will verify the all of the information gained during the counseling session such as pathology reports and other parts of the medical records. This part is essential because patients are often inaccurate in their recollection of family history. Once the history is taken and verified, then risk assessment may be calculated. There are several programs available that help calculate risk. Genetic counseling is important because it helps patients and families understand the medical and psychological implications of knowing that they may have an inherited predisposition to the development of a cancer.

It is critically important that counseling be done both before and after testing. Appropriate counseling will provide the following:

- Informed consent
- Psychological assessment and support
- Purpose of the test and who should be tested
- General information about the genes and the mutations to be tested for
- Possible test results and implications of these results
- Accuracy of the tests and the likelihood of finding a mutation
- Cost of testing
- Possible consequences of testing (i.e., genetic discrimination)
- Importance of sharing results with family members
- Banking DNA for future testing
- Options for treatment if testing is declined
- Management strategies if the test is positive. This will include surveillance, prevention and prophylaxis

Ordering the Tests

The test is usually performed on blood. DNA is extracted from the white cells of the buffy coat. Full sequence testing of the BRCA1 and BRCA2 genes are around $3500 dollars. Site-specific testing is around $400, and testing for the Ashkenazi founder mutations is about $500 dollars.

Interpreting the Test Results

There are four possible test results that one can get from genetic testing. The first is a positive test for a deleterious mutation. This then requires counseling for increased surveillance, medical management for prevention, or surgical prophylaxis. The second possibility is that there is a known mutation in the family and site-specific testing is performed and the mutation is not found in this relative, this patient assumes the risk of the general population for developing breast or ovarian cancer. Another possibility is that the test is negative. This individual should be followed carefully depending on family history, and general screening should be followed. Records need to be kept of these encounters in case information becomes available in the future that puts this patient at risk. Finally, there can be a mutation of uncertain significance. This is an uncertain result, and this patient also needs to be followed should it be revealed in the future that this mutation is actually a deleterious mutation. This is a more common result in minority patients than in white patients because of the lack of information available on minority patients.

It is important to maintain records on these patients and continually update them with new information as it becomes available. The impact of genetic information on patients and their families can be tremendous. Making sure that further counseling is available in the future is critical. The algorithm is for the various possible test results can be seen in Figures 19-39 and 19-40.

Lynch Syndrome (Hereditary Nonpolyposis Colon Cancer)

Endometrial cancer is the most common gynecologic cancer in the United States and accounts for 6% of all gynecologic cancers in women. This accounts for around 40,000 cancers per year, around 5% of which are inherited. The primary syndrome through which this occurs is through a germline MMR defect known as Lynch syndrome. Endometrial cancer is significantly elevated in women with Lynch syndrome such that the risk is around 60% and is elevated in many other cancers also (see Figure 19-31).

Lynch syndrome is a hereditary cancer predisposition syndrome that predisposes individuals to a variety of cancers. It is the result of germline mutations in one of several MMR genes (*MLH1, MSH2, MSH6,* and *PMS2*; there may be others but these are the major genes known thus far). Loss of function in any one of these genes leads to genetic instability during replication and can result in loss of cellular control and the development of cancer. As stated previously, endometrial cancer can be inherited in other syndromes and counseling will need to reflect this.

The average age of onset of endometrial cancers in women with Lynch syndrome varies but is usually thought to be around 45 to 55 years of age. Although we lump the MMR defects together, there is significant variability within the syndrome based on the affected gene. *MSH2* seems to carry a higher risk of developing cancer than those with a *MLH1* mutation. *MSH6* mutations seem to be disproportionately associated with endometrial cancer and less so with colon cancer. It is important to identify women with Lynch syndrome so that they can be screened for other cancers. Identification of this syndrome within the family will also allow for increased awareness, diagnosis, screening, and early treatment of other members of the family.

One can look for several features that would suggest the likelihood that an inherited problem is present. One of these features is the presence of multiple primary tumors in a single individual. Up to 20% of individuals with both colon and endometrial cancer will have a germline mutation in either *MLH1* or *MSH2*. Any woman with both colon and endometrial cancer should undergo evaluation for Lynch syndrome regardless of age. The risk of ovarian cancer in Lynch syndrome may be as high as 12%, although most reports estimate it to be around 5%. Women with both endometrial and ovarian cancer may have a risk of Lynch syndrome in the 7% to 10% range. Therefore women with both ovarian and endometrial cancer should also be considered for evaluation for Lynch syndrome. Soliman and the group from MD Anderson found synchronous ovarian and endometrial cancers in 7 of 102 patients with Lynch syndrome.

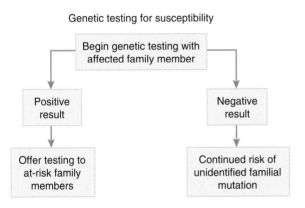

Genetic testing for susceptibility

FIGURE 19-39 Algorithm for testing and management of an affected individual.

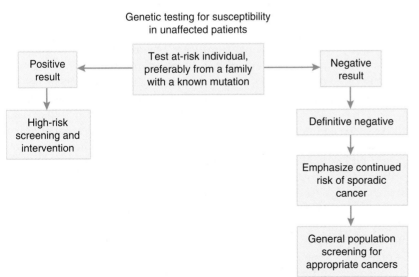

Genetic testing for susceptibility in unaffected patients

FIGURE 19-40 Algorithm for testing and management in individuals who are not affected but have a family history.

The risk of Lynch syndrome in women with endometrial cancer based on their personal history can be seen in Table 19-10. Early age of onset of endometrial cancers is also an indicator of Lynch syndrome. The prevalence of the disease markedly increases if the cancer presents before the age of 50. However, one must be careful in this setting because obesity also increases the likelihood of developing endometrial cancer. Cancer family history in conjunction with personal history of cancer can help assess risk of predisposition for the development of a cancer. The most commonly used criteria are Amsterdam II criteria. This follows the rule of 3,2,1: (1) three relatives with a Lynch-associated cancer (at least one first-degree relative); (2) two successive generations; and (3) one diagnosis under the age of 50. Other computer-based models can be used to assess risk of Lynch syndrome. These include MMRpro and PREMM; they have been validated on very large sample sizes. Obviously, the greater and more complete the family history, the more accurate the model. Family history is a valuable tool in identifying individuals and families at risk. However, one must consider that families are now smaller than in the past, there may be poor communication between parts of families, and misattributed paternity, to name a few. If testing is undertaken on the basis of family history alone, then complete molecular evaluation is necessary to assure that that individual is not at risk.

Lynch syndrome is interesting among inherited diseases in that it has some very characteristic molecular features that are useful in determining risk of disease and can help in the screening process. MSI is a hallmark feature of mismatch repair. This is the result of DNA slippage and can be detected on an NCI-established panel of five microsatellites (see Figure 19-33). Two or more positive microsatellite markers classify the cancer as MSI-high (MSI-H). One marker classifies the tumor as MSI-low (MSI-L) and no positive marker as MSI-stable (MSI-). Around 20% of colon cancers and 30% of endometrial cancers are MSI positive. The problem with MSI evaluation is that most MSI is due to silencing of *MLH1* because of promoter methylation and therefore is not the result of inherited disease but is a sporadic occurrence. Although it is a feature of the cancer, it is not a hereditary component.

IHC is useful in helping determine if an individual cancer is due to a MMR defect and can determine which gene is responsible for the problem. The Ohio State group has developed a reasonable algorithm for screening patients for inherited Lynch-associated endometrial cancer (see Figure 19-37). More research needs to be undertaken to determine the most cost-effective way to evaluate patients for inherited disease. Some institutions evaluate all patients for inherited disease but recently some reasonable guidelines were established for screening the general population. All patients with endometrial cancer younger than age 50 should be screened with MSI or IHC. Patients with synchronous primary endometrial and colon cancer should be screened and screening should be considered if a first-degree relative has any Lynch-associated cancers. Also, one should consider screening and hysterectomy with bilateral salpingo-oophorectomy should be considered.

The gold standard for determining if someone has an inherited disease is still molecular genetic sequencing of the MMR proteins. Even with direct sequencing some types of mutations such as large rearrangements can still go undetected, but this technology is improving. Hence, the sensitivity for detecting a MMR mutation is not 100%. Once a mutation is identified, then site-specific analysis can be performed on the relatives. It is expensive to test each gene, around $1000 per gene, but site-specific testing is only about $300 to $400. If a negative or variant of uncertain significance occurs, the family history must always be considered and those patients should always have follow-up screening when there is suspicion of Lynch syndrome.

This is why genetic counseling is so important. Both pre-test and post-test counseling and ongoing counseling should be routinely offered as more data become available. Counseling should include discussion of risks of testing, interpretation of the results, and interpretation of risk based on family history alone irrespective of the results of any tests. Screening and risk reducing surgery should also be discussed. These issues are important for the individual's future management. Remember that one cannot forget the impact on the rest of the family and counseling should also focus on this group with regard to testing, screening, surveillance, testing, and risk-reducing surgery.

LEGAL ASPECTS OF GENETIC TESTING

Concern over the legal aspects of genetic evaluation is one of the most significant barriers patients and health care providers express with regard to using this technology. There is fear over genetic discrimination in health insurance, life insurance, and disability insurance procurement and even discrimination with regard to employment. These fears include the individual but also affect other family members and are a major reason for not undergoing recommended testing.

Almost all states have passed legislation preventing discrimination on the basis of genetic information. Unfortunately, there is wide opinion as to what constitutes genetic information and this opinion varies from state to state. Some states consider family history as "genetic information," whereas others narrow this definition to include only information from genetic testing.

There is some increased protection to individuals under the Health Insurance Portability and Accountability Act (HIPAA). This law offers protection of those who are members of group insurance plans, including the federal group plans Medicare and Medicaid. Under HIPAA individuals are offered protection against being denied insurance coverage or even have their individual rates raised because of knowledge of genetic information. However, the insurance company can raise the rate of an entire group if there is enough risk within that group. It could even deny coverage to an entire group. Hence, federal law offers some important protection for patients, but this area still needs to be better defined by the courts. Despite the ambiguities in the law, incidents of health care discrimination are very few.

There is currently proposed legislation that would broaden protection of individuals with increased genetic risk. Many argue against the legislation as unnecessary because there are currently no data to suggest that any discrimination exists. The Genetic Information Nondiscrimination Act (GINA) of 2008 offers expanded protection of individuals and groups. GINA expands on the protection offered by HIPAA to further limit the ability of insurance carriers to raise rates or deny coverage to individuals and groups. Again, the actual impact of these laws need to be tested in court and it is therefore difficult to predict exactly what effect these laws will ultimately have on genetic discrimination. Several important points should be considered here: (1) the actual incidence of genetic discrimination is exceedingly small, with few cases nationwide that address this issue, and (2) national sympathy clearly sides with those with the possibility of genetic disease. Nonetheless, part of counseling should include the possibility of discrimination with information gained from the test.

It is the duty and obligation of the physician to inform the patient of the risks of a positive genetic test. However, there is also a duty of the physician to inform other family members who are at risk for the disease. Case law at this time generally falls on the side of favoring the individual's right to privacy over the physician's obligation to inform other family members. However, there is a case litigated in 1996, *Safer v Estate of Pack*, in which an individual with familial adenomatous polyposis died from colon cancer. He requested that his family not be informed. His daughter developed colon cancer at the age of 36 and sued her father's physician's estate claiming that he had an obligation to warn those at risk and that he had failed to fulfill these obligations. The case was dismissed, but this was later reversed by the New Jersey Court of Appeals, which ruled that a physician's obligation may extend beyond that of the immediate family and that the physician had an obligation to tell the patient that he had an obligation toward the health of his children.

Genetic tests are unique in that they affect not only the individual, but may also affect the offspring and other relatives. This further confuses the issue of patient confidentiality and is an issue that will continue to be sorted out as time progresses and other genetic issues are defined by scientific discovery. Guidelines published by the AMA and ASCO encourage physicians to educate family members regarding inherited disease. This is an important part of the counseling process and is one of the reasons most centers recommend counseling before testing.

Finally, there is a duty by physicians to meet the standard of care. This is defined as what is reasonable or what a reasonable physician should do for his or her patient. Genetic testing and counseling is quite new, and therefore clear standards have not been established. However, it is clear that it is important to take a family history and inform patients of diseases for which they may be at risk and offer testing for these diseases when available. Although there are no universally established standards, most specialties, such as the American Society of Clinical Oncology and the American Medical Association, have their own guidelines. This information provides a reasonable template for clinicians to follow.

CONCLUSION

Focused cancer family history should be part of the initial evaluation of all patients. Maternal and paternal pedigrees should be constructed to include at least three generations (the patient's, her parents', and her grandparents') if genetic disease is suspected. Information regarding the family member's age at diagnosis and additional details such as bilaterality of breast cancer are very helpful. Updates of the family history should be asked about at annual examinations because additions and new diagnoses may alter the initial recommendation regarding genetic testing.

Indicators of a possible hereditary cancer syndrome include early age at diagnosis, multiple primary cancers (such as breast and ovarian cancer, or colon and endometrial cancer, or bilateral breast cancer), cancer in two or more close relatives on the same side of the family, and/or rare cancers such as male breast cancer or ureteral cancer. If after review of the patients' pedigree a hereditary cancer syndrome is suspected, the patient should be referred for genetic counseling and possibly testing. The counselor may expand upon the pedigree and request confirmatory documents such as pathology reports, operative reports, and/or death certificates. Tumor blocks may be obtained to perform MSI and IHC testing if HNPCC is suspected. After a discussion of the individual patient's risk and benefits that may be expected from the genetic testing results, informed consent should be obtained and 20 to 30 mL of blood drawn for genetic testing. It usually takes 2 to 4 weeks for these results to return; the findings are then presented to the patient and the clinical recommendations are discussed.

The American Society of Clinical Oncology offers guidelines for cancer predisposition testing that are followed by most cancer geneticists. Genetic testing is recommended when the individual has a personal history or family history suggestive of a cancer susceptibility syndrome, when the test can be adequately interpreted, and when the test result will influence medical management.

The benefits of genetic testing include a more precise estimation of cancer risks for the individual and her family and the identification of those individuals who should participate in risk-reducing interventions. Families should be reminded, however, that the finding of a genetic mutation only predicts an elevated risk of cancer developing. A negative genetic test result does not guarantee that the individual will not get cancer, but rather that the person shares the general population risk rather than an elevated risk because of a hereditary predisposition. Most health insurance companies cover the costs of genetic testing when these guidelines are followed. Furthermore, current legislation, including HIPAA prohibits discrimination based on genetic information and specifically states that genetic information in the absence of a diagnosis of cancer does not constitute a pre-existing condition. Once a genetic abnormality is identified, the patient can be counseled regarding optimal future prevention, surveillance, and prophylactic surgery.

GLOSSARY

Allele Alternative forms of the same gene. Because of the paired nature of chromosomes, every gene exists in two copies. Each is an allele.

Antioncogene See tumor suppressor gene.

c-erb-b2 **protooncogene** Also referred to as HER-2 or neu, this gene encodes a protein that is structurally similar to the receptor for epidermal growth factor. When it is amplified, the gene is of prognostic significance in breast and ovarian neoplasms.

Capping: The addition of 7-methylguanosine residues to the 5' end of most eukaryotic mRNA.

Chromosome One mechanism for activating oncogenes.

Chromosome translocation Exchange of genes or a portion of genes between different.

Cloning An in vivo method to produce unlimited quantities of specific DNA fragments from as little as a single DNA molecule. Also, the process by which a DNA molecule is joined to another DNA molecule that can replicate autonomously in a specially designed host, usually a bacterium or yeast.

Codon A group of three nucleotides forming a base-coding message in the gene sequence. In ras genes, for example, the 12th, 13th, or 61st codon is often mutated, leading to oncogene activation.

Complementary DNA (cDNA) DNA synthesized from mRNA template such that the DNA sequence is complementary to the mRNA.

Contig The sequence of DNA created by use of YACs, BACs, and cosmids to fill an unknown region of DNA suspected of having a candidate gene.

Cosmid Used for large-scale analysis of the human genome when large DNA fragments of known sequence are needed (40 kb).

Cytoplasmic signal transduction molecules Proteins within the cytoplasm of cells responsible for transmitting signals from one event to the next event.

DNA probe A short segment of DNA in which the base sequence is specifically complementary to a particular gene segment. The probe is used, for example, on the Southern blot assay to determine whether a certain gene is present in a tumor sample undergoing DNA analysis.

Exons The coding portion of genes.

Gel electrophoresis A molecular biology laboratory technique in which DNA, RNA, or proteins are separated according to molecular weight, charge, and spatial characteristics in an electric field applied to a gel. For example, because DNA is negatively charged, it migrates toward the positively charged electrode.

Gene amplification The presence of multiple copies of a gene within a cell that is normally present in only two copies per somatic cell. An increased number of copies of an individual gene, usually a protooncogene, per cell.

Gene deletion The deletion of part or all of a gene through removal of DNA sequences by any of several mechanisms.

Gene expression The active transcription of a gene into an RNA molecule followed by translation of the protein product.

Gene rearrangement The process by which part or all of a gene is moved from its normal location in the genome to another site within the genome.

Genomic imprinting An epigenetic modification of a parental allele of a gene that leads to differential expression of that allele.

Growth factor Protein that acts on cells to promote cell growth.

Growth factor receptors Proteins that interact with growth factors and transmit the growth signal to the cell.

HER-2 See *c-erb-b2* protooncogene.

Heteronuclear RNA A form of RNA, a pre-mRNA, that exists before splicing and consists of both introns and exons.

Heterozygosity Two different forms of the same gene in a cell. An oncogene is generally heterozygous. For example, one allele may be mutated while the other copy remains normal. In addition, different forms of a gene may be normal variants. Variations in the exact base sequence within DNA are common in the genome among humans. These are called polymorphisms and are often responsible for the heterozygous state.

Informative A term used to describe the situation in which two homologous chromosomes from an individual can be distinguished from one another at a given locus; heterozygous is an alternative term.

Insertion The addition of a DNA sequence into the genome.

Introns Portions of genomic DNA that are interspersed between exons and are transcribed along with the exons into heteronuclear RNA.

Locus A general term to describe a defined chromosome region.

Loss of heterozygosity Losses of specific regions of DNA from one copy of a given chromosome that can be distinguished from the region retained on the other chromosome.

Messenger RNA (mRNA) The mature form of processed RNA used as a template for directing translation of proteins.

Myc protooncogenes The protooncogene family that includes *c-myc, N-myc, L-myc,* and *R-myc.* They encode nuclear-associated DNA-binding proteins that affect DNA replication and transcription.

Neu See *c-erb-b2* protooncogene.

Nonsense mutation A nucleotide substitution that results in a truncated protein product by generating a stop codon specifying premature cessation of translation within an open reading frame.

Nuclear transcription factors Proteins involved in regulating the expression of genes by controlling transcription. Some factors enhance and others repress gene expression and others do both, depending on the intracellular environment.

Oncogenes Genes that regulate cell growth in a positive fashion (i.e., promote cell growth). Oncogenes include transforming genes of viruses and normal cellular genes (protooncogenes) that are activated by mutations to promote cell growth.

Open reading frame A sequence of DNA representing at least some of the coding portion of a gene that is transcribed and subsequently translated into a protein because it does not contain any internal translation termination codons.

Palindrome (inverted repeats) These are sequences that look the same if read forward or backward. This

allows the sequence to fold back on itself, and it is particularly susceptible to mutation.

Point mutation The replacement of one nucleotide in the DNA sequence of the wild type with another nucleotide.

Polymorphism Variation in the exact base sequence of DNA that makes up the genome. These occurrences are normal and common in humans. Polymorphisms are used in the study of molecular genetics because they are inherited. Ones found near or within disease genes can be used to study linkage in genetics.

Primers Short DNA pieces that are complementary to portions of specific DNA sequences.

Promoter The DNA sequence of a gene to which RNA polymerase binds and initiates transcription.

Protooncogenes Any of a number of genes that encode various proteins involved in normal cell growth and proliferation, including growth factors, growth factor receptors, regulators of DNA synthesis, and phosphorylating modifiers of protein function. These are cellular genes that are the normal counterparts of transforming viral oncogenes.

ras **gene** A family of genes that encode similar cell membrane-bound proteins involved in signal transduction. Three types, *K-ras, N-ras,* and *H-ras,* are the widely studied ras genes in human tumors. Their protooncogene becomes activated by point mutations, most often in specific codons, of the gene sequence.

RB The first tumor suppressor gene to be discovered. It is a 4.7-kilobase gene, located on chromosome 13q14, and encodes a 110,000-dalton nuclear phosphoprotein that suppresses the cell cycle. Absence of RB is the cause of retinoblastoma, and research is revealing that it is involved in the pathogenesis of many other neoplasms.

Reverse transcriptase An enzyme discovered in retroviruses that has the unique ability to transcribe DNA from an RNA template. This is the reverse of the normal physiologic process.

Tp53 **gene** A tumor suppressor gene that encodes a nuclear phosphoprotein that arrests cells from entering the S-phase of the cell cycle. Located on chromosome 17(p13), *Tp53* is postulated to contribute to diverse tumorigenesis.

Transcription The process of converting the DNA code into a complementary mRNA segment.

Translation The process by which specific amino acids are incorporated into a protein as dictated by the sequence of the mRNA template.

Translocation Nonhomologous recombination.

Tumor suppressor gene A gene that suppresses cellular growth and proliferation. Therefore, when its protein products are absent, it contributes to tumor development or progression. Also known as antioncogenes, these normal cellular genes encode proteins that are thought to normally regulate growth in a negative fashion.

Uninformative The term used to describe the situation when the two homologous chromosomes from an individual cannot be distinguished from one another at a given locus; homozygous is an alternative term.

Vector A DNA vehicle that can be propagated in living cells (e.g., bacteria and yeast) into which foreign DNA can be inserted and propagated with the vector DNA. Examples of vectors include bacterial plasmids, cosmids, bacteriophages, and, most recently, yeast artificial chromosomes.

Wild type The term used to describe the normal gene or gene product. In contrast, a gene that has had its DNA sequence altered is referred to as a mutant gene, and its resultant product is a mutant protein. A gene that encodes a protooncogene, for example, is a wild-type gene because it is unaltered.

For full reference list, log onto www.expertconsult.com ⟨http://www.expertconsult.com⟩.

Palliative Care and Quality of Life

Dana M Chase, MD, Siu-Fun Wong, Lari Wenzel, PhD,
and Bradley J. Monk, MD

EVOLUTION OF PALLIATIVE CARE

Once viewed as limited and focused care during the final days of life, the scope of palliative medical care and quality of life (QOL) research has evolved since the 1990s. Although several definitions of palliative care exist, it is broadly defined as interdisciplinary care that seeks to prevent, relieve, or reduce the symptoms of a disease or disorder without affecting a cure. "Palliative care" and the related term "palliative medicine" are being used with increasing frequency in the United States and have become the labels of choice throughout the world to describe programs based on the hospice philosophy. When approaching death, including care at the end of life, the Institute of Medicine (IOM) recommends the following:

> Palliative care should become, if not a medical specialty, at least a defined area of expertise, education and research.

Palliative care overlaps with "terminal care," "death and dying," "hospice," "end-of-life care," "comfort care," and "supportive care." The term "supportive care," which is often used by oncologists, is particularly

TABLE 20-1　Issues in Palliative and End-of-Life Care

Emphasis on the trajectory
Symptom control and psychological support
Comprehensive assessment
Cancer pain management
Communicating effectively
Diagnosis and prognosis
Symptoms
Negotiating goals of care
Clinical trials
Withdrawing and withholding therapy
Advanced care planning
Cancer doctors and burnout

TABLE 20-2　Improving End-of-Life Care: Recommendations of the Institute of Medicine

1. Reliable and skillful supportive care
2. Effective use of knowledge to prevent and relieve pain and other symptoms
3. Policymakers, consumers, health practitioners, and organizations:
   - Measure quality of life (QOL) and other outcomes
   - Develop tools for improving QOL and hold health care organizations accountable
   - Revise payment mechanisms to encourage good end-of-life care
   - Reform laws and regulations that impede effective use of opioids
4. Change medical education to ensure relevant attitudes, knowledge, and skills
5. Recognition of palliative care as a defined area of expertise, education, and research
6. Research establishment to strengthen knowledge base
7. Promote public education

BARRIERS TO OPTIMAL END-OF-LIFE CARE IDENTIFIED BY THE AMERICAN SOCIETY OF CLINICAL ONCOLOGY

1. Inappropriate attitudes of health care professionals and patients (e.g., reluctance to discuss death and dying)
2. Ineffective communication about the prognosis
3. Unrealistic expectations and treatment options
4. Failure of physicians to recognize and emphasize the importance of symptom management and psychosocial support
5. Social attitudes (e.g., fear of opioid addiction)
6. Economic barriers, including lack of universal access to care and underfunding of end-of-life care
7. Fear of the attending physician losing control of the patient's care; hospice teams to work more closely with attending physicians
8. Lack of systematic education for physicians about clinical and psychosocial aspects of care

Modified from the Institute of Medicine's Report and ASCO Task Force.

ill defined and sometimes refers to comfort care or palliative support of the critically ill patient, particularly those suffering from the adverse effects of cancer treatment. All these terms have a number of meanings and are often unfamiliar to clinicians. They outline the relationships of health care professionals with patients and family members during the terminal stages of life and the treatment of advanced malignancies (Table 20-1).

QOL is a concern in all areas of medicine and of primary importance in the palliative care setting. Within the clinical setting, assessment of a patient's QOL begins with an understanding of a patient's knowledge about his or her condition and potential management strategies, their values, and their personal cost–benefit calculations. Certain therapies have no chance of improving survival end points but may have an acceptable therapeutic index based on a reasonable balance between the toxicity of the intervention and the resolution of symptoms secondary to the condition being treated. With this concept in mind, investigators and clinicians have begun to collectively measure QOL in clinical trials and community-based practices in an attempt to define alterations in QOL and to prospectively ascertain interventions that might improve "survivorship." It is no longer appropriate to simply survive one's illness, but rather one must avoid the "killing cure," allowing patients to enjoy life and function productively while interacting with their environment during multimodality cancer treatment.

The gynecologic oncologist is in a unique position to function collectively as a primary care provider, surgeon, radiation oncologist, and chemotherapist allowing, comprehensive transfer of treatment with an emphasis on the patient's QOL. Reports from the IOM's Committee on Care at the End of Life and the American Society of Clinical Oncology (ASCO) Task Force on Cancer Care at the End of Life, both published in 1998, clearly acknowledge the physician's responsibility in caring for patients throughout the continuum of their illness (Table 20-2). The ASCO document asserts as follows:

In addition to appropriate anti-cancer treatment, comprehensive care includes symptom control and psychosocial support during all phases of life.

Gynecologic oncologists are not only faced with the challenge of providing end-of-life care, but they must also explore ways to integrate palliative care throughout the continuum of illness. Indeed, recent literature suggests that gynecologic oncologists recognize the growing importance of their role as the patient's disease progresses. It is in this role, when the challenges of effective, compassionate care and communication are heightened, that an understanding of the principles and the clinical practice of palliative medicine are critical. A review of the recommendations for and barriers to effective palliative and end-of-life care as outlined by the IOM and ASCO is listed in Table 20-2.

Palliative care is differentiated from other medical specialties by its fundamental philosophy of care delivery; care is collaboratively provided by an interdisciplinary team prompted by issues and concerns of the patient and family. "Family" as defined by the patient and staff may include friends and relatives. Palliative care is, by definition, care delivered through the coordinated efforts of the team that is collectively confident and skilled when assessing and addressing the physical, psychosocial, and spiritual needs of the patient and family. It differs from more traditional "multidisciplinary" care that is directed by a physician, which allows team members to simply focus on their own areas of expertise. In contrast, the palliative care "intradisciplinary" team recognizes that all information about the patient and family is relevant. Thus the home health aide or the pharmacist may have a point of view that would be helpful for the care plan. Common members of these multidisciplinary teams include medical social workers, pastoral caregivers, nutritionists, radiation oncologists, medical oncologists, pain specialists, psychologists, physical therapists, and caseworkers. Early in the treatment of a gynecologic cancer, side effects of therapy should be anticipated and treated prophylactically. Later, some symptoms may be dealt with without the extensive evaluation associated with the assessment of tumor response or disease status. However, the development of symptoms often indicates disease progression, and appropriate laboratory or radiographic studies may lead to an alteration of treatment. As the cancer progresses, making cytotoxic therapy less likely to be effective, the workup of new symptoms must be tailored to the individual patient based on the prognosis and on the desires expressed by the patient and family. In end-of-life care, there is no room for long-term evaluation or a "wait and see" attitude. As a result, control of annoying symptoms may be pursued more aggressively, and management may resemble that given in an intensive care situation but without an extensive diagnostic evaluation. Control of symptoms is not an end in itself, but it should be sought to allow the patient time to optimize QOL and to support the patient in reaching peace with self and closure with important people in the patient's life.

QUALITY OF LIFE IN GYNECOLOGIC CANCERS

The Food and Drug Administration requires that QOL is monitored and reported in all cancer therapy clinical trials. However, although researchers and oncologists may recognize the futility of advanced and/or recurrent cancer therapy in the setting of reduced QOL, patients might not concur. Specifically, in gynecologic cancers, there are a wide range of outcomes and patient characteristics to be considered. In ovarian cancer, the majority of patients present in their sixties with advanced metastatic disease. These patients experience a rapid decline of QOL, perhaps prediagnostic nor preclinical. QOL before therapy in these patients might be low, and

perhaps aggressive treatment with chemotherapy only builds on these deficits. Most advanced ovarian cancer patients have a recurrence, and despite poor outcomes, patients are often treated with multiple rounds of chemotherapy. In contrast, cervical cancer patients may present at a younger age with minimal symptoms in perhaps earlier stages. However, whether it be fertility-terminating surgery and/or chemotherapy and radiation, the therapy can be life-altering and/or toxic. These side effects suffered, however, may be acceptable in event of likely cure. However in advanced cases, when the disease recurs in these women, their already-low QOL combined with new symptoms related to recurrence makes further treatment difficult in the setting of often ineffective therapy. Furthermore, cervical cancer patients are often of lower socioeconomic status and present with unique social and/or emotional challenges, especially in the setting of cancer diagnosis. Finally, in many situations, endometrial cancer patients have the most favorable prognosis in terms of QOL in that they frequently present in early stage and are often treated with surgery alone. One might theorize that, in some of these patients, their medical comorbidities, including obesity and diabetes, make treating their likely chronic, instead of terminal, cancer diagnosis challenging.

Quality of Life in Ovarian Cancer

Because the majority of ovarian cancer patients present in advanced stages, most women enter treatment with some QOL dysfunction likely related to symptom severity at presentation. The study of QOL in ovarian cancer therefore must take into consideration this baseline level of dysfunction and monitor the effect of surgery and/or chemotherapy. Because the prognosis is generally poor for those with advanced ovarian cancer, the goal of therapy is perhaps to extend life without greatly compromising one's QOL. In clinical trials, great attention is now paid to measuring QOL throughout the study of cancer therapeutics. QOL has also been monitored post-therapy to document the needs and deficiencies of these women. In the measurement of QOL, a standardized and validated measure, the FACT-O, is frequently used in clinical trials. The FACT-O is a combination of the FACT-G (General) plus additional questions related specifically to ovarian cancer (Tables 20-3 and 20-4). The FACT-G is composed of four subscales: the physical, social/family, emotional, and functional well-being. Patients can answer on a scale of 0 to 4, with 0 being not at all and 4 being very much. In the physical well-being subscale, the patient is asked to elaborate on pain, nausea, lack of energy, and how these physical symptoms affect their life and/or how bothered by these symptoms the patient is. The social/family well-being

TABLE 20-3   The FACT-G Versus the EORTC QLQ-CS

FACT-G	QLQ-C30
PHYSICAL WELL-BEING	
Lack of energy	Short of breath
Nausea	Pain
Trouble meeting the needs of family	Need to rest
Pain	Trouble sleeping
Side effects of treatment	Felt weak
Ill feeling	Lacked appetite
Forced to spend time in bed	Felt nauseated
	Vomited
SOCIAL/FAMILY WELL-BEING	Constipation
	Diarrhea
Close to friends	Fatigue
Emotional support from family	Staying in bed or chair
Support from friends	Strenuous activity
Family acceptance of illness	Long walk
Satisfaction with family	Short walk
communication about illness	Help with daily functions
Feeling close to partner	Limited in work or daily
Satisfaction with sex life	activities
	Limited in leisure activities
EMOTIONAL WELL-BEING	Difficulty concentrating
	Feeling tense
Sadness	Worry
Satisfaction with coping with illness	Irritable
Losing hope in the fight against illness	Depressed
Feeling nervous	Difficulty with memory
Worry about dying	Physical condition affect
Worry that condition will get worse	family life
	Physical condition affect
FUNCTIONAL WELL-BEING	social life
	Physical condition affect
Ability to work	financial status
Work is fulfilling	
Enjoying life	
Accepting illness	
Sleeping well	
Enjoying the things I usually do for	
fun	
Content with quality of life	

TABLE 20-4   Additional Concerns Scales

	Cervical	Ovarian	Endometrial
Bleeding or discharge	X		X
Odor	X		
Fear of sex	X		
Sexually attractive	X		
Narrow or short vagina	X		
Fertility concerns	X	X	
Fear of harms of treatment	X		
Interest in sex	X	X	
Body appearance	X	X	X
Constipation	X		X
Appetite	X		
Urinary incontinence/ dysuria/discomfort with urination/frequency	X		X
Ability to eat foods that are liked	X		
Swelling in stomach		X	X
Weight loss		X	
Control of bowels		X	
Vomiting		X	
Hair loss		X	
Appetite		X	
Ability to get around		X	
Feel like a woman		X	
Stomach cramping		X	X
Discomfort of pain in stomach			X
Hot flashes			X
Cold sweats			X
Fatigue			X
Pain with intercourse			X
Trouble with digestion			X
Shortness of breath			X
Discomfort or pain in pelvis			X

subscale addresses the amount of emotional support the patient has from her friends, family, and/or partner. The emotional well-being subscale targets the patient's feelings and emotions regarding the illness and how anxious she about dying from this disease. Finally, the functional well-being subscale concerns the patient's ability to function in society, such as her ability to work, sleep, and enjoy life. This subscale looks at the patient's ability to accept illness and move on to live a "normal" life again. In the final section of the FACT-O, there is an additional concerns scale that targets specific symptoms, life-altering changes, and chemotherapy in ovarian cancer.

Only a few prospective randomized trials have utilized this measure to assess QOL. The Gynecologic Oncology Group (GOG) has used the FACT-O in several prospective phase III randomized trials to monitor QOL during various experimental treatment protocols (Table 20-5). The first ovarian cancer GOG trial using the

FACT-O was published by Wenzel and colleagues in 2005. They published the QOL results for a randomized trial of interval secondary cytoreduction in advanced ovarian cancer patients. In this trial (GOG protocol 152), 424 patients were enrolled and 380 (90%) of those women completed the initial and midtreatment questionnaires. Roughly 80% of the patients continued to complete the measures at the second though fourth assessment points. In this study a higher QOL as measured by the FACT-O was associated with improved overall survival. Although the FACT-O results did not differ between the groups receiving or not receiving this surgical intervention, this trial did emphasize that improvements in QOL existed for women in both arms at 6 and 12 months after therapy. Then in 2007 Wenzel colleagues reported the QOL results of a second ovarian cancer clinical trial. This trial compared the use of intraperitoneal (IP) vs intravenous (IV) chemotherapy for optimally debulked ovarian cancer patients. Despite the reported benefits of IP therapy for progression-free and overall survival, this study demonstrated physical and functional well-being deficits both

TABLE 20-5 Prospective GOG Trials Including QOL Measurements

Cancer Site	GOG Protocol Number	Study Title
Ovarian	GOG 152 (2005)	A randomized trial of interval secondary cytoreduction in advanced ovarian carcinoma
	GOG 172 (2007)	A randomized trial of interval secondary cytoreduction in advanced ovarian carcinoma
Cervical	GOG 169 (2006)	A randomized trial of cisplatin vs cisplatin plus paclitaxel in advanced cervical cancer
	GOG 179 (2005)	A randomized trial of cisplatin with or without topotecan in advanced carcinoma of the cervix
	GOG 204 (pending publication)	A randomized trial of paclitaxel plus cisplatin vs vinorelbine plus cisplatin vs gemcitabine plus cisplatin vs topotecan plus cisplatin in stage IVB, recurrent or persistent carcinoma of the cervix
Endometrial	GOG 122 (2007)	A randomized trial of whole abdominal irradiation and combination chemotherapy in advanced endometrial carcinoma
	LAP-2	A randomized clinical trial of laparoscopy (scope) vs open laparotomy (open) for the surgical resection and staging of uterine cancer

during and after therapy in the IP arm. Neurotoxicity and abdominal discomfort were also more prevalent in the IP arm. Although the QOL scores improved over time, specifically at 12 months out from initial treatment, this manuscript perhaps prompted physicians to reconsider this treatment modality. In 2009 von Gruenigan and colleagues combined the results from the previously described trials and reported the specific line items in the FACT-O that were reported between cycles. For example, the authors report significant differences in concerns such as pain, nausea, feeling ill, and side effects of treatment. Because significant functional well-being deficits were also reported, they suggest interventions aimed at specific side effects as a means to improve patient's functional status. Social well-being went relatively unharmed except for satisfaction with one's sex life. Emotional deficits were also noted across all items except for acceptance of illness. This study demonstrated that when broken down into individual line items, perhaps interventions can be designed to target improvement in these various areas.

Quality of Life in Cervical Cancer

Although cervical cancer patients may present with pelvic pain and/or bleeding in more advanced stages, it may also be detected based on screening tests alone. The usual treatment involves surgery for early stage followed by possible radiation and/or chemotherapy for high-risk cases versus chemotherapy and radiation alone for more advanced stages. Cervical cancer presents unique issues for QOL research perhaps not addressed in the ovarian cancer research. Cervical cancer patients present with a unique set of symptoms, side effects from treatment, and socioeconomic issues not seen in ovarian cancer patients. For example, these women usually have a lower median age at presentation; are more likely to be Latina and/or nonwhite, and often have lower income. Furthermore, the chemotherapy and specifically the radiation received by these women causes such symptoms as sexual dysfunction and urinary and bowel dysfunction that perhaps affect women in unique ways.

In the measurement of QOL for cervical cancer, there are, as for ovarian cancer, two tools that are most widely used: the FACT-Cx and the QLQ-CX24. The FACT-Cx is composed of the same physical, social, functional, and emotional well-being subscales as the FACT-G but in addition has a seven-item scale for concerns related specifically to cervical cancer. These concerns involve vaginal discharge, bleeding, odor, narrowing or shortening, constipation, and dysuria. The GOG has published three studies in advanced cervical cancer that have used the FACT-Cx. These patients have a poor median survival, typically less than 6 months, and therefore it is still debatable whether treatment is futile in this setting. This is especially of concern in such advanced cancer cases in which symptomatology can be debilitating and further aggressive treatment perhaps does more harm than good. This is an ideal patient population to study QOL because if QOL decreases with treatment, then one might argue against treatment in a disease in which overall survival is so poor.

In 2006 GOG protocol 169 was published by McQuellon and colleagues and reported QOL end points in a randomized trial that compared cisplatin versus cisplatin plus paclitaxel in advanced cervical cancer (Table 20-5). Despite the impressive deficits in QOL compared to the general population, these two treatment regimens did not differ with regard to QOL. The cisplatin and paclitaxel arms did demonstrate improvements in response rate and progression-free survival and because of this, the QOL data help to promote this regimen. In 2005 the QOL data from GOG 179 were published by Monk and colleagues. This randomized trial studied cisplatin as compared to cisplatin and topotecan in advanced or recurrent cervical cancer cases. The FACT-Cx was used to document QOL between these two regimens, in addition to the exploring its relation to prognosis. There were statistical differences in QOL between the two regimens, but of interest was the relationship of the FACT-Cx to overall survival. As the FACT-Cx score increased so did overall survival, and this was statistically significant. Finally, in GOG protocol 204, which studied multiple platinum-doublets in this population, it demonstrated again no difference in QOL scores between these regimens. The specific QOL data have yet to be published.

Quality of Life in Endometrial Cancer

Endometrial cancer usually presents with vaginal bleeding and at an early stage. Treatment is surgical and occasionally involves postoperative chemotherapy and/or radiation. Likely as a result of the less invasive or aggressive treatment, with the majority of patients presenting at an early stage, there are not as many studies that focused exclusively on QOL in endometrial cancer patients. For example, in the GOG there are only two published reports of QOL in endometrial cancer patients and there has yet to be an endometrial cancer–specific subscale incorporated into this research. In 2007 Bruner and colleagues published the results of the QOL components of GOG protocol 122, which compared whole abdominal irradiation (WAI) and combination chemotherapy in advanced endometrial cancer patients (Table 20-5). In this study using the FACT-G in addition to the Fatigue Scale (FS), Assessment of Peripheral Neuropathy (APN), and Functional Alterations due to Changes in Elimination (FACE), QOL was measured before and after therapy. The WAI arm suffered greater deficits in the FS and FACE scores, but these scores somewhat improved over the varying time points. Conversely, the neuropathy scores were worse in the chemotherapy arm. Of note, the FACT-G scores did not differ between the two arms at any time point. The data generated in this study provide patients with the risks and benefits of each therapy and can perhaps shed light on whether QOL concerns in patients can overshadow the potential survival benefits of one modality.

In 2009 the QOL data were published from Europe's Post Operative Radiation Therapy in Endometrial Cancer (PORTEC-2) trial, in which patients received external beam radiation versus vaginal brachytherapy. This study used the QLQ-C30 measure in addition to subscales from the prostate cancer and ovarian cancer module, which included both bowel and bladder symptoms and sexual functioning symptoms from those scales. Despite the lack of significant differences between groups, there was a low level of sexual functioning in the two groups. The vaginal brachytherapy group overall reported better social functioning, fewer bowel symptoms, and less limitation in activity from those side effects. These results suggest the use of a treatment modality potentially as effective with less impact on QOL. In another GOG trial, Kornblith and colleagues published the results of the QOL component of the LAP-2 protocol, which compared patients undergoing laparoscopic staging versus laparotomy. The measures used included the FACT-G and a six-item scale consisting of items related to surgical side effects. In addition, they used the Physical Functioning Subscale of the Medical Outcome Study-Short Form (MOS-SF36;PF), which was developed to assess activities of daily living. The differences in QOL between these two groups favored the laparoscopy group, but this difference was modest. The authors very eloquently describe that in order to spare one patient the short-term QOL decline with laparotomy, 10 patients would have to be offered laparoscopy. In fact, only better body image persisted in the laparoscopy group at 6 months, all other measurements becoming comparable by that time point. QOL data can be complex in analysis and interpretation but can shed light on misconceptions regarding the benefits of one therapy or intervention over another.

MANAGEMENT OF COMMON PHYSICAL SYMPTOMS

Even when cancer can be treated effectively and a cure or life prolongation can be achieved, there are always physical, psychosocial, or spiritual concerns that must be addressed to maintain function and to optimize the QOL. Symptoms are a reminder to the patient and caregivers of the cancer and the potentially devastating effects of treatment. Symptoms related to cancer and its treatment have not attracted much notice in the past when patients and physicians alike felt that pursuing them might detract from the "real" goal of controlling the tumor. Consequently, symptoms have been taken for granted by the medical profession. Successful and appropriate management of physical symptoms can allow the care team to focus on the psychosocial closure of life and provide the patient an opportunity to participate more fully in the decisions of care and to rebuild or establish stronger relationships with family, friends, and co-workers.

Many physicians and nurses find symptom management in patients with advanced disease to be a frustrating experience because the symptoms may persist or progress. Although the symptoms are not always completely controlled, acknowledgment of the problem and working toward its relief offer invaluable support to the patient. Reliance on medical and drug therapies has been the traditional method to control symptoms. There is increasing recognition that nonpharmacologic approaches have significant benefits for individual patients. Nontraditional approaches such as acupuncture, biofeedback, aromatherapy, massage, and herbal medicine may have a role in the management of symptoms. Each of the following four physical symptoms is addressed in detail: fatigue, pain, nausea/vomiting, and diarrhea/constipation.

Fatigue

Fatigue is the most prevalent (60% to 96%) and one of the least understood symptoms that affect cancer patients. Several factors are implicated in the causes of fatigue (e.g., anemia, pain, poor nutrition, insomnia, and psychological distress). Fatigue has been reported by gynecologic patients as severe, distressing, and uncontrollable. Unfortunately, cancer-related fatigue is not relieved by rest and might not improve post-therapy. Patients have identified fatigue with cancer as the major obstacle to normal functioning and good quality of life. Although almost a universal symptom of patients undergoing primary antineoplastic therapy or treatment with biologic response modifiers, it is also extremely common in populations with persistent or advanced cancer. Perhaps this is the result of inadequate attention on the part of health-care professionals coupled with a patient's reluctance to discuss their fatigue.

Given the prevalence and impact of cancer-related fatigue, there have been remarkably few studies of the phenomenon. Its epidemiology has been poorly defined, and the variety of clinical presentations remains anecdotal. Perhaps this is secondary to the inability of fatigue to be measured in any way other than subjectively. The existence of discrete fatigue syndromes linked with predisposing factors or potential etiologies has not been confirmed, and clinical trials to evaluate putative therapies for specific types of cancer-related fatigue are almost entirely lacking.

Patients and practitioners can generally differentiate "normal" fatigue experienced by the general population from clinical fatigue associated with cancer or its treatment. The term "asthenia" has been used to describe fatigue in oncology patients but has no specific meaning apart from the more common term. This condition is inherently subjective and multidimensional. Typically, it develops over time and is characterized by diminishing energy, mental capacity, and psychological condition of cancer patients (Table 20-6). It is also linked with lethargy, malaise, and asthenia in the revised National Cancer Institute (NCI) Common Toxicity Criteria. These classifications may enhance awareness of fatigue and improve reporting of the condition.

When fatigue is primarily related to a treatment, there is generally a clear temporal relationship between the condition and the intervention. In patients receiving cytotoxic chemotherapy, for example, it often peaks within a few days and declines into the next treatment cycle. During the course of fractionated radiotherapy, it

TABLE 20-6 Proposed Criteria for Cancer-Related Fatigue

The following symptoms commonly present almost daily during the same 2-week period in the past month:
- Significant fatigue, diminished energy, or increased need to rest disproportionate to any recent change in activity level
- Plus five (or more) of the following:
  - Complaints of generalized weakness or limb heaviness
  - Diminished concentration of attention
  - Decreased motivation or interest in engaging in usual activities
  - Insomnia or hypersomnia
  - Experience of sleep as unrefreshing or nonrestorative
  - Perceived need to struggle to overcome inactivity
  - Marked emotional reactivity (e.g., sadness, frustration, or irritability) when feeling fatigued
  - Difficulty completing daily tasks attributed to feeling fatigued
  - Perceived problems with short-term memory
  - Postexertional malaise lasting several hours
  - The symptoms cause clinically significant distress or impairment in social, occupational, or other important areas of functioning
  - There is evidence from the history, physical examination, or laboratory findings that the symptoms are a consequence of cancer or cancer-related therapy
  - The symptoms are not primarily a consequence of a comorbid psychiatric disorders, such as major depression, somatization disorder, or delirium

Modified from Cella D et al: Oncology 12:369-377, 1998.

is often cumulative and may peak over a period of weeks. Occasionally, it persists for a prolonged period beyond the end of chemotherapy or radiation treatment. The relationship between fatigue and demographic characteristics, physiologic factors, and psychosocial factors is not well defined. The specific mechanisms that precipitate or sustain the syndrome are unknown. Fatigue may present a final common pathway to which many predisposing or etiologic factors contribute (Table 20-7). The pathophysiology in any individual may be multifactorial. Proposed mechanisms include abnormalities in energy metabolism related to increased nutritional requirements (e.g., as a result of tumor growth, infection, fever, or surgery), decreased availability of metabolic substrate (e.g., as a result of anemia, hypoxemia, or poor nutrition), or the abnormal production of substances that impair metabolism or normal function of muscles (e.g., cytokines or antibodies). Other proposed mechanisms link fatigue to the pathophysiology of sleep disorders and major depression. Further research is necessary to determine mediating mechanisms and optimal interventions.

A detailed characterization of fatigue combined with an understanding of the most likely etiologic factors is necessary to develop a therapeutic strategy (Figure 20-1). The initial approach to fatigue should involve a screening tool. The recommended screen for cancer-related fatigue begins with a simple question: How would you

TABLE 20-7 Potential Predisposing Factors with Cancer-Related Fatigue

---

PHYSIOLOGIC

Underlying disease
Treatment for the disease
   Chemotherapy
   Radiotherapy
   Surgery
   Biologic response modifiers (e.g., interferon)
Intercurrent systemic disorders
   Anemia
   Infection
   Pulmonary disorders
   Hepatic failure
   Heart failure
   Renal insufficiency
   Malnutrition
   Neuromuscular disorders
   Dehydration or electrolyte disturbances
Sleep disorders
Immobility and lack of exercise
Chronic pain
Use of centrally acting drugs (e.g., opioids)

PSYCHOSOCIAL

Anxiety disorders
Depressive disorders
   Stress-related
   Environmental reinforcers

Modified from Portenoy RK: Principles and Practice of Supportive Oncology. Philadelphia, Lippincott-Raven, 1998, pp 109-118.

rate your fatigue on a scale of 0 to 10 over the past 7 days? The score generated from this scale can drive the approach to treatment. A score of 0 to 3 is considered mild, 4 to 6 is moderate, and greater than 6 is severe. Those in the moderate to severe range should be evaluated immediately, whereas mild fatigue may be re-evaluated. Fatigue can then be approached differently depending on the patient's being in active treatment, remission, or the end of life. Those screened positive for moderate to severe fatigue then undergo a comprehensive assessment that includes the description of fatigue-related phenomena, a physical examination, and a review of laboratory and imaging studies that may allow a possible hypothesis concerning pathogenesis, which, in turn, may suggest appropriate treatment strategies. Patients may describe fatigue in terms of decreased vitality or lack of energy, muscular weakness, dysphoric mood, insomnia, impaired cognitive functioning, or some combination of these disturbances. Although this variability suggests the existence of fatigue subtypes, this has not yet been confirmed. Regardless, the patient's history should clarify the spectrum of complaints and attempt to characterize features associated with each component. This information may suggest specific etiologies (e.g., depression) and influence the choice of therapy. Neurologic and psychological evaluation may also help further clarify potential etiologies and fatigue in some patients. Other characteristics are similarly important. Onset and duration, for example, distinguish acute and chronic fatigue. Acute fatigue of recent onset is anticipated to end in the near future. Chronic fatigue is persistent for a prolonged period (weeks to months or longer), and it is not expected to remit in a short time. Patients perceived to have chronic fatigue typically require more intensive evaluation and a management approach focused on both short- and long-term goals. Other important descriptors of fatigue include the severity, daily pattern, course over time, exacerbating and palliative factors, and associated distress. An assessment of cancer-related fatigue should also include consideration of broader concerns, including global QOL, other symptoms, and disease status. Fatigue may be only one of numerous factors that influence QOL. Among these factors are progressive physical decline, psychological disorders, social isolation, financial concerns, and spiritual distress. Optimal care of the cancer patient includes a broader assessment of these factors and should be directed toward maintaining or enhancing QOL. Successful strategies should ameliorate fatigue within a broader approach of patient care. Evaluation of the patient regarding the nature of fatigue, options for therapy, and anticipated outcomes is an essential aspect of the therapy. Unfortunately, results of a patient survey indicate that patients and their oncologists seldom discuss fatigue.

An initial approach to cancer-related fatigue includes efforts to correct potential etiologies, if possible and appropriate. This may include elimination of nonessential centrally acting drugs, treatment of a sleep disorder, reversal of anemia or metabolic abnormalities, or management of major depression. Referring to the NCCN guidelines for the approach to pain, emotional distress, anemia, and nutrition may prove helpful. Perhaps sleep disturbances, interventions aimed at increasing activity levels, and the management of comorbidities may be more straightforward. Many of these initial interventions are relatively simple and pose minimal burdens to the patient, health care provider, and caregiver.

In general, education and counseling are advised in the initial treatment of cancer-related fatigue. Patients and family may be requested to document fatigue levels in a diary or on a scale and to describe associations or exacerbations and timing of the symptom. Much like the approach to urinary incontinence, patients may be counseled toward behavior modifications or adjustments to help avoid this symptom such as eliminating nonessential potentially "tiring" behaviors that may call for unnecessary expenditure of energy. Conversely, increasing physical activity has been proposed as a treatment for cancer-related fatigue. A Cochrane analysis

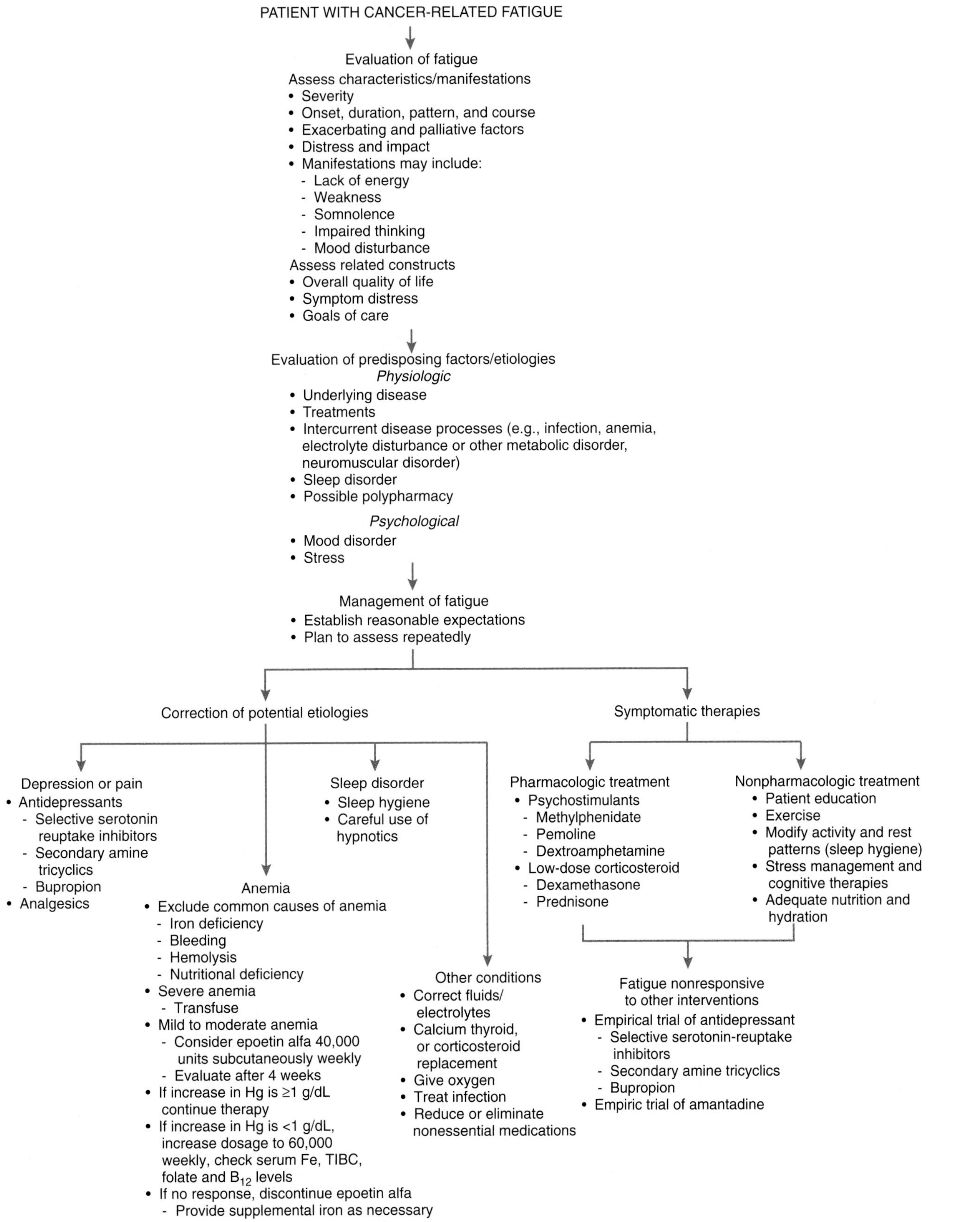

PATIENT WITH CANCER-RELATED FATIGUE

↓

Evaluation of fatigue

Assess characteristics/manifestations
- Severity
- Onset, duration, pattern, and course
- Exacerbating and palliative factors
- Distress and impact
- Manifestations may include:
  - Lack of energy
  - Weakness
  - Somnolence
  - Impaired thinking
  - Mood disturbance

Assess related constructs
- Overall quality of life
- Symptom distress
- Goals of care

↓

Evaluation of predisposing factors/etiologies

Physiologic
- Underlying disease
- Treatments
- Intercurrent disease processes (e.g., infection, anemia, electrolyte disturbance or other metabolic disorder, neuromuscular disorder)
- Sleep disorder
- Possible polypharmacy

Psychological
- Mood disorder
- Stress

↓

Management of fatigue
- Establish reasonable expectations
- Plan to assess repeatedly

Correction of potential etiologies

Depression or pain
- Antidepressants
  - Selective serotonin reuptake inhibitors
  - Secondary amine tricyclics
  - Bupropion
- Analgesics

Anemia
- Exclude common causes of anemia
  - Iron deficiency
  - Bleeding
  - Hemolysis
  - Nutritional deficiency
- Severe anemia
  - Transfuse
- Mild to moderate anemia
  - Consider epoetin alfa 40,000 units subcutaneously weekly
  - Evaluate after 4 weeks
- If increase in Hg is ≥ 1 g/dL continue therapy
- If increase in Hg is <1 g/dL, increase dosage to 60,000 weekly, check serum Fe, TIBC, folate and B_{12} levels
- If no response, discontinue epoetin alfa
  - Provide supplemental iron as necessary

Sleep disorder
- Sleep hygiene
- Careful use of hypnotics

Other conditions
- Correct fluids/electrolytes
- Calcium thyroid, or corticosteroid replacement
- Give oxygen
- Treat infection
- Reduce or eliminate nonessential medications

Symptomatic therapies

Pharmacologic treatment
- Psychostimulants
  - Methylphenidate
  - Pemoline
  - Dextroamphetamine
- Low-dose corticosteroid
  - Dexamethasone
  - Prednisone

Nonpharmacologic treatment
- Patient education
- Exercise
- Modify activity and rest patterns (sleep hygiene)
- Stress management and cognitive therapies
- Adequate nutrition and hydration

Fatigue nonresponsive to other interventions
- Empirical trial of antidepressant
  - Selective serotonin-reuptake inhibitors
  - Secondary amine tricyclics
  - Bupropion
- Empiric trial of amantadine

FIGURE 20-1   Evaluation and approach to management of the patient with cancer-related fatigue. (*Adapted from Portenoy RK, Itri LM: Oncologist 4[1]:1-10, 1999. Copyright 1999 AlphaMed Press. All rights reserved.*)

demonstrated improvements in fatigue with an exercise intervention. Adherence to the U.S. Surgeon General recommendations for 30 minutes of exercise on most days of the week may thus be advisable to cancer patients in recovery. Physical therapy referrals should be made in certain patients, and caution with activity should be obvious in certain patients such as those with bone metastasis, neutropenia, anemia, thrombocytopenia, or active infection. Therapies such as massage, acupuncture, or psychosocial interventions are also described in the National Comprehensive Cancer Network guidelines.

In patients with fatigue-associated major depression, treatment with an antidepressant is strongly indicated. As many as 25% of cancer patients develop major depression at some point during their illness. Patients at greatest risk are those with advanced disease, uncontrolled physical symptoms (e.g., pain), or a previous history of a psychiatric disorder. Although the relationship between depression and fatigue is not well understood, they often occur together and both adversely affect QOL. Despite the high prevalence in the cancer population, depression is often underdiagnosed and consequently undertreated. A trial with an antidepressant is usually warranted in a patient with fatigue associated with any significant degree of depressed mood and similarly can be therapeutic when concurrent anxiety or pain exists. In addition, brief, focused psychological counseling can be helpful for several reasons when a mood disorder (e.g., depression and/or anxiety) and a physical symptom (e.g., pain and/or fatigue) co-occur. First, counseling offers the patient an opportunity to identify and express her fears, which are often driving the depressed or anxious mood. Second, the depressed or anxious mood can exacerbate existing physical symptoms such as pain. Therefore provision of counseling has the dual benefit of reducing the mood disorder, which by extension reduces fatigue and pain. Third, brief, focused counseling can offer the patient important behavioral modifications such as time and energy management strategies, which permits and teaches the patient to conserve energy physically and emotionally for the priorities in her life. This is useful to address the practical challenges associated with fatigue and pain management.

Anemia may be a major factor in the development of cancer-related fatigue. Anecdotally, transfusion therapy for severe anemia has often been associated with substantial improvement in fatigue. As compared to other cancers, gynecologic cancers are especially known for being associated with severe anemia, with hemoglobin levels less than 9.9 in many cases. Not only does anemia have a significant correlation with poor performance status, but it also may be implicated in tumor sensitivity to radiation and chemotherapy. It has been suggested that an optimal oxygen level for tumors to respond to therapy is reflected by a hemoglobin level between 12 and 14 g/dL.

New data demonstrate the association between chemotherapy-induced mild to moderate anemia and both fatigue and QOL impairment. For example, combined data from 413 patients and three randomized placebo-controlled trials of epoetin alfa, the recombinant form of human erythropoietin, reveal that treated patients experienced a significant increase in hematocrit, a reduced need for transfusion, and a significant improvement in overall QOL. Those patients with an increase in hematocrit of more than 6% also demonstrated significant improvement in energy level and daily activities. Additional studies in patients treated with chemotherapy and radiation therapy for various gynecologic tumors confirm that epoetin alfa has positive effects on hemoglobin levels. Two large, prospective, randomized, multicenter community trials have demonstrated that patients experience significant improvement in energy levels, activity level, functional status, and overall QOL when epoetin alfa is administered as an adjunct to cytotoxic chemotherapy.

Blood transfusion is an option for the treatment of cancer-related anemia; however, transfusions are associated with poor outcomes and QOL as a result of infections, allergies, and/or dependence on medical centers. For those reasons, many practitioners rely on growth factors, including epoetin alfa (rHuEPO—Epogen or Procrit) or darbepoetin alfa (Aranesp) to treat anemia. Kurz and colleagues concluded that rHuEPO increases hemoglobin levels and decreases transfusions in patients with gynecologic malignancies undergoing polychemotherapy without compromising QOL. It has even been suggested that rHuEPO may be given prophylactically in older patients (>65) and those with baseline hemoglobins of less than 10.5 who are going to be given chemotherapy consisting of carboplatin and paclitaxel. Whereas Aranesp has a longer half-life and therefore may be given at shorter intervals, there are few clear advantages compared to Procrit. Unfortunately this therapy is not without risks and there are concerns that the risk of VTE is increased for these patients. It remains unclear whether there is a definite survival advantage with rHuEPO use great enough to counterbalance its VTE risk. QOL effects must also be taken into account. More recently, research has shown that survival may be decreased in women receiving rHuEPO for correction of anemia for hemoglobin levels over 12. Therefore, currently, patients with cancer may be counseled about the risks and benefits of the use of growth factors for the correction of anemia and now a potential progression and survival disadvantage needs to be included.

Many of the pharmacologic therapies for fatigue associated with medical illness have not been rigorously evaluated in controlled trials. Nonetheless, there is evidence to support the use of several drug classes. Psychostimulants, such as methylphenidate, pemoline, and dextroamphetamine, have been well studied for the treatment of opioid-related somnolence and cognitive impairment and depression in elderly and medically ill patients. There are no controlled studies of these drugs for cancer-related fatigue, but empiric administration may yield favorable results in some patients.

A clinical response to one drug does not necessarily predict a response to the others, and sequential trials may be needed to identify the most beneficial therapy. Methylphenidate has been more extensively evaluated in the cancer population than other stimulant drugs and is often the first drug to be administered. Pemoline has less sympathomimetic activity than other psychostimulants but has a low risk of severe hepatotoxicity compared with similar agents. It is available in a chewable formulation that can be absorbed through the buccal mucosa for patients who are unable to swallow or take oral medications.

Adverse effects associated with the psychostimulants include anorexia, insomnia, tremulousness, anxiety, delirium, and tachycardia. To ensure safety, slow and careful dose escalation should be undertaken to minimize potential adverse effects. A regimen of methylphenidate, for example, usually begins with a dose of 5 to 10 mg once or twice daily (morning and, if needed, midday). If the drug is tolerated, the dose is increased. Most patients appear to require less than 60 mg/day, but some require much higher doses.

Extensive anecdotal observations and very limited data from controlled trials support the use of low-dose corticosteroid therapy in fatigued patients with advanced disease and multiple symptoms. Dexamethasone and prednisone are most commonly used. There have been no comparative trials.

The selective serotonin-reuptake inhibitors, secondary amine tricyclics (e.g., nortriptyline and desipramine), or bupropion are sometimes associated with the experience of increased energy that appears disproportionate to any change in mood. For this reason, these agents have also been tried empirically in nondepressed patients with fatigue. Given the limited experience in the use of these drugs for this indication, an empirical trial should be considered only in severe and refractory cases.

Amantadine has been used to treat fatigue in patients with multiple sclerosis, but it has not been studied in other patient populations. This drug is usually well tolerated, and an empirical trial may be warranted in selected patients with severe refractory cancer-related fatigue.

Nonpharmacologic approaches for the management of cancer-related fatigue are supported mainly by favorable anecdotal experience (Table 20-8). Patient

TABLE 20-8 Nonpharmacologic Interventions for the Management of Cancer-Related Fatigue

Patient education
Consider the patient's preferences, education level, and readiness to learn
Use of a patient's diary
Exercise
Individualize exercise program
Use of rhythmic and repetitive types of exercise
Initiate gradually
Modification of activity and rest patterns
Assess sleep hygiene
Establish routine sleep patterns
Avoid use of stimulants before sleep
Regular exercise
Stress management and cognitive therapies
Use of stress reduction techniques or cognitive therapies
Use of relaxation therapy, hypnosis, or distraction
Adequate nutrition and hydration
Proper diet
Monitor weight and hydration status regularly
Referral to a dietitian

Modified from Portenoy RK: Principles and Practice of Supportive Oncology. Philadelphia, Lippincott-Raven, 1998, pp 109-118.

preferences should be considered in the selection of one or more of these approaches. In particular, sleep hygiene principles should be tailored to the individual patients and might include the establishment of a specific bedtime, wake time, and routine procedures before sleep. Patients should also be instructed to avoid stimulants and central nervous system depressants before going to sleep. Regular exercise performed at least 6 hours before bedtime may improve sleep, whereas napping in the late afternoon or evening may worsen it.

Cancer and its treatment can also interfere with dietary intake. With aggressive approaches to management, the patient's weight, hydration status, and electrolyte balance should be monitored and maintained to every extent possible. Regular exercise may improve appetite and increase nutritional appetite. Referral to a dietitian for nutritional guidance and suggestions for nutritional supplements may be useful.

Pain

Cancer pain can be managed effectively through relatively simple means in up to 90% of the 8 million Americans who have cancer or a history of cancer. Unfortunately, pain associated with cancer is often undertreated. Although cancer pain or associated symptoms cannot always be eliminated, proper use of available therapies can effectively relieve pain for most patients. Management of pain extends beyond pain relief and encompasses the patient's QOL and the ability to work productively, to enjoy recreation, and to function normally in the family and society.

TABLE 20-9　Barriers to Cancer Pain Management

PROBLEMS RELATED TO HEALTH CARE PROFESSIONALS
Inadequate knowledge of pain management
Poor assessment of pain
Concern about regulation of controlled substances
Fear of patient addiction
Concern about side effects of analgesics
Concern about patients becoming tolerant to analgesics
Problems related to patients
Lack of cultural competency and communication
Reluctance to report pain
　Concern about distracting physicians from treatment of underlying
　　disease
　Fear that pain means disease is worse
　Concern about not being a "good" patient
Reluctance to take pain medications
　Fear of addiction or of being thought of as an addict
　Worries about unmanageable side effects
　Concern about becoming tolerant to pain medications
Problems related to the health care system
Low priority given to cancer pain treatment
Inadequate reimbursement
　The most appropriate treatment may not be reimbursed or may be
　　too costly for patients and families.
Restrictive regulation of controlled substances
Problems of availability of treatment or access to it

*Modified from Management of Cancer Pain: Adults. Washington, D.C., U.S. Dept of
Health and Human Services, March 1994.*

TABLE 20-10　Recommended Clinical Approach

A	Ask about pain regularly.
	Assess pain systematically.
B	Believe the patient and family in their reports of pain and what relieves it.
C	Choose pain control options appropriate for the patient, family, and setting.
D	Deliver interventions in a timely, logical, coordinated fashion.
E	Empower patients and their families.
	Enable patients to control their course to the greatest extent possible.

*Modified from Management of Cancer Pain: Adults. Washington, D.C., U.S. Dept of
Health and Human Services, March 1994.*

State and local laws often restrict the medical use of opioids to relieve cancer pain, and third party payers may not reimburse for a noninvasive pain control treatment. Thus clinicians should work with regulators, state cancer pain initiatives, or other groups to eliminate these health care system barriers to effective pain management (Table 20-9).

Flexibility is the key to management of cancer pain. Thorough discussions with patients and their families encouraging them to be active in pain management are critical (Table 20-10). Effective treatment strategies exist, but patients often need reassurance to report pain. Failure to assess pain is a critical factor leading to undertreatment. Thus a simple screening tool should be used to inquire about the patient's pain level. This is described as "universal screening" by the NCCN. The goal of the initial assessment of pain is to characterize the pain by location, intensity, and etiology. This can be accomplished through a detailed history, physical examination, social assessment, and diagnostic evaluation. The mainstay of pain assessment is patient self-reporting. To enhance pain management across all settings, clinicians should teach patients to use pain assessment tools in their homes. The clinicians should listen to the patient's descriptive words about the quality of the pain, inquiring about its location, severity, aggravating or relieving factors, and the patient's cognitive response to the discomfort. Finally, goals for pain control should be clear.

Continued assessment of cancer pain is crucial. Changes in pain patterns and the development of new pain should trigger diagnostic evaluation and modification of the treatment plan. Persistent pain indicates the need to consider other etiologies (e.g., related to disease progression or treatment, and alternative—perhaps more invasive—treatment; Figure 20-2). Pain related to an oncologic emergency should be addressed immediately. This includes pain resulting from a bone fracture or impending fracture, brain or epidural metastases, infection, or obstructed or perforated viscous.

Drug therapy is the cornerstone of cancer pain management. It is effective, relatively low risk, and inexpensive and usually works quickly. Even within the same family of analgesic drugs, individual variations in tolerability and side effects are well recognized. Recommendations for pharmacologic therapy begin with the World Health Organization (WHO) ladder (Figure 20-3), a three-step hierarchy for analgesic pain management. Substitution of drugs within a category should be tried before switching therapy. The simplest dosage and schedule and the least invasive pain management modality should be attempted first. For mild to moderate pain, nonsteroidal anti-inflammatory drugs (WHO ladder step 1) are often effective (Table 20-10). When pain persists or increases (Table 20-11), opioids can be added (WHO ladder step 2). Moderate to severe pain requires opioids of higher potency and dose (WHO ladder step 3) (Table 20-12). Dosing should be on a regular schedule (i.e., "by the clock") to maintain a level of drugs that would help prevent the recurrence of pain. Ask for patient and family cooperation in establishing the effective level when administering medications to prevent long-term cancer pain on an around-the-clock basis with additional doses ("as needed" and usually required).

Oral administration is preferred because it is convenient and usually cost effective. When patients cannot take oral medications, other less invasive (e.g., rectal or transdermal) routes should be offered. Parenteral methods should be used only when simpler, less

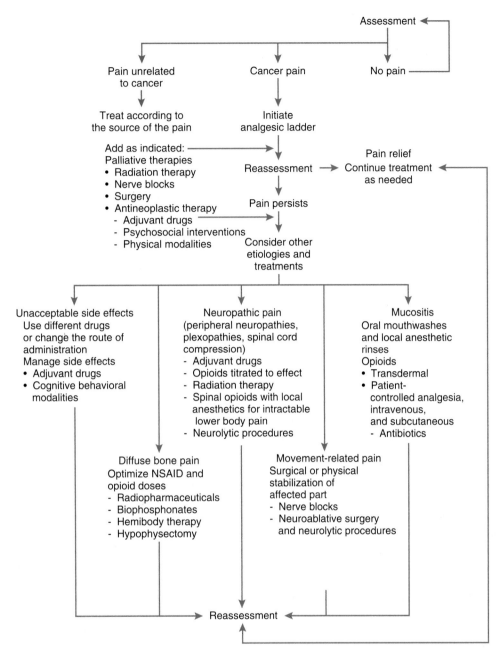

FIGURE 20-2 Continuing pain management. *(Modified from U.S. Dept of Health and Human Services: Management of Cancer Pain: Adults. Washington, D.C., U.S. Dept of Health and Human Services, March 1994.)*

demanding, less costly methods are inappropriate or ineffective. An assessment of the patient's response to several different oral opioids is usually advisable before abandoning the oral route in favor of parenteral, neurosurgical, or other invasive approaches. Rectal administration is a safe, inexpensive, and effective route for the delivery of opioids and nonopioids when patients have nausea or vomiting. Rectal administration is inappropriate for the patient who has diarrhea, anal/rectal involvement, or mucositis; who is neutropenic; who is physically unable to place the suppository in the rectum; or who

prefers other routes. Transdermal administration is also feasible but does not allow rapid dose titration. Patient-controlled analgesia (PCA) devices can be used both on an inpatient or outpatient basis. The opioid may be administered orally or via a dedicated portable pump to deliver the drug intravenously, subcutaneously, or epidurally (intraspinally). Intraspinal administration should be considered for the patient who develops intractable pain or intolerable side effects from other routes of administration. Use of this route requires skill and expertise that may not be available in certain

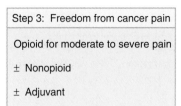

FIGURE 20-3 World Health Organization three-step analgesic ladder. *(Modified from World Health Organization: Cancer pain relief and palliative care. Geneva, Switzerland, World Health Organization, 1990.)*

settings. Table 20-13 presents the advantages and disadvantages of regional administration. This route is often efficacious because gynecologic tumors often affect the pelvis, making profound analgesia frequently possible without motor or sympathetic blockade. Drugs and routes of administration that are not recommended for the management of cancer pain are summarized in Table 20-14.

The general principles to pain management are described by the NCCN. This includes a dose of medication that sustains pain relief for the full time period before the next dose. The dose should be calculated based on the patient's requirements for the previous 24 hours. A sustained dose with an around-the-clock medication should be started in addition to an as-needed medication. The around-the-clock and as-needed doses are increased based on the severity of the uncontrolled pain. Of note, pure opioid preparations are preferred to eliminate the risk of overdosing acetaminophen or ibuprofen. The "as-needed" medication should be about 10% to 20% of the sustained total 24-hour dose. Of note, before converting to a transdermal approach, the pain should be relatively well-controlled by an oral short-acting opioid. The maximum patch dose is 100 mcg/hour; however, if a patient requires a higher dose, multiple patches may be used. An IV dose of 20 mg/day of IV morphine or 60 mg/day of oral morphine is equivalent to 25 mcg/hr of transdermal fentanyl. Although the patch typically lasts for 72 hours, being thin, fever, or

heat from external sources such as electric blankets may increase the absorption of the transdermal fentanyl and thus may be contraindications to patch use.

Clinicians who follow patients during long-term opioid treatment should watch for potential side effects and administer agents to counteract them. Constipation and nausea and vomiting, common side effects to opioid analgesics, are discussed later. Drug-induced sedation should be treated by a reduction in dose and by increasing the frequency of opioid administration. Central nervous system stimulants as described earlier may also decrease opioid-related sedation. Patients receiving long-term opioid therapy generally develop tolerance to the respiratory depressant effects of these agents. When indicated for reversal of opioid-induced respiratory depression, administration of naloxone is indicated with titration in small increments to improve respiratory function without reversing analgesia. Careful monitoring is mandatory until the episode of respiratory depression resolves. For more subacute respiratory depression, simply withholding one or two doses until the symptoms resolve followed by restarting at 25% of the total dose is often effective. Dry mouth, urinary tension, pruritus, myoclonus, altered cognitive function, dysphoria, euphoria, sleep disturbances, sexual dysfunction, physiologic dependence, tolerance, and inappropriate secretion of antidiuretic hormone are also reported side effects of opioid agents.

Adjuvant drugs are valuable during all phases of pain management to enhance the analgesic efficacy, to treat concurrent symptoms, and to provide independent analgesia for specific types of pain. These adjuvants include corticosteroids, anticonvulsants, antidepressants, neuroleptics, local analgesics, hydroxyzine, and psychostimulants. Corticosteroids provide a range of effects, including mood elevation, anti-inflammatory activity, antiemetic activity, and appetite stimulation and may be beneficial in the management of cachexia and anorexia. They also reduce cerebral and spinal cord edema and are essential in the emergency management of elevated intracranial pressure and epidural spinal cord compression. Anticonvulsant agents are used to manage neuropathic pain, especially lancinating or burning pain. They should be used with caution when administered to patients undergoing marrow suppressant therapy such as chemotherapy and radiation. Antidepressants are useful in the pharmacologic management of neuropathic pain. These drugs have innate analgesic properties and may potentiate the analgesic effects of opioids. Perhaps the most widely reported experience has been with amitriptyline; therefore this drug should be viewed as the tricyclic agent of choice. Neuroleptics, particularly methotrimeprazine, have been used to treat chronic pain syndromes. Methotrimeprazine lacks opioids' inhibiting effects on gut motility and may be useful for treating

TABLE 20-11   Dosing for Acetaminophen and Common NSAIDs

Medications	Common Proprietary (Trade) Name	Usual Daily Dose (Adults)		Usual Daily Dose or Maximum Dose (Adults)
		Dosage and Route	Frequency	
Acetaminophen	Tylenol, others	325-650 mg PO	q 4 hr	4000 mg (>2 weeks)
		650-1000 mg PO	qid	6000 mg (<2 weeks)
		650 mg PR	q 4 hr	
SALICYLATES				
Aspirin (acetylsalicyclic acid)	Others	600-1500 mg PO	qid	6000 mg
Same for buffered and enteric-coated oral formulations		300–600 mg PR	q 4 hr	
Magnesium salicylates	Doan's, others	600 mg PO	qid	4000 mg
Choline magnesium trisalicylate	Trilisate	500-1000 mg PO	tid	4000 mg
		750-1500 mg	bid	
Diflunisal	Dolobid	500-750 mg PO	bid	1500 mg
Salsalate	Disalcid	750-1500 mg PO	bid	3000 mg
PROPIONIC ACID DERIVATIVES				
Fenoprofen	Nalfon, others	200-600 mg PO	qid	3200 mg
Flurbiprofen	Ansaid, others	50-75 mg PO	qid	300 mg
Ibuprofen (OTC and Rx)	Motrin, Advil, others	200-800 mg PO	qid	3200 mg
Ketoprofen	Others	25-75 mg PO	tid-qid	300 mg
		200 mg XR PO	Daily	200 mg XR
Naproxen	Aleve, Anaprox Naprosyn, EC-Naprosyn, others	200-500 mg PO	bid-tid	1500 mg
Oxaprozin	Daypro, others	600-1200 mg PO	Daily	1800 mg
ACETIC ACID DERIVATIVES				
Diclofenac	Voltaren, Voltaren-XR, Cataflam, Flector (transdermal), others	50-75 mg PO	bid-tid	200 mg (PO)
		100 mg XR	Daily-bid	
		1 patch (180 mg) TDS	bid	
Indomethacin	Indocin, Indocin SR	25-50 mg PO	tid-qid	200 mg (both PO and PR)
		75 mg-SR PO	bid	150 mg-SR
		50 mg PR	bid-tid	
Sulindac	Clinoril, others	150-200 mg PO	bid	400 mg
Tolmetin	Others	400-600 mg PO	tid	1800 mg
PYRANOCARBOXYLIC ACID				
Etodolac	Others	200-400 mg PO	tid-qid	1000 mg
		400-600 mg XR PO	Daily-bid	1200 mg XR
PYRROLIZINE CARBOXYLIC ACID				
Ketorolac	Others	10 mg PO	qid	40 mg
		15-30 mg IM/IV	qid	120 mg IM/IV
FENAMATES (ANTHRANILIC ACIDS)				
Meclofenamate	Others	50-100 mg PO	tid-qid	400 mg
Mefenamic acid	Ponstel	250 mg PO	qid	4000 mg
ENOLIC ACID DERIVATIVES				
Meloxicam	Mobic, others	7.5-15 mg PO	Daily	15 mg
Piroxicam	Feldene, others	10-20 mg PO	Daily	20 mg
NAPHTHALAKANONES				
Nabumetone	Others	1000-2000 mg PO	Daily	2000 mg
COX-2 SELECTIVE				
Celecoxib	Celebrex	100-200 mg PO	bid	400 mg
		200 mg PO	Daily	

References: (1) Pain Management for Primary Care Clinicians. Arthur G. Lipman, editor. 2004. (2) Guideline for the Management of Cancer Pain in Adults and Children. American Pain Society 2005. (3) Facts and Comparisons®E Answers, 2010 Wolters Kluwer Health.

PO, Oral; PR, rectal; SR, sustained-release; TDS, transdermal; XR, extended release.

TABLE 20-12 Dosing of Opioid Analgesics for the Management of Persistent Cancer Pain[1,2,3]

Medication	Proprietary (Trade) Name	Usual Starting Dose for Moderate to Severe Cancer Pain in Adults ≥50 kg of Body Weight			Usual Starting Dose for Moderate to Severe Cancer Pain in Adults <50 kg of Body Weight			Approximate Equianalgesic Dosing of Opioid Analgesics in Adults		
		Oral	Parenteral	Rectal	Oral	Parenteral	Rectal	Oral	Parenteral	Rectal
Codeine[4]		30-60 mg q4h	30 mg q4h	NA	0.5-1 mg/kg q4h	0.5 mg/kg q4h	NA	200 mg	120 mg	NA
Codeine combination products[5]	Tylenol #2, #3, #4; others	1-2 tablets q4h (max: acetaminophen 4000 mg/day)	NA	NA	Codeine: 0.5-1 mg/kg q4h Acetaminophen: 10-15 mg/kg q4h	NA	NA	Per codeine recommendations above		
Hydrocodone combination products[5]	Vicodin, Lorcet, Lortab, Norco others	1-2 tablets q4h (max: acetaminophen 4000 mg/day)	NA	NA	Hydrocodone: 0.135 mg/kg q4h; Acetaminophen: 10-15 mg/kg q4h	NA	NA	30 mg	NA	NA
Fentanyl[6]	Duragesic (TDS); Sublimaze (IV); [Fentora (buccal); Actiq (Lozenge); Onsolis (soluble buccal film—**for breakthrough pain only**]; others	Buccal 100-200 mcg/dose prn Lozenge 200 mcg/dose prn Buccal Film 200 mcg/dose prn	Transdermal 25 mcg/h q72h mcg/kg IV 20-50 mcg/h	NA	NA	Transdermal 12 mcg/h q72h for opioid tolerant pts IV 1-3 mcg/kg/h	NA	NA	mg TDS and IV	NA
Hydromorphone	Dilaudid; Exalgo (ER tablet)	2-4 mg q4h; 8-24 mg—ER daily	1-2 mg q4h; 0.2-0.5 mg/h	3 mg q6h	0.03-0.08 mg/kg/dose q4h	0.015 mg/kg/dose q4h; 0.003-0.005 mg/kg/h (max 0.2 mg/h)	NA	7.5 mg	1.5 mg	3 mg
Levorphanol	Levo-Dromoran, others	2 mg q6h	1 mg q4h	NA	NA	NA	NA	4 mg	2 mg	NA
Meperidine[7]	Demerol, others	50-150 mg q4h	50-150 mg q4h	NA	1.1-1.5 mg/kg q4h	1.1-1.5 mg/kg q4h; 0.3 mg/kg/h	NA	300 mg	75 mg	NA
Methadone	Dolophine, others	2.5-10 mg q8h	1.5-5 mg q8h	NA	0.1 mg/kg q4h (max 10 mg/dose)	0.05 mg/kg q4h	NA	20 mg	10 mg	NA

Drug	Brand									
Morphine immediate-release	Others	10 mg q4h	2.5-5 mg q4h; 1 mg/hr	10-20 mg q4h	0.3 mg/kg q4h	0.1-0.2 mg/kg q4h; 0.03 mg/kg/hr	NA	60 mg	10 mg	60 mg
Morphine controlled-release products	Kadian (ER); Avinza (ER); MS Contin (CR); others	MS Contin 15-30 mg q12h / Kadian 10-20 mg daily / Avinza 30 mg daily	10-15 mg x1 *DepoDur (liposomal) for epidural use only*	MS Contin 15-30 mg q12h	0.3-0.6 mg/kg q12h	NA	NA	30 mg	NA	30 mg
Oxycodone	Others	5-10 mg q4h	NA	NA	0.2 mg/kg q4h	NA	NA	NA	NA	60 mg
Oxycodone controlled-release products	Oxycontin; others	10-20 mg q12h	NA	10 mg q12h	NA	NA	NA	13 mg	NA	20 mg
Oxycodone combination products	Percocet; Tylox; others	5 mg q6h (max APAP 4000 mg/day)	NA	NA	0.1-0.2 mg/kg q4h (5 mg/dose; max APAP 90mg/kg/day)	NA	NA	NA	NA	NA
Tramadol	Ultram; Ultram ER; Ryzolt (ER); Rybix ODT	25-50 mg q6h (NTE 400 mg/day); ER 100 mg daily (NTE 300 mg/day)	NA	NA	1-2 mg/kg q6h (NTE 400 mg/day)	NA	NA	NA	NA	NA
Tramadol 37.5 mg + APAP 325 mg	Ultracet; others	2 tablets q6h	NA	NA	NA	NA	NA	NA	NA	NA

[1]Caution: Recommended doses do not apply for adult patients with body weight less than 50 kg. For recommended starting doses for adults <50 kg body weight, see Table 21-10.

[2]Caution: Recommended doses do not apply to patients with renal or hepatic insufficiency or other conditions affecting drug metabolism and kinetics.

[3]Caution: For morphine, hydromorphone, and oxymorphone, rectal administration is an alternative route for patients unable to take oral medications. Equianalgesic doses may differ from oral and parenteral doses because of pharmacokinetic differences. Note: A short-acting opioid should normally be used for initial therapy of moderate to severe pain.

[4]Caution: Codeine doses above 65 mg often are not appropriate because of diminishing incremental analgesia with increasing doses but continually increasing nausea, constipation, and other side effects.

[5]Caution: Doses of aspirin and acetaminophen in combination opioid/NSAID preparations must also be adjusted to the patient's bodyweight.

[6]Transdermal fentanyl dosage is not calculated as equianalgesic to a single morphine dosage. See the package insert for dosing calculations. Doses above 25 μ/hr should not be used in opioid-naïve patients.

[7]Not recommended. Doses listed are for brief therapy. Switch to another opioid for long-term therapy.

Note: Published tables vary in the suggested doses that are equianalgesic to morphine. Clinical response is the criterion that must be applied for each patient; titration to clinical responses is necessary. Because there is not complete cross-tolerance among these drugs, it is usually necessary to use a lower than equianalgesic dose when changing drugs and to retitrate to response.

IM, intramuscular; N/A, not available; N/R, not recommended; SC, subcutaneous; q, every.

Modified from Management of Cancer Pain: Adults. Washington, D.C., U.S. Dept of Health and Human Services, March 1994.

TABLE 20-13   Advantages and Disadvantages of Intraspinal Drug Administration

System	Advantages	Disadvantages
Percutaneous temporary catheter	Used extensively both intraoperatively and postoperatively Useful when the prognosis is limited (<1 month)	Mechanical problems include catheter dislodgment, kinking, or migration
Permanent silicone-rubber epidural	Catheter implantation is a minor procedure Dislodgment and infection are less common than with temporary catheters Bolus injections, continuous infusions, or PCA (with or without continuous delivery) can be given	
Subcutaneous implanted injection port	Increased stability, less risk of dislodgment Can deliver bolus injections or continuous infusions (with or without PCA) Useful when the prognosis is limited (<1 month)	Implantation more invasive than external port catheters Approved only for epidural catheter in the United States Potential for infection increases with frequent injections Need for more extensive operative procedure
Subcutaneous reservoir	Potentially reduced infection in comparison with external system	Difficult to access, and fibrosis may occur after repeated injection
Implanted pumps (continuous and programmable)	Potentially decreased risk of infection	Need for more extensive operative procedure; need for specialized, costly equipment with programmable systems

Modified from Management of Cancer Pain: Adults. Washington, D.C., U.S. Dept of Health and Human Services, March 1994.
PCA, Patient-controlled analgesia.

opioid-induced intractable constipation or other dose-limiting side effects. It also has antiemetic and anxiolytic effects. Local analgesics have been used to treat neuropathic pain. Side effects for these may be greater than with other drugs used to treat neuropathic pain. Hydroxyzine is a mild anxiolytic agent with sedating and analgesic properties that is useful in treating anxious patients who are in pain. This antihistamine also has antiemetic and antipruritic properties. Psychostimulants, as discussed earlier, may be useful in reducing opioid-induced sedation when opioid dose adjustment (e.g., reduced dose and increased dose frequency) is not effective.

Patients should be encouraged to remain active and participate in self-care when possible. Noninvasive physical and psychosocial modalities can be used concurrently with drugs and other interventions to manage pain during all phases of treatment. The effectiveness of these modalities depends on the patient's participation and communication concerning which methods best alleviate pain. Generalized weakness, deconditioning, and aches and pains associated with cancer diagnosis and therapy may be treated by cutaneous stimulation such as heat or cold, massage, pressure, and vibration. Unfortunately, these modalities sometimes increase pain before relief occurs. Massage should not be substituted for exercise in ambulatory patients. Exercise is useful for treating subacute and chronic pain because it strengthens weak muscles, mobilizes stiff joints, and helps to restore coordination and balance, thus enhancing patient comfort and providing cardiovascular conditioning. Physical therapists may be consulted to increase

weightbearing exercise. Repositioning is also effective to maintain correct body alignment and prevent or alleviate pain and possibly prevent ulcers. Immobilization has been effective only to stabilize fractures or otherwise compromised limbs or joints. Finally, acupuncture, which involves inserting small solid needles into the skin, may be an effective alternative to more standard therapies.

Cognitive behavioral interventions are an important part of a multimodal approach to pain management. They help to give the patient a sense of control and to develop appropriate skills to deal with pain. These skills include relaxation and imagery, cognitive distraction and reframing, patient education, psychotherapy, biofeedback, structured support, and support groups and pastoral counseling.

With rare exception, a less invasive analgesic approach should precede invasive palliative approaches. However, for a few patients in whom behavioral, physical, and drug therapy do not alleviate pain, invasive therapies are useful. These include radiation therapy to destructive bone metastasis, palliative surgical approaches, and nerve blocks.

Because vulvar cancers and occasionally ovarian or endometrial cancers occur in elderly patients, they especially require comprehensive assessment and aggressive management when cancer pain occurs. Older patients are at risk for undertreatment of pain because of underestimation of their sensitivity to pain, the expectation that they tolerate pain well, and the misconceptions about their ability to benefit from the use of opioids. Careful consideration should be given to elderly patients

TABLE 20-14 Drugs and Routes of Administration Not Recommended for Treatment of Cancer Pain

Class	Drug	Rationale for Not Recommending
Opioids	Meperidine	Short (2-3 hour) duration; repeated administration may lead to CNS toxicity (tremor, confusion, or seizures) as a result of accumulation of neurotoxic active metabolite, normeperidine; high oral doses required to relieve severe pain (especially >800 mg/day and in the presence of renal dysfunction), may further increase the risk of CNS toxicity
Miscellaneous	Cannabinoids	Side effects of dysphoria, drowsiness, hypotension, and bradycardia preclude its routine use as an analgesic
	Cocaine	Has demonstrated no efficacy as an analgesic or coanalgesic in combination with opioids
Opioid agonist–antagonists	Pentazocine Nalbuphine Butorphanol	Risk of precipitating withdrawal in opioid-dependent patients; analgesic ceiling; possible production of unpleasant psychomimetic effects (e.g., dysphoria, hallucinations)
Partial agonist	Buprenorphine	Analgesic ceiling; can precipitate withdrawal
Antagonist	Naloxone Naltrexone	May precipitate withdrawal; limit use to treatment of life-threatening respiratory depression
Combination preparations	Brompton's cocktail	No evidence of analgesic benefit to using Brompton's cocktail over single opioid analgesics
	DPT (meperidine, promethazine, and chlorpromazine)	Painful; absorption unreliable; should not be used for short (2-3 hour) duration
Anxiolytics alone	Benzodiazepine (e.g., alprazolam)	Efficacy poor compared with that of other analgesics; high incidence of adverse effects
		Analgesic properties not demonstrated except for some cases of neuropathic pain; added sedation from anxiolytics may limit opioid dosing
Sedative/hypnotic drugs alone	Barbiturates (benzodiazepine)	Analgesic properties not demonstrated; added sedation from sedative/hypnotic drugs limits opioid dosing

ROUTES OF ADMINISTRATION		RATIONALE FOR NOT RECOMMENDING
Intramuscular (IM)		Painful; absorption unreliable; should not be used for children or patients likely to develop dependent edema or in patients with thrombocytopenia
Transnasal		The only drug approved by the FDA for transnasal administration at this time is butorphanol, an agonist-antagonist drug, which generally is not recommended. (See opioid agonist-antagonists above.)

Modified from Management of Cancer Pain: Adults. Washington, D.C., U.S. Dept of Health and Human Services, March 1994.

FIGURE 20-4 Evaluation and approach to management of patients with chemotherapy-induced emesis.

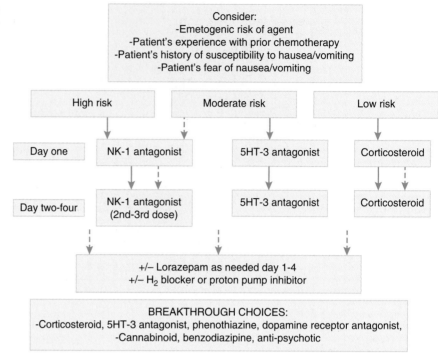

who are in pain and who have multiple chronic diseases that increase their risk for drug–drug and drug–disease interactions. In addition, visual, hearing, motor, and cognitive impairments may require simpler pain assessment scales and more frequent pain assessments. Nonsteroidal anti-inflammatory drugs are more likely to cause gastric and renal toxicity and other drug reactions such as cognitive impairment, constipation, and headaches in older patients. Alternative nonsteroidal anti-inflammatory drugs (e.g., choline magnesium trisalicylate) or coadministration of misoprostol should be considered to reduce gastric toxicity. Older persons tend to be more sensitive to the analgesic effects of opioids. In addition, the peak opioid effect is higher and the duration of pain relief is longer. Drug clearance may also be slower, thus making cautious initial dosing and subsequent titration and monitoring necessary. Elderly patients may not be able to physically place rectal suppositories or activate PCA devices.

Nausea and Vomiting

Nausea and vomiting also have a high prevalence in advanced cancer patients. The cause may be divided into physiologic, treatment-related, metabolic, and psychological causes. As is the case in many symptoms of advanced cancer, the causes of nausea are often multifactorial. More than 50% of patients receiving opioids experience nausea in the first 10 to 14 days of therapy until they develop tolerance to this side effect. Many palliative specialists may prescribe antiemetics for the first weeks of opioid therapy. The most successful therapy is given orally and prophylactically. Nausea and vomiting tend to be the most feared symptom related to cancer treatment. Chemotherapy-induced nausea and vomiting (CINV) may occur in 70% to 80% of patients receiving chemotherapy. Even after antiemetic therapy patients prefer to experience other toxicities and side effects rather than withstand nausea and vomiting. CINV can be divided into four subcategories. The NCCN defines *acute nausea* as occurring shortly after chemotherapy administration but resolving within the first 24 hours. *Delayed nausea* occurs after 24 hours, peaks 48 to 72 hours, and resolves by 6 to 7 days. *Anticipatory nausea* is described as a learned or conditioned response before chemotherapy; finally, *breakthrough CINV* can occur when a patient experiences symptoms despite appropriate therapy.

An evaluation and approach to management of patients with chemotherapy-induced emesis appears in Figure 20-4. Agents used to control nausea and vomiting have different mechanisms of action and may be used in combination for better control (Table 20-15). There are basically three main classes of drugs for CINV: 5-HT serotonin receptor antagonists, corticosteroids, and the NK1 antagonist aprepitant. ASCO recently updated their guidelines for the use of antiemetics in oncology, and their recommendations, with some additions, are detailed in Figure 20-5. All have a high therapeutic index for CINV and should be considered first-line therapy. The 5-HT3 antagonist blocks serotonin receptors of the

TABLE 20-15   Antiemetic Agents (Adult Dosages)

Medications	Common Proprietary (Trade) Name	Usual Daily Dose (Adults)		
		Oral Dose	Parenteral Dose	Rectal Dose
*ANTIDOPAMINERGICS**				
Phenothiazines				
Chlorpromazine	Thorazine	10-25 mg q4h	25-50 mg IM/slow IV q4h	NA
Perphenazine	Trilafon	2-6 mg q6h	NA	NA
Prochlorperazine	Compazine	5-10 mg q6h	5-10 mg IM/slow IV q3h (max: 40 mg/day)	25 mg bid
Promethazine	Phenergan	12.5-25 mg q4h	12.5-25 mg IM/slow IV q4h	12.5-25 mg q4h
Others				
Metoclopramide	Reglan, Metozolv ODT	0.5 mg/kg q6h	1-2 mg/kg q2h up to 5 doses	NA
ANTICHOLINGERICS†				
Scopolamine	Transderm Scop	NA	NA	1 patch (1.5 mg) TDS q72h
Trimethobenzamide	Tigan	300 mg q6h	200 mg IM q6h	NA
ANTIHISTAMINES				
Diphenhydramine	Benadryl‡	25-50 mg q6h	25-50 mg q6h	NA
BENZODIAZEPINES				
Lorazepam	Ativan	0.5-2 mg PO/SL q4h	0.5-2 mg IV q4h	NA
CORTICOSTEROIDS				
Dexamethasone	Decadron	10 mg ×1 or 4 mg q4h	10-20 mg ×1 or 4 mg q4h	NA
5-HT3 (Serotonin) Receptor Antagonists				
Dolasetron	Anzemet	100 mg daily	1.8 mg/kg or 100 mg daily	NA
Granisetron	Kytril, Sancuso (TDS)	2 mg daily or 1 mg bid	10 mcg/kg/dose or 1 mg daily or bid	TDS:1 patch (3.1 mg/day) up to 7 day per application
Ondansetron	Zofran, Zofran ODT	24 mg daily or 8 mg bid Radiation tx: 8 mg tid	0.15 mg/kg q4h ×3 or 24-32 mg daily	NA
Palonosetron	Aloxi	0.5 mg × 1	0.25 mg IV × 1	NA
SUBSTANCE P/NEUROKININ 1 RECEPTOR ANTAGONIST				
Aprepitant (oral) or fosaprepitant (IV)	Emend	125 mg day #1 then 80 mg daily on day #2 and #3	115 mg day #1	NA
CANNABINOIDS				
Dronabinol	Marinol	5-10 mg qid	NA	NA
Nabilone	Cesamet	1-2 mg tid	NA	NA

If extrapyramidal symptoms occur, administer 50 mg diphenhydramine IM or IV.

†*Also Scopolamine transdermal patch—use one patch every 3 days.*

‡*Also has antihistamine properties.*

GABA, *Gamma-aminobutyrate;* NA, *not available;* q, *every.*

chemoreceptor trigger zone (CTZ) to prevent vomiting. Corticosteroids are often used to enhance the effect of other agents, yet they have an unclear antiemetic action. Dexamethasone (20 mg intravenously) is most effective when administered with a 5-HT3 antagonist. There are several 5-HT serotonin receptor antagonists, which all have similar therapeutic and side effect profiles. There is some suggestion that palonosetron performs superior to other agents in this class; however, further studies are warranted. 5-HT receptor antagonists in addition to dexamethasone and aprepitant are indicated for the control of CINV in high-dose chemotherapy regimens. Aprepitant (Emend), a neurokinin-1 receptor antagonist, is the newest agent and has an important role in both

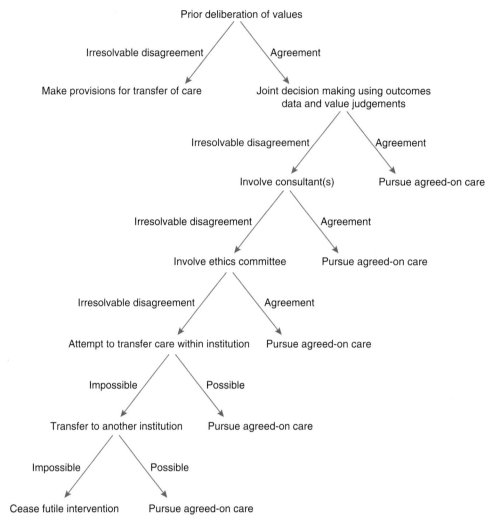

FIGURE 20-5   Fair process for considering futility cases. *(Modified from Medical Futility in End-of-Life Care: Report of the Council on Ethical and Judicial Affairs. JAMA 281:939, 1999.)*

acute and delayed CINV. For breakthrough CINV, the following agents may be considered when first-line therapeutics fail: metoclopramide, phenothiazines, butyrophenones, and cannabinoids. Metoclopramide has its effect locally in the gut and is excellent to control vomiting because of gastric stasis. In chemotherapy prophylaxis, it can be combined safely with corticosteroids or benzodiazepines. Phenothiazines partially inhibit the CTZ and are the drugs of choice for radiation-induced nausea and vomiting and symptoms induced by mild or moderately emetogenic agents. Benzodiazepines are appropriate for refractory anticipatory vomiting that may occur with only a mention of chemotherapy. The amnesic effects of benzodiazepines are helpful to many patients. It has been postulated that corticosteroids overcome the adrenal insufficiency that causes nausea and vomiting in patients with advanced cancer. Patients who describe around-the-clock nausea, not just intermittent with meals, may have a central nervous system lesion or a proximal small bowel obstruction that must be evaluated. Cannabinoids are best used in younger patients and have equivalent or superior activity compared with the phenothiazine and prochlorperazine agents. Specifically, the cannabinoids dronabinol and nabilone, both approved by the U.S. Food and Drug Administration, are indicated for refractory CINV and, despite dysphoric side effects hindering their prescription, patients have been shown to prefer the use of these agents for subsequent chemotherapy cycles. In anticipatory CINV, the most important concept is the prevention of acute and delayed emesis with the aforementioned drugs. However, ultimately when one is faced with controlling anticipatory CINV, benzodiazepines and behavioral therapy are suggested. Finally, when CINV proves to be refractory, one must consider other etiologies for nausea and vomiting.

TABLE 20-16   Antidiarrheal Agents (Adult Dosages)

Medications	Common Proprietary (Trade) Name	Dosing Regimen	Comments
ANTISECRETORY			
Bismuth Subsalicylate	Kaopectate, Pepto-Bismol, Kao-Tin, Maalox Total Stomach Relief Liquid	2 tablets or 30 mL q1h up to 8 doses per day (regular strength) or 4 doses/day (maximum strength)	Contains aspirin. Watch for max daily dose of aspirin; may cause Reye syndrome; interferes with radiologic examinations of GI tract (Bismuth is radiopaque); stool may appear gray-black in color
Octreotide	Sandostatin, others	0.1-0.5 mg SC 2-3 times per day (max: 2.4 mg/day) LAR: 20-40 mg IM per month	50% dose reduction in patients requiring dialysis or with liver cirrhosis
ANTI-PERISTALTIC			
Loperamide	Imodium A-D, others	4 mg then 2 mg after each stool (max: 8 mg/day OTC; 16 mg/day Rx) Maintenance: 2-4 mg q6h	
Diphenoxylate 2.5 mg/atropine 0.025 mg	Lomotil , lonox, others	2 tablet or 10 mL (5 mg diphenoxylate) qid (max: 20 mg per day)	Use with extreme caution in pts with hepatorenal disease or abnormal liver function, may cause hepatic coma
Difenoxin 1 mg/ atropine 0.025 mg	Motofen	2 tablets then 1 tablet after each loose stool Maintenance: 1 tablet q3-4h (max: 8 tabs per day)	Use with extreme caution in pts with hepatorenal disease or abnormal liver function, may cause hepatic coma
Opium	Opium Tincture (C-II), Paregoric (C-III)	Opium tincture: 0.6 ml qid Paregoric: 5-10 ml qid	
Codeine	Codeine sulfate	15-60 mg q4h	

Last, an important concept in CINV is the selection of therapy based on the risk assessment of the chemotherapeutic agents used, a concept highlighted in the recent ASCO guidelines. The emetogenicity of these antineoplastic drugs is separated into four categories: high, moderate, low, and minimal risk. For example, a high-risk drug such as cisplatin requires treatment with 5-HT receptor blockers, dexamethasone, and aprepitant followed by dexamethasone and aprepitant for delayed CINV. Low emetogenic drugs (e.g., paclitaxel) may require only dexamethasone, without additional agents for delayed CINV.

Diarrhea and Constipation

Diarrhea is a common complication of pelvic radiation. It can generally be managed with anticholinergic drugs such as atropine sulfate (Lomotil). Rarely, tinctures of opium or serotonin antagonists are required for refractory or secretory diarrhea (Table 20-16). Patients who have been previously treated with antibacterial therapy or are immunocompromised should be tested for *Clostridium difficile* (e.g., enzyme-linked immunosorbent assay [ELISA] for enterotoxin) before antidiarrheal therapy. When detected, metronidazole or vancomycin therapy is usually effective. Rarely, cholestyramine resin is needed to control the symptoms of *C. difficile* infectious diarrhea. A search for more unusual infectious etiologies such as salmonella, shigella, *Escherichia coli*, and parasites has not been cost effective among gynecologic oncology patients in the absence of foreign travel or other data, that might suggest these etiologic agents.

Constipation is highly prevalent in patients with advanced cancer. Close to 90% of patients receiving opioids have difficulty passing stool or pass stool infrequently. One cardinal rule of palliative care is "the hand that writes the opioids writes the laxative at the same time." Other causes of constipation are advanced disease, other medications such as anticholinergic agents, inability to eat a high-fiber diet, insufficient fluid intake, and lack of activity.

A specific discussion regarding opioid-induced constipation is warranted here. Of note, a tolerance to the opioid used with regard to constipation does not occur. In general, a stimulant laxative and a stool softener should be used (for example, senna with docusate). Adequate fluid intake and physical activity should be encouraged. Agents such as Metamucil that increase fiber content in the stool are not recommended. If constipation persists, secondary etiologies, such as bowel obstruction, should be considered. Impaction should be ruled out and then secondary anticonstipation agents should be considered. These agents include magnesium hydroxyl, bisacodyl, lactulose, sorbitol, magnesium citrate, or polyethylene glycol. Various enemas or agents such as metoclopromide may also be added. A general approach should be to begin patient on a stool softener and stimulant and, if in 48 hours no bowel movement results, then additional agents should be started such as milk of magnesia or lactulose. If no bowel movement in 72 hours, then fecal impaction should be assessed and treated. If no impaction, then such interventions as an enema, mineral oil, or magnesium citrate should be tried. If impacted, a glycerine suppository or oil retention enema should be used.

Metabolic causes of constipation include hypercalcemia and hypokalemia. Evaluation of complaints of constipation should include consideration of bowel obstruction and spinal cord compression. A manual rectal examination is critical when evaluating this complaint.

Several treatment options are now available for the nonsurgical candidate with bowel obstructions secondary to advanced cancer. A discussion of these treatments follows.

Cachexia and Malnutrition

Cachexia is defined by Femia and Goyette as loss of more than 5% of bodyweight over 2 to 6 months. Clearly cachexia is related to nutritional status because the cancer itself causes metabolic alterations such as increased muscle protein breakdown and glucose metabolism and the treatment of cancer affects appetite and food intake. The literature supports the fact that the patient's body habitus, and therefore QOL, is altered by these changes. Furthermore, it is evident that malnutrition contributes to poor outcome in gynecologic oncology patients. Clearly oncologists need to be aware of the implications of malnutrition in patients receiving therapy because poor nutritional status may negatively affect a patient's response to therapy and her QOL during therapy.

Nutritional support using dietary supplements and shakes (e.g., Ensure) along with the oncologist's attention to this issue may improve the response to treatment for some patients. Nutritional counseling, oral nutritional supplementation, and home parenteral nutrition have also been linked to improved QOL. Finally, although appetite stimulants such as megestrol acetate (Megace) are thought to improve cancer-related anorexia–cachexia, they have not been shown to affect survival and/or global QOL. However, of note, Megace is thought to be more effective than either eicosapentaenoic acid (alpha 3-omega fatty acid) or marijuana derivatives, and only corticosteroids may perform as effectively as Megace. Unfortunately, Megace carries the risk of venous thromboembolism, perhaps as high as a sixfold increase, and this might limit its use in the gynecologic oncology patient population.

On the contrary, oncologists and patients may differ when it comes to nutrition and hydration in the supportive and/or palliative care setting. Brown and colleagues found that the majority (63%) of patients would like nutrition and hydration to be continued even though the use of respiratory supports, such as oxygen or ventilators, might be limited. The authors state that patients may not consider nutritional support "heroic." Even though patients might not agree with discontinuation of nutritional support, the management of malnutrition in the palliative setting remains controversial. For example, although total or home parenteral nutrition (TPN, HPN) is considered by many to be unnecessary in terminally ill patients, there is some evidence that it has a positive impact in certain patient populations, including patients with a life expectancy of greater than 3 months. TPN carries its own risks and discomfort and therefore strong QOL studies need to address this issue.

PSYCHOSOCIAL AND SPIRITUAL NEEDS OF PATIENTS AND FAMILIES

Management of only the physical symptoms of cancer is now considered to be an inadequate approach to oncologic care. It is well recognized that physical and psychological symptoms are intertwined and patients can benefit from a multidisciplinary approach to care. A growing body of literature suggests that tailored psychosocial interventions can enhance not only QOL for cancer survivors but also may have the additional benefit of improving neuroendocrine and immune functioning, which could positively affect disease states. If proved effective, this complementary and cost-efficient approach could significantly improve patient care, QOL, and aspects of survival. The effect of cancer on the family and patient is profound and touches every area of their lives. Effective care of the patient requires that these needs be addressed. A team of professionals is needed to foster effective communication in the patient–physician relationship, to assess the effect of disease and its treatment on the patient's psychosocial and spiritual well-being; and to achieve optimal care for the patient and family.

Strategies for Breaking Bad News and Preserving Hope

Perhaps the most important tool in caring for patients and their families is effective communication. Transferring information about the diagnosis, prognosis, risks, and benefits of treatment and progression of disease is a difficult and unavoidable responsibility. Sharing bad news and responding to the questions presented by the patient and family require compassion, empathy, and skill. Unfortunately, development of these skills has not historically been emphasized in medical training despite the fact that powerful medical institutions and societies (e.g., ASCO, IOM, ACS, NCI) demand excellence and vigilance when caring for people with progressing cancer. The absence of an integrated formal palliative care curriculum throughout medical training continues to promote a skill set gap.

Identification of cancer progression, or progressive cancer-related symptoms, is often the catalyst for planning alterations in care and readdressing issues about the patient's and family's goals and objectives. Breaking bad news is a difficult and emotionally laden task for the physician. Thoughtful planning and delivery of such information, however, can shape the patient's subjective experience of the physician and perception of his or her degree of support and caring.

The individual's response to news is often determined by the following:

1. The adequacy of information given
2. Whether the person delivering the information showed and responded to the patient's concerns

Although wishes vary from one individual to another, most patients (80%) want to know their diagnosis, their chance of cure, and adverse effects of any treatments. Significantly, patients do vary in the degree of information that they are able to assimilate at one time. Traditionally, men with advanced disease, older patients, and individuals from lower socioeconomic backgrounds are likely to want to hear fewer details and may comfortably defer to the physician and/or family with regard to decision-making. In most cases, patients want to hear the diagnosis from the physician who will be responsible for their care.

When breaking bad news, it is critical to project reasonable hope and confidence. Despite the most sensitive and effective communication style, patients are left with major concerns about their situation as it relates to their physical, social, psychological, and spiritual well-being. Open communication should be maintained, and these concerns should be explored throughout the continuum of care using expertise and support from other team members. Excessive concern about the need to preserve hope can lead to false optimism or less than full disclosure over time. This approach leads to poor coping skills and failed expectations. Lending strength does not require that the physician be less than honest but that the truth be disclosed over a period of time, in a setting in which the patient has the support required, and with repetition so that information can be assimilated and understood in small amounts. Patients should be encouraged and nurtured to develop their own coping strategies and defense mechanisms in dealing with their illness. This strategy brings hope against all odds. For

example, if asked, "Doctor, I know I am dying, but can there still be a miracle?" The answer is, "Yes, there can be." This suggests that the medical information is clearly understood but demonstrates confidence to overcome suffering and despair. However, it is unusual for patients to so clearly articulate their inevitable demise; more likely they would ask, "Is there still hope?" The physician's capacity to appropriately convey hope through articulation of a comprehensive care plan will help the patient to recognize that quality time is a reasonable expectation. Forcing a patient to adopt the physician's view of the odds (chance of a cure) does not take into consideration what can generally harm the personal framework that patients must deal with. It also corrodes the patient–physician relationship that must endure through the palliative therapy or future care. Thus, maintaining hope is best achieved through honesty, cautious optimism, compassion, and acceptance of the vulnerability experienced by all cancer patients.

Timing is critical to breaking bad news. Judging what portion of the information should be disclosed is an art. Conveying a balance of honesty and maintaining hope can sometimes seem impossible, often because physicians tend to project their own concerns onto patients and assume that they will give up hope. In reality, hope is an innate characteristic that is rarely abandoned by open and compassionate discussion of the prognosis and treatment options. When there are no remaining viable cytotoxic treatment options, there are still many palliative options that can achieve meaningful therapeutic ends, thus preserving hope and avoiding a sense of helplessness. It is useful for patients to hear such optimism in the face of a generally poor prognosis. As the patient's illness advances, feelings of helplessness as a result of loss of control and fear of dying may resurface. At this point, the physician can openly recognize the patient's fear and grief and externally acknowledge his or her own attitudes toward death. Unfortunately, doctors and other staff tend to spend less time with patients as the disease progresses and patients deteriorate into a terminal condition. This is presumably because the health care professionals feel helpless (and perhaps even threatened) when confronted with the imminence of death. Many health care professionals fail to realize the importance of compassion and active palliative care. Actively participating in symptom management and compassionate listening helps to ease the patient's mind, thus allowing the patient to ask questions that help plan realistically for the future and maintain a sense of control. Although most patients know when they are dying and can verbalize this realization, they also retain hope. The physician is uniquely poised to encourage and reinforce the patient's hope without giving false or insincere reassurance. One study that focused on end-of-life preferences of gynecologic cancer patients reported that only

5% of 108 patients would stop fighting after receiving a poor prognosis with no medically recommended treatment options left. Most (70%) of these patients expressed their resolve to continue fighting against their disease, even under the poorest prognostic circumstances. Proper management involves directing resources to assist with this fight and fostering this hope among dying patients. The involvement of other professionals familiar with care for the dying can relieve the physician of being the sole provider of hope with sensitive attention to incurable problems.

MANAGEMENT OF PSYCHOSOCIAL AND SPIRITUAL DISTRESS

Approaching "the person, not the disease" is a prerequisite to understanding the patient's experience and providing appropriate physical, psychosocial, and spiritual care. A cancer diagnosis creates a profound sense of loss of control and fear for many individuals. Changes in physical function and the effect on psychosocial issues may further compound this sense. Stressors commonly experienced by patients undergoing cancer treatment may be as problematic for the patient as the physical decline. Table 20-17 highlights the complex challenges faced by patients.

Patients are often reluctant to disclose struggles, including feelings of depression, and anxiety if they do not perceive this disclosure to be relevant to their physical care. Recent research has shown that many individuals are fearful of burdening their family members emotionally, physically, and financially during their final days. A recent prospective study examining the prevalence of depressed mood and request for

TABLE 20-17 Psychosocial Challenges Experienced by Cancer Patients

THREAT OF OR ACTUAL:

Loss of ability to engage in employment because of side effects or symptoms

Loss of ability to participate in all social activities previously enjoyed because of symptoms of side effects or infection concerns

Guilt feeling about the impact of the diagnosis on people about whom the patient cares

Diminished sense of self-esteem and self-worth

Changes in body image

Discrimination or stigmatization by others

Role conflicts (e.g., meeting the demands of multiple responsibilities including those of being a patient)

Loss of comfort with sexual intimacy with a significant other

Fear of the dying process and concerns about symptoms that conjure up images of physical suffering (e.g., pain, cachexia, and shortness of breath)

Modified from Portenoy RK: Principles and Practice of Supportive Oncology. Philadelphia, Lippincott-Raven, 1998, pp 109-118.

TABLE 20-18 Tasks of the Dying Patient

PRACTICAL

Complete a family trust

Put affairs in order

Complete advanced directives

Communicate wishes regarding funeral/burial arrangements

Plan for the future of surviving family members

PSYCHOSOCIAL

Grieve the loss of dreams for the future

Accept the reality of the prognosis and impending death

Use medical intervention and own internal resources to cope with physical deterioration

Express thanks and love to family and friends

Find closure around interpersonal conflicts ("I forgive you, please forgive me")

Say goodbye to family and friends

SPIRITUAL

Engage in life review, reflect on the past and present

Make meaning of one's life

Resolve existential/spiritual conflict

Modified from Loscalzo M, Zabora J: Care of the cancer patient: Responses of family and staff. In Bruera E, Portenoy R (eds): Topics in Palliative Care, Vol 2. New York, Oxford University Press, 1998. © Oxford University Press. Reproduced by permission of Oxford University Press, Inc., www.oup.com.

euthanasia among terminally ill cancer patients noted that of 138 patients, 32 patients (22%) had depressed mood and made an explicit request for euthanasia. The risk to request euthanasia for patients with depressed mood was 4.1 times higher than that of patients without depressed mood at inclusion (95% CI, 2.0 to 8.5). This information heightens our awareness to formally evaluate depression in terminally ill cancer patients and provide timely intervention as indicated.

Discussions about resources available to assist patients and families, including the role and function of community agencies, support groups, and hospice programs, are critical. There are many tasks that a patient should have the opportunity to accomplish in the time before death. These tasks are summarized in Table 20-18.

Identification and treatment of psychosocial problems, including depression and anxiety, should involve interventions and expertise that will offer optimal care to the patient and family. As noted earlier, pharmacologic interventions are often necessary but should be considered in combination with psychological counseling, supportive interventions, and education for the patient and family. Determination of the appropriate referral depends in large part on the type and magnitude of the psychosocial or psychological disruption and the extent to which this diagnosis interfaces with physical symptomatology such as pain or fatigue. Optimal programs include a team consisting of psychiatry, psychology, social work, and chaplain services. In

TABLE 20-19 Interventions for Bereaved Individuals

Provision of information/education: Offers education to surviving family members about grief response, explaining death to children, practical information to facilitate problem-solving and arranging for disposition of the body (e.g., funeral and burial arrangements) and future memorial activities

Bereavement follow-up: Offers formalized contracts by the staff or volunteers at identified intervals to provide support, monitor for difficulties, and arrange for intervention as needed

Individual/family grief counseling: Offers counseling for bereaved individuals experiencing grief; some individuals may require long-term psychotherapy or psychiatric care if bereavement-related depression or risk of suicide exists

Bereavement support groups: Offers a forum for the mutual support among bereaved individuals; may have a special purpose (e.g., for parents who have lost a child) or have a particular religious affiliation

Memorial or remembrance services: Offered by the hospital or hospice to acknowledge the grief process

Note: Families of patients who die in hospital would not necessarily have knowledge of or access to any follow-up if a bereavement program is not in place at the institution. Bereavement follow-up is typically a part of hospice services, and institutions may successfully partner with local hospices to make this service accessible for these families.

Modified from Portenoy RK: Principles and Practice of Supportive Oncology. Philadelphia, Lippincott-Raven, 1998, pp 109-118.

addition, novel programs are acknowledging if not incorporating aspects of complementary and alternative medicine (CAM) based on recognition that a substantial proportion of cancer patients seek out various CAM methodologies.

Psychosocial care must continue to address the needs of the family as death imminently approaches and after death occurs. The health care team has an opportunity through the period of anticipatory grieving to assess and monitor the family and to identify risk factors indicating the need for more intensive intervention. An understanding of the spectrum of grief and the nature of "normal" grief is essential for providers to effectively support grieving families, identify abnormal reactions, and intervene. Table 20-19 illustrates the range of bereavement services that may be available for family members.

QUALITY OF LIFE ISSUES IN ADVANCED AND RECURRENT OVARIAN CANCER

Pleural Effusion

Dyspnea is the subjective feeling of respiratory distress and thus is often an interplay between anxiety and hypoxia from tumor burden. Some have suggested that supportive care of this symptom should include the provider's ability to address the patient's subjective breathlessness. As dyspnea may indicate poorer prognosis and shorter interval to death, addressing this symptom is paramount to enhancing QOL in the time period near death.

Dyspnea may result from a combination of three different complications: first, obstructive pathology such as pleural effusions; second, cancer cachexia or malnutrition and weakness; and, third, an increase in ventilator requirements such as metabolic acidosis or anemia. Perhaps gynecologic oncologists most frequently encounter this tumor effect in the ovarian cancer patients because the dyspnea may be secondary to pleural effusions. It is suggested that thoracocentesis and chemical pleurodesis be reserved for palliative situations in which chemotherapy or other treatments are not likely to reverse the effusions. For symptomatic control and/or when mechanical control of the pleural effusion is not an option, most advocate opioids and/or oxygen therapy. Benzodiazepines and oxygen therapy may also have a role in control of dyspnea, although evidence is lacking. Finally, some have advocated activity modifications to prevent the onset of dyspnea, which may involve caregiver instruction to tailor activities of daily living.

Small Bowel Obstruction

Although epithelial ovarian cancer is a surface-spreading disease that rarely invades vital organs, partial or complete bowel obstruction is often seen at the time of initial diagnosis or, more frequently, in association with recurrent disease. Obstruction may be secondary to extrinsic compression of the small bowel or hypoperistalsis as a result of mesenteric and bowel surface implants. The symptoms, which are almost always present, are intestinal colic, continuous abdominal pain, nausea, and vomiting. In most cases, nausea and vomiting can be relieved by conservative measures, and intestinal symptoms usually resolve after primary cytoreductive surgery and multiagent cisplatin-based cytotoxic chemotherapy. Despite the high objective response rate of primary epithelial ovarian cancer to several platinum-based combination chemotherapeutic regimens, most patients with advanced disease often develop intraperitoneal recurrences and require a salvage regimen for palliation of symptoms. Several therapeutic strategies have been used in these patients, such as including re-treatment with cisplatin or carboplatin or the use of paclitaxel, hexamethylmelamine, oral etoposide, tamoxifen, gemcitabine, liposomal doxorubicin, vinorelbine, or topotecan. Multiple clinical factors must be considered when selecting the most appropriate salvage therapy. Unfortunately, in patients previously treated with cisplatin, other therapeutic agents are not likely to be effective in relieving symptoms of bowel obstruction or ascites.

For most patients who present with bowel obstruction secondary to recurrent intraperitoneal cancer, initial management should include proper radiographic documentation of the obstruction, hydration, correction of any electrolyte abnormalities, parenteral alimentation, and intestinal intubation and decompression. There is a fair representation of various treatment options in the literature. A recent retrospective study found that surgery carries a higher morbidity, although chemotherapy and surgery had similar outcomes in terms of reobstruction. Of note, conservative management alone has much earlier reobstruction rates. In some patients the obstruction may be relieved with this conservative approach. However, palliative surgery is usually considered in almost every patient at some time before disease progression and death. When surgery is indicated, the type of surgery depends on the extent of the disease and on the number and location of obstructions. If the obstruction is mainly contained in one area, this area can be either resected (if secondary cytoreduction is indicated) or bypassed. Because the success of secondary cytoreduction depends on the chemosensitivity of the residual disease present after debulking surgery, intestinal bypass is generally preferable rather than resection because most patients present after multiple failed attempts at cytotoxic therapy resulting in chemotherapy-resistant cancer. In addition, intestinal bypass surgeries such as enterocolostomy are usually associated with reduced morbidity when compared with a radical resection. At the time of operation, the balloon at the end of a long intestinal tube can often be palpated and used to identify the small bowel proximal to the obstruction. This small bowel can then be anastomosed in a side-to-side fashion to the most appropriate area of colon, thus bypassing the site of obstruction. Obviously, it is critical to obtain a preoperative Gastrografin enema to ensure that there is no obstruction of the lower colon beyond the bypass site. In rare cases, the colon may be encased in tumor, necessitating a colostomy with or without bypass surgery. Sadly, multiple sites of obstruction are common in patients with recurrent epithelial ovarian cancer. When multiple sites of obstruction are present, resection of several segments of intestine is usually not indicated. In the inoperable cases or situations in which the patient and/or oncologist decide to proceed with medical or conservative management, several options exist. A percutaneous endoscopic gastrostomy allows patients to hydrate themselves by mouth. By decreasing intestinal secretions, octreotide improves QOL and lessens hospitalization. Moretti and colleagues used temporary nasogastric drainage with the simultaneous use of octreotide and antiemetic and analgesics in a terminal patient. Critical in their algorithm is fluid management because they stress keeping daily water intake between 0.5 to 1.5 liters. In the last month of her life, this combined medical and conservative approach decreased pain, nausea, dry mouth, thirst, dyspnea, feeling of

abdominal distention, and drowsiness in the palliative setting. In such cases, an ileostomy or even a proximal jejunostomy may be necessary to provide adequate intestinal diversion. On the contrary, if the extent of disease is so great that the morbidity of intestinal surgery seems excessive, stomach decompression with a gastrostomy may be effective in palliating symptoms of obstruction and ascites such as pressure, nausea, vomiting, and pain. When the stomach or anterior abdominal wall is not involved with tumor, drainage tubes can often be placed percutaneously, thus avoiding the morbidity of a laparotomy.

With careful attention to nutrition, chemosensitivity/resistance of disease, and the sites of intestinal obstruction, some degree of palliation can generally be obtained with surgery, chemotherapy, or gastric decompression. Careful attention to each of these factors is necessary to avoid unnecessary morbidity and unindicated surgery in these debilitated terminal patients with recurrent or refractory ovarian cancer.

Many have attempted to define the prognostic factors that predict benefit after surgery; some of the key factors include: age older than 65, nutritional status, tumor burden, rapidly reaccumulating ascites, poor nutritional status, carcinomatosis, previous chemotherapy for recurrence, and radiation therapy to the whole intestine. Krebs and Goplerud used a predictive index by scoring patients with a value of 0, 1, or 2 in six of the aforementioned categories and found that patients who scored higher than six had worse outcome with surgery. However, if surgery is chosen, the patient must understand the possibility of living with an ileostomy in roughly 50% of cases with potential complications of fistula(s) for the balance of the patient's life. In a study by Mangili and colleagues, only surgical treatment was a prognostic factor for improved survival; however, it is likely that those patients who were offered surgery had other qualities that predisposed them to improved survival.

Ascites

Because malignant ascites are almost always the result of intraperitoneal cancer, treatment of these effusions generally involves therapy directed against the associated malignant neoplasm. However, treatments are occasionally directed specifically toward the palliation of symptoms related to malignant ascites, particularly when the intraperitoneal cancer is refractory to all known treatments. The traditional treatment with diuretics and salt and fluid restriction is rarely effective. Therefore patients usually undergo therapeutic paracentesis, resulting in an imbalance of protein and electrolytes. For this reason, novel therapies such as intraperitoneal immunotherapy and drainage using a

Denver peritoneal venous shunt have been proposed to palliate symptoms associated with malignant ascites. One series involved 42 patients who were treated over a 5-year period with a peritoneal venous shunt, which diverted peritoneal fluid into the vascular space. This treatment relieved symptoms with neither hematogenous metastasis nor evidence of disseminated intravascular coagulation. Of note, the median survival time of patients with breast and gynecologic cancer after surgery was significantly longer than that of patients with primarily gastric and intestinal neoplasms, resulting in an improvement in QOL.

Management approaches with diuretics with or without serial paracentesis versus permanent indwelling catheters are case-dependent. A recent Phase I/II trial using monoclonal antibodies against ascites-specific malignant cells, and specifically EpCAM on the surface of ascitic tumor cells, resulted in the control of ascites but randomized controlled studies are still lacking. Other approaches suggested include the use of VEGF antagonists to reduce ascites because VEGF may be implicated in the formation of ascites by increasing vascular permeability. A hope for cure is no longer possible once a woman develops recurrent disease associated with symptomatic bowel obstruction and ascites. However, a sense of optimism and hope are still common, not for a cure but toward a goal of symptom relief and palliation with chemotherapy, surgery, tube drainage, or supportive care. Only through careful patient selection and insight into the toxicity associated with these therapies can hope for acceptable QOL be realized. A Cochrane review published in 2010 failed to support or refute the use of drains for ascites because they did not find any eligible trials to review.

Role of Palliative Surgical Procedures

The role of surgery to palliate bowel obstruction was discussed earlier. Surgery can be useful in the palliation of pain or fistula during the terminal phase of ovarian cancer progression. The advantages and disadvantages of these procedures must be continually weighed. Cytoreductive surgery for debulking as a means to palliate pain is indicated when effective chemotherapy exists to treat unresected residua.

QUALITY OF LIFE ISSUES IN ADVANCED AND RECURRENT UTERINE AND CERVICAL CANCER

Ureteral Obstruction

The patient with bilateral ureteral obstruction and uremia secondary to the extension of cervical or uterine cancer presents a serious dilemma for the clinician.

Management should be divided into two subsets of patients:

1. Those who have not received prior radiation therapy
2. Those who have recurrent disease after pelvic radiation

Ureteral obstruction resulting from endometrial cancer differs from obstruction secondary to cervical cancer in that it is more frequently associated with disease outside of the pelvis and because it is more difficult to cure. In addition, adequate doses of radiation are more difficult to deliver to the corpus than to the cervix using standard brachytherapy techniques, thus contributing to the lower rate of pelvic control among patients with endometrial cancer after radiation therapy.

Patients with bilateral ureteral obstruction from untreated cancer or from recurrent pelvic disease after surgical therapy should be seriously considered for urinary diversion followed by appropriate radiation therapy. However, because the salvage rate in this clinical situation is low, supportive care alone allowing progressive uremia and demise must be considered as an alternative to more aggressive therapy. Placement of retrograde ureteral stands using cystoscopy should be attempted first if supportive care alone is declined. When this is not possible, a percutaneous nephrostomy should be placed followed by an attempt at antegrade stent placement. A third option is surgical urinary diversion such as a urinary conduit and anastomosing both ureters into an isolated loop of ileum (Bricker procedure) or creating a continent pouch from a segment of bowel. When necessary, urinary diversion is usually performed before the radiation has begun, thus allowing for surgical assessment of the extent of the disease. If extra pelvic disease is discovered at laparotomy, therapy is altered because the chance of a cure is greatly diminished.

The patient with a bilateral ureteral obstruction after a full dose of pelvic radiation therapy presents a more complicated problem. Less than 5% of these patients will have obstruction caused by radiation fibrosis, and often this group is difficult to identify. To identify patients whose obstruction is a result of recurrent disease, an examination under anesthesia, cystoscopy, and proctoscopy with multiple biopsies are recommended. When recurrent cancer is absent, simple diversion of the urinary stream can be lifesaving, and therefore all patients must be considered to belong to this category until the recurrent malignancy is found.

When the presence of recurrent disease is established as the cause of bilateral ureteral obstruction, the decision process becomes difficult and somewhat philosophical. Numerous studies suggest that "useful life" is not achieved by urinary diversion in this subset of patients. Brin and colleagues reported on 47 cases (5 with cervical cancer) with ureteral obstruction secondary to advanced pelvic malignancy undergoing diversion. The results of this report are discouraging. The average survival time was 5.3 months; only 50% of the patients were alive at 3 months and only 20% were alive at 6 months. After the diversion, 63.8% of the survival time was spent in the hospital. Delgado also reported on a group of patients with recurrent pelvic cancer and renal failure that were treated with urinary conduit diversion. Delgado's results show an insignificant increase in survival time, and he suggests that these patients should never undergo urinary diversion because a more preferable method of expiration (uremia) is then eliminated from the patient's future. Obviously, this decision should be made in consultation with the family and even with the patient, if possible. When urinary diversion is performed, accentuation of the other clinical manifestations of recurrent pelvic cancer (i.e., severe pelvic pain, repetitive infections, and hemorrhage) is generally observed, leading to increased suffering. Pain control and progressive cachexia burden the physician and the patient. Episodes of massive pelvic hemorrhage are associated with difficult decisions concerning transfusion. An extension of the inpatient hospital stay is inevitable, and the financial impact of the patient on her family is often considerable.

Fistula

Urinary or colon fistulas are common sequelae of progressive cervical cancer and uterine corpus cancer. Because both urinary and intestinal fistulas have a great impact on QOL, consideration should always be given to diversion of either the urinary or fecal stream in order to reduce symptomatology. Bladder drainage can often sufficiently reduce the incontinence associated with a urinary fistula without the need for surgical urinary diversion. Ureteral ligation with percutaneous nephrostomy drainage is another option. However, urinary conduit or other surgical procedures are often necessary to adequately divert the urinary stream. Surgical repair of a urinary fistula secondary to recurrent cancer or radiation is rarely successful with existing surgical techniques.

Colovaginal fistulas can generally be palliated with a colostomy. Although controversial, a loop colostomy often provides adequate fecal stream interruption to prevent further fistula drainage. However, some surgeons argue that an end colostomy with Hartmann pouch is necessary to completely interrupt the fecal stream. In either situation, a mini-laparotomy is generally all that is required to adequately accomplish the palliative goal.

Sexual Dysfunction

The treatment of women with gynecologic malignancies may result in vaginal abnormalities that interfere with sexual function. Disturbances in sexuality are more common after the treatment of vulvar, vaginal, and cervical carcinoma compared with corpus and ovarian cancer. This is a result of the frequent use of radical surgery and radiotherapy to treat the three former malignancies. The reported frequency of sexual dysfunction after surgery, radiotherapy, or both varies considerably. Of women, 4% to 100% report a shortened vagina after a radical hysterectomy, whereas 17% to 58% have reduced lubrication. However, until recently, there were no reliable data on reductions in vaginal elasticity or genital swelling during sexual stimulation after radical hysterectomy. A report from Sweden published in *The New England Journal of Medicine* in 1999 demonstrated a statistically significant decrease in vaginal elasticity (23%) among women treated for early cervical cancer compared to a control group (4%). In addition, this study of 256 patients with cervical cancer, who were retrospectively surveyed and compared with 350 controls, also showed a decrease in lubrication during arousal and a reduction in perceived vaginal length after treatment. Furthermore, a large number of women indicated that these changes and their effects on sexual intercourse distressed them. Of note, the frequency of orgasms and orgasmic pleasure was similar in the two groups, although dyspareunia was more common in the women who had cervical cancer. Finally, this study did not show any significant difference among those women treated with radical surgery versus radiotherapy, although other retrospective comparisons have documented a significant increase in sexual dysfunction among those patients treated with radiation versus surgery. A direct comparison between radiation and surgery in the treatment of cervical cancer emphasizing not only outcome but also QOL and sexual function is needed. Regular vaginal dilatation is widely recommended to those women treated with radiation as a way to maintain vaginal length and elasticity. Again, this intervention has never been tested in a prospective fashion. The appropriate use of hormone replacement therapy and lubricants may also improve coital function.

Dyspareunia resulting from gynecologic cancer therapy should be evaluated and treated because dyspareunia can lead to loss of desire and can cause women to become sexually avoidant. This often leads to difficult interpersonal relationships between the woman and her partner. Loss of sexual desire in the postcancer population is common and represents a challenging problem. Long after ordinary physical health has been regained, women may describe feeling little or no sexual desire.

Counseling and support groups may be helpful in overcoming this frustration.

Anxiety and Depression

The prevalence of depressive and anxiety disorders among women with gynecologic cancers approached 50%. In a study by Fowler and colleagues, depression and anxiety symptoms were high (42% and 30%, respectively) in women who had sought consultation by a gynecologic oncologist. The severity and prevalence of these psychological symptoms correlated highly with the number of gynecologic symptoms. Of note, older women and those women without a partner were more likely to suffer from depression and anxiety.

The prevalence and severity of symptoms may fluctuate during the patient's treatment course. Chan and Woodruff tracked the psychosocial state in gynecologic cancer patients to identify risk factors for maladjustment during treatment. Although most patients adjusted well in their sample of 74 women, those with lower socioeconomic status and those without family support or religious belief suffered more from adjustment disorders. Furthermore, pain, health-related QOL, and poor performance status have been shown to affect these psychological disorders.

There is limited evidence reporting the optimal pharmacologic and psychosocial interventions in depressive disorders among cancer patients. Four classes of drugs have been used: tricyclic antidepressants (TCA), serotonin reuptake inhibitors (SSRI), neuroleptics, and benzodiazepines. It has been suggested that TCAs may be particularly helpful in patients with insomnia and cachexia and that SSRIs may be indicated for patients with low energy, although the evidence regarding dosages and drug choice are heterogeneous. The neuroleptics, such as haloperidol, or the benzodiazepines are not only indicated in patients with anxiety but can ameliorate nausea and vomiting simultaneously. Apart from medical therapy, it has been shown that actively seeking support for psychological concerns enhances QOL and mood. It is not surprising that treatment of depressive and anxiety disorders in these patients might require medical therapy combined with such psychosocial therapy as can be found in cancer support groups.

END-OF-LIFE DECISION-MAKING

As summarized in the American College of Obstetrics and Gynecology Committee Opinion published in May 1995, the moral character of medicine is based on three values central to the human relationship:

1. Patient benefit
2. Patient self-determination
3. Ethical integrity of the health care professional

Patient Benefit

The obligation to promote the good of the patient is a basic presumption of medical care and the defining feature of a physician's ethical responsibility. To promote the patient's good is to provide care in which benefits outweigh burdens or harms. Benefits, in turn, are understood only relative to the goals that the patient and physician hope to achieve through medical care.

Patient Self-Determination

The inherent value of individual autonomy or self-determination is one of the fundamental bases of democracy in the United States and provides certain protection during end-of-life decision-making. In health care, the value of individual autonomy is as firm in the ethical and legal doctrines as in informed consent. Under this doctrine, the patient has a right to control what happens to her body. This means the following:

1. No treatment may be given to the patient without her consent (or if she lacks decision-making capacity, the consent of her surrogate).
2. The patient (or her surrogate) has the right to refuse unwanted medical treatment. This right is not contingent on the presence or absence of a terminal illness, on the agreement of family members, or on the approval of physicians or hospital administrators.

In the medical context, physician respect for patient self-determination consists of an active inclusion of the patient in decisions regarding her own care. This involves frank discussion of the diagnosis and prognosis; the relative risks and benefits of alternative treatments; and, based on these discussions, the identification or the operative goals of care.

Legal Developments That Bear on End-of-Life Decision-Making

In the 1990s several developments in the law influenced end-of-life decision-making. First, in June 1990, in a decision on the *Cruzan* case, the United States Supreme Court affirmed that patients have a constitutionally protected right to refuse unwanted medical treatments. The ruling reaffirms states' authority to adopt procedural requirements for the withdrawal and withholding of life-prolonging medical interventions. A second legal development was the passage of the federal Patient

Self-Determination Act (PSDA), which took effect on December 1, 1991. The PSDA requires Medicaid and Medicare participating health care institutions to inform all adult patients of their rights "to make decisions concerning medical care, including the right to accept or refuse medical or surgical treatment and the right to formulate an advance directive." Under the PSDA, institutions are legally required to provide this information to patients upon admission for care or upon enrollment in health maintenance organizations. The institution must note in the chart the existence of an advance directive and must respect such a directive to the fullest extent under state law.

An advance directive is the formal mechanism by which a patient may express her values regarding her future health status. It may take the form of a proxy directive or an instructional directive, or both. Proxy directives, such as the durable power of attorney for health care, designate a surrogate to make medical decisions on behalf of the patient who is no longer competent to express her choices. Instructional directives, such as "living wills," focus on the types of life-sustaining treatments that a person would or would not choose in various clinical circumstances.

A patient's goals of care are very likely to change with time in different clinical circumstances. As a static expression of the patient's wishes, an instructional directive may thus be a limited tool that could conceivably undermine a patient's most current desires. With this in mind, the patient's appointment of a proxy who knows her interest and accepts the role of surrogate decision-maker may be the best way of ensuring that her wishes will be carried out (proxy directive).

Surrogate Decision-Making

If the patient who lacks decision-making capacity has not designated a health care proxy, state law may dictate the order in which relatives should be asked to serve as surrogates. The person selected should be one who knows the patient's values and wishes and will respect them in his or her role as a surrogate decision-maker. If there is conflict regarding the decision of a surrogate, it may be appropriate to seek the advice of an ethics committee or consultant or, possibly, the courts.

In proxy decision-making for the dying patient, surrogates and health care providers should be aware that there is documentation and gender disparity in clinical medicine and research in court decisions surrounding the right to refuse life-sustaining treatment. In review of "right to die" cases, it was found that courts honored the previously stated treatment decisions of men in 75% of cases, whereas they respected the prior choices of female patients in only 14% of cases. Given the

persistence and pervasiveness of social attitudes to take women's moral choices less seriously than those of men, gynecologists and patient surrogates must prevent these vices from undermining their advocacy for female patients. Likewise, this evidence should further motivate women to make a treatment decision as explicit as possible.

Futility

Treatments that offer no benefit to patients are clearly not obligatory. However, there is no single point at which all patients will conclude that they have completed a certain number of therapeutic interventions, thus making further control of their disease impossible. Although the cancer is increasingly less likely to respond to second-, third-, or fourth-line agents, this is not necessarily an indication of their potential efficacy in that individual patient. Ovarian cancer, in particular, is a disease entity that requires treatment individualized to the needs and presentations of each patient in ways that other disease practices do not.

The American Medical Association (AMA) Council on Ethical and Judicial Affairs to date has not defined an approach to determine what treatment is and is not medically futile, although the council has discussed related issues concerning end-of-life care in many reports. For example, it has affirmed the ethical standing of withdrawing and withholding unwanted interventions, noted the constructive role that advanced care planning can play in preempting difficult and conflicting situations, and advised the use of a range of orders not to intervene. The council has also opposed physician-assisted suicide out of concern that recent calls from citizens and professionals for physician-assisted suicides are a response to experiences of excessive and futile interventions at the end of life. Because definitions of futile care are value laden, universal consensus on futile care is unlikely to be achieved. Rather, a process-based approach has been proposed that includes four distinguishable steps aimed at deliberation and resolution, two steps aimed at securing alternatives in case of irresolvable differences, and a final step aimed at closure when all alternatives have been exhausted (Figure 21-5). This has been outlined by the report of the Council on Ethical and Judicial Affairs of the AMA published in its journal in March 1999.

First, earnest attempts should be made to deliberate over and negotiate a prior understanding between patient, proxy, and physician about what constitutes futile care for the patient and what falls within acceptable limits for the physicians, family, and possibly also the institution. This prior understanding is best achieved before critical illness occurs. If serious disagreement is irresolvable, provisions can be made for a sensitive and orderly transfer of care at such a time that it can pre-empt later conflicts.

Second, joint decision-making should also be made at the bedside between patient or proxy and physician. This joint decision-making should do the following:

- Make use of outcome data whenever possible
- Incorporate the physician's and patient's or proxy's intent or goals for treatment
- Abide by established standards of deliberation and informed consent

Third, the assistance of an individual consultant or a patient representative is a further step and is often helpful to reach a resolution within all parties' accept-able limits. The role of this individual consultant is not to singlehandedly resolve the conflict but rather to facili-tate discussions that help to reach that end.

Fourth, an institutional committee, such as an ethics committee, may be involved if disagreements are irre-solvable. A final step may occur if the outcome of the institutional process coincides with the patient's desire, but the physician remains unpersuaded. In such a case, arrangements may be needed for transfer to another physician within the institution.

Alternatively, arrangements for transfers to another institution may be sought if the physician's position does not agree with that of the patient. Finally, if transfer is not possible because no physician and no institution can be found to follow the patient's or the proxy's wishes, it may be because the request is consid-ered offensive to medical ethics and professional stan-dards in the eyes of a majority of the health care profession. In such cases, by ethics standards, the inter-vention in question should not be provided, although the legal ramifications of this course of action are uncertain.

As a result of the complicated nature of these proceedings, the AMA Council recommends that all health care institutions, whether large or small, adopt the policy of medical futility and those policies on medical futility follow their process approach presented earlier.

Hospice

Palliative care programs often foster identification with hospice, and some have integrated hospice home care or inpatient programs. In the United States, hospice has come to mean primarily a government-regulated orga-nization or program for dying persons and their families that typically focuses on home care and is limited to the following patients and situations:

1. Life expectancy of 6 months or less
2. A focus on comfort measures. This is sometimes (but not always) defined by hospice programs as a desire to forgo various "aggressive" and often expensive management approaches. These approaches may usually include cardiopulmonary resuscitation; blood product replacement; and some forms of radiotherapy, surgery, chemotherapy, and acute care hospitalization, at least insofar as these treatment modalities are used to try to cure or prolong life rather than to palliate symptoms
3. A general preference for care at home (except where inpatient hospice is available and specifically sought)
4. A willingness to sign a form acknowledging the desire to enter a hospice program and to focus on comfort care
5. Health insurance that covers hospice

Many hospice programs also require a primary care-giver to be either in the home or regularly available. Another requirement reported by patients or family members is that they had to agree to forgo cardiopulmo-nary resuscitation, calls for emergency services, or future hospitalization. This requirement is not embodied in federal hospice regulations or the PSDA.

Although hospice staff may be perceived as more knowledgeable and empathic than conventional home care workers, hospice may actually provide much fewer hours of formal care, particularly home health aide time. This finding was recently documented for home care patients with amyotrophic lateral sclerosis. Thus patients and families are often forced to choose between hospice care with insufficient home health aide support and a conventional home care approach that includes signifi-cantly more hours of home health aide time. Hospice programs in the United States are increasingly con-stricted by the eligibility requirements created by Medi-care and other insurers and by the limits of reimbursement, thus making it difficult to cover expensive treatments or provide as much home health aide time as conventional programs. Many programs have become extremely cau-tious about admission or recertification in the face of the threat posed by an unsympathetic and perhaps ill-conceived government audit that scrutinizes long-stay patients and those with diagnoses other than cancer. At the same time, health maintenance organizations and insurers have attempted to "unbundle" hospice services, providing and paying for only part of the hospice package (e.g., home nurses without social service, chap-lains, volunteers, or bereavement care).

Throughout the world, palliative care is developing as an area of special clinical expertise. It is a recognized specialty in Great Britain and Australia and has been the subject of national attention in the Canadian undergraduate medical curriculum. Although a fledging field, it can boast of multiple clinical centers and training programs; various fine textbooks, journals, and educational conferences; and a small body of research expertise. The challenge that palliative care faces today is to avoid orthodoxy while moving toward greater unanimity about the nature of the field, with improved standards for palliative care professionals and programs.

For full reference list, log onto www.expertconsult.com ⟨http://www.expertconsult.com⟩.

Role of Minimally Invasive Surgery in Gynecologic Malignancies

Jeffrey M. Fowler, MD, David E. Cohn, MD, and Robert S. Mannel, MD

LAPAROSCOPIC SURGERY IN GYNECOLOGIC ONCOLOGY

Recent advances in the techniques of minimally invasive surgery (MIS) have greatly expanded its role in the management of gynecologic malignancies. Before the 1990s, MIS was mostly limited to laparoscopy for diagnosis of pelvic disease and for tubal sterilization procedures. The great majority of gynecologic oncology procedures for definitive surgical management were performed via large midline abdominal incisions in order to accomplish appropriate extirpation of the malignancy and surgical staging. The laparotomy causes significant trauma to the patient with many potential associated morbidities, which are increased in incidence and severity in patients with comorbid conditions. The potential applications for MIS in patients diagnosed with a gynecologic malignancy have gradually expanded over the past 20 years with improvements in video-laparoscopic instrumentation and surgical training. Since 2005 advances in robotic surgery led to the increased use of MIS for comprehensive surgical management of patients with

gynecologic cancers. Most gynecologic oncologists now offer MIS as an option for surgical management of patients diagnosed with cervical, endometrial, and ovarian neoplasia.

Advanced laparoscopic procedures have been an option for a subpopulation of gynecologic oncology patients since the late 1980s. The goal of MIS is to decrease patient discomfort, hospital stay, and short- and long-term morbidity while at the same time providing an overall improvement in quality of life (QOL) and allowing for earlier implementation of other adjuvant therapies if necessary. Incorporating laparoscopic procedures into the comprehensive management of gynecologic oncology patients has been only moderately successful secondary to limitations of the available technology; a difficult and long learning curve; variability in surgeon training and experience; longer operative times; and patient factors limiting the use of MIS such as prior surgeries, extent of disease, and obesity. Technologic limitations to rapid implementation of complicated laparoscopic surgery in gynecologic oncology include a limited two-dimensional field of vision, counterintuitive motions often required for the surgeon and assistant, limited degrees of freedom of the instruments, and ergonomic disadvantages for the surgeon. Advanced robotic technologies have improved most of these limitations, allowing for expansion of the role of MIS in patients with gynecologic cancer.

As illustrated in other chapters in this textbook, there is a long history in the evolution of surgery in patients with gynecologic cancers. These include incorporation of modifications to radical surgical procedures that reduce the toxicities of treatment with the goal of obtaining the optimal oncologic outcome while improving overall patient QOL. It is important that the goals of cancer control and patient safety are not compromised by a given surgical approach. In other words, MIS serves as another tool to achieve these goals, rather than a separate end itself. The historical advantages of laparotomy compared to laparoscopy include maximal surgical exposure, three-dimensional vision, direct tissue palpation and manipulation, and ease of suturing and other instrument use. The previously mentioned disadvantages of MIS related to these factors are balanced by potential patient outcome–related improvements. A disadvantage of a given surgical approach should not translate into an accepted compromise. Regardless of surgical approach, it is still imperative that the surgeon adhere to the primary surgical principles of optimal exposure, meticulous tissue dissection, expert knowledge of anatomy, and an understanding of the natural history of the diseases being treated in order to overcome any potential compromise.

LAPAROSCOPIC SURGICAL STAGING OF GYNECOLOGIC MALIGNANCIES

The cornerstone of appropriate surgical staging is an accurate pelvic and para-aortic lymph node dissection. Incorporation of MIS into the surgical management of patients with gynecologic cancer was not feasible until a technique for adequate laparoscopic lymph node dissection was made possible. Pioneering descriptions of laparoscopic procedures for pelvic lymph node dissection came from Europe in the late 1980s by Dargent and Queurleau. Although exciting in terms of the prospects of MIS, there were concerns regarding adequacy of lymph node dissection, operative risks, and ability to access the para-aortic nodes. Since that time, laparoscopic skills evolved and this approach has been demonstrated to be feasible with many descriptions of the surgical technique and outcomes of the laparoscopic pelvic and para-aortic lymph node dissections now reported. Data concerning the laparoscopic approach in the surgical treatment of the gynecologic oncology patient are primarily nonrandomized and retrospective

aiming to establish the feasibility of MIS lymphadenectomy in highly selected patients. Only a few multicenter prospective randomized clinical trials have been completed regarding the feasibility of comprehensive laparoscopic management in patients with gynecologic cancer.

ROBOTIC SURGERY IN GYNECOLOGIC MALIGNANCIES

Robotic surgery overcomes many of the technologic limitations of laparoscopy. The robotic platform provides the surgeon superior high-definition 3-D vision, magnification, wristed instruments, and motion scaling. The surgeon has much more ability to directly control the operative field compared to laparoscopy, thus eliminating many important disadvantages of laparoscopy. The operator of the robotic platform not only has improved vision, but also controls the direction and distance of the camera from the operative field without relying on the assistant. In addition, the surgeon has three other port sites to use for a dissector, cutting instrument, and another retracting instrument. Loss of haptic feedback is a potential disadvantage; however, the experienced surgeon is able to overcome loss of this sense with heightened visual feedback and meticulous surgical technique. In addition, there are no significant ergonomic disadvantages and risk of injury to the surgeon and much less risk of fatigue. These significant technological improvements have allowed the gynecologic surgeon to perform much more complicated surgeries via MIS on a heterogeneous group of patients. The published experience for robotics in gynecologic oncology is limited, but it is rapidly expanding. Multiple series now exist describing major and complicated gynecologic oncology procedures such as hysterectomy, adnexectomy, pelvic and para-aortic lymph node dissection, and radical hysterectomy.

MINIMALLY INVASIVE SURGERY LEARNING CURVE

Recent advances in the techniques of MIS have greatly expanded its role in the management of gynecologic malignancies. Several recent studies have shown an increasing use of laparoscopy as a treatment modality in gynecologic malignancies. Although advanced laparoscopic technology has been available for more than two decades, the incorporation of MIS into surgical management of the gynecologic oncology patient has been relatively slow. Whether this relative lack of mainstream adaptation of LS into the practice is a result of technology or training limitations is unclear, although strong biases support both potential causes. Although difficult to quantify, there is a long and difficult learning curve related to laparoscopy and advanced pelvic operations. The availability of the robotic surgery platform is rapidly expanding the role and adaptation of MIS in the surgical management of women with gynecologic cancer. Nevertheless, these procedures remain major surgeries performed through small incisions and therefore offer unique challenges to the surgeon. Appropriate patient selection, along with a comprehensive understanding of surgical techniques and contraindications, allows for optimal utilization of MIS in the gynecologic oncology patient population.

Little information exists to define the learning curve for laparoscopy and gynecologic oncology surgical procedures. Eltabbakh reported on 75 consecutive patients for laparoscopic management of women with endometrial cancer undergoing laparoscopic-assisted vaginal hysterectomy (LAVH), bilateral salpingo-oophorectomy (BSO), and pelvic lymph node (PLN) sampling. There was both a significant decrease in operating time and significant increase in the number of pelvic lymph nodes harvested with increasing surgeon experience. The experience of the operative assistant has also been shown to be important in major laparoscopic procedures for gynecologic malignancies. Scribner reported a significant difference in successful completion of laparoscopic lymphadenectomies when the first assistant was a skilled attending surgeon compared to a resident or fellow in training. The primary surgeon's experience is the most important factor in improving outcomes in gynecologic oncology laparoscopic surgery. Melendez and colleagues noted improvement in operating room time and a decrease in complications over time in patients with endometrial cancer; however, it required 12 years to gain this experience in 124 patients with endometrial cancer, which reflects a highly selected population of patients. Based on this report and others it likely requires roughly 20 to 25 laparoscopic endometrial cancer cases to gain proficiency in this procedure, but individual surgeon experience and outcomes are quite heterogeneous. In the largest single-institution report on transperitoneal laparoscopic pelvic and para-aortic lymph node dissection, Schneider and colleagues estimated 20 operations were required to gain the needed experience for laparoscopic pelvic lymphadenectomy and up to 100 for para-aortic lymphadenectomy.

The robotic platform is being more rapidly adapted by gynecologic oncologists to perform extrafascial and radical hysterectomies with pelvic and para-aortic lymph node dissections and is similarly associated with a learning curve. Seamon and colleagues determined that proficiency for hysterectomy with pelvic and para-aortic lymph node dissection in women with endometrial cancer is achieved at 20 cases (approximately 10 cases per surgeon), and further efficiency continues to improve over time. Holloway and colleagues demonstrated improved operating room times and ability to perform aortic node dissections in a similar group of patients with improvement in patient safety over time. The learning curve for the robotic radical hysterectomy has not been defined but likely is longer than the extrafascial hysterectomy because this is a more complicated surgical procedure. Patient selection based on previous surgical history and, most important, level of obesity significantly influence the learning curve (in addition to surgeon experience in both laparoscopic and robotic MIS.)

The laparoscopic surgical technique is principally different from open laparotomy in the loss of three-dimensional vision, counterintuitive movements, subtle tactile sensation, limitations of instrumentation, and a heavy reliance on skilled surgical assistance. The surgeon needs to compensate for these losses with a thorough understanding of abdominal and pelvic anatomy when operating laparoscopically. In a prospective, randomized trial, Coleman reported significant improvement in laparoscopic proficiency in residents exposed to a laboratory-based skills curriculum. Training specifically geared toward laparoscopic surgery using models, cadavers, and animal labs is important in gaining proficiency in advanced laparoscopic surgery. The learning curve for robotics does appear to be distinctly different from that for laparoscopy as investigators have demonstrated that surgical drills and suturing are performed with enhanced precision and dexterity when comparing robotic technologies to laparoscopy in a training labaratory. In a survey of laparoscopy training among Society of Gynecologic Oncology members, 85% reported receiving none or limited laparoscopic training during their fellowship. Among active fellows, 67% report performing fewer than five laparoscopic surgeries per month. These data confirm the need for improved training during residency and fellowship programs and continuing medical education and mentoring for established surgeons. The transition from laparoscopy to robotic surgery for the MIS management of gynecologic cancers will likely further diminish experience in laparoscopic surgery in this population. There may be an advantage to the robotic platform for novice minimally invasive surgeons given the ability for higher magnification and three-dimensional vision. However, any novel technology does not obviate the need for sound surgical principles and technique, knowledge of anatomy, and understanding of the natural history of the diseases being treated.

MINIMALLY INVASIVE SURGICAL TECHNIQUE

Positioning of the patient is critical in advanced MIS. For most gynecologic procedures, the appropriate position

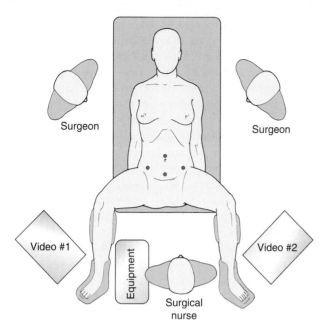

FIGURE 21-1   Operating room setup for laparoscopic surgery. Positioning of patient for laparoscopic gynecologic surgery. Note: Arms tucked (1); two video monitors toward foot of table (2); and modified dorsal lithotomy position with adjustable stirrups (3).

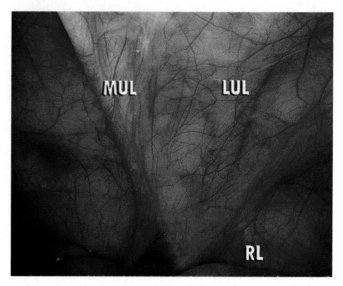

FIGURE 21-2   Anterior abdominal wall. *LUL,* Lateral umbilical ligament; *MUL,* medial umbilical ligament; *RL,* round ligament.

is in a dorsal lithotomy position with adjustable Allen stirrups to allow for manipulation of the uterus and LAVH as indicated. In patients who do not have a uterus or in whom the uterus is not anticipated to be removed, placement in a supine position may be appropriate. The patient's arms should be tucked by her side to allow mobility and ergonomic comfort for the operating surgeon and assistant. Care should be used in protecting both the upper and lower extremities with appropriate padding to prevent pressure points and nerve injuries. For laparoscopic surgery, video monitors should be placed on each side of the table across from the operating surgeon and the assistant and located toward the foot of the table. This allows for comfortable positioning of the surgeon in a natural angle of viewing the video monitor and minimizing of counterintuitive surgical movement. Placement of the monitors toward the patient's head can be considered in situations in which extensive upper abdominal surgery will be undertaken (Figure 21-1).

Number, position, and size of trocars for laparoscopic surgery will depend on the surgery anticipated. In cases that require removal of an adnexal mass or lymph nodes, a 10- to 12-mm accessory port will be needed for extraction of the specimen. Most LS can be accomplished successfully with the placement of a 5- or 10-mm port at the level of the umbilicus for camera placement, a 10- to 12-mm port suprapubically, and a 5-mm port in each of the lateral lower quadrants. Gynecologic oncologists will usually use a total of 4 to 6 ports to obtain adequate exposure and accomplish advanced pelvic procedures.

Safe placement of the primary port, or camera port, is the most critical part of the procedure in terms of minimizing major surgical complications. A number of surgical approaches have been described and accepted for placement of the primary port. A nasogastric tube should be used to achieve gastric decompression before placement of the Verres needle or primary trochar. Lateral ports can safely be placed in a line one third of the distance from the anterior superior iliac spine to the umbilicus. Care should be taken when placing the lateral port and to do so under direct visualization with inspection of the deep inferior epigastric vessels lying along the lateral boundary of the rectus abdominis muscles. These can be directly identified lateral to the obliterated umbilical ligaments (Figure 21-2). Transillumination will not reliably reveal the location of these vessels.

The port-site setup for robotic surgery is different than for laparoscopic procedures because ports are generally placed above the umbilicus (Figure 21-3). Various port setups have been described for robotic gynecologic oncology surgery. Most gynecologic oncologists will use four 8-mm robotic ports and two additional laparoscopy ports to be controlled by the bedside assistant. In addition, the robot must be "docked" or attached to the ports, which is accomplished between the legs of the patient or from the side. Once the surgical procedure commences, the experienced robotic surgeon can efficiently alternate (swap) control of the various robotic ports through a unique clutching system using both hand and foot controls, can operate all instruments in real time, and has direct control of both monopolar and bipolar electrosurgical energy sources. Although there is less reliance on the bedside assistant, that person is still instrumental in facilitating the case through robotic

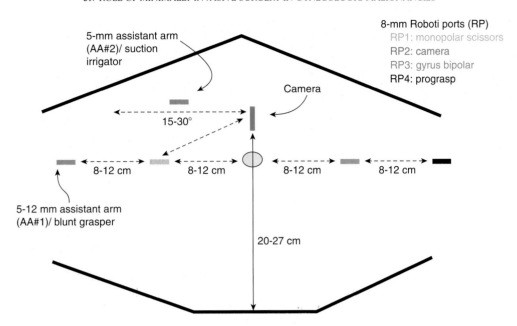

FIGURE 21-3 Robotic port setup for endometrial cancer staging. Trocar placement for hysterectomy, pelvic and aortic lymphadenectomy. Note the robotic ports *(RP)* are 8 mm, assistant arm *(AA)* #1 is 5-12 mm, and AA#2 is a 5-mm port. Although the placement of RP#1 and 3 corresponds to approximately the midclavicular line, AA#1 and RP#4 are at the midaxillary line. *(From Seamon LG, Cohn DE, Valmadre S, et al: J Robotic Surg 2:71, 2008.)*

instrument changes, manipulation of vaginal instruments, suction-irrigation, and use of an additional grasping instrument for retraction.

Once the ports are placed, actual surgical technique varies little except for the surgical steps required to complete various aspects of the procedure. Once successful insufflation and placement of the trocars are accomplished, visual inspection of the abdominal cavity is undertaken and the patient is placed in a steep Trendelenburg position. As in any surgical procedure, excellent exposure should be accomplished initially and maintained throughout the case. Use of steep Trendelenburg is necessary, in lieu of packing the bowel, to achieve adequate visualization of the pelvis and lower abdominal region. Lysis of any adhesions holding the small bowel or omentum into the pelvis or lower abdomen should occur before beginning the pelvic and upper abdominal dissection. The small bowel is carefully placed in the upper abdomen by flipping the bowel from a caudad to a cranial position, exposing the mesentery of the small bowel and the aortic bifurcation (Figure 21-4). Care should be taken with this maneuver by using blunt instruments and gentle technique. In obese patients, body habitus may not allow steep Trendelenburg because of unacceptably high peak inspiratory pressure. In addition, obesity may prevent adequate mobilization of the small bowel out of the pelvis and upper abdomen to allow for retroperitoneal dissection. Some authors have advocated use of additional port sites to help circumvent this problem.

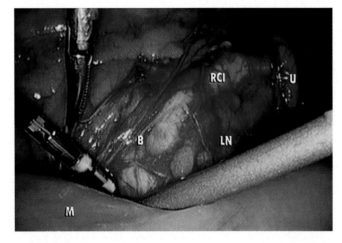

FIGURE 21-4 Para-aortic area. *B*, Aortic bifurcation; *LN*, right para-aortic lymph nodes; *M*, bowel mesentery; *RCI*, right common iliac artery; *U*, ureter.

The key to successful advanced laparoscopic surgery is the same as that for open laparotomy: access to the retroperitoneum. In the pelvis, this is accomplished by dividing the round ligament laterally or opening the pelvic peritoneum lateral and parallel to the infundibulopelvic ligament. Some surgeons prefer to keep the round ligament intact so they can retract against it to keep the paravesical space open while dissecting tissue. Dissection is then carried down to the level of the external iliac artery, which is then followed in a cephalad and medial direction to the common iliac artery. At this

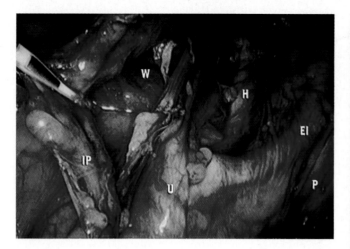

FIGURE 21-5   Pelvic sidewall. *EI,* External iliac artery; *H,* hypogastric artery; *IP,* infundibulopelvic ligament; *P,* psoas muscle; *U,* ureter; *W,* peritoneal window.

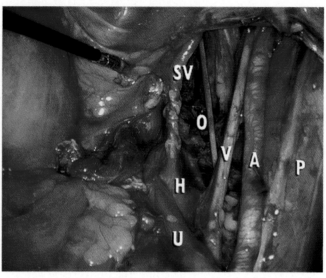

FIGURE 21-6   Pelvic sidewall retroperitoneal anatomy. *A,* External iliac artery; *H,* hypogastric artery; *O,* obturator nerve; *P,* psoas muscle; *SV,* superior vesicle artery; *U,* ureter; *V,* external iliac vein.

point, the ureter can be found crossing the pelvic brim and a window can be created between the ovarian vessels and the ureter (Figure 21-5). Development of the pararectal space is under direct visualization after identification of the bifurcation of the common iliac vessel and the ureter. The surgeon places traction on the ureter medially developing the pararectal space between the hypogastric artery laterally and the ureter and rectum medially. Care must be taken during this dissection to avoid disrupting the cardinal web deep in the retroperitoneum. Because of the positive pressure environment of MIS resulting from the pneumoperitoneum, the boundaries of the paravesical space can be identified visually during laparoscopic surgery. The superior vesicle artery and umbilical artery are clearly visible as the medial umbilical ligament (see Figure 21-2). Dissection is carried along the external iliac artery to the level of the superior vesicle artery. At this point the superior vesicle artery is retracted in a medial direction and the paravesical space is easily developed with the bladder and superior vesicle artery medially and external artery and obturator node bundle laterally. Once this is accomplished, the uterine artery can be clearly identified at the origin of the superior vesicle artery from the hypogastric artery. This retroperitoneal pelvic dissection is the cornerstone of any laparoscopic surgery performed in the pelvis, including removal of an adnexal mass, laparoscopic-assisted vaginal hysterectomy, laparoscopic radical hysterectomy, and pelvic lymph node dissection (Figure 21-6). Dissection can be facilitated with a variety of energy sources and clip appliers, each with their own advocates.

Extension of the incision along the peritoneum overlying the right common iliac artery and then along the aorta to the level of the duodenum allows for exposure of the para-aortic retroperitoneum (Figure 21-7). During

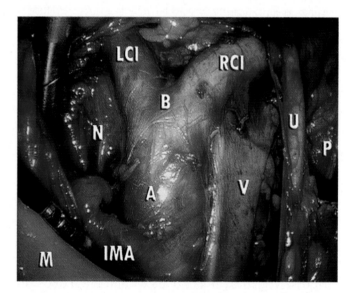

FIGURE 21-7   Para-aortic retroperitoneal anatomy. *A,* Aorta; *B,* aortic bifurcation; *IMA,* inferior mesenteric artery; *LCI,* left common iliac artery; *M,* bowel mesentery; *N,* sympathetic nerve; *P,* psoas muscle; *RCI,* right common iliac artery; *U,* right ureter; *V,* inferior vena cava.

this dissection, the peritoneum attached to the base of the cecum can be elevated in an anterior-cephalad direction providing excellent exposure to the right para-aortic lymph node region. Margins of resection are identical to an open approach and can be extended to the level of the renal vessels. The left-sided para-aortic lymph node dissection requires dissection underneath the inferior mesenteric artery mobilizing the descending colon and rectosigmoid off the left common iliac artery and retracting the inferior mesenteric artery and ureter laterally and cephalad. This gives excellent exposure to the left para-aortic lymph nodes inferior to the inferior mesenteric artery. Dissection can be continued above the inferior mesenteric artery in a similar manner. Some authors have advocated sacrificing the inferior mesenteric artery in order to get enhanced exposure to the upper left para-aortic nodes.

Unfortunately, the potential limitations previously described for MIS compared with laparotomy lead to the potential for inherent compromises in surgical technique. Therefore the surgeon needs to obtain experience over time in order to optimize patient outcomes and emphasize excellent surgical technique. Knowledge of anatomy, the disease process, and surgical technique is key during these complicated surgical procedures. In order to minimize complications that are possible with any major surgical procedure, vigilance and meticulous surgical technique are required.

APPLICATIONS OF MINIMALLY INVASIVE SURGERY IN GYNECOLOGIC ONCOLOGY

Cervical Cancer

The pioneering reports describing the use of advanced laparoscopic techniques in gynecologic oncology were initially described in patients with cervical cancer in which laparoscopy was used for pelvic lymph node dissection in patients with early-stage disease to assess the feasibility for abdominal radical hysterectomy. One of the initial concerns about MIS in cervical cancer was that the laparoscopic approach would not be as thorough as laparotomy in assessing metastatic cancer and performing a comprehensive lymphadenectomy. Early studies in patients undergoing initial laparoscopic lymphadenectomy before laparotomy confirmed that a thorough pelvic and para-aortic lymphadenectomy is possible via LS, with no positive nodes discovered at laparotomy performed following laparoscopic lymphadenectomy. Nevertheless, the completeness of laparoscopic dissection was dependent on the experience of the surgeon, and the most common area for missed lymph nodes was lateral to the common iliac bifurcation. Once the feasibility of laparoscopic lymphadenectomy was established, the use of MIS for radical surgery in patients with early-stage cervical cancer and for preradiation surgical assessment in patients with advanced disease was made possible.

Early-stage cervical cancer—radical hysterectomy

The establishment of the feasibility of laparoscopic lymphadenectomy led to the renewed interest in radical vaginal hysterectomy with laparoscopic lymphadenectomy and the development of novel minimally invasive radical hysterectomy techniques. Several groups worldwide have demonstrated the feasibility of the Schauta radical vaginal hysterectomy, laparoscopic-assisted radical vaginal hysterectomy (LAVRH), and total laparoscopic radical hysterectomy (LRH) with the goals of maintaining a high level of cancer control with improved patient outcomes in women with early-stage cervical cancer. The Schauta radical vaginal hysterectomy, described more than 100 years ago, and its subsequent modifications are performed completely vaginally; however, the surgeon does not have the opportunity to perform a retroperitoneal lymph node dissection. The LAVRH has many descriptions but usually involves a laparoscopic phase that includes the lymphadenectomy followed by developing the pararectal and paravesical spaces, dividing the parametria and paravaginal pedicles, and completing the remainder of the procedure vaginally. For the LRH, the entire radical pelvic operation is completed with MIS techniques. One advantage of the LAVRH over the LRH is the ability to precisely define the vaginal incision. Additionally, the performance of LAVRH allows for the development of the MIS skills required to perform a fertility-sparing radical vaginal trachelectomy. Currently, the favored laparoscopic approach is the LRH because there is no need for a perineal phase for the performance of a vaginal incision, exposure is improved, visualization of critical anatomy and surgical planes is better, and anatomic limitations are fewer as a result of a narrow pelvis or lack of uterine descensus. Most important, however, is the fact that LRH mimics the well-established steps of an abdominal radical hysterectomy, thereby making LHR easier to adopt.

There is no doubt that the LARVH and LRH are feasible for patients with early-stage cervical cancer. It has been demonstrated that these techniques can accomplish the oncologic goals of the surgery, allowing for the identification of critical anatomy, performance of a thorough lymph node dissection, and completion of the radical resection of the primary tumor with adequate margins. The traditional abdominal radical hysterectomy and the LRH/LARVH procedures have never been compared in prospective randomized studies. The initial series describing laparoscopic radical hysterectomies were primarily investigating operative feasibility and perioperative outcomes. More recent series are larger and report recurrence and survival data, which compare favorably with matched historical patients undergoing a traditional radical hysterectomy for cervical cancer. It is not likely that the laparoscopic and open radical hysterectomy will be compared in a large multi-institutional prospective trial considering recent changes in MIS technology (robotics) and the fact that the incidence of invasive cervical cancer continues to trend downward in developed countries.

TABLE 21-1   Representative Sample of Single-Institutional Series on Laparoscopic Radical Hysterectomies

Study	N	Operating Room Time (hours)	Blood Transfusion (%)	Intraoperative Complications (%)	Postoperative Complications (%)	Chronic Genitourinary (%)	Length of Stay (days)
Argentina, 1999	56	4.5	NR	2	6	2	4
Quebec, 2000	54	4.5	4	7	10	0	5
France, 2002	50	4.5	2	4	16	4	8
France 2, 2002	95	4.0	NR	NR	12	2	NR
WCC, 2002	78	3.5	1.3	9	9	1.3	3
Germany, 2003	200	5.5	19	13	15	3.5	NR
MSKCC, 2003	19	6.0	5	11	5	0	4.5
Toronto, 2004	71	3.5	7	13	14	3	1
MDA, 2007	35	5.75	11.0	11	>20	0	2
China, 2007	90	4.5	NR	9	40	3	NR
Italy, 2009	65	3.25	0	5	10	1.5	4

Most reports on LARVH and LRH demonstrate rates of complications comparable to those seen with the traditional open approach. A number of single-institution series reveal that the operative time is longer for LRH but associated with a decreased length of hospital stay (Table 21-1). Compared to the abdominal radical hysterectomy, LRH is associated with fewer postoperative complications, less blood loss, and reduced rates of blood transfusion. Nevertheless, major intraoperative complications have been reported in almost all of the series on LRH and include injuries to vascular structures, bladder, ureter, and bowel and the development of postoperative fistulae. The rates of these serious complications appear to be at least equivalent to those seen with laparotomy. Most authors stress that there is a lengthy learning curve for LRH and that complications decrease and overall operative efficiency improves as the surgeon gains experience. Therefore these procedures should be performed by highly skilled and experienced surgeons in selected patients in order to obtain optimal outcomes. Of note, improvements in subspecialty training, collective and individual experience in performing the traditional abdominal radical hysterectomy, better perioperative care, and a general trend toward decreased hospital stay have demonstrated an overall improvement in the outcomes of patients undergoing the open abdominal approach. In fact, the shortest average length of hospital stay reported in many of the laparoscopic radical hysterectomy series is not dissimilar to that reported in contemporaneous series of open radical hysterectomy. There is a lack of prospective data to compare cost and morbidity between the two approaches and retrospective data do not definitively establish a significant advantage for the laparoscopic approach. Currently, it appears that with appropriate training and experience, LARVH and LRH are comparable to the open technique with regard to cost, morbidity, other perioperative outcomes, and survival.

Although the feasibility of LRH has been established, there continues to be disadvantages to this MIS technique, including suboptimal ergonomics and less surgeon control over the operative field (which can be associated with an increased rate of bladder and ureteral complications compared to the traditional open approach). The robotic platform represents a significant improvement in MIS technology by affording the surgeon advantages over laparoscopy, as previously discussed in this chapter. This approach has been rapidly adapted by many gynecologic oncologists, which has led to publications describing the technical aspects of the procedure and the comparison of perioperative outcomes to the traditional open procedure. Whereas the radical hysterectomy, in general, remains a difficult procedure, the robotic platform allows for a significant shortening of the learning curve for MIS radical pelvic procedures. Initial series comparing robotic radical hysterectomy to open radical hysterectomy demonstrate that the procedures can be performed in a reasonable length of operating room time and may be associated with less severe intraoperative complications, less blood loss, fewer postoperative complications, and a decreased length of stay (Table 21-2). Boggess and colleagues have compared their experience in robotic radical hysterectomy in early-stage cervical cancer to historical controls undergoing abdominal radical hysterectomy and revealed similar survival outcomes among patients treated with these procedures. Most surgeons who use robotic techniques feel that the superior vision and wristed instruments provide optimal MIS capacity to perform the meticulous dissection required for the radical hysterectomy.

Early-stage cervical cancer—fertility-sparing surgery

The ability to perform an adequate laparoscopic lymphadenectomy combined with the revival of the radical

TABLE 21-2 Comparison of Robotic Abdominal Radical Hysterectomy to the Traditional Open Radical Hysterectomy

Study	N	Operating Room Time (hours)	Blood Transfusion (%)	Intraoperative Complications (%)	Fistulae (%)	Postoperative Complications (%)	Length of Stay (days)
ROBOTIC							
Boggess	51	3.5	0	0	0	8	1.0
Ko	16	4.5	6	0	6	19	1.7
Magrina	27	3.2	4	NR	0	7	1.7
Estepe	32	2.4	3	3	0	29	2.6
Mangioni	40	4.5	8	5	0	NR	3.7
LAPAROTOMY							
Boggess	49	4.2	8	0	0	16	3.2
Ko	32	3.4	31	3	0	22	4.9
Magrina	35	2.7	9	6	0	9	3.6
Estepe	14	1.9	36	0	0	19	4.0
Mangioni	40	3.3	23	13	0	—	5.0

vaginal hysterectomy have led to the development of novel techniques for fertility preservation in young patients with early-stage cervical cancer. The laparoscopic vaginal radical trachelectomy (LVRT) is one of the most exciting applications of MIS in gynecologic oncology. In an effort to define the potential number of patients in whom this procedure would be considered, Sonoda reported on 435 patients undergoing radical hysterectomy. Eighty-nine of these patients were younger than 40 years of age and had tumors that met the criteria for fertility-sparing radical trachelectomy (which represented 20% of their early-stage population) (Table 21-3). This study clearly shows that there is a substantial population of patients who may benefit from this approach.

The LVRT technique combines laparoscopic pelvic and common iliac lymph node dissection with a radical vaginal trachelectomy (with preservation of the uterine fundus and creation of a neocervix). This procedure was initially described by Dargent in 1987; since then, several centers have reported preliminary results on fertility-sparing radical trachelectomy with laparoscopic lymphadenectomy. Survival and fertility follow-up reports have been encouraging. To date, more than 300 cases have been reported with a recurrence rate of 4.1% and a death rate of 2.5%, which falls well within the range of survival seen with traditional radical hysterectomy in similar populations. Randomized prospective comparisons are not available, but case-control studies in matched patients reveal equivalent oncologic outcomes when comparing radical hysterectomy with radical trachelectomy. Plante reported on the obstetric outcomes of 72 patients undergoing the surgery over a 12-year time span. A total of 50 pregnancies occurred in 31 women. Infertility rates and first and second trimester pregnancy loss did not appear to be increased. Of the patients reaching the third trimester, 22% had preterm

TABLE 21-3 Suggested Clinical Eligibility Criteria for Laparoscopic Radical Vaginal Trachelectomy

1. Confirmed invasive cervical cancer: squamous, adenocarcinoma, or adenosquamous
2. FIGO stage Ia1 with lymphovascular space involvement, FIGO Ia2 to Ib1
3. Desire to preserve fertility
4. No clinical evidence of impaired fertility
5. Lesion size <2 cm
6. Patient is a candidate for a vaginal hysterectomy
7. Estimated cervical length ≥2 cm clinically
8. Adequate resolution of acute inflammation postcone

delivery (although only 8% were delivered before 32 weeks.) There appears to be enough data now published to consider fertility-sparing radical trachelectomy a viable option for select and motivated patients. Recently, the fertility-sparing radical trachelectomy has been described robotically, in which the entire procedure is performed minimally invasively without a perineal or vaginal phase.

Advanced-stage cervical cancer—surgical staging

Patients with advanced-stage disease or bulky early-stage cervical cancers are generally treated with definitive radiotherapy and concurrent chemotherapy. For this group of patients, laparoscopy has been used for surgical staging and to assist radiation oncologists in the safe placement of interstitial brachytherapy implants. Unfortunately, as many as 30% to 50% of these patients are inaccurately staged by clinical or radiologic methods. Even positron emission tomography/computed tomography scans will not identify all patients with extrapelvic disease. Although controversial, surgical staging has been advocated to accurately define the extent of disease and guide the subsequent radiation fields. In patients with gross evidence of lymph node metastasis, their removal has been demonstrated in retrospective studies to improve survival compared with radiation of these nodes without debulking.

Before advanced MIS techniques, retroperitoneal lymphadenectomy for surgical staging of cervical cancer was performed at the time of extraperitoneal laparotomy. This approach afforded the surgeon excellent exposure to both the pelvic and para-aortic nodes with the ability to debulk grossly positive nodes. A transperitoneal laparotomy approach is not recommended because it is associated with a significant increase in the rate of severe postirradiation enteric morbidity compared to extraperitoneal laparotomy, presumably secondary to adhesion formation. Both transperitoneal and extraperitoneal laparoscopic approaches have been described for surgical staging of cervical cancer. Initially, there was concern that transperitoneal laparoscopic lymph node dissection would be associated with increased adhesion formation as experienced with transperitoneal laparotomy for lymphadenectomy. The extraperitoneal laparoscopic approach avoids this risk, but the surgeon only has access to the common iliac and para-aortic lymph nodes and is unable to perform a PLN dissection. However, transperitoneal laparoscopy, in general, is associated with fewer intraperitoneal adhesions when compared to laparotomy. Blinded studies in animal models reveal a similar rate and severity of adhesions between transperitoneal laparoscopic lymph node dissection and extraperitoneal laparotomy; however, transperitoneal laparoscopic lymphadenectomy is associated with significantly fewer adhesions compared to transperitoneal laparotomy.

Multiple single-institutional series exist describing laparoscopy for pretreatment lymphadenectomy for advanced cervical cancer. The procedure is feasible with acceptable morbidity when compared to laparotomy. A significant advantage for the laparoscopic approach is avoiding potential complications of a large abdominal incision and quicker postoperative recovery, allowing the patient to proceed to definitive radiation therapy more quickly. Although laparoscopic resection of nodes grossly involved with metastatic disease is technically feasible, it is definitely more difficult compared to laparotomy, especially when the nodes are fixed to vessels. Therefore some surgeons prefer extraperitoneal laparotomy in case they encounter nodes that require debulking. The robotic platform obviates many of the inherent disadvantages of laparoscopy. As in laparoscopy, the robotic approach can be used for pelvic and para-aortic lymph node dissection. In addition, the three-dimensional magnified vision, enhanced surgeon control over the operative field, and precision afforded by the wristed instruments enable the surgeon to perform the more complicated debulking surgeries if necessary.

Endometrial Cancer

Laparoscopy

In the population of patients diagnosed with a gynecologic malignancy, MIS is most often applied for those diagnosed with endometrial cancer. Before the availability of advanced laparoscopic procedures, vaginal hysterectomy was a less invasive option for definitive surgical therapy, especially in patients with severe comorbidities and increased risk of complications secondary to laparotomy. In fact, assuming the disease is confined to the uterus, the curative potential of the hysterectomy should be equivalent regardless of the surgical approach. The disadvantages of the vaginal hysterectomy in endometrial cancer include the inability to fully inspect the peritoneal cavity and retroperitoneum (lymph nodes) for metastatic disease and potential inability to complete BSO. The addition of laparoscopy to the vaginal hysterectomy essentially eliminates these disadvantages. Most patients with endometrial cancer present with apparent early-stage disease. Approximately 15% to 25% will be upstaged as a result of surgical staging. The majority of patients with extrauterine disease have occult (without gross evidence) spread. Current disease assessment modalities such as preoperative imaging, intraoperative palpation, gross inspection, and frozen section of the uterus all are inaccurate when compared to comprehensive surgical staging that includes bilateral pelvic and para-aortic lymph node dissection. Comprehensive surgical staging with lymphadenectomy provides the best definition of the biologic nature of the disease and allows the oncologist to make informed postoperative treatment decisions. Laparoscopic-assisted vaginal hysterectomy bilateral salpingo-oophorectomy (LAVH-BSO) or total laparoscopic hysterectomy (TLH) can be substituted for total abdominal hysterectomy bilateral salpingo-oophorectomy (TAH-BSO) in the algorithm presented earlier in this book for the management of endometrial cancer.

The overall management of patients with apparent early-stage endometrial cancer continues to evolve. Endometrial cancer remains the least uniformly managed gynecologic malignancy, even among gynecologic oncologists. It remains controversial whether all patients should have surgical lymph node assessment and, in those undergoing lymphadenectomy, the extent to which lymph node dissection should be performed. Nevertheless, until laparoscopic lymph node dissection was described, comprehensive surgical staging of endometrial cancer by MIS was not feasible. The earliest series published on MIS management of endometrial cancer primarily described pelvic lymphadenectomy with a minimum of patients undergoing a para-aortic lymph node dissection. The ability to perform laparoscopic lymphadenectomy evolved from pelvic nodes to right-sided para-aortic nodes to a bilateral para-aortic lymph node dissection to the level of the inferior mesenteric artery. Although controversial, recent reports on surgical staging of endometrial cancer recommend that selected patients at high risk for extrauterine disease have a bilateral para-aortic dissection to the level of the renal vessels. This technique has been described laparoscopically but is technically difficult and likely currently applied to a small minority of patients undergoing MIS management of endometrial cancer.

Until recently, most data describing the experience of laparoscopy in management of EC came from single institutions and are primarily retrospective studies. It is clear that advances in MIS technology, training, and experience allow the surgeon the opportunity to ensure removal of the uterus and adnexae, inspect the peritoneal cavity, define the retroperitoneal anatomy, and perform a thorough pelvic and para-aortic lymph node dissection. The reported benefits of a laparoscopic approach in endometrial cancer are lower blood loss and transfusion rates, shorter hospital stay, faster postoperative recovery, and superior short-term quality of life, albeit at the expense of longer operative times. However, these studies are biased by the fact that they represent only selected patients (such as those with low body mass index [BMI]) compared to an institution's entire population of endometrial cancer patients. Additionally, these series vary as to whether comprehensive surgical staging was performed and, if so, as to the extent of lymph node dissection (Table 21-4). Surgeon experience and patient factors such as obesity and/or previous abdominal surgery contribute to the many disadvantages of the laparoscopic approach in endometrial cancer, especially if the goal is comprehensive surgical staging. In a study of two California databases from 1997 to 2001, only 7.7% of patients diagnosed with endometrial cancer underwent surgery via a laparoscopic approach. A recent survey of members of the Society of Gynecologic Oncologists (29% responding) revealed that use of laparoscopy as a surgical treatment option for endometrial cancer is increasing; however, only 8% of all respondents

use this approach in more than 50% of their cases. Therefore the majority of patients who present with endometrial cancer will undergo definitive surgical management via laparotomy rather than laparoscopy. Barriers to the incorporation of MIS into the management of patients with endometrial cancer likely include the difficult learning curve and inherent technologic disadvantages of the laparoscopic approach.

Until recently, there was no prospective randomized trial reporting the surgical outcomes comparing laparoscopy and laparotomy in the management of endometrial cancer. The Gynecologic Oncology Group (GOG) recently completed analysis of the LAP-2 trial, which enrolled 2531 patients with apparent early-stage endometrial cancer. All patients in this study were to undergo complete surgical staging and were randomly assigned in a 2:1 ratio of laparoscopy to laparotomy. Of the 1678 patients on the laparoscopy arm, 25.8% required conversion to laparotomy. More than half of these conversions were a result of poor visualization (exposure), 16% were from metastasis, and 11% were from bleeding. Figure 21-8 graphs the likelihood of converting from laparoscopy to laparotomy as a function of BMI, age, and evidence of metastatic disease. In this landmark study, there was no significant difference in rate of node positivity between the two groups; however, significantly fewer patients in the laparoscopy arm (78.5%) compared with the laparotomy arm (86.4%) had lymph nodes histologically identified from all four primary nodal regions (which include the right and left periaortic and bilateral pelvic lymph nodes). The incidence of intraoperative complications, reoperations, and readmissions was similar, but significantly fewer Common Toxicity Criteria grade II or greater postoperative complications ($P < 0.0001$) occurred on the laparoscopy arm (14.3%) compared to the laparotomy arm (21.1%). Similar transfusion rates were seen between the groups (7% to 9%). Consistent with other studies in the literature, operative time was significantly longer for the laparoscopic arm (203 minutes) versus the laparotomy arm (136 minutes). For those patients successfully completing laparoscopic surgery, the average length of hospital stay was 2 days

TABLE 21-4   Single-Institution Reports on Laparoscopy in Endometrial Cancer

Study	N	Body Mass Index	Hysterectomy Only (%)	Pelvic Nodes (%)	Aortic Nodes (%)	Operating Room Time (min)	Conversion (%)	Hospital Stay (days)
Eltabbakh	100	28	14	86	24	NR	6	2
Gemangini	69		84	16	NR	214	3	2
Gil-Mareno	55	28	9	100	51	192	0	4
Frigerio	55	25	0	100	NR	220	5.4	4
Malur	37	30	32	68	54	177	0	9
Kim	74	40	17	83	?	147	NR	10
Zullo	40	NR	0	100	10	NR	12.5	3
Fleisch	124	27	17	83	55	148	16	NR

FIGURE 21-8 Predicted probability curve for risk of conversion by body mass index (BMI), age, and metastatic disease. *(From Walker JL, Piedmonte MR, Spirtos NM, et al: J Clin Oncol 27:5331, 2009.)*

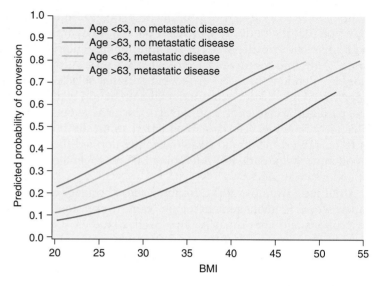

versus 4 days for laparotomy (P <0.0001). During the perioperative period, the LAP-2 study revealed significantly better overall quality of life, pain scores, resumption of normal activities, and time until return to work in the laparoscopy arm. By 6 months after surgery, no significant quality of life differences were found except in that of body image. Previously reported but small single-institution studies reveal no differences in survival between laparoscopy and laparotomy for the surgical management of endometrial cancer. LAP-2 is the only large, multi-institutional randomized study to examine this most important survival end point. The estimated 3-year overall survival from this study is 89.8% for laparoscopy and 89.9% for laparotomy, with similar rates of recurrence and death from disease.

Laparoscopy offers selected patients with endometrial cancer the potential benefits of shorter hospital stay, less need for blood transfusion, and decreased postoperative complications with a similar risk of intraoperative complications. Nevertheless, laparoscopic hysterectomy with pelvic and para-aortic lymph node dissection remains difficult to learn and is least likely to be offered or successful in patients with obesity, the group of patients most likely to benefit from MIS. Although morbid obesity is the most common risk factor for developing endometrial cancer, it is also the major limitation to successful laparoscopic surgical management. Most studies reporting the use of MIS for the treatment of endometrial cancer describe a population of patients with a mean BMI lower than that typically seen in the overall population of patients with endometrial cancer. Even the LAP-2 study represents a selected group of patients because the median BMI was 28 kg/m^2 in both arms. The rate of conversion from laparoscopy to laparotomy ranges quite widely between single-institution reports. Variables such as intent to perform

comprehensive staging, adhesions, intraoperative complications, discovery of metastatic disease, and surgeon experience have all been reported as important factors. In the LAP-2 study, the overall conversion rate was 25.8% and strongly influenced by BMI (with a rate of 17.5% in patients with a BMI 25 kg/m^2 and a rate of 57% in patients with a BMI greater than 40 kg/m^2.)

Robotics

Although it has been advocated that laparoscopy should be the surgical approach of choice for patients with endometrial cancer, this is yet to be realized secondary to the inherent disadvantages of this technology. As previously mentioned, recent developments in robotic technology have allowed the surgeon to gain advantages compared to laparoscopy and is rapidly being adopted by gynecologic oncologists independent of their prior laparoscopic experience. Relatively large single-institution and pooled reports reveal that the robotic surgical staging of patients with endometrial cancer is feasible and that the patient experiences the typical benefits of MIS compared with laparotomy. Furthermore, these reports have shown that robotic surgery is likely applicable to a larger portion of patients diagnosed with endometrial cancer compared with laparoscopy, including patients who are morbidly obese (Table 21-5). Seamon and colleagues demonstrated that comprehensive surgical staging is feasible in a relatively heavy group of patients (mean BMI 34 kg/m^2), as robotic pelvic and para-aortic dissection was performed in 85% of the patients overall and in 67% of the patients with BMI more than 45 kg/m^2. Gehrig and co-workers compared their robotic and laparoscopic experience in obese patients (BMI >30 kg/m^2) with endometrial cancer and demonstrated a significant difference in hospital stay, blood loss, and operating room time in favor of the

TABLE 21-5 Case Series of Surgical Outcomes with Robotic Surgery and EC

Author	N	Age	Body Mass Index	OR Time	Estimated Blood Loss	LOS	Δ	LN	IOC	POC
Lowe	405	62	32	170	88	2	7	16	4	15
Seamon	105	59	34	262	99	1	12	29	NA	NA
Boggess	103	62	32	191	75	1	3	33	1	10
Denardis	56	59	29	177	105	1	5	19	4	16
Bell	40	63	33	184	166	2	NA	17	0	8
Hoekstra	32	62	29	195	50	1	3	17	6	13
Veljovich	25	53	26	283	67	2	NA	18	NA	NA
Summary	**766**	**60**	**30**	**200**	**100**	**1**	**7**	**21**	**3**	**10**

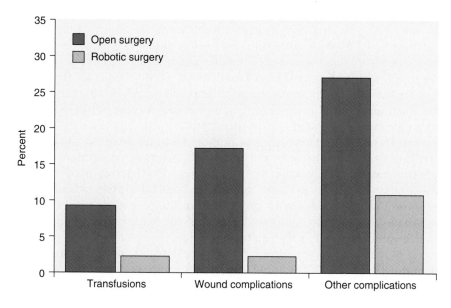

FIGURE 21-9 Transfusion rates, postoperative complications, and wound complications for laparotomy compared with robotic hysterectomy lymphadenectomy for endometrial cancer. The blood transfusion rate (9% compared with 2%, OR 0.22, 95% CI 0.05-0.97, P = 0.046), wound problems (17% compared with 2%, OR 0.10, 95% CI 0.02-0.43, P = 0.002), and complications (27% compared with 11%, OR 0.29, 95% CI 0.13-0.65, P = 0.003) were reduced for robotic surgery. *(From Seamon LG et al: Obstet Gynecol 114:16, 2009.)*

robotic group. Seamon and colleagues compared 105 patients with endometrial cancer undergoing robotic surgery to 76 patients managed laparoscopically and revealed a similar ability to complete surgical staging. However, comprehensive surgical staging was able to be performed in heavier patients compared with laparoscopy (BMI 34 kg/m² vs 29 kg/m²), and with significantly shorter length of stay (LOS), lower conversion to laparotomy, and shorter operating room time in favor of the robotic group. Compared to laparotomy, the advantages of the robotic approach are more dramatic in obese patients with endometrial cancer. In a matched cohort study in patients with a median BMI of 40 kg/m² and multiple comorbidities, patients managed robotically experienced a decreased LOS (1 vs 3 days) and significantly lower rates of overall complications (OR = 0.29), blood transfusion (OR = 0.22), and wound complications (OR = 0.10) compared with laparoscopy (Figure 21-9). Although it is most critical that the surgeon have expertise in the management of patients with endometrial cancer, it appears that the learning curve for comprehensive robotic staging of endometrial cancer is not as

difficult as laparoscopy. It is very likely that the robotic platform will evolve into the dominant MIS approach, if not the preferred overall surgical approach in patients with endometrial cancer.

Adnexal Mass

One of the most common clinical scenarios presented to the gynecologic surgeon is that of the suspicious adnexal mass. Because most masses are asymptomatic, the major reason for surgical removal is to determine if a malignancy is present. The finding of a persistent ovarian mass represents a major reason for surgery in gynecology. Killackey reported that 17% of laparotomies in gynecology are performed primarily for this indication. It has been reported that 5% of persistent premenopausal ovarian masses and 20% to 50% of those in postmenopausal women will be malignant. This risk of malignancy (and potential need for surgical staging or cytoreduction) has led to the recommendation that suspicious ovarian masses be removed through a vertical midline incision. This recommendation, however, is made with the assumption that a gynecologic oncologist or other trained surgeon will be available to provide surgical support if required. This surgery may include radical pelvic or upper abdominal dissection, retroperitoneal lymphadenectomy or lymph node debulking, or bowel resection. Most gynecologists do not have such assistance on standby for every surgery performed for a pelvic mass. Potential advantages of minimally invasive approaches to the pelvic masses are cost savings and decreased morbidity in those women without cancer and early diagnosis and referral for appropriate surgical management in those who are found to have malignancies.

Postmenopausal women undergoing laparotomy for ovarian masses have a much greater likelihood of malignancy than premenopausal women. Postmenopausal patients with ovarian masses differ from premenopausal patients with respect to the predictive value of CA-125. An elevated CA-125 has a positive predictive value for malignancy of 80% to 98% in this population. Postmenopausal patients with an adnexal mass and an elevated CA-125 are presumed to have a malignancy and should have surgery by an ovarian cancer specialist regardless of the ultrasound findings. Pelvic ultrasonography, tumor markers, menopausal status, and clinical presentation all contribute to risk stratification for ovarian cancer. Using these and other tests, multiple scoring systems have been devised to provide the surgeon with a predictive value of ruling in or ruling out a malignancy.

The ability to identify patients preoperatively at highest risk for cancer (with the appropriate selection of surgical approach and consultation or referral for surgical management of this potential cancer) is often challenging. Although pelvic ultrasonography, tumor markers, and clinical presentation all contribute to risk stratification for ovarian cancer, the definitive evaluation of a mass is determined at surgery. However, multiple scoring systems have been devised to provide the surgeon with a preoperative probability of a mass being malignant. The Society of Gynecologic Oncology and the American College of Obstetrics and Gynecology jointly published referral guidelines and management recommendations for patients who present with a pelvic mass. Chapter 10 includes a comprehensive discussion of risk assessment of an adnexal mass in both premenopausal and postmenopausal women. In general, if a surgeon stratifies the risk of an adnexal mass into low-, medium-, and high-risk categories for malignancy, then the risk of finding an "unexpected" ovarian cancer at the time of surgery should be extremely low.

Minimally invasive surgery management

Several authors have reported on the LS management of suspected benign ovarian masses. In 1992 Nezhat reported 1209 adnexal masses managed laparoscopically. The majority of patients had endometriosis or functional cysts. However, 64 patients had benign ovarian tumors and 4 were malignant. There were no reported major complications in removing masses up to 25 cm in diameter and clearly demonstrated the technical feasibility of managing ovarian masses laparoscopically. Since then, multiple authors have reported on the use of laparoscopic oophorectomy in both premenopausal and postmenopausal women. The complication rates in these nonrandomized reviews of laparoscopic surgery vary from 0% to 18% and include bowel injury, ureteral injury, wound infection, hematoma, and hemorrhage. A consensus of these retrospective reviews and small randomized trials is that laparoscopic management of adnexal masses is associated with decreased or similar operating time and decreased perioperative morbidity including pain, infection, and blood loss compared with laparotomy. These studies also show a decreased length of stay and potential cost savings; however, major complications are still possible.

More recently, authors have reported on using laparoscopy in the initial management of ovarian masses suspicious for malignancy. Dottino reported on 160 patients with suspicious adnexal masses who had no evidence of gross metastases or extension above the umbilicus. No distinction was made based on other risk factors for malignancy; however, all of these patients were referred for gynecologic oncology consultation. One hundred forty-one patients were successfully managed laparoscopically. Invasive ovarian cancer was discovered in 9 patients, borderline ovarian tumors in 8, and nongynecologic cancer in 4. Dottino reported a 3% incidence of intraoperative complications requiring conversion to laparotomy and only one incidence of intraoperative spillage of tumor. This was a sex cord–stromal tumor, which did recur locally. Canis reported on 230 adnexal masses suspicious or solid at ultrasound evaluated initially by laparoscopy. Twenty percent of the invasive cancers and 50% of the borderline tumors had cyst puncture or rupture at time of diagnosis. One case of tumor dissemination occurred with morcellation of an immature teratoma. These studies highlight the need to prevent tumor spill and/or morcellation for all suspicious masses. There is concern that the positive pressure carbon dioxide environment established during pneumoperitoneum may predispose the patient to intraperitoneal seeding. Animal studies have shown an increased seeding rate in the pneumoperitoneum group compared to controls. This may be explained by peritoneal damage and exposure of the underlying basal lamina, which could facilitate implantation. No clear conclusions can be drawn regarding the risk to humans, but these studies suggest cyst rupture or spillage should be avoided in all ovarian masses that could possibly be malignant.

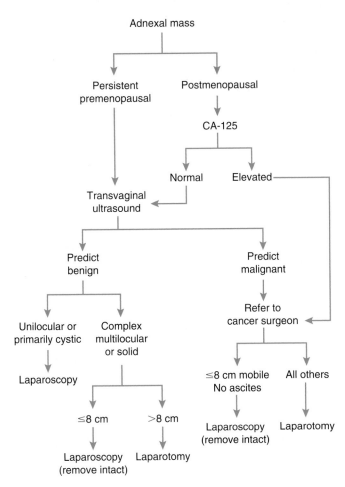

FIGURE 21-10 $\quad$ Suggested management of adnexal mass.

through the anterior abdominal wall trocar site. More complex cysts that are felt to be benign can be removed through a colpotomy or by extending the midline port-site incision at the end of the case. Some multilocular ovarian neoplasms greater than 8 cm in size that are felt to be benign based on ultrasound have a large dominant cyst. These can be managed through a posterior colpotomy with transvaginal drainage of the dominant cyst and subsequent removal of the ovary through the colpotomy. Suspicious masses should not be intentionally aspirated or morcellated outside of a controlled situation that prevents tumor spill and intraperitoneal dissemination.

If known ultrasound criteria are used, the negative predictive value for ovarian malignancy in premenopausal women should be greater than 95%. If the schema is adhered to, those few women with malignancies should have their tumor removed with no intra-abdominal spillage (see Figure 21-10). The rare finding of malignancy will still allow for appropriate timely referral, surgical staging, and treatment. Because the majority of premenopausal women will have masses with benign characteristics, this approach could substantially reduce the number of laparotomies performed for ovarian masses.

When the transvaginal ultrasound is consistent with probable malignancy, a different approach is recommended (see Figure 21-10). The positive predictive value of ultrasound alone ranges from 30% to 80%. Patients should have primary therapy by a physician trained to deal with ovarian cancer surgery and staging. These tumors can be managed with MIS if they are 8 cm or smaller and can be removed intact through a colpotomy or mini-laparotomy. If malignancy is documented, these patients should have further surgery by appropriately trained physicians. Patients with ovarian masses greater than 8 cm that are suspicious for malignancy or those that cannot be removed without controlled rupture by laparoscopy should undergo laparotomy by ovarian cancer specialists. Patients who are found to have disease spread beyond the ovary at time of MIS should have a confirmatory biopsy and referral for definitive therapy and staging.

Ovarian Cancer

Diagnosis of ovarian cancer

As a result of the relatively poor ability to predict malignancy with existing preoperative technology, a number of studies have looked at using laparoscopy to assess the presence or absence of ovarian cancer. Aspiration cytology of ovarian cyst fluid has a poor negative predictive value in the range of 58% to 80%. Case reports have raised the possibility that aspiration or biopsy of malignant ovarian cysts may lead to peritoneal tumor

The algorithm presented in Figure 21-10 is based on a strategy of maximal use of MIS combined with minimal risk of unexpected finding of ovarian cancer or intra-abdominal tumor spill. The presence of a unilocular cystic mass in premenopausal women is rarely malignant regardless of size. This fact is important because most of these patients are candidates for ovarian conservation with cystectomy. The same criteria for conservative management can be used with MIS as is already being done with laparotomy. Cystectomy has been described using a variety of techniques using MIS. Equipment such as needle aspirators and intra-abdominal bagging devices can allow for cyst decompression without spillage. Techniques have been described for either transabdominal or transvaginal cyst aspiration and removal. Large cysts can be aspirated transvaginally and removed via a posterior colpotomy with no intra-abdominal spillage. Size limits for removal of unilocular cysts seem to be related to safety of trocar insertion, surgical exposure, and experience of the surgeon. If oophorectomy is to be performed, the aspiration of the unilocular cyst will allow most of these to be removed implantation, limiting its application for diagnostic purposes. Also, use of therapeutic aspiration is ineffective for resolution of an ovarian cyst, with a recurrence rate as high as 67%. Therefore routine or intentional cyst aspiration is not recommended, especially in the presence of a suspicious mass. Reports of success are likely to include functional cysts because aspiration does nothing to interrupt the pathologic process of an ovarian neoplasm or endometrioma. When laparoscopic biopsy is highly suspicious for malignancy, definitive surgery should be performed if a trained ovarian cancer surgeon is available; otherwise, the surgery should be aborted and the patient should be referred immediately to such a specialist.

Ovarian cyst rupture

The main concern about managing a suspicious adnexal mass with MIS, especially when a cancer is apparently confined to the ovary, is that rupture may cause dissemination of malignant cells into the peritoneal cavity and adversely affect surgical stage and thus survival. MIS is more likely than laparotomy to result in capsular rupture because it potentially includes more tumor manipulation and masses often must be drained before removal from the peritoneal cavity. It is certainly possible that the robotic approach may result in less chance of cyst rupture than laparoscopy. In an assessment of outcomes in the laparoscopic management for adnexal masses, both benign and malignant, mass rupture occurred in 25% of the cases. Therefore use of laparoscopy has been discouraged because of the potential for rupture of a malignant ovarian cyst. However, the prognostic impact of cyst rupture in an encapsulated stage I ovarian cancer remains controversial. Some reports indicate a decrease in survival in patients in whom cyst rupture occurs at the time of open oophorectomy. This has led to the incorporation of cyst rupture in the staging of early ovarian cancer. Tumors otherwise assigned to stage Ia or Ib would be upstaged to Ic if rupture occurs during surgery, and this may have an impact on recommendations for adjuvant therapy. Other authors, however, were not able to demonstrate worsening of prognosis based on cyst rupture. Dembo reviewed more than 500 cases of stage I ovarian cancer, reporting that dense ovarian adhesions, grade, and the presence of ascites were predictors of relapse; however, cyst rupture was not shown to be associated with the risk of recurrence. Masses that are noted to have ruptured before surgery may be more likely to be associated with recurrent disease than those ruptured at the time of surgery. It seems likely that the majority of cysts ruptured at the time of surgery are secondary to dense adhesions and difficult surgical excision, which may result in rupture regardless of the surgical approach. Cyst rupture may just be an indicator of these tumors being more aggressive early ovarian malignancies rather than a surgical event affecting prognosis. Until the true effects of spillage of cyst contents are known, the surgical goal should be to remove high-risk ovaries intact. Any spillage should be managed with copious irrigation, as is the case with open surgery.

Another concern regarding MIS for ovarian cancer has been the possible effects of a delay in referral for subsequent definitive surgery and staging after an initial diagnosis of cancer. In an early report by Maiman of 42 patients referred for malignant ovarian neoplasms excised laparoscopically, the mean interval to laparotomy was 5 weeks and more than 10% of these patients did not undergo subsequent exploratory surgery. The impact of this delay on survival is not known. In a review of 48 cases of surgical staging following laparoscopic removal of malignant ovarian masses, Lehner reported that a delay of more than 17 days was associated with an increased risk of advanced-stage disease for malignant and low-malignant-potential tumors on univariate analysis. These concerns are heightened by Kindermann's retrospective survey of 192 cases of ovarian malignancy initially diagnosed laparoscopically. Those patients with a delay of more than 8 days between laparoscopic biopsy and definitive surgery had an increased risk of port-site metastasis and progression to stage III disease. In this report, only 7% of the apparent stage I tumors were removed intact as a result of biopsy, capsule rupture, and morcellation, making interpretation of these data difficult. These findings suggest that all efforts should be made to avoid intraoperative spillage from the ovary and to limit delay until definitive surgery. If patients are managed according to Figure 21-10, the unexpected finding of ovarian malignancy should be less than 5%. The few malignant masses that are managed with MIS should be removed without intra-abdominal rupture and survival is unlikely to be negatively affected. Managing patients according to this schema allows for appropriate and timely referral of patients with ovarian malignancy to physicians appropriately trained to manage these patients.

Early-stage ovarian cancer

The location and frequency of subclinical metastasis in patients with presumed early-stage ovarian cancer have encouraged investigation of the use of laparoscopic surgery for this patient population. Many areas traditionally evaluated during open laparotomy can be adequately assessed via MIS, including peritoneal cytology, diaphragm, omentum, pelvic and para-aortic lymph nodes, and pelvic peritoneum. Areas that are less likely to be fully visualized laparoscopically include the abdominal peritoneum and the bowel mesentery and serosa secondary to less ability to "run the bowel" and the inability to palpate. Review of the literature would indicate that the most common sites of subclinical metastasis in ovarian cancer include peritoneal cytology, pelvic and para-aortic lymph nodes, the diaphragm, and the pelvic peritoneum, all of which can be adequately evaluated laparoscopically or robotically (see Table 11-16). The inability to thoroughly evaluate the abdominal peritoneum and bowel mesentery could potentially lead to a 3% to 5% risk of understaging. Laparoscopic staging may be particularly helpful in patients who have undergone a recent exploratory laparotomy for removal of an adnexal mass found to be malignant who did not have appropriate staging. In 1995 Childers reported on the technical feasibility of laparoscopic staging of presumed stage I ovarian cancer. He found metastatic disease in 8 of 14 patients, including 3 with positive para-aortic nodes, 3 with pelvic disease, and 2 with positive cytology. Following this report, several small series of laparoscopic staging in this patient population have been published. In a case-controlled series, Chi demonstrated equivalent node counts and omental size removed in patients undergoing laparoscopic versus open procedures. There was no significant difference in rate of metastatic disease between the groups, although the numbers are too small to provide adequate power. Leblanc has recently reported on 42 patients who underwent laparoscopic restaging for ovarian and fallopian tube cancers. Eight were found to have metastatic disease. The remaining 34 patients had stage Ia grade I to II disease and had no follow-up chemotherapy. There were three reported recurrences in this group with a median follow-up of 54 months. To date there are no randomized trials looking at surgical staging or survival outcomes in early-stage ovarian cancer managed laparoscopically.

Advanced ovarian cancer

MIS surgery has had a limited role in the management of advanced ovarian cancer. Authors have reported its use in confirming the origin of abdominal carcinomatosis prior to neoadjuvant chemotherapy. Since the early 1980s, authors have reported its role in second-look laparotomy. Initial studies from the early 1980s utilizing laparoscopy followed by immediate laparotomy indicated a false-negative predictive value of 29% to 55% for laparoscopic surgery. With advances in video equipment and surgical technology there has been a resurgence of use of laparoscopic surgery in this setting. In more recent nonrandomized trials reporting on technical feasibility it appears laparoscopy is comparable to laparotomy in terms of complications, with a range of 1% to 5%. Unfortunately these studies were not controlled with immediate postlaparoscopy laparotomy, so the false-negative rate cannot be adequately assessed. Clough did report on 20 patients undergoing initial laparoscopy followed by immediate laparotomy using modern minimally invasive technology. The negative predictive value was

86%, indicating continued deficiencies in the technique. This information, in combination with the fact that second-look surgery has been determined to be of no therapeutic value, relegates this surgery to limited application in the setting of research protocols. Some investigators have recently reported on the use of hand-assisted laparoscopy for radical intraperitoneal tumor debulking and cytoreductive surgery. These studies lack conclusive data for adequacy of surgery or comparison with open technique for morbidity and survival and should be considered investigational. Laparoscopy can be useful for determining extent of disease in order to assess the feasibility of cytoreductive surgery or neoadjuvant chemotherapy. Ports for intraperitoneal chemotherapy can be placed with laparoscopic guidance in patients without such access before initiating primary chemotherapy.

COMPLICATIONS OF LAPAROSCOPIC SURGERY

An evaluation of MIS indicates that adverse events can be categorized into two broad groups—those complications that are part of laparoscopic abdominal surgery in general and those that are related to a specific surgical procedure or disease process. Advantages to a MIS technique include smaller incisions, less tissue manipulation and damage, and decreased adhesion formation. Many postoperative complications associated with laparotomy also are decreased. Nevertheless, these are still major surgical procedures performed via minimized access and therefore major surgical complications are possible, some unique to MIS. Many complications related to the specific surgical procedures will occur at least at a minimum rate and can vary with complexity of the procedure and surgeon experience. General complications such as trocar insertion, injuries to bowel or vessels, CO_2 pneumoperitoneum extravasation, and port-site herniations are unique to MIS. Major intraoperative complications during MIS are fortunately uncommon. Approximately 50% of serious intraoperative complications in laparoscopy occur with trochar insertion. In general gynecology major vascular injuries are almost exclusively related to trochar insertion; however, in gynecologic oncology such injuries may also occur during retroperitoneal dissection. Gastrointestinal (GI) and urologic injuries are more common than major vascular injuries. Most GI injuries will be related to placement of ports, mobilization of the bowel to gain exposure, adhesiolysis, thermal damage, port-site hernias, and occasionally secondary directly to the surgical dissection. Prevention of GI injuries is most important because these types of complications often go unrecognized and may be more difficult to identify during an MIS case. Vigilance is required in addressing serious and subtle signs or symptoms that may indicate an occult GI injury resulting from MIS. There should be a high index of suspicion and the expectation should be continuous improvement postoperatively. In gynecologic MIS, most urologic complications result from adnexectomy and/or hysterectomy. A marked increase in major genitourinary complications was noted after the advent of advanced gynecology MIS procedures. Genitourinary complications are prevented by meticulous dissection, wide mobilization of the bladder off of the lower uterine segment and cervix, and skeletonization of the uterine vessels.

As noted previously in this chapter, a number of studies have reported on complications associated with laparoscopic pelvic and para-aortic lymphadenectomy and radical pelvic dissection. Most series of MIS in gynecologic oncology report a decrease in perioperative and postoperative complications compared to laparotomy. In early series there appeared to be an increased number of ureteral, bladder, and vascular injuries compared to open technique. Prevention of complications begins long before the actual operative procedure with appropriate treatment selection and preoperative counseling. Selection of a surgical route will often be based on a surgeon's formal training and experience. It is recommended that surgeons develop a careful accumulated experience of increasingly complex MIS procedures. Further analysis almost uniformly indicates that there is a learning curve associated with advanced MIS, and larger, more mature series have intraoperative complication rates comparable to an open approach.

The overall incidence of MIS complications is difficult to quantitatively define because it is primarily based on retrospective reports and very likely to be underreported. The data on MIS complications are mostly anecdotal, based on single institutional experience and even less commonly based on meta-analysis and rarely prospective and/or randomized studies. This is not unique to MIS because most data on surgical complications are retrospective and therefore biased and imprecise. Various series on MIS in gynecology and gynecologic oncology report the incidence to be <1% to >10%. The actual rate of surgical complications that occur in MIS will depend on institutional/surgeon experience, types and mix of surgical procedures, and associated patient comorbidities. Chi reported on the risk factors for complications and conversion to laparotomy in 1451 patients undergoing a wide variety of laparoscopic procedures by a gynecologic oncology division over a 10-year time frame. Significant complications occurred in 2.5% of the patients and were associated with increased age, previous radiation, and malignancy. The complication rates reported in this series fall within the accepted range using an open technique. Likewise, the need to convert to laparotomy has been associated with prior abdominal surgeries,

obesity, bleeding, and adhesive disease. Conversion rates decrease with increased surgeon experience and should not be considered a complication but rather sound intraoperative judgment. Similar conclusions can be drawn from the experience with LAVH compared to abdominal or vaginal hysterectomy.

In general, MIS offers many potential advantages and disadvantages to the surgeon (and therefore the patient) but introduces additional layers of technological, human, and procedural complexity for any given surgical procedure traditionally performed via laparotomy. There is no substitution for knowledge of anatomy, steps in the surgical procedure itself, and the natural history of the patient's disease or condition. Counterintuitive movement, depth perception, and blind aspects to the surgical field are all unique potential compromises to MIS, especially laparoscopy. Major complications in MIS can often be attributed to misperception rather than a pure technical error. These are all obviated, especially earlier in the surgeon's experience, by deliberate camera work and meticulous dissection, which eventually becomes more instinctual and automatic as the surgeon gains experience. There is no substitute for continued practice and accumulated experience, which allows for development of innate skills in avoiding potential problems. Knowledge of energy sources used is critical in preventing MIS surgical complications. Meticulous skeletonization of pedicles and mobilization of adjacent structures away from the field of dissection reduce the chance of unintended thermal damage. Laparoscopy gives partial loss of haptic feedback and loss of three-dimensional vision, whereas the current robotic technology gives no haptic or touch feedback but allows for high-definition three-dimensional vision. Both limitations in sensory feedback can be overcome with practice and experience while maintaining rigorous surgical discipline.

Port-Site Recurrences

Since 1978 port-site recurrences have been reported in multiple carcinomas, including gynecologic malignancies. Concern has been expressed that incisional seeding may be increased in laparoscopic surgery potentially leading to a reduction in overall survival. A review of the literature by Ramirez in 2003 found 31 articles describing port-site metastases in 58 gynecologic cancer patients. These included 33 invasive ovarian cancers, 7 low malignant potential tumors of the ovary, 12 cervical cancers, 4 endometrial cancers, and 1 each of fallopian tube and vaginal cancer. In the ovarian cancer patients, 83% had advanced-stage disease with most reporting carcinomatosis and ascites. The median time to diagnosis was 17 days, and it is unclear how this affected survival. Reports of abdominal wall metastasis after paracentesis in a similar population are common. It appears that proper preoperative assessment may have spared many of these patients a laparoscopic procedure. The 12 cervical cancer patients reported with port-site metastasis are cause for concern given that there are only a few isolated reports of metastases to an abdominal scar. Of these 12 patients, 75% had laparoscopic lymphadenectomy and the majority had positive nodes. Half the patients had recurrence in the port used for placement of the laparoscope. The median time to port-site recurrence was 5 months, and of the 11 patients for whom data were given, only 27% were without evidence of disease with a median 12-month, follow-up. Of the 4 patients reported to have port-site recurrences in endometrial cancer, only 1 had disease limited to the uterus. The small number of port-site recurrences makes it difficult to document any benefit to clipping the fallopian tubes or minimizing uterine manipulation as a way to prevent these complications.

A number of factors have been proposed to explain the etiology of port-site metastasis. Studies have suggested that the risk may be increased with the use of carbon dioxide when compared to other insufflating agents. The positive pressure associated with a pneumoperitoneum has been associated with increased tumor growth and a high incidence of port-site metastasis when compared to gasless laparoscopy. Some investigations have shown the potential aerosolization of viable tumor cells and efflux with gas through the trocar sites. Also theorized is a diminution of inflammatory response using minimally invasive versus open laparotomy incisions. Childers reported port-site metastasis to be 0.3% per trocar site, which is comparable with the 0.1% risk of abdominal wall seeding with percutaneous biopsy of abdominal malignancies. As a result of the advanced stage of most of the reported cases, it is not clear whether port-site metastases occur because of the aggressive nature of the disease or because of risk factors uniquely associated with laparoscopic surgery. To date, use of laparoscopy has not been associated with a decrease in survival for cancer patients. There is, however, a lack of large prospective randomized trials comparing laparotomy to laparoscopy at the current time.

CONCLUSIONS

The laparotomy causes significant trauma to the patient with many potential associated morbidities, which are increased in incidence and severity in patients with comorbid conditions. In an attempt to reduce surgical morbidity, advanced laparoscopic procedures are an option but only for a subpopulation of patients undergoing major pelvic procedures. Incorporating laparoscopy into the comprehensive management of gynecologic oncology patients has been only moderately successful secondary to a difficult and long learning curve, variability in surgical experience, longer operative times, and patient factors such as surgical history and obesity. Whether this relative lack of mainstream adaptation of laparoscopy into the practice is a result of technology or training limitations is unclear, although strong biases support both potential causes. Technologic limitations to rapid implementation of complicated laparoscopic surgery in gynecology include a limited two-dimensional field of vision, counterintuitive motions often required for the surgeon and assistant, limited degrees of freedom of instruments, difficulty suturing, and ergonomic disadvantages for the surgeon. In some settings, major operative complications have been noted to be increased via laparoscopy compared to laparotomy.

Robotics overcomes many of the technologic limitations of laparoscopy. The robotic platform provides the surgeon superior high-definition three-dimensional vision, magnification, wristed instruments, and motion scaling. The surgeon has much more ability to directly control the operative field compared to laparoscopy, thus eliminating many important disadvantages of laparoscopy. The technological improvements offered by robotic surgery have allowed the gynecologic surgeon to perform much more complicated surgeries via MIS on a heterogeneous group of patients. Surgeons at the beginning of their learning curve will need to build their case complexity appropriately and consider operating room duration along with other potential surgical risks. Previous laparoscopic experience is very helpful, at least in the initial phase of adapting to robotics; however, the robotic platform translates quite nicely from laparotomy because surgeons are able to mimic the procedure robotically from their laparotomy experience. As technology continues to improve, a higher proportion of patients diagnosed with a gynecologic malignancy is eligible for MIS. Technology advances do not substitute for subspecialty training, surgical experience and judgment, and knowledge of disease and anatomy. The minimum number of cases to be appropriately credentialed and then proficient is yet to be determined but will vary with surgeon training, experience and skill, and type and complexity of the procedure. Nevertheless, it is very likely that robotics will become the minimally invasive surgical approach of choice for comprehensive surgical management of gynecologic oncology patients and many general gynecology patients in the near future. It is also a certainty that the technology will continue to change and improve and hopefully will become less expensive.

For full reference list, log onto www.expertconsult.com <http://www.expertconsult.com>.

Epidemiology of Commonly Used Statistical Terms and Analysis of Clinical Studies

Wendy R. Brewster, MD, PhD

EPIDEMIOLOGY

Epidemiology is the study of distribution of disease and the factors that determine disease occurrence in populations. The focus is on groups as compared to the individual. Persons within a population do not have equal risk for disease occurrence, and the risk of a disease is a function of personal characteristics and environmental exposures. Patterns of disease occurrence within specific populations can be evaluated to determine why certain groups develop illness when others do not. The impact of epidemiology on gynecologic oncology is evidenced by the significance of studies such as the association with infection of oncogenic HPV and cervical cancer, obesity and the risk of endometrial cancer, and the risk factors for gestational trophoblastic neoplasia. Epidemiologic studies are unique in their focus on human populations and its reliance on nonexperimental observations. Epidemiological methods are used in searching for causes of disease, disease surveillance, determining the cause of disease, diagnostic testing, searching for prognostic factors, and testing new treatments.

Because the quality of epidemiologic evidence varies greatly among studies, the scientific community endorses the principles of Sir Austin Bradford Hill, an eminent British statistician, when attempting to identify causal associations. A cause of a specific disease is an antecedent event or characteristic that is necessary for the occurrence of the disease (Table 22-1).

EVIDENCE-BASED MEDICINE

As much as possible, medical decisions should be based on quality evidence. The best evidence is a properly designed randomized controlled trial. Evidence from nonrandomized but well-designed control trials is of lesser quality. Next in reliability is well-designed cohort or case-control studies, which have been repeated by several investigators. Opinions of respected authorities and extensive clinical experience are least reliable.

Physicians are currently encouraged to practice evidence-based medicine. This means that clinical trial evidence must pass statistically valid tests for conclusions to have meaning. Good science depends on accurate (i.e., statistically significant and meaningful) data from clinical trials. The best trials are usually experimental, powered, randomized, and blinded. Patients randomly assigned to a treatment group or a control group must have an equal probability of being assigned to either group. This prevents selection bias (e.g., putting

TABLE 22-1   Strength of Association

1. Temporality. Exposure must precede the onset of the disease
2. Dose-response. Risk increases as exposure increases
3. Replication. The association is observed repeatedly
4. Coherence. The association is consistent with other scientific knowledge and does not require that established facts be ignored
5. Exclusion of the role of chance. Appropriate statistical tests demonstrate that the observed association is extremely unlikely to have arisen by chance

Modified from Hill AB. Proc Roy Soc Med 58:295, 1965.

TABLE 22-2   Mathematical Definitions of Statistical Terms

Terminology	Mathematical Definition
Prevalence rate	Number of persons with disease/total number in the group
Incidence rate	Number of new cases/total number at risk per unit of time
Kappa	(Pobs − Pchance)}/(1 − Pchance)
Sensitivity	True positive/(True positive + False negative)
Specificity	True negative/(True negative + False positive)
Predictive value positive	True positive/(True positive + False positive)
Predictive value negative	True negative/(True negative + False negative)

healthier or better prognosis patients in one group and those with a poor prognosis or high likelihood of disease risk in another group). Blinding prevents patients, investigators, and/or statisticians from knowing who is in the control group and experimental group; thus bias actions are avoided.

Retrospective and observational studies are descriptive and do not involve either an intervention or a manipulation, whereas an experimental study does. A prospective trial poses the question before the data are collected, thus allowing better control of confounding variables, unlike a retrospective study, which poses the question after the data are collected.

MEASURES IN EPIDEMIOLOGY

In order to describe and compare groups in a meaningful manner it is important to find and enumerate appropriate denominators and statistical terms (Table 22-2).

Incidence rate: Measures the new cases of a specific disease that develop during a defined period of time and the approximation of the risk for developing the disease. The incidence rate focuses on events. Incidence measures the probability of developing a disease.

Kappa coefficient: Kappa indicates how much observers agree beyond the level of agreement that could be expected by chance. Kappa is estimated as (Pobs − Pchance)}/ (1 − Pchance). Thus the kappa coefficient is the observed agreement, corrected for chance as a fraction of the maximum obtainable agreement, also corrected for chance. Landis and Koch have suggested useful categorizations. Kappa = 0.00 should be taken as representing "poor" agreement, 0.00 ± 0.20 as "slight" agreement, 0.21 ± 0.40 as "fair" agreement, 0.41 ± 0.60 as "moderate" agreement, 0.61 ± 0.80 as "substantial" agreement, and 0.81 ± 0.99 as "almost perfect" agreement. A kappa coefficient of 1 represents perfect agreement.

Mean: The average of a sample of observations.

Median: The middle value when the values are arranged in order from the smallest to the largest.

Meta-analysis: The statistical process of pooling the results from separate studies concerned with the same treatment or issue is frequently used in the context of medical statistics and provides the quantitative backbone of the evidence-based medicine program. A large number of meta-analyses are undertaken with the broad aim of combining divergent outcomes into a single estimate of treatment effect. For example, The Cochrane Collaboration endeavors to collate and synthesize high-quality evidence on the effects of important health-care interventions for a worldwide, multidisciplinary audience and publishes these in the Cochrane Database of Systematic Reviews. Meta analyses serve the following purposes: increases the statistical power by increasing the sample size, resolves uncertainty when reports do not agree, and improves the estimates of effect size. The bias of publication only of positive results is a concern for those using results of meta-analysis because, if statistically significant or "positive" results are more likely to be published, a meta-analysis based on the resulting literature will be biased. The quality of the studies included is important to the quality of the final result.

Pearson's correlation r: The degree to which two variables are related is called correlation. Pearson's correlation is represented by the value r and varies between −1 and +1. It is usually presented as a scatter point graph. A value of −1 suggests a perfect negative linear relationship; a value of 0 reflects no linear relationship; and a value of one reflects a perfect linear relationship. Values of −1, 0, and +1 are rare.

Person time: The sum of the observation period of risk for the persons in a group being studied.

Predictive value positive: The proportion of positive test results that is truly positive (i.e., the probability that someone classified as exposed is truly exposed). This value only refers to positive tests.

Predictive value negative: The proportion of negative test results that is truly negative. The predictive value of a negative test result refers to the proportion of patients with a negative test result who are free of disease.

These values, unlike sensitivity and specificity, indicate the reliability of the test in the determination of presence or absence of disease.

Prevalence rate: The amount of disease in a population. Prevalence measures the proportion of diseased individuals at a particular time and represents a snapshot of the disease. Other commonly used terminology is prevalence proportion and point prevalence. It is a measure of status and includes individuals with newly diagnosed disease and those surviving with disease. The numerator is the number of affected individuals in a specific time period. The denominator is the total number of persons in the group. Prevalence rates range between 0 and 1.

QALY (quality adjusted life year): The QALY was developed as an attempt to combine the value length of life and quality of life into a single index number. One year of perfect health is given a value of 1. Death is given a value less than 0. A year of less than perfect health will have a value less than 1. States of health considered worse than death can be argued to have a negative value. The QALY value is determined by multiplying the utility value associated with that state of health by the years lived in that state. QALY is a metric used to compare the benefit of health-care interventions. Combination of QALYs with the cost of an intervention (cost/QALY) can provided an economic framework for comparisons of therapies. QALYs have several limitations and should not be used alone in decision making.

Sensitivity: The proportion of truly diseased persons who are classified as diseased by the test. The sensitivity of a test is therefore the probability of a test being positive when the disease is present. The sensitivity of test may also be called the true-positive rate. In Figure 22-1 it is evident that the cutoff point of a test can affect the sensitivity. If the cutoff point is moved to the left, more diseased persons will be identified. At the same time, more healthy persons will be erroneously

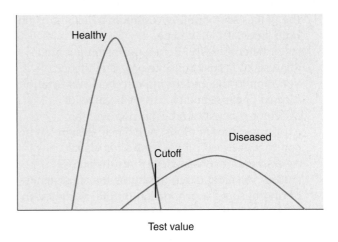

FIGURE 22-1 Effects of shifting cutoff point on sensitivity and specificity.

classified as sick. However, as the cutoff value for normal is moved to the right the test will become less sensitive because fewer diseased persons will be classified as such.

Specificity: The proportion of a population of disease-free individuals who are classified as undiseased by a test. In contrast to the sensitivity of a test, the specificity of a test is the probability that a test will be negative when the disease is absent. The cutoff point of a test for normality influences the specificity. As the value of normality or cutoff moves to the left the test becomes less specific because fewer health individuals are recognized as such. In contrast, moving the cutoff values to the right increases the specificity (Figure 22-1). In the best scenario, a test would be able to discriminate between diseased and healthy individuals without any overlap. More often the scenario is as presented in Figure 22-1, in which there is significant overlap and whatever the cutoff value healthy persons may be classified as diseased and sick persons classified as healthy. When we set the cutoff point for a test we must be attentive to the purpose of the test. If the disease is treatable and missing the disease has serious ramifications, then we must favor sensitivity over specificity. Alternatively, if it is more important to correctly identify healthy individuals, then specificity is prioritized. Published reports of the performance of tests usually just provide sensitivity and specificity results. Variations of these measures occur under many conditions and will also produce variations in predictive values.

Standard deviation: A measure of the variability within each group. If there is a normal (bell-shaped curve) distribution, approximately 95% of the values are within two standard deviations on both sides of the average.

Tests of heterogeneity: Before performing a meta-analysis, it is customary to assess evidence of variation in the underlying effects. This variation, termed "heterogeneity," arises because of differences across studies in populations, exposures/interventions, outcomes, design, and/or conduct. A forest plot is useful for visual assessment of consistency of results across studies. A statistic that measures the consistency of findings as the proportion of total variation in point estimates attributable to heterogeneity is now widely used.

ANALYSIS OF CLINICAL TRIALS

Null hypothesis: This hypothesis, symbolized by H0, is a statement claiming that there is no difference between the experimental and population means. The alternative hypothesis (H1) is the opposite of the null hypothesis. Often in research we need to be able to test for both the positive and adverse outcomes; therefore a two-tailed hypothesis is chosen, even though the expectation of the experiment is in a particular direction.

Significance level: A level of significance termed the alpha value is determined before the study has begun. The alpha value is the likelihood that a difference as large or larger that occurred between the study groups could be determined by chance alone. The alpha level is established by those designing the study and becomes the level of statistical significance. The most typical alpha level is 0.05.

One-tail test: A test to determine a difference in only one direction (e.g., to determine if drug A is better than drug B).

Two-tail test: A test to determine any difference between the variable (e.g., if either drug A or drug B is superior to the other). It is usually considered that in a two-tail test more trust can be placed in the statistically significant results than with a one-tail test. When in doubt, the two-tail test is preferred.

Confidence interval (CI): The range of values that is believed to contain the true value within a specific level of certainty.

Alpha error: The rejection of the null hypothesis when it is, in fact, correct. Also called a Type I error.

Beta error: Failure to reject the null hypothesis when it is, in fact, incorrect. Also called a Type II error.

Power: The probability that a study will be able to correctly detect a true effect of a specific magnitude. The statistical power refers to the probability of finding a difference when one truly exists or how well the null hypothesis will be rejected. The power is usually specified beforehand in prospective studies. The values of 0.8 (80%) or 0.9 (90%) are typical. The higher the value, the less chance there is of a type II error. A 0.9 value means that a type II error would be avoided 90% of the time.

Risk: The proportion of unaffected individuals who, on average, will contract the disease of interest over a specified period of time. Results of a trial are often expressed as absolute or relative risk reductions. The absolute difference is the actual difference between the units of the difference. In relative risk, the differences are the percentage change. Relative risk reductions often sound much more dramatic than do the absolute values. One must consider the prevalence of a disease when evaluating risk reductions. Where there is a low prevalence of a disease process, small risk reductions become unimpressive and must be evaluated in terms of the benefits of a particular mode of therapy.

Odds ratio (OR): The ratio of the odds that an event will occur in one group compared with the odds that the event will occur in the other group. In an osteoporosis study (OR), if 14 of 22 people who are thin, in an osteoporosis study, have fractures, the odds of having a fracture are 14 in 22 or 0.64. If 5 of the 33 nonthin people fracture bone, the odds are 5 in 33 or 0.15. The odds ratio (OR) is 0.64 divided by 0.15 or 4.2, meaning that thin people are 4.2 times more likely to receive fractures. An OR of 1 means that both groups have a similar likelihood of having an event.

Cox proportional hazard regression analysis: Cox regression analysis is a technique for assessing the association between variables and survival rate. The measure of risk provided for each variable is the risk ratio (RR). An RR of 1 means that the risk is the same for each participant. An RR greater than 1 indicates increased risk; a ratio less than 1 indicates less risk. A ratio of 5.4 means that the patients with a variable are 5.4 times more likely to have the outcome being studied. Confidence intervals can also be provided with risk ratios. This type of analysis is usually presented in a table.

Actuarial (life table) survival: This technique uses grouped information to estimate the survival curve. The data are grouped into fixed time periods (e.g., months, years) that include the maximum follow-up. The survival curve is estimated as a continuous curve and gives an estimate of the proportions of a group of patients who will be alive at different times after the initial observation. The group includes patients with incomplete follow-up.

Chi square ($\chi2$): The primary statistical test used for studying the relationship between variables. This is a test used to compare proportions of categorical variables.

Multivariate analysis: A technique of analysis of data that factors many variables. A mathematical model is constructed that simultaneously determines the effect of one variable while evaluating the effect of other factors that may have an influence on the variable being tested. The two most common algorithms developed to accomplish this task are the step-up and step-down procedures. Variables are added to an initial small set or deleted from an initial large set while testing repeatedly to see which new factor makes a statistical contribution to the overall model.

Univariate analysis: Analyses may be univariate or multivariate as they examine one or more variables at a time, respectively.

Receiver operator characteristics (ROC): These curves are the best way to demonstrate the relationships between sensitivity and specificity. They curves plot sensitivity (true-positive rate) against the false-positive rate (1-specificity) (Figure 22-2). The closer the curve is to the upper lefthand corner, the more accurate it is because the true-positive rate is closer to 1 and the false-positive rate is closer to 0. Along any particular ROC curve one can observe the impact of compromising the true-positive and false-positive rates. As the requirement that a test have a high true-positive rate increases, the false-positive rate will also increase. The closer the curve is to the 45-degree diagonal of the ROC area under the curve, the less accurate the test (Figure 22-2).

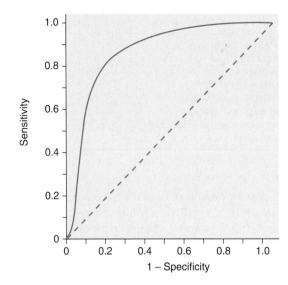

FIGURE 22-2   A hypothetical example of an ROC curve. The solid line represents the performance of the diagnostic test of interest; the dashed diagonal line serves as a reference of a test with no diagnostic value. *(From Greenberg RS et al: Medical Epidemiology (3rd ed). Lange Medical Books/McGraw-Hill, 2001, p 84, Fig. 6-6. Reproduced by permission of The McGraw-Hill Companies.)*

TYPES OF CLINICAL TRIALS

Clinical trials are experiments in which the investigator intervenes rather than observes and is the best test of a cause-and-effect relationship. A properly conducted experiment requires that when the intervention is applied to one group, there be a control group or some other suitable standard by which subjects of the clinical experiment or their guardians must give informed consent. The gold standard of clinical trials is the randomized experiment. With randomization each subject has an equal chance of being in either of the arms of the trials. Randomization is important because it equalizes baseline characteristics of the subjects so that the comparison of the treatments is fair. If randomization is not feasible, possible nonrandom standards of comparison must include patients similar to the treated group. Randomization is the current norm for demonstrating efficacy and safety of investigational methods. The advantages of randomization are numerous:

- Decreases investigator's bias in assigning patients to treatment groups
- Permits certain statistical methods to be used in the resulting data
- Allows for blinding of the patient and investigator
- Is the current norm for demonstrating efficacy and safety of investigational medicines

Unacceptable methods of randomization include the following:

- Alternate assignments
- Alternate day assignments
- Birthday assignments
- Coin tosses
- Initials of a patient

Single-patient clinical trials are indicated only in specific situations. They are generally used to evaluate

TABLE 22-3   Types of Clinical Trials

Single-patient clinical trials
Multicenter trials
National clinical trials
Continuation trials
Compassionate plea trials
Pharmacoeconomic trials
Trials to evaluate medical devices
Pharmacokinetic trials

TABLE 22-4   Bias and Confounding Factors: Examination of the Literature in the Field

Specifying and selecting the clinical trial sample
    Popularity bias
    Referral filter bias
    Diagnostic/access bias
    Wrong sample size
    Migrator/nonrespondent/volunteer bias
Executing the exposure
    Contamination/withdrawal/compliance/therapeutic bias
Information bias
Observer bias
Interviewer bias
Use of nonvalidated instruments
Active control bias
Analyzing the data
    Post hoc significance bias
    Fishing expeditions
Interpreting the analysis
Publishing the results

rare diseases when other types of trials are inappropriate or when only a small percentage of patients respond to a specific treatment. Single-patient clinical trials are useful to determine the response of a particular patient is a result of placebo or if an adverse reaction is related to a specific medication. The disease should be chronic and the disease severity must be stable during the clinical trial duration. It should be expected that the effect of the treatment should be measurable in a short time and the effect should be rapidly reversible once the treatment has stopped. The investigator and patient should be blinded and the patient's condition should return pre-existing baselines between treatment legs.

Multicenter trials are advantageous because they offer more rapid patient accrual and allow for greater protocol complexity. Multicenter trials reduce the opportunity for an individual's bias to influence the conduct of the trial; they increase the likelihood for the inclusion of a more representative study population and facilitate a higher standard for data processing and analysis. Disadvantages of multicenter trials are the administrative considerations that underlie the management and administrative arrangements (e.g., IRB/Ethics committees). Considerations must be delineated for criteria for patient enrollment, diagnostic classification, and assessment of treatment outcome. These trials are inherently more costly (Table 22-3).

EVALUATION OF CLINICAL TRIALS

Many factors must be considered when evaluating a clinical trial. The most important is the clinical trial objective or aim. Whether the objectives of the trial are adequately assessed depends on the presence and extent of bias and confounding factors. Bias is a nonrandom error in a study that can alter the outcome. Types of bias to consider when evaluating a manuscript are listed in Table 22-4.

Specifying the sample size or number of participants in the study needed to detect a difference or an effect of a given magnitude depends on many variables. The most important is the magnitude of the effect desired or

expected. Other important considerations are the desired probability of the study to identify the correct outcome (power), the variability of the variables being analyzed, the number of parts of the clinical trial, the magnitude of the placebo effect, and the number of dependent parts of the clinical trials. When determining the sample size, one must consider if the size of the treatment groups will be equal or nonequal (e.g., 2:1 ratio). An advantage of using groups of unequal size is that more information will be gained about patient responses in the larger arm. A disadvantage is the loss in study power; however, this detraction is not usually substantial if the ratios are kept under 3:1.

Placebo Treatment Groups

Placebo treatment groups control for the psychological aspects of being in a treatment trial. They also control for adverse events being attributed to a medicine when they result from spontaneous changes in the disease or from other causes and allow a stronger interpretation of the data. Placebo treatment groups are considered ethical if the following occur:

- No standard treatment exists.
- The standard treatment has been proven ineffective.
- Standard treatment is inappropriate for the particular clinical trial.
- Placebo has been reported to be effective in treating the condition.
- The disease is mild and lack of treatment is not considered to be medically important.
- The disease process is characterized by frequent spontaneous exacerbations and remissions.

Controls Used in Clinical Trials

Control groups in clinical trials may be obtained by many different methods. Randomized control groups are the most traditional and accepted and only chance should determine who enters any of the study arms. Nonrandom control groups may also be used. Subjects in these nonrandom control groups should have similar characteristics to that of the "treatment arm" and may include historical data obtained on the same patients on no therapy, the same therapy, or different therapy. Subjects in the control arm may be assigned to a placebo, an active medication, or concurrent use of nontreatment; use a different dose of the same medication; or receive usual care.

Dropouts from clinical trials are inevitable. The simplest reasons may be that the subjects declined to participate after enrollment or that the clinical course during the trial required a change in therapy. Whatever the reason for noncompliance or dropout, these subjects should be followed because it is essential to analyze the outcomes of the groups as intent to treat. Inclusion of these data provides a conservative estimate of the differences in treatment.

Studies of Therapy

There are many different types of clinical trials and in general they are categorized into categories or phases. Phase I trials are usually to screen the safety of the intervention or drug. These trials can be inclusive of multiple doses of a new medicine or evaluation of an old medicine in a new therapeutic area. These trials usually consist of 10 to 100 subjects.

Phase II trials clarify and establish the protocol and elucidate the experimental conditions that will allow the most important phase of the trial to give a definitive result. These trials are valuable because they establish protocols and the experimental conditions that will allow the final phase of the trial to give a definitive result. They allow for the following:

1. The evaluation of a variable related to the clinical pharmacology of a medicine
2. Development of clinical experience by research personnel under open label conditions before initiation of a double-blind trial

Aims of phase II trials are to assess how many people should be included in the final phase of testing, determine the end points of the trial, and provide preliminary estimates of effective dose and duration of treatment.

Phase III trials are for comparison to standard therapy or placebo if ethically justifiable. These trials are more commonly randomized and are regarded as the best way to obtain unbiased data.

Blinding

Blind refers to the lack of knowledge of the investigational agent by the patients, investigators, ancillary personnel, data review committees, and statisticians. Blinding is used to decrease the biases that may occur during a clinical trial. An open-label trial indicates that no blind is used. Examples of open-label trials are as follows:

- Pilot trials
- Case studies in life-threatening situations
- Unusual studies in which definitive data may be obtained (e.g., coma patients)
- Clinical trials in which ethical considerations do not permit blinding

In single-blind clinical trials, either the patient or investigator is unaware of the treatment received. Single-blind trials provide a degree of control when a double-blind trial is impossible or impractical and provides a degree of assurance of the data's validity compared with open-label trials. In double-blind trials neither the investigator nor the patient is aware of what treatment the patient is receiving. This allows for strong data interpretation if all other aspects of the trial were properly designed and conducted, the blind remained intact, the protocol was not seriously breached, the power of the trial was adequate, and the patients were compliant. Tripleblind trials are situations in which anyone who interacts with either the patient of physician is blinded. These studies allow for the strongest interpretation of data if the conditions can be met.

If blinding is to be used, then the study should be designed so that it is very difficult to break the blind. Unblinding may occur based on any of the following:

- Adverse reactions
- Lack of efficacy
- Efficacy
- Changes in laboratory values
- Errors in labeling
- Comments from unblinded study personnel
- Information presented in correspondence or reports
- Intentionally looking for clues (Table 22-5)

When to Stop a Clinical Trial

The decision to stop a clinical trial has many important ramifications. The ethical dilemmas include the needs of the next eligible patient insomuch that a subject should

TABLE 22-5   Types of Blinds

Open label
Single blind
Double blind
Full double blind
    Keeping blind everyone who interacts with the patient
Full triple blind
    Keeping blind anyone who interacts with the patients and the
        investigators

never be randomly assigned to an established inferior treatment. This must be balanced by the collective needs of society that terminating a trial will still result in the correct policy for the future and the need for sufficient data to change clinical practice for the better.

Early termination of a trial has its disadvantages. If the trial is stopped after recruitment of a small number of subjects, the results may lack credibility. The assumed treatment difference may be the result of chance and a false-positive result. The early stopping of trials can result in imprecision and wide confidence intervals for treatment effect. Finally, the treatment recommendation that results from stopping a trial early may be unduly enthusiastic.

Statistical stopping guidelines should be determined before the clinical trial begins. A sufficiently small P value for treatment difference on a trial's primary end point can be a guideline for when it is ethically desirable to stop a trial. It is most acceptable to have a limited number of preplanned interim analyses. Multiple repeated looks at the data can guard against the risk of a false-positive result.

For full reference list, log onto www.expertconsult.com ⟨http://www.expertconsult.com⟩.

Basic Principles in Gynecologic Radiotherapy

Catheryn M. Yashar, MD

A basic understanding of the principles of radiation oncology is essential to the gynecologic oncologist. Radiation therapy is used in the curative treatment of locoregionally advanced cervical and vaginal carcinoma. It is often an adjuvant therapy prescribed for uterine or vulvar carcinoma and in inoperable patients may be the only definitive therapy available. Last, it can be used for the palliative treatment of gynecologic carcinomas.

INTRODUCTION TO ELECTROMAGNETIC RADIATION

Radiant energy or radiation is an essential component of life on earth. For example, sunlight provides heat, light, and energy for plant photosynthesis and radio waves provide a method of communication. This electromagnetic radiation physically consists of photons, or "packets" of energy without mass or charge. The primary difference between the radiations is the energy of the photons. The energy is proportional to frequency ($E = h\nu$, where h is Planck's constant and ν is frequency) and inversely proportional to wavelength (Table 23-1). A common analogy is to compare wavelength with the length of a person's stride when walking; the number of strides per minute is the frequency of the wave.

Photons, a nonparticulate radiation, are only one form of radiation. Another form of radiation is particulate radiation. Particulate radiation consists of subatomic particles such as electrons, protons, α particles, and neutrons.

Radiation is not harmful in ordinary quantities and is actually helpful to life processes. In fact, exposure to radiation is a constant phenomenon (Tables 23-2 and

TABLE 23-1   Electromagnetic Spectrum

	Wavelength (M)	Frequency (Hz)	Energy (J)
Radio	$>1 \times 10^{-1}$	$<3 \times 10^{9}$	$<2 \times 10^{-24}$
Microwave	$1 \times 10^{-3} - 1 \times 10^{-1}$	$3 \times 10^{9} - 3 \times 10^{11}$	$2 \times 10^{-24} - 2 \times 10^{-22}$
Infrared	$7 \times 10^{-7} - 1 \times 10^{-3}$	$3 \times 10^{11} - 4 \times 10^{14}$	$2 \times 10^{-22} - 3 \times 10^{-19}$
Visible	$4 \times 10^{-7} - 7 \times 10^{-7}$	$4 \times 10^{14} - 7.5 \times 10^{14}$	$3 \times 10^{-19} - 5 \times 10^{-19}$
Ultraviolet	$1 \times 10^{-8} - 4 \times 10^{-7}$	$7.5 \times 10^{14} - 3 \times 10^{16}$	$5 \times 10^{-19} - 2 \times 10^{-17}$
X-ray	$1 \times 10^{-11} - 1 \times 10^{-8}$	$3 \times 10^{16} - 3 \times 10^{19}$	$2 \times 10^{-17} - 2 \times 10^{-14}$
Gamma ray	$<1 \times 10^{-11}$	$>3 \times 10^{19}$	$>2 \times 10^{-14}$

TABLE 23-2   General Population Radiation Exposure

Radiation Source	Average Annual Whole Body Dose (millirem/year)
Natural: Cosmic	29
Terrestrial	29
Radon	200
Internal (^{40}K, ^{14}C, etc.)	40
Manmade (diagnostic radiograph, nuclear medicine, consumer products such as smoke detectors)	64
All others (fallout, air travel, occupational)	2
Average annual total	360 mrem/year
Tobacco smokers add ~280 mrem	

TABLE 23-3   Radiation Associated with Common Activities

Activity	Typical Radiation Dose
Smoking	280 mrem/year
Chest radiograph	8 mrem/single radiograph
Drinking water	5 mrem/year
Cross-country airplane trip	5 mrem/year

TABLE 23-4   Radioactive Isotopes Used in Radiation Oncology

Element	Isotope	E_{max} (MeV)	$T_{1/2}$	Clinical Use
Radium	^{236}Ra	3.26	1600 y	Historical
Cesium	^{137}Cs	0.514, 1.17	30 y	Temporary intracavitary implants
Iridium	^{192}Ir	0.38_{ave}	74.2 d	Temporary interstitial implants and source for high dose rate machine
Iodine	^{125}I	0.028_{ave}	60.2 d	Permanent interstitial implants
Phosphorus	^{32}P	None	14.3 d	Permanent intracavitary placement
Palladium	^{103}Pd	20KV	17 d	Permanent prostate seed implant

23-3). However, high-energy, or "ionizing" radiation, is not entirely harmless, although it is commonly used for both diagnostic and therapeutic purposes. High-energy radiation can be injurious to biologic material, and its use in oncology depends on the ability of normal tissue to recover from the effects more effectively or efficiently than malignant tissue. Radiation causes both reversible and irreversible changes in normal tissue, and these effects are placed into two categories: acute effects (apparent during or shortly after the radiation course) and long-term effects (apparent from 6 months to years after completion of therapy). Radiation effects may not be initially apparent except by careful chemical or microscopic study. Indeed, the effects may not be apparent for many years or may manifest only in the offspring of the irradiated organism. The accepted position regarding radiation exposure is that incidental environmental radiation, diagnostic tests, and therapeutic radiation can all be detrimental. Although in many cases

the chance of injury from diagnostic or environmental radiation is slight, the possibility of damage from a known exposure must always be weighed against the importance of the information to be gained or the effect desired. Incidental exposure must be avoided through control of environmental hazards whenever possible by following the ALARA principle (*As Low As Reasonably Achievable*).

There are many forms and sources of radiation, including natural isotopes and manmade radiations. The natural radiation emissions (gamma and beta rays) of isotopes such as iridium, iodine, and cesium are used for therapeutic purposes in many human malignancies (Table 23-4). In addition, during the past four decades increasingly sophisticated machines have been manufactured to produce high-intensity, directed radiation to treat both malignant and benign conditions. Modern machines emit energies greater than 1 million electron volts (1 MeV) and are termed supervoltage or megavoltage machines (Table 23-5). The most commonly available are called linear accelerators (linacs). Even these have recently become more sophisticated to allow increasingly precise delivery of radiation in the form of intensity modulated radiation therapy (IMRT). The newest generation models allow for real-time computed tomography (CT) for position verification, termed

TABLE 23-5   Radiation Delivery by Energy

Modality	Voltage	Source
Low voltage (superficial)	85–150 keV	X-ray
Medium voltage (Orthovotage)	180–400 keV	X-ray
Supervoltage	500 keV–8 MeV	Linear accelerator, ^{60}Co machine
Megavoltage	Above supervoltage energy	Betatron, linear accelerator

TABLE 23-6   Historical and Si Units of Radiation

Quantity	Historical Unit	SI Unit	Conversion Factor
Exposure	R	C/kg	2.58×10^{-4} C/kg/R
Absorbed dose	Rad	Gray (Gy)	10^{-2} Gy/rad
Dose equivalent (used in radiation protection)	Rem	Seivert (Sv)	10^{-2} Sv/rem
Activity	Curie (Ci)	Becquerel (Bq)	3.7×10^{10} Bq/Ci

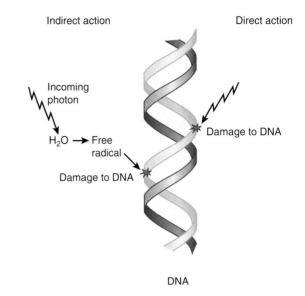

FIGURE 23-1   Direct and indirect actions of radiation. DNA, the most lethal target of radiation is schematically shown in the center. In direct action the incident photon displaces an electron from the target (DNA) molecule. In indirect action, another molecule, such as water, is ionized and the displaced electron diffuses to the target and damages the DNA.

image-guided radiation therapy, or IGRT. Image guidance is also more commonly used in brachytherapy, which historically used only two-dimensional imaging. With the advent of computed tomography (CT) and magnetic resonance imaging (MRI) compatible brachytherapy applicators, imaging modalities are used to more precisely direct the radiation to the tissues at risk while simultaneously avoiding normal, uninvolved tissues. The acceleration in technology has paralleled the advances in computer technology. In addition, simulations that combine radiation delivery planning with positron emission tomography (PET) and MRI imaging are currently being used at several centers.

RADIATION UNITS

Those in training and in practice must familiarize themselves with the international system (SI) of weights and measures used today. The SI units and appropriate conversions are shown in Table 23-6.

When a radiation exposure occurs, the resultant ionizations deposit energy in the air. If a patient lies in the path of the beam, energy will be deposited in the patient. This deposition of energy by radiation exposure is called radiation-*absorbed dose*, measured in the acronym rad. One rad is equivalent to the deposition of 100 ergs of energy into each gram of the irradiated object. The SI unit of radiation absorbed dose is the gray (Gy), and 1 Gy = 1 cGy =100 rads = 1 joule/kg. The erg and joule are units of energy.

RADIATION PHYSICS

Energy Deposition

Radiation energy is deposited into the tissue in one of two ways: direct or indirect ionization. Ionization is when an outer shell electron is stripped from an atom leaving a positive charge. Direct ionization is the predominant mechanism of action of particles that possess charge, but photons can also cause direct ionization. Examples of directly ionizing particles include particulate radiation such as protons and neutrons. Indirect ionization produces free radicals of other molecules, namely water, which diffuse and damage critical targets (Figure 23-1). A free radical has an unpaired outer shell electron that is chemically unstable and very reactive. The hydroxyl free radical (made by the lysis of H_2O) diffuses only about 1 nm and breaks the chemical bonds in cellular proteins and other key substances such as DNA. Either form of energy deposition results in ionization of target molecules. Scientists estimate that about two-thirds of cell biologic damage is from indirect action by ionizing radiation, from sources such as x-rays or gamma rays.

The electrons generated by penetrating photons lose their energy slowly, resulting in a low energy deposition along the electron track, or low linear energy transfer (LET; defined as energy transferred per unit length of track – keV/μm). High LET radiations (neutrons,

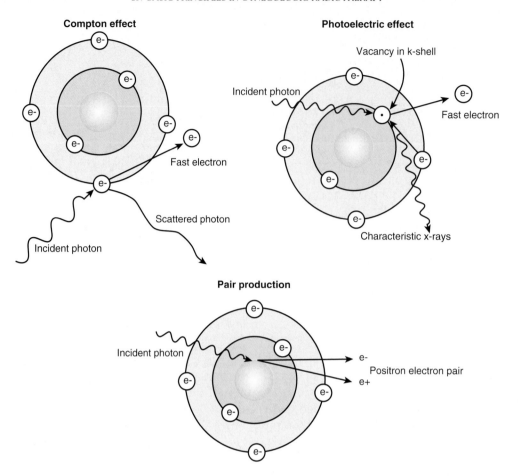

FIGURE 23-2   The major photons interactions important in therapeutic and diagnostic radiation oncology.

negative π mesons, or alpha particles) deposit more energy per unit length, are more commonly directly ionizing, and are less susceptible to perturbations such as oxygen tension. This means that for the same reaction produced in healthy cells by all radiation modalities, high LET radiation has a higher probability (1.5 to 2.5 times that of x-rays) of killing those cells in less than ideal circumstances (i.e., hypoxic tumor cells, cells in a resistant part of the cell cycle, etc.).

Sources of Radiation

Gamma rays are the photons emitted from the atomic nuclear decay of radioactive isotopes—for example, ^{137}Cs (cesium) or ^{60}Co (cobalt). *X-rays* are photons electrically generated by bombarding a target such as tungsten with electrons (how a linear accelerator works). When these fast-moving electrons approach the tungsten nuclear field, they are attracted to the nucleus and thus veer from their original path. This change in direction causes deceleration and kinetic energy is converted to x-rays in the form of bremsstrahlung photons. These emitted x-rays, or photons, vary in energy from zero to a maximum determined by the kinetic energy of the

bombarding electrons. Machines such as the betatron and linear accelerator generate electrons with high kinetic energy and thus produce high-energy x-rays. In addition to bremsstrahlung photons, characteristic photons are also produced as atoms seek to fill electron orbital vacancies (see later discussion). Gamma rays and x-rays can be collectively called *photons*, and what is of medical importance is the energy and delivery of the photon, not the source.

Photon Interactions

The interaction of photons with matter is accomplished through six mechanisms: (1) Compton scattering, (2) photoelectric absorption, (3) pair production, (4) triplet production (5) photodisintegration, and (6) coherent scattering (no energy transfer). The Compton effect is the major interaction of photons in tissue used in modern radiotherapy (Figure 23-2). When the photon from the linear accelerator interacts with outer orbital atomic electrons, part of the photon energy transfers to the electron as kinetic energy. The photon is deflected with reduced energy. The ejected electron is propelled forward and sets up a cascade of increasing energy deposition by displacing more electrons. As a result of this initiation and subsequent *buildup effect,* megavoltage photon beams have a skin-sparing effect not seen in older machines and therefore produce less superficial tissue change.

The photoelectric effect is seen at lower energies. This effect is the most important in diagnostic radiology. In this interaction, the incident photon is absorbed completely by an inner shell electron. The inner shell electron is ejected with kinetic energy equal to the incident photon energy less the electron-binding energy. An outer shell electron then drops into the vacancy. As this electron changes orbit its energy is reduced and the excess energy is given off in the form of a photon, called a "characteristic photon."

In pair production, photon energies greater than 1.02 MeV interact with the strong electric field of the nucleus and lose all incident energy. The incident photon energy is converted into matter in the form of a positron–electron pair. If this happens in the field of an orbital electron, three particles are produced in the interaction and the interaction is called triplet production.

Last, in photodisintegration the high-energy photon enters the nucleus and ejects a neutron, proton, or alpha particle. This is important for shielding considerations in linear accelerators that operate at energies above 15 MeV.

Radioactive Decay

Naturally radioactive substances decay to more stable substances by several methods: (1) beta decay (^{32}P, ^{18}F), (2) electron capture (^{125}I), (3) alpha decay (^{226}Ra), and (4) isomeric transition (gamma emission and internal conversion). "Decay" is the manner in which an isotope releases, or gains, matter and/or energy to become a more stable substance. The rate of decay of a radionuclide is exponential and is termed the "activity." The old unit for activity was the Curie (Ci). The SI unit is the becquerel (Bq) defined by 1 Bq = 1dps (disintegration per second). The half-life ($T^{1/2}$) is the time required to disintegrate to half the original activity. $T^{1/2}$ of commonly used radioactive substances is in Table 23-4.

^{137}Cs (Cesium-137), used in low dose rate (LDR) applications, is a by-product of the fission process in a nuclear reactor and decays via beta and gamma emission. In beta decay a neutron from the nucleus converts into a proton (positively charged) and an electron. Again, to increase stability a photon is released and the ^{127}Cs becomes the more stable ^{137}Ba (Figure 23-3). ^{137}Cs decays approximately 2%/year.

^{192}Ir (Iridium 192) is also produced in a nuclear reactor and decays via beta decay (see earlier) and electron capture. In electron capture the nucleus "captures" an orbital electron and converts a proton into a neutron. ^{192}Ir

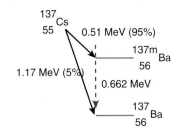

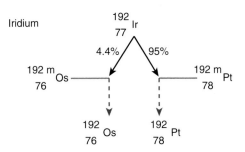

FIGURE 23-3   Decay diagram of ^{137}Cs and ^{192}Ir.

then becomes the excitable ^{192m}Pt and ^{192m}Os, which release gamma rays to stabilize. ^{192}Ir is the primary isotope used for high dose rate (HDR) applications and interstitial implants. It decays approximately 1%/day.

Inverse Square Law

Another important physics concept in radiotherapy is the inverse square law. This law states that the dose of radiation at a given point is inversely proportional to the square of the distance from the source of radiation (dose $\propto$ 1/distance^2). This rapid decrease in dose is very important in brachytherapy. It underscores why the bladder and rectum can be relatively protected from the high intracavitary doses of radiation—especially with good vaginal packing to maximize the distance from the source to the normal organ. It also underscores why good geometry is critical when performing implants. Last, it explains the reasoning behind standing at the door (increasing the distance) while conversing with a brachytherapy patient. As a simplistic example consider the following. The dose at point A is 4. Two feet away the dose would be 4 divided by the square of the distance (2^2) or 4/4 = 1. Another 2 feet away the dose would be 1/4 ($4/4^2 = 4/16 = 1/4$).

Depth Dose Characteristics of Radiation

The last physics concept to master is variation in radiation beam characteristics based on energy. To that end it is important to realize that the energy and penetrating

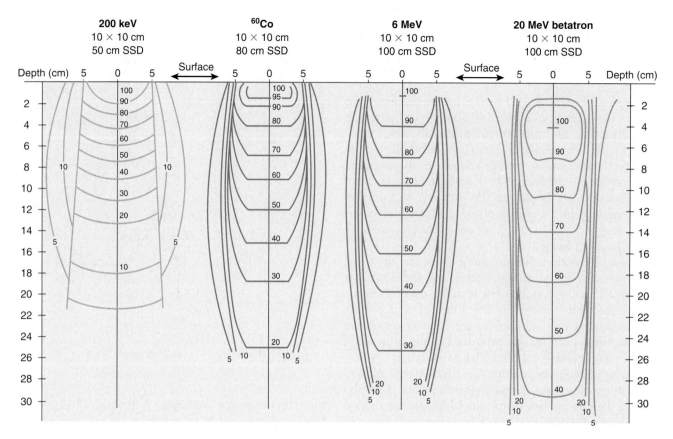

FIGURE 23-4   Comparison isodose curves and depth-dose distribution through a single field. Each machine is delivering photons of different energies. Note that higher-energy machines deliver radiation to a greater depth for the same surface dose. Note also the skin sparing with 6-MV and 20-MV equipment. Last, note the difference in lateral scattering—higher energy photons are more "forward-moving" with less lateral scatter.

power of ionizing radiation increase as the photon frequency increases and wavelength decreases. In addition, as energy increases, the depth of maximum dose increases (D_{max}; remember the *buildup effect* discussed earlier). For low energies, such as 250 keV, the maximum dose is at the skin surface. For a 4 MeV (4 million electron volts) accelerator the D_{max} is approximately 1 cm, for 6 MeV D_{max} is at 1.5 cm, and for 22 MeV D_{max} is at 3.5 cm, and so on. Knowing this, one can see why higher-energy beams are more suited to treat deeply seated tumors, such as in the uterine or cervix. These higher energy beams will differentially spare more superficial tissues. Depth of maximum dose curves and isodose distributions (areas receiving similar dose) for various energies are shown in Figure 23-4.

The reduced effect on skin of supervoltage radiation, compared with orthovoltage (keV range) radiation, is based on a physical characteristic of radiation. With higher energy, forward movement of the energy cascade (in the direction of the primary beam) is greater with reduced lateral scattering. As the energy increases, it becomes more penetrating and the photons and resultant liberated electrons travel a greater distance into the absorbing material. Therefore the percentage of

radiation at any specific depth, compared with the surface dose, increases as the energy increases.

In summary, above the energy of 400 to 800 keV, the advantages to higher energy photons are less damage to the skin at the portal of entry, greater radiation at depth relative to the surface, and reduced lateral scatter of radiation in the tissues. In addition, there is less photoelectric effect at higher energies and therefore less absorption in bone.

RADIOBIOLOGY

The selective destruction of tissues forms the basis of therapeutic radiation. Neoplastic cells are preferentially killed by radiation compared to the surrounding normal tissues, primarily as a result of differences in repair capabilities. This differential radiosensitivity between normal and cancerous tissues determines in large part whether a radiated neoplasm is eradicated. The ratio that defines the dose necessary to effect tumor kill with the dose likely to cause normal tissue damage is the therapeutic ratio, and modern radiotherapy is striving to maximize this ratio (Figure 23-5).

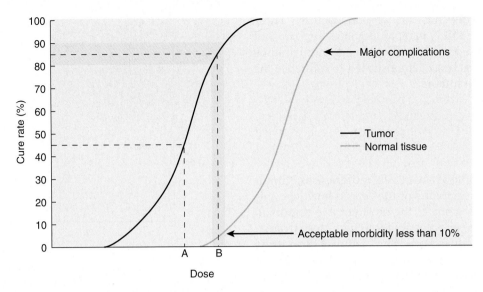

FIGURE 23-5 Therapeutic ratio. Diagrammatic representation of a parallel tumor response and normal tissue tolerance curve demonstrating the relationship between increasing dose, increasing cure rate, and increasing morbidity. Under ideal circumstances *(B)*, an 80% to 90% cure rate can be achieved with 5% to 10% morbidity. Pushing the cure rate carries with it an increase in morbidity. However, attempts to avoid all morbidity *(A)* significantly reduce the ability to cure. Although the shape of these curves varies for various tumor types and dose rates, general concepts are valid whenever radiotherapy is used to treat malignant lesions.

Structural Changes

Deposition of radiation energy in the cell can lead to a variety of changes that alter normal function. Degradation, or breaking into smaller units, and crosslinking are examples of structural damage that can affect proteins, enzymes, and nucleic acids. The initial chemical change occurs in a fraction of a second and is rarely detected directly. Some changes are repaired almost immediately, whereas others can never be repaired. Although various morphologic and functional changes occur in irradiated cells, the bulk of direct and indirect evidence suggests that the biologic effects of radiation result principally from DNA damage. For example, it has been calculated that 1 million cGy are required to inactivate cell cytoplasmic enzyme systems, and doses of 1000 cGy are required to damage cell membranes. In contrast, chromosomal aberrations and mutations can be produced by very low doses of radiation. Because only a few hundred cGy are needed to produce a high degree of lethality in cell tissue culture, it seems logical that nuclear changes are responsible for cell death.

Radiation-induced DNA damage destroys the cell by one of several mechanisms. It may stimulate cell apoptosis, called interphase death, which is visible by several methods, including light microscopy and Western blot. Radiation may also cause mitotic death. In this form of damage the cell outwardly appears normal but is sufficiently damaged so that cell division is not possible. Actual death of the cell does not occur, however, until cell division is attempted. This is why tumors may continue to regress after completion of radiation.

A variety of DNA lesions are produced by radiation including base damage, DNA–protein crosslinking, single-strand breaks, and double-strand breaks (DSB). Repairing even a single nucleotide requires many genes and a series of steps. The most toxic cellular lesion inflicted by ionizing radiation is the DSB. In fact, the proficiency of repair of DSB correlates well with radiation-induced lethality. The repair of DSB can occur by several mechanisms. Religation of complementary DSB ends, homologous recombination (HR), is efficient and cells can usually survive. The Mre11 protein is attracted when a DSB occurs and may be the first sensor of the break and primarily involved in repair through nuclease activity, unwinding DNA, or removing hairpin loops. When the ends are not complementary, nonhomologous end joining (NHEJ) is used and can be complicated by small DNA deletions or insertions. These errors in turn can lead to cell death or mutation. Some of the necessary proteins for NHEJ are Ku70, Ku80, DNA ligase IV, and XRCC4. The Ku70/Ku80 complex binds to the DSB and unwinds the strand while the DNA ligase IV/XRCC4 complex repairs DSBs. Mammalian cells seem to repair more by NHEJ than HR.

Radiosensitivity

Radiosensitivity is the response of the tumor to irradiation that can be measured by the extent of regression, rapidity of response, and response durability.

Radiosensitivity depends on several factors. These factors include the ability to repair damage, hypoxia, cell cycle position, and growth fraction. In addition, volume of initial tumor has been demonstrated to influence the ability to eradicate tumors.

Understanding that radiosensitivity and radiocurability are not identical in meaning is essential. Relatively radioresistant tumors accessible to high-dose local radiation therapy can be cured, whereas radiosensitive tumors that are widely metastatic can only be controlled locally. An excellent example of a relatively radioresistant tumor is squamous cell carcinoma of the cervix; however, this malignancy remains one of the most curable tumors in humans because of its accessibility to high-dose irradiation and the relatively radioresistant nature of the hosting normal tissues (e.g., cervix and vagina). The ability to place radium or cesium in juxtaposition to the malignancy within dose ranges tolerable to the surrounding normal tissue is the key to success.

Many attempts have been made to develop an assay to predict tumor radiosensitivity. However, no assay yet developed accurately predicts the outcome in a given tumor. This is likely secondary to tumors containing mixed cell populations with differing sensitivities to chemotherapy and radiation. Sensitive cells are eliminated, whereas resistant cells continue to grow. This explains why many tumors initially respond to therapy but are ultimately incurable.

In vitro models have been developed to predict and study tumor cell radiosensitivity. Cellular radiosensitivity is generally quantified by measuring the loss of reproductive capacity, which can be plotted in a survival curve. Survival curves are characterized by an initial slope, α, and the terminal slope, β. Alpha (α) represents irreparable damage to the cell, whereas β represents the repairable damage (Figure 23-6). The α/β ratio is the dose where the contribution from alpha equals the contribution from beta and is a measure of radiosensitivity. Large ratios are seen with rapidly dividing cells and help predict the response of tumors and the early effects of radiation. Low ratios characterize late responding tissues.

In addition, the size of the shoulder (Dq) on a survival curve relays valuable information as it represents the magnitude of repair of sublethal damage (SLD). Broad shoulders have small α/β ratios and good repair of SLD. This repair of sublethal damage takes several hours (2-6 hours) to complete. The ability of cells to repair SLD forms the basis for the use of fractionated doses in clinical radiation therapy, in which differential capacities between normal tissue and tumor to repair a sublethal injury can be exploited (Figure 23-7). This differential repair capacity also forms the basis for accelerated fractionation or hyperfractionation in which the dose is given twice a day. This approach works very well with

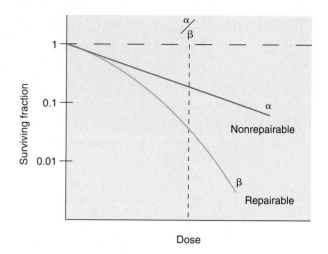

FIGURE 23-6   Cell survival curve. The initial slope, α, represents irreparable damage, whereas the terminal slope, β, represents reparable damage. The α/β ratio is the point on the curve where the two are equal.

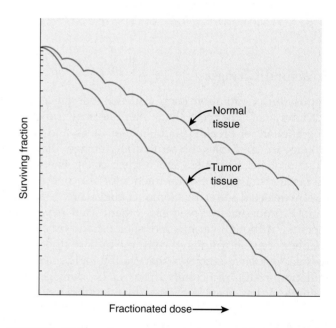

FIGURE 23-7   Different capacities between normal tissue and tumor to accumulate and repair sublethal injury from fractionated doses result in differential survival. The normal tissue is able to repair more efficiently and effectively.

rapidly growing tumors. Treated twice a day, the normal tissues have sufficient time to repair but the tumor tissues, less organized, efficient, and accurate, are differentially killed. Some cells have almost no shoulder indicating a limited ability to repair sublethal damage, and these cells can be eradicated with relatively low doses of radiation. For example, dysgerminomas are highly curable with relatively low doses of radiation

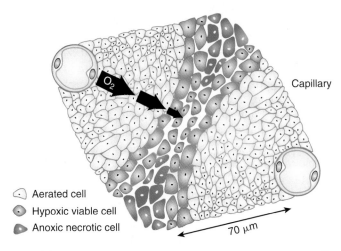

FIGURE 23-8 As distance from blood supply increases, cells become hypoxic and even anoxic. Hypoxic cells are more radioresistant and, therefore, harder to sterilize. Oxygen diffuses about 70 μm from the capillary.

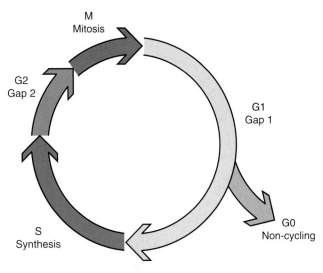

FIGURE 23-9 Cell cycle.

(20-30 Gy) compared with cervical cancer tumors, which may require more than 70 Gy to obtain cure.

The availability of oxygen is of vital importance to the radiosensitivity of the cell also. As radiation enters the cell, it interacts with organic molecules (DNA). This molecule may repair itself unless an oxygen molecule becomes attached, thereby "fixing" the damage. The addition of O_2 will enhance low LET radiation (photons) but does not similarly affect high LET radiation. The ability of oxygen to enhance radiation is measured by the oxygen enhancement ratio, or OER (OER = dose of XRT without O_2 for a given effect/dose of XRT with O_2 for the same effect). It takes at least 2% (17 mm Hg) tissue O_2 to see the full oxygen effect.

Tumor cells with potentially unlimited capacity for growth are limited as they outgrow the blood supply. In fact, tumors above 200 μm have necrotic cores secondary to a limited diffusion distance for oxygen. Oxygen may effectively penetrate approximately 70 μm from the blood vessel (Figure 23-8). Outside this distance, tumor cells become deficient and enter a noncycling phase. They may become hypoxic or even anoxic and necrotic. This is important from a radiobiologic standpoint because noncycling cells exhibit a greater capacity to repair radiation injury. Hypoxic cells are more resistant to the effects of radiation than are cells with normal oxygen tension. Thus large tumors can be difficult to control with radiation therapy, not only because there is a greater number of cells to sterilize, but also because a proportion of these cells are hypoxic, noncycling, and radioresistant. As a clinical example, experience notes that exophytic friable cervical lesions that hemorrhage easily on contact respond better and more quickly than infiltrative lesions. The blood supply and oxygenation varies considerably between these two lesions, with the friable lesion better vascularized and oxygenated and therefore more radiosensitive. Unfortunately, attempts to overcome this differential sensitivity by mechanisms such as hyperbaric oxygen and radiosensitizers have been less than optimal to date.

Another factor important in radiosensitivity is the proportion of mitotic or clonogenic cells in the tumor. Cycling cells are more radiosensitive. In fact, mitotic counts have been shown to correlate with the prognosis in many tumors. The position in the cell cycle is also important (Figure 23-9). Cells in late G2 and mitosis (M-phase) are the most sensitive to radiation, and cells in late synthesis (S-phase) are the most resistant (Figure 23-10). This is exploited with chemotherapies such as paclitaxel, which arrests cells in mitosis and is a profound radiation sensitizer.

Finally, the initial tumor volume greatly influences the ability to sterilize a site. Generally, the smaller the tumor volume, the less radiation is required to destroy all cells. As the volume increases, the dose to obtain local control is increased. The concept of treating with "shrinking" fields is to serially reduce the size of the radiation portals to give a higher dose of radiation therapy to the central portion of the tumor where presumably more hypoxic, radioresistant cells are present.

Historically, clinicians attempted to correlate radiation tumor response and local tumor control. Generally, the faster and more complete the tumor response at the completion of the therapy, the greater long-term control, assuming that no distant metastasis occurs. Although this is not uniformly true, it has been shown in cervical cancer that there is a good correlation between local tumor control and complete or partial regression of the cancer at the completion of radiation. In addition, Grigsby has correlated post-treatment PET tumor

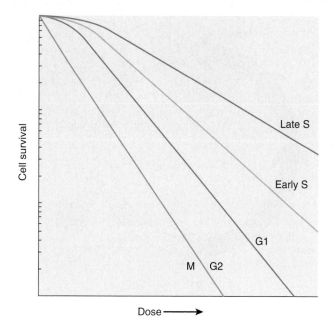

FIGURE 23-10　The survival curve for cells in mitosis and G2 is steep and has no shoulder. The curve for cells late in S phase is shallower and has a large shoulder. G1 and early S are intermediate in sensitivity.

response (which measure glucose metabolism) with survival.

Another factor limiting radiocurability is the normal tissue toxicity with increasing radiation doses. Normal tissue effects depend on total dose, dose fraction size, volume, and inherent tissue radiosensitivity. The ultimate goal is to obtain maximal curability with minimal side effects. Combining radiation therapy with surgery or chemotherapy decreases normal tissue tolerance to a given dose. Well-established port size, total dose, and fractionation schemes have been identified but cannot remain static. Variations are being investigated to increase curability and decrease complications, including new chemotherapeutic radiosensitizers, technological advances in the delivery of radiation such as IMRT, and radioprotectors such as ethyol.

RADIOSENSITIZERS, HYPOXIC CELL SENSITIZERS, AND RADIOPROTECTORS

Radiation sensitizers and protectors are being actively investigated to increase the effectiveness of radiation or allow dose escalation while minimizing side effects. Radiation sensitizers increase the ability of radiation to cause permanent, lethal damage. This therapeutic gain may be from a variety of mechanisms including selective uptake, targeting, or activation. To be effective, sensitizers must have acceptable normal tissue side effects. Known radiation sensitizers include chemotherapeutic agents such as cisplatin, 5-fluorouracil, paclitaxel, adriamycin, and gemcitabine. Hypoxic cell sensitizers include the imidazole drugs such as misonidazole and bioreductive agents such as tirapazamine. Endogenous sulfhydryl compounds and ethyol afford radioprotection to normal tissues.

The advantages afforded by chemoradiation can be by several mechanisms. Some agents inhibit the repair of radiation damage, such as cisplatin, whereas others block cells in a radiosensitive cell cycle phase, such as paclitaxel. Adriamycin, docetaxel, and paclitaxel have unique effects when combined serially with radiation, as "radiation recall" is an uncommon but distressing phenomenon. After a course of radiation the normal tissue sensitization can be "recalled" when the chemotherapy is initiated—this phenomenon is a re-emergence of a prior radiation burn that conforms exactly to the prior radiation portal. The mechanism of this is unknown but well described for these chemotherapies.

The nitroimidazoles such as metronidazole, misonidazole, etanidazole, and nimorazole are electron affinic and increase the sensitivity of radioresistant hypoxic cells to XRT. They mimic oxygen and can diffuse into hypoxic areas. Unfortunately, clinical studies to date have demonstrated significant toxicity and little clinical utility with these drugs.

Tirapazamine is entering clinical trials as an adjunct to radiotherapy. GOG trial 219 randomized chemoradiation for cervical cancer with and without tirapazamine. Tirapazamine is bioactivated intracellularly to a cytotoxic, active free radical that causes extensive chromosomal breaks and inhibits DNA repair. The reaction is driven by low tissue oxygen tension and when combined with radiation may allow more effective destruction of tumors with hypoxic cores. The Gynecologic Oncology Group published a phase II trial for advanced or recurrent cervical carcinoma utilizing tirapazmine and cisplatin and concluded that the combination was fairly well tolerated. A subsequent phase III trial randomizing stages Ib2-IVa between standard cisplatin and radiation versus cisplatin, radiation and tirapazamine was opened but closed for accrual in 2009.

Radioprotection has been proved in several sites with the use of ethyol. Amifostine (ethyol; WR-2721) is an organic thiophosphate extensively studied by Walter Reed Army Institute of Research. Normal tissues noted to be protected included the salivary glands, bone marrow, immune system, skin, oral mucosa, esophagus, intestinal mucosa, kidney, and testes. It is dephosphorylated to the active metabolite (WR-1065) in the tissues.

It is believed that tissue versus tumor alkaline phosphatase concentration variations provide the differential protective effect. In addition, tissue pH differences afford selective tissue versus tumor uptake of ethyol. When given intravenously the plasma half-life is less than

10 minutes, but there is prolonged retention of the drug in normal tissue. In the first 30 minutes, drug uptake into normal tissues has been shown to be 100 times that of tumor tissues. Once inside the cell, the metabolite scavenges oxygen free radicals and provides an alternative target for alkylating agents, like cisplatin.

There have been numerous studies of the protective effect of ethyol with no reported decrease in antitumor efficacy. A phase III trial in head and neck cancer unequivocally established its role in salivary gland protection, confirming earlier studies. Other clinical trials have shown ethyol protects from cisplatin-induced renal, neurologic, and bone marrow toxicity. Liu published a phase III randomized trial in rectal cancer patients treated with pelvic radiation with and without ethyol (340 mg/m^2). The toxicity in the mucous membranes and genitourinary and gastrointestinal tract was reduced by 50% in the ethyol arm. Moderate to severe late toxicities were seen in 14% of those treated without ethyol compared to zero in the ethyol-treated patients. Athanassiou and colleagues randomly assigned 205 patients with pelvic radiation plus or minus ethyol and demonstrated a significant decrease in bladder and gastrointestinal toxicity. Complete responses to therapy and median survival were not significantly different between the arms. The RTOG (Radiation Therapy Oncology Group 0116) completed a two-arm trial utilizing ethyol with chemoradiation for pelvic and para-aortic radiation with concomitant cisplatin in cervical carcinoma. Arm 1 consisted of cisplatin chemotherapy concomitant with para-aortic radiation and demonstrated significant acute and late toxicity. Arm 2 again demonstrated significant acute and long-term toxicity, with no significant benefit demonstrated with the addition of ethyol, although compliance to the medication was disappointing. Ethyol has been found to be useful in reducing early and late toxicity with hypofractionated accelerated conformal radiation by Koukourakis. Toxicities with intravenous administration include hypotension and nausea. Data on subcutaneous administration demonstrate less hypotension, but treatable nausea and skin effects persist. There have been rare reports of Stevens-Johnson syndrome.

Genetic Effects

It is not possible to generalize and assign a specific mutation rate to a given radiation dose. Gene loci differ greatly in their mutability, and the random damage exerted by irradiation on any particular chromosome makes predictability impossible. The mitotic stage, cell type, sex, species, and dose rate influence the mutation rate as studied in lower animals and bacteria. Data from lower animals are difficult to extrapolate to humans, and therefore prediction of mutation rates cannot be expected

TABLE 23-7 Radiation Doses to Low Pelvis from Diagnostic Scans

Examination	Dose to Fetus (First Trimester) and Maternal Gonads (mcGy)
Lower-extremity radiograph	1
Cervical spine radiograph	2
Chest radiograph	8
Chest fluoroscopy	70
Lumbar spine radiograph	275
Hip radiograph	100
IVP	585
Upper GI	330
Lower GI	465
Chest CT	8
Abdominal CT	800
Pelvic CT	2300

Modified from DiSaia PJ: In Scott JR, DiSaia PJ, Hammond CB, Spellacy WN (eds): Danforth's Obstetrics and Gynecology, 8th ed. Philadelphia, JB Lippincott, 1999.

from the evidence that has been accumulated from various types of radiation exposure. Direct evidence of radiation-induced mutation in humans is lacking, although there is strong anecdotal evidence for carcinogenesis in those exposed to radiation. A few examples are excess skin cancers seen in those exposed to x-rays before safety standards were established, lung cancer in pitchblende miners, bone tumors in radium dial painters, and liver tumors in those exposed to Thorotrast contrast. The largest groups of humans available for study are survivors and descendants of those exposed in Hiroshima and Nagasaki. Although there has been no detectable effect on the frequency of prenatal or neonatal deaths or on the frequency of malformations in subsequent generations, this does not mean that no hereditary effects were produced. The number of exposed parents was small, and dosages were so low that it would have been surprising if an increase in mutation had been detected in such a brief period. There has not been sufficient time for the several generations needed to reveal recessive damage.

Radiation does not produce new and unique mutations but increases the incidence of spontaneous mutations. Based largely on experiments in mice, it is estimated that the doubling dose (i.e., the dose that will double the spontaneous mutation rate) for humans is probably 100 cGy based on DR exposure. Between 1% and 6% of spontaneous mutations in humans can be ascribed to background radiation. With the use of image intensifiers, improved radiographic film, and appropriate shielding to prevent scatter, it is possible to attain satisfactory radiographic visualization of internal structures with reduced exposure. The average dose of irradiation to the gonads of some common diagnostic techniques is given in Table 23-7. The use of diagnostic radiographs and CT scans has increased and fueled concerns that toxic radiation effects may emerge, especially among children exposed to increased diagnostic medical irradiation. Current recommendations stress the use of ionizing radiation only when necessary, and substitution of alternate sources of imaging, such as magnetic resonance imaging, which relies on magnetic fields, when possible.

In general, most mutations are harmful and there is no known threshold dose for the genetic effect. Permanent sterility in females is estimated to have a threshold of 250 to 600 cGy to acute exposure and 0.2 Gy/year for protracted exposure. The threshold dose for sterility varies based on the age of the patient, with younger patients being more resistant to the deleterious effect.

Fetal Effects

The classic effects of radiation on the mammalian embryo are as follows: (1) intrauterine and extrauterine growth restriction; (2) embryonic, fetal, or neonatal death; and (3) gross congenital malformations. Dose, gestational age, and dose rate are all important factors influencing radiation damage. The recommendation for fetal dose during the entire gestation is 0.5 rem or less (roughly 0.5 cGy). Monthly exposures should not exceed 0.05 rem. If a pregnant patient receives 10 cGy in the sensitive period of 10 days to 26 weeks, therapeutic abortion should be considered to avoid radiation effects including malformations, microcephaly, and mental retardation.

The peak incidence of gross malformations occurs during early organogenesis (10-40 days of gestation in the human), although cellular, tissue, and organ hypoplasia can be produced by radiation throughout the fetal and neonatal period with sufficient dose. Diagnostic x-ray procedures should be avoided in the pregnant woman unless there is overwhelming urgency. In women of childbearing age, possible damage to an early conceptus can be prevented by performing tests immediately after the commencement of a menstrual period and obtaining a negative pregnancy test result. Compelling evidence that radiation may be a causative agent in childhood cancer after prenatal exposure comes from several studies in Great Britain and the United States.

Some concrete information is available from the Japanese survivors of the atom bomb attacks in 1945. Examination of children born to survivors demonstrates the primary effect from in utero radiation was microcephaly and mental retardation. The most sensitive phase for mental retardation was from 8 to 15 weeks of gestation. In addition, permanent growth restriction was also observed, especially in those embryos exposed less than 1500 m from the center of the explosion. Hall reached the following conclusions:

1. Moderately large doses of radiation (>200 cGy) delivered to the human embryo before 2 to 3 weeks of gestation are unlikely to produce severe abnormalities in most children born, although a considerable number of embryos may be reabsorbed or aborted (all-or-none phenomenon).
2. Significant irradiation between 4 and 11 weeks of gestation leads to severe abnormalities in many organs.
3. Irradiation between 11 and 16 weeks of gestation may produce some eye, skeletal, and genital organ abnormalities; however, stunted growth, microcephaly, and mental retardation are often present.
4. Irradiation of the fetus between 16 and 20 weeks of gestation may lead to a mild degree of microcephaly, mental retardation, and stunting of growth.
5. Irradiation after 30 weeks of gestation is unlikely to produce gross structural abnormalities leading to a serious handicap but could cause functional disabilities.

PRINCIPLES OF CLINICAL RADIATION THERAPY

The technical modalities used in modern radiation therapy may be divided into two major categories:

1. **External irradiation**. This applies to irradiation from sources at a distance from the body (e.g., teletherapy with ^{60}Co, linear accelerator, betatron, or orthovoltage radiograph machines).
2. **Local irradiation** (brachytherapy). This applies to irradiation from sources in direct proximity to the tissue or tumor. Brachytherapy can be delivered with either a low dose rate system or a high dose rate system. LDR systems require hospital admission to a shielded room and dose delivery at roughly 50 to 100 cGy/hour. HDR systems are commonly done on an outpatient basis and deliver doses of 120 cGy/hr.
   a. **Intracavitary irradiation** is done with applicators loaded with radioactive materials such as cesium or iridium (e.g., vaginal ovoids, vaginal cylinder, intrauterine tandem, tandem and ring, or, historically, Heyman capsules).
   b. **Interstitial irradiation** (endocurie therapy) is usually delivered in the form of removable needles containing cesium, or iridium. The term also applies to permanent isotope implants, such as ^{125}I (iodine) seeds or ^{103}Pd (palladium).

c. **Direct therapy** was historically delivered by means of cones from an orthovoltage machine (e.g., transvaginal) but is rarely available today.

d. **Intraperitoneal or intrapleural** instillation of radioactive colloids, such as ^{32}P, is yet another local therapy but is infrequently used.

External Beam Radiation (Teletherapy)

External radiation is radiation therapy that is delivered from outside the body. It is most commonly delivered with photons, electrons, or protons. Machinery to deliver the radiation includes ^{60}Co units, orthovoltage machines, or linear accelerators, although linear accelerators are the overwhelming majority. Except in the developing world, ^{60}Co units are unusual. Typically a patient will need planning done before initiation of radiation, called simulation. Marks and/or permanent tattoos are applied to the skin to allow for daily setup and, commonly, a planning CT is performed replacing the traditional fluoroscopic simulation. The use of MRI, CT, or PET images to fuse with treatment planning CT data is widely available to better delineate tumor targets and normal tissue and in many centers are part of the standard simulator machine. Three areas must be targeted. The gross tumor volume requires the highest radiation dose. Microscopic extensions into surrounding tissues must be targeted but generally require a lesser dose for sterilization. Subclinical disease presumed to be present in postoperative beds or regional nodes must also be treated to prevent marginal failures.

Local Radiation (Brachytherapy)

Local application of radiation (also known as brachytherapy) permits very high doses to restricted tissue volumes. In this situation, the physical principle (inverse square law) that the intensity of irradiation rapidly decreases with distance from the radiation source is used to advantage. Brachytherapy is well suited to treat small tumors with well-defined limits and a clinical situation where it is desirable to restrict the volume of tissue irradiated. Larger volumes of tissue that need radiation therapy are best treated with external irradiation. Historically, radium (^{226}Ra) had been the most common isotope used for local application, but because of storage, risk of leaks, and extremely long half-life it is rarely used in this country. Sources used today are often converted to mg-Ra-equivalents. Brachytherapy sources such as ^{125}I, ^{137}Cs, ^{192}Ir, and ^{103}Pd are more commonly used today (Table 23-4).

Although conventional LDR intracavitary brachytherapy has produced very good results in cervical cancer, remote afterloading HDR intracavitary brachytherapy is becoming more widespread. The treatment results of LDR and HDR appear to be similar both for local control and survival, although there are no large American randomized trials. Retrospective studies, however, mirror the results of the randomized studies. There remain concerns over potential differences in late complications resulting from the different biologic mechanisms between the continuous low dose rate of LDR and the intermittent high dose rate of HDR. The increased interest in HDR arises from cost of inpatient hospitalization, the risks of prolonged bed rest, and radiation exposure to medical personnel with LDR systems. In both LDR and HDR, it is very important to keep the doses to normal tissues as low as possible by proper placement of radiation carriers and the use of shielding and packing/retraction techniques. HDR units use computer technology to "optimize" the dwell time of a single source to give the required distribution. The American Brachytherapy Society has published consensus guidelines on the administration of HDR for both cervical and uterine carcinomas. Also in use as an alternative to LDR or PDR is pulsed dose rate (PDR), although randomized trials on this method are lacking and published reports are few but increasing.

The term *dosimetry* is applied to the measurement and calculation of dose that the patient receives. In brachytherapy, as radiation intensity rapidly decreases with increasing distance from the source, tissue adjacent to the radiation source is treated to a high dose while relatively sparing surrounding tissue. The effectiveness of this distribution of irradiation depends on meticulous application of these sources. Interstitial application of radioactive sources is more difficult than intracavitary application. It is essential that the gynecologic oncologist be able to critically assess the placement of tandem and ovoids/cylinder/ring to assess the optimal placement of brachytherapy sources (Figures 23-11 and 23-12). Increased use of computer planning to optimize the dose to the tumor and minimize the dose to the normal tissues is under active clinical investigation and is likely to replace the current two-dimensional dosing guidelines and restrictions based on calculated doses to points (e.g., points A, B, bladder and rectal points) with three-dimensional, volume-directed, image-guided brachytherapy (IGBT). The European collaborative group Groupe Européen de Curiethérapie and the European Society for Therapeutic Radiology and Oncology (GEC-ESTRO) has published extensive work on this subject and an international trial. EMBRACE (*M*ri-guided *BR*achytherapy in *CE*rvical cancer) is open to test the utility and applicability of the new guidelines.

Normal Tissue Tolerance

The tolerance of any tissue (normal or tumor) to irradiation therapy depends on several characteristics of radiation, including (1) fractionation technique, (2) field

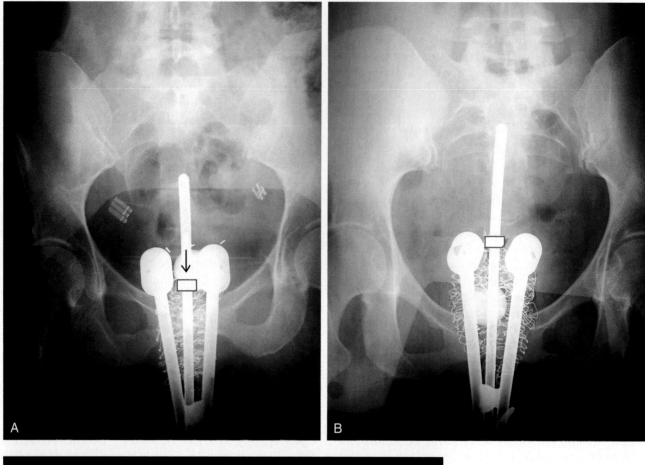

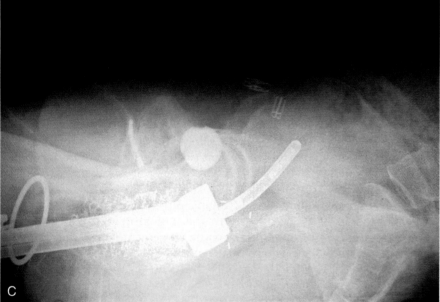

FIGURE 23-11 Assessing proper placement of tandem and ovoids. In both photos small interstitial silver seeds mark the cervix. Note that in **A** the cervical stop, outlined in red, has dropped away from the cervix compromising the dose delivery to the tumor and increasing the complications. In **B,** this has been corrected. Also note that the vaginal packing (delineated by radiopaque string) lies below the ovoids and that the tandem is midline and bisects the ovoids. In **C,** a lateral radiograph, the tandem again bisects the ovoids and lies beneath the bladder (Foley balloon is filled with contrast material) and does not lie too close to the sacrum.

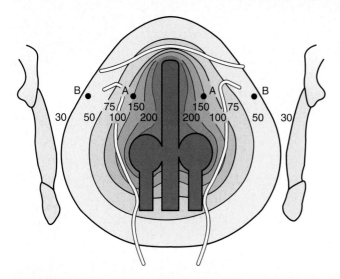

FIGURE 23-12 Isodose curves surrounding a typical Fletcher-Suit intracavitary application (tandem plus ovoids) for cervical cancer. Note the location of points *A* and *B* and the relative dose rates at distances from the system.

arrangement, (3) total dose, (4) dose rate, and (5) volume irradiated.

Fractionation is the number of treatments to deliver the total dose. Pelvic radiation delivered to a patient for a total dose of 5000 cGy given in five daily fractions of 200 cGy each week for 5 weeks is well tolerated in most cases. However, if that same total dose of 5000 cGy were given in five fractions of 1000 cGy every Monday for 5 consecutive weeks, tolerance would be low.

In addition, multiple fields are used to minimize toxicity by dividing the exposure of normal tissue into multiple different regions. Three-dimensional conformal therapy (3DCF), IMRT, and IGRT are areas of active investigation to further maximize dose to tumor and minimize toxicity to the surrounding normal tissues (Figure 23-13). With external irradiation, the patient is treated to all fields 5 days/week.

As is seen in LDR brachytherapy versus HDR brachytherapy dose rate affects tolerance. The final dose in HDR is necessarily lower to compensate for normal tissue tolerance concerns with the markedly higher dose rate in HDR. Conversion of doses to a 2-Gy dose equivalent is recommended by the GECT-ESTRO guidelines and is becoming more common (see later).

Finally, the volume of tissue irradiated is also an integral factor in tolerance. For example, a 1-cm circular field of skin would easily tolerate the fractionation and dose rate of 1000 cGy each Monday for 5 consecutive weeks. However, for a larger volume, such as whole-pelvis radiation, such a treatment plan is intolerable.

Patient factors also affect normal tissue tolerance. Previous surgery affects the morbidity of radiation therapy. In both cervical and uterine cancer, surgery identifies adverse surgical pathologic findings that direct radiation therapy. In cervical cancer, surgical evaluation of possible lymph node metastases, particularly in advanced cancers, may be done, or a radical hysterectomy may be aborted because on inspection the tumor is more advanced than originally indicated. Transperitoneal lymph node dissection followed by pelvic and possibly para-aortic radiation increases radiation-induced complications, particularly to the bowel. Radiation complications can be severe, including fistula formation, bowel obstruction, and perforation. The retroperitoneal approach to lymph node dissection has a decreased complication rate and is the preferred method of surgically evaluating lymph node status in cervical cancer. Medical conditions that affect blood flow such as diabetes, hypertension, and peripheral vascular disease can decrease normal tissue tolerance also.

Pelvic Organ Tolerance

Irradiation tolerance of the normal organs of the pelvis varies from one patient to another and is subject to the factors previously mentioned, such as volume, fractionation, and total dose of irradiation. As is illustrated in many areas of oncology, the more advanced lesions require higher doses for tumor eradication, and hence the possibility of morbidity increases. This, combined with the fact that advanced cancer often already compromises the integrity of the bladder and rectum, means that serious sequelae can develop in patients with advanced cervical, vaginal, and corpus lesions when curative therapy is sought. New advances in radiation delivery will, hopefully, decrease these adverse effects.

The normal tissues of the cervix and the corpus of the uterus can tolerate very high doses of radiation. In fact, they withstand higher doses better than any other comparable volume of tissue in the body; surface doses of 20,000 to 30,000 cGy in about 2 weeks are tolerated. This remarkable tolerance level permits a large tumor dose and allows a very high percentage of central control of cervical cancer. The unusual radiation tolerance of the uterus, and the vagina, stemming from an unusual ability to recover from radiation injury, accounts for the success of brachytherapy in the treatment of cervical lesions.

In contrast, the sigmoid, rectosigmoid, and rectum are more susceptible to radiation injury than are other pelvic organs. The frequency of injury to the large bowel often depends on the total dose administered by both the external beam and the intracavitary system. With external beam radiation alone, the large bowel is the most sensitive of pelvic structures. The bladder tolerates slightly more radiation than does the rectosigmoid, according to most authorities. Acceptable maximal point doses are 75 Gy and 70 Gy to the bladder and rectum, respectively. Fletcher proposed a rule that gives the upper limits of

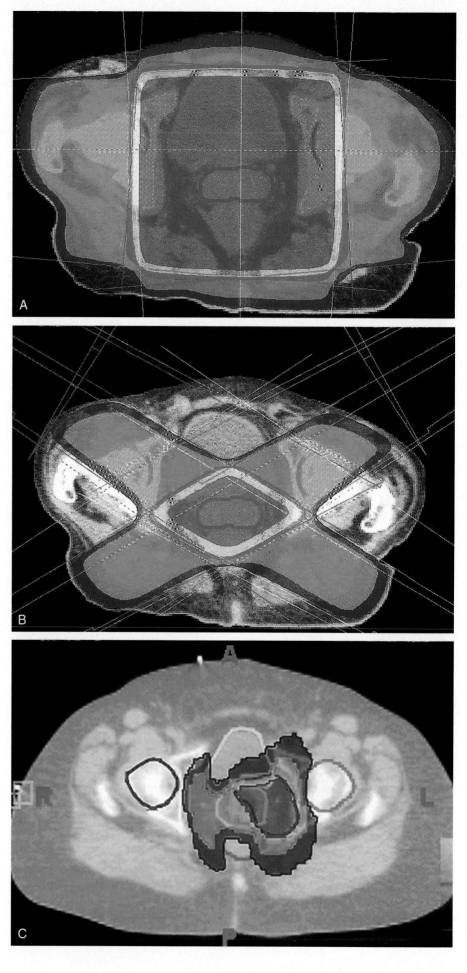

FIGURES 23-13 Comparison of normal tissue irradiated with four field box technique, **(A)** three-dimensional conformal therapy **(B)** and intensity modulated radiation therapy **(C)**. The red represents areas that receive 100% of the prescription dose, yellow 90%, green 50%, and blue 40%. Notice how the normal tissue volume receives less dose as the treatment is delivered more conformally.

pelvic irradiation and indirectly gives the tolerance of the bladder and rectum. The guidelines limit the sum of the central dose, stating that external beam radiation dose plus the number of milligram-hours of cesium administered by brachytherapy should never exceed 10,000. There is a parallel time guideline also critical to this limit. This is a necessary safety to prevent compact systems from exceeding vaginal/cervical tolerance. This guideline is valid only when the Fletcher-Suit brachytherapy systems are used. Most of this is applicable to therapy for the uterus, cervix, and vagina. In general, if a large dose of intracavitary irradiation is applied centrally for a small lesion, the amount of external beam applied centrally must be reduced. Conversely, if a lesion is large and the vaginal geometry is poor, a smaller intracavitary dose can be given and the dose administered by external beam may be raised (6000-7000 cGy).

GEC-ESTRO dose/volume guidelines limit the bladder to 90 Gy_{EQD2} and rectum/sigmoid to 70 to 75 Gy_{EQD2} for a calculated 2-cc volume combining doses from both external beam irradiation and brachytherapy. In this system doses from HDR brachytherapy are converted by a formula to a 2-Gy equivalent to allow the doses to be added (EQD2 – equivalent dose at 2Gy). The formula for conversion is EQD2 = D X [(d + α/β)/2 + α/β], where D is total dose, d is dose/fraction, and α/β is 3 for late-responding tissues and 10 for tumor/acute-responding tissues. Certain assumptions are made in this model, such as the same 2 cc of bladder, rectum, and sigmoid receive the maximal amount of irradiation with each fraction of brachytherapy. Especially in the mobile sigmoid colon, this assumption may be erroneous but models the worst-case scenario. A recent paper by Georg and colleagues demonstrated that the 5-year actuarial rectal toxicity was 20% if the dose exceeded 75 Gy_{EQD2} and 5% if the 2-cc dose remained below 75 Gy_{EQD2}. For bladder the 5-year actuarial toxicity was 13% versus 9% if a value of 100 Gy_{EQD2} was used. Insufficient events occurred in the sigmoid colon in this study for definitive analysis, but recommendations remain to keep the sigmoid less than 70 to 75 Gy_{EQD2}. It is hoped that further study will refine these guidelines.

Pelvic radiation spares a significant portion of the small bowel, because bowel is normally in episodic motion. This tends to prevent any one segment from receiving an excessive dose. However, if loops of small bowel are immobilized as a result of adhesions caused by previous surgery, they may be held directly in the path of the radiation beam and thus injured (Fig. 23-14). The result of such an injury is usually not manifested for at least 6 months or longer after completion of radiation. Studies demonstrate that the use of IMRT in the postoperative setting can decrease the acute effects of irradiation on the bladder and bowel, but definitive randomized studies are not available to date (see later).

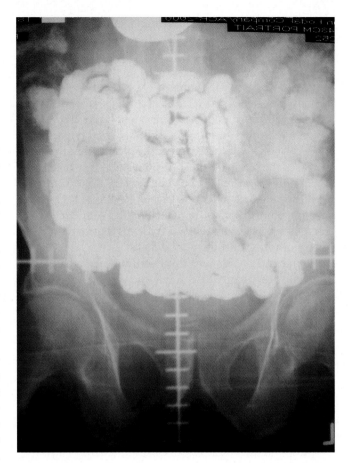

FIGURE 23-14 Small bowel in the pelvis demonstrated by small bowel contrast.

Long-Term Effects

Finally, it is important to understand the permanent nature of radiation injury. When any area of the body is subjected to tumoricidal doses of radiation, the normal tissues of that area suffer an injury that is only partially repaired. The tumor tissue disappears but the normal tissue bed remains, and residual radiation changes must be seriously considered should other disease processes ensue. Radiobiologists estimate that in the case of injury to normal tissues, only 5% to 20% of the damage is repaired. If a second malignant neoplasm arises in that same area many years later, additional tumoricidal radiation is frequently impossible because of permanent radiation changes. In addition, any surgical procedures performed within a previously irradiated field are at higher risk for poor healing, fistula formation, and so forth.

Radiation-induced soft tissue necrosis can be a significant complication. This is usually a result of a progressive obliterative endarteritis that leads to decreased blood flow and a resultant hypoxic tissue bed. This causes increased fibrosis, poor healing, and chronic ulceration. Local conservative management (e.g., hydrogen peroxide douche, estrogen therapy) will resolve the problem in many cases. A small group of patients has significant tissue breakdown that may be painful and may lead to fistula formation. The use of hyperbaric oxygen has been shown to enhance healing in these radiation-induced injuries. Treatment with hyperbaric oxygen requires entering a tank where one breathes 100% oxygen at an increased atmospheric pressure. This increases the oxygen concentration in all body tissues up to 20 times normal. This treatment is done daily for 6 to 8 weeks and side effects include nausea, claustrophobia, painful pressure on the ears—similar to the changes experienced with airline pressure changes—pneumothorax, and oxygen toxicity.

Permanent changes to the genitourinary and gastrointestinal tract can cause signs and symptoms such as decreased bladder capacity, hematuria, ureteral or urethral stricture, hematochezia, bowel obstruction, chronic diarrhea, tenesmus, fecal incontinence, and fistula formation. Gynecologic changes include dryness and shortening of the vagina, dyspareunia, and decreased orgasm. All of these long-term effects should be addressed by the oncology team to maximize the patient's quality of life.

NEW RADIATION MODALITIES

Protons

Protons result in an excellent physical dose distribution. The dose increases slowly with depth and reaches a sharp maximum near the end of the particle's range called the Bragg peak. This sharp dose peak allows for extremely precise, circumscribed delivery. Other than the physical distribution advantage, protons have biologic properties similar to x-rays. Protons are ideal for specific clinical situations, such as spinal cord tumors and eye melanomas, in which a sharp dose delivery is critical to avoid normal tissue damage. Reports also describe the utility in more common tumors, such as prostate cancer. Although useful in several clinical situations, cost of delivery from a cyclotron or special linear accelerator makes it currently available in a few cities, although interest is mounting and new centers are being built or contemplated in other areas.

Electrons

Most modern linear accelerators can produce high-energy electron beams. Electrons lose energy rapidly as they travel in tissue and interact with tissue atoms, and ultimately their kinetic energy is reduced to zero. Therefore, unlike photons, electrons have a specific range dependent on energy and the tissue traversed. Transvaginal electron irradiation can be used for a copiously bleeding exophytic cervical lesion to induce hemostasis. The dosimetry is such that most of the energy delivered transvaginally is absorbed into the malignant lesions itself. Lesions of the vulva and inguinofemoral lymph nodes are also treated with electron beams in many institutions. The limitations of electron therapy are related to the strengths. Because it loses energy rapidly it cannot be used for deep-seated tumors and the applicator must rest very close to the tumor itself, so only fairly superficial, shallow lesions are appropriately treated with electrons.

Fast Neutrons

Neutrons interact in tissue to produce recoil protons, α particles, and other nuclear particles. Their potential usefulness stems from a reduced OER (this translates into decreased hypoxic cell resistance), reduced differential killing by cell cycle, reduced ability for cells to repair sublethal damage, and higher effectiveness for slowly cycling tumors.

Although randomized controlled trials demonstrated that neutron therapy provided improved local control in some tumors, its utility was limited by higher morbidity and cost. Overall, use is limited by the cost of the cyclotron, limited depth penetrations, high surface entrance dose, lack of sharp beam boundaries, and variable intensity modulation.

Negative Pi Mesons and Other Heavy Ions

Negative pi mesons, or pions, are negatively charged particles that have a mass 273 times that of an electron. These are produced in a cyclotron or linear accelerator using 400 to 800 MeV protons that bombard a beryllium target. Pions exhibit a Bragg peak produced by elicited protons, neutrons, and α particles. Other heavy ions such as neon, argon, and carbon have been studied, but equipment to produce these special particles is expensive and not widely available. Use is limited to experimental therapy only. As with neutrons, these forms of radiation have a high biologic effectiveness and a low dependence on oxygen.

NEW RADIATION DELIVERY TECHNOLOGY

Intraoperative Radiation

Several centers throughout the world are investigating the utility of large-fraction intraoperative external irradiation. Patients are subjected to operative procedures in which the area of involvement is carefully defined and radiation fractions of 1500 to 2500 cGy are delivered directly to the area identified. Applications of this technique in gynecologic oncology have been in the treatment of biopsy-proven positive para-aortic or pelvic nodes and marginally resectable recurrences. Electron beam radiation is delivered with one high-dose fraction with the bowel and other sensitive normal tissues packed to the side, thus minimizing the probability of visceral injuries. For best results, external beam radiation is often combined with intraoperative therapy. Because the intraoperative accelerators only deliver electrons, it is subject to the same limitations as all electron beams (see previous discussion). Experience in both primary and recurrent tumors has been reported. The results are limited but have shown increased local control when used selectively. The role of intraoperative radiation in gynecology is not widespread and is limited to a few institutions that are capable of providing this specialized therapy. New techniques involving intraoperative low-energy radiation sources in the kV range are being investigated in other sites such as breast, but there are no reports of use in gynecologic cancers as yet.

Hyperthermia

As discussed previously, solid tumor masses often have hypovascular centers, which are poorly penetrated by antineoplastic drugs and have hypoxic, radioresistant cell fractions. Hyperthermia is another method used to overcome these relatively radioresistant tumors. Although several anecdotal clinical observations have been made, current interest in hyperthermia is based mainly on careful biologic studies on cells and transplantable tumors performed in the 1980s. Although there is no evidence that tumor cells are consistently more sensitive to heat than normal cells, several factors may contribute to a therapeutic gain. Tumor hypoxic cell populations have an acidic pH and are nutritionally deprived. These factors increase sensitivity to heat. Therapeutic gain is also derived from selective heat retention in the tumor. The hypoxic core is maintained at a higher temperature than the normal tissues, which more efficiently remove heat secondary to better-organized vasculature. Ultimately, cell death is dependent on the temperature achieved and is time dependent. Hyperthermia is combined with radiation as each modality preferentially kills a separate part of the tumor; in addition, heat increases the cell kill of external radiation by inhibiting sublethal and potentially lethal damage repair. Late S phase is the most sensitive phase to hyperthermia but the most resistant to low LET (photon) radiation, and thus the two modalities complement one another. The first notable use of hyperthermia in gynecologic oncology has been with interstitial hyperthermia for deep tumors of the pelvis. Increased survival has been demonstrated, although reports are mixed and the therapy is not commonly available.

Three-Dimensional Conformal Radiation Therapy

Three-dimensional conformal radiation therapy is linked to a multiplicity of imaging modalities, especially CT. Beam placement using a CT simulator replaces the conventional simulator (fluoroscopic planning machine) for plan design to the extent that the term "virtual simulation" is used to describe it. The digitally reconstructed radiographs link the plan to the treatment unit in a manner that is rapidly replacing the conventional simulator. 3DCF entails shaping of the beam to conform to the target as seen by CT imaging. The physician arranges the beams to maximize dose to the tumor and minimize dose to normal tissues. Patient, tumor, and normal target movement demand patient immobilization and that adequate margin be placed around the targets to prevent a "marginal miss."

Intensity Modulated Radiation Therapy

IMRT, compared to 3DCF therapy, uses the power of computers to perform hundreds to thousands of iterations of planning to maximize and shape tumor dose and minimize normal tissue dose (Fig. 23-15). This form of planning, called forward planning, gives the computer instructions on what dose to deliver to the targets and also sets limitations on normal structures. Both 3DCF therapy and IMRT use small collimator "leaves" to finely shape the beam. These "leaves" are mobile and block portions of the generated x-rays. If the collimator "leaves" move while the radiation beam is on and vary the beam intensity, areas of tumor and normal tissue can receive a spectrum of doses, hence the term *intensity modulated*. These collimator "leaves" also allow for irregular shapes to be treated. This technology has demonstrated similar local control with reduced complications in several sites such as prostate and head and neck. In gynecologic cancer decreased radiation to normal tissues including bowel, bladder, and bone marrow has been demonstrated, especially in the postoperative setting. Papers have been published on the use of IMRT in postoperative uterine and cervical carcinoma, vulvar carcinoma, whole abdominal radiotherapy, vaginal carcinoma, and intact cervical carcinoma. Because of the daily variation in bladder and rectal filling, the mobility of the upper vagina and cervix, and the change in cervical volume over the span of treatment in intact cervical cancer, use of IMRT should be undertaken with extreme caution and special attention should be given to assure that the target is accurately delineated and treated with

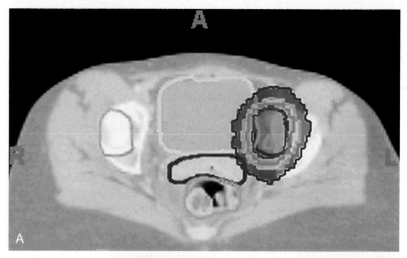

FIGURE 23-15 In **A** and **B,** note how little normal tissue is treated to accomplish the sidewall nodal boost. In **C,** note how the renal parenchyma and spinal cord are relatively spared in treating the para-aortic recurrence.

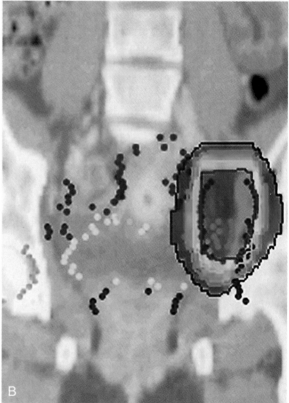

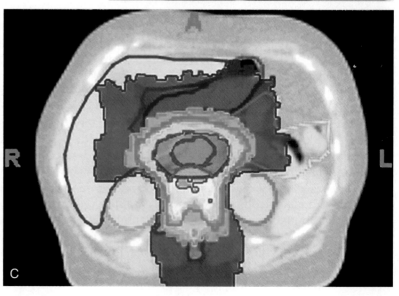

each fraction. Randomized, prospective trials evaluating IMRT are anticipated, and consensus guidelines for clinical target volume delineation have been recently published by Lim and colleagues. Introduction of new technology such as tomotherapy (a linear accelerator linked to an online CT scanner), cyberknife (a linear accelerator capable of fiducial imaging to target radiation), and cone-beam CT (CT scan mounted to the linear accelerator) for image-guided radiotherapy assists in daily target and normal tissue localization but in gynecologic cancer is still investigational. Other concerns regarding this technology include the enormous physician and physics time used for planning, increased cost, and the unknown long-term consequences of lower dose but increased volume of tissue exposed to radiation.

Stereotactic Radiotherapy

Stereotactic radiation and gamma knife radiation are similar to IMRT and 3DCF radiation because they allow precise, high-dose delivery of external radiation. It is commonly used for both primary and metastatic brain tumors, small lung tumors, and an increasing number of other sites. Stereotactic radiation uses a modification of the linear accelerator, whereas gamma knife is a separate machine with 201 separate ^{60}Co sources used to focus on the target.

Immune-Tagged Radiation Therapy

Recently, several products that tag a radioisotope to a monoclonal antibody have entered the market. This modality of radiation allows delivery of the radioactive isotope to the unique antibody target. It has been used successfully in lymphomas and awaits the identification of a unique target prior to development for a gynecologic use.

GLOSSARY

absorbed dose The energy imparted to matter by ionizing radiation per unit mass of irradiated material. The unit is the gray (Gy), defined to be an energy absorption of 1 joule/kg. The old unit was the rad, which was defined as an energy absorption of 100 ergs/g.

brachytherapy Treatment of malignant tumors by radioactive sources that are implanted close to (intracavitary) or within (interstitial) the tumor.

dosimetry The term applied to the measurement and calculation of dose that the patient receives.

electron volt (eV) The energy of motion acquired by an electron accelerated through a potential difference of 1 volt.

excitation The moving of an electron to a more distant orbit within the same atom.

gamma rays Electromagnetic irradiation (originating inside the nucleus) emitted by excited nuclei. The gamma rays from an isotope will have one or several sharply defined energies.

Gray (Gy) The special name for the unit of absorbed dose and specific energy impacted; 1 Gy = 1 joule/kg = 100 rads.

half-life The time in which half the atoms of a radioactive species disintegrate.

image-guided brachytherapy (IGBT) the use of imaging for three-dimensional, volume directed planning.

image-guided radiation therapy (IGRT) use of images taken before, during, or after treatment while in the treatment room to allow visualization of target, fiducial markers, and/or organs at risk.

intensity modulated radiation therapy (IMRT) computer technology that allows variable fluence across the beam and increased conformance to target relative to normal tissues.

inverse square law The intensity of radiation from a point varies inversely as the square of the distance from the source. Thus the dose rate at 2 cm from a source is one fourth that at 1 cm. At 3 cm, the dose rate is one ninth that at 1 cm.

ionization The removal of an electron from an atom, leaving a positively charged ion.

ionizing radiation Radiation capable of causing ionization.

isotope Nuclides having an equal number of protons but a different number of neutrons (excitable situation).

keV 1000 eV.

linear energy transfer (LET) The energy lost by the particle or photon per micron of path depth. High LET radiations are more effective against hypoxic cells.

meV 1,000,000 eV.

oxygen enhancement ratio (OER) The ratio of the dose required for a given level of cell killing under hypoxic conditions compared with the dose needed in air.

penumbra The radiation outside the full beam, which is often caused by scatter or incomplete collimation.

rad A unit-absorbed dose of ionizing radiation equivalent to the absorption of 100 erg per gram of irradiated material.

relative biologic effectiveness (RBE) A ratio of the absorbed dose of a reference radiation to the absorbed dose of a test radiation to produce the same level of biologic effect, other conditions being equal.

rem The old unit of dose equivalent. It is the product of the absorbed dose in rads and modifying factor and is being replaced by the sievert.

roentgen (R) An internationally accepted unit of radiation quantity: It is the quantity of "x-ray or gamma irradiation such that the associated corpuscular emission per 0.001293 g of air produces, in air, ions carrying 1 esu of quantity of electricity of either sign." X-rays originate outside the nucleus.

Sievert (SU): The unit of dose equivalent in the SI system (1 Sv = 100 rem).

x-rays: Rays emitted by a particular generator will emit a spectrum of energies.

For full reference list, log onto www.expertconsult.com ⟨http://www.expertconsult.com⟩.

ABSTRACT

A

Staging:

Staging of Cancer at Gynecologic Sites

For the complete details of anatomy, staging classification, and rules for classification by sites of malignant tumors of the female pelvis, please, go to expertconsult.com. To access your account, look for your activation instructions on the inside front cover of this book.

Cervix Uteri, Corpus Uteri, Ovary, Vagina, Vulva, Gestational Trophoblastic Tumors, and Fallopian Tube

In 1976 the American Joint Committee adopted the classification of the International Federation of Gynecology and Obstetrics (FIGO), which is the format used in the *Annual Report on the Results of Treatment in Carcinoma of the Uterus, Vagina and Ovary*, which is published every 3 years. This report has used the FIGO classification with periodic modifications since 1937, the last being 2009. Numerous institutions throughout the world contribute their statistics for inclusion in this voluntary collaborative presentation of data.

The cervix and corpus uteri were among the first anatomic sites to be classified by the TNM system. This utilizes extent of primary tumor (T), nodal metastasis (N), and distant metastasis (M) status to stage cancers. This system has been approved by the American Joint Committee on Cancer (AJCC) and the International Union Against Cancer (UICC). FIGO has worked closely for many years with the AJCC and UICC in the classification of cancer at gynecologic sites. Staging of malignant tumors is essentially the same, and stages are comparable in the two (FIGO and TNM) systems regarding categories and details.

B

Modified from Common Terminology Criteria for Adverse Events (CTCAE)*

(version 4.0)
U.S. Department of Health and Human Services
National Institutes of Health, National Cancer Institute
Published May 28, 2009 (v4.03: June 14, 2010)

For the complete table containing common terminology criteria for adverse events, please go to expertconsult.com. To access your account, look for your activation instructions on the inside front cover of this book.

Quick Reference

The NCI Common Terminology Criteria for Adverse Events is a descriptive terminology that can be utilized for Adverse Event (AE) reporting. A grading (severity) scale is provided for each AE term.

Components and Organization

System Organ Class

System Organ Class (SOC), the highest level of the MedDRA hieracrhy, is identified by anatomic or physiologic system, etiology, or purpose (e.g., SOC

Investigations for laboratory test results). CTCAE terms are grouped by MedDRA Primary SOCs. Within each SOC, AEs are listed and accompanied by descriptions of severity (Grade).

CTCAE Terms

An AE is any unfavorable and unintended sign (including an abnormal laboratory finding), symptom, or disease temporally associated with the use of a medical treatment or procedure that may or may *not* be considered related to the medical treatment or procedure. An AE is a term that is a unique representation of a specific event used for medical documentation and scientific analyses. Each CTCAE v4.0 term is a MedDRA LLT (Lowest Level Term).

Definitions

A brief definition is provided to clarify the meaning of each AE term.

Grades

Grade refers to the severity of the AE. The CTCAE displays Grades 1 through 5 with unique clinical descriptions of severity for each AE based on this general guideline:

---

*CTCAE v4.0 incorporates certain elements of the MedDRA terminology. For further details on MedDRA, refer to the MedDRA MSSO website (http://www.meddramsso.com).

Blood Component Therapy

Despite the recent increase in the use of hematopoietic growth factors, transfusion therapy plays an important role in caring for oncology patients, particularly now that more effective treatment regimens have led to longer survivals. In many instances the patient with cancer behaves like a patient with a chronic disease requiring frequent blood components caused by disorders secondary to the disease and/or treatment. Whole blood is separated into cellular and non-cellular components including red cells, platelets, and plasms.

1. Blood component: A portion of blood is separated by physical and mechanical means, such as differential centrifugation (Figure C-1). Cell separation technology, capable of collecting platelets, plasma, granulocytes, peripheral blood stem cells, and red cells, has an increasingly important role in transfusion medicine. Anticoagulants and other additives used in blood collection containers allow storage of liquid red cells for up to 42 days.
   a. Packed red blood cells (RBCs): These cells are prepared from whole blood by centrifugation and subsequent removal of plasma.
      (1) Hematocrit: 60%-80%
      (2) Indications
         (a) Replacement of hemoglobin-containing cells in an anemic patient with heart failure, renal failure, burns, or bone marrow failure
         (b) Debilitated patients
         (c) Elderly patients
         (d) Patients with liver disease
      (3) Recommend to use packed RBCs for losses of blood less than 1000-1500 mL/70 kg; with greater losses, whole blood probably should be used
      (4) Therapeutic effect: In a 70-kg adult, each unit should increase the hematocrit by 3%-4%.
   b. Frozen RBCs: Long-term preservation of frozen RBCs without damage can be accomplished by the addition of glycerol; before transfusion, the RBCs should be thawed and washed to remove glycerol
      (1) Advantages
         (a) Blood of rare types can be stored for long periods
         (b) 2, 3-diphosphoglycerol and adenosine triphosphate levels remain the same as they were on the day that the blood was frozen
         (c) Free of plasma protein, platelets, white blood cells, and fibrin
         (d) Has been claimed to reduce the incidence of hepatitis acquired from a blood transfusion
      (2) Disadvantages
         (a) Expensive
         (b) Outdated in 24 hours after thaw
         (c) Takes time to thaw and deglycerolize
   c. Buffy coat: poor erythrocytes; would reduce the incidence of febrile transfusion reaction
      (1) Indication
         (a) Patients with repeated febrile nonhemolytic transfusion reaction caused by leukocyte antibody
         (b) Hematopoietic growth factors applied to oncologies from transfusion therapy is designed to limit the exposure of patients to allogenic blood with its innate risks. The synthesis of erythropoietin (EPO) by recombinant technology was a very important advance in decreasing red cell transfusions. EPO has also been used to increase the yield of autologous donations and also to stimulate erythropoiesis after surgery.

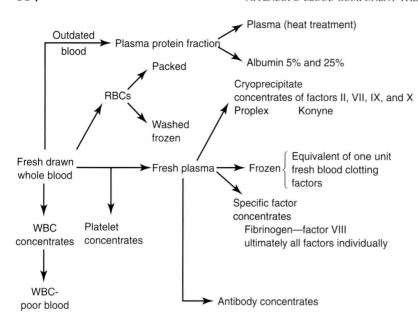

d. Platelet concentrates
   (1) One unit of platelet concentrate contains 5.5×10^{10} platelets suspended in 30–50 mL of plasma
   (2) Shelf-life: 72 hours at room temperature
   (3) Thrombocytopenia does not usually produce serious bleeding unless the platelet count is <20,000, except if there is a platelet function defect, a coagulation defect, or local cause of hemorrhage (e.g., trauma, surgery)
e. Fresh frozen plasma
   (1) Contains albumin, globulin, active coagulation factors, complement, and electrolytes
   (2) Should be type-specific
   (3) Shelf life: 12 months at –20 to –30°C; should be used within 2 hours after thawing
   (4) Indications
      (a) Deficiency in coagulation factors
      (b) Situation with plasma loss
      (c) Rapid reversal of oral anticoagulant therapy
f. Cryoprecipitate: Cold insoluble precipitate remains when fresh frozen plasma is allowed to thaw at 4° C; it contains factor VIII with fibrinogen and factor XIII
   (1) Indications
      (a) von Willebrand disease
      (b) Replacement of fibrinogen, factor XIII
2. Plasma fraction: Derivatives of plasma are obtained by a chemical process such as alcohol precipitation
   a. Coagulation factor concentrates
      (1) Factor VIII concentrates
      (2) Factor IX concentrates

      (3) Prothrombin complex (factor II, VII, IX, X concentrates)
      (4) Fibrinogen concentrates
   b. Immunoglobulin concentrates
   c. Albumin: Filtered and pasteurized by heating for 10 hours at 60° C to eliminate the risks of viral hepatitis
      (1) 5% albumin: isosmotic, sodium 145 mEq/L; for rapid expansion of vascular volume
      (2) 25% albumin: sodium 145 mEq/L; given intravenously; one volume of 25% albumin will draw about four volumes of additional fluid from the extravascular space into the circulation; used for treatment of hypoalbuminemia
   d. Plasma protein factor: 5% solution of selected human plasma protein in buffered saline solution; heat-treated to eliminate the risk of hepatitis; indicated for rapid expansion of vascular volume
3. Stroma-free hemoglobin solution
   a. Advantages
      (1) No need for blood typing
      (2) Longer storage capacity
      (3) Maintains better microcirculation
      (4) Potentially improved oxygenation of ischemic myocardium
      (5) No antigenicity
4. Autologous blood: The collection and reinfusion of the patient's own blood by preoperative autologous blood donation or intraoperative blood salvage. For autologous blood donation, the blood should be taken at least 2 weeks before the surgical procedure, and the patient must maintain a hemoglobin level

TABLE C-1   Risk of Infection

Agent risk	Unit
Hepatitis B	1:50,000
Hepatitis C	1:100,000
Human immunodeficiency virus	1:150,000–1:1,000,000
Human T cell lymphotropic virus	1:50,000

From ACOG, Technical Bulletin 199, Nov. 1994, and Management of Hepatitis C. NIH Consensus Statement Online 15(3):1, 1997.

of 11 g/dL or more. If large amounts of blood are required, frozen cells are another option. Many patients can donate as often as once a week. Intraoperative blood salvage requires the sterile collection and reinfusion of shed blood that is free of infecting agents such as malignant cells. The RBCs are collected in sterile plastic bags, washed, and concentrated before being reinfused into the patient.

5. Complications: Infection, transfusion reactions, and alloimmunization are the major complications associated with the transfusion of blood components (Table C-1).

Once in each 6000 units of blood transferred, an acute hemolytic reaction will occur, with a mortality rate of 1:17. These reactions are usually due to ABO incompatibility and resultant intracellular hemolysis. Patients develop fever, chills, chest pain, nausea, hypotension, and disseminated intravascular coagulation. Mild reactions to leukocyte and platelet antigens are usually associated with a febrile episode alone. Hemolytic reactions to other blood groups such as Kidd, Duffy, and Kell can be associated with fever, anemia, hyperbilirubinemia, and a positive direct Coombs test. Some of these milder transfusions reactions manifest themselves 7 to 10 days after the transfusion.

Hematopoietic growth factors are designed to limit the exposure of oncology patients to blood and blood products. Red cell substitutes are currently in development, and some are in phase II and III clinical trials. None are currently approved for clinical use in the United States. They consist of artificially derived products that have oxygen-carrying properties and are structurally similar to hemoglobin. Their development has been hampered by relatively short half-life in the circulation.

The isolation and then synthesis of erythropoietin has been very helpful in limiting red cell transfusions. Granulocyte colony-stimulating factor (G-CSF) has been proven to decrease infection rates in neutropenic patients after chemotherapy. The limitations of platelet transfusions have stimulated the research into agents that can stimulate platelet production, and such products are now available. In addition, thrombopoietic growth factors have the potential to stimulate platelet apheresis donors and increase stem cell harvest yields, thus expanding progenitor cells.

For full reference list, log onto ⟨www.expertconsult.com⟩.

D

Suggested Recommendations for Routine Cancer Screening

Cervical Cancer

Cervical cancer screening should begin at age 21 years. Cytologic screening is recommended every 2 years for women ages 21 to 29 years with either conventional or liquid-based cytology. Women ages 30 years and older who have had three consecutive cervical cytology test results that are negative for intraepithelial lesions and malignancy may be screened every 3 years. Women with any of the following risk factors may require more frequent cervical cytology:

- Women who are immunosuppressed.
- Women who are infected with human immunodeficiency virus (HIV).
- Women who were exposed to diethylstilbestrol in utero.
- Women who were previously treated for CIN2, CIN3, or cancer.

Co-testing using the combination of cytology plus HPV DNA testing is appropriate screening for women older than 30 years. Co-testing in women younger than 30 years is not recommended.

In women who have had a total hysterectomy for benign indications with no prior history of high-grade CIN, routine cytology testing should be discontinued.

It is reasonable to discontinue cervical cancer screening between 65 and 70 years of age in women who have had three or more negative cytology test results in a row and no abnormal test results in the past 10 years.

Women who have been immunized against HPV-16 and HPV-18 should be screened by the same regimen as nonimmunized women.

Breast Cancer

Mammography should be performed every year for women 40 years of age and older.

Evidence from several studies indicates that there is a decrease in mortality for all women when appropriate screening by mammography is instituted and performed by qualified personnel. The efficacy of mammography is not in doubt. The question that remains is the optimal screening frequency, and the answer may be provided by data now being compiled. Safety is no longer a concern, but it is recognized that mammography is the most costly of all screening modalities. Dedicated equipment is essential, and considerable skill and experience are required to interpret the films. It is important, therefore, to determine the most prudent utilization of resources. Until the optimal screening frequency is determined, it appears reasonable to follow recommendations of the American College of Obstetricians and Gynecologists, the American Cancer Society, and the National Cancer Institute.

Endometrial Cancer

Total population screening for endometrial cancer and its precursors is neither cost-effective nor warranted. High-risk patients may require endometrial sampling.

The cost-effectiveness of screening asymptomatic women for endometrial cancer and its precursors is very low; therefore the practice is unwarranted. On the other hand, perimenopausal and postmenopausal women with a history or evidence of abnormal vaginal hemorrhage are at high risk for endometrial cancer, and their symptoms should be investigated by endometrial biopsy or curettage. Dilatation and curettage are recommended when endometrial hyperplasia or questionable endometrial carcinoma is present and when there is insufficient tissue for diagnosis by endometrial biopsy.

If estrogen-progestin therapy is instituted, endometrial biopsy is not required before treatment is begun unless there are reasons (e.g., abnormal bleeding) to place the patient at high risk for endometrial neoplasia. If unexpected breakthrough bleeding occurs during therapy, endometrial biopsy is recommended to rule out the development of abnormal endometrial histology. Endometrial biopsy by aspiration curettage performed in the office is diagnostically reliable and cost effective in symptomatic patients. The timing of further biopsies, if needed, is a clinical decision that should be based on previous histologic results and the patient's history.

Ovarian Cancer

No available techniques are currently suitable for routine screening. Many different techniques, including peritoneal fluid profiles, investigation of tumor-associated antigens, and ultrasonography, have been or are being investigated as possible screening tools for ovarian cancer. To date, none of these techniques has proved to be practical or effective.

Colorectal Cancer

Beginning at 50 years of age, one of three screening options should be selected: (1) yearly fecal occult blood testing plus flexible sigmoidoscopy every 5 years, (2) colonoscopy every 10 years, or (3) double-contrast barium enema (DCBE) every 5 to 10 years. A digital rectal examination should be performed at the time of each screening sigmoidoscopy, colonoscopy, or DCBE.

Available data do not substantiate the cost-effectiveness of various screening recommendations. Because colorectal cancer is a significant risk to women, the task force suggests that the recommendations of the American Cancer Society (ACOG) and the National Cancer Institute be used as a guide.

Lung Cancer

No available techniques are currently suitable for routine screening. The only effective way to reduce mortality from lung cancer is to promote a "stop smoking" message to the public. Although some support is evolving for annual radiographic screening for those at risk (i.e., women 50 years and older who smoke more than one pack of cigarettes daily), neither the American Cancer Society nor the National Cancer Institute has adopted this guideline. This information is based on the ACOG Committee Opinion, No. 247, December 2000.

Nutritional Therapy

In the cancer patient, malnutrition may appear simultaneously with the disease. Cancer patients often exhibit anorexia because of decreased nutritional intake with resultant weight loss. There may be an increased nutritional requirement because of the increased demands of the patient and the tumor. Resting metabolic rates can vary greatly, but in as many as 60% of patients the rate may be elevated. The stage of malnutrition in the cancer patient can lead to cachexia with weakness and tissue wasting. The extent of malnutrition in the patient may be greater than can be explained by decreased nutritional intake. Metabolic abnormalities include an abnormal response to glucose tolerance testing, increased gluconeogenesis (which can result in decreased muscle protein synthesis), and abnormalities in protein and fat metabolism. A patient with a malignancy may need additional nutritional support while that patient undergoes intensive treatment, which can include surgery and chemotherapy. Parenteral nutrition seems to improve a patient's tolerance of the treatment and improves her nutritional state; however, parenteral nutrition has not been shown to improve survival.

The malnutrition seen in cancer patients is commonly referred to as *cancer cachexia*. Nutritional depletion is seen as a protein-calorie malnutrition with a loss of body cell mass. The importance of protein-calorie nutrition is its association with increases in postoperative complications, deficiencies in immune function, and poorer tolerance of therapy.

Dietary nutrients required for good health include water, protein, fat, carbohydrates, vitamins, and minerals. Energy is required for normal body function, growth, and repair. Protein is necessary for growth and development to maintain body structures and function. It is the source of the essential amino acids and nitrogen needed for the synthesis of nonessential amino acids. Dietary protein replaces the essential amino acids and nitrogen that are lost through protein turnover and normal body functions. During illness, protein requirements increase. Nitrogen balance is essential for good health and requires intake of protein and energy. At higher energy intakes,

less protein is needed to achieve nitrogen balance. Nitrogen is lost continuously in the body through normal body functions. Fat is the food substance with the highest concentration of calories.

The visual protein compartment is best measured by assessment of the plasma albumin, transferrin, and total lymphocyte count. Albumin is the major determinant of plasma colloidal osmotic pressure because its large size does not permit it to pass the capillary membrane. The appearance of edema is often a sign of low serum albumin. Serum levels lower than 3.0 g/dL are reflective of nutritional deficiency. Transferrin is a protein of hepatic origin and transports iron. The level is reflective of the patient's ability to make serum protein. Transferrin levels are more sensitive than albumin levels because of its shorter half-life (8 days compared to 20) and it is preferable to evaluate the efficacy of nutritional therapy. The response of a patients total lymphocyte count to nutritional therapy may also be a favorable prognostic sign during the first 7 to 14 days of therapy. (Table E-1)

Linoleic acid is the only essential fatty acid required in the diet; it is necessary for the synthesis of arachidonic acid, which is a major precursor of prostaglandin. Linoleic acid comes mainly from polyunsaturated vegetable oils. A deficiency of essential fatty acids results in poor wound healing, hair loss, and dermatitis. Fatty acids and cholesterol make up most of the fat in our diets. Carbohydrates include sugar, starch, and fibers. When carbohydrates are not included in the diet, ketosis begins to occur, and there is excessive breakdown of protein as amino acids are used for gluconeogenesis. Water-soluble and fat-soluble vitamins cannot be synthesized in adequate amounts by the body. Fat-soluble vitamins are required for absorption, transport, metabolism, and storage. They are not excreted in the urine like the water-soluble vitamins, and an excess accumulation can lead to well-known toxic conditions. Major minerals, as well as trace elements, are important in human nutrition.

Lack of appetite with reduction in food intake is a key factor in cancer cachexia. The role of the neurotransmitter serotonin appears to be central to appetite. Inhibition

TABLE E-1   TPN Indications

Severely malnourished patients undergoing surgery
Patients with postoperative complications that require nutritional
support
Therapy-induced complications that require nutritional support
Note: Routine use of TPN in patients with cancer is not indicated.

TPN, Total parenteral nutrition.

of serotonin increases appetite and food intake in animals. Cancer patients also report a loss of taste and smell with a resulting loss of appeal of most foods. Weight loss may also be greatly influenced when the location of the tumor affects the ability to take nutrition (e.g., a mass causing a partial bowel obstruction). Cytokines produced by the patient in response to a growing neoplasm may result in nutritional derangements. Cytokines can regulate appetite and metabolic rate, so they can be very important factors. Dudrick suggests that patients who have a 10-lb weight loss or a 10% decrease in body weight 2 months before assessment, serum albumin of less than 3.4 g/dL, anergy to four of five standard skin test antigens, and a low total lymphocyte count, and who cannot or will not eat enough are candidates for nutritional assessment. Nutritional history, with a 24-hour dietary recall, can be used to assess nutritional intake. Anthropometric measurements are useful when assessing the patient's nutritional status. Relative body weight is probably the most useful of these measurements, because rapid weight loss is usually an indication of protein-calorie undernutrition. The triceps skinfold test assesses fat stores, and mid-arm circumference tends to assess protein status. Edema, which is often seen with protein-calorie deficiency, can mask true weight loss and muscle wasting. Serum albumin is probably the single most important test for determining protein calorie undernutrition. Albumin is the main plasma protein needed to maintain plasma osmotic pressure as well as other functions. In a patient with low albumin, morbidity and mortality are increased. Albumin can be influenced by conditions other than malnutrition and may be affected by hydration status. Transferrin binds and transports iron in the plasma and is a good indicator of protein nutritional status. The extent of malnutrition depends on the type and site of the cancer. Cancers such as ovarian cancer, with its potential effect on the gastrointestinal (GI) tract, appear to contribute to malnutrition to a greater degree than does cervical cancer. As expected, malnutrition becomes worse as the cancer progresses. The mechanism of cancer-related malnutrition is unknown. There are probably multiple contributing factors. Decreased food intake because of anorexia, early satiety, nausea, and vomiting can play a role. Poor absorption of nutrients can also be a contributing factor. Food aversion, particularly in patients undergoing chemotherapy or irradiation, is well known. Change of taste and smell can contribute to decreased intake. Generalized weakness may also contribute to decreased food intake. Decrease in total lymphocyte count (<1200) is also suggestive of malnutrition. Creatinine height index (CHI) may be helpful, because urinary creatinine excretion is proportional to total body muscle mass. As muscles become depleted, creatinine excretion falls. A CHI of 80% or more usually indicates a normal lean body mass. A CHI between 60% and 80% indicates moderate depletion; a CHI of less than 60% indicates severe depletion.

Eternal Nutrition

Numerous clinical trials have been published using aggressive eternal nutritional support as a supplement during cancer therapy in patients who would not eat well. The trials are not consistent in demonstrating benefit of eternal nutrition. However, it is a well-accepted concept that eternal therapy is the preferred route for feeding cancer patients when the GI tract is not obstructed. Methods of eternal nutrition vary from frequent snack between meals to the insertion of a comfortable nasogastric feeding tube on a continuous drip of nutritional supplements. Others have used gastrostomy or jejunostomy feeding tubes.

The role of total parenteral nutrition (TPN) in the patient with cancer has yet to be determined. TPN can correct nutritional deficits that commonly occur in the cancer patient. TPN can also improve nitrogen balance and decrease catabolism. Glucose turnover and clearance rates are increased; gluconeogenesis is suppressed; and free fatty acid oxidation is increased. TPN can increase body weight and reverse serum markers of malnutrition; however, as an adjuvant to cancer therapy, the results have not been encouraging. TPN has not added to lean body mass or eliminated the GI or hematologic toxicity associated with chemotherapy. In patients treated with chemotherapy, response rates and survival have not been increased with TPN. Although irradiation can contribute to poor nutrition (e.g., diarrhea, enteritis, and malabsorption), particularly to the GI tract when gynecologic cancers are treated, TPN has not produced a significant improvement regarding treatment response, tolerance to treatment, local control, survival, or decreased complications of therapy. Nutritional support for the cancer patient requiring surgery is also ill defined. Malnourished patients undergoing surgery have a higher postoperative morbidity and mortality compared with well-nourished patients. Whether TPN can affect morbidity and mortality in the cancer patient is undetermined, and the concern that TPN may stimulate tumor growth is unfounded. Although routine use of TPN in the cancer patient is not warranted, it may be indicated in severely malnourished patients undergoing surgery or for those with postoperative complications. Nutritional supports are of two main types: enteric and parenteral. For the patient with a functional GI tract, enteric nutrition may be considered through the use of a naso-enteric tube. A gastrostomy or jejunostomy tube may also be used. Obviously, GI dysfunction is a contraindication to this method. Nevertheless, this method appears to be cost effective; it probably maintains the GI mucosa integrity, provides a normal sequence of intestinal and hepatic metabolism before systemic distribution, appears to preserve normal hormonal patterns, and avoids the risk of sepsis. Enteric solutions differ in composition, calorie content, and multiple other factors. These solutions are usually complete, because they contain a full supplement of nutrient requirements, or incomplete, when they are designated to contain a specific macronutrient such as fat, protein, or carbohydrate. Most solutions contain 1000 calories and 37 to 45 g/L of protein. Elemental diets consist mainly of amino acids and simple sugars. They are extremely hypertonic and may induce diarrhea, which may be corrected with a formula of lower osmolarity. Electrolyte imbalance and glucose intolerance can also occur.

Many cancer patients who require nutritional supplementation will need TPN. In some cases, TPN can be administered through a peripheral vein, particularly if TPN is to be given for only a short amount of time. Although adequate protein can usually be infused peripherally, high-caloric supplementation is usually given centrally. Fat solutions, which can account for a high caloric intake, can be given peripherally. Major complications of peripheral TPN are thrombophlebitis and infiltration. In most cases, TPN is given through a central vein—either the subclavian vein or a major neck vessel. The catheter can be inserted in the superior vena cava, which allows rapid infusion of hypertonic solutions without difficulty. Infusion of parenteral solution should be started slowly to prevent hyperglycemia. If glucose intolerance develops, a small amount of insulin is used to control blood sugars. Meticulous care must be taken of the central catheter, because this site can be a major source of infection. Frequent changing of IV tubing and filters and also the catheter is required routinely. TPN is usually managed as a team endeavor, with the attending physician, nutritionist, nurse, pharmacist, and dietitian. Daily requirements must be standardized regarding calories, proteins, fat, minerals, vitamins, and trace elements. These should be varied as the situation demands. Metabolic complications may include hyperglycemia or hypoglycemia, hyperosmolarity, azotemia, hyperchloremic metabolic acidosis, mineral electrolyte disorder, liver enzyme elevations, and anemia. In many hospitals, standard hyperalimentation solutions with appropriate nutrients have been formulated, and adjustments are made for specific needs. Intense metabolic monitoring is required in these patients, and established hospital protocols are now available in many institutions.

Today, both enteric and parenteral nutritional support can be implemented successfully on an outpatient basis. Indications are not uniformly agreed on for this method of nutrition. In the cancer patient, nutritional support may be indicated to help satisfy nutritional needs while toxicity of treatment is abating. Most authorities do not believe that home nutritional support is needed for the terminally ill cancer patient.

A typical nutritional guideline for the adult patient is shown in Table E-2 (see the Expert Consult website). Many institutions have nutritional protocols in place. Although there may be variations on the theme, these guidelines have become relatively standardized.

Additional therapies can also be considered along with nutritional support to alleviate cancer cachexia. Synthetic progestins (megestrol acetate and medroxyprogesterone acetate) in high doses decrease production of cytokines and serotonin and thus improve appetite and a sense of well-being. Responses often are seen within 15 to 30 days of therapy, and side effects are minimal. Some authors have reported more thromboembolic events with megestrol acetate, but not in placebo-controlled studies.

For full reference list, log onto ⟨http://www.expertconsult.com⟩.

Index